INTERNAL MEDICINE BOARD CERTIFICATION REVIEW

AN EXCELLENT GUIDE

AN ESSENTIAL TOOL FOR BOARD CERTIFICATION

FIRST EDITION

by

D. KANJILAL, M. D.

A CD-ROM EDITION OF THIS GUIDE IS ALSO AVAILABLE

RIVERCROSS PUBLISHING, INC.
NEW YORK • ORLANDO
for
DURGA PUBLISHERS, INC.

First Edition - 1998

ISBN: 1-58141-028-X
Library of Congress Catalog Card Number: 98-24053

Available from all Barnes & Noble Bookstores. To contact Barnes & Noble in New York call (212) 807-0099 or FAX (212) 633-2522; in Pennsylvania call (215) 707-3157. From other book and library dealers, such as Campus Book Store (216) 743-1101, J. A. Majors Co., Rittenhouse Book Distributors, and any of the Matthews Medical Bookstores.

This book and the CD-ROM are available for purchases by libraries, hospitals or other educational institutions. Please contact Rivercross Publishing, Inc. 6214 Wynfield Ct, Orlando, FL 32819. Phone: (407) 876-7720, Fax: (407) 876-7758.

INTERNAL MEDICINE BOARD CERTIFICATION REVIEW is distributed by Login Brothers in the United States and Canada. Phone: (800) 680-2889; Fax: (312) 432-7801.

Library of Congress Cataloging-in-Publication Data

Kanjilal, D., 1954-
Internal medicine board certification review / by D. Kanjilal. - 1st ed.
p. cm.
Includes index.
ISBN 1-58141-028-X
1. Internal medicine--Examinations, questions, etc. I. Title.
[DNLM: 1. Internal Medicine examination questions. 2. Medicine examination questions. WB 18.2 K161 1998]
RC58.K36 1999
616'.0076--dc21
DNLM/DLC
for Library of Congress 98-24053
CIP

Dedication

Devoted to Srimod Durga Prasanna Paramhansa Dev, Lokenath Baba, and Jesus Christ

Dedicated to my parents Bimalendu and Asha Kanjilal, to my wife Debjani, to my children Nivedita, Anirban, to my brothers Debabrata, Subrata, Asoke, to my sister Shibani

Dedicated to all the readers.

INTRODUCTION

This is the first edition of the Internal Medicine Board Certification Review (IMBCR). This book is written to help the candidates not only to pass the Board examination but also to obtain top scores.

This book contains over four thousand indirect itemized questions, 291 diagrams and pictures (X-rays, sonograms, CT scan, various syndromes, and skin lesions), 83 graphs, 16 hematological diagrams, 35 EKG's, flow volume curves, dissociation curves, pressure-volume dissociation curves, tympanometry, audiometry, BAER studies, flowmetry or urodynamic studies, cystograms, normal pressure-flow curves, oxygen saturation and pressure gradient in the heart, calculations of the cardiac outputs and shunts, left ventricular function curves, relationships between right atrial pressure and cardiac output or venous return, water deprivation and urine osmolality curves. In addition to that, all the important chapters discussed are pertinent to the Board examination.

I am confident that in no other single volume can one find so much information of this type. (If more in depth discussion of a topic is needed, by all means, consult your textbooks! This book complements them, not replace them.)

Since everyday brings new discoveries in the world of Internal Medicine, books like these can become outdated quickly. I will not be able to print a new edition every month, but I can assure you that an electronic edition will be available every six months or so. All items in the software version have been indexed for fast and accurate searches from a keyboard.

My fellow physicians should note that this book presupposes a baseline knowledge of Internal Medicine.

I extend my sincere thanks to L. Janacek for the clear diagrams, to Preeti Agarwal and Atul Kumar for their desktop publishing expertise, Josh Furman and Dr. Ram S. Verma Ph.D. for their continued support, and Login Brothers for their marketing excellence.

Good luck to those who apply themselves diligently to this book!

D. Kanjilal, M.D.

TABLE OF CONTENTS

TABLE OF CONTENTS

TABLE OF CONTENTS

TABLE OF CONTENTS

TABLE OF CONTENTS

TABLE OF CONTENTS

TABLE OF CONTENTS

TABLE OF CONTENTS

TABLE OF CONTENTS

TABLE OF CONTENTS

TABLE OF CONTENTS

TABLE OF CONTENTS

TABLE OF CONTENTS

TABLE OF CONTENTS

TABLE OF CONTENTS

TABLE OF CONTENTS

TABLE OF CONTENTS

TABLE OF CONTENTS

TABLE OF CONTENTS

ABBREVIATED TERMS

AVM	arterio-venous malformation
H/O	History of
R/O	ruled out
BAL	bronchoalveolar lavage
CXR	chest X-ray
↓	decreased
↑	increased
→	normal
BP	blood pressure
RR	respiratory rate
HR	heart rate
T	temperature
CNS	central nervous system
HIV	human immunodeficiency virus
I.M.	intramuscular
GC	gonococcal
IV	intravenous
IL	interleukin
Prn	if needed
PG	prostaglandins
SI	small intestine
STAT	immediately
Hb	hemoglobin
hct	hematocrit
WBC	white blood cells
RBC	red blood cells
ER	emergency room
p	phosphorous
Ca	calcium
Na	sodium
K	potassium
Gl	glucose
CO	carbon monoxide
DLco	diffusing lung capacity of carbon monoxide
TB	tuberculosis
U/A	urinalysis
DKA	diabetic keto acidosis

TIPS FOR THE EXAMINATION

1. The first answer, which comes into your mind, is probably the right answer.

2. Any definite statement is usually the wrong answer.

3. When there is a choice between either observation or refer to a subspecialist (e.g., orthopedic or surgeon), then observation is probably the right answer.

4. Any eye injury should be referred to ophthalmologist; any acute surgical condition should be referred to surgeon.

5. All the masses or swelling need not be examined by a surgeon.

6. When there is a choice between either observation (i.e., do not do anything) or has something, to be done, observation is the right answer.

7. Always try to remember what is normal in different clinical conditions.

8. You must know the following in every disease condition:
   a. Most common cause.
   b. Most common organism in an infection.
   c. Most common clinical presentation.
   d. Preferred investigation of choice.
   e. Preferred treatment of choice.
   f. Prophylactic treatment.
   g. Most common prognostic sequela.
   h. Most common pathological findings in tumors.
   i. Isolation precautions in communicable diseases.

9. The following are not very important:
   a. Epidemiology
   b. Incidence
   c. Dosage of antibiotics and other medicines.

10. In the examination there are several questions, each of which have long descriptions followed by four or five questions: First find out whether all the questions given have any relation with the description. If there is no relation then don't read the lengthy description, just answer the questions. But if there is a relation, then underline the abnormal findings and try to make a diagnosis. Once you know the diagnosis, then you will be able to answer those questions. Remember that questions given are very tricky but every disease has its own characteristics.

11. In some questions you might see that out of the five choices in the answer, one answer you have never heard of and the other choices do not match with the description. The answer you never heard of is probably the right answer.

12. Very few questions are repeated from the first half to the second half of the test or from the first day to the second day. If you don't know certain answers, please refer to standard textbooks of Medicine.

13. Have a good night sleep before the examination.

PICTURES

In this section we have provided pictures of both the radiological and of the clinical presentations of different diseases as well as brief descriptions. Description numbers correspond to picture numbers (e.g., item no.1 is the description of picture no.1). All the pictures are placed at the end of this section.

Picture number	Description
D-1.	CT scan of the chest shows empyema in (L) thoracic cavity.
D-2.	Ileofemoral deep vein thrombosis: (L) leg is swollen and edematous.
D-3.	Atrophy of the hand muscles: It may be due to nerve injury.
D-4.	Cavernous sinus thrombosis: Swollen, red, edematous face around the eyes plus fever, headaches and rigors.
D-5.	Islet cell cancer of the pancreas: MRI shows mass in the body of the pancreas.
D-6.	Large (R) renal cyst: MRI shows large cystic cavity in (R) kidney and crescent shaped compressed kidney tissue are present medially.
D-7.	Hematoma in the (R) kidney: MRI shows lucent areas around the kidney. It is due to trauma or injury.
D-8.	Bone cyst in (L) humerous: X-ray picture shows lucent cystic mass in upper part of (L) humerous.
D-9.	Traumatic asphyxia result in hemorrhage and petechiae over the face and upper part of the body.
D-10.	(R) trapezius muscle paralysis due to accessory nerve damage. The patient is unable to lift the (R) shoulder during shrugs.
D-11.	Tongue fasciculations due to motor neuron disease.
D-12.	Herpes zoster in the (L) upper chest: Painful maculo-papulo-vesiculo-crusted lesions along the dermatome.
D-13.	Rhinophyma: Hyperplasia of the sabaceous glands and connective tissue of the nose.
D-14.	Thyroid nodule: Thyroid mass moves with swallowing.
D-15.	Hypertrichosis: It is due to use of diazoxide for hypertension.
D-16.	Psoriasis in both legs: The patient has psoratic lesions in both legs.
D-17.	Small bowel obstruction: Plain abdominal x-ray shows multiple air-fluid levels.
D-18.	Ulcerative colitis: It involves from cecum to descending colon. Loss of normal haustral markings, pseudopolyps (nodular ulcerations), small cecum and colon are due to scarring. Reflux of barium enema into the terminal ileum.
D-19.	HIDA scan of the liver: Normal HIDA scan (a, b, c, d): a= Isotope is in the liver initially. b, c= Isotopes are in the biliary tree. d=Isotope is concentrated in the gallbladder.

Abnormal HIDA scan (e,f):
e and f= No isotope is in the gallbladder after 60 minutes and 120 minutes respectively, indicates obstruction of the cystic duct which may be due to acute cholecystitis.

D-20. Pancreatic abscess: CT scan shows accumulation of gas shadows over the pancreatic area due to abscess.

D-21. Keratoacanthoma of the back: Ulcerating tumor with central keratin plug. Tumor grows rapidly and resolves spontaneously.

D-22. Chronic rheumatiod arthritis: Polyarthritis with deformed both hands.

D-23. Gout (L) big toe: Red, swollen, tender, painful joint.

D-24. Prolapsed intervertebral disc between L5 and S1: It causes compression on the nerve roots, results in low back pain and neurological abnormalities.

D-25. Holmes-Adie syndrome (or myotonic pupil): Pupil are of different size but regular, right pupil sluggishly react to direct light and accommodation. It is more common in women than men. It has **no pathological significance** but may be associated with hypo or areflexia, so the patients can be reassured.

D-26. Anthrux or malignant pustule in the back of the neck: It is more common in veterenarian, grows very rapidly,ulcerated lesion with adherent black scab at the base, Gram stain shows Gram-positive rods, and penicillin is the drug of choice.

D-27. Xanthoma in both hands :It is due to high cholesterol and the patient may be susceptible to have myocardial infarction .

D-28. Skin necrosis of hemorrhagic type: It is found in patients with C deficiency. Protein-C is produced in the liver and it is a coagulation protein. Use of warfarin causes further reduction of protein-C production result in microthrombosis and skin necrosis.

D-29. Chronic pancreatitis: Plain x-ray shows irregular calcifications over the pancreatic area.

D-30. Carcinoma of the colon: MRI shows metastases of the liver.

D-31. Gastric ulcer: Barium study shows ulcer crater projecting from the lesser curvature.

D-32. Carcinoma of the transverse colon: Barium enema shows filling defect near the hepatic flexure.

D-33. Osteoarthritis (L<R): Swollen, deformed joints with effusion.

D-34. Cerebellar cyst: MRI shows large cerebellar cyst.

D-35. Tuberous sclerosis: Adenoma sebaceum of the face.

D-36. Liver disease: Palmer erythemas in both hands.

D-37. Lung metastases: X-ray picture shows pulmonary metastases from primary lesions may be originated from thyroid, kidney, testis, breast, or ovaries.

D-38. Penile cancer :Irregular lesion at the tip of the penis in a HIV-positive patient. It may be associated with human papilloma virus types 16 and 18.

D-39. Diabetic neuropathy: Picture shows ulcer in the (R) foot.

D-40. Hypothyroidism: Large goiter in the front and both sides of the neck.

D-41. Enlarged prostate: Intravenous urography shows filling defect due to enlarged prostate and thickened bladder.

D-42. Breast cancer :Mammography shows lesion in the breast.

D-43. Cerebral arteriovenous malformation (AVM): CT scan with contrast shows AVM.

D-44. Skull fractures: Both depressed and linear fractures in the (R) side of the skull due to trauma.

D-45. Diabetes neuropathy (Charcot joint): Painless, swollen, deformed (L) ankle and the foot.

D-46. Graves' disease: Pretibial myxedema of the leg and the foot.

D-47. Horner syndrome: Ptosis and constricted pupil of the (L) side.

D-48. Sturge-Weber syndrome: Diffuse capillary hemangiomas along the distribution of the branches of trigeminal nerve.

D-49. Oculomotor nerve palsy: Ptosis and deviation of the (R) eye due to paralysis.

D-50. Paget disease of the tibia: Bowed and thickened tibia, increased bone density, loss of normal bony architecture, but absence of fracture.

D-51. Gluten induced steatorrhea: The patient has H/o diarrhea abdominal distension, weight loss, poorly developed secondary sexual characters. Diagnosis is made by small bowel biopsy. Gluten free diet is the treatment.

D-52. Lymphogranuloma venereum: It is a sexually transmitted disease caused by chlamydia trachomatis.

D-53. Pulmonary embolisms: Pulmonary angiogram shows balloon occlusion.

D-54. Pleural thickening (R) side: Thickened and calcified (R) sided pleura.

D-55. Lung cancer: Plain x-ray shows mass in the (R) lung.

D-56. Right upper lobe collapse: It is due to mass obstructing the (R) upper lobe bronchus.

D-57. Wilson disease: Kayser-Fleishcher ring in the cornea.

D-58. Gynecomastia: Enlargement of both breast in a patients who had cirrhosis and hepatocellular cancer.

D-59. Subarachnoid hemorrhage: It is due to rupture of the aneurysm of anterior communicating artery. CT scan shows blood in the interhemispheric fissure.

D-60. Local thrombophlebitis: It is due to small emboli which may have originated from the heart (abscesses). It is common in IV drug users.

D-61. Senile purpura in an elderly patient: It is more common on the extensor surfaces of the upper extremities. It is due to rupture of small superficial venules in a thin, atrophic skin. There are **normal** function of the platelets and coagulation factors.

D-62. Stevens-Johnson syndrome: The patients has fever, conjuctivitis, ruptured vesicobullous lesions over the skin and mucosa.

D-63. Xanthomas: It is more prominent in the lower eyelids. It is associated with hyperlipidemias.
D-64. Hepatic lacertation: It is due to trauma. CT scan shows intrahepatic hepatoma.
D-65. Hepatic metastases: MRI shows metastases to the liver from the primary colon cancer.
D-66. Obstruction of the common bile duct (CBD): It is due to tumor at the papilla of Vater.
D-67. Renal mass (L) side: Intravenous pyelography shows displaced calyces due to renal mass.
D-68. Raynaud syndrome: Painful necrotic ulcer in the tip of the finger.
D-69. Hypopituitarism: The patients has enlarged breasts, short stature, and small genitalia due to low gonadotrophic hormones.
D-70. Porphyria cutaneous tarda: Pigmented scarring and blister formation due to photosensitivity.
D-71. Apthous ulcer: It is commonly found inside the mouth particularly lower lip.
D-72. Right sided facial palsy: It is due to acute thrombotic stroke.
D-73. Alcaptonuria: Picture shows accumulation of homogentesic acid in the sclera. It is due to deficiency of the enzyme homogentesic acid oxidase.
D-74. Candida nail infection: It causes chronic destruction of the nails.
D-75. Pulmonary asbestosis: X-ray shows multiple pleural calcified plaques due to asbestosis. H/O exposure to asbestos, and higher incidence of pleural mesotheliomas.
D-76. Bilateral hydronephrosis: Voiding cystourethrogram shows bilateral hydronephrosis due to pelvic tumor.
D-77. Bilateral polycystic kidneys: CT scan shows bilateral polycystic kidneys.
D-78. Renal cell cancer: Inferior vena cavagram shows (R) renal mass invading the IVC.
D-79. Osteogenic sarcomas: X-ray shows bony erosions and sun-ray appearance of the lower end of the femur.
D-80. Oral candida infections: It is common in HIV positive patients .
D-81. Molluscum contagiosum: It can be found in normal or HIV positive individuals.
D-82. Granuloma annulare: It is a ring shaped papular lesion which may be present in normal or diabetic individuals.
D-83. Tuberculous infection in the knee joint: A patient has swollen, tender, painful knee joint. He also has positive PPD test.
D-84. Non-Hodgkin lymphoma: The patient appears with low grade fever, enlarged lymph nodes in cervical, axillary, and inguinal regions, anemia, enlarged spleen. Picture shows rapidly growing lesion in the back.
D-85. Neurofibromatosis (or von Recklinghausen's disease): The patients appear with neurofibromas and cafe-au-lait spots.

D-86. Bell's palsy: It is due to lower motor neuron paralysis of the facial nerve. It may be due to viral or unknown etiology.

D-87. Pelvic metastases form prostate cancer: Metastatic lesions in the pelvic bones but the bone is **not** enlarged like Paget's disease.

D-88. Cerebral infarctions: CT scan was done 12 hours after the (L) middle cerebral artery embolism. It shows hypodense areas in left cerebral region.

D-89. Discoid dermatitis: Weeping lesion secreting serous fluid.

D-90. Pitting edema due to cardiac failure: Both feet is swollen, nontender.

D-91. Stones in (R) ureter: Plain x-ray shows single stone in (R) ureter.

D-92. Thyrotoxic nodule causing hyperthyroidism: The patient appears with small thyroid mass, signs and symptoms of hyperthyroidism.

D-93. Barber's rash: It is a vesiculo-crusted lesions over the face due to **Streptococcus pyogenes**.

D-94. Nephoric syndrome: The patient appear with periorbital and facial edemas, proteinuria, hypoalbuminemia.

D-95. Optic atrophy: Optic disc is pale and flat. It has well-defined margin. It may be due to pituitary tumor compressing on the optic pathway.

D-96. Right subdural hematoma: CT scan shows (R) subdural hematoma plus cerebral atrophy and dilated ventricles.

D-97. Metastatic lesion in the brain: Primary cancerous lesion is in the lung.

D-98. Interstitial pneumonias in both lungs: The patient is HIV positive or has immunosuppressive disease.

D-99. Pleural effusion in (R) lung: Larger amount of fluid is accumulated in (R) lung.

D-100. Pneumothorax: Plain x-ray shows pneumothorax and collapsed lung in the left side of the chest.

D-101. Erysipelas: The patient appears with red, hot, tender skin over the face and neck. It has well-defined margin and is due to Streptococcus pyogenes.

D-102. Acanthosis nigricans: Dark brown or black hyperpigmented areas. Rule out adenocarcinoma of the stomach. It may be present in Cushing's syndrome, Stein-Leventhal syndrome, obese patients with or without insulin resistance syndromes.

D-103. Migrating thrombophlebitis: Rule out carcinoma of the pancreas. The patient appears with ischemia of the skin and atrophy of the muscles of the leg.

D-104. Teretoma of the anterior mediastinum: Plain x-ray shows large mass in the anterior mediastinum.

D-105. Thallium scan:

(a) Normal- Doughnut shaped ring of ventricular myocardium.

(b) Coronary artery stenosis- Defect in the septum and inferior wall of the ventricular myocardium.

D-106. Uterine leiomyomas: X-ray shows large calcified mass attached to the uterus. The patients H/O constipation, dysuria, and mestrual irregulatities.

D-107.Abdominal ascites: Free fluid in the peritoneal cavity and paucity of the bowel gas pattern.
D-108.Fibrotic chronic lung disease: Bilateral clubbing of the fingers.
D-109.Lichen planus: Papular, itchy lesions with dystrophic nails.
D-110.Cerebral abscesses: CT scan shows occipital abscesses in a HIV-positive patient due to toxoplasma infection.
D-111.Peutz-Jeghers syndrome: Pigmentations on the buccal mucosa, palate, lips, rarely in hands and feet. Rule out multiple intestinal polyposis.
D-112.DIC (disseminated intravascular coagulation): The patient appears with purpuric rashes, ecchymosis, neutropenia, thrombocytopenia. It is most commonly due to systemic bacterial infections.
D-113.Common bile duct stones and dilated common bile duct: Endoscopic retrograde cholangiopancreatogram shows dilated CBD but normal intrahepatic duct in patients with CBD stones.
D-114.Leukonychia: White nails, rule out nephrotic syndrome or chronic liver disease.
D-115.Carcinoma of the stomach: Barium study shows filling defect due to cancerous lessions.
D-116.Colonic polyps: Barium enema shows filling defects. The patient appears with abdominal pain and bloody stool.
D-117.Renal cell cancer: CT scan shows large renal mass with central necrotic areas.
D-118.Left frontal meningiomas: CT scan shows large mass in the frontal lobe area.
D-119.Bilateral enlarged parotid glands: The patient with alcoholic cirrhosis shows bilateral enlarged parotid glands.
D-120.Rheumatoid arthritis: Deep ulcerations in the foot due to vasculitis.
D-121.Temporal arteritis: Dilated, tortuous temporal arteries. The patient appears with headaches, visual disturbances, and tenderness over the arteries.
D-122.Genital herpetic lesions: Picture shows multiple ulcerated lesions over the shaft of the penis.
D-123.Diabetic neuropathic ulcers: Deep penetrating ulcers under the first metatarsal head which is a pressure point. Ulcers are well-defined with surrounding thickened skin.
D-124.Blue hand: It is due to methemoglobinemia. It may be due to use of dapsone. The patients may have underlying gluten induced enteropathy.
D-125.Osteolytic bony lesion due to metastases: Primary lytic lesions may by in the kidney, thyroid, lung, or breast. Breast cancer metastases may also be blastic or mixed type.
D-126.Brain metasteses: Primary lesions may be in the lung, breast, colon, or other sites.
D-127.Primary lung cancer: X-ray shows mass in the (L) lung.
D-128.Miliary pulmonary tuberculosis: Bilateral diffuse lesions have shown in x-ray.
D-129.Pemphigoid: Multiple blisters with or without inside hemorrhages.

D-130.Malignant melanoma: Rapidly growing black color ulcerative lesions in the hand. The biopsy confirms the diagnosis.

D-131.Unilateral proptosis: It could be due to retroorbital mass or even in thyrotoxicosis which is usually bilateral.

D-132.Autoimmune pernicious anemia: The patient appears with premature gray hair. Autoimmune pernicious anemia may be associated with gastric cancer..

D-133.Erythema nodosum: The patients appear with painful, tender, purplish-red erythematous nodules over the pretibial regions. Rule out systemic diseases, infections, and drug use.

D-134.Anal cancer: H/O painful defecation for last several months. The biopsy confirms the diagnosis.

D-135.Osteoarthritis: Deformed interphalangeal joints, presence of Heberden's nodes at the distal and Bouchard's nodes at the proximal interphalangeal joints.

D-136.Drug rashes: It may appear as symmetric erythematous maculopapular rashes in the lower extremities or any other part of the body.

D-137.Multiple rheumatoid nodules in the lungs: Chest x-ray shows multiple nodular lesions and bilateral fibrotic changes.

D-138.Systemic lupus erythematosus: Butterfly appearance of the rashes over the nose.

D-139.Pulmonary embolism: The ventilation scan is normal in both lungs but the perfusion scan shows defects in both lungs.

D-140.Bilateral hydronephrosis due to enlarged prostate: IVP shows hydronephrosis, hydroureter, and enlarged urinary bladder.

D-141.Bilateral renal scarring due to obstructive uropathy: DMSA scan shows defect in both kidneys.

D-142.Hypertensive retinopathy: Fundoscopic examination shows retinal hemorrhages, exudates, narrowed blood vessels.

D-143.Right sided cerebral infarction due to acute stroke: CT scan shows hypodense areas in (R) parieto-occipital regions.

D-144.Bronchopulmonary aspergillosis: Bilateral pulmonary fibrosis and bronchiectasis.

D-145.Erythema multiforme: Initially it may begins as target like lesions in the hands and feet, then erythematous lesions spread proximally into the body.

D-146.Multiple bone metastases: Bone scan shows increased uptake of the metastatic bony lesions. Primary cancer may be originated from lungs, Kidneys, prostate or breasts.

D-147.Ankylosing spondylitis: X-ray shows severely demineralized bony changes of the cervical vertebrae which has lost its normal curvature.

D-148.Diabetic retinopathy: Proliferation of new blood vessels, exudates, and hemorrhages.

D-149.Lung abscesses: It is due to aspiration, secondary infections (pneumonia), and followed by abscess formation.

D-150.Spider nevi: It due to defective liver functions, particularly estrogen metabolism.

D-151.Ramsay Hunt syndrome: It is due to herpes zoster infections of the VII cranial nerve.

D-152.Pyoderma gangrenosum: Large, necrotic painful ulcer with slough formation. Rule out ulcerative colitis.

D-153.Hereditary hemorrhagic telangiectasia: Red spot on the lips, gum, nose, tongue, and inside the GI tract. It blanches on pressure. The patients may have epistaxis or GI bleeding.

D-154.Syringomyelia: Wasted hand muscles in both hands.

D-155.Contact dermatitis: It is due to the earring.

D-156.COPD (Chronicsobstructive pulmonary diseases): Blue bloaters means cyanosis and peripheral edema due to right heart failure.

D-157.Thrombus inside the (L) atrium: The patient has rheumatic mitral stenosis with atrial fibrillations.

D-158.Thrombocytopenic purpura: Purpuric lesions over the body may be due to drug use .

D-159.Psudohypoparathyroidism: The patient has a short third finger which is due to short third metacarpal bone.

D-160.Toxic megacolon: X-ray abdomen shows dilated colon. The patient has been suffering from ulcerative colitis.

D-161.SVC (superior vena cava obstruction): The patient has puffy face, dilated veins of upper chest areas, chronic cough, loss of weight. Rule out bronchial carcinoma obstructing the SVC.

D-162.Infective endocarditis: The patient has subconjucntival hemorrhages due to septic emboli.

D-163.Lumphoma of the testis: Swollen testis in an elderly patient.

D-164.Right subdural hemorrhage: It is due to trauma .

D-165.Myasthenia gravis: The patients has bilateral ptosis and facial weakness.

D-166.Kaposi's sarcoma: It is found in HIV-positive patients.

D-167.Genital warts: It may sessile filiform or hyperplastic. It is a STD.

D-168.Tinea infections or ringworm: Lesions are itchy and scaly.

D-169.Severe alopecia areata: Bald areas over the scalp.

D-170.COPD (chronic obstructive pulmonary disease): This patient has well maintained oxygenation and low $Paco_2$, so it is called pink puffer.

D-171.Left bronchial cancer: It causes collapse of the upper lobe due to bronchial obstruction.

D-172.Left ventricular thrombus: Echocardiogram shows (L) ventricular mass.

D-173.Cystic fibrosis: Bronchiectatic changes, hyperinflated lungs, and flattened diaphragm.

D-174.Staphylococcal pneumonias: The patient is extremely sick .

D-175.Tuberculous pleural effusion: Extensive effusion in (R) pleura.

D-176.Sarcoidosis: Bilateral hilar lymph nodes enlargement.

D-177.Boutonnier deformity: It may be present in advanced stage of rheumatoid arthritis. It is due to rupture of the central portion of extensor tendon but lateral portions are displaced to each side to maintain the deformity.

D-178.Polyarteritis nodosa: Purpuric rashes over the feet are due to vasculitis.

D-179.Horner syndrome: (R) eye ptosis and constricted pupil; normal (L) eye.

D-180.Benign mole (or melanocytic nevus): It may change into malignancy.

D-181.Swan neck deformity of the finger: It is found in advanced stage of rheumatoid arthritis. It is due to disruption of the palmer plate of proximal interphalangeal joint, may be associated with rupture of the insertion site of flexor sublimis tendon.

D-182.Dermatomyositis: Erythema and edema of the face.

D-183.Kyphosis in COPD-emphysema patients: Hyperinflated lungs and kyphosis are found in COPD patients.

D-184.Unilateral lymphedama: The patients has swollen, nontender, heavy (L) leg.

D-185.Simple obesity : Excessive fat deposition in upper arm, breasts, abdomen, buttocks, and thighs.

D-186.Budd-Chiari syndrome: It is due to hepatic venous obstruction. The patients appear with dilated veins of the abdominal wall.

D-187.Anorexia nervosa: Excessive loss of body weight plus secondary amenorrhea.

D-188.Colonic diverticulum: Multiple colonic diverticulm. The patient has abdominal pain and lower GI bleeding.

D-189.Esophagitis and ulcers: Endoscopy picture shows inflammed and ulcerated esophagus due to reflux.

D-190.Gallstones**:** The patient has severe upper right abdominal pain.

D-191.Metastasis in the (R) adrenal gland: Primary cancerous lesion from another part of the body which needs to be determined.

D-192.Degenerative arthritis: X-ray shows narrowed, irregular hip joint space, and damaged cartilage inside.

D-193.Pemphigus vulgaris: Ruptured blisters and crusted lesions all over the body.

D-194.Ehlers-Danlos syndrome: Hyperextended fingers and hyperelasticity of the skin.

D-195.Hyperthyroidisms: Bilateral proptosis in both eyes.

D-196.Mitral value prolapse: Echocardiogram shows prolapse of mitral valve into the left ventricle (LV).

D-197.Esophageal varices: Barium swallow shows varices in the lower esophagus.

D-198.Left hypoglossal nerve paralysis: It is due to lower motor neuron lesion in the 12th cranial nerve. The tongue has fasciculations and is deviated to the paralysed side during protrusion.

D-199. Abdominal aortic aneurysms: Angiogram shows dilated abdominal aorta. It can rupture easily.

D-200. Silicosis: Chest x-ray shows bilateral silicotic nodules and inflitrative granulomas.

D-201. Fractures tibia and fibula: It is due to fall with the outstretched hands.

D-202. Esophageal cancer: Barium swallow shows filling defects in the lower esophagus.

D-203. ARDS (adult respiratory distress syndrome): Chest x-ray shows pulmonary edema due to increased capillary permeability.

D-204. Pneumoconiosis: Chest x-ray shows fibrotic changes in both lungs.

D-205. **Right facial nerve palsy** due to upper motor neurone lesion: Weakness in the **lower facial muscles, e**specially around the mouth and eye. The forehead is supplied from both sides, so wrinkling of the brow remains intact (remember, **wrinkling is asymmetric in lower motor neurone lesion, such as Bell's palsy).** It is due to thrombotic stroke of the **left carotid artery**.

D-206. Acute surgical emphysema following pneumothorax: Acute onset of chest pain following cough in a patient with chronic obstructive pulmonary disease. Pneumothorax is revealed in chest x-ray. The patient suddenly developes acute swelling of the face, neck, and upper part of the chest.

D-207. Bell's palsy (lower motor neuron lesion of the VII cranial nerve): The patient has weakness in the muscles of the forehead, around the eye and mouth (remember, forehead muscles remain normal in upper motor neurone lesions) .

D-208. Obstructive bullous emphysema of the left lung: Dark lucent shadow in the left lung, shifting of the mediastinum to the right.

D-209. Left lower lobe collapse: Visible wedge-shaped shadow behind the heart shadow.

D-210. Massive pleural effusion in (R) side: Mediastinum is shifted to the left, cardiac border and size cannot be measured.

D-211. Pompholyx: It is a variant of eczema. It appears with vesicular lesions over the palms, soles, and fingers. It is characterized by remission and relapse, the relapse could be due to emotional stress or heat exposure.

D-212. Reiter's disease (or circinate balanitis): The patient appears with macular ulcerative lesions over the penis, vesicular rashes inside the buccal mucosa, redness of both eyes, and knee joints swelling.

D-213. Cardiac failure: The patients appears with distended external jugular veins during physical examination.

D-214. Pneumonia in (R) upper lobe: Chest x-ray shows consolidation and infiltrates in right upper lobe.

D-215. Left pneumothorax: Left lung is almost completely collapsed due to left pneumothorax.

D-216. Completely collapsed left lung: It results in compensatory emphysema of the right lung which is deviated toward the left side of the chest.

D-217. Mediastinal hemorrhage: Chest x-ray shows wide mediastinal shadow.

D-218. Acne vulgaris: Papulo-pustular lesions over the face and other parts of the body.

D-219. Leukocytoclastic vasculitis: It is due to deposition of immune complexes in the post-capillary venules. The patient appears with painful, purpuric lesions over the lower extremities.

D-220. Down syndrome: The patient appear with characteristic facial features such as hypertelorisms upward and outward slanting of both eyes, epicanthic folds. The patient is very friendly in nature.

D-221. Achalsia of the esophagus: Lower esophageal sphincter fails to relax. The patients appears with H/O dysphagia and food retention in the lower end of esophagus.

D-222. Retinitis pigmentosa: The patient appears with progressive peripheral loss of vision, night blindness. The fundoscopic examination shows retinal pigmentations, pallor of the optic disc, and attenuation of retinal arteries.

D-223. Pneumonia of the left lower lobe: Chest x-ray shows consolidation of the left lower lobe and absence of adjacent diaphragmatic shadow.

D-224. Pan-acinar emphysema with bullae formations: Bullae formations (white demarcated lines) in both lungs in a patients with chronic bronchitis plus emphysema.

D-225. Alzheimer's disease: Cerebral atrophy results in dilation of sulci, fissures, ventricles and poor demarcation between grey and white matters.

D-226. Irritant dermatitis: It is due to exposure of the hand with the chemical irritants.

D-227. Fournier's gangrene: It is due to bacteroides infection, usually B.frgilis.

D-228. Cirrhosis of the liver: CT scan shows cirrhotic (small) liver, ascites, and enlarged spleen.

D-229. Renal artery stenosis: The patient has hypertension due to renal artery stenosis which is shown by aortogram.

D-230. Bladder rupture due to trauma: Cystogram shows tear drop urinary bladder.

D-231. Addison disease: The patient has generalized hyperpigmentations specially over the extensor surfaces.

D-232. Klinefelter's syndrome: The patient appears with small genitalia, enlarged breast, and may be unusually tall in stature.

D-233. Primary hepatocellular carcinoma of the liver: CT scan shows enlarged liver with tumor mass plus enlarged spleen.

D-234. Right fourth cranial nerve palsy: The patient is asked to look down and to the left. The patient's right eye is **unable to go down** due to superior oblique muscle paralysis which is supplied by the fourth cranial nerve. The patient complains of double vision.

D-235. Tinker's Tartan (erythema ab igne): It is due to exposure to an excessive local heat (application of hot water bottle or sitting in front of a fire).

D-236. Collapse of right middle lobe: Chest x-ray shows RML collapse.

D-237.Congestive heart failure: Chest x-ray shows increased vascular markings, fluid in the horizontal fissure, and Kerley's B-lines.

D-238.Paralytic ileus: Abdominal x-ray shows distended both large and small intestine. It is due to accidental injury.

D-239.Duodenal ulcer: Barium study shows central ulcer crater in the duodenal cap.

D-240.Chronic sarcoidosis: The patient appears with lupus pernio which is dusky purple infiltrations of the nose.

D-241.Hodgkin disease: The patients has massive enlargement of the submandibular, cervical, and supraclavicular lymph nodes. He also has splenomegaly and mediastinal lymph adenopathies.

D-242.Free peritoneal air due to rupture of the intestine: It is due to trauma to the intestine, probably stab wound injury.

D-243.Hepatoma of the liver: CT scan shows large hepatoma in the left lobe of the liver.

D-244.Subcapsular splenic hematoma: It is due to traumatic injury in the spleen.

D-245.Squamous cells carcinoma: The cancerous lesion has thick edges and an irregular granular base.

D-246.Postoperative pneumonia: Chest x-ray reveals consolidation in right lower lobe, probably due to aspiration and /or diaphragmatic movements.

D-247.Dermatitis herpetiformis: It is due to IgA deposits in the dermal papillae. The patient appears with itchy blisters with or without rupture.

D-248.Infectious mononucleosis: The patient appears with acute tonsillitis, purpuric spots over the palate, sore throat , and develops rashes with ampicillin use.

D-249.Right kidney laceration and hematoma: It is due to trauma. CT scan is the best investigation of choice.

D-250.Epidural hematoma: CT scan shows biconvex lesion in the (R) frontal region. The patient should have characteristic lucid interval and it is due to trauma.

D-251.Deep vein thrombosis: The patient appears with acutely swollen leg, which is painful.

D-252.Acromegaly: The patient appears with prognathism, prominent supraorbital ridge and nose, thickene soft tissue and skin.

D-253.Turner syndrome: The patients has short stature, web neck, small breasts, increased carrying angle at the elbow (cubitus valgus), infertility, but normal mental development.

D-254.Acute hemarthrosis of the knee joints: It is a complication of hemophillia and von-Willebrand disease.

D-255.Bullous pemphigoid: Subepidermal tense blisters which is preceeded by itching, may be associated with eczematous eruption. It is due to IgG deposits at the dermal-epidermal junction.

D-256.Renal staghorn calculi: The patient had recurrent UTI and E.coli infections.

D-257.Aortic arch aneurysm: Barium filled esophagus is pushed to the (R) side by the large aortic aneurysm.

D-258.Pericardial cyst: X-ray shows round mass at the right cardiophrenic angle.

D-259.Atherosclerotic right coronary artery: The patient appears with chest pain, coronary angiogram shows narrowing and intraluminal thrombus formations.

D-260.Bladder calculi: X-ray picture shows layers of stone inside the urinary bladder.

D-261.Multiple basal cell carcinoma (Rodent ulcer): Different stages of lesion, characteristically over the bridge of the nose.

D-262.Psoriatic arthritis: The patient appears with swollen finger joints.

D-263.Eczema herpeticum: The patient develops herpetic lesions over the existing eczematous lesions.

D-264.Vitamin B_{12} deficiency: The smooth, red tongue with absence of filiform papillae.

D-265.Pulmonary artery hypertension: The arteriogram shows very narrow pulmonary artery branches.

D-266.Right middle lobe atelactasis: The lateral x-ray shows wedge-shaped density over the heart shadow.

D-267.Collapsed left lung: Chest x-ray shows almost complete absence of left pulmonary shadow plus mediastinal shift to the left.

D-268.Right upper lobe collapse: It is due to bronchogenic carcinoma of the upper bronchus.

D-269.Multiple sclerosis: MRI shows bilateral multiple high-signal (very white) lesions.

D-270.Holmes-Adie pupil: (R) eye slowly responds to light and accomodation but no response with rapid testing.

D-271.Myotonic dystrophy: The patient has facial weakness, frontal baldness, atrophic temporal and sternomastoid muscles.

D-272.Gum hypertrophy: It is due to chronic use of phenytoin.

D-273.Pericardial effusion: Chest x-ray shows enlarged heart shadow.

D-274.Left shoulder dislocation: X-ray shows anterior dislocation of the head of the humerous. It is due to trauma to the shoulder.

D-275.Acute pancreatitis: CT scan shows many small cyst formation which may coalesce to form large pseudocyst.

D-276.Cryoglobinemia: The patient has skin necrosis and ulcerations due to vascular blockage and capillary leak.

D-277.Cold nodule in right sided thyroid gland: Thyroid scan shows cold nodule which is decreased areas of uptake in (R) lobe of the thyroid gland and it is also enlarged. Left lobe is normal. Cold nodular areas have decreased blood supply and may have cancer.

D-278.Larger intracerebral bleed in right side: CT scan shows ventricles are displaced to the left side. It is due to traumatic injury.

D-279. Cerebral tumor in left side: CT scan shows mass in the anterior portion of cerebral hemisphere.

D-280. Cerebral aneurysm (R) side: CT scan shows large aneurysm just to the right side of sphenoidal sinuses.

D-281. CMV retinitis in AIDS patients: Typical cottage cheese-like retinal exudates and associated hemorrhages.

D-282. Roth's spots in subacute bacterial endocarditis: Retinal hemorrhages with central white spots.

D-283. Preretinal hemorrhages or subhyaloid hemorrhages: It may be due to difficult intubations, subarachnoid hemorrhages, or diabetic retinopathies.

D-284. Occlusion of inferior branches to retinal artery: Pale areas in an otherwise normal retina with visual defects.

D-285. Marfan syndrome: The tall thin patient has superior subluxation or dislocation of the lens, MVP, arachnodactyle, and aortic dissection leads to rupture.

D-286. Pityriasis rosea (christmas tree pattern): It is a benign condition that may be preceeded by URI symptoms. First lesion is 'herald patch' which is solitary, round, or oval lesion located over the trunk. It is followed by oval or round, tannish pink or salmon colored, scaling papules and plaques over the trunk, neck, and upper arms.

D-287. Tuberous sclerosis: Hypopigmented skin spots, adenoma sebaceum, periungula fibromas, cafe-au-lait spots, shagreen patches, tuber (granulomas) inside the brain appeared as irregular calcifications.

D-288. Janeway lesions in bacterial endocarditis: Painless hemorrhagic macules on the sole.

D-289. Male pseudohermaphroditism (androgen insensitivity): 46, XY chromosome; a patient with large breasts, absence of pubic and axillary hairs, amenorrhea, absence of uterus, ovary; presence of testes inside the abdomen or in labia majora.

D-290. Male pseudohermaphroditism (5 alpha-reductase deficiency): 46 XY chromosome; prepubertal virilization but normal male breast.

D-291. Klinefelter syndrome: A patient appears with enlarged breast, small male genitalia.

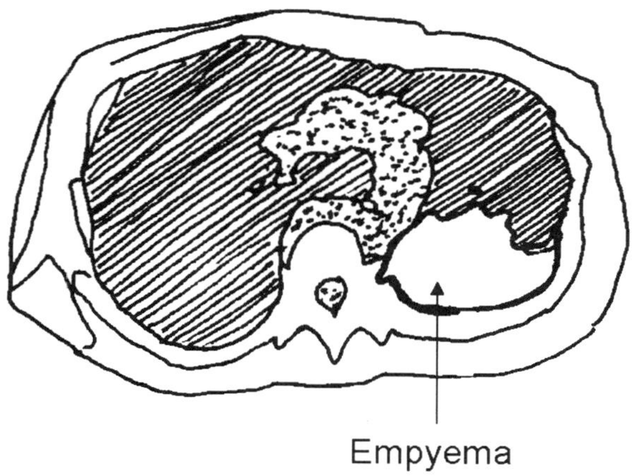

D-1: Empyema (L) thoracic cavity (CT scan)

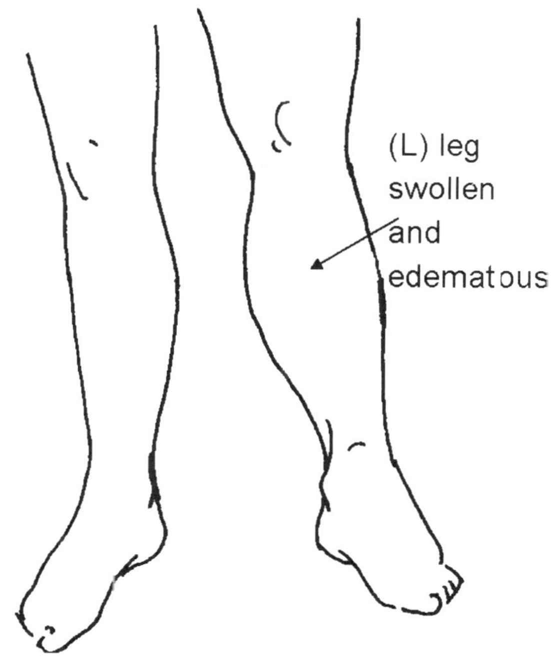

D-2: Ileofemoral deep vein thrombosis

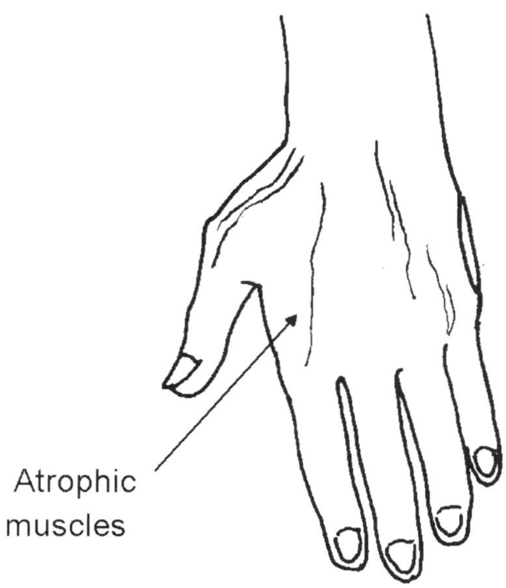

D-3: Atrophy of the hand muscles

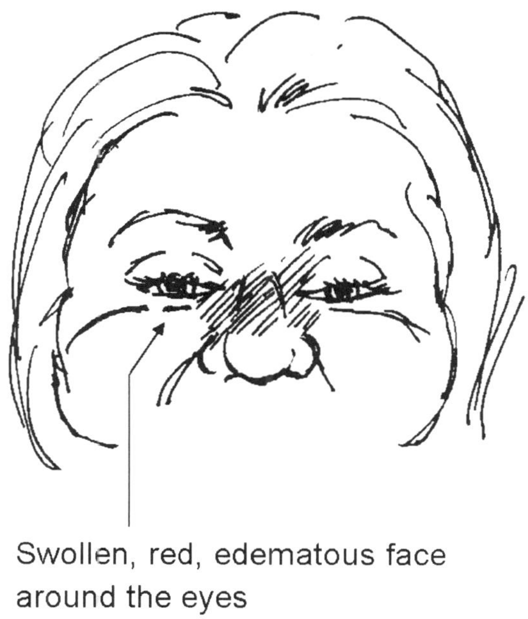

D-4: Cavernous sinus thrombosis

Picture 16

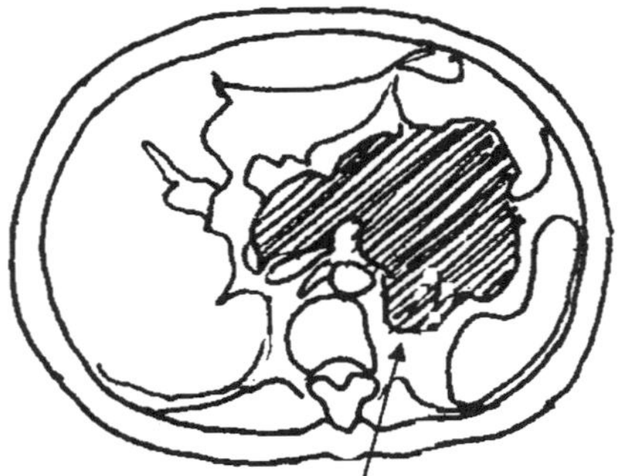

D-5: Islet cell cancer of the pancreas (MRI)

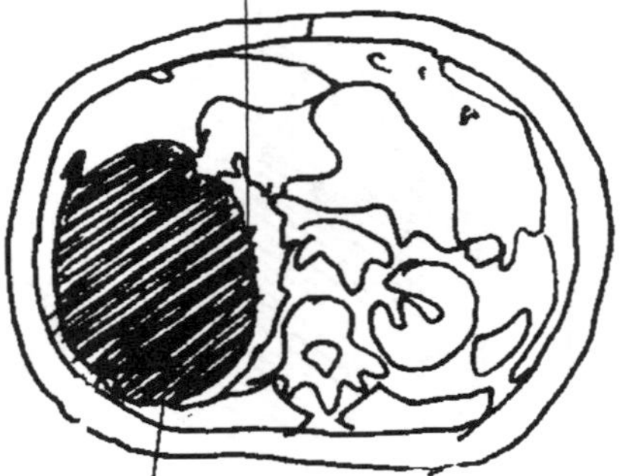

D-6: Large renal (R) cyst (MRI)

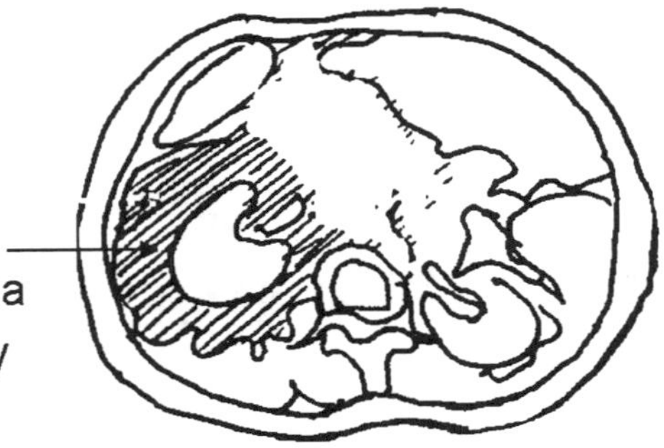

D-7: Hematoma (R) kidney (MRI)

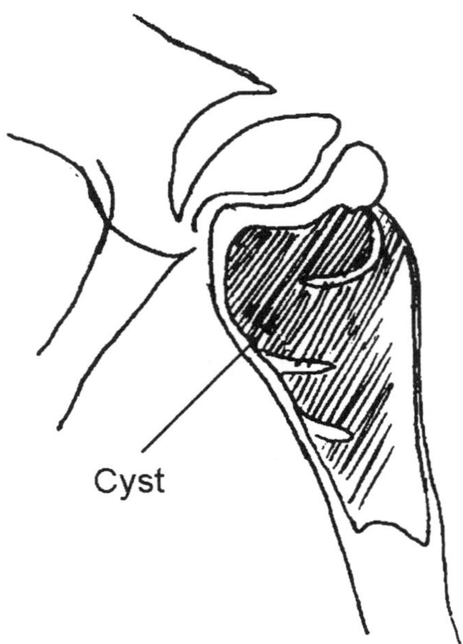

D-8: Bone cyst in (L) humerus (X-ray)

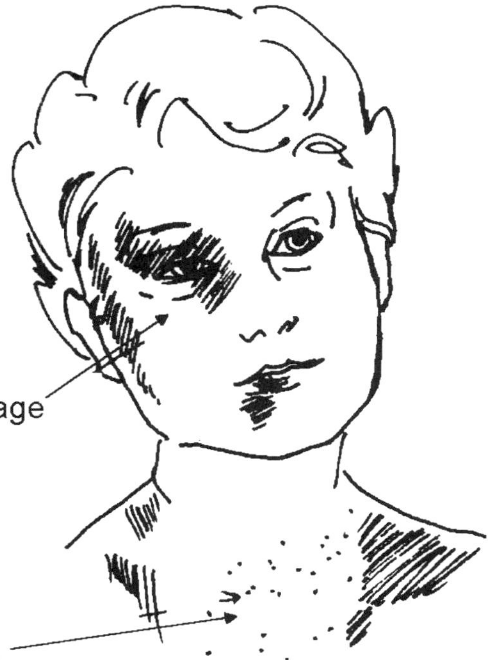

D-9: Traumatic asphyxia causing hemorrhage and petechiae

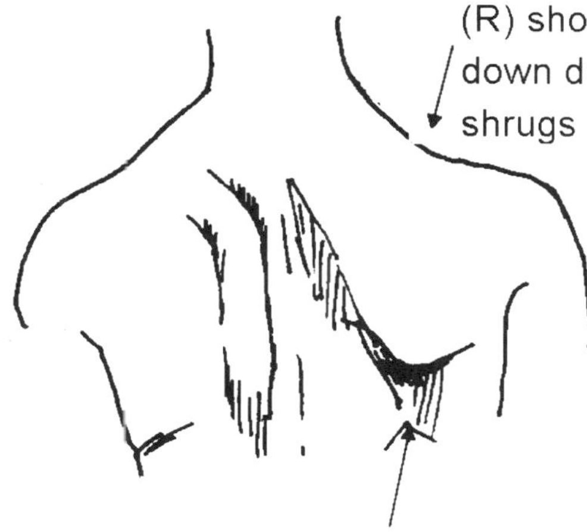

D-10: (R) trapezius muscle paralysis due to accessory nerve damage

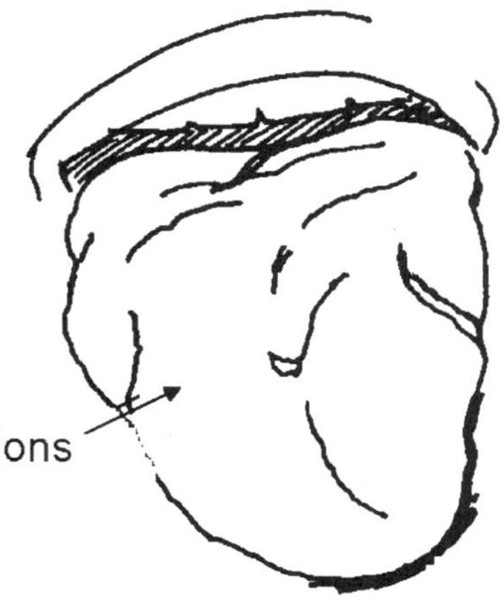

D-11: Tongue fasciculations due to motor neuron disease

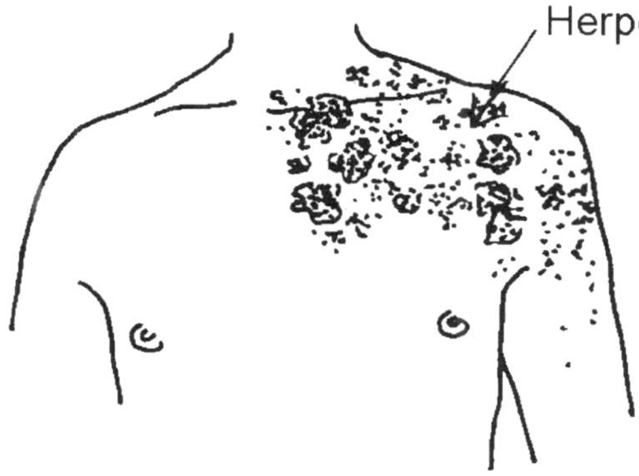

D-12: Herpes zoster

Picture 18

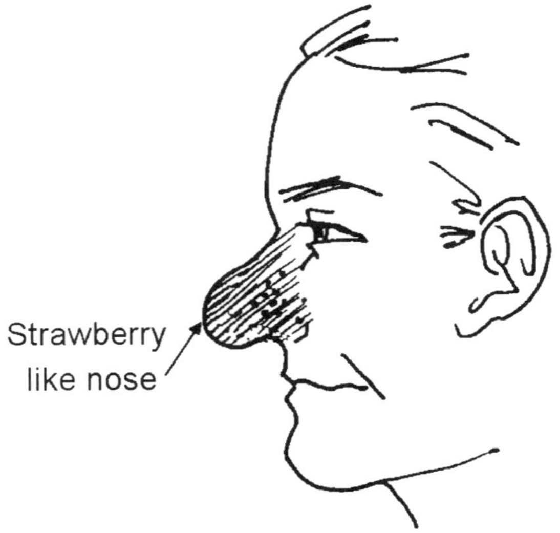

D-13: Rhinophyma

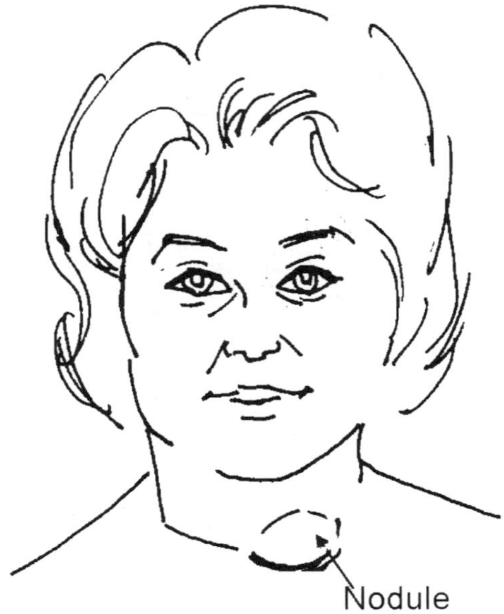

D-14: Thyroid nodule

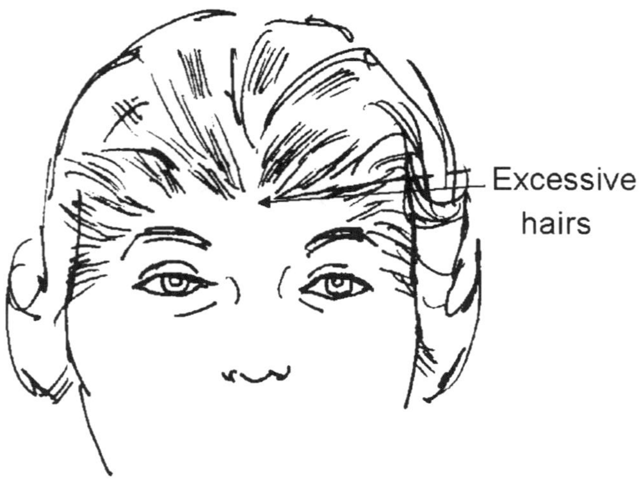

D-15: Hypertrichosis

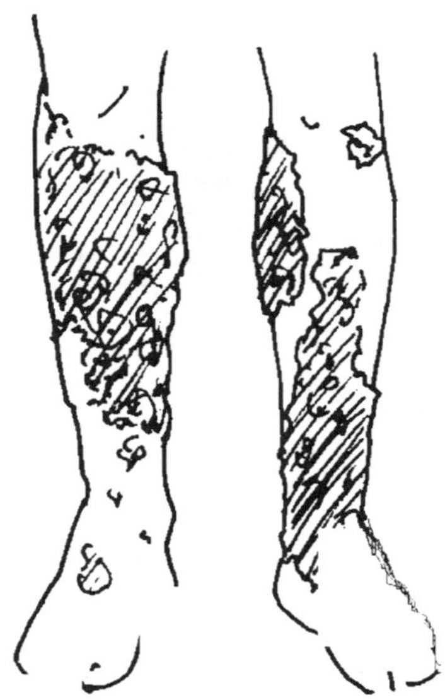

D-16: Psoriasis in both legs

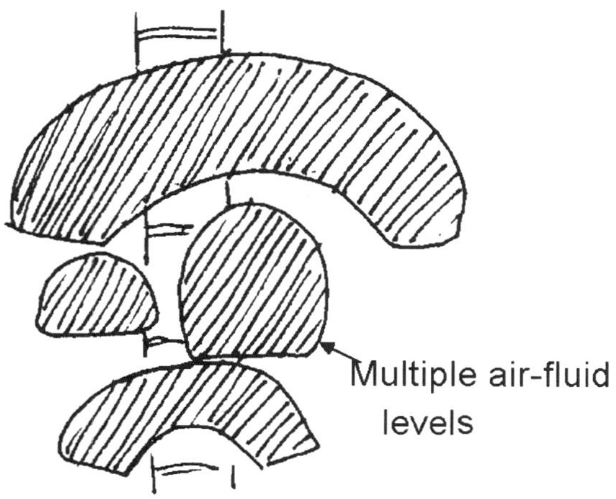

D-17: Small bowel obstruction (X-ray)

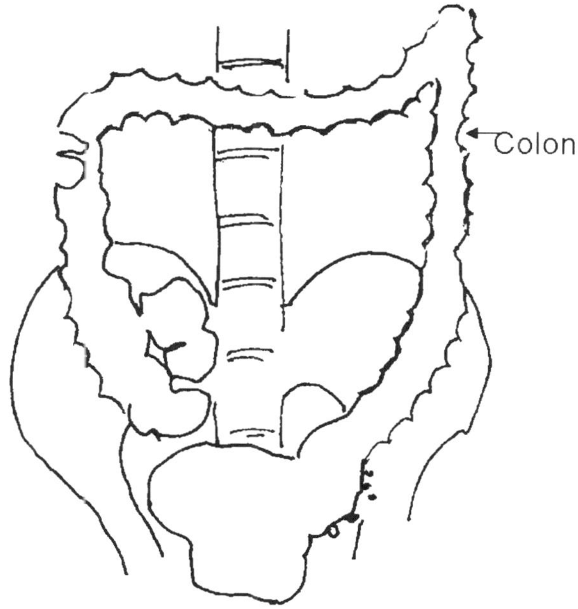

D-18: Ulcerative colitis (Barium enema)

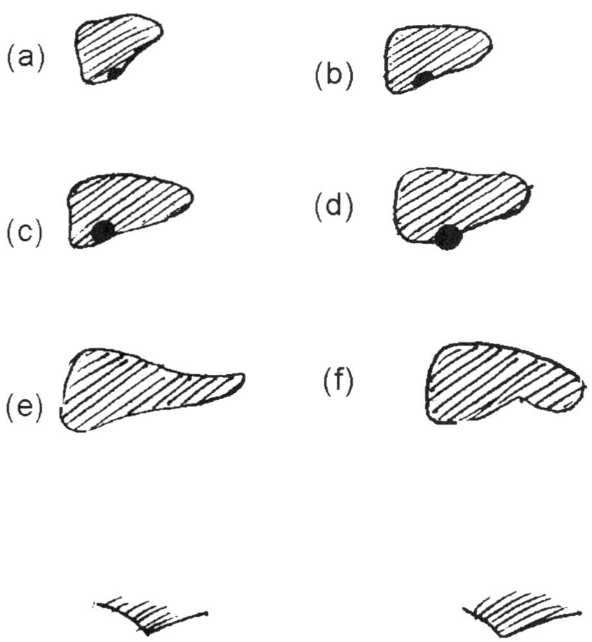

D-19: Normal HIDA scan (a,b,c,d)
Abnormal HIDA scan (e,f) due to obstruction of the cystic duct

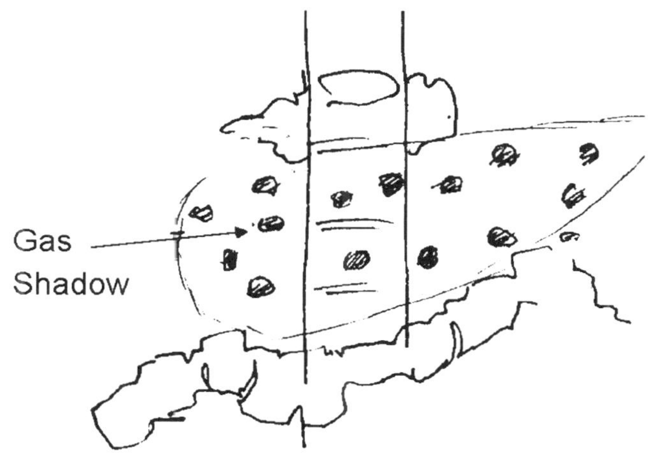

D-20: Pancreatic abscesses (CT scan)

Picture 20

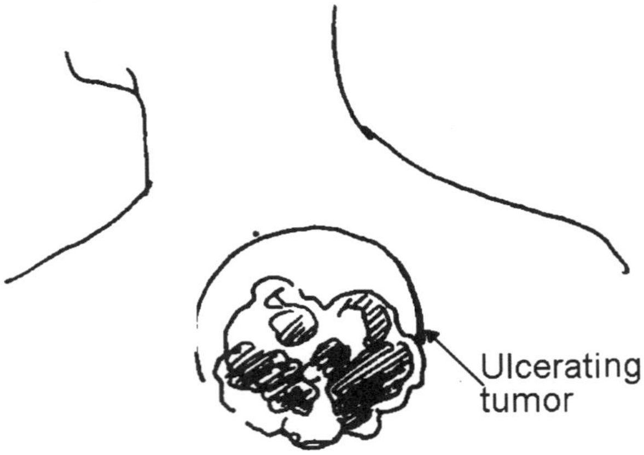

D-21: Keratoacanthoma of the back

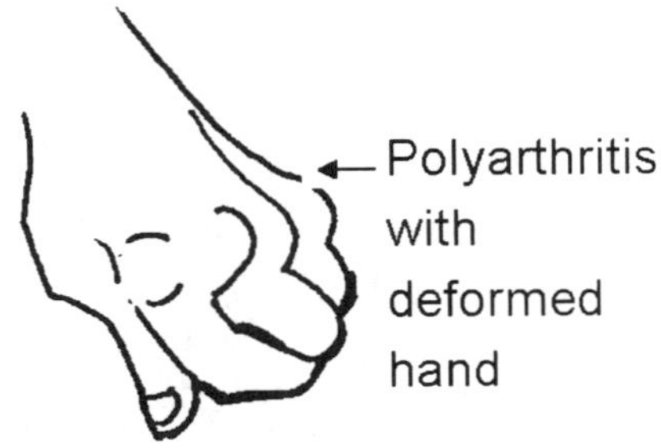

D-22: Chronic rheumatoid arthritis

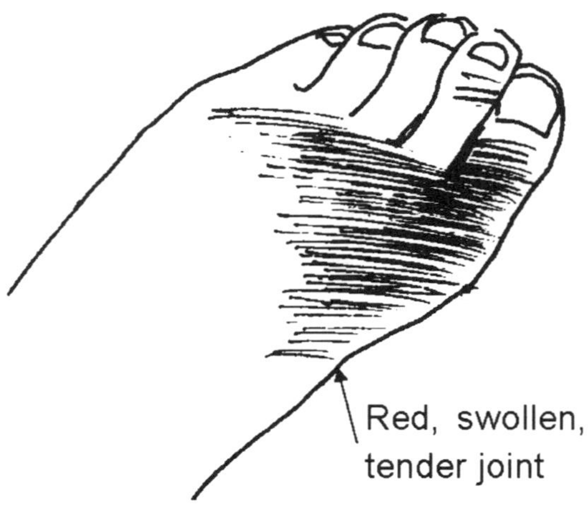

D-23: Gout (L) big toe

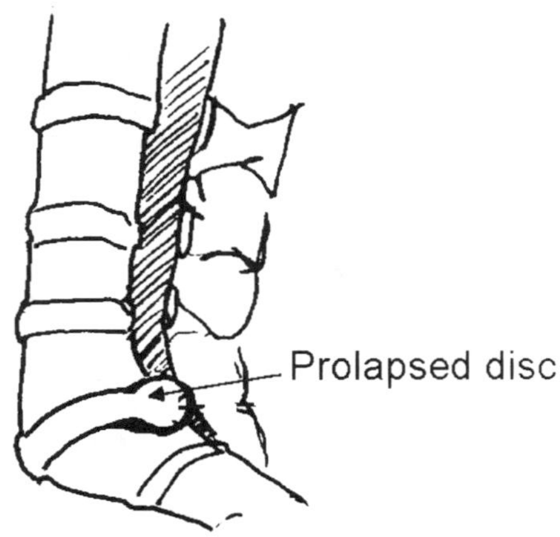

D-24: Prolapsed intervertebral disc between L_5 and S_1 (MRI)

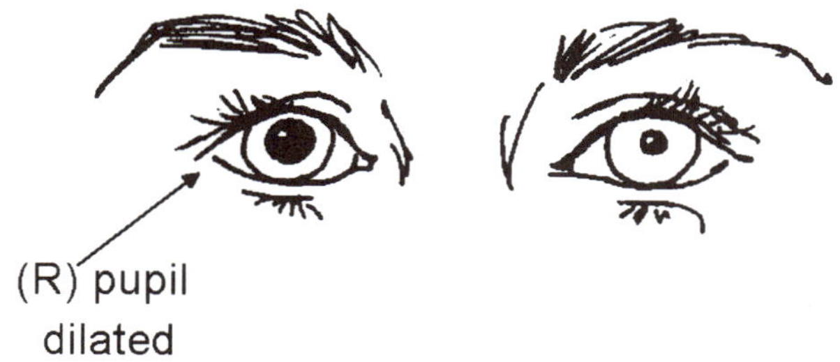

D-25: Holmes-Adie syndrome

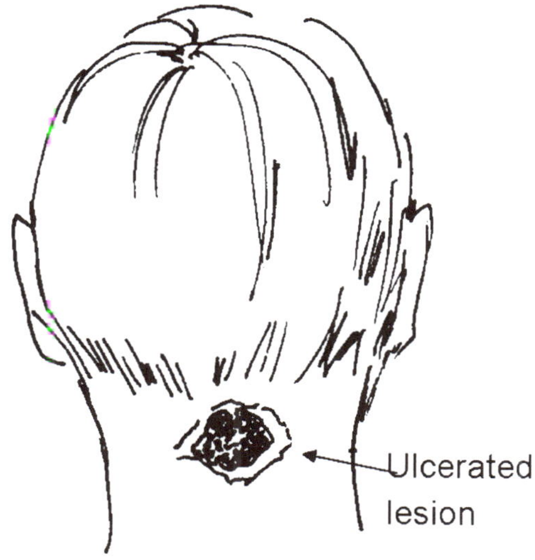

D-26: Anthrux or malignant pustule

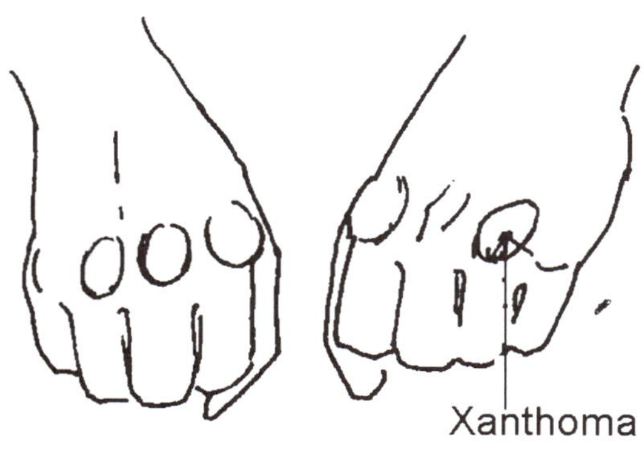

D-27: Xanthoma in both hands

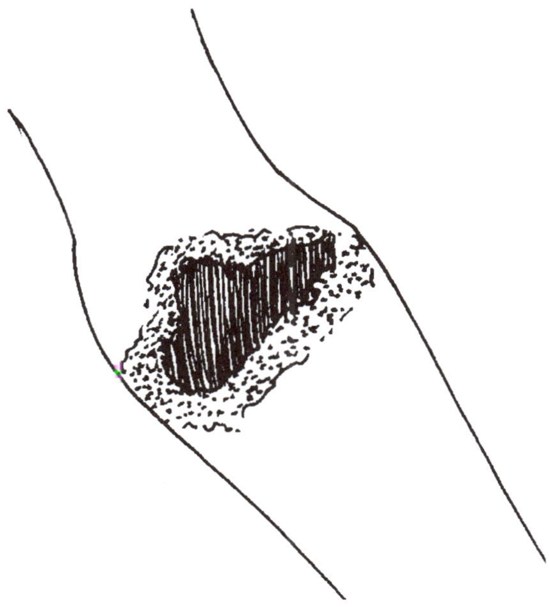

D-28: Skin necrosis due to protein C deficiency

Picture 22

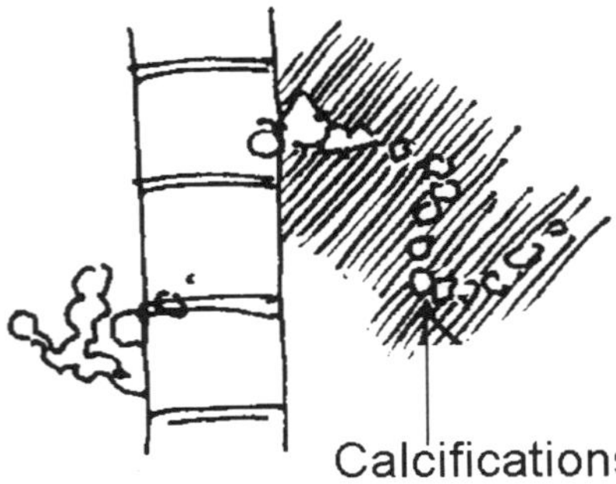

D-29: Chronic pancreatitis (x-ray)

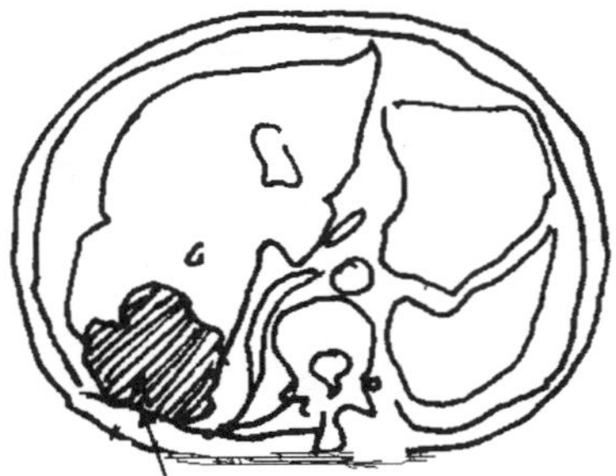

D-30: Carcinoma of the colon (MRI)

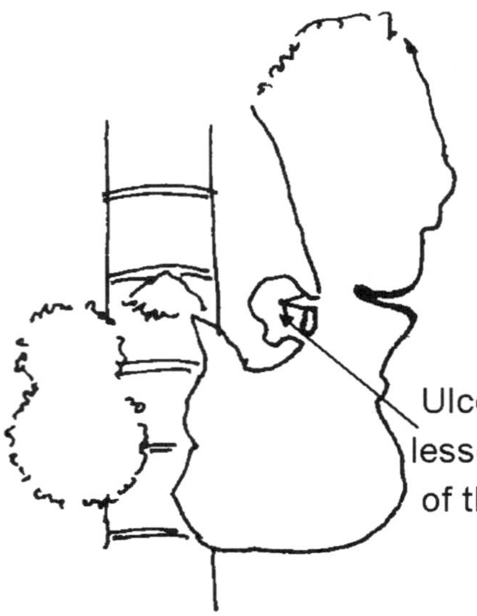

D-31: Gastric ulcer (Barium study)

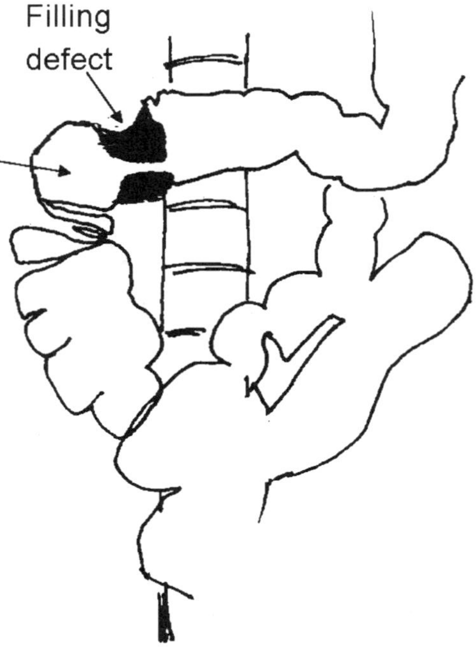

D-32: Carcinoma of the transverse colon (Barium enema)

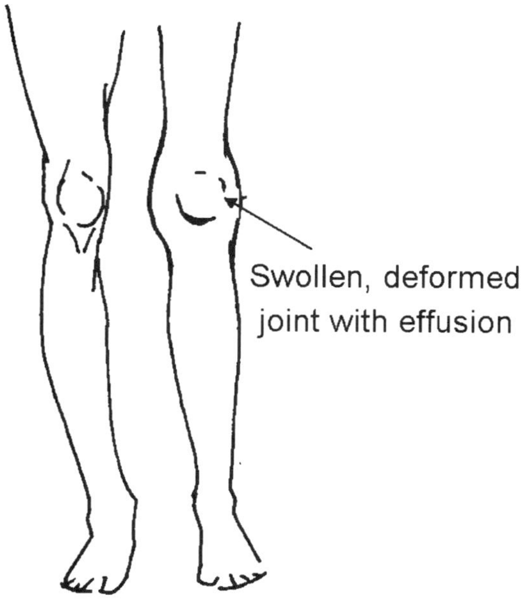

D-33: Osteoarthritis (L > R)

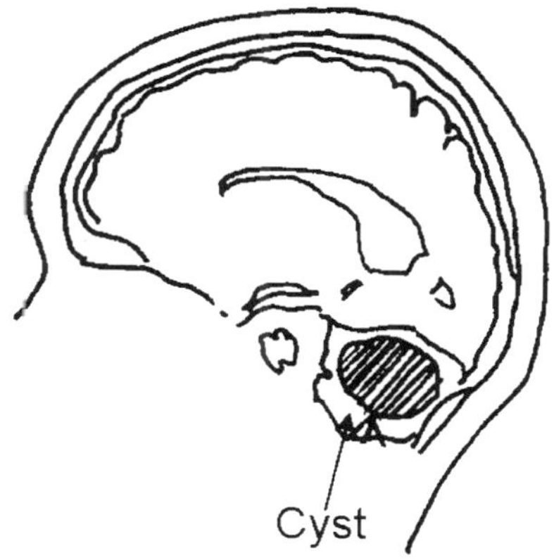

D-34: Cerebellar cyst (MRI)

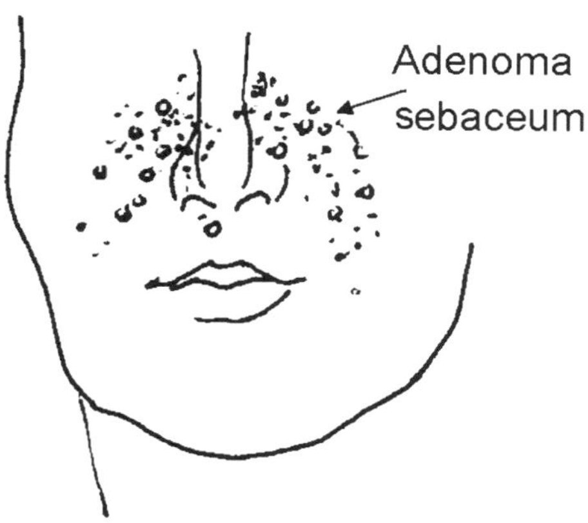

D-35: Tuberous sclerosis

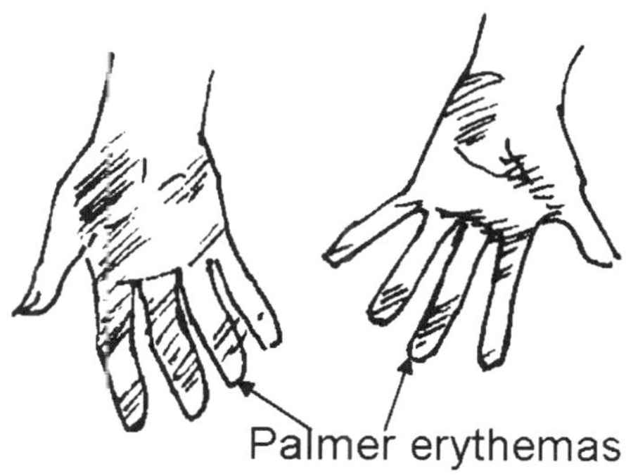

D-36: Liver disease

Picture 24

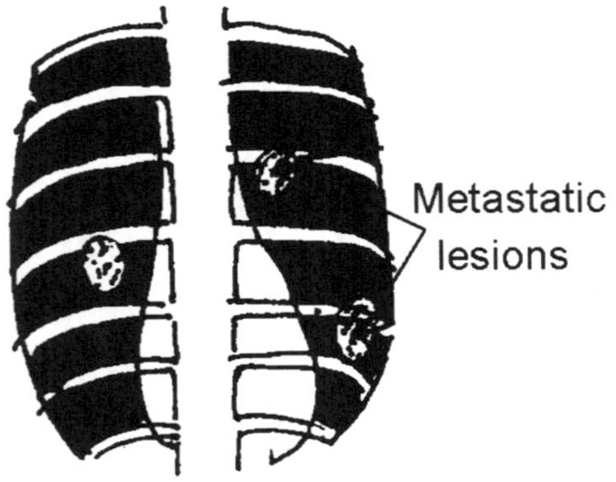

D-37: Lung metastases (X-ray)

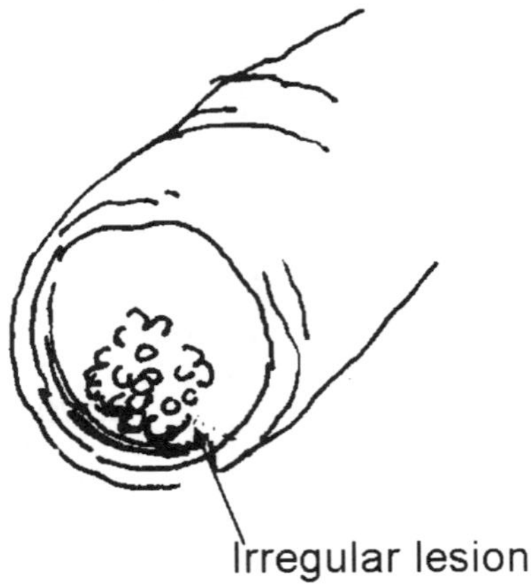

D-38: Penile cancer

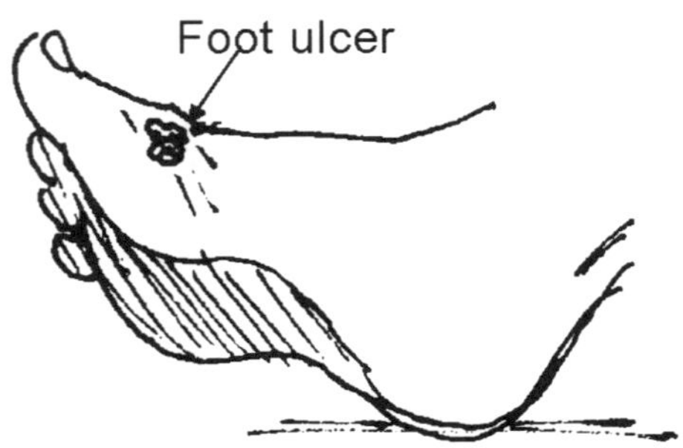

D-39: Diabetic neuropathy

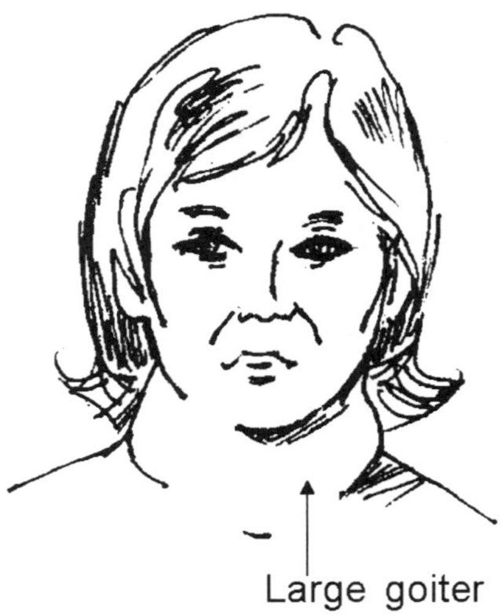

D-40: Hypothyroidism

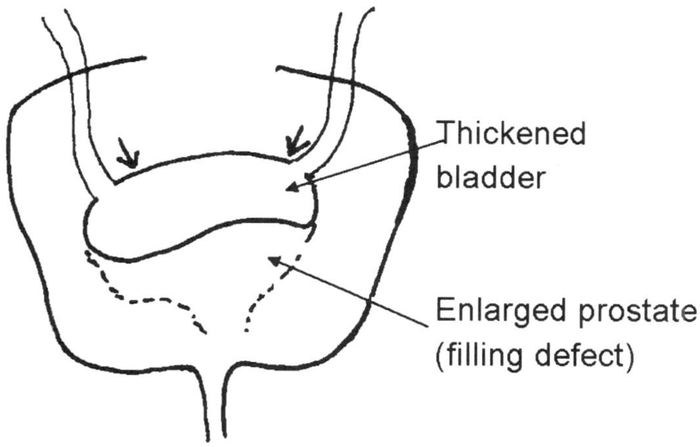

D-41: Enlarged prostate (Intravenous urography)

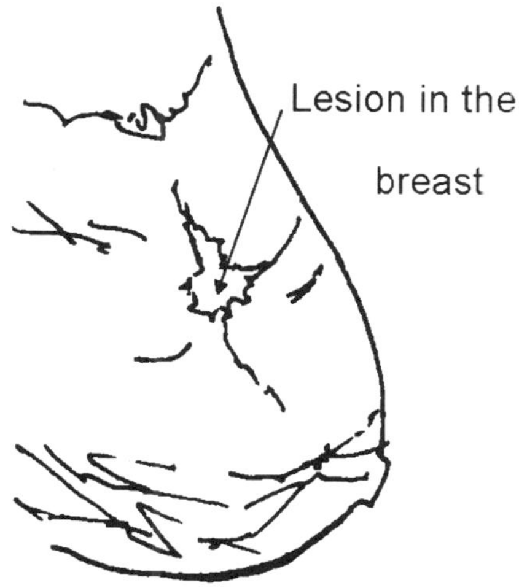

D-42: Breast cancer

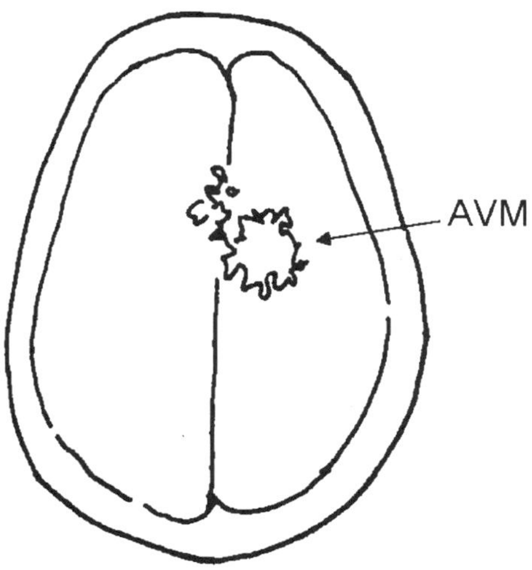

D-43: Cerebral arteriovenous malformation (AVM) (CT with Constrast)

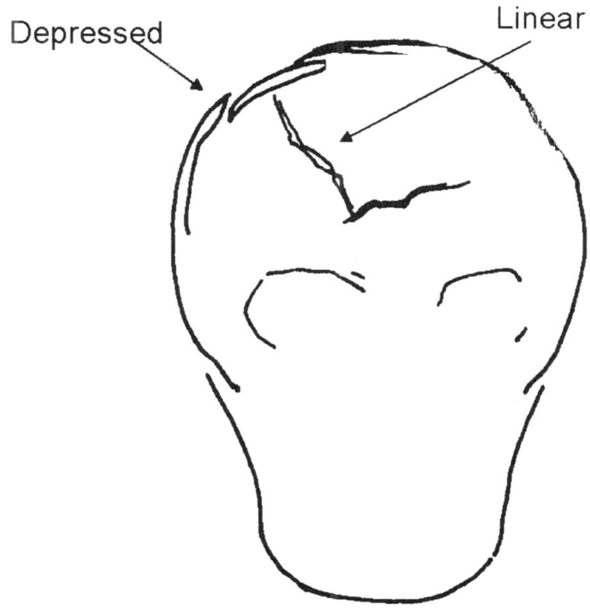

D-44: Skull fractures (X-ray)

Picture 26

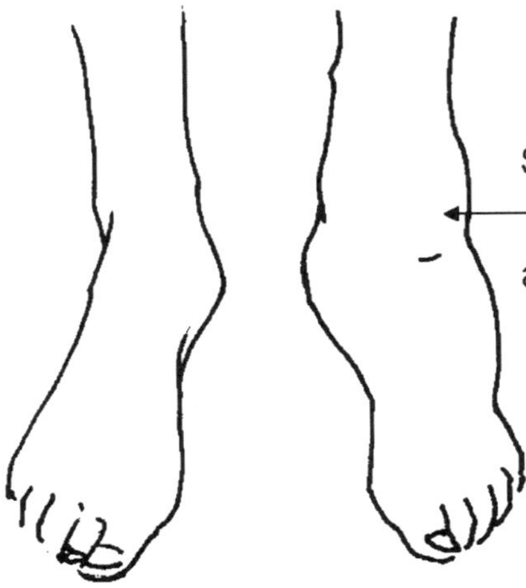

D-45: Diabetes neuropathy (Charcot joint)

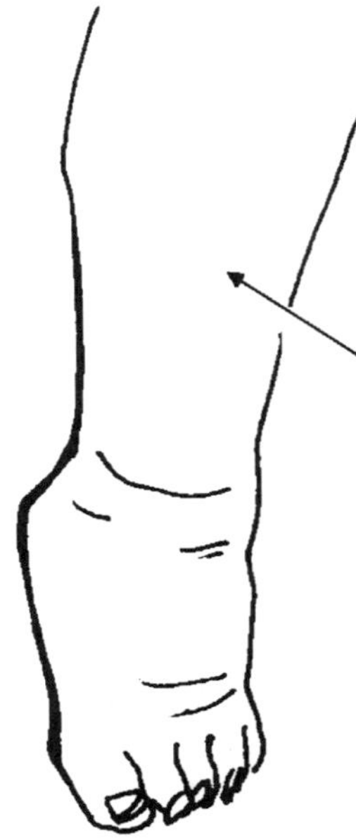

D-46: Grave's disease

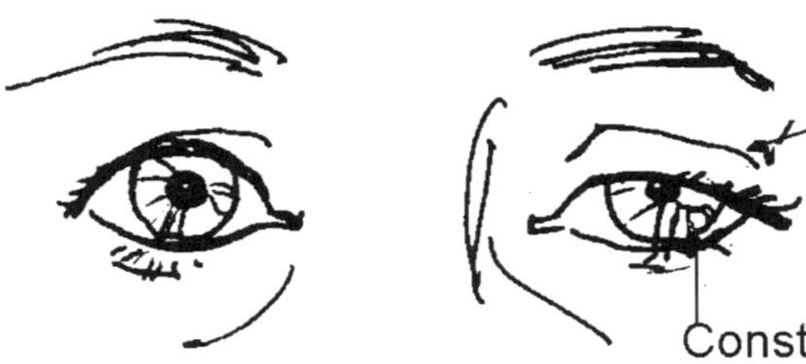

D-47: Horner's syndrome

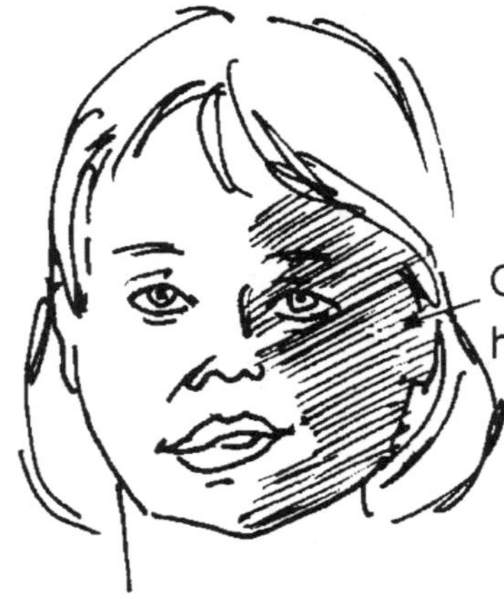

D-48: Sturge-Weber syndrome

Picture 27

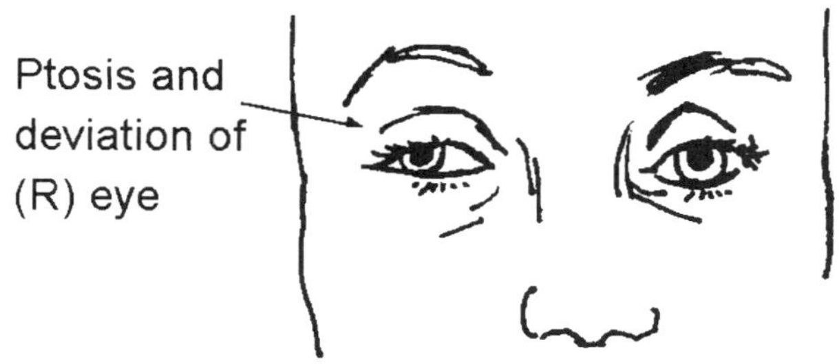

D-49: Oculomotor nerve palsy (R) eye

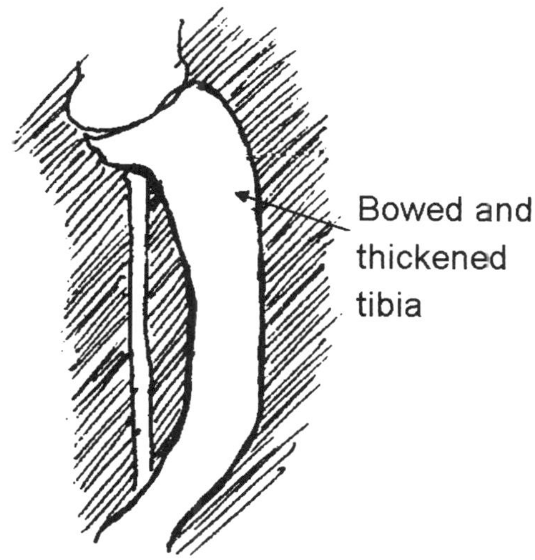

D-50: Paget's disease

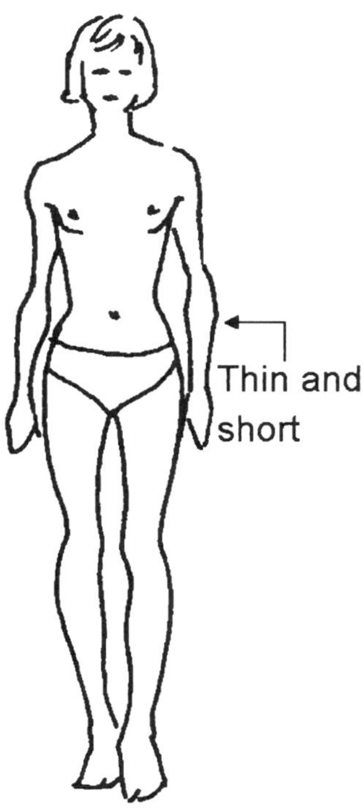

D-51: Gluten induced steatorrhea

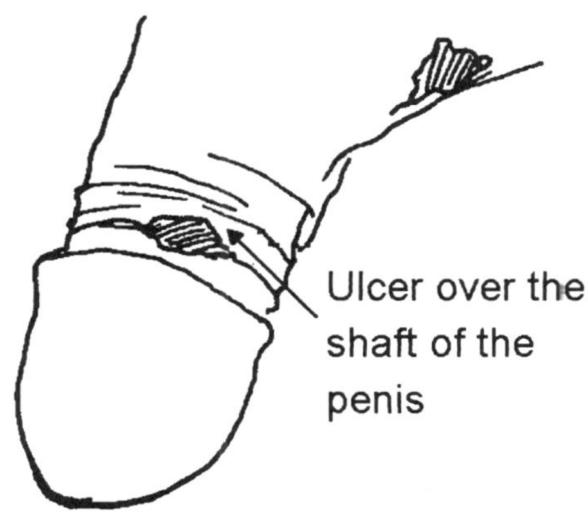

D-52: Lymphogranuloma venereum

Picture 28

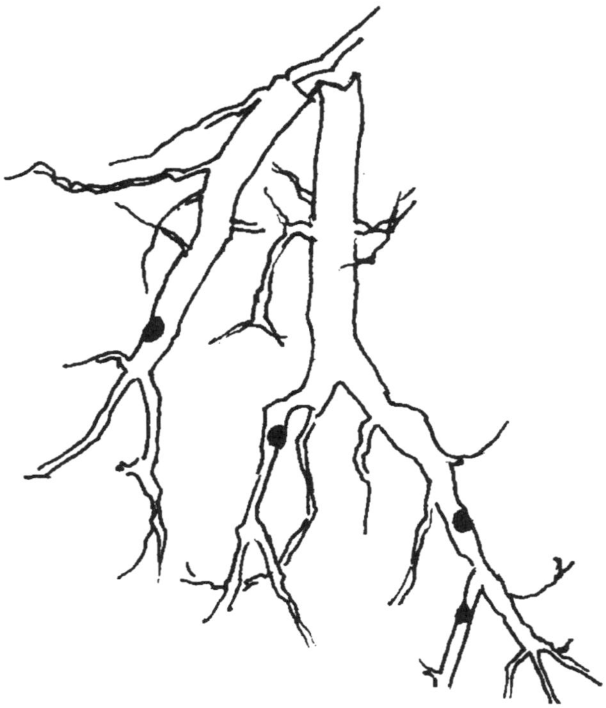

D-53: Pulmonary embolisms (angiogram)

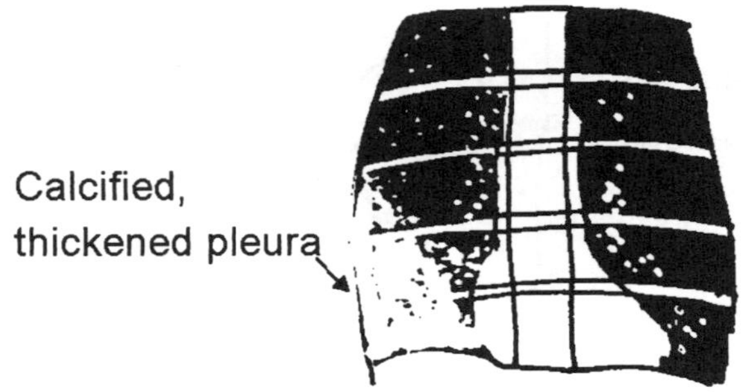

D-54: Pleural thickening (R) side

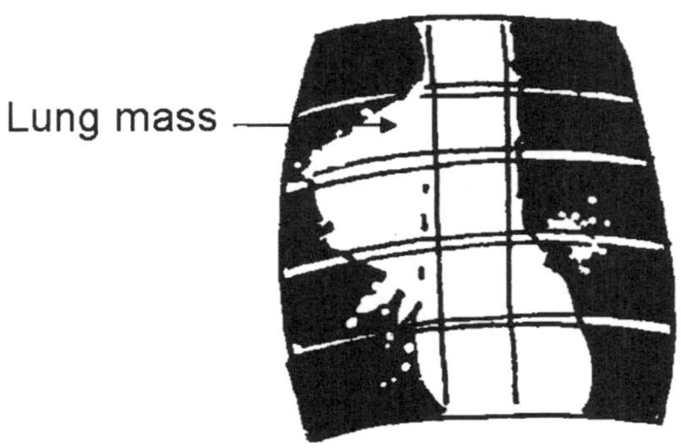

D-55: Lung cancer (R) side (X-ray)

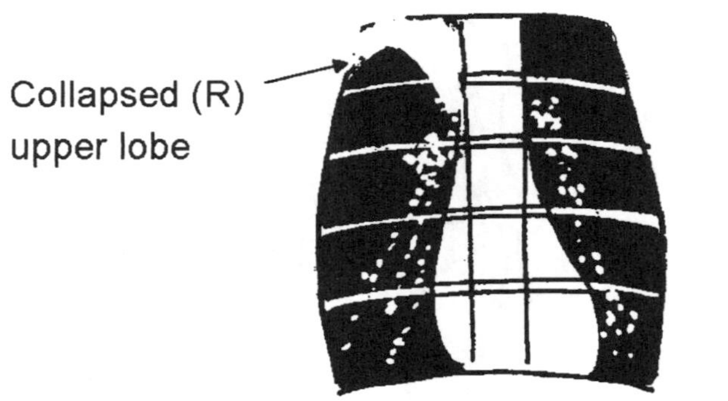

D-56: (R) upper lobe collapse

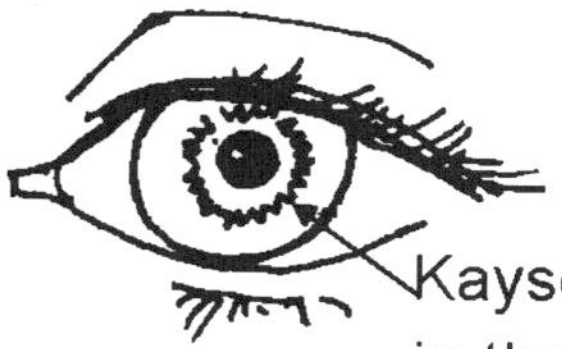

D-57: Wilson's disease

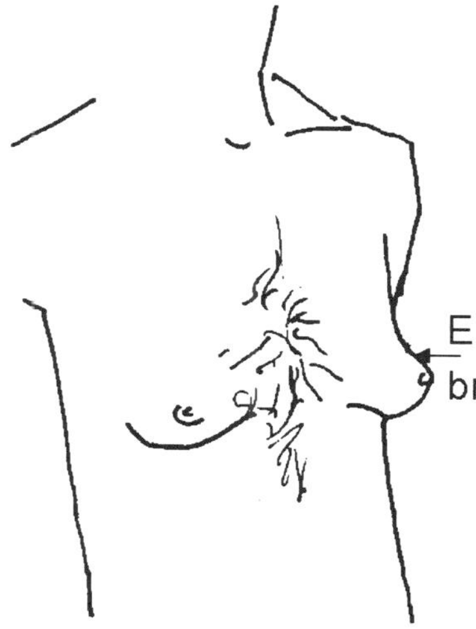

D-58: Gynecomastia in a male patient

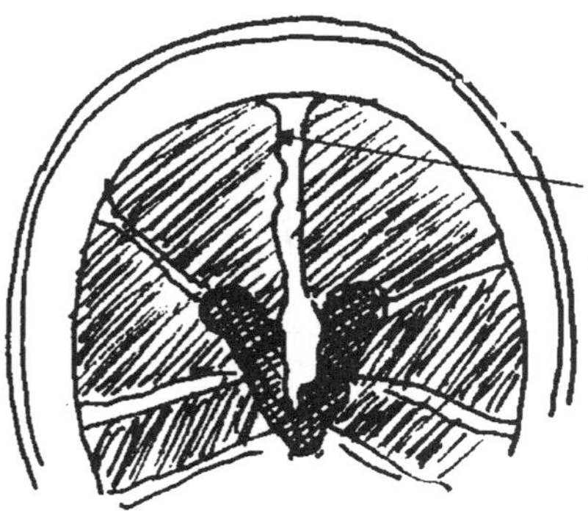

D-59: Subarachnoid hemorrhage (CT scan)

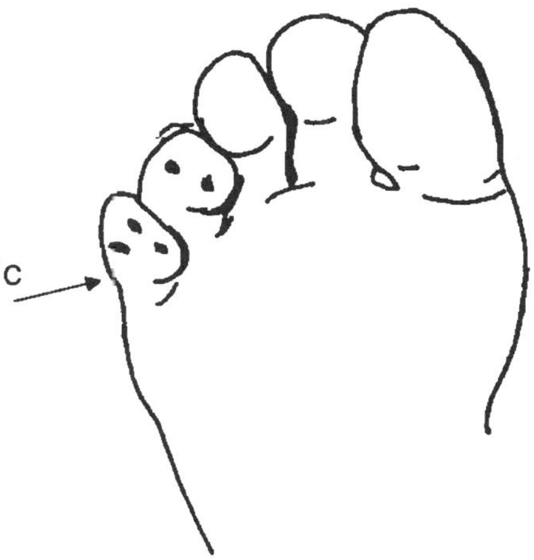

D-60: Local thrombophlebitis (R) foot

Picture 30

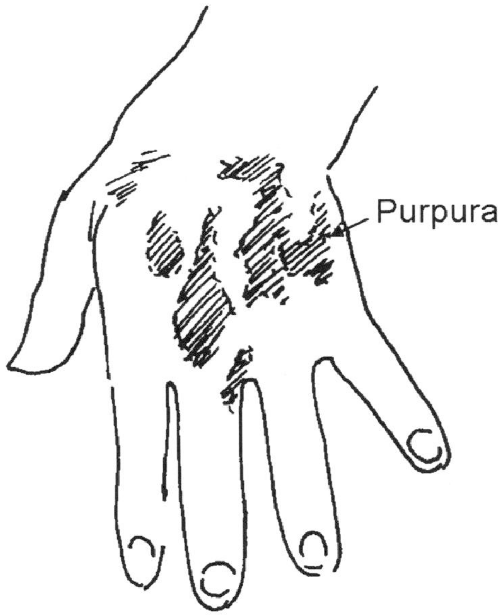

D-61: Senile purpura in an elder patient

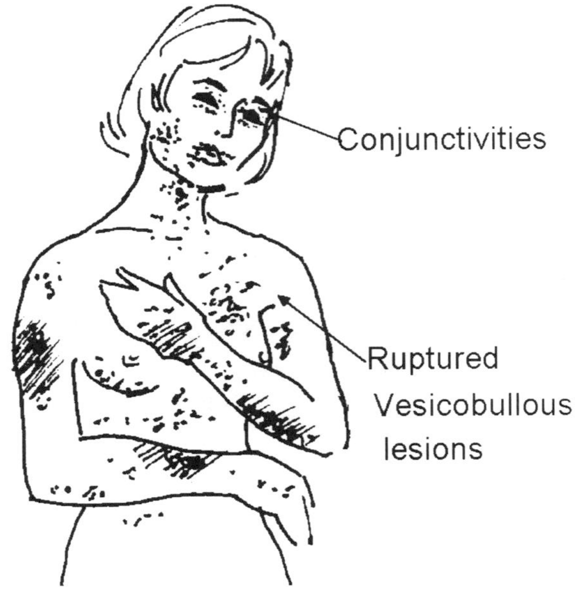

D-62: Stevens-Johnson syndrome

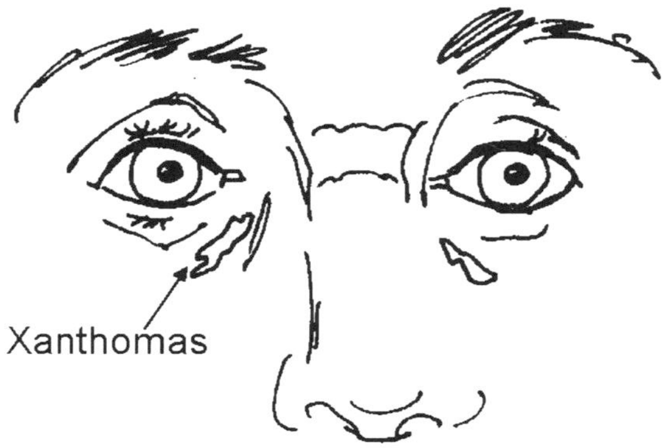

D-63: Xanthomas

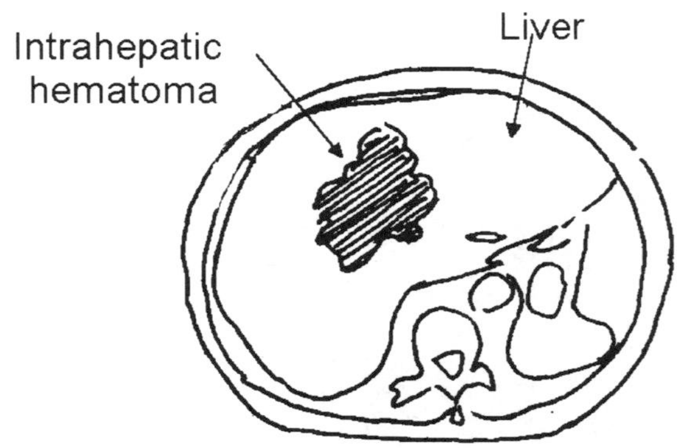

D-64: Hepatic laceration (CT scan)

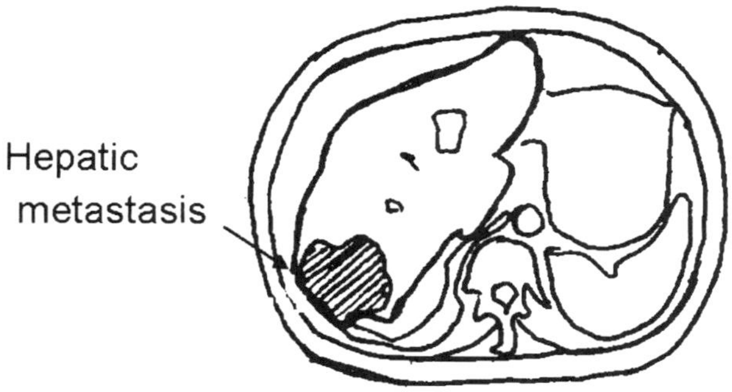

D-65: Hepatic metastasis (MRI)

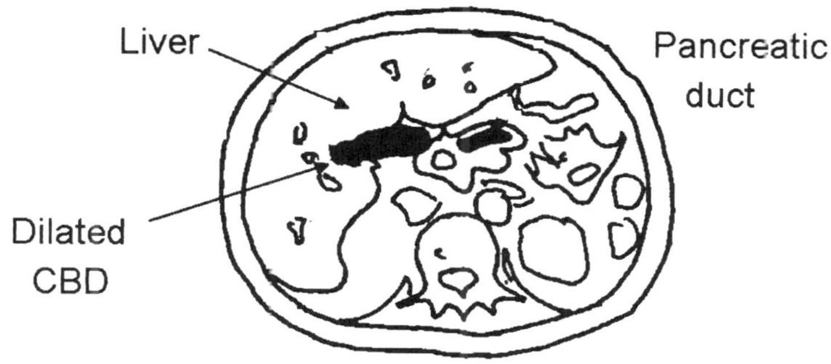

D-66: Obstruction of common bile duct (CBD) (CT scan)

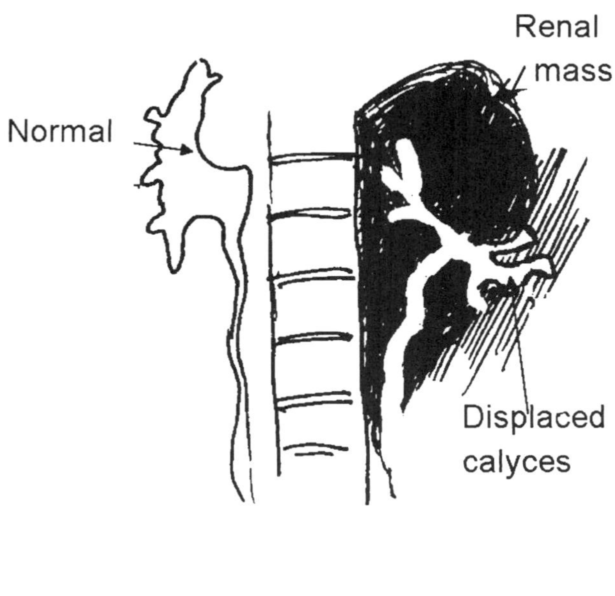

D-67: Renal mass (IVP)

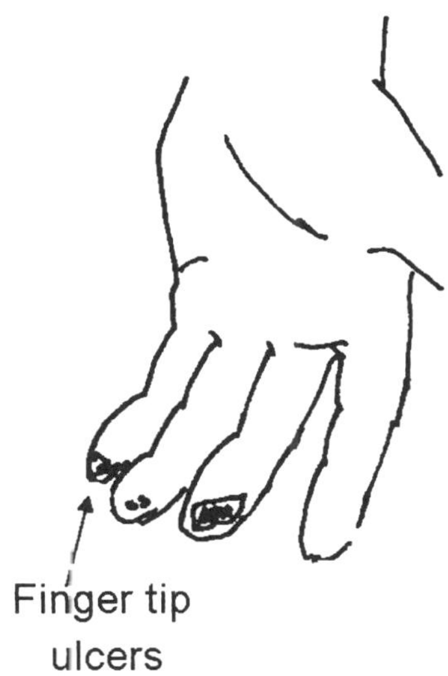

D-68: Raynaud syndrome

Picture 32

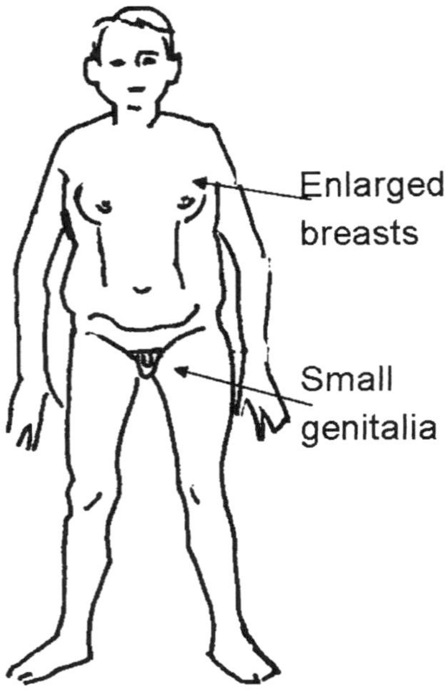

D-69: Hypopituitarism

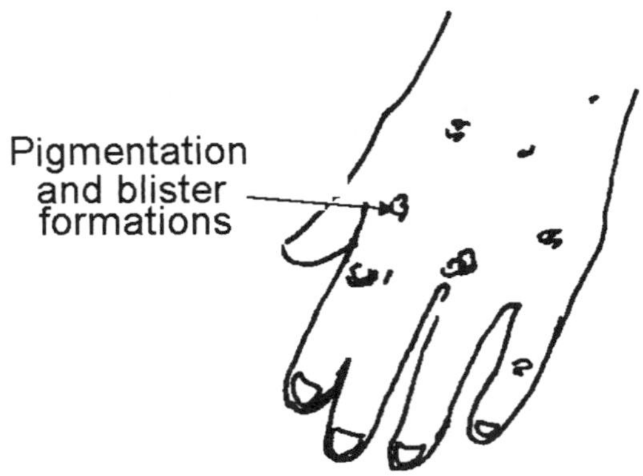

D-70: Porphyria cutaneous tarda

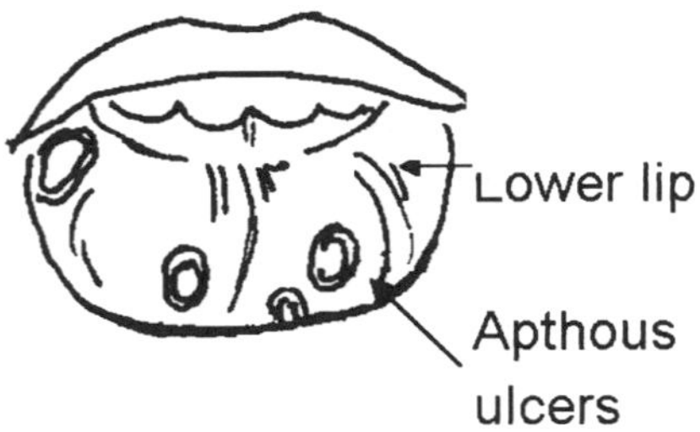

D-71: Apthous ulcers

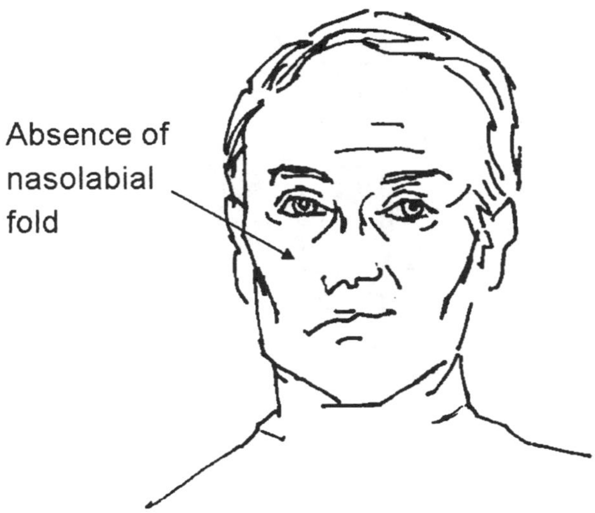

D-72: (R) facial palsy

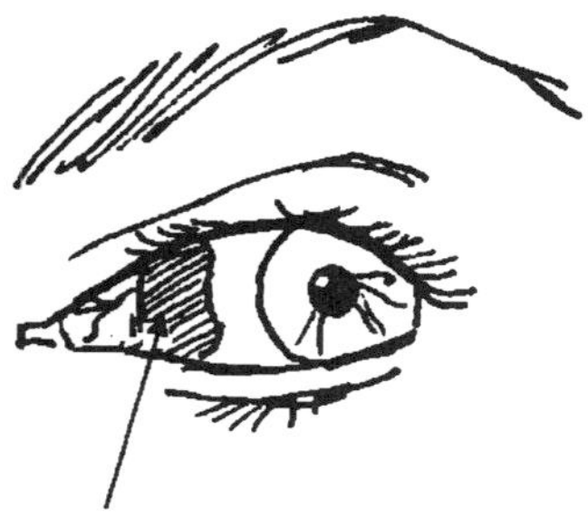

D-73: Alcaptonuria

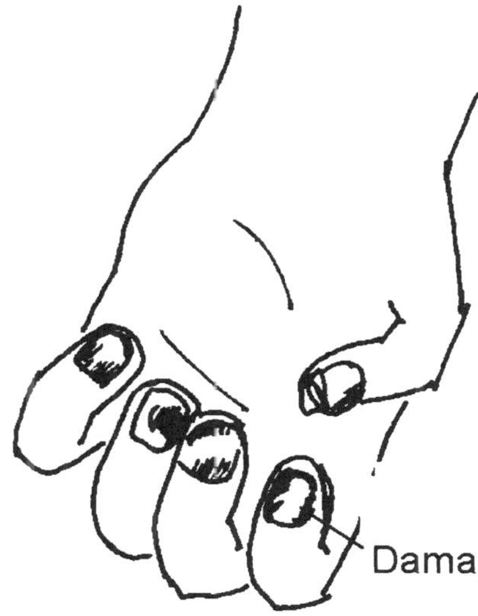

D-74: Candida nail infections

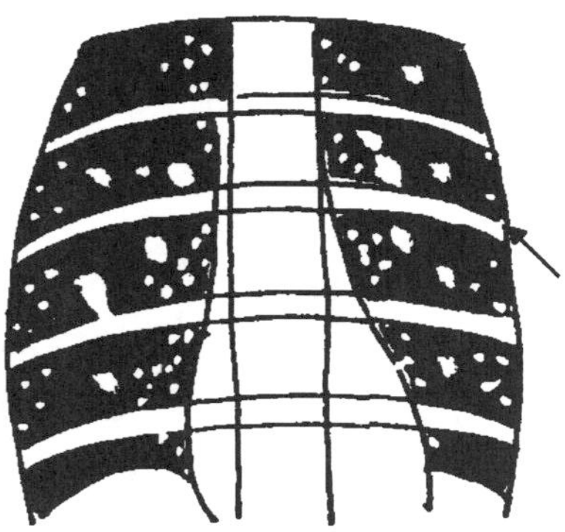

D-75: Pulmonary asbestosis (x-ray)

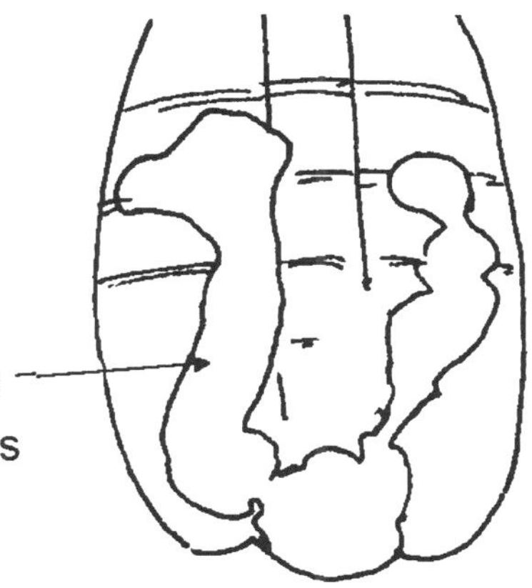

D-76: Bilateral hydronephrosis (VCUG)

Picture 34

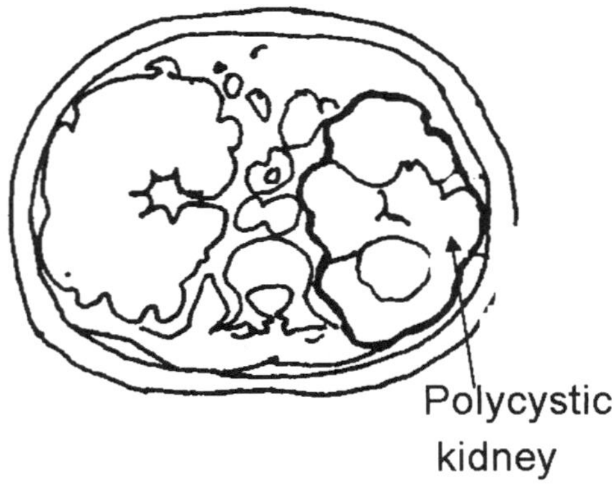

D-77: Bilateral polycystic kidneys (CT scan)

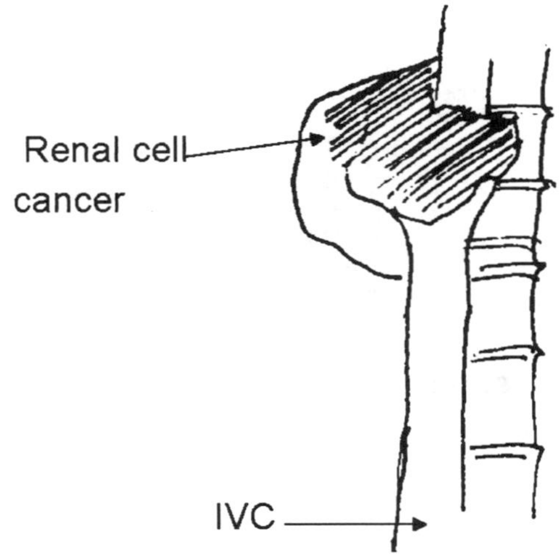

D-78: Renal cell cancer invades the inferior vena cava (IVC gram)

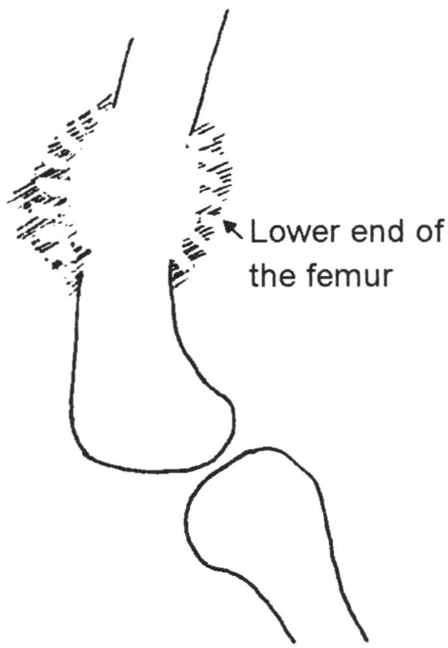

D-79: Osteogenic sarcomas (x-ray)

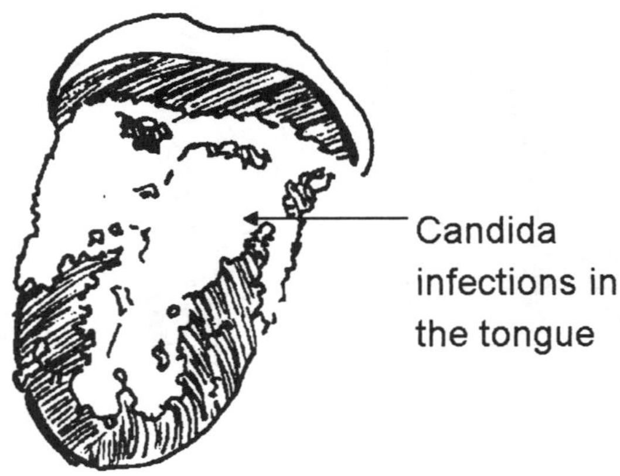

D-80: Oral candida infections

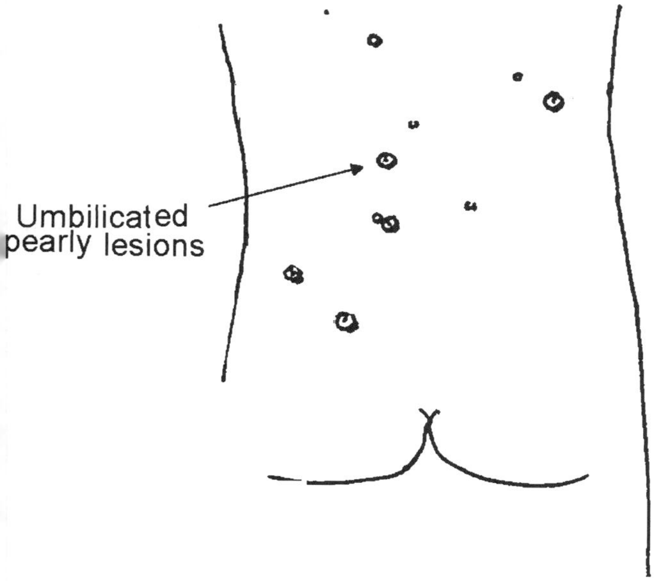

D-81: Molluscum contagiosum

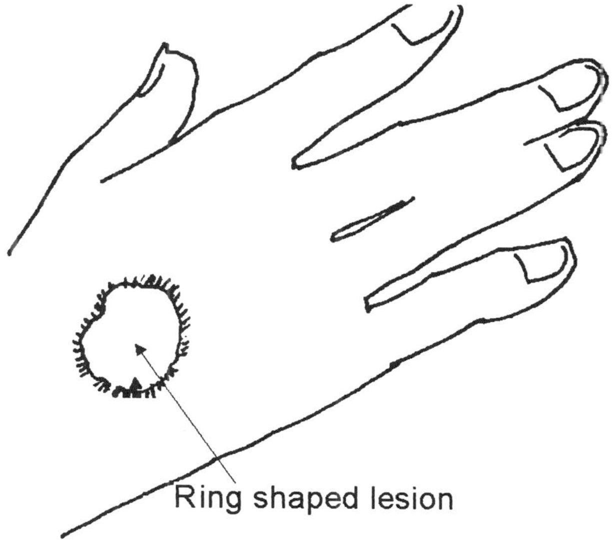

D-82: Granuloma annulare

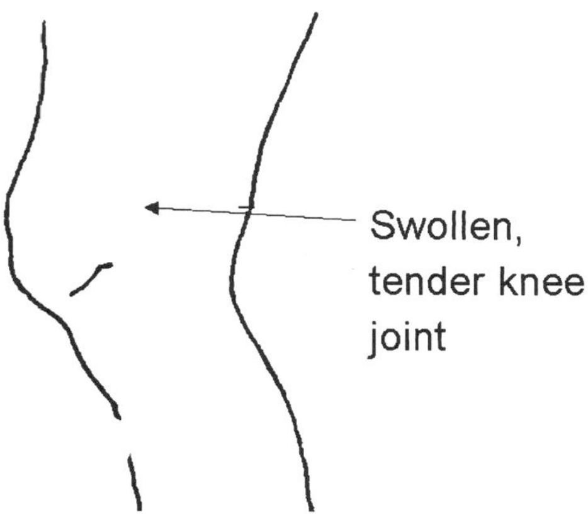

D-83: TB infection in the knee joint

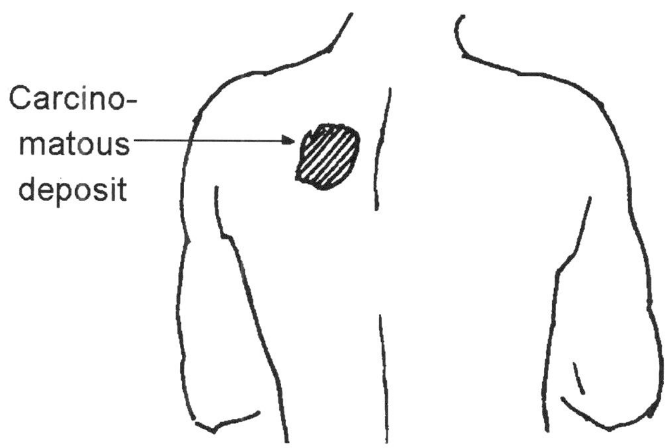

D-84: Non-Hodgkin lymphoma

Picture 36

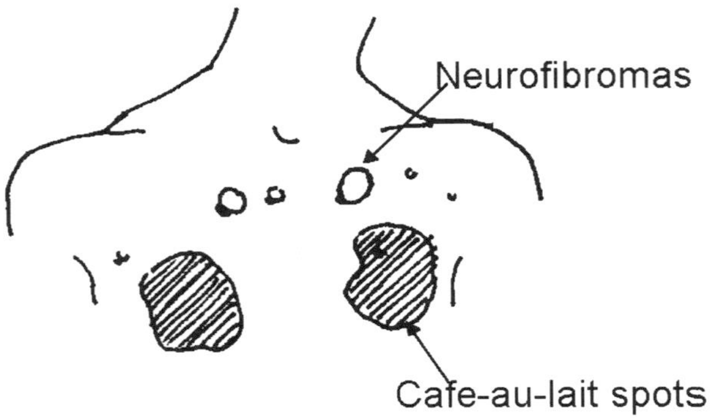

D-85: Nerofibromatosis (Von Recklinghausen's disease)

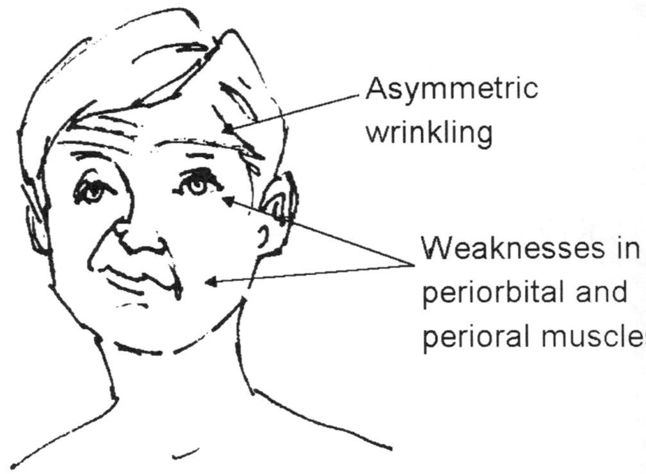

D-86: Bell's plasy (L) side of the face

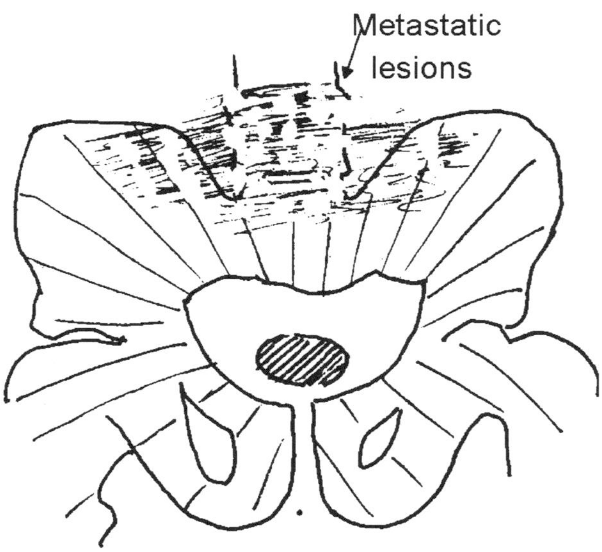

D-87: Pelvic metastases from prostate cancer

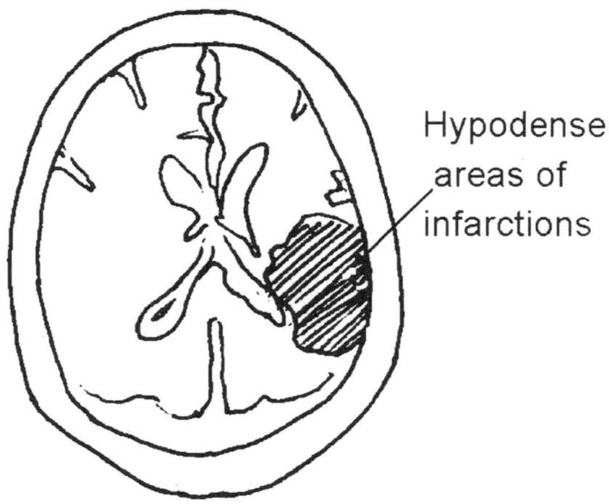

D-88: Cerebral infarctions due to embolus in left middle cerebral artery (CT-Scan)

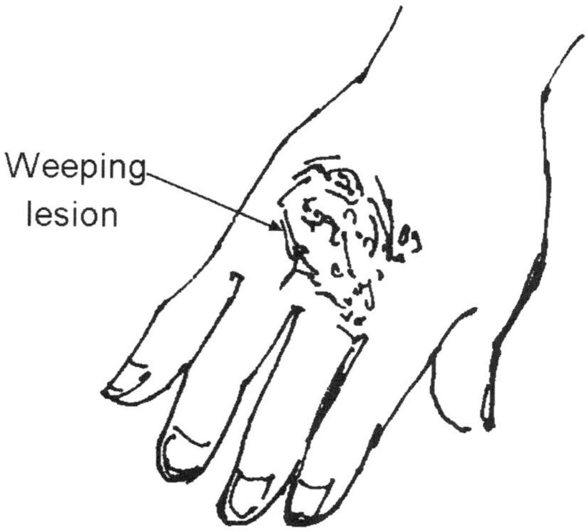

D-89: Discoid dermatitis in (R) hand

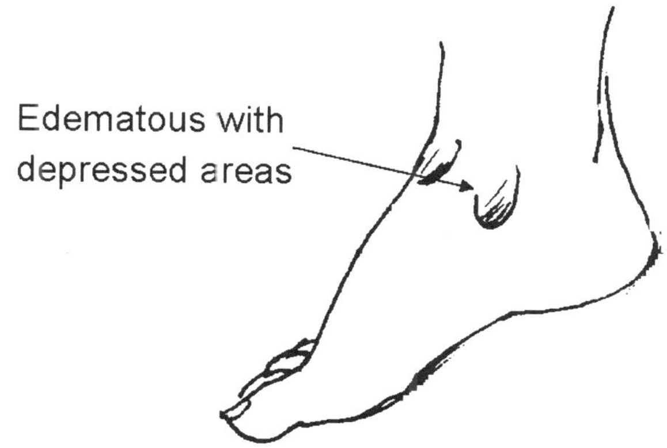

D-90: Pitting edema due to cardiac failure

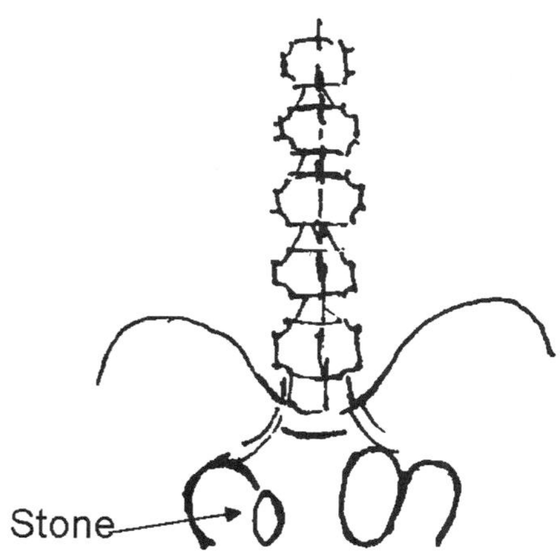

D-91: Stone in the (R) ureter (x-ray)

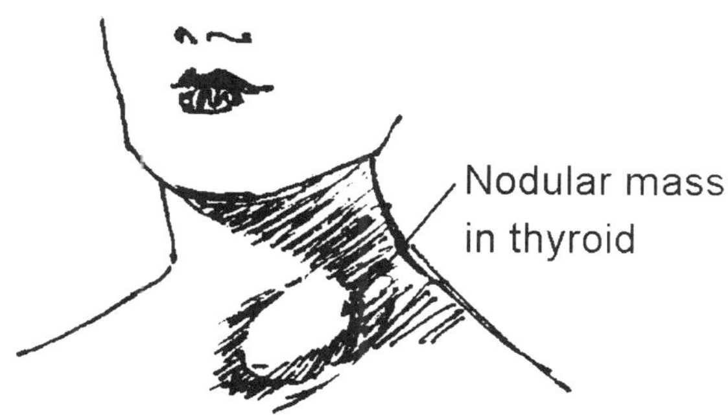

D-92: Thyrotoxic nodule

Picture 38

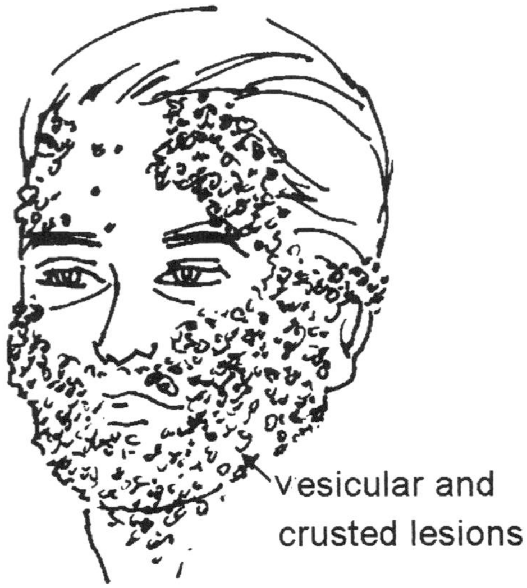

D-93: Barber's rash

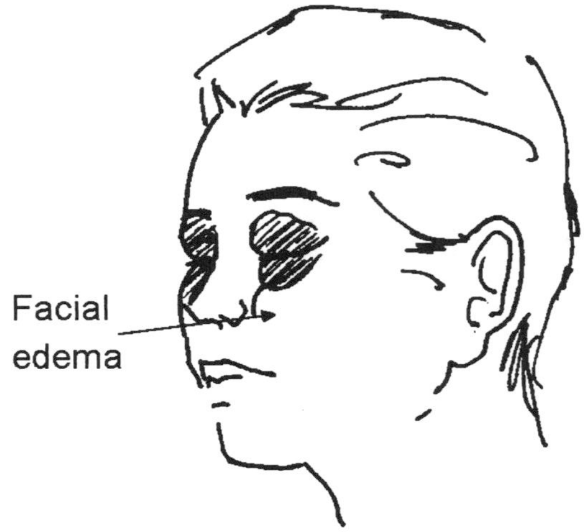

D-94: Nephrotic syndrome

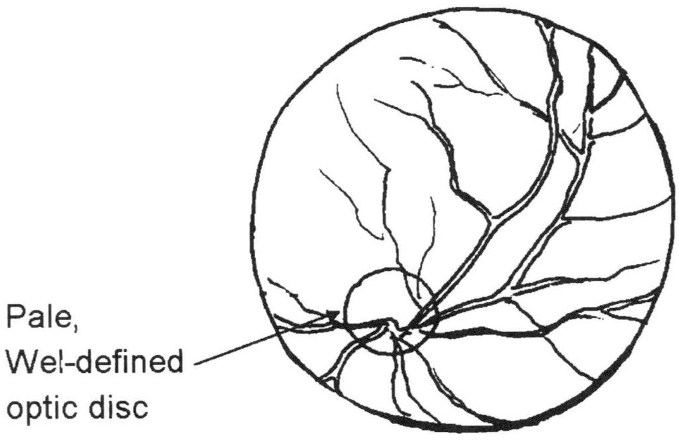

D-95: Optic atrophy (Fundoscopy)

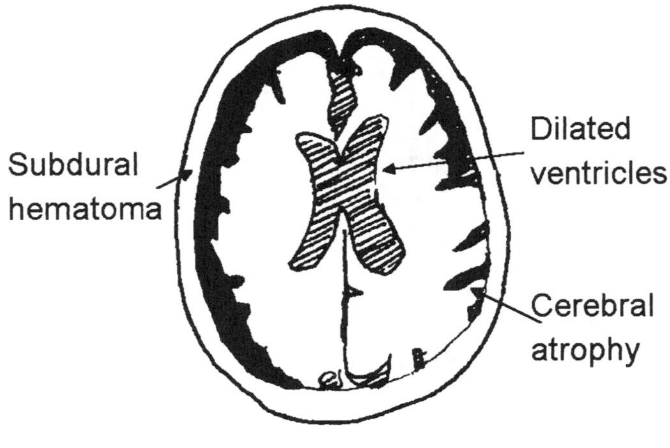

D-96: (R) Subdural hematoma (CT scan)

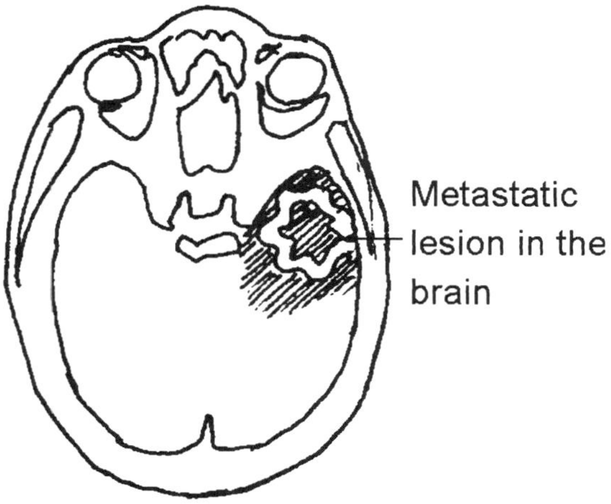

D-97: Metastatic lesion in the brain
from primary lung cancer
(CT scan)

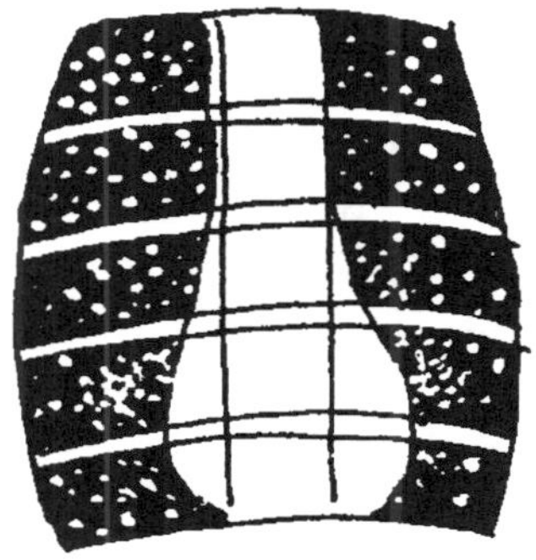

98: Interstitial pneumonias in both lungs

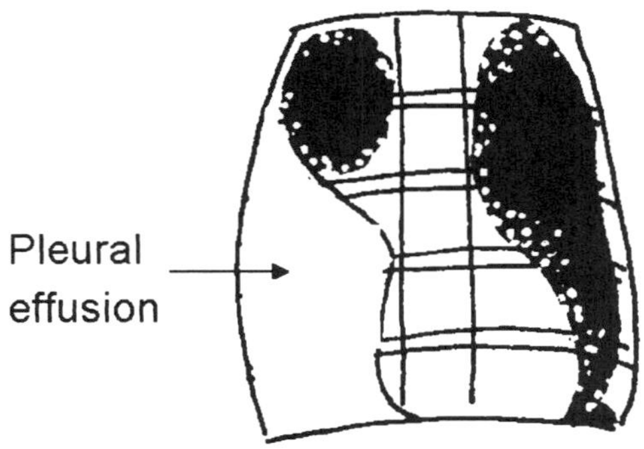

D-99: Pleural effusion in (R) lung

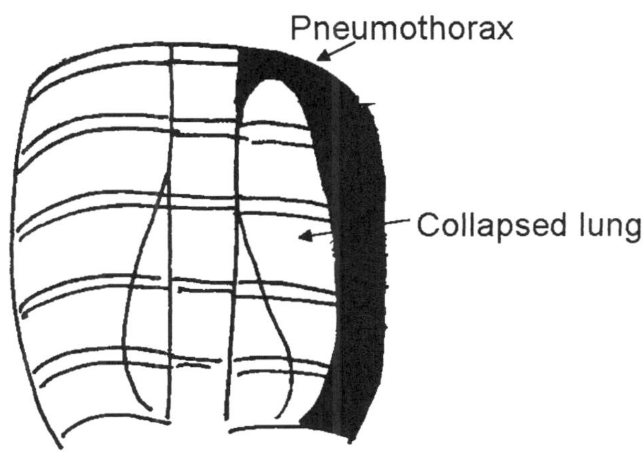

D-100: Left pneumothorax (X-ray)

Picture 40

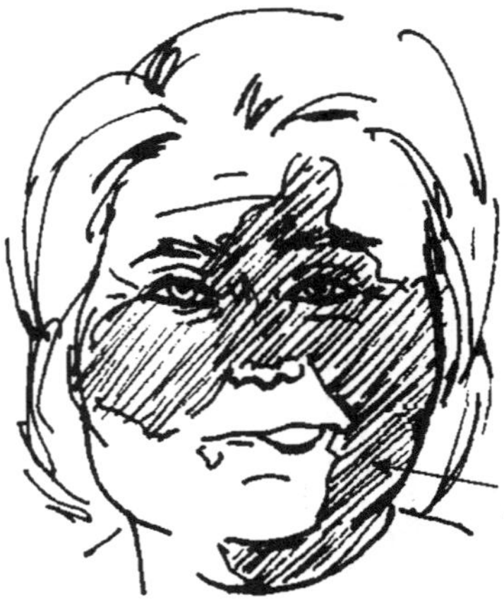

D-101: Erysipelas

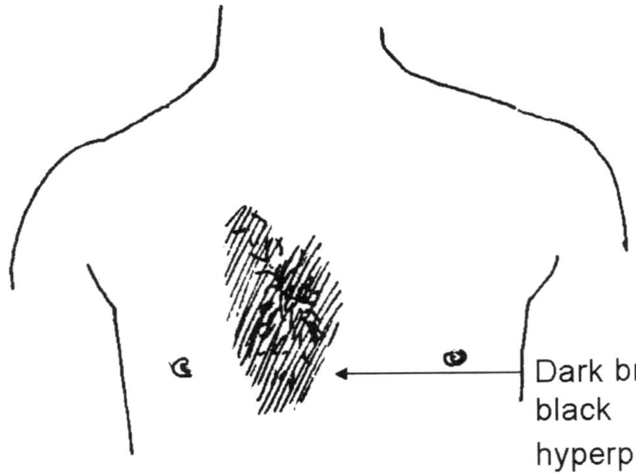

D-102: Acanthosis nigricans

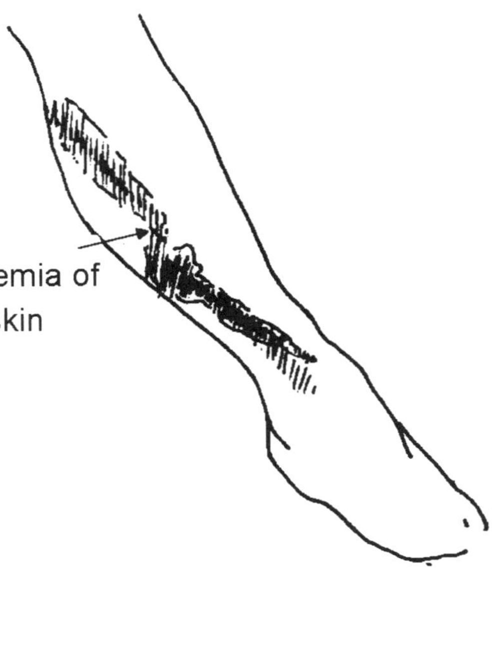

D-103: Migrating thrombophlebitis

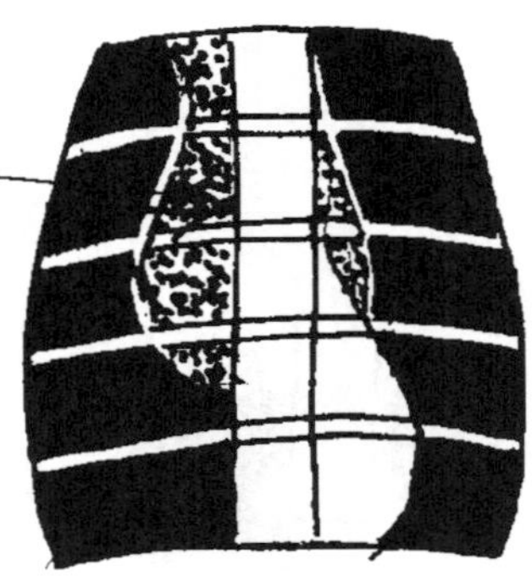

D-104: Teratoma of the anterior mediastinum (X-ray)

Picture 41

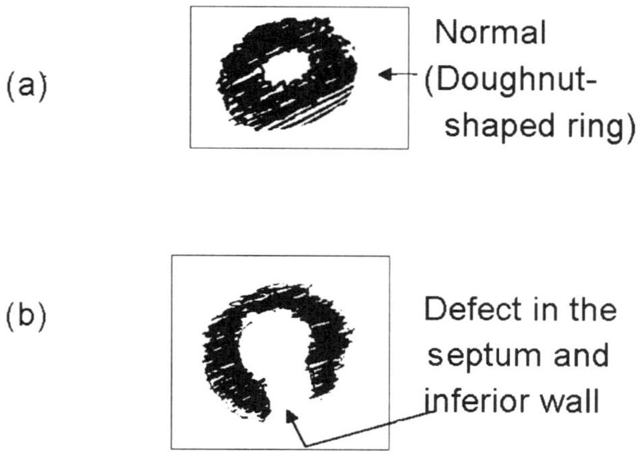

D-105: (a) Normal thallium scan
(b) Coronary artery stenosis

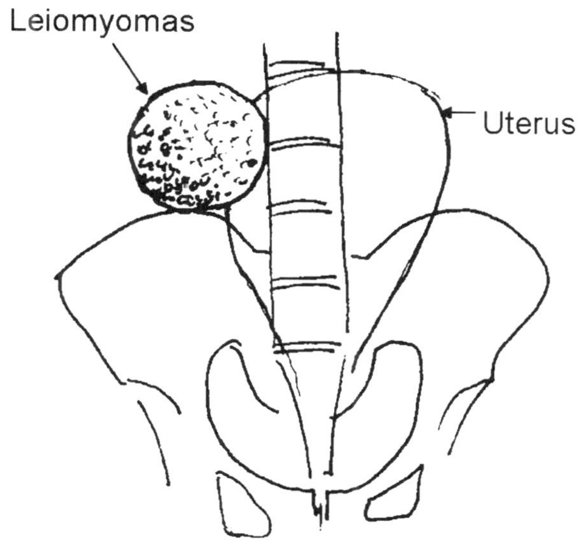

D-106: Uterine leiomyomas (X-ray)

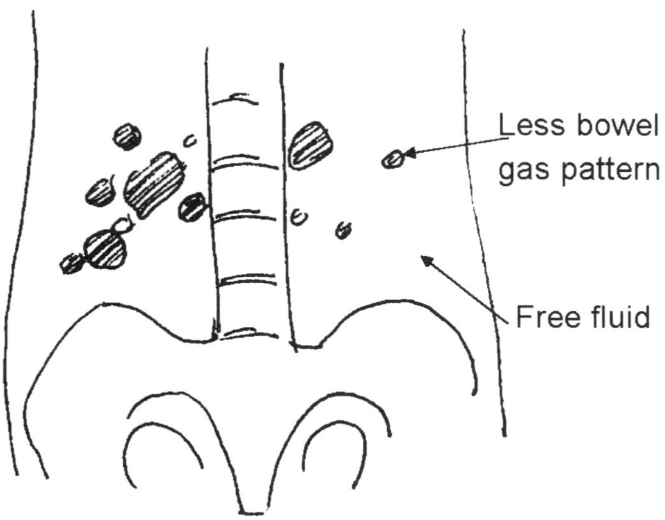

D-107: Abdominal ascites (x-ray)

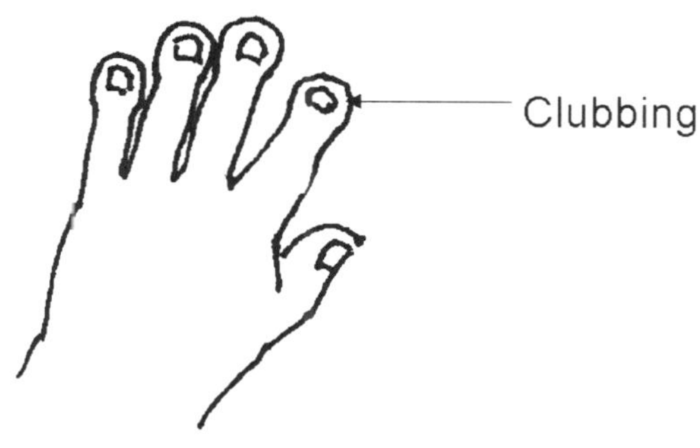

D-108: Fibrotic chronic lung disease

Picture 42

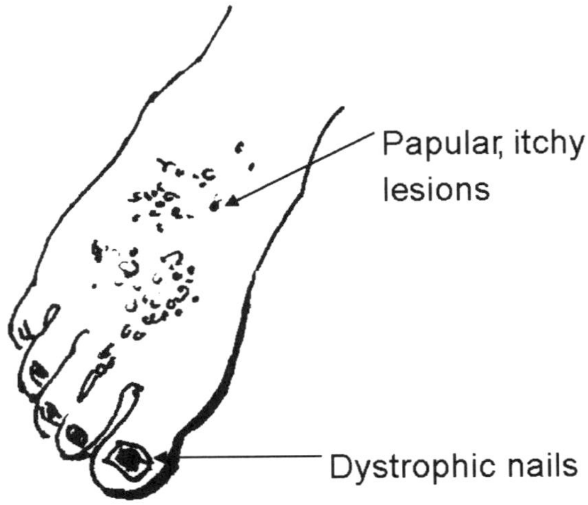

D-109: Lichen planus

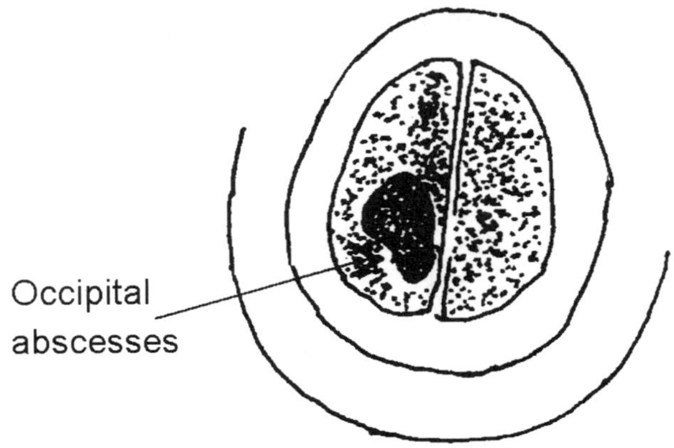

D-110: Cerebral abscesses (CT scan)

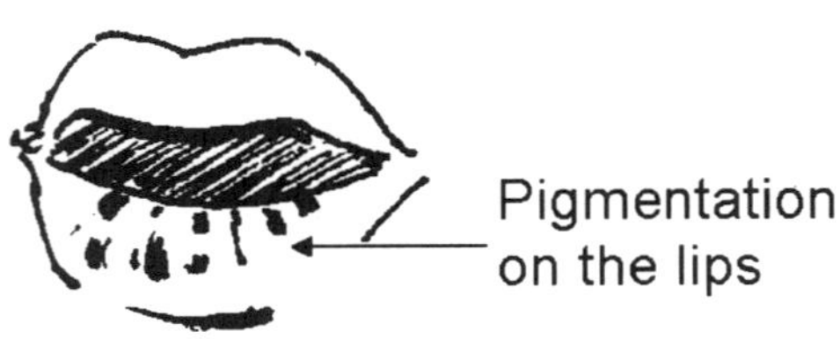

D-111: Peutz-Jeghers syndrome

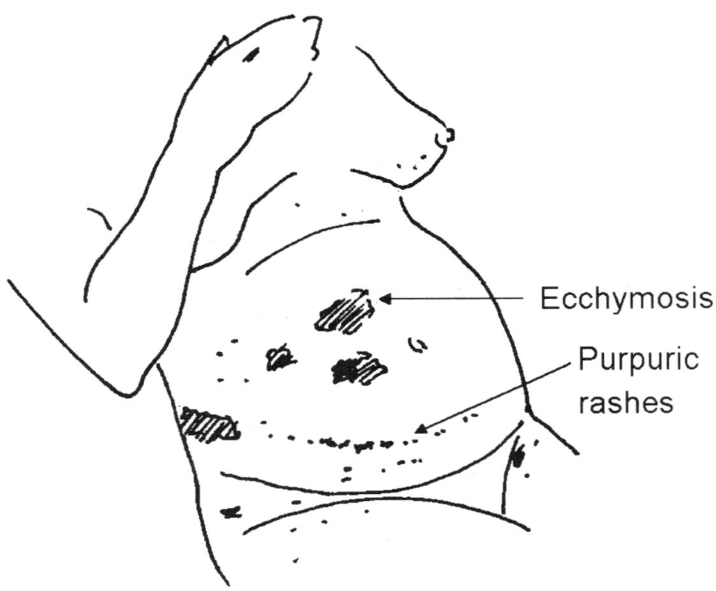

D-112: DIC

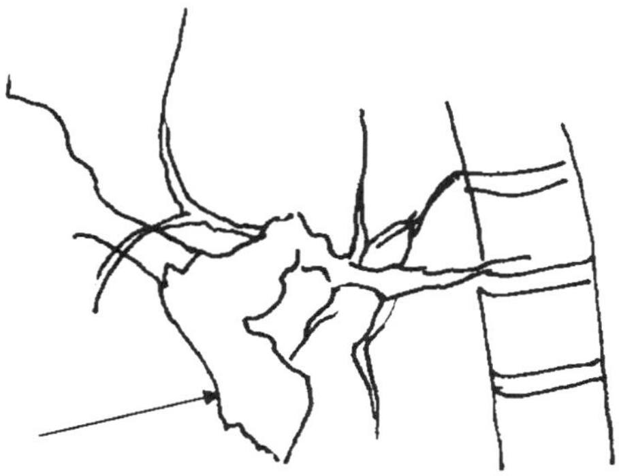

D-113: Common bile duct stones (ERCP study)

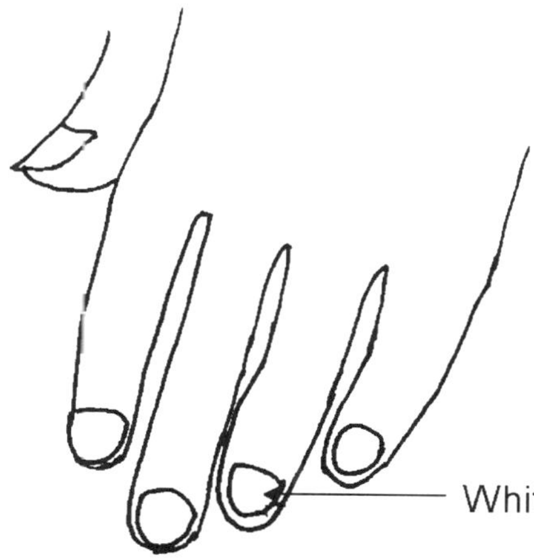

D-114: Leukonychia

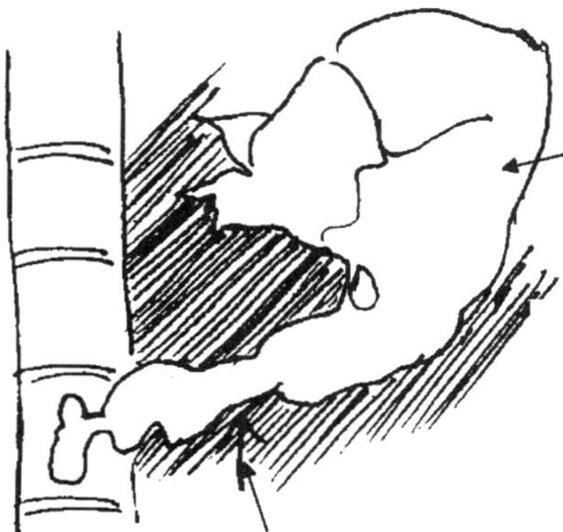

D-115: Carcinoma of the stomach (Barium study)

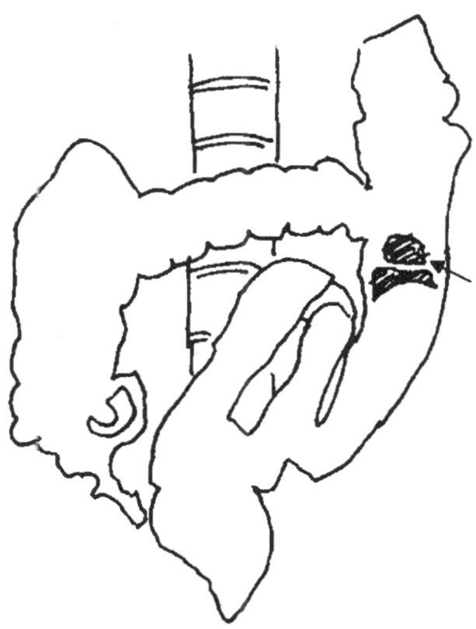

D-116: Colonic polyps (Barium enema)

Picture 44

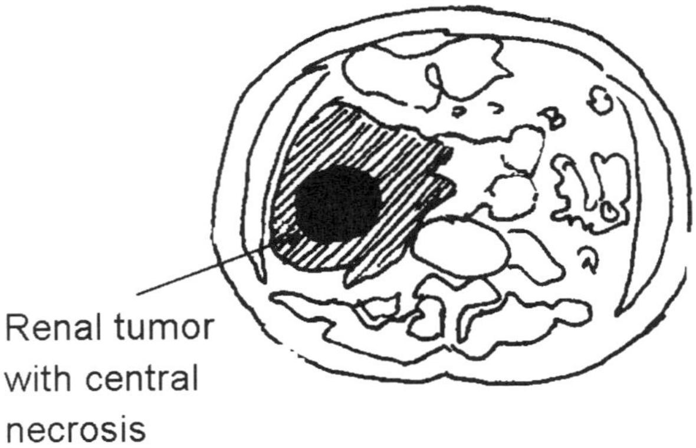

D-117: (R) Renal cell cancer (CT scan)

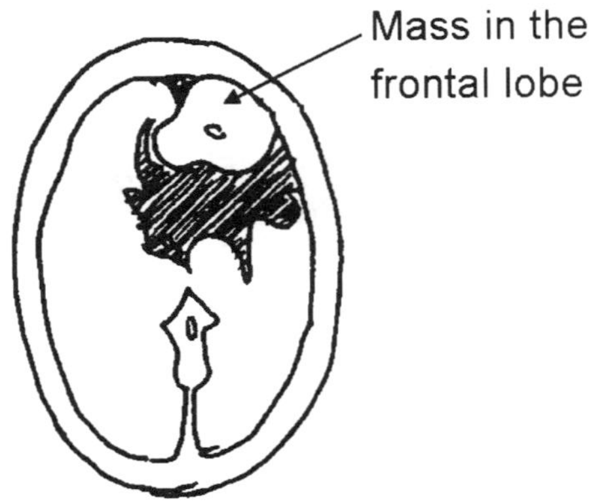

D-118: (L) Frontal meningiomas (CT scan)

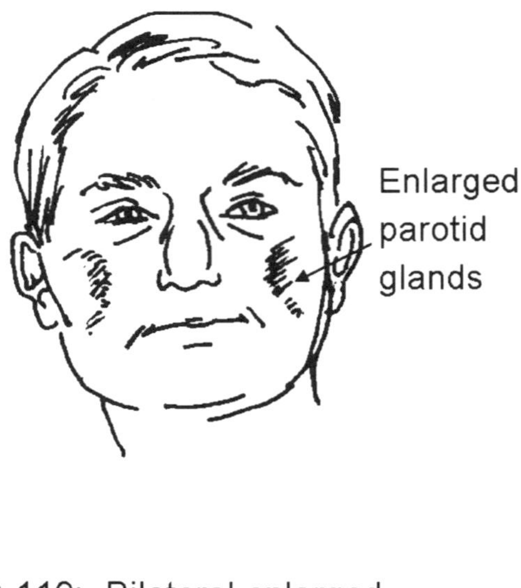

D-119: Bilateral enlarged
parotid glands

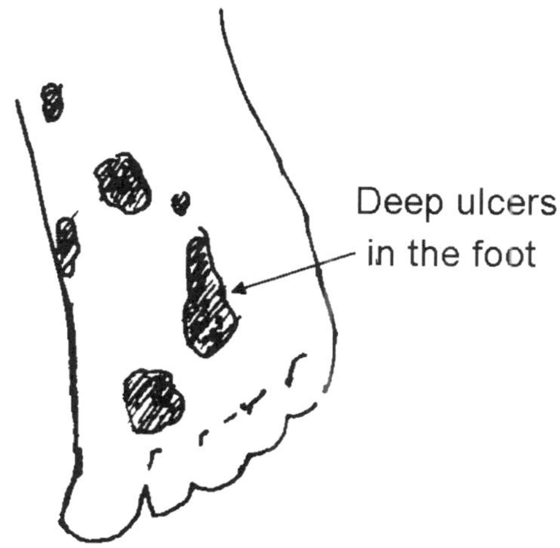

D-120: Rheumatoid arthritis

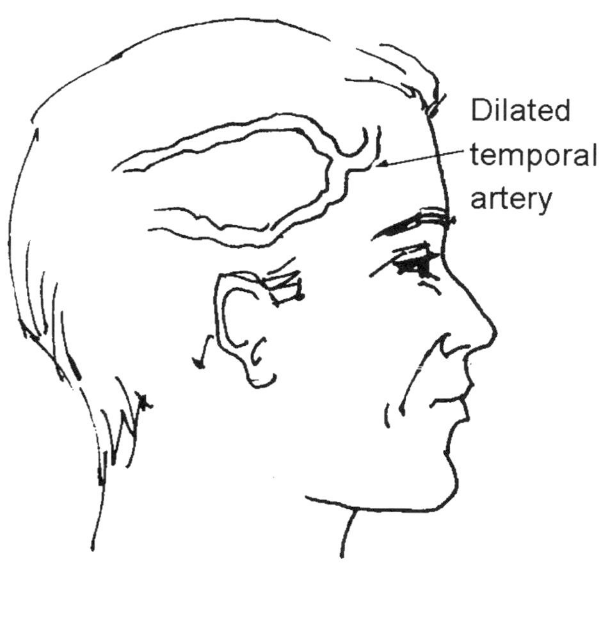

D-121: Temporal arteritis

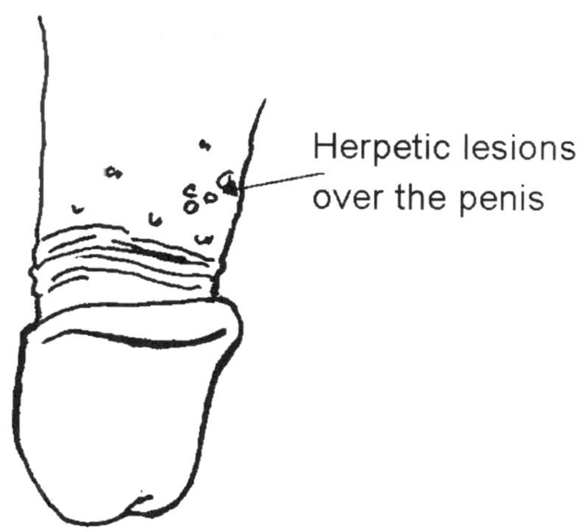

D-122: Genital herpes simplex

Picture 46

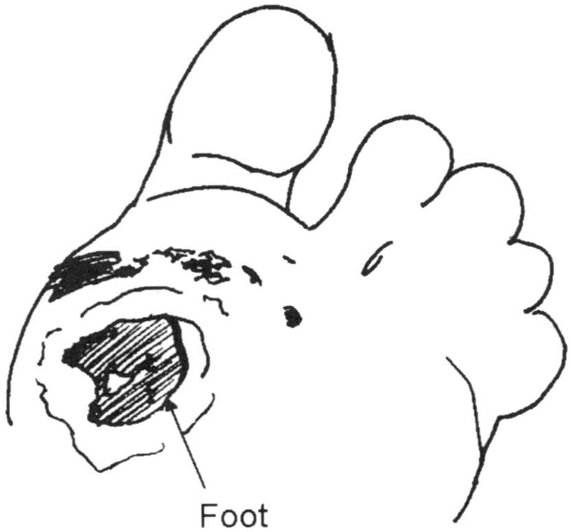

D-123: Diabetic neuropathic ulcers

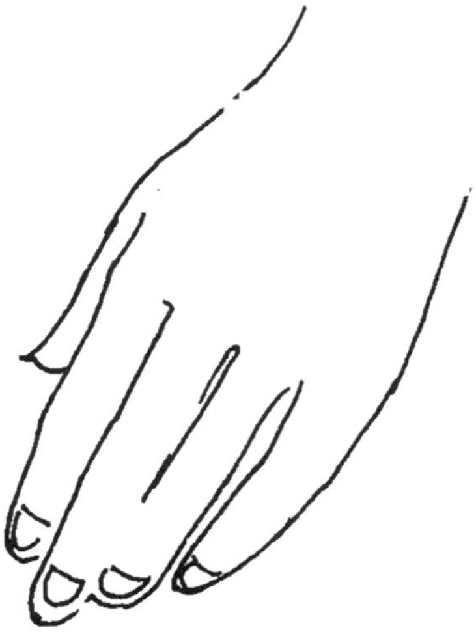

D-124: Blue hand

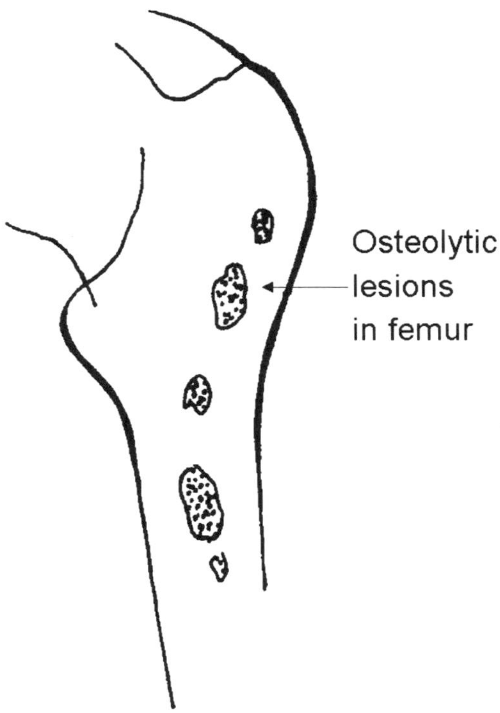

D-125: Osteolytic bony metastases (x-ray)

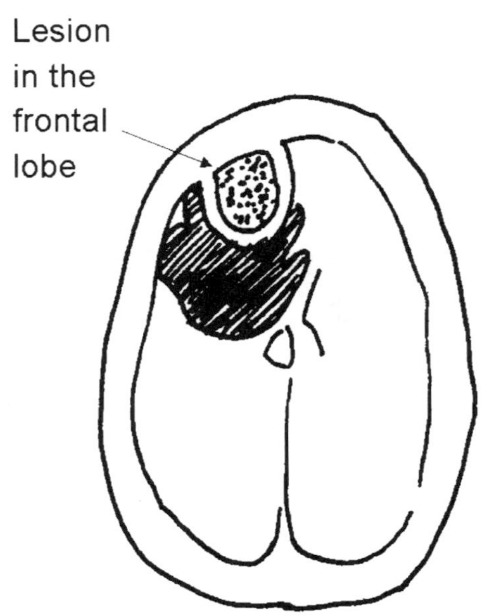

D-126: Brain metastasis (CT scan)

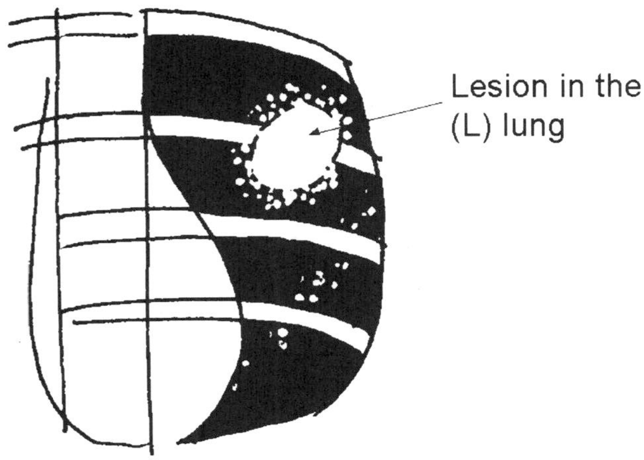

D-127: Primary lung cancer (x-ray)

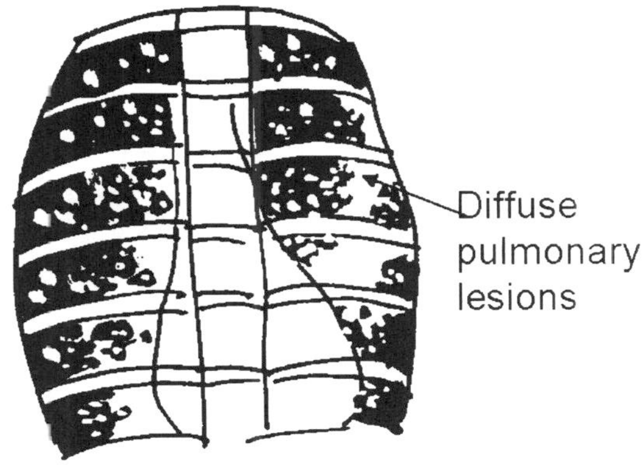

D-128: Miliary pulmonary TB (X-ray)

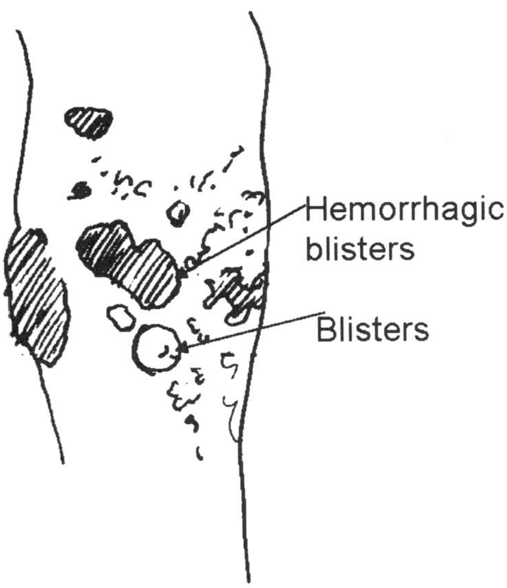

D-129: Pemphigoid

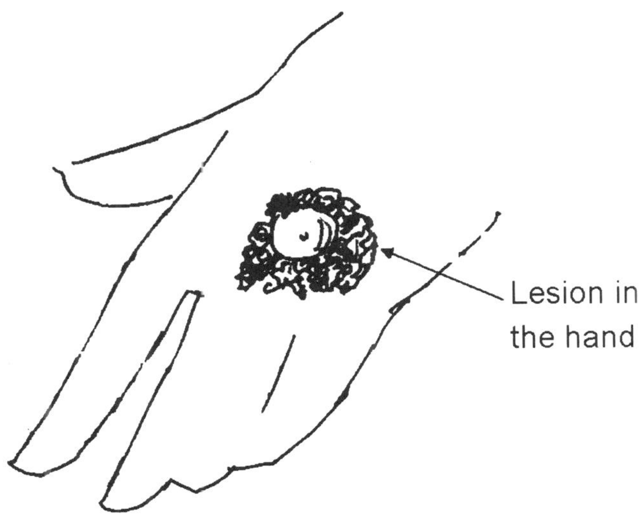

D-130: Malignant melanoma

Picture 48

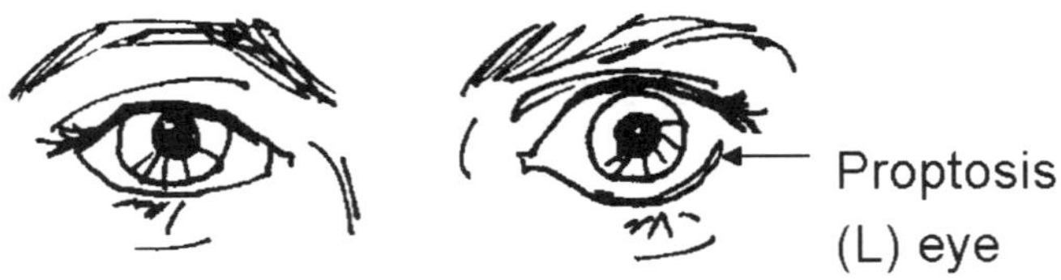

D-131: Unilateral proptosis

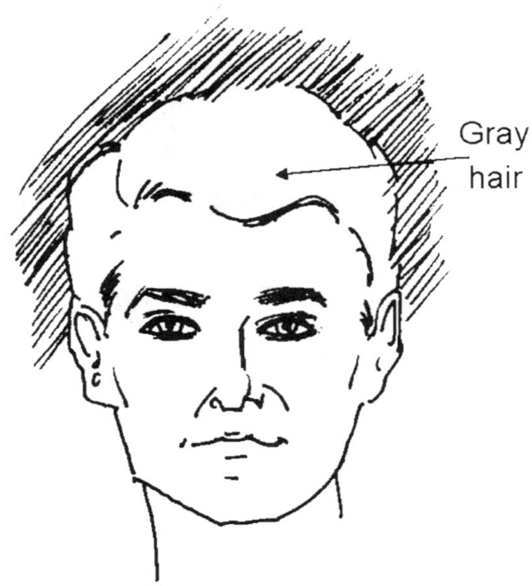

D-132: Premature gray hair (Autoimmune pernicious anemia)

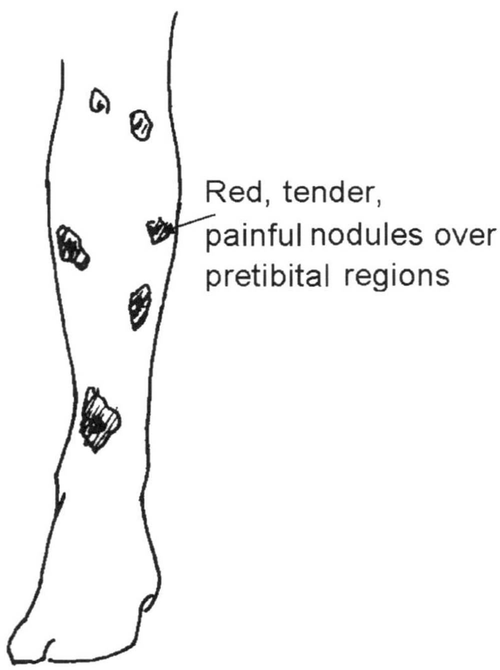

D-133: Erythema nodosum

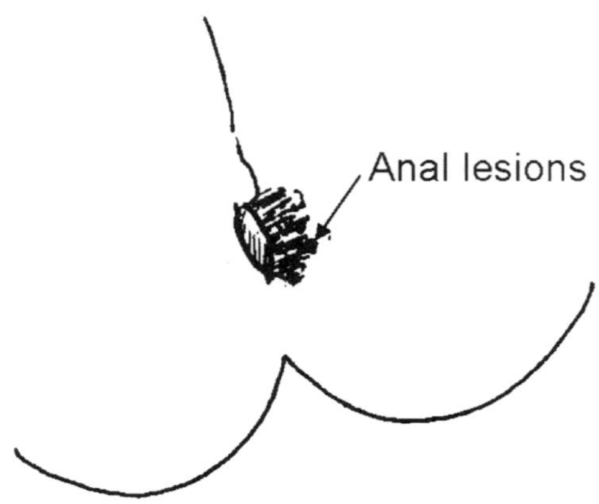

D-134: Anal cancer

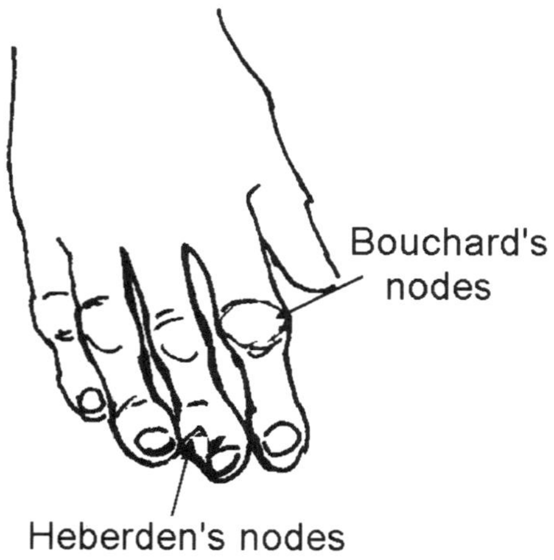

D-135: Osteoarthritis

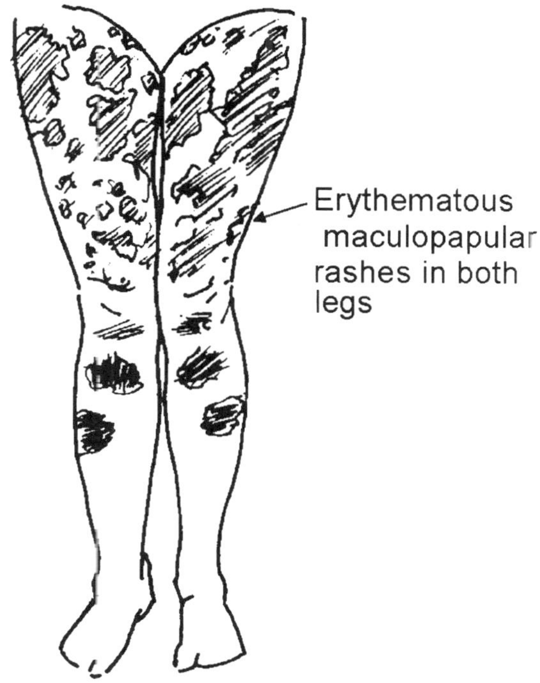

D-136: Drug rashes

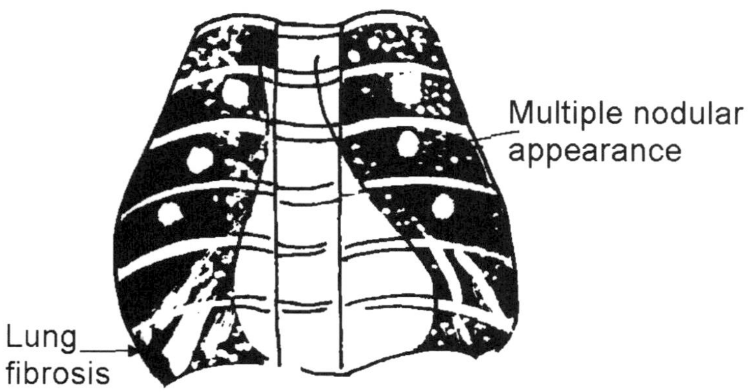

D-137: Multiple rheumatoid nodules in the lungs (X-ray)

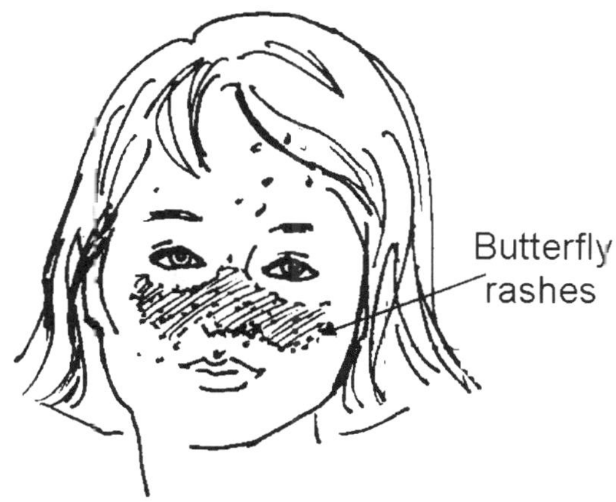

D-138: SLE (Systemic lupus erythematosus)

Picture 50

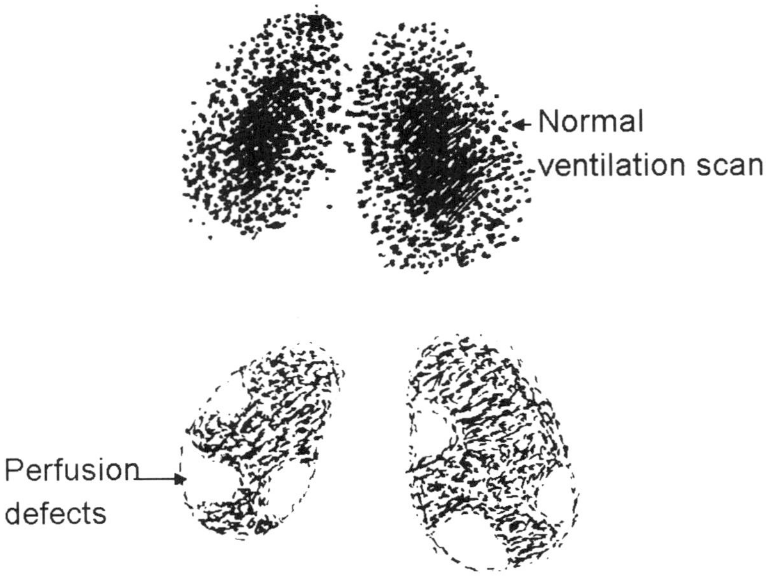

D-139: Pulmonary embolisms (Ventilation-perfusion scan)

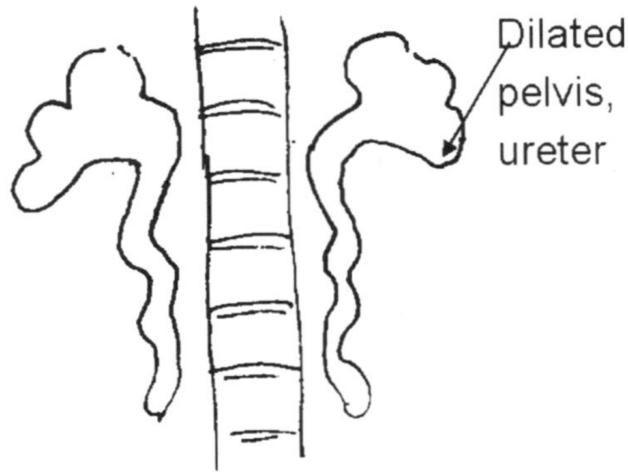

D-140: Bilateral hydronephrosis due to enlarged prostate (IVP)

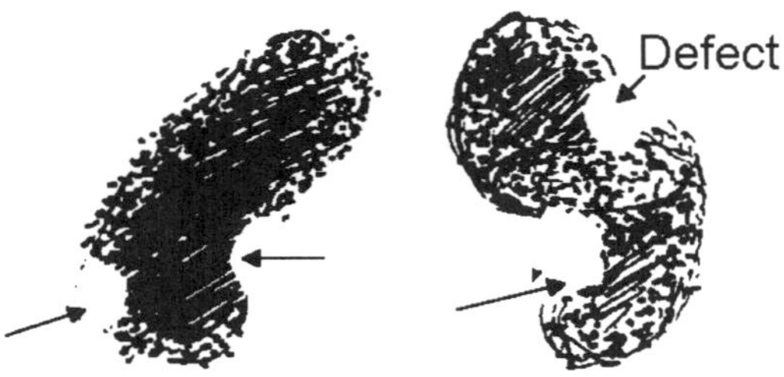

D-141: Renal scarring due to reflux nephropathy (DMSA Scan)

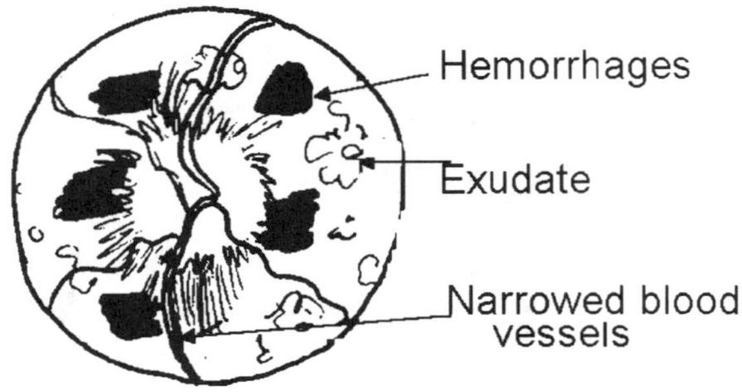

D-142: Hypertensive retinopathy (fundoscopic examination)

Picture 51

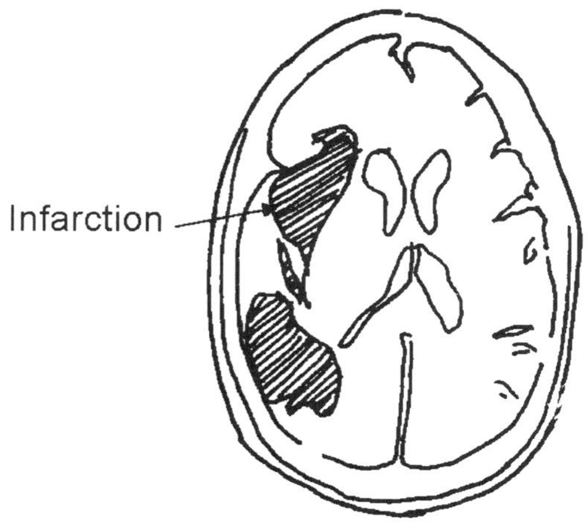

D-143: (R) Cerebral infarction (CT scan)

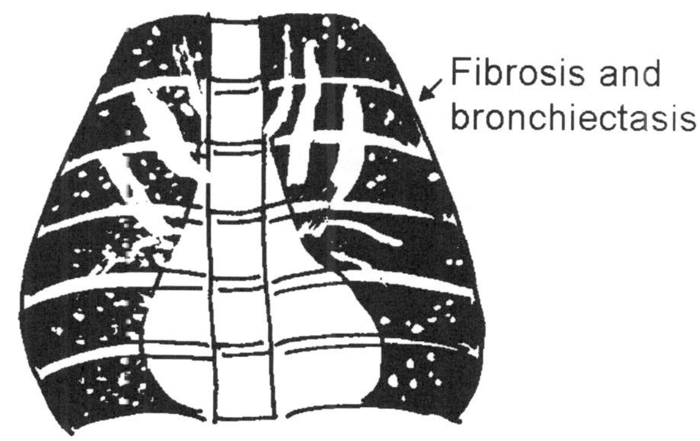

D-144: Bronchopulmonary aspergillosis (X-ray)

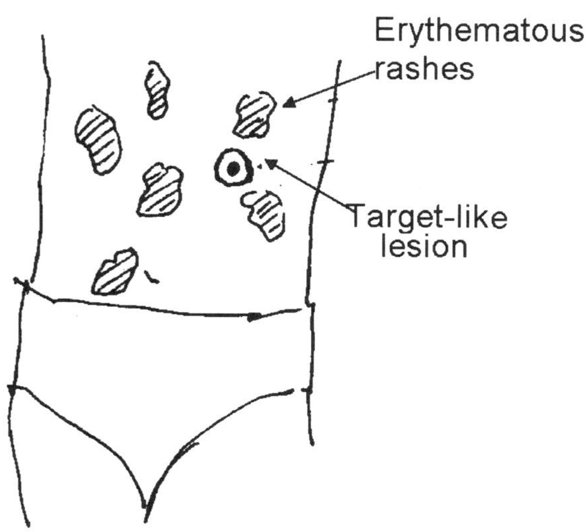

D-145: Erythema multiforme

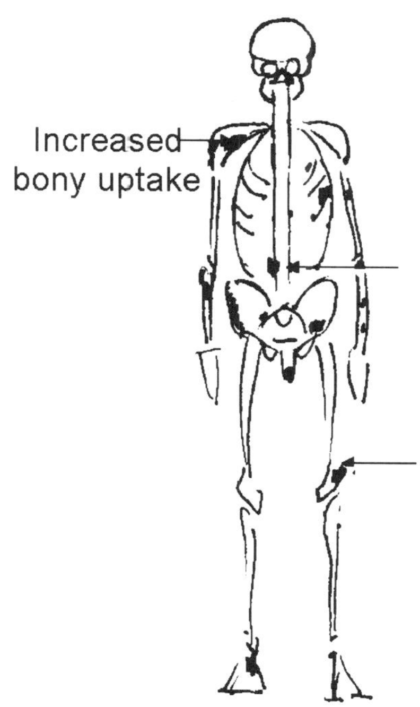

D-146: Multiple bone metastases (Bone scan)

Picture 52

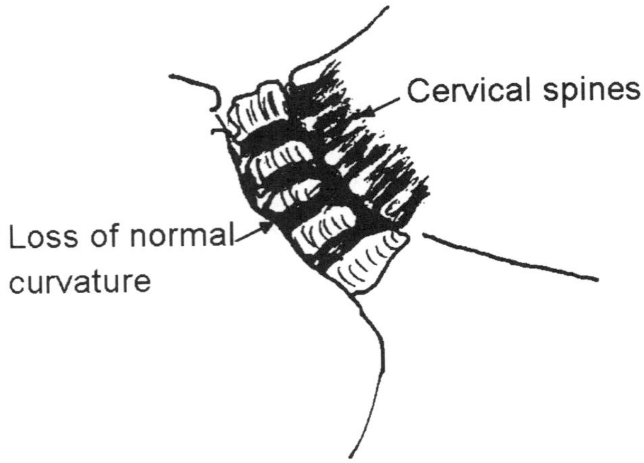

D-147: Ankylosing spondylitis (x-ray)

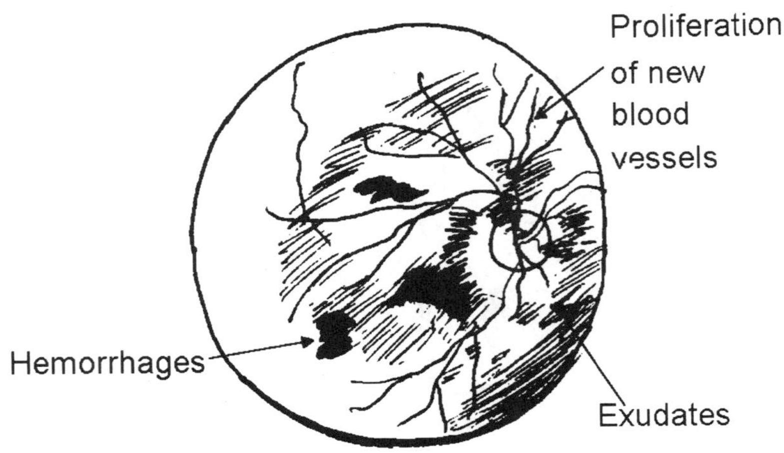

D-148: Diabetic retinopathy (Fundoscopic examination)

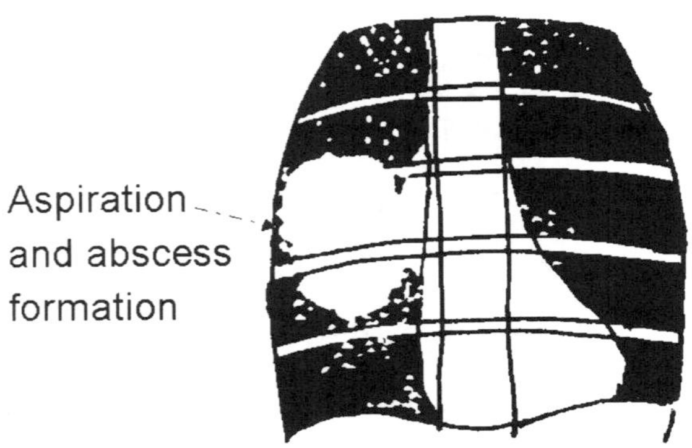

D-149: Lung abscesses (x-ray)

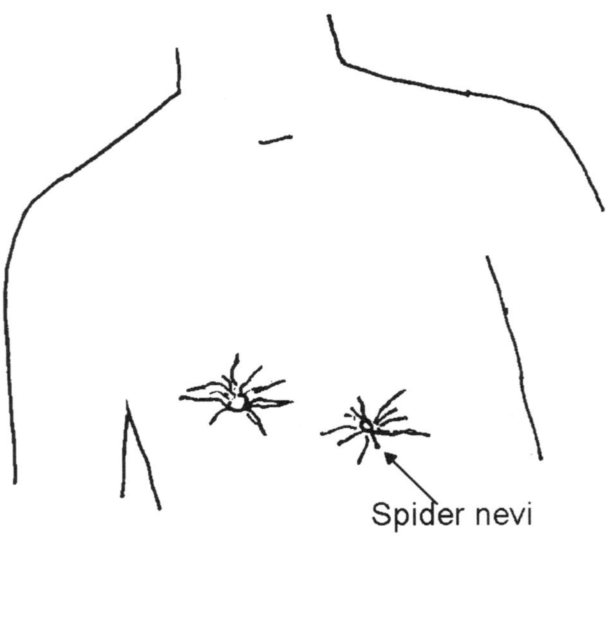

D-150: Spider nevi

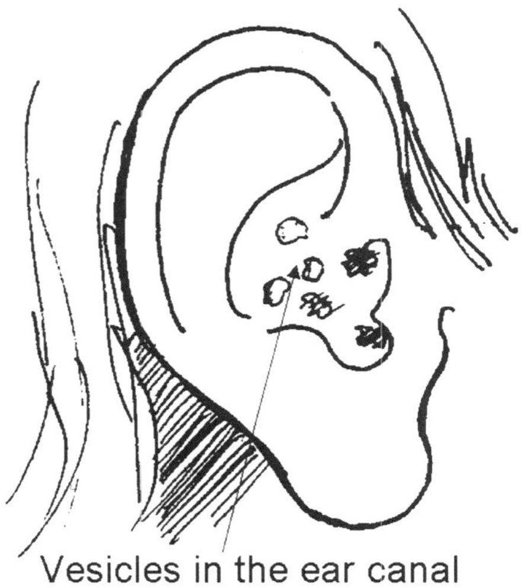

D-151: Ramsay Hunt syndrome due to herpes zoster

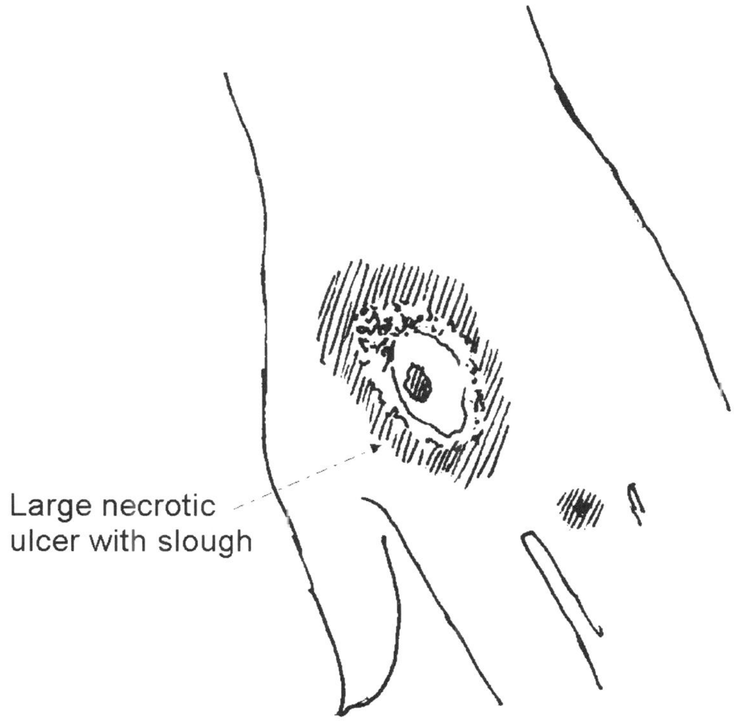

D-152: Pyoderma gangrenosum

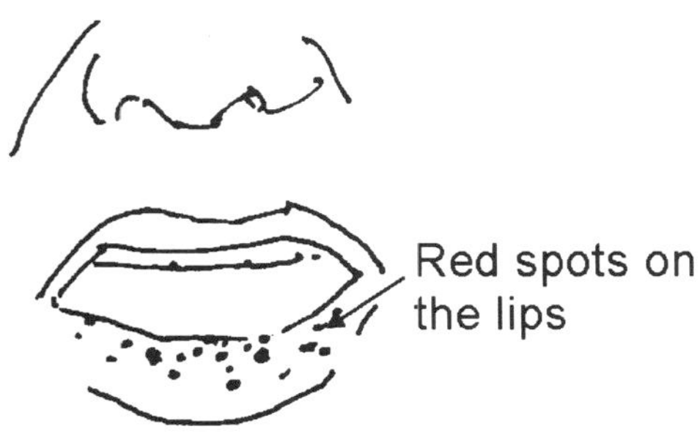

D-153: Hereditary hemorrhagic telangiectasia

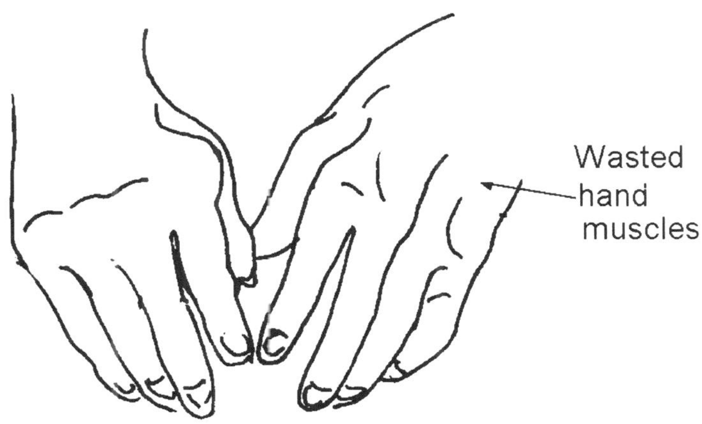

D-154: Syringomyelia

Picture 54

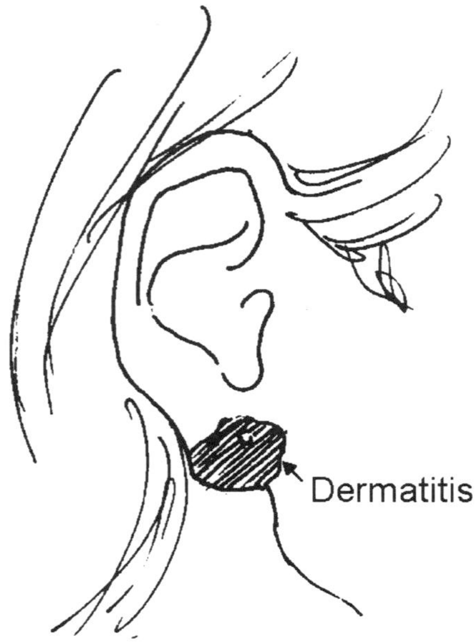

D-155: Contact dermatitis due to earring

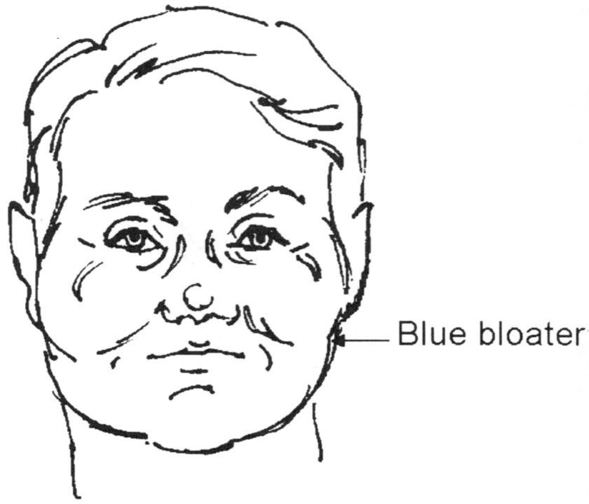

D-156: COPD

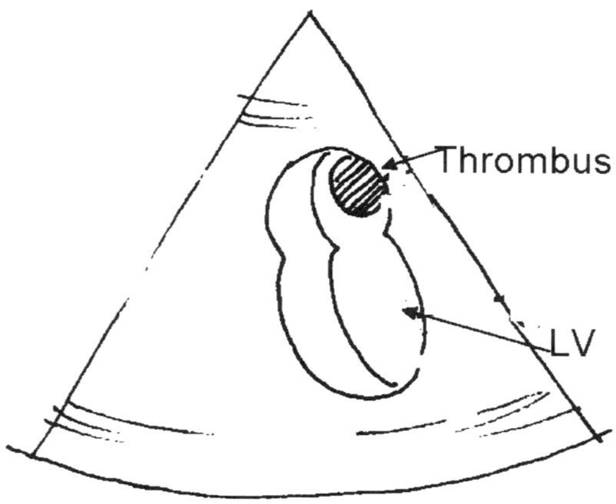

D-157: Thrombus inside the (L) atrium (Echocardiogram)

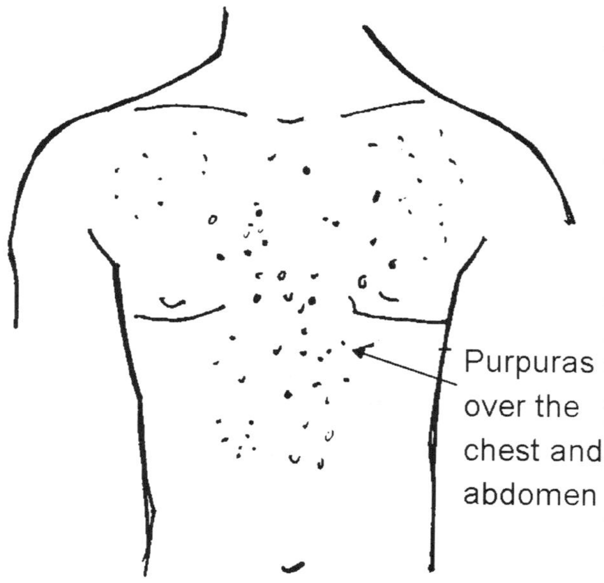

D-158: Thrombocytopenic purpura

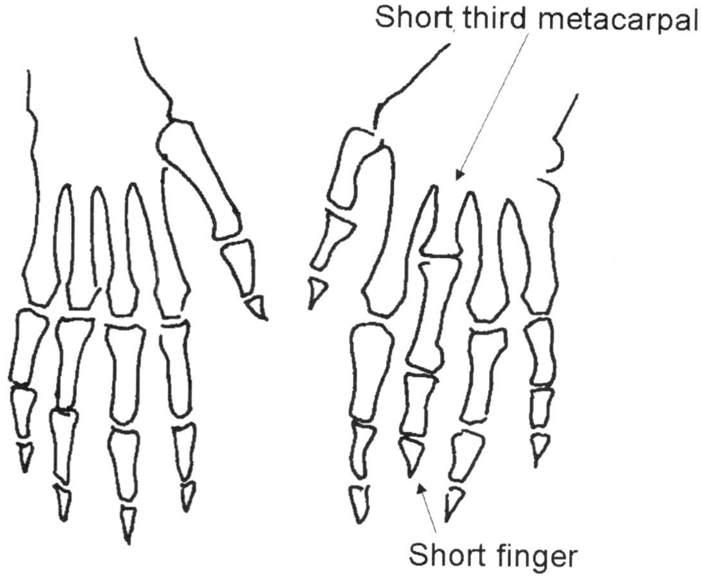

D-159: Pseudohypoparathyroidism

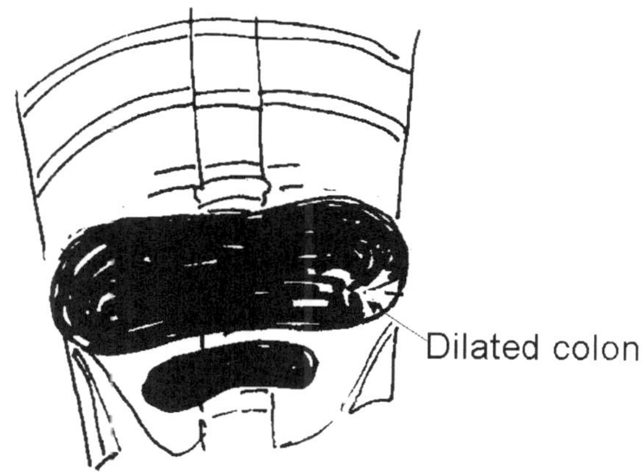

D-160: Toxic megacolon (x-ray)

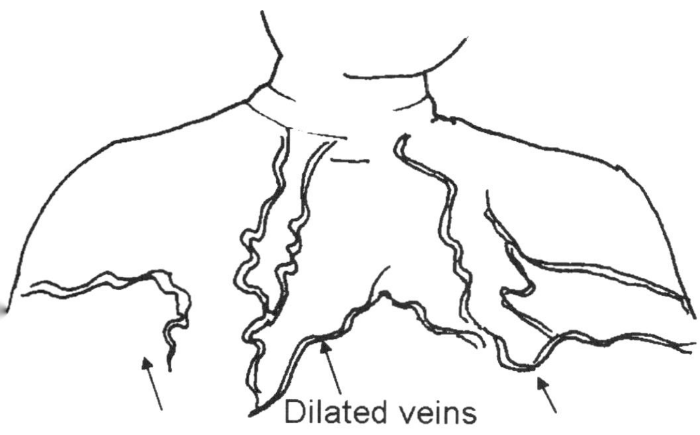

D-161: SVC obstruction

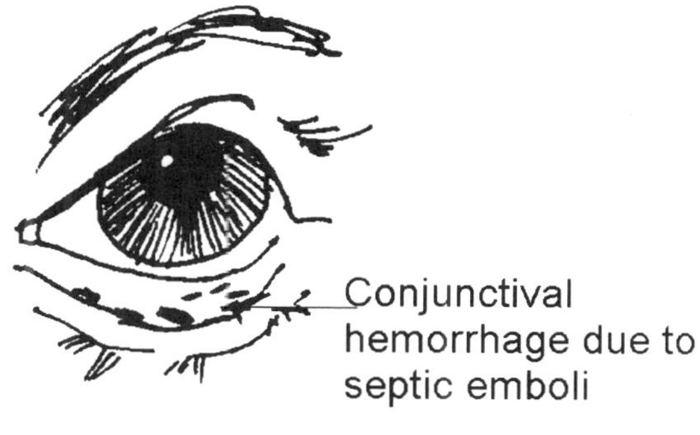

D-162: Infective endocarditis producing septic emboli

Picture 56

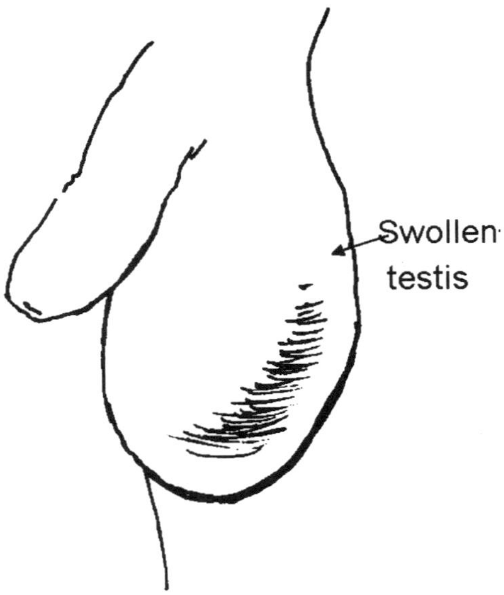

D-163: Lymphoma of the testis

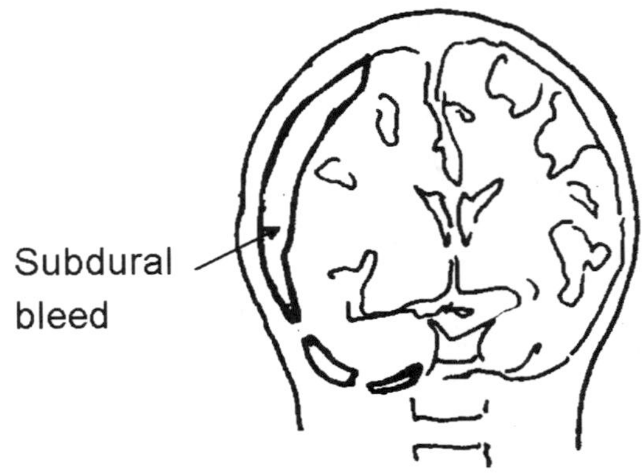

D-164: (R) subdural hemorrhage (MRI)

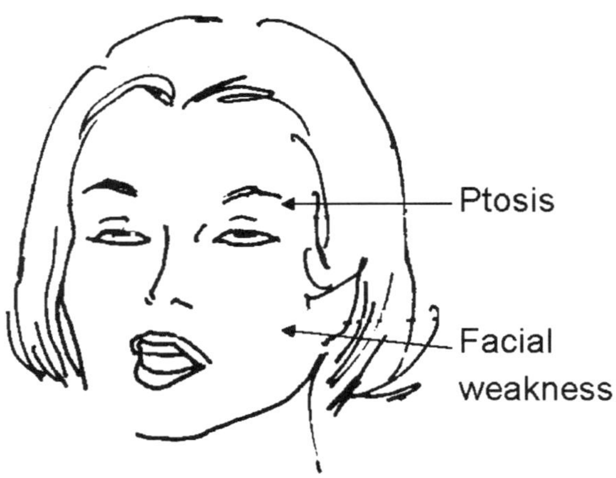

D-165: Myasthenia gravis

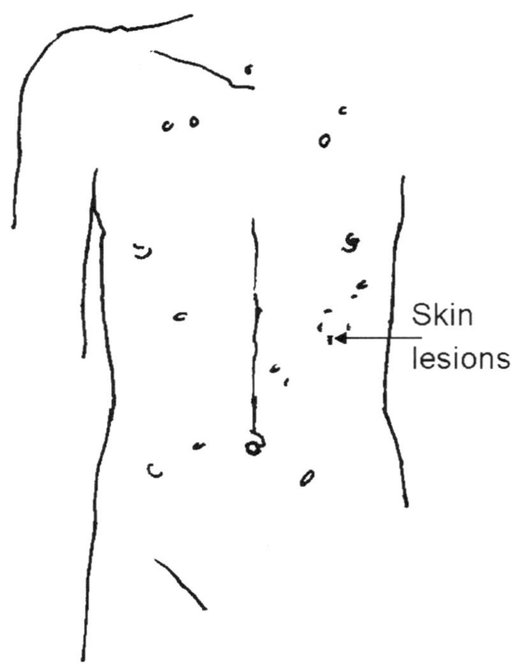

D-166: Kaposi's sarcoma

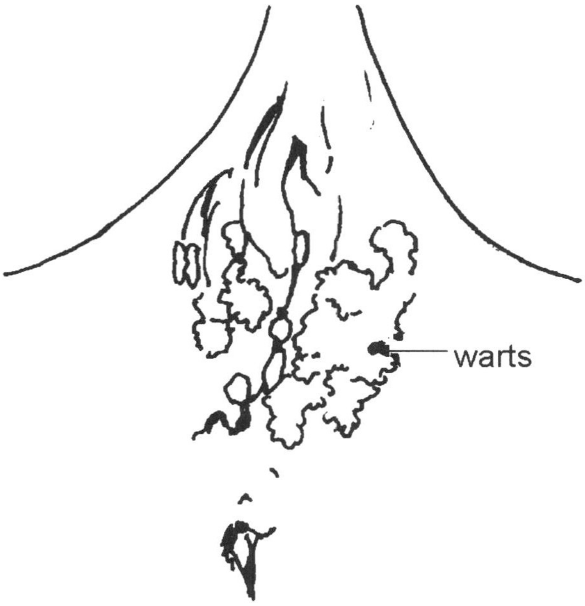

D-167: Genital warts

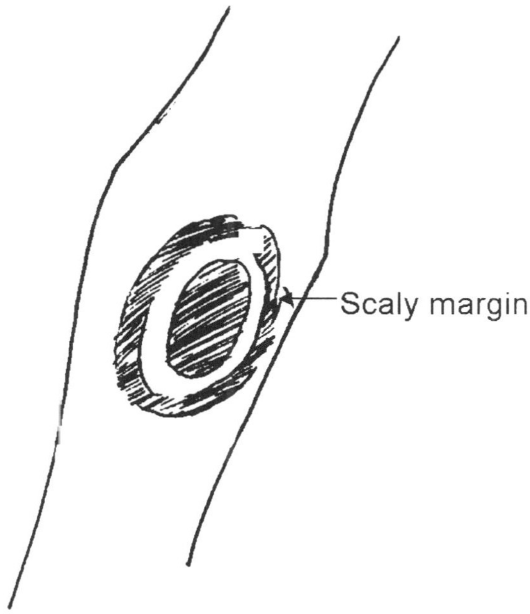

D-168: Tinea or ringworm

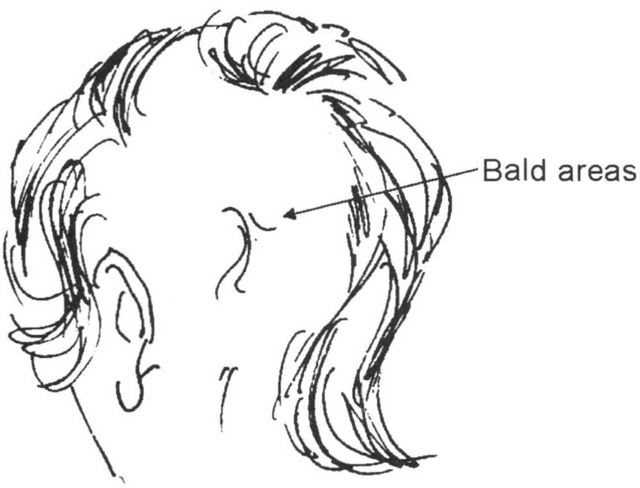

D-169: Severe alopecia areata

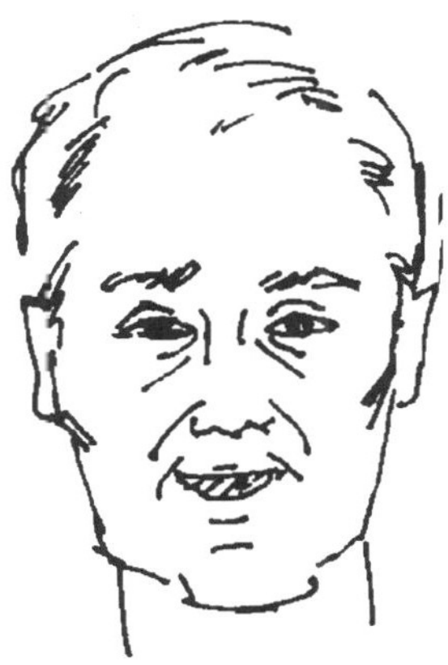

D-170: COPD (pink puffer)

Picture 58

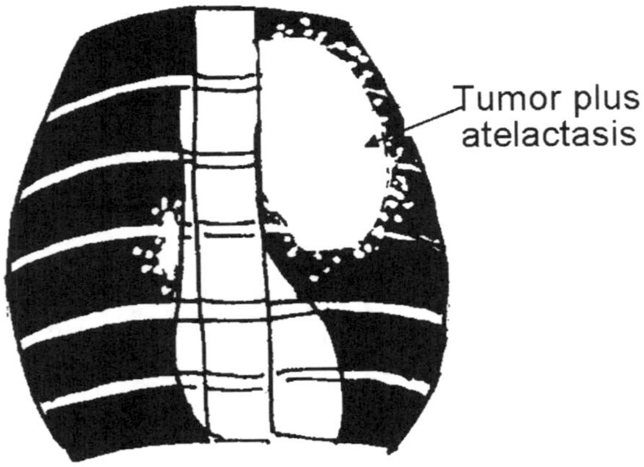

D-171: (L) bronchial cancer (X-ray)

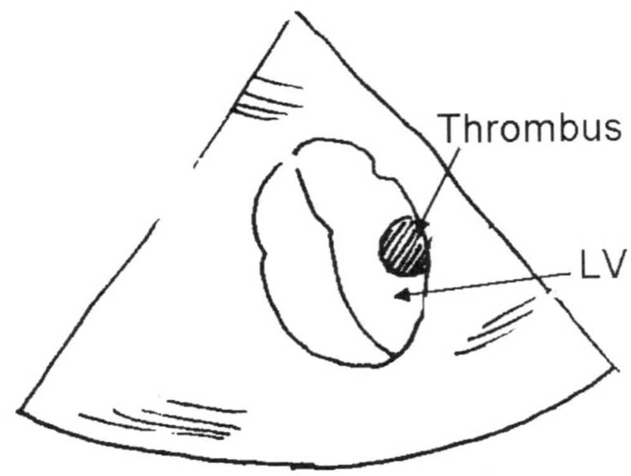

D-172: (L) ventricular thrombus (Echocardiogram)

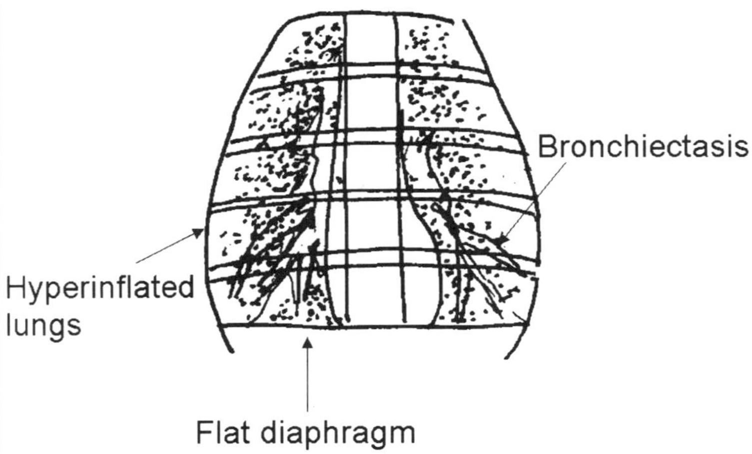

D-173: Cystic fibrosis (x-ray)

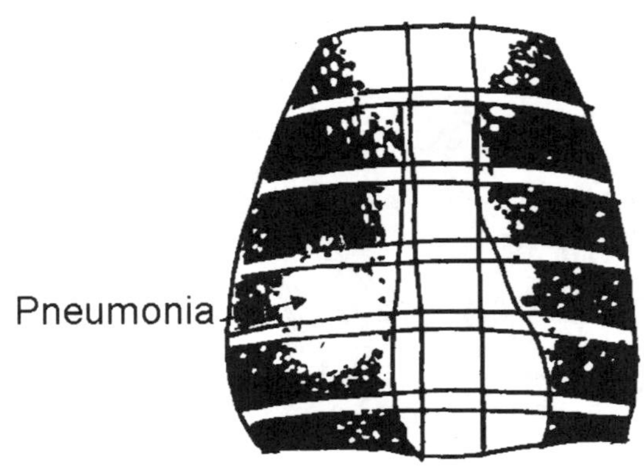

D-174: Staphylococcal pneumonias

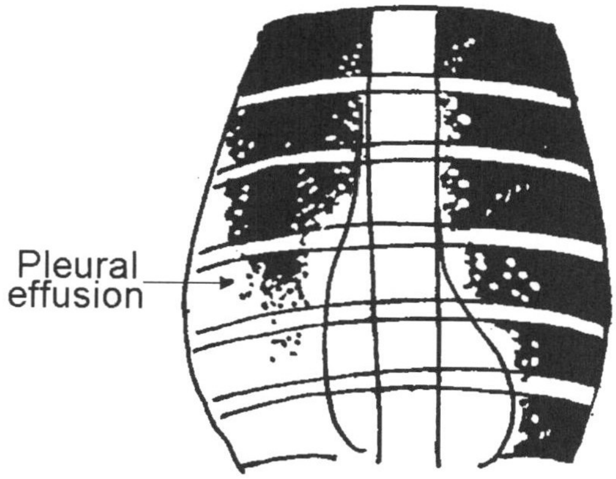

D-175: TB pleural effusion

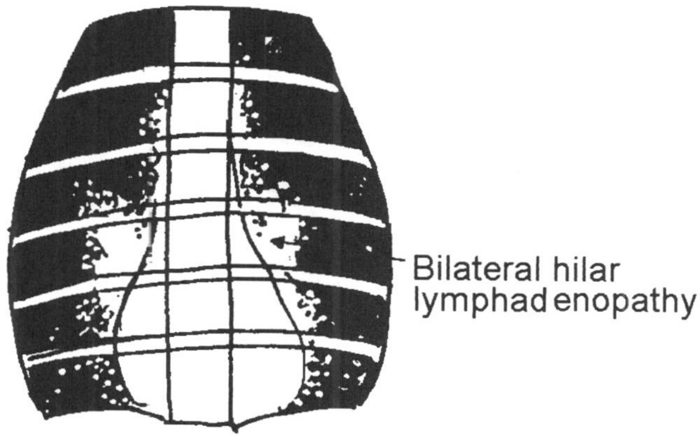

D-176: Sarcoidosis (x-ray)

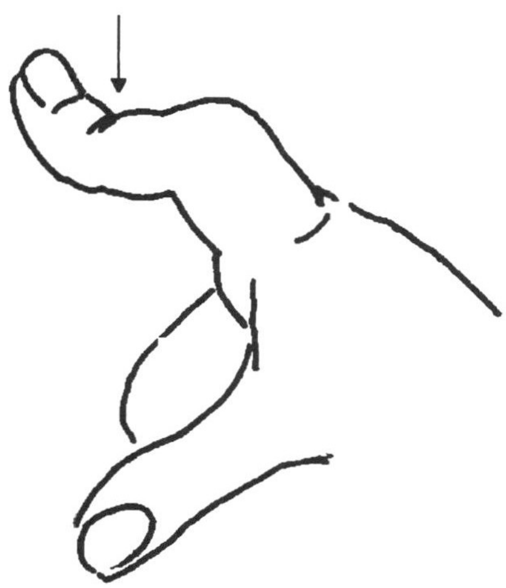

D-177: Boutonniere deformity (advanced rheumatoid arthritis)

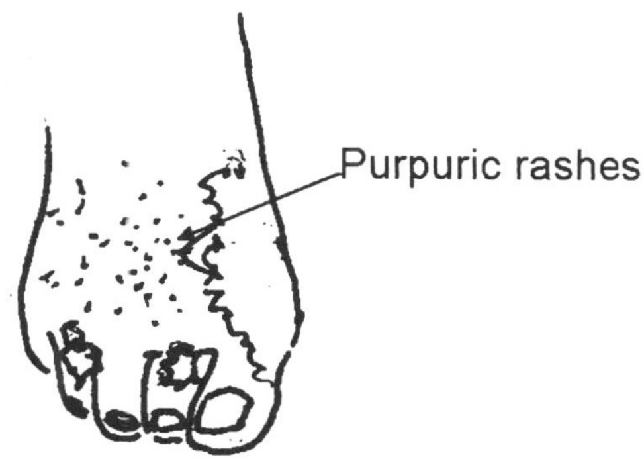

D-178: Polyarteritis nodosa

Picture 60

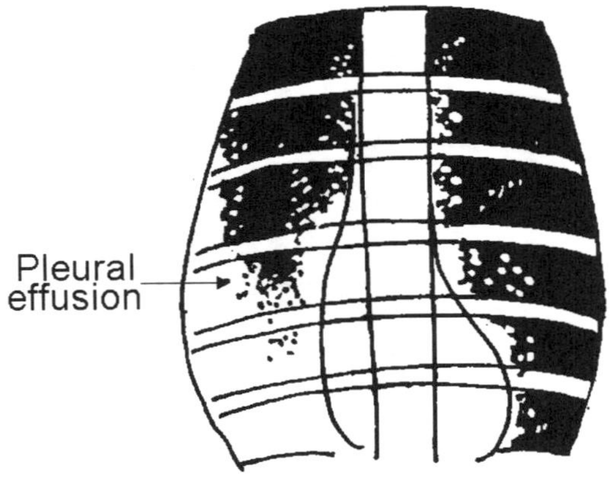

D-175: TB pleural effusion

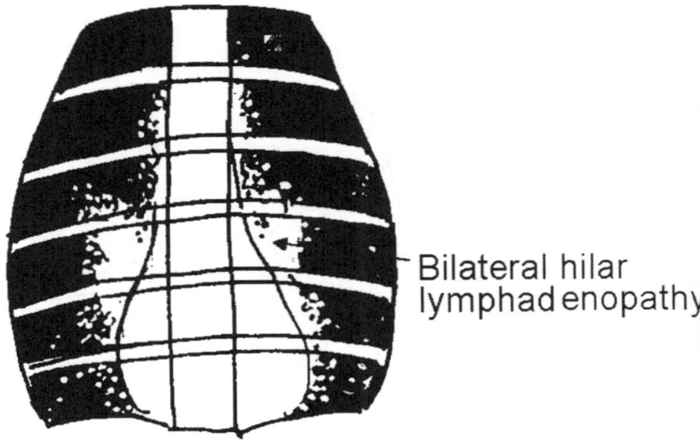

D-176: Sarcoidosis (x-ray)

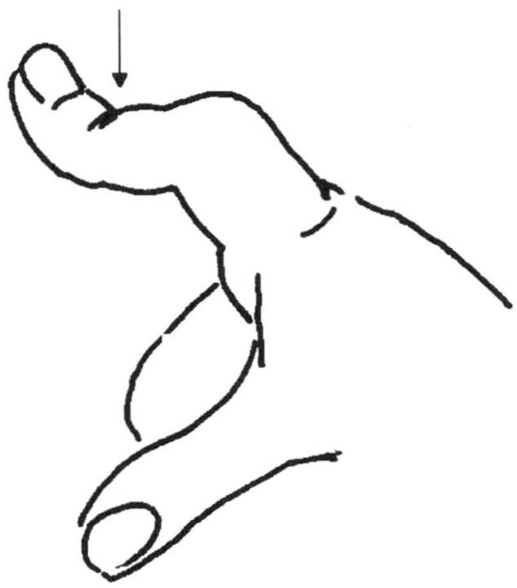

D-177: Boutonniere deformity (advanced rheumatoid arthritis)

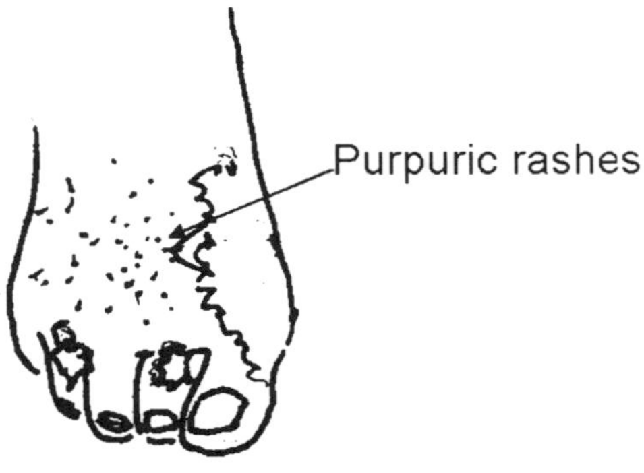

D-178: Polyarteritis nodosa

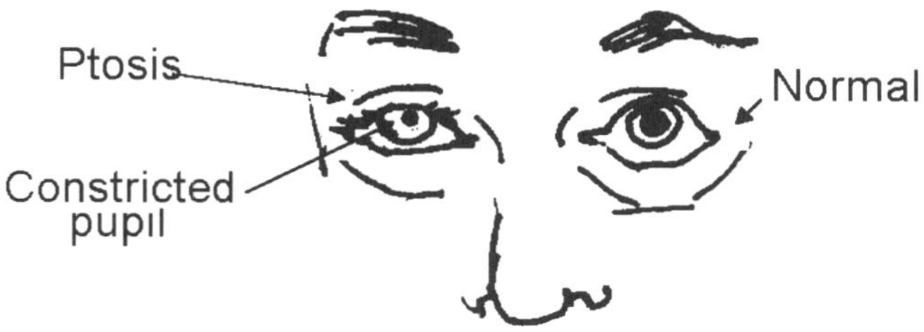

D-179: Horner Syndrome

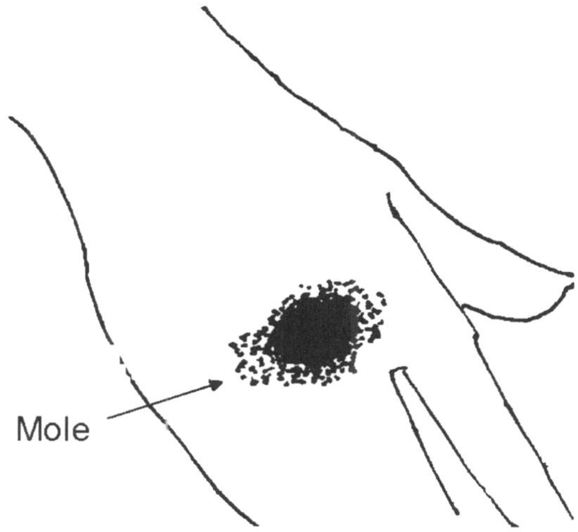

D-180: Benign mole (melanocytic nevus)

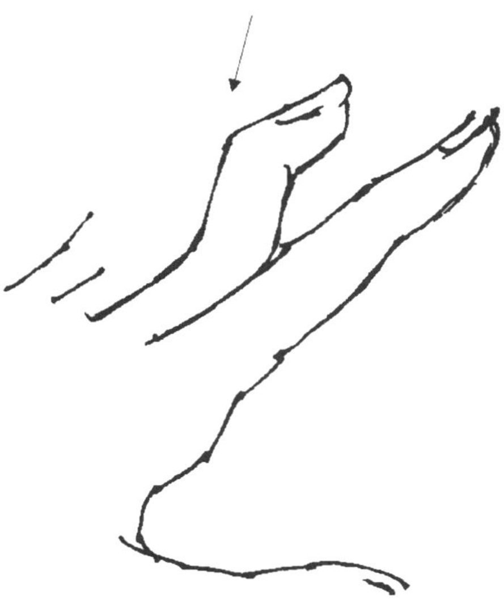

D-181: Swan-neck deformity

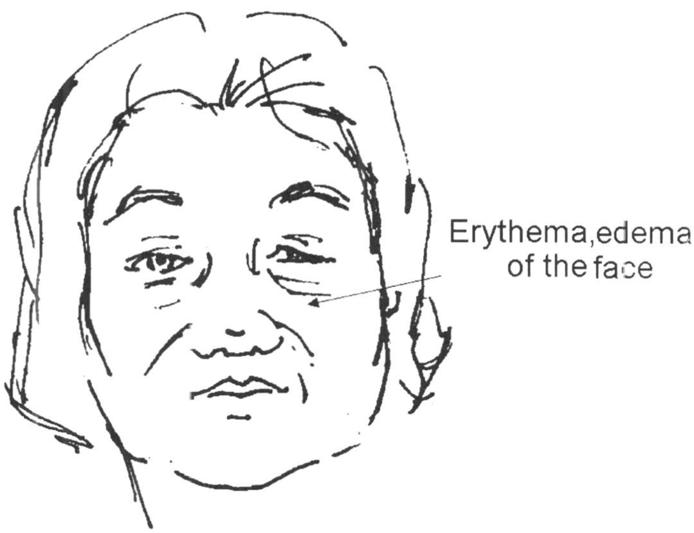

D-182: Dermatomyositis

Picture 62

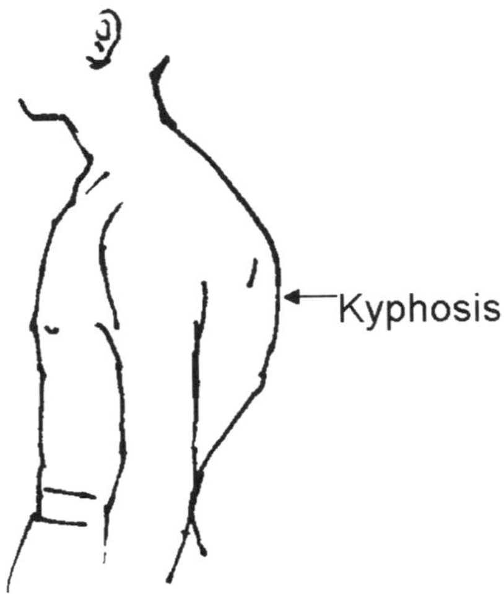

D-183: Kyphosis in COPD-emphysema patient

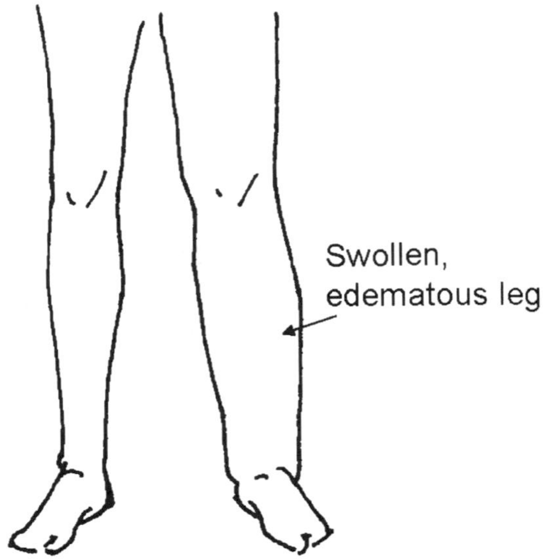

D-184: Unilateral lymphedema

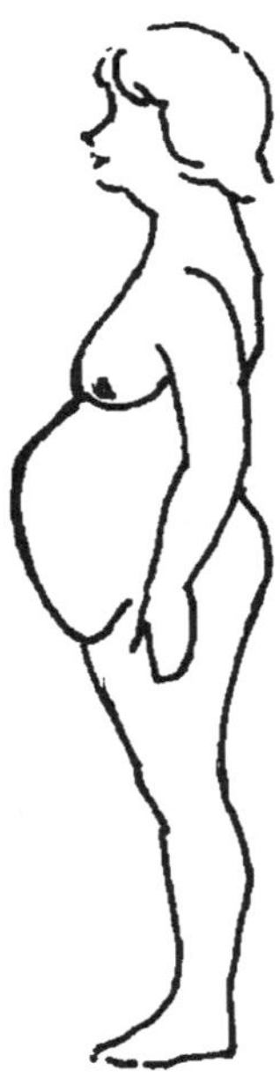

D-185: Simple obesity

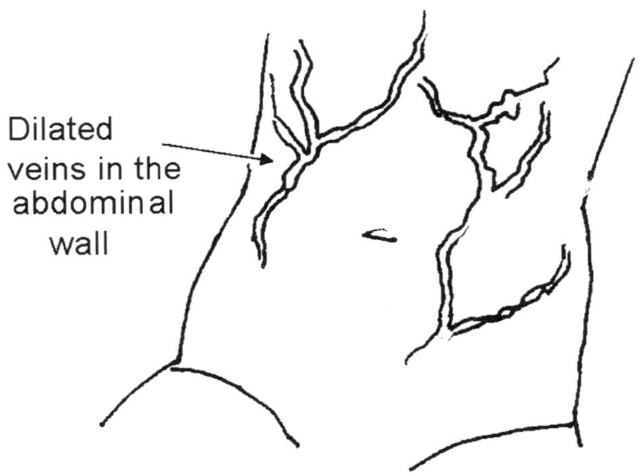

D-186: Budd-Chiari syndrome

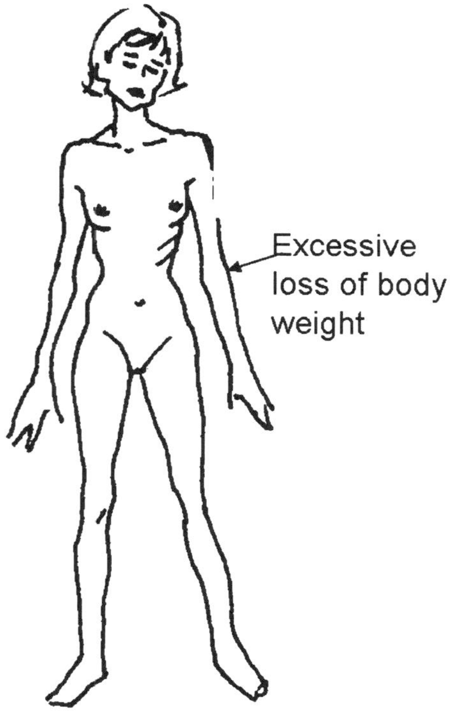

D-187: Anorexia nervosa

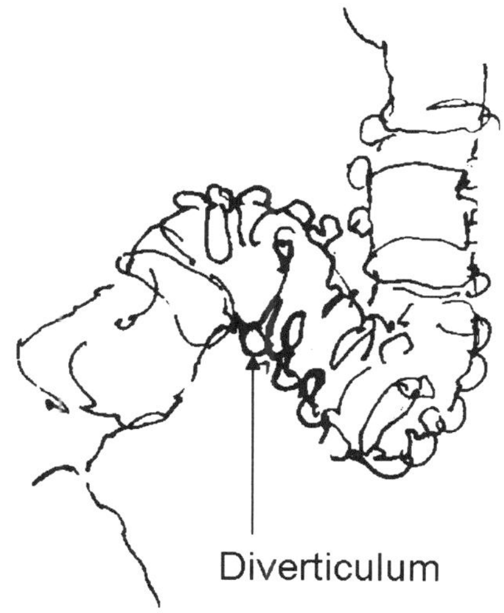

D-188: Diverticulum in Colon (Barium enema)

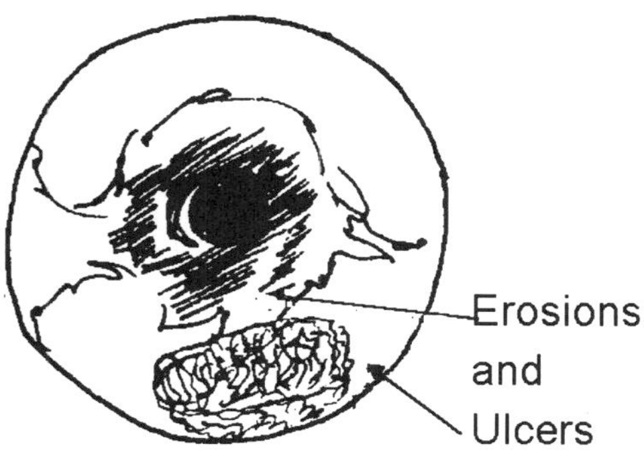

D-189: Esophagitis (Endoscopy) and ulcers

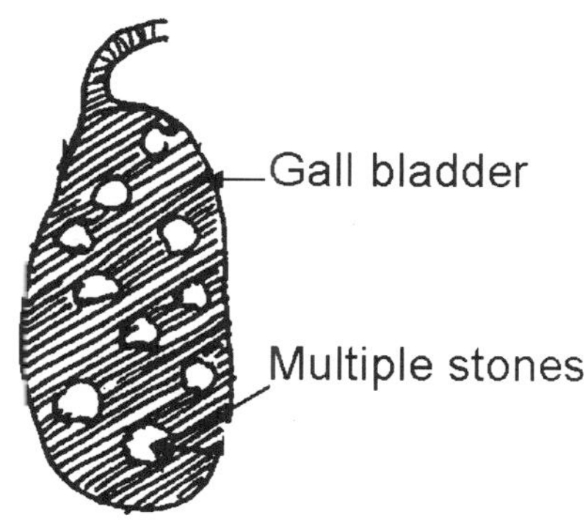

D-190: Gallstones (X-ray)

Picture 64

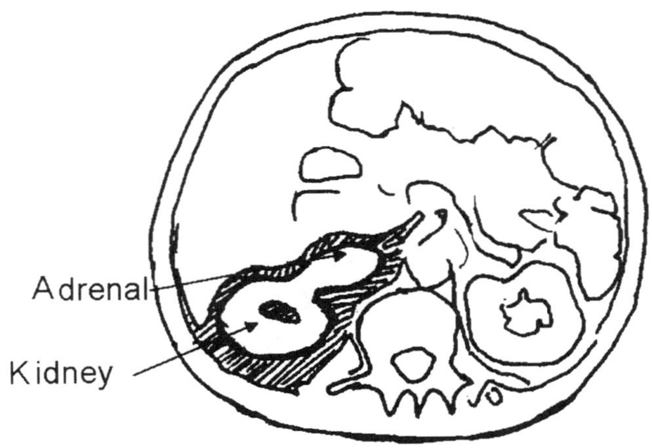

D-191: Metastasis in the (R) adrenal gland (CT Scan)

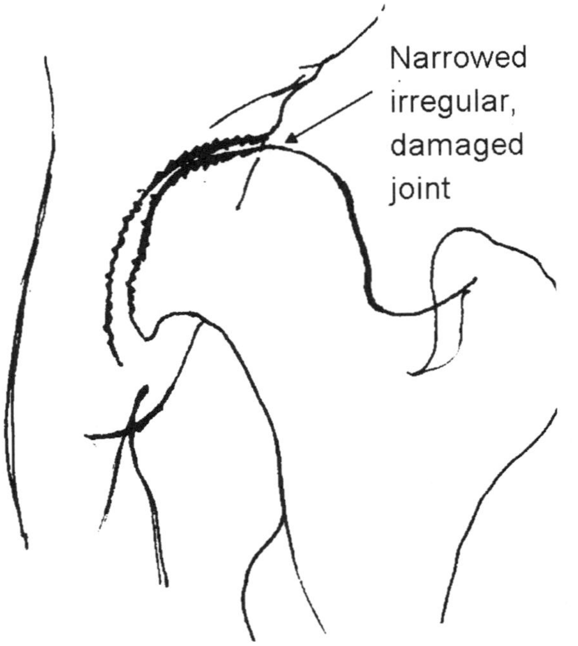

D-192: Degenerative arthritis in hip joint (X-ray)

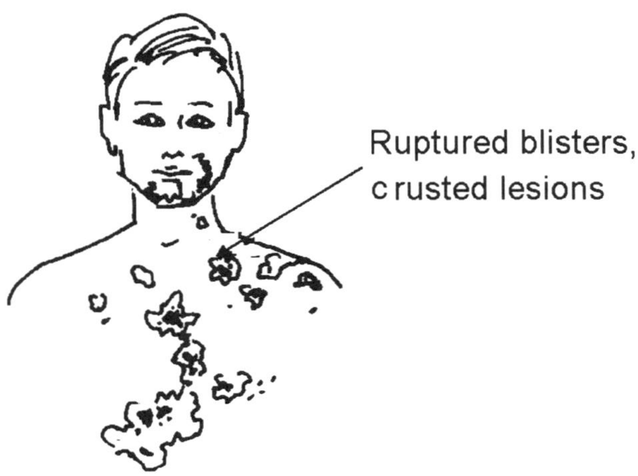

D-193: Pemphigus vulgaris

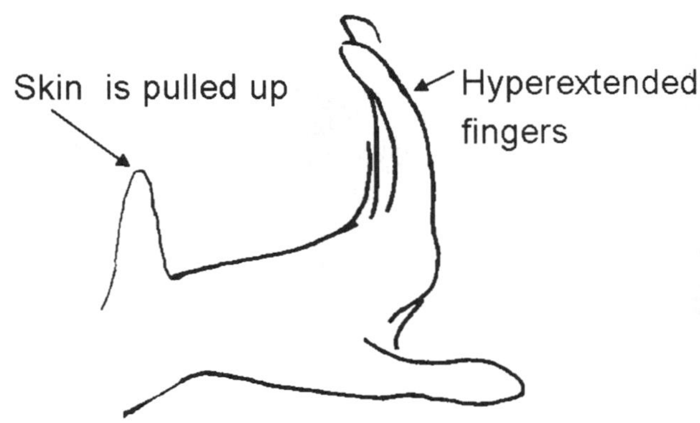

D-194: Ehlers-Danlos syndrome

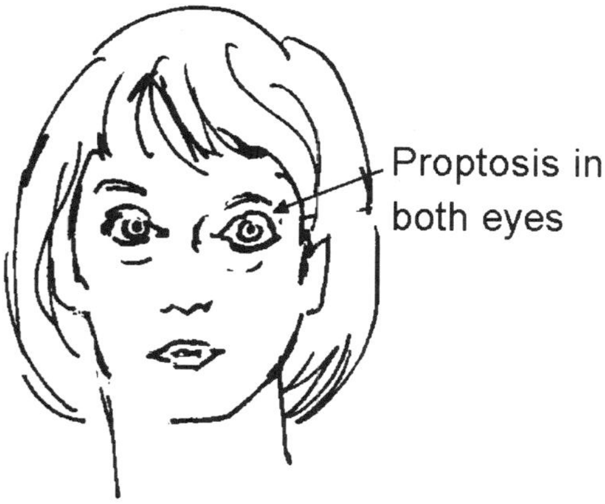

D-195: Hyperthyroidism

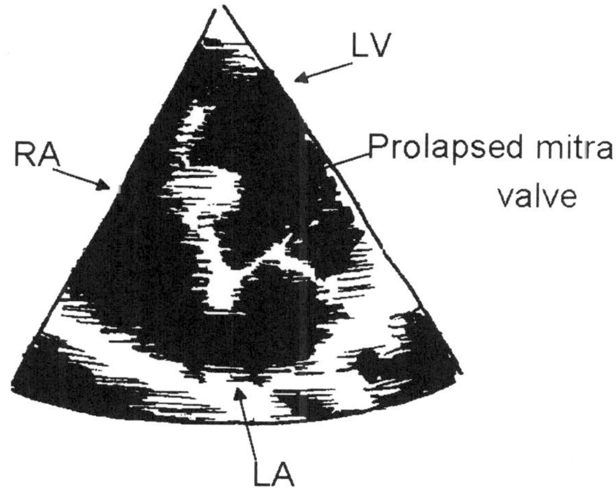

D-196: Mitral valve prolapse (Echocardiogram)

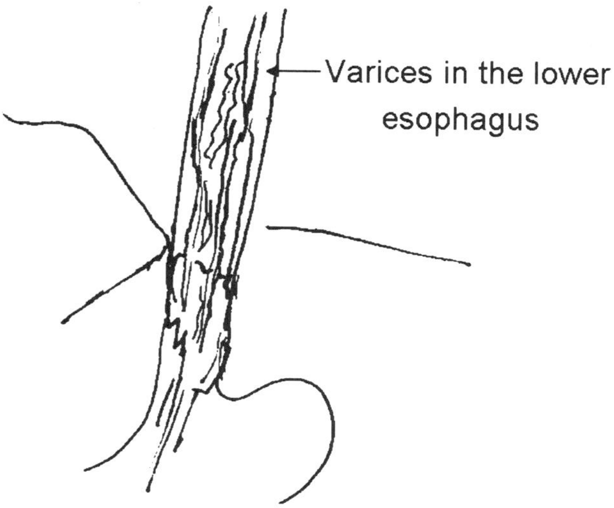

D-197: Esophageal varices (Barium swallow)

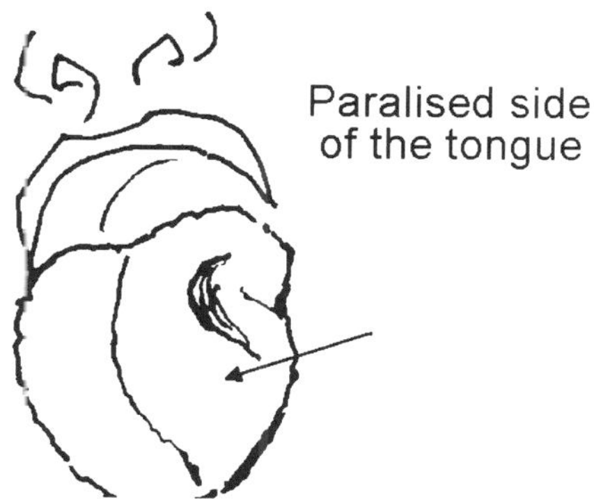

D-198: (L) Hypoglossal nerve paralysis

Picture 66

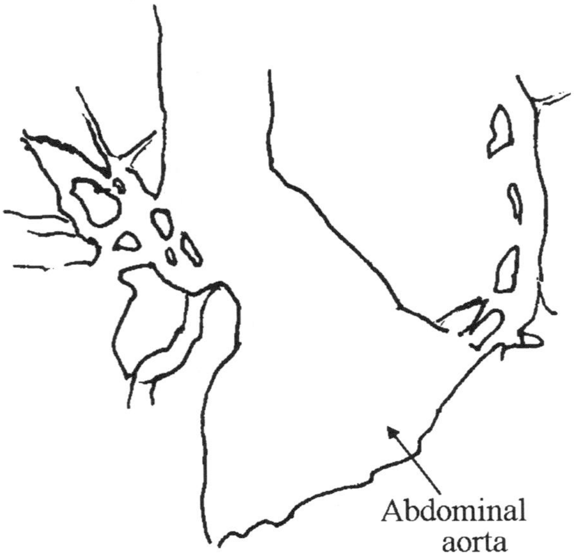

D-199: Abdominal aortic aneurysm (Angiogram)

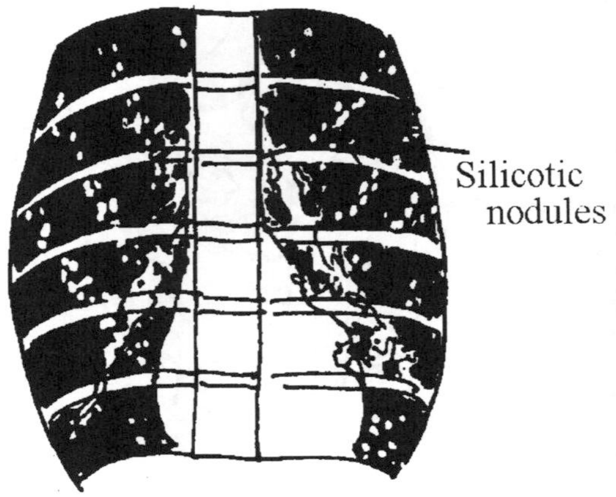

D-200: Silicosis (X-ray)

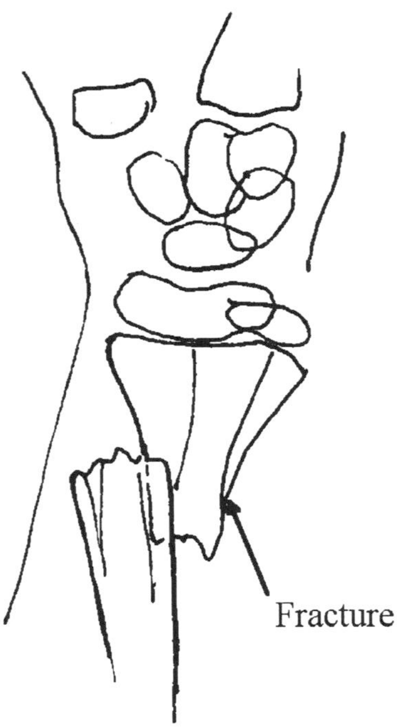

D-201: Fractures tibia and fibula (X-ray)

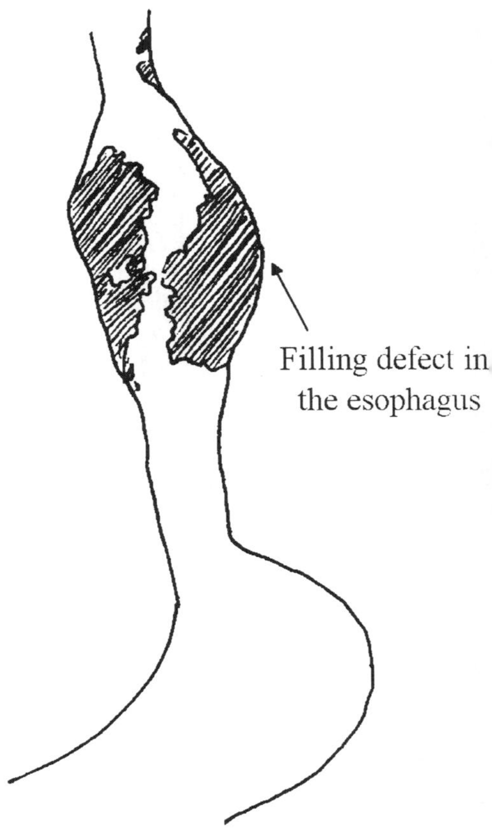

D-202: Esophageal cancer (Barium study)

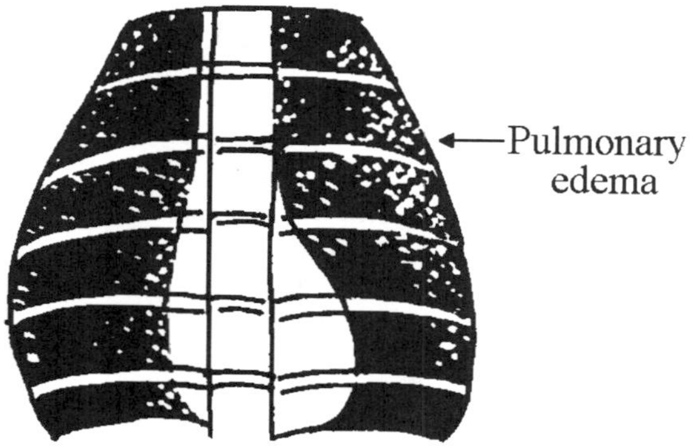

D-203: ARDS (X-ray)

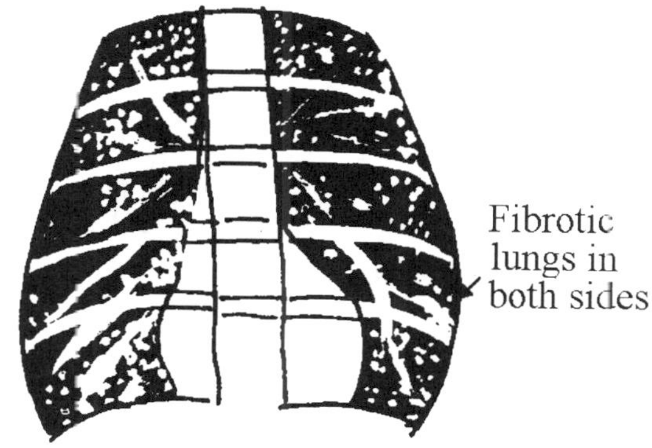

D-204: Pneumoconiosis (X-ray)

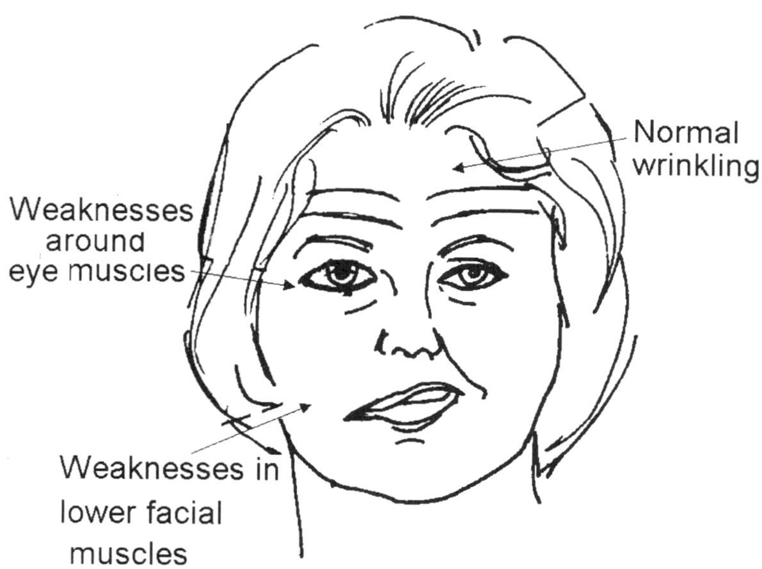

D-205: (R) Facial nerve palsy (upper motor neuron lesion, left carotid artery thrombosis)

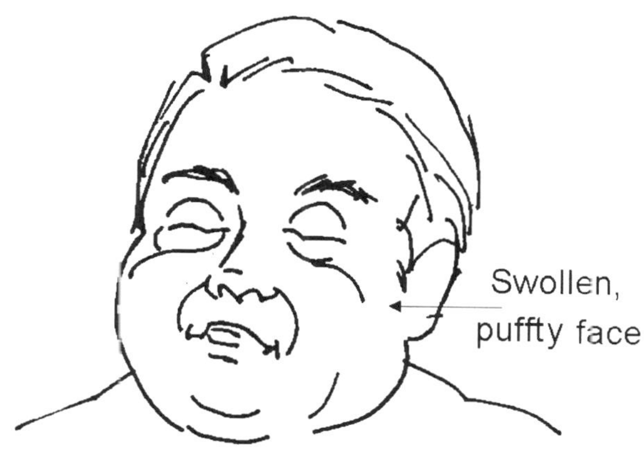

D-206: Acute surgicalemphysema following pneumothorax

Picture 68

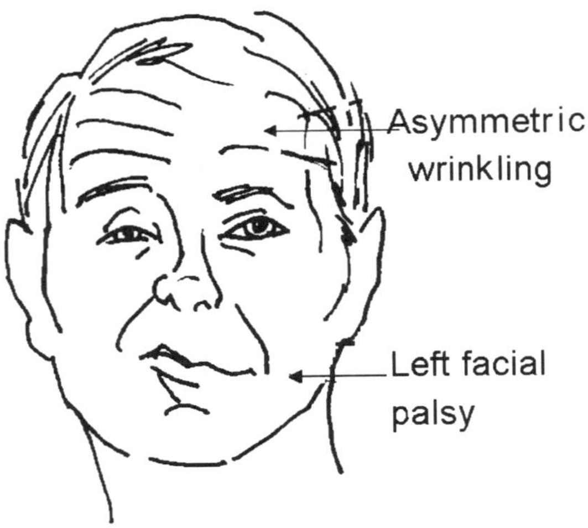

D-207: Bell's palsy (lower motor neuron lesion)

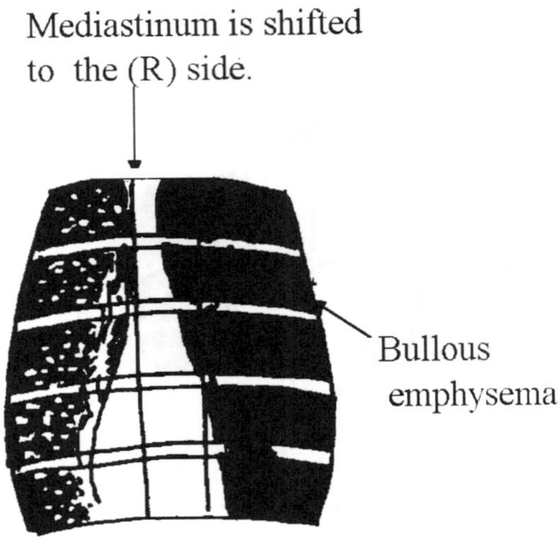

D-208: Obstructive bullous emphysema (L) lung (X-ray)

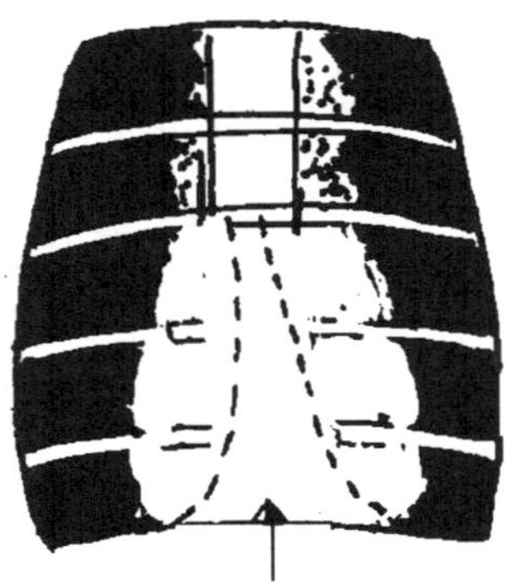

D-209: Left lower lobe collapse (X-ray)

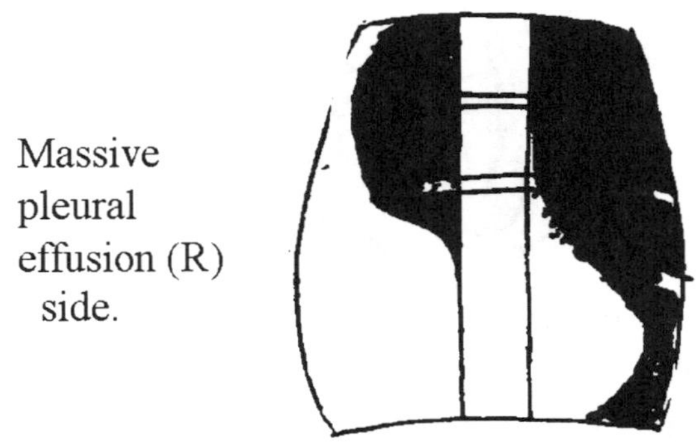

D-210: Massive pleural effusion (R) side

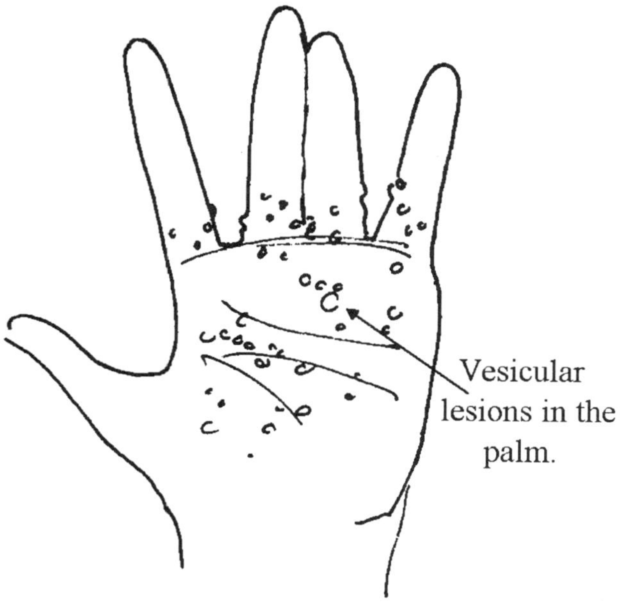

D-211: Pompholyx (a variant of eczema)

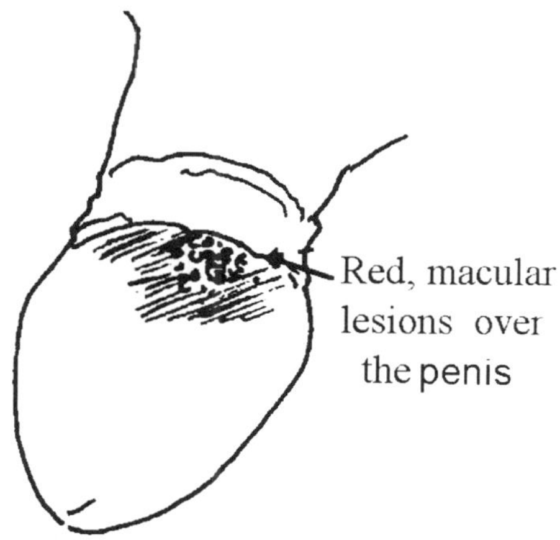

D-212: Reiter's disease

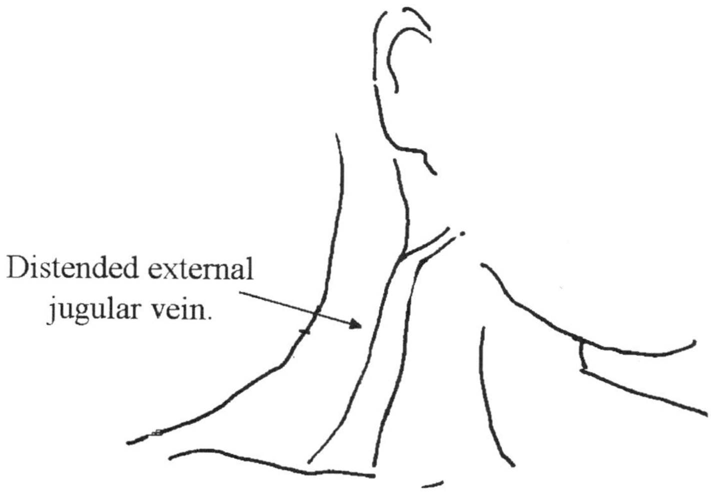

D-213: Cardiac failure

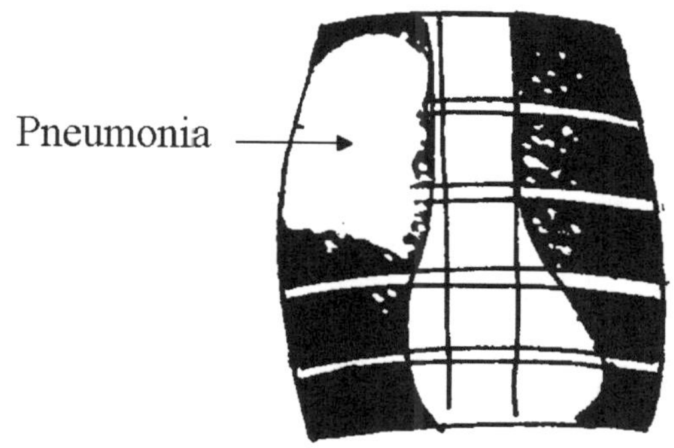

D-214: (R) upper lobe pneumonia (X-ray)

Picture 70

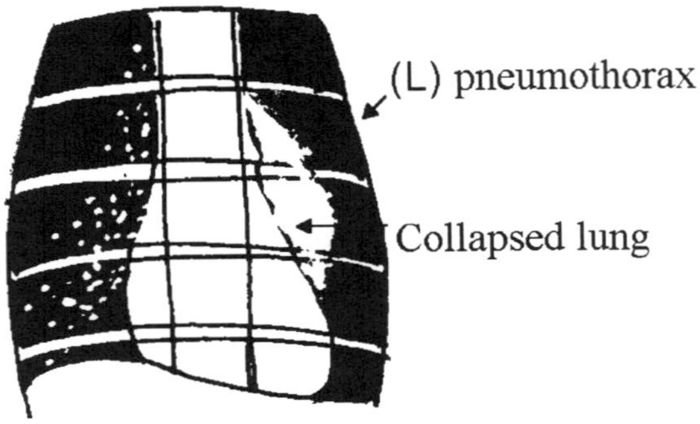

D-215: Left pneumothorax and collapsed lung

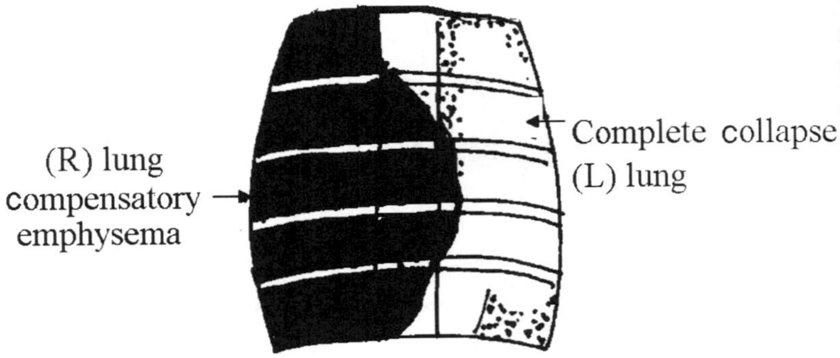

D-216: Completely collapsed (L) lung plus compensatory emphysema of (R) lung (X-ray)

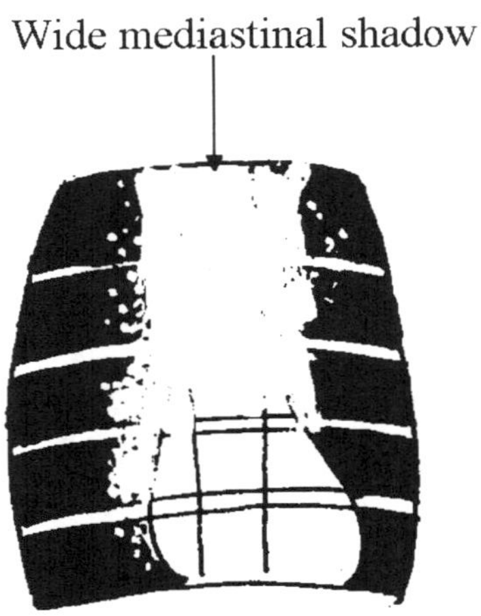

D-217: Mediastinal hemorrhage

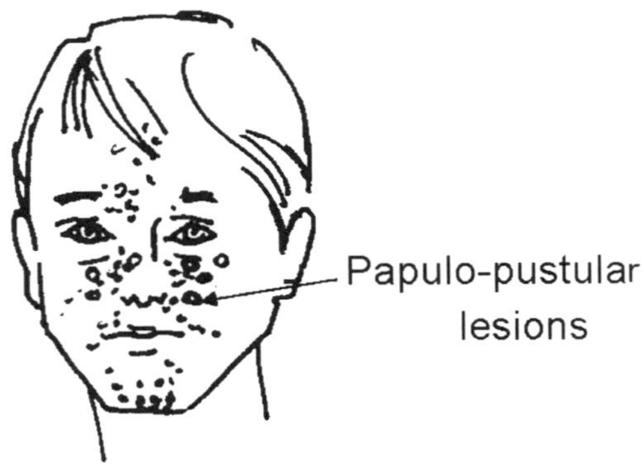

D-218: Acne vulgaris

Picture 71

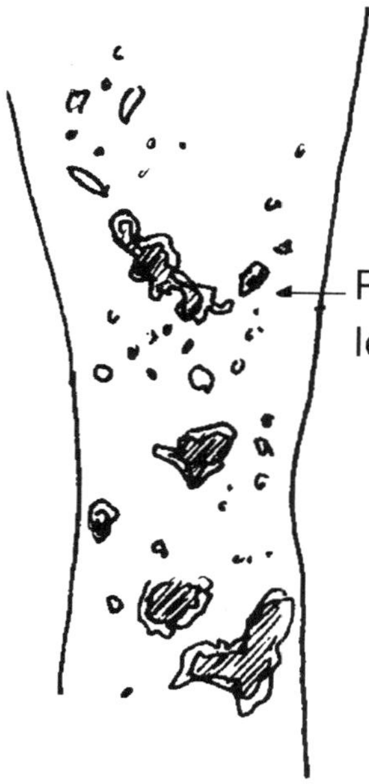

D-219: Leukocytoclastic vasculitis

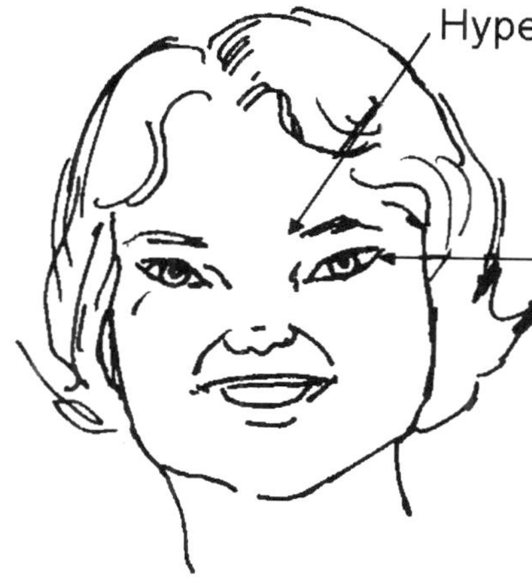

D-220: Down syndrome

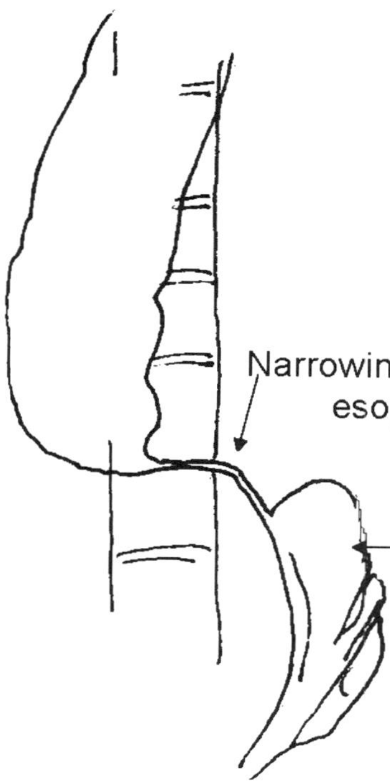

D-221: Achalasia of the esophagus
(Barium swallow)

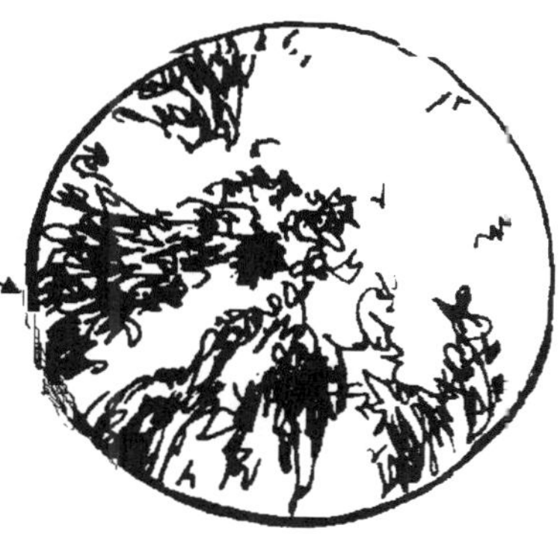

D-222: Retinitis pigmentosa (Fundoscopy)

Picture 72

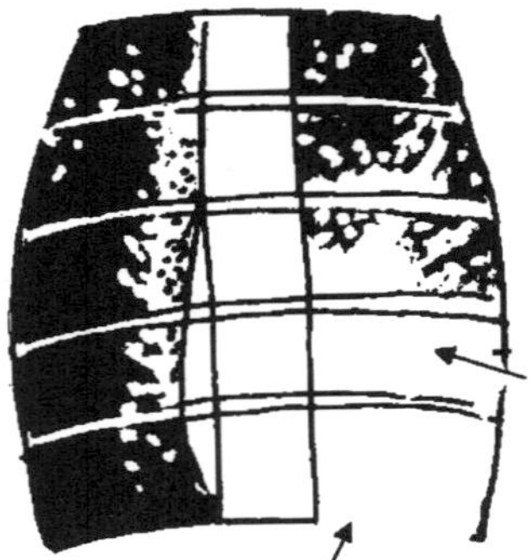

D-223: Left lower lobe pneumonia (X-ray)

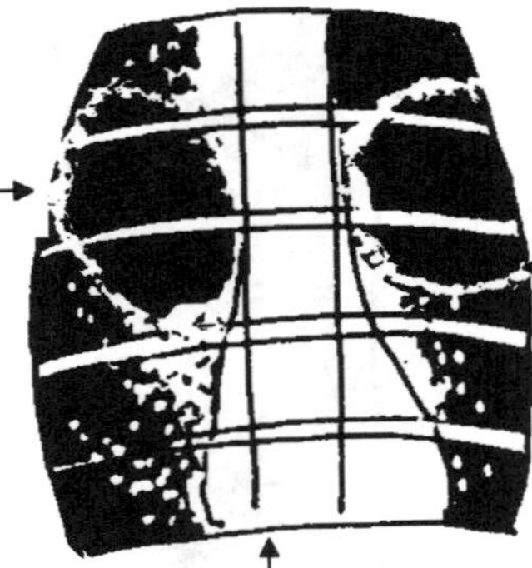

D-224: Pan-acinar emphysema with bullae formation.

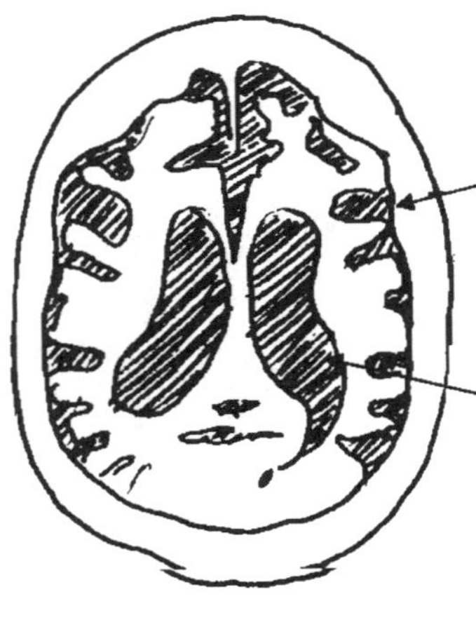

D-225: Alzheimer's disease (CT scan)

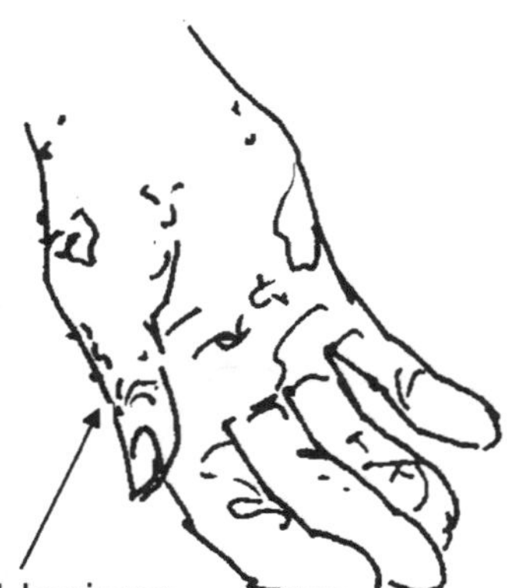

D-226: Irritant dermatitis

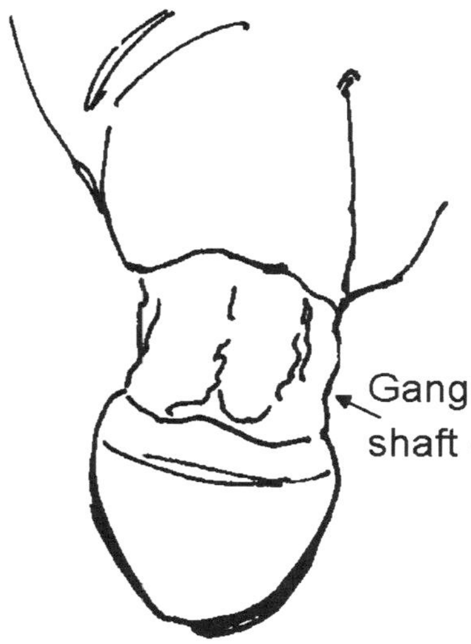

D-227: Fournier's gangrene

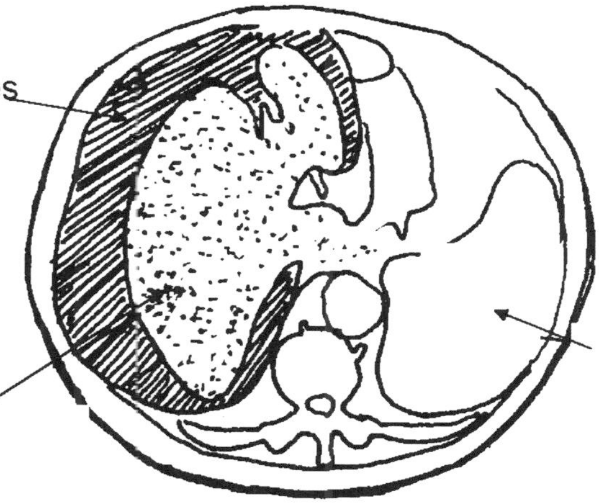

D.228: Cirrhosis of the liver (CT scan)

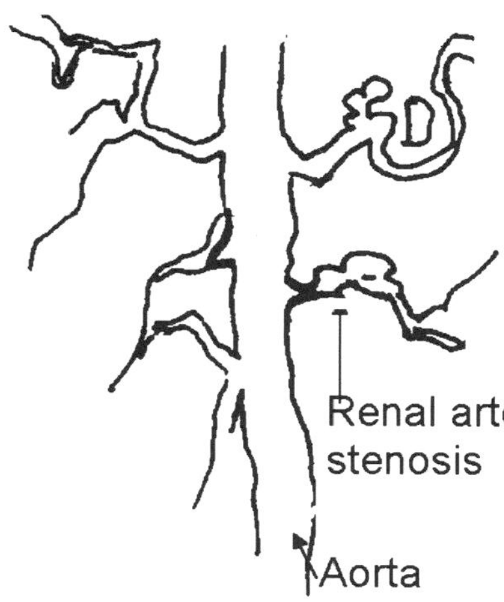

D-229: Renal artery stenosis (Aortogram)

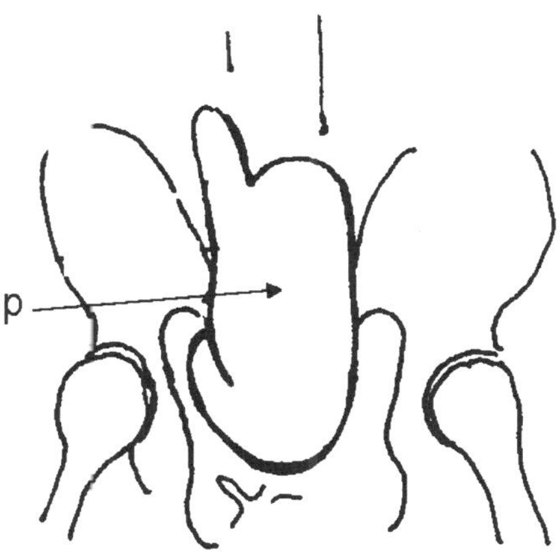

D 230: Bladder rupture due to trauma (Cystogram)

Picture 74

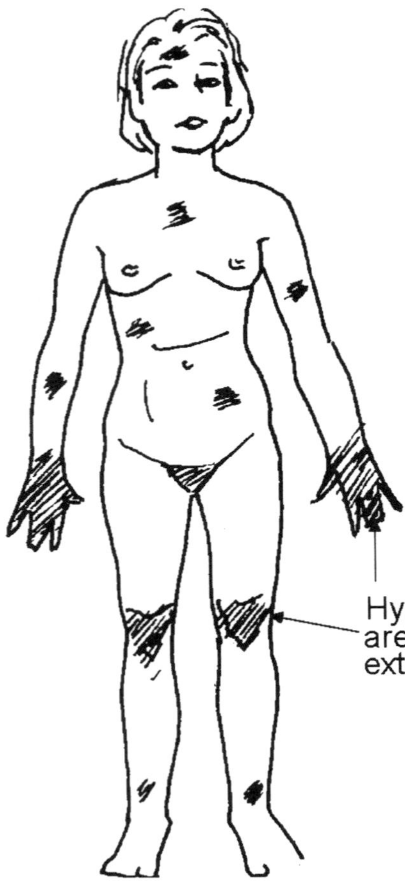

D-231: Addison disease

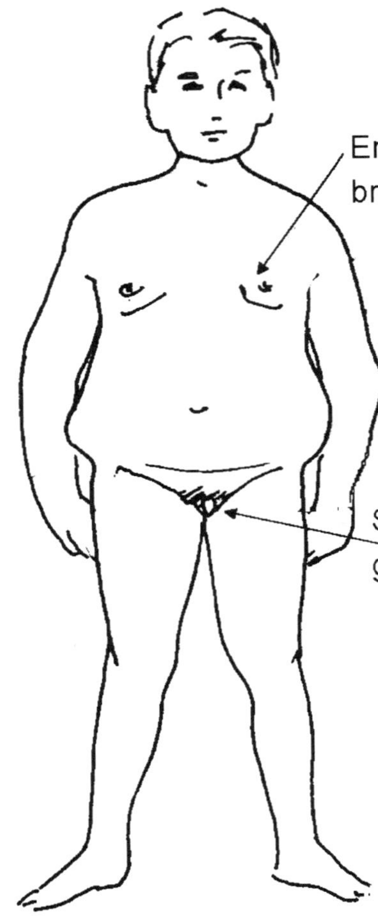

D.232: Klinefelter syndrome

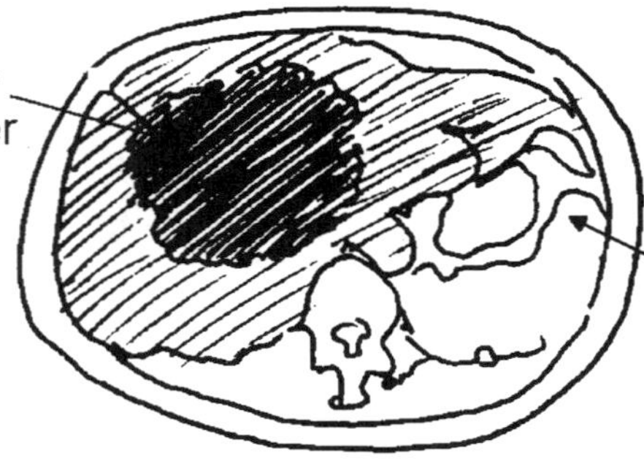

D-233: Primary hepatocellular carcinoma (CT Scan)

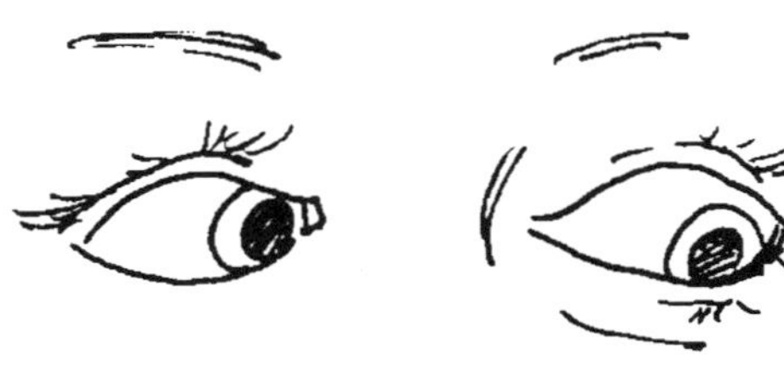

D-234: Right fourth cranial nerve palsy

Picture 75

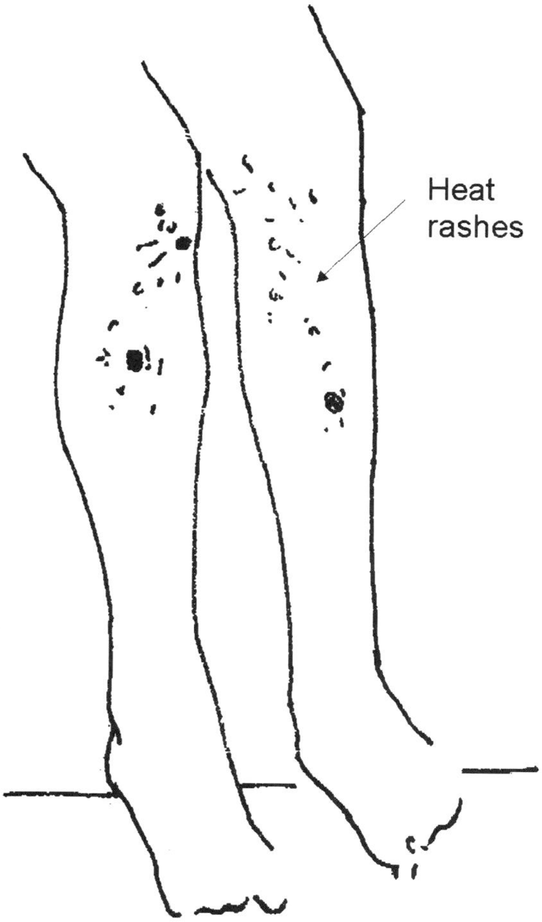

D-235: Tinker's Tartan (erythema ab igne)

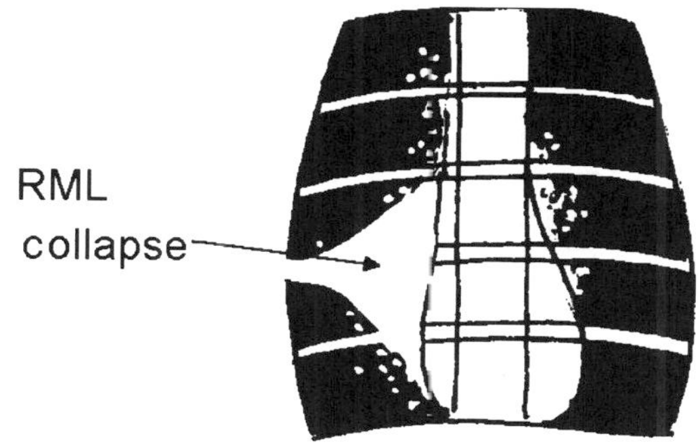

D-236: Collapse of (R) middle lobe

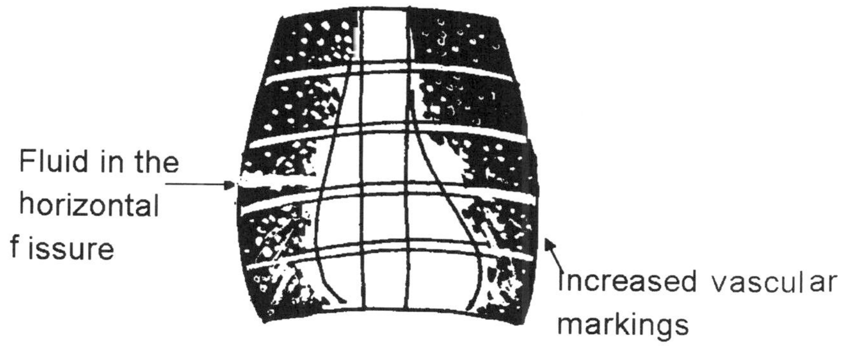

D-237: Congestive heart failure (x-ray)

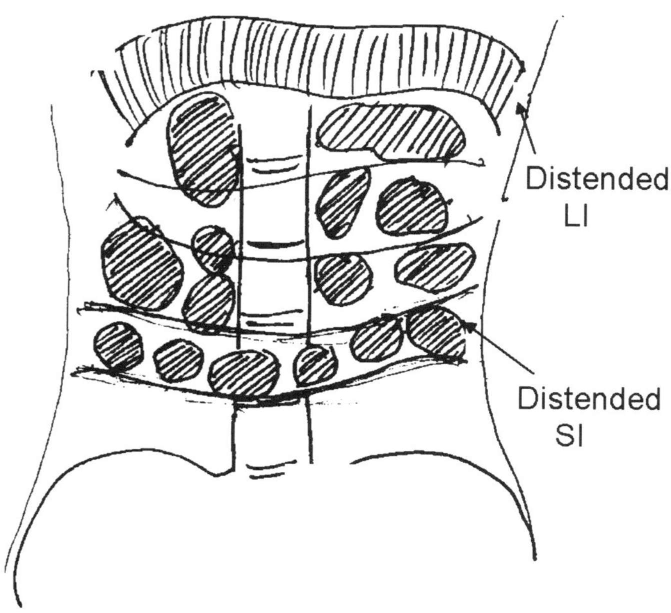

D-238: Paralytic ileus (x-ray)

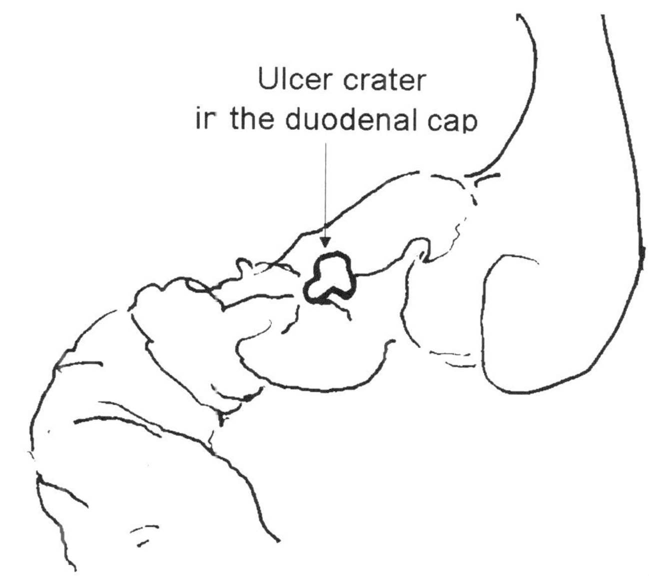

D-239: Duodenal ulcer (Barium study)

Picture 76

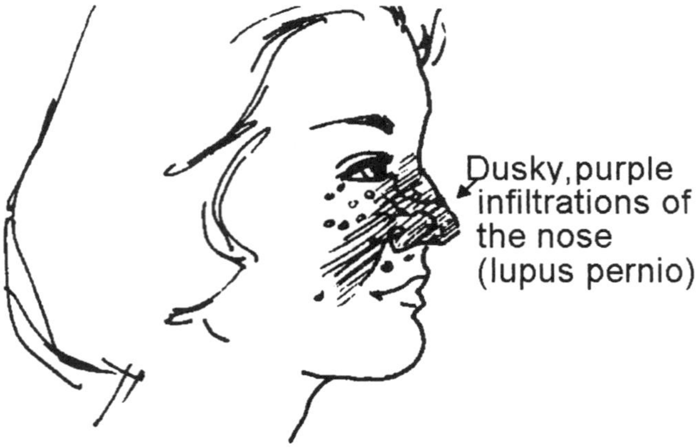

D-240: Chronic sarcoidosis

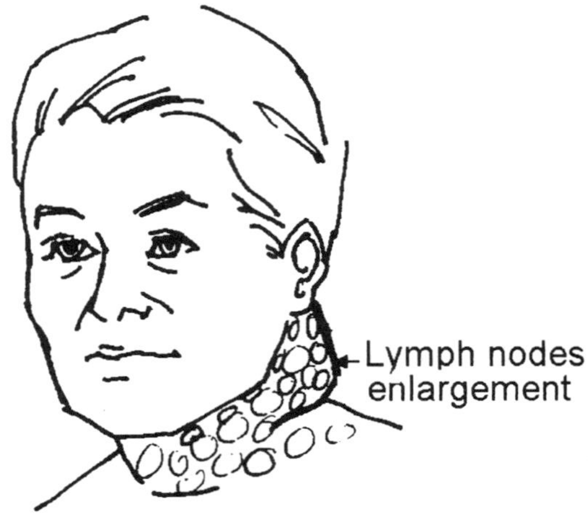

D-241: Hodgkin disease

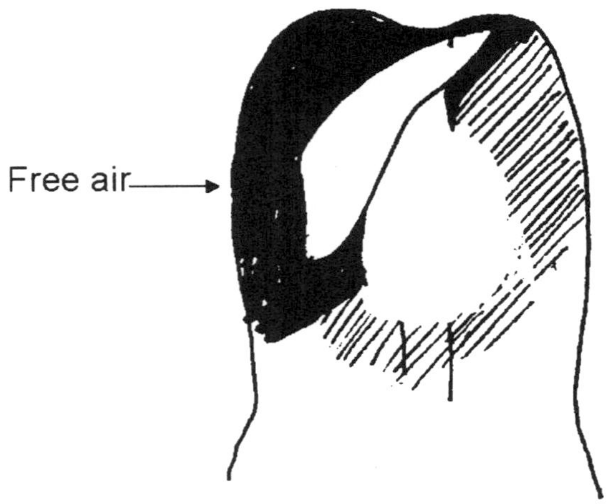

D-242: Free peritoneal air due to rupture intestine (x ray)

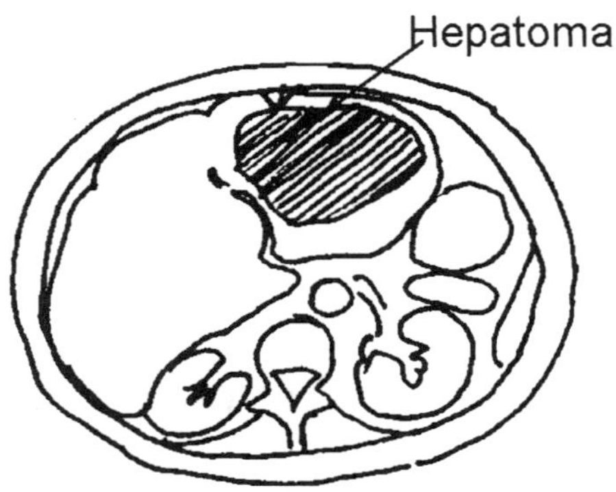

D-243: Hepatoma of the (L) lobe of the liver (CT scan)

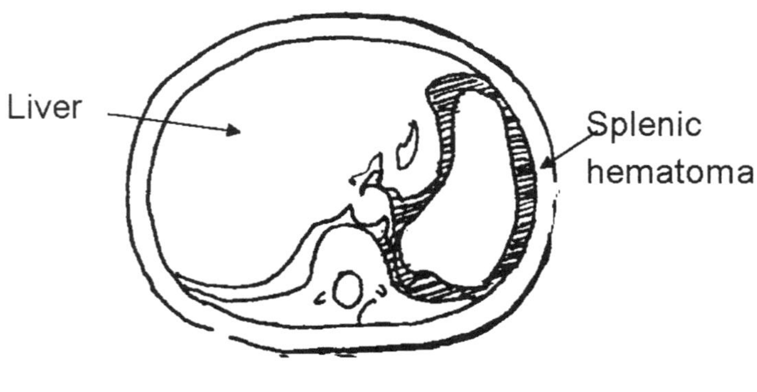

D-244: Subcapsular splenic hematoma

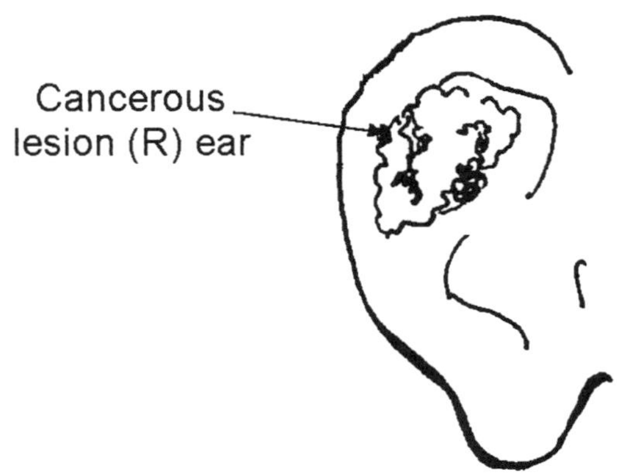

D-245: Squamous cell cancer

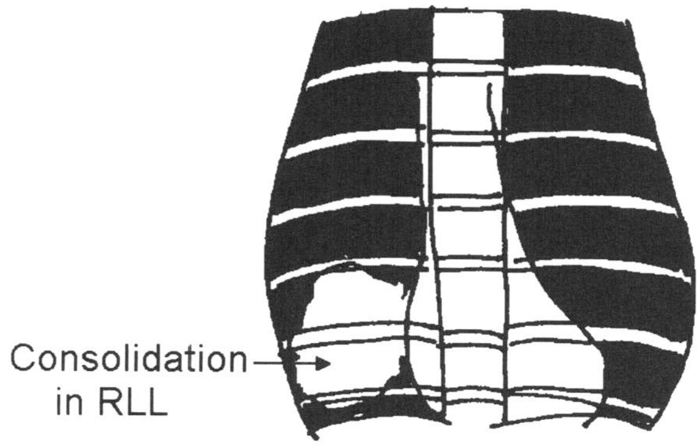

D-246: Postoperative pneumonia

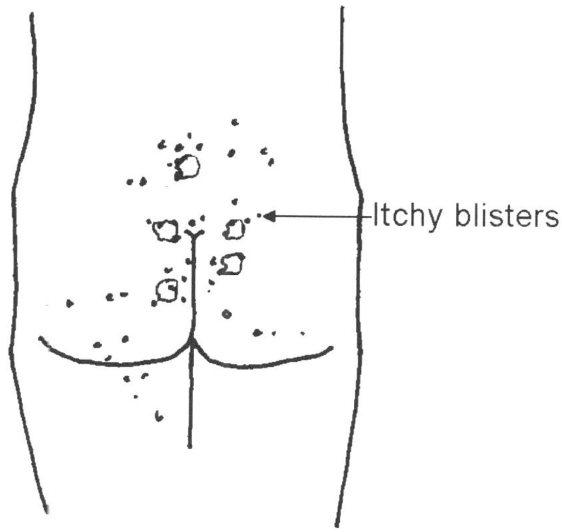

D-247: Dermatitis herpetiformis

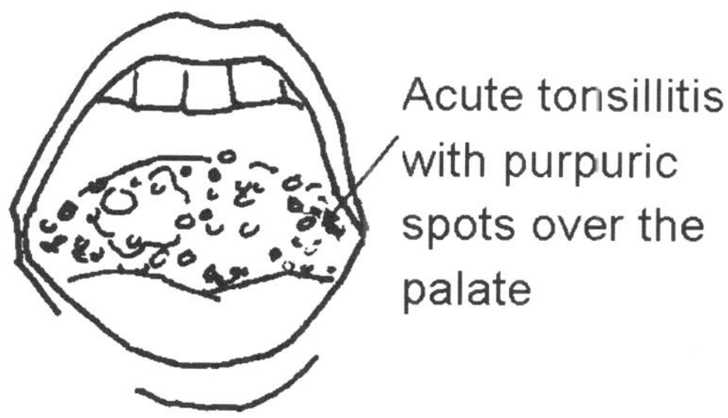

D-248: Infectious mononucleosis

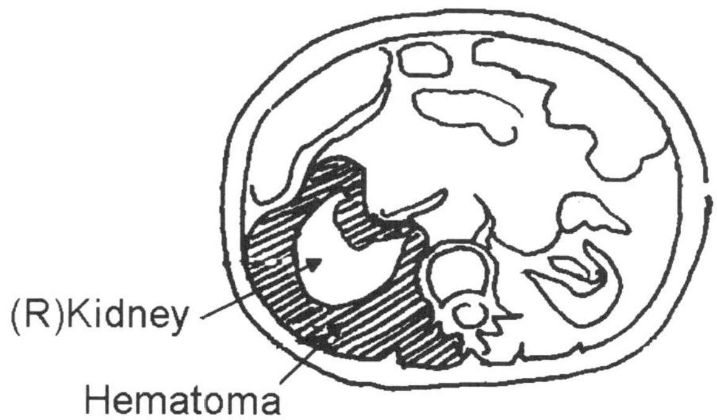

D-249: (R) kidney laceration and hematoma (CT scan)

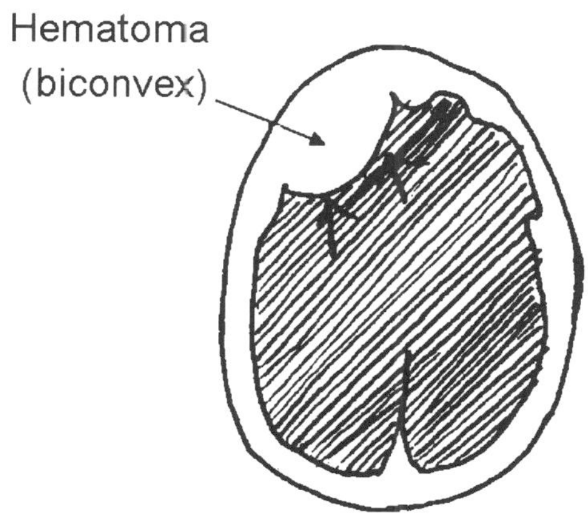

D-250: Epidural hematoma (CT scan)

Picture 78

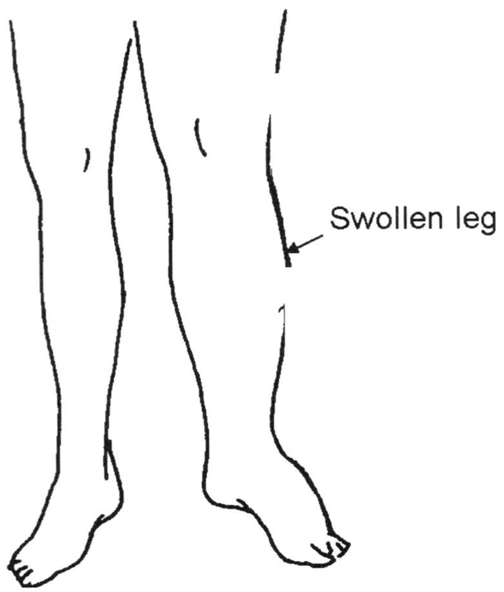

D-251: Deep vein thrombosis

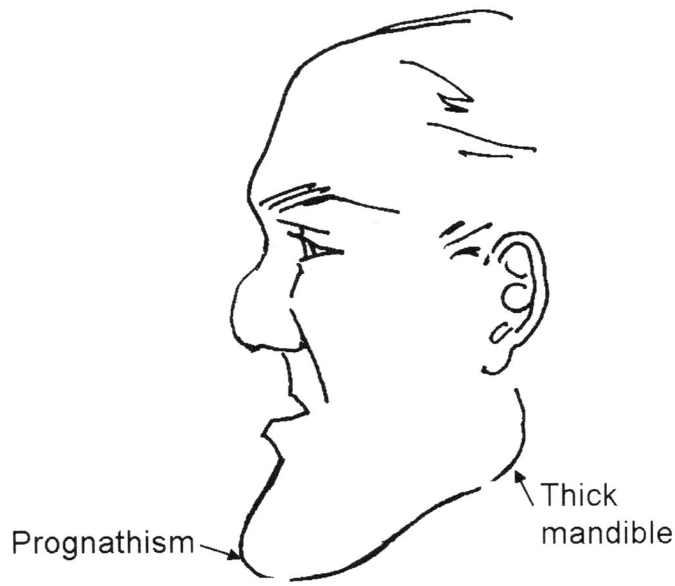

D-252: Acromegaly

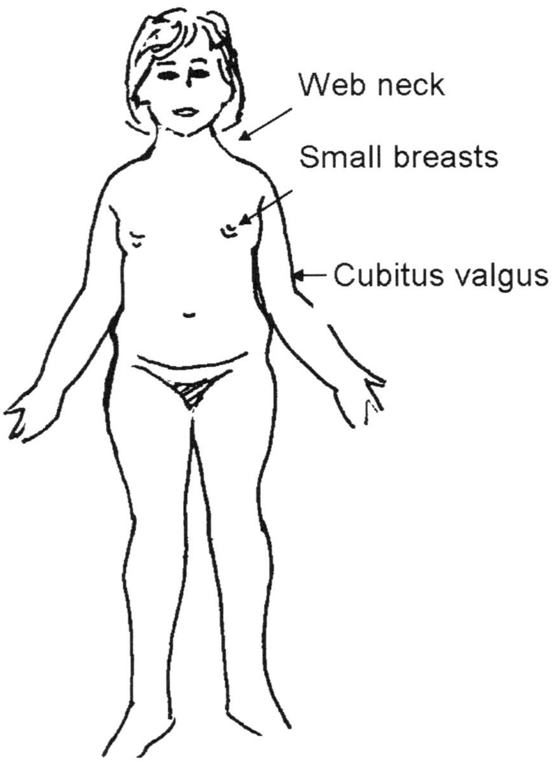

D-253: Turner's syndrome

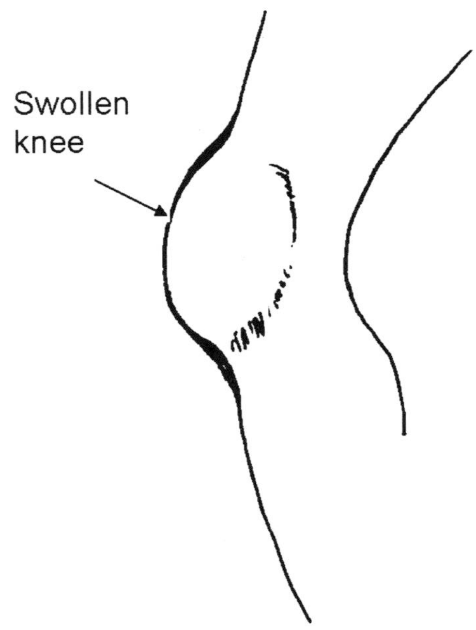

D-254: Acute bleeding in to the knee joint

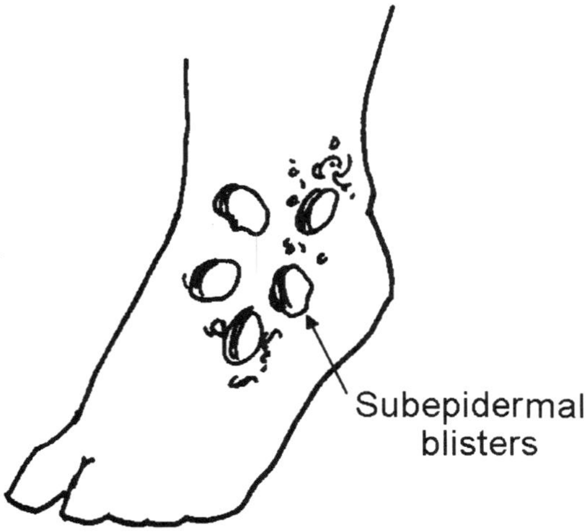

D-255: Bullous pemphigoid

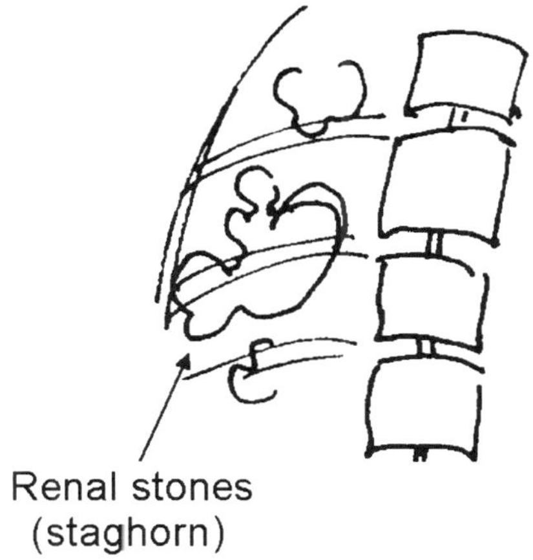

D-256: Renal stones (X-ray lateral view)

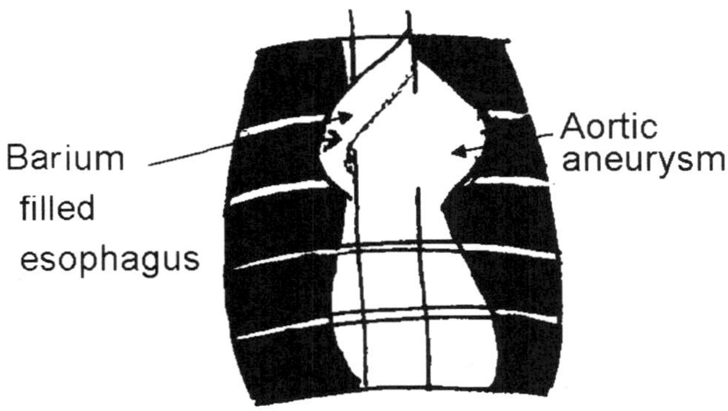

D-257: Aortic arch aneurysm (Barium filled esophagus then x-ray)

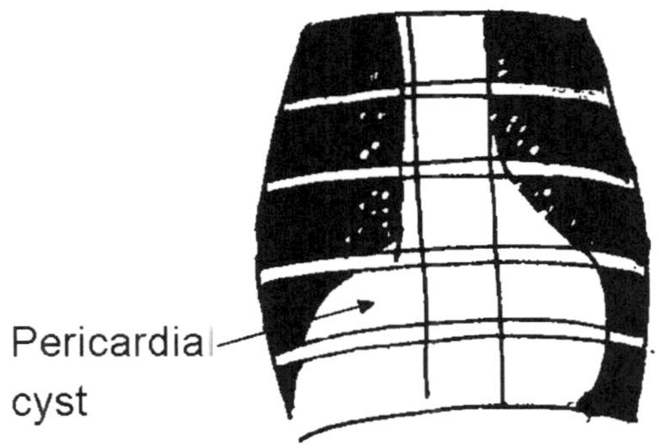

D-258: Pericardial cyst (X-ray)

Picture 80

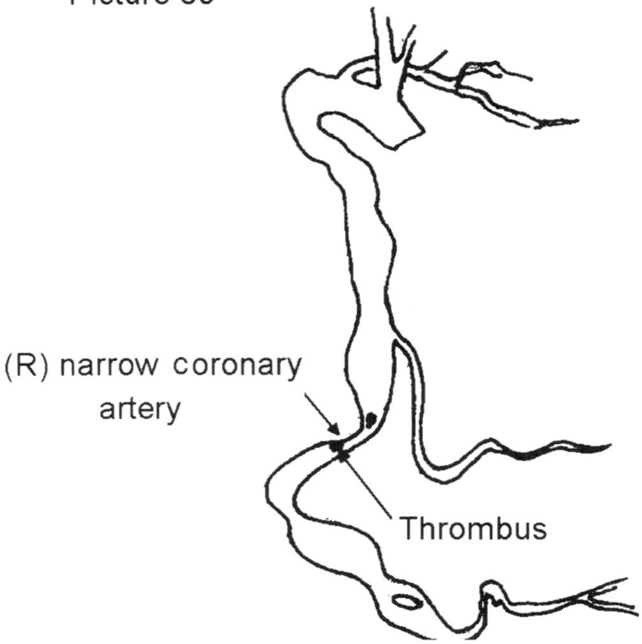

D-259: Atherosclerotic (R) coronary artery (Angiogram)

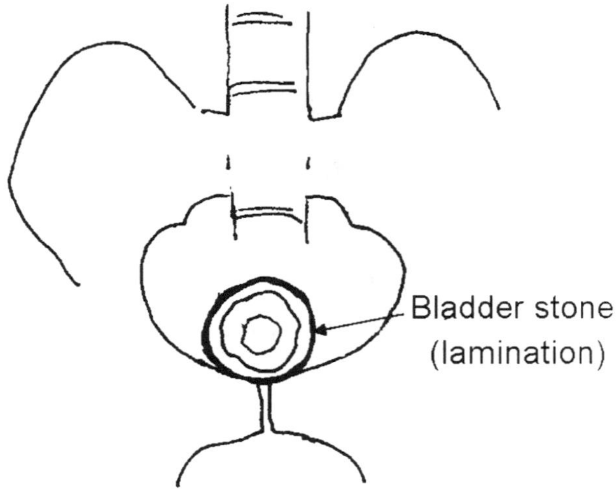

D-260: Bladder calculus (X-ray)

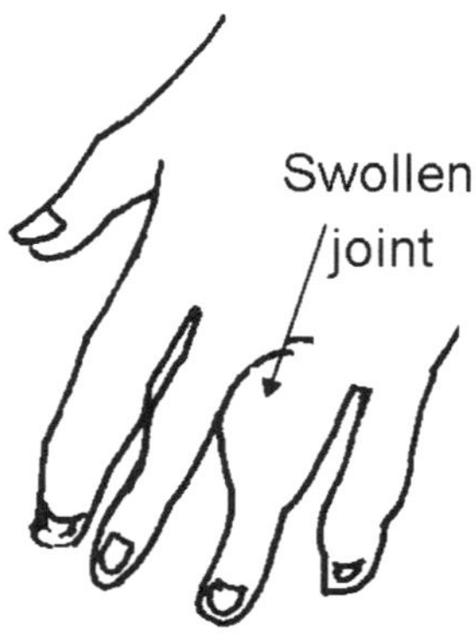

D-262: Psoriatic arthritis

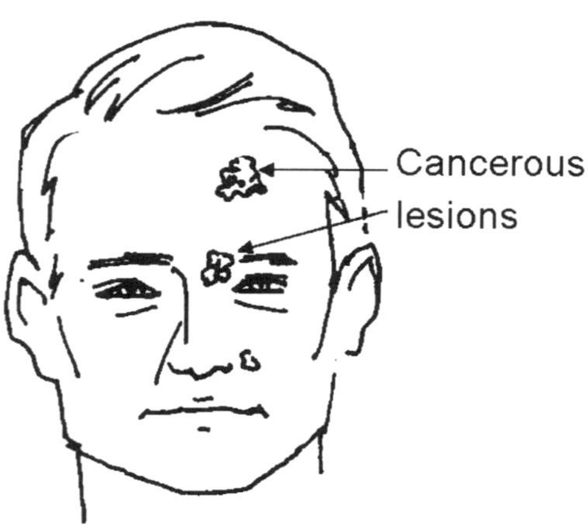

D-261: Multiple basal cell carcinoma

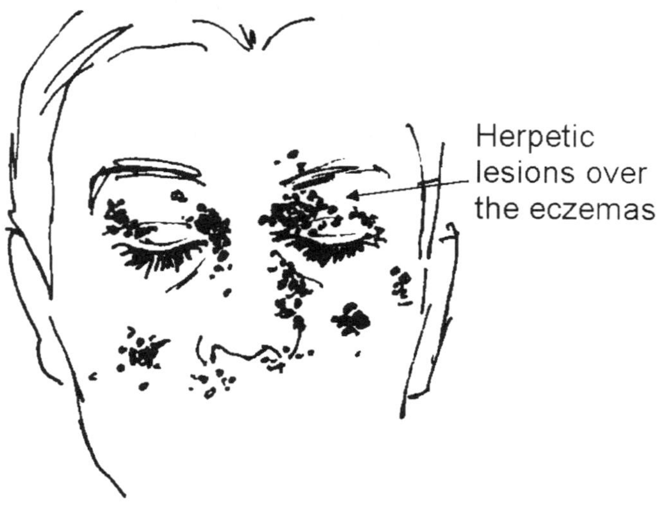

D-263: Eczema herpeticum

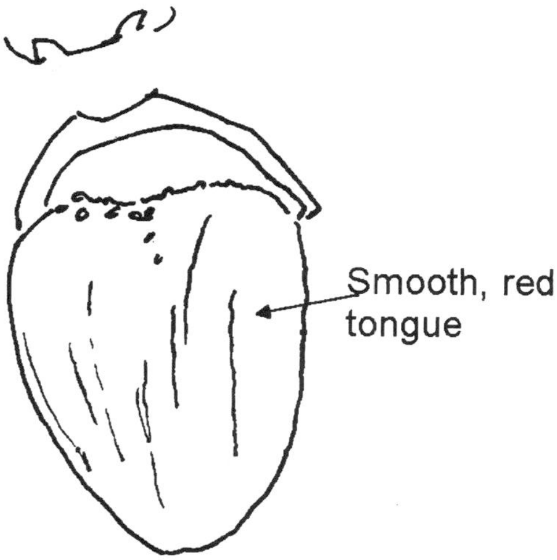

D-264: Vitamin B_{12} deficiency

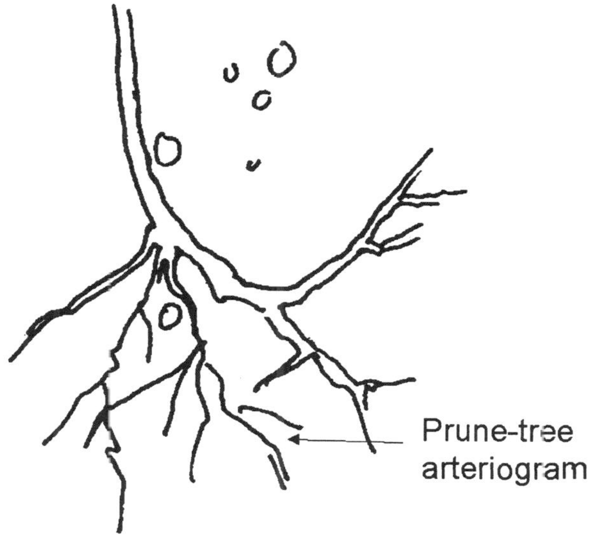

D-265: Pulmonary artery hypertension (Angiogram)

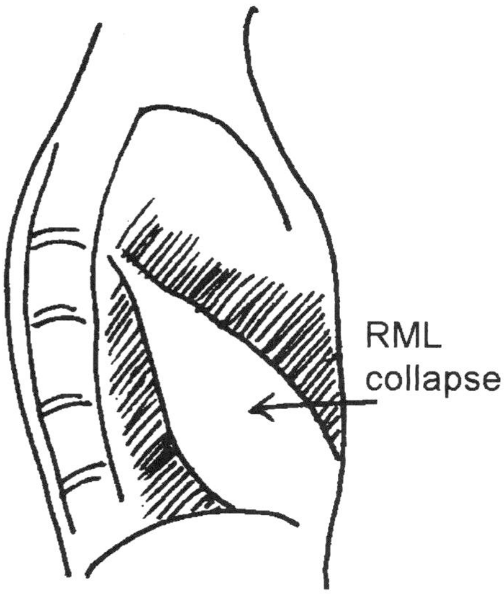

D-266: Right middle lobe (RML) collapse (lateral X-ray)

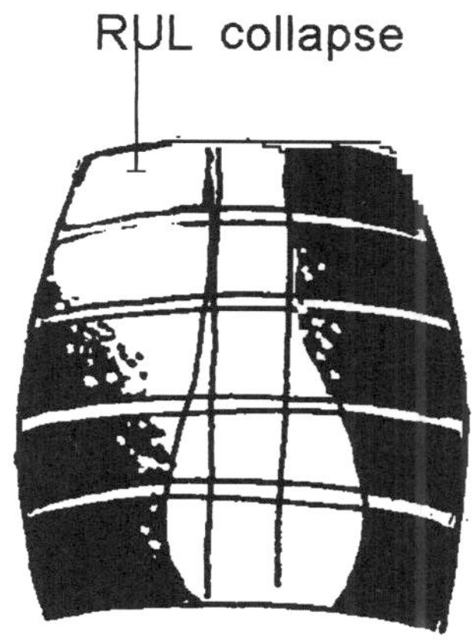

D-268: Right upper lobe (RUL) collapse (X-ray)

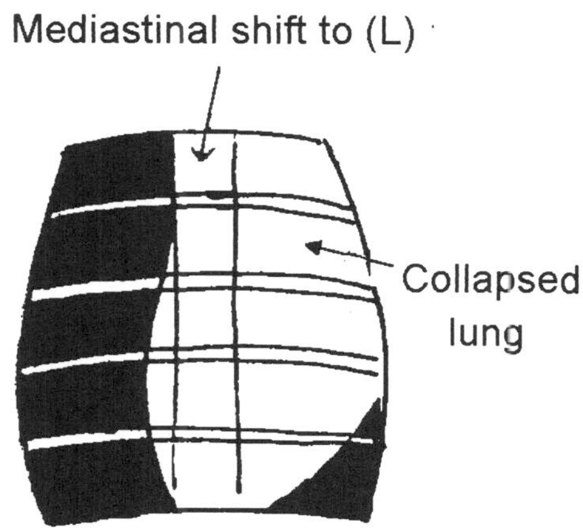

D-267: Severe collapse of left lung (X-ray)

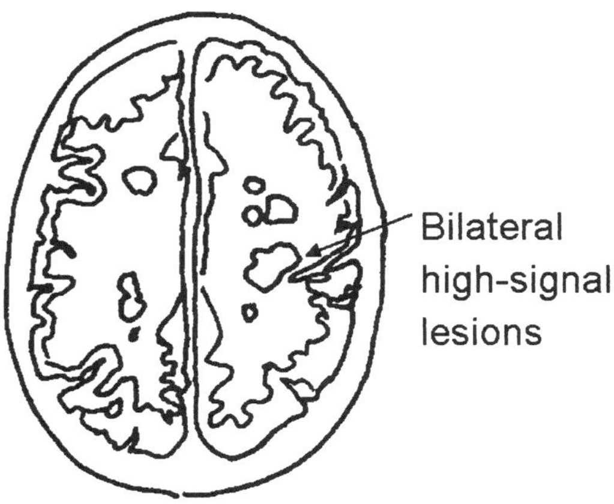

D-269: Multiple sclerosis (MRI)

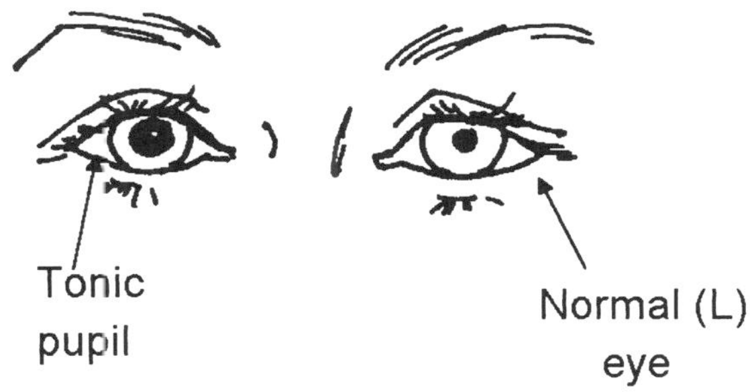

D-270: Holmes-Adie pupil

Picture 82

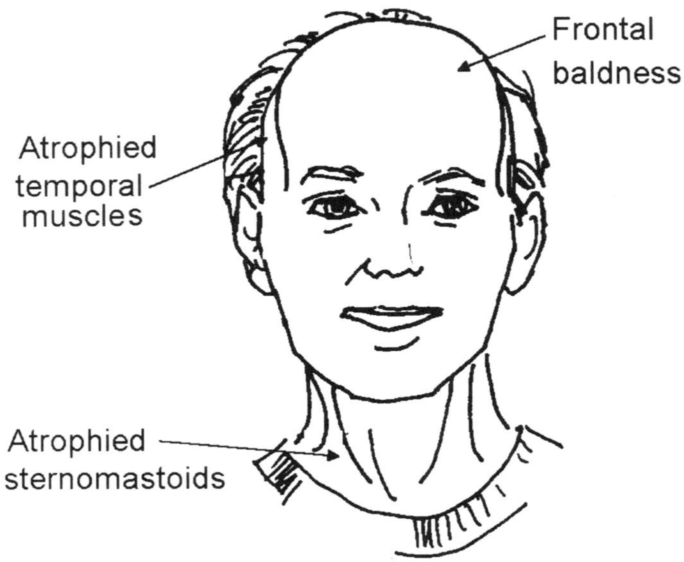

D-271: Myotonic dystrophy

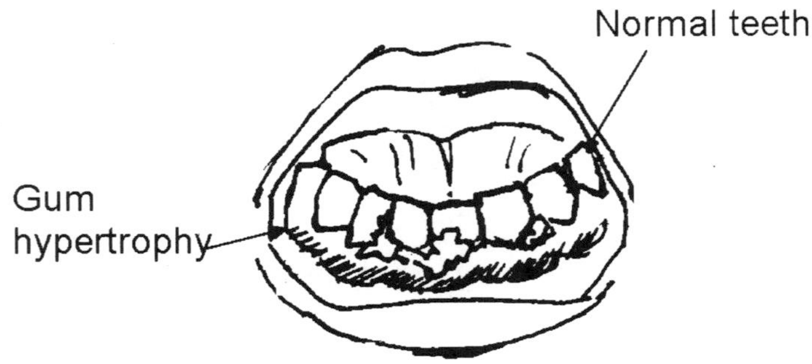

D-272: Gum hypertrophy (use of phenytoin)

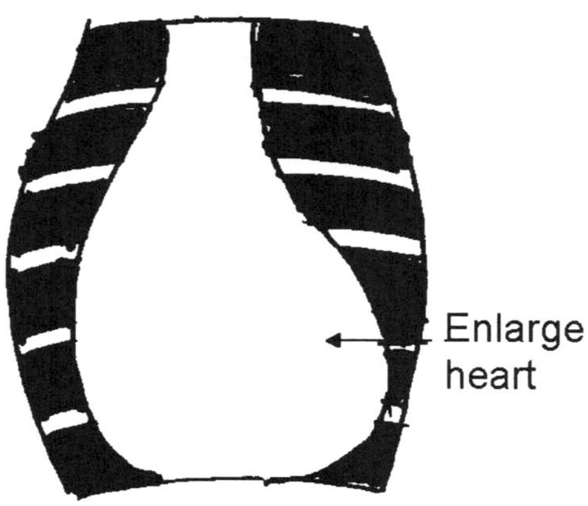

D-273: Pericardiac effusion (X-ray)

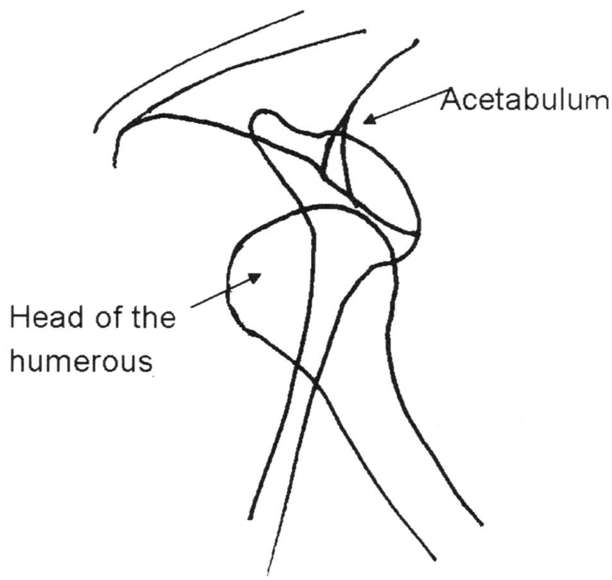

D-274: Shoulder dislocation (anterior)
(x-ray)

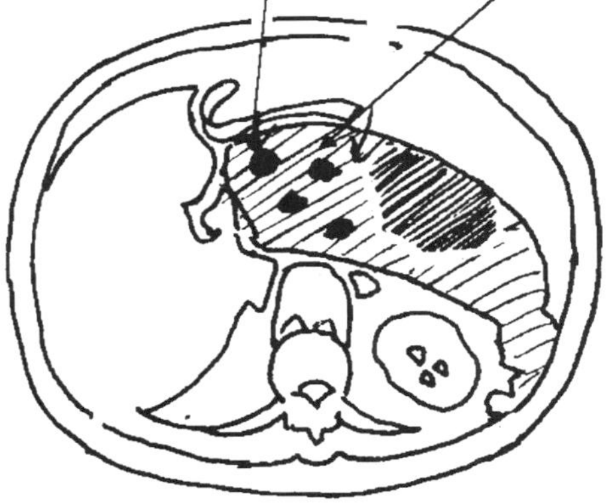

D-275: Acute pancreatitis (CT scan)

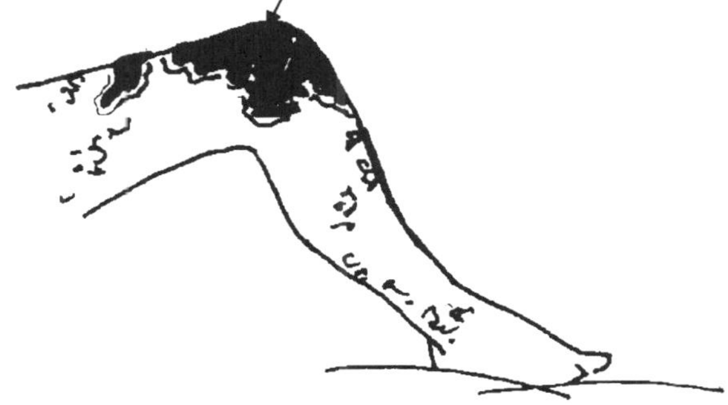

D-276: Cryoglobulinemia

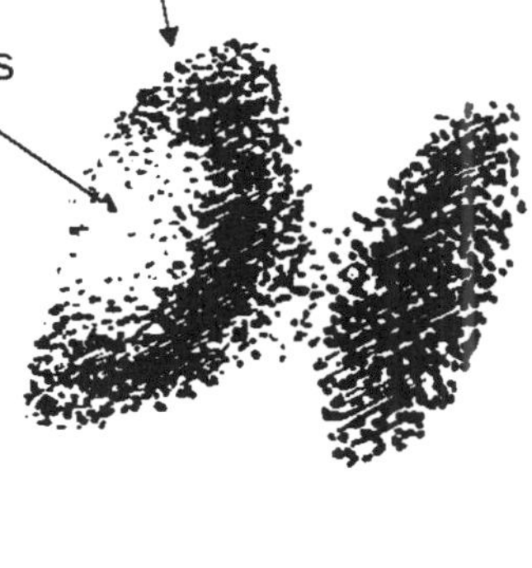

D-277: Cold nodule in (R) of the thyroid (Thyroid scan)

Picture 84

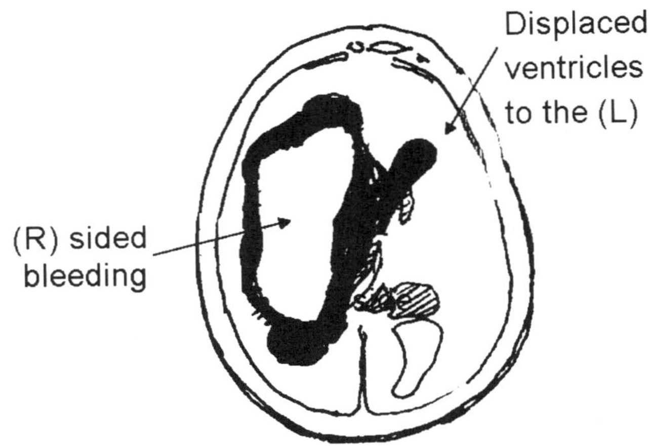

D-278: Large intracerebral bleed (R) side
(CT scan)

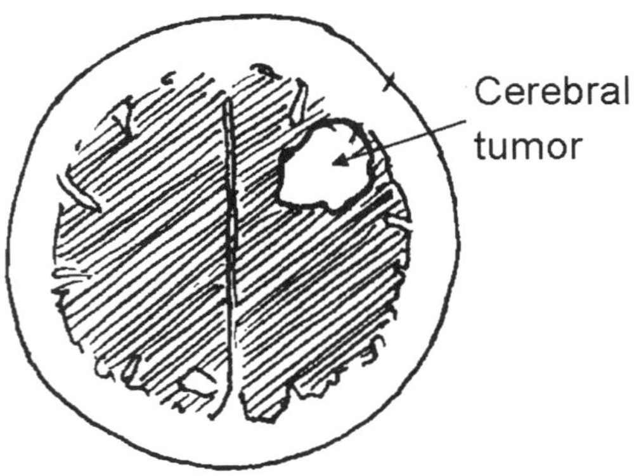

D-279: Cerebral tumor (L) side (CT-scan)

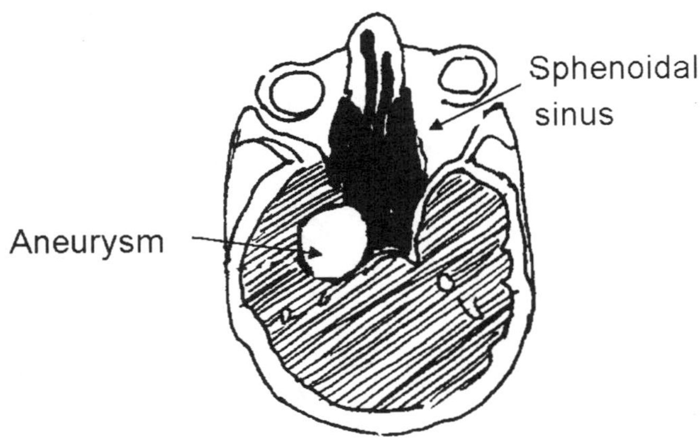

D-280: Cerebral aneurysm (CT scan)

Picture 85

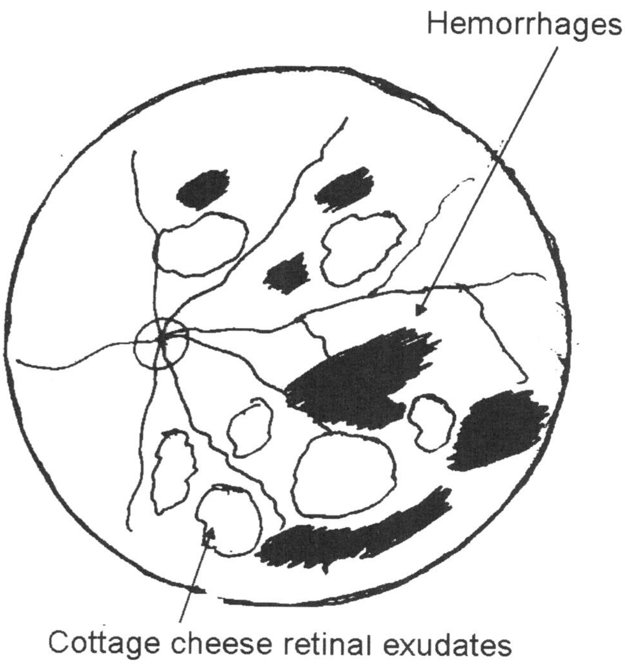

D-281: CMV retinitis in AIDS patient

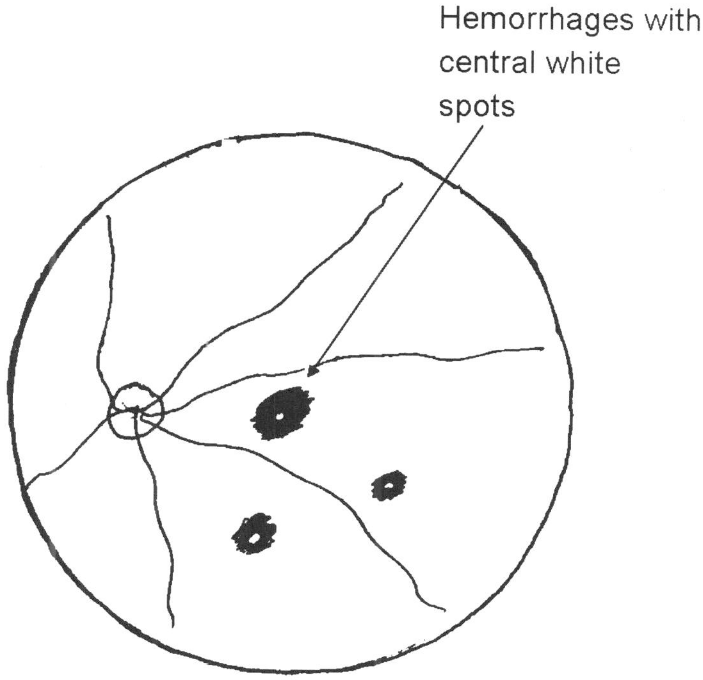

D-282: Roth's spots in subacute bacterial endocarditis

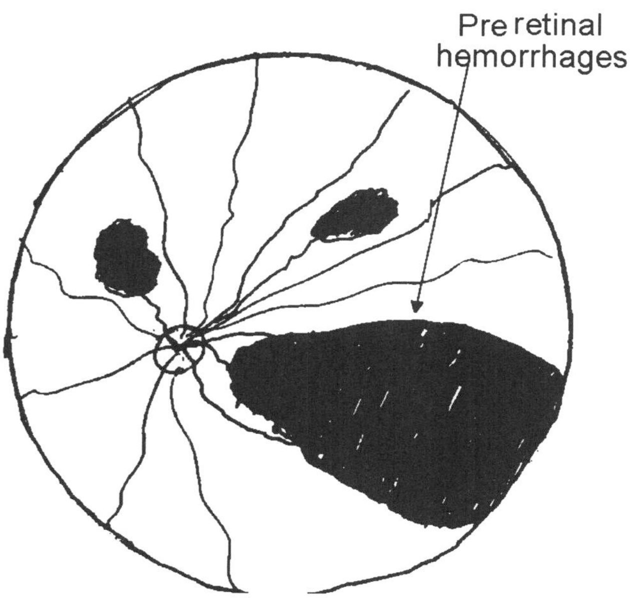

D-283: Preretinal hemorrhages (Postintubation)

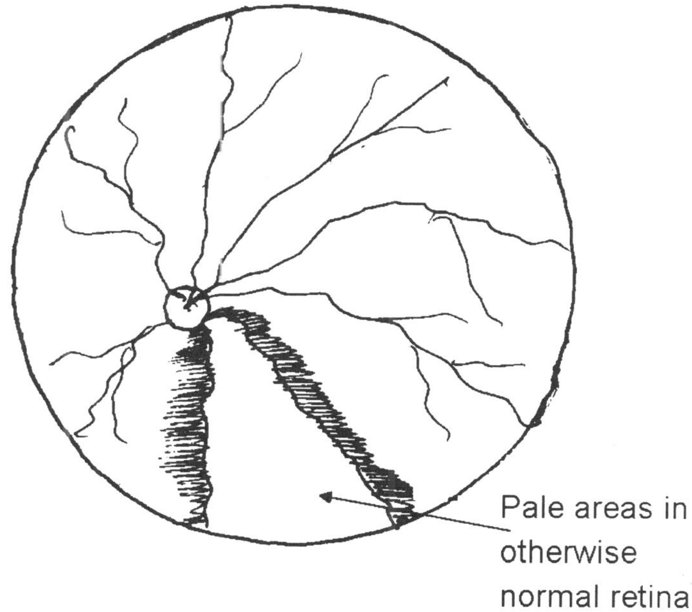

D-284: Occlusion of a branch of retinal artery due to emboli

Picture 86

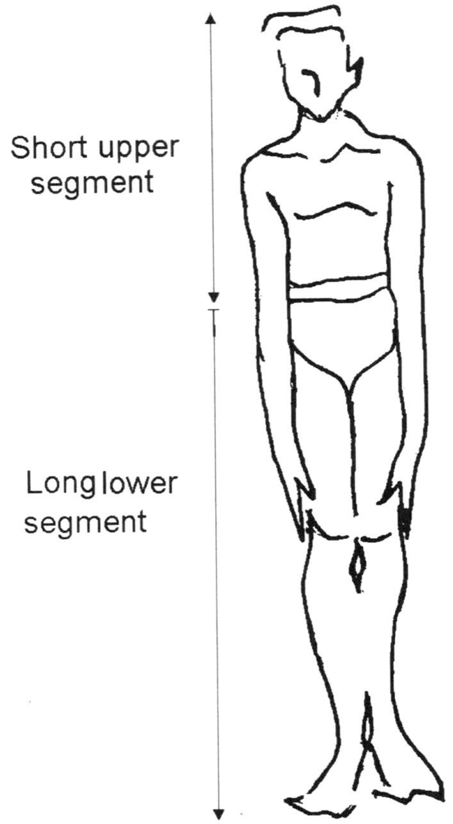

D-285: Marfan syndrome

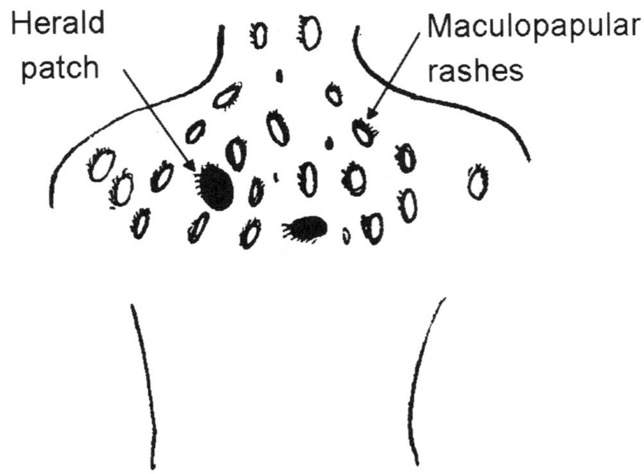

D-286: Pityriasis rosea (Christmas tree pattern)

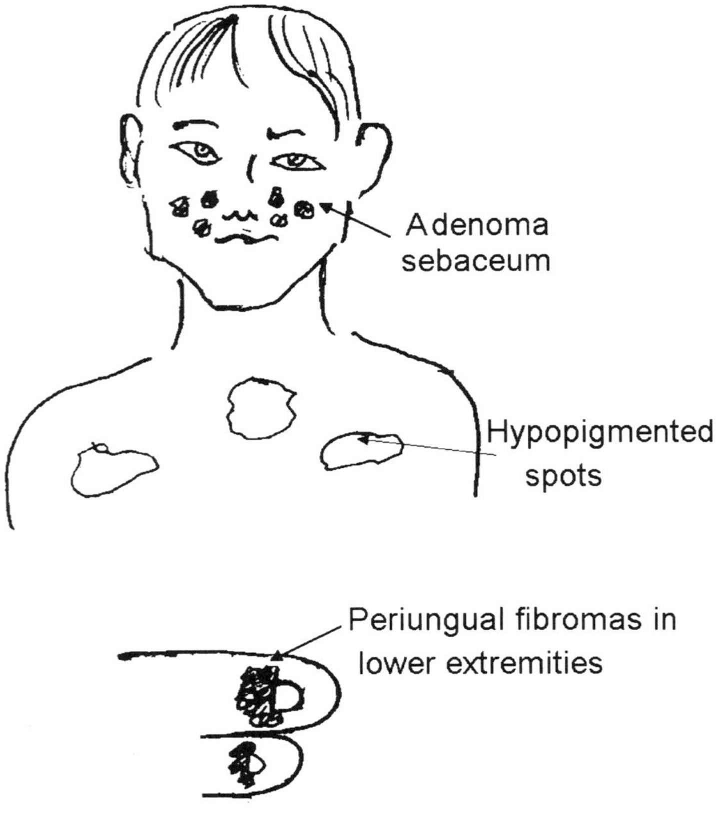

D-287: Tuberous sclerosis

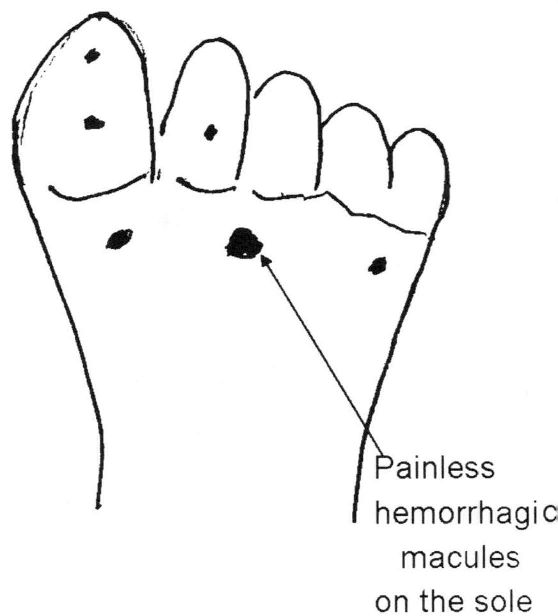

D-288: Janeway lesions

Picture 87

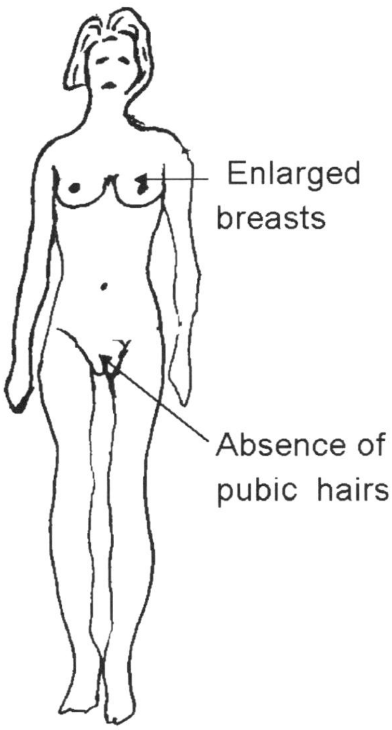

D-289: Male pseudohermaphroditism (Complete androgen insensitivity)

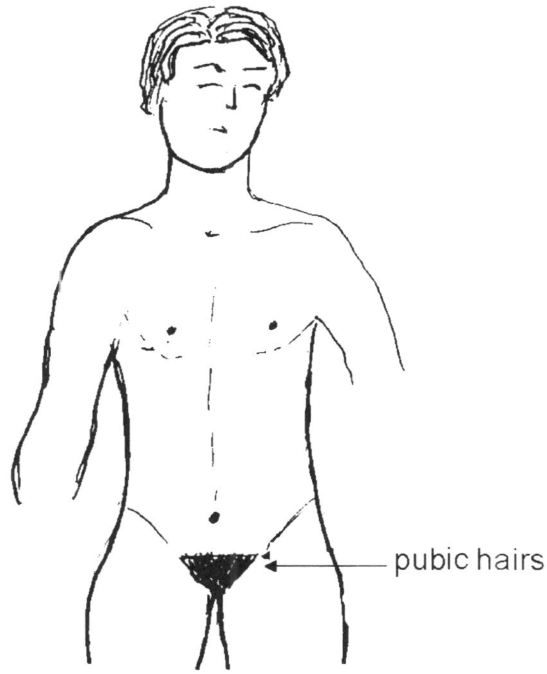

D-290: Male pseudohermaphroditism (5 alpha reductase deficiency)

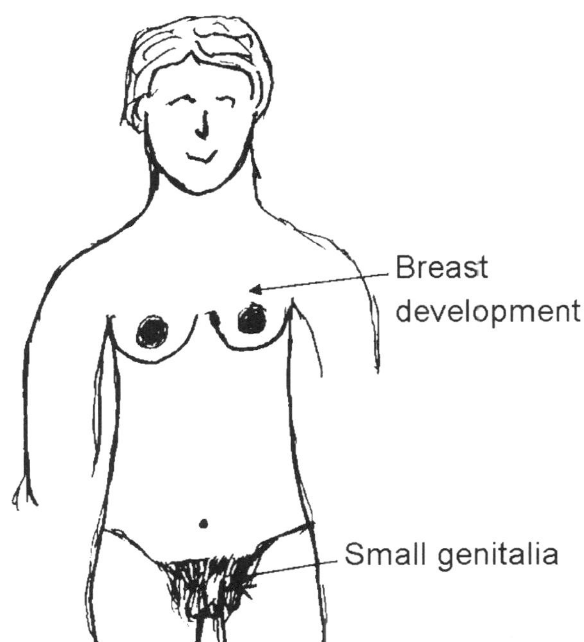

D-291: Klinefelter syndrome (47, XXY)

DIAGRAMS

1. Flow-volume curve in different diseases of the respiratory tract:
   (A) **Normal: (Normal inspiration and expiration phases)**

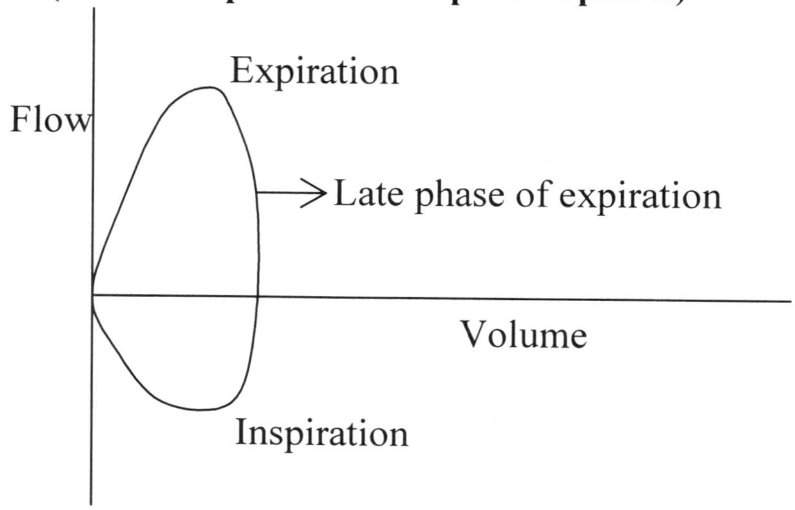

   (B) **Obstructive: (Prolonged expiration phase)**
   (e.g., Asthma, emphysema, bronchiolitis, Chronic bronchitis, bronchiectasis, cystic fibrosis)

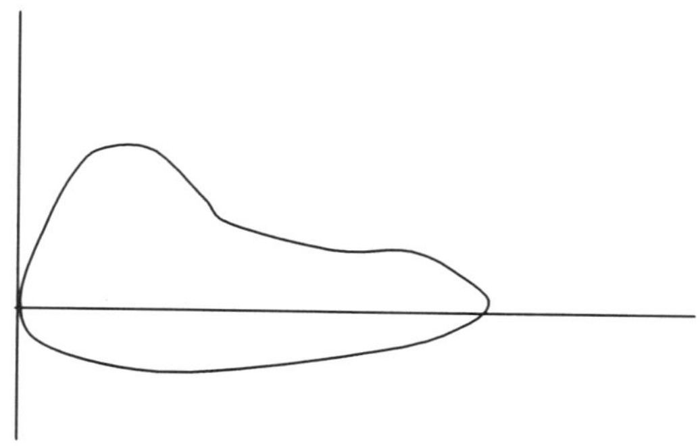

   (C) **Restrictive lung diseases: (Two types)**
   (i) **Parenchymal (Reduced both inspiration and expiration phases):**
   (a) Idiopathic pulmonary fibrosis
   (b) Sarcoidosis
   (c) Drug or radiation induced lung injury
   (d) Pneumoconiosis
   (ii) **Extraparenchymal (Reduced mostly inspiration or both inspiration and expiration)**
   (a) **Chest wall:**
   - Obesity
   - Kyphoscoliosis
   - Ankylosing spondylitis

(b) **Neuromuscular:**
- Myasthenia gravis
- Muscular dystrophies
- Cervical spine injury
- Guillain- Barre syndrome
- Diaphragmatic paralysis or weakness

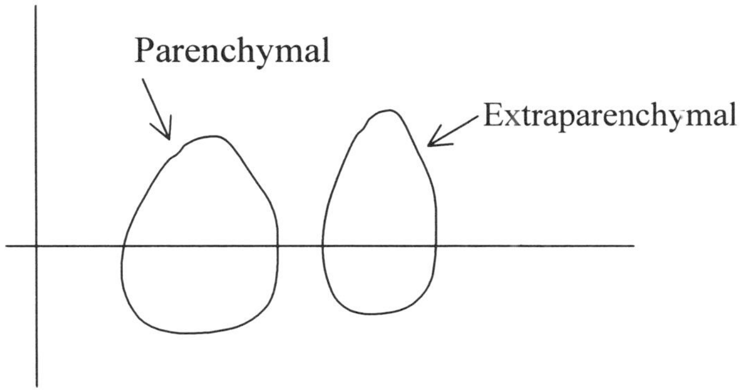

(D) **Variable extrathoracic obstruction (it gets worse during inspiration than expiration):**

(i) **Pharyngeal obstruction are due to the following:**Trauma, foreign body, deep neck or pharyngeal abscess, enlarged tonsils, sleep apnea.

(ii) **Laryngeal obstruction are due to the following:**External trauma, foreign body, angioneurotic edema, vocal cord paralysis, tumor.

(iii) **Tracheal obstruction are due to the following:**Tumor, trauma, enlarged thyroid gland.

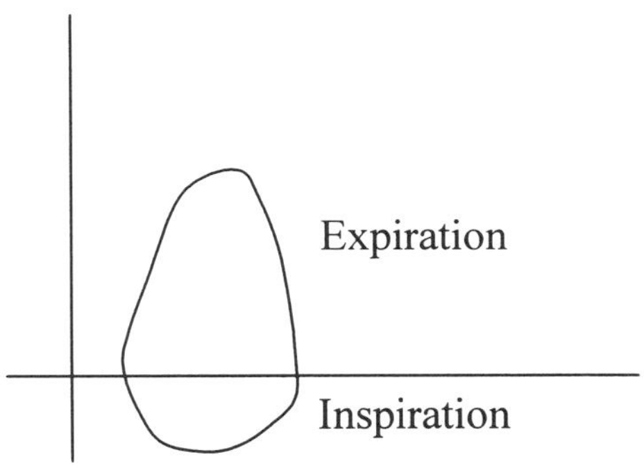

(E) **Variable intrathoracic obstruction (it gets worse during expiration than inspiration):**

(i) **Tracheal obstruction are due to the following:Tumor, trauma, enlarged lymph nodes, aortic aneurysm, mediastinal fibrosis.**

Diagram **90**

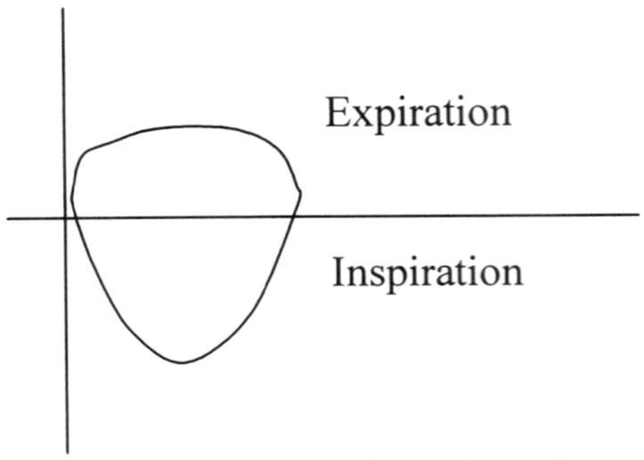

(F) **Fixed upper airway obstruction (it gets worse during both inspiration and expiration):**

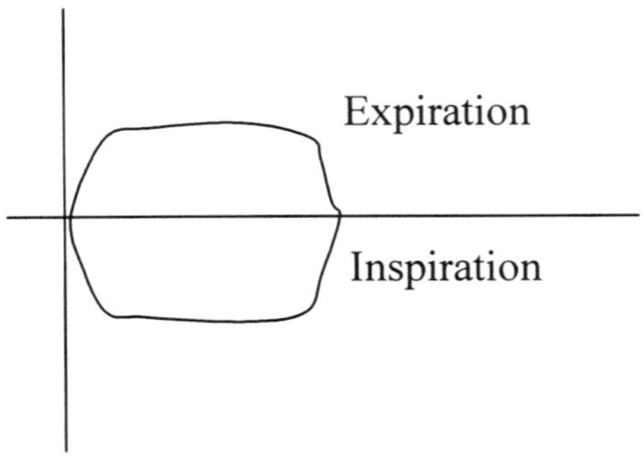

2. **Dissociation curves for Carbon monoxide (CO) and oxygen (O_2):**

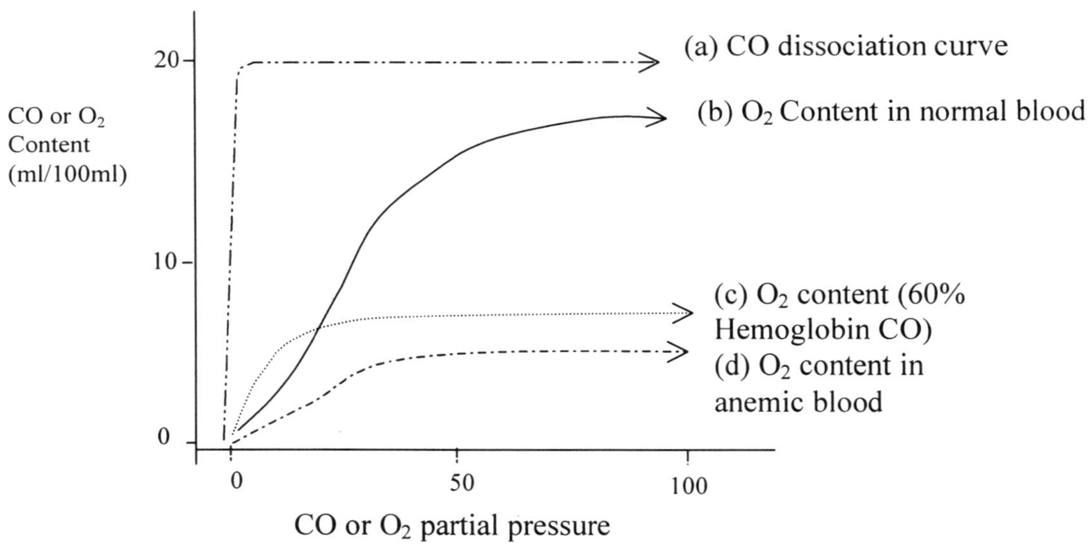

(a) At low partial pressure hemoglobin (Hb) is completely saturated with CO. **This is extreme shift to the left**. In carbon monoxide poisoning Hb binds with CO very strongly, enough Hb will not be available to carry O_2 and also the release of O_2 to the tissues. Patients will have normal Po_2 and Hb but severely reduced O_2 content.

Treatment:

(i) **Hyperbaric oxygen**: It increases the inspired Po_2 to 2000 mm Hg, all the oxygen will be carried by the blood in dissolved form.

(ii) **Combination of 95% O_2 and 5% CO_2 to breathe:** Addition of 5% CO_2 will increase the rapid washout of CO from the blood.

(b) **O_2 content in normal blood:** Normal release of O_2 to the tissues.

(c) **CO dissociation curve for 60% Hb CO:** It is more shift to the left than oxygen dissociation curve in anemic blood (curve d).

(d) **O_2 dissociation curve in anemic blood:** It is shift to the right to release oxygen to the tissue.

3. Alveolar sizes and collapses: (P=2T/R)

P= Pressure
T= Surface tension
R= Radius of the alveoli

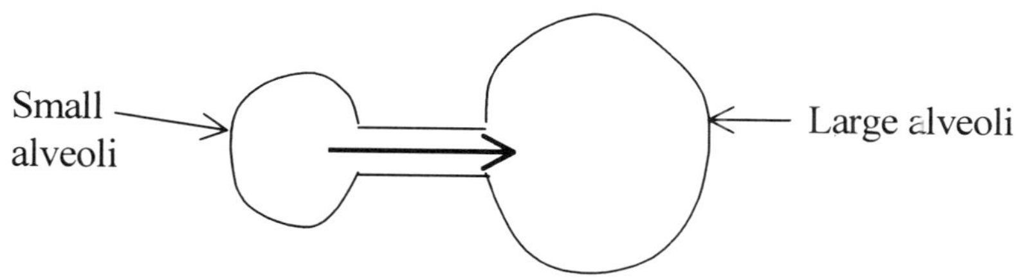

Remember, small alveoli collapses to the larger alveoli

4. **Work done on the lung demonstrated in pressure-volume curve:**

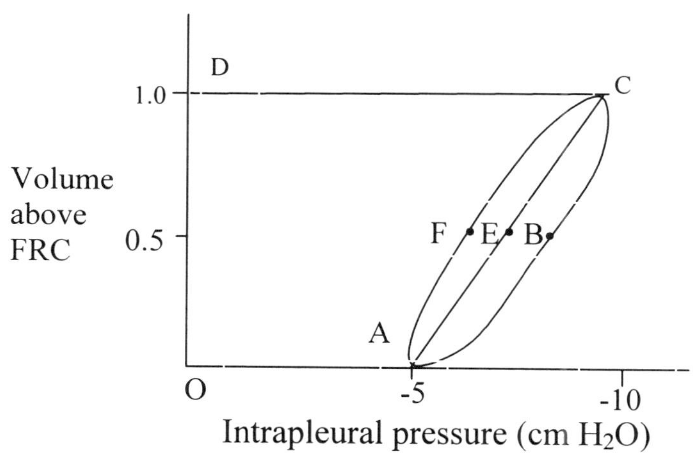

Diagram **92**

(i) ABC: Inspiration
(ii) CFA: Expiration
(iii) OABCD: Total work of breathing by the lungs
(iv) OAECD: Work required to overcome the **elastic forces**
(v) ABCEA: Work required to **overcome viscous (airways and tissues) resistance**

5. **Glucose filtration, reabsorption and excretion curve:**
   (a) Maximum tubular reabsorption (TmG)= 2 mmol/minute
   (b) Maximum rate of excretion when plasma level is 16 mmol/(PG)

ABC:	Glucose filtration
AB:	Glucose reabsorption and filtration
BC:	No reabsorption, only filtration
BEG:	No reabsorption
B:	Maximum reabsorption point
AD:	No glucose excretion, all reabsorption
DEF:	All glucose excretion

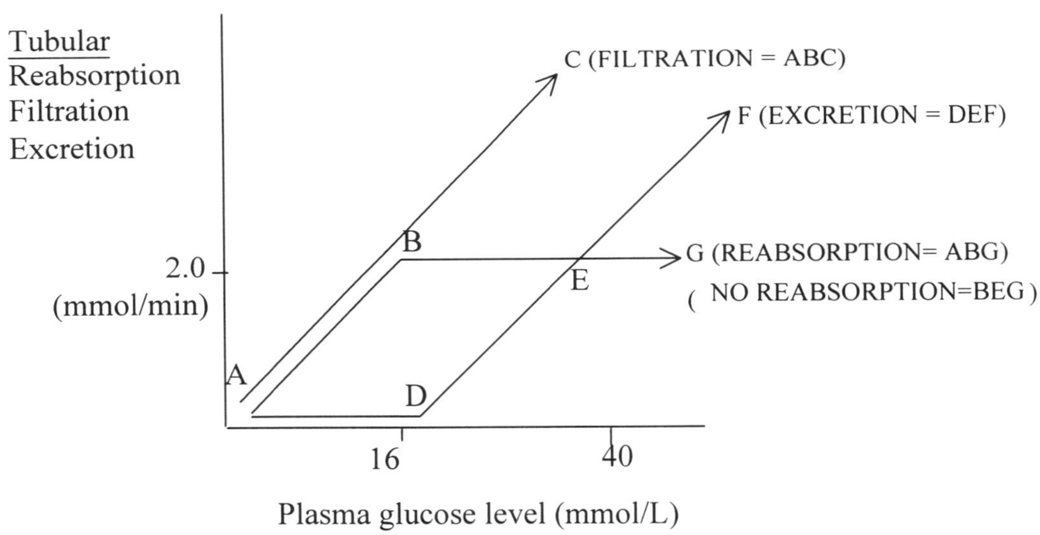

6. **Different types of resistance to hormone action:**

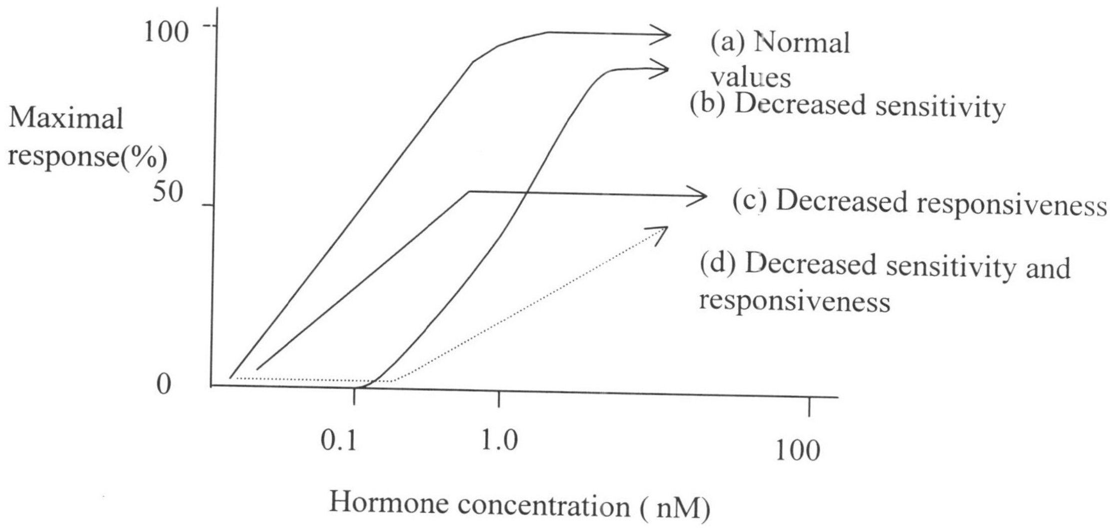

7. **Tympanometry and different disease conditions:**

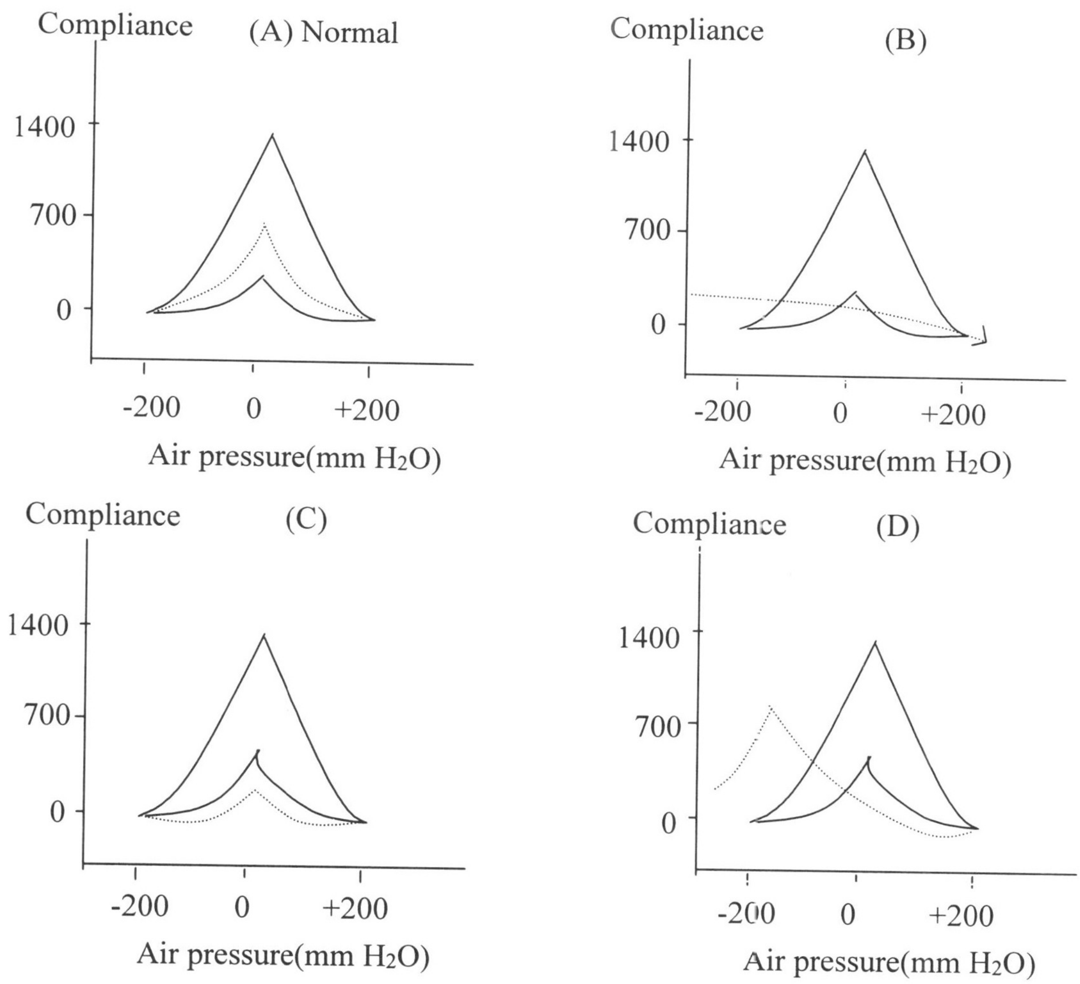

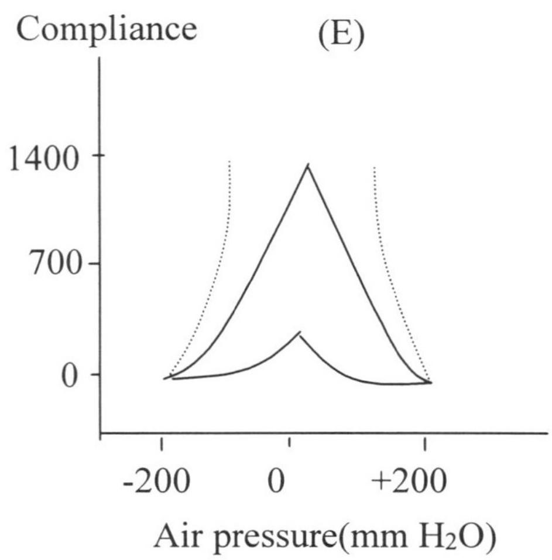

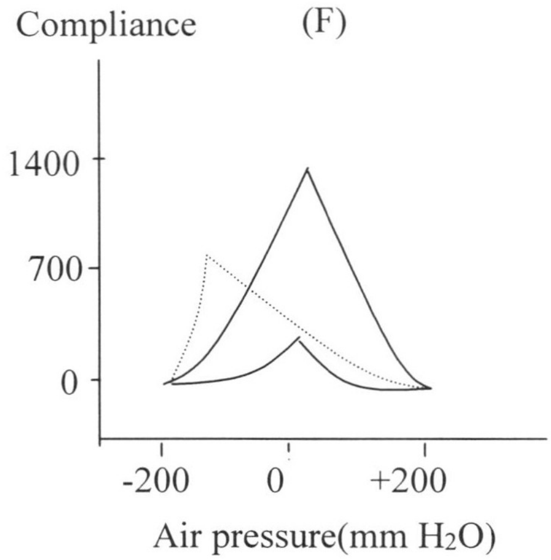

(A) Normal: See dotted line following the normal curve. Normal curve is found in normal individual, acoustic neuroma, presbycusis, excessive exposure to loud noice, and Meniere's disease.

(B) Otitis media (acute, chronic; serous, adhesive), perforated ear drum, creumen occluding patent ventilating tube in ear drum, fluid in middle ear or effusion.

(C) Otosclerosis, thickened ear drum, scar ear drum, tympanosclerosis.

(D) Poor eustachian tube function, URI (upper respiratory tract infection)

(E) Discontinuation of ossicular chain (trauma), flaccid ear drum.

(F) Near normal.

8. **Audiometry in different disease conditions:**

(A) Normal (AC>BC)

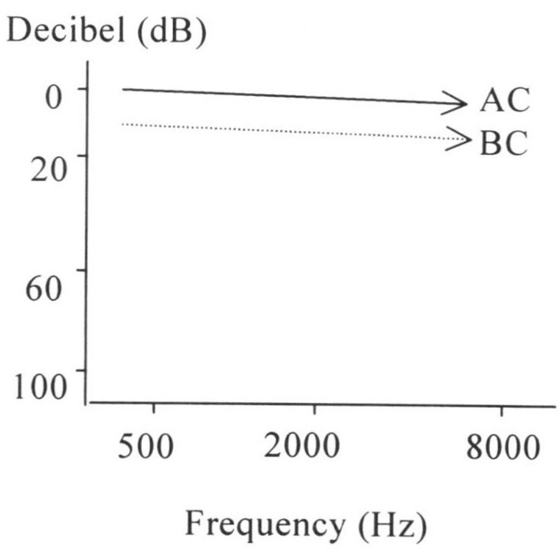

(B) Conductive loss

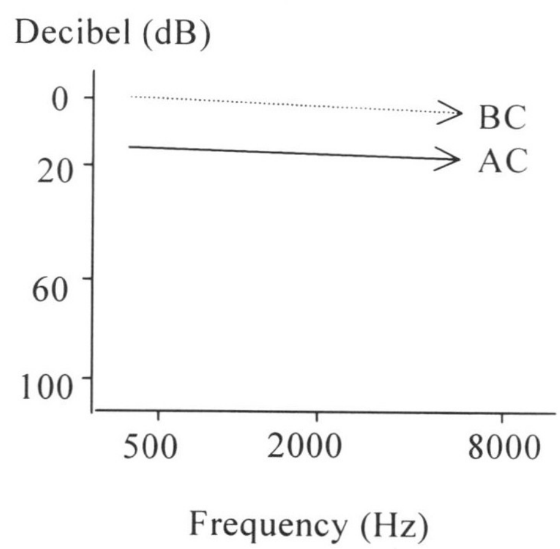

(C) Sensorineural loss

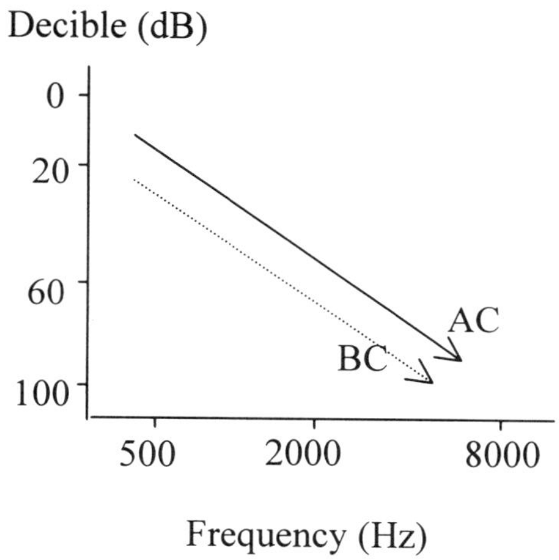

(D) Mixed loss

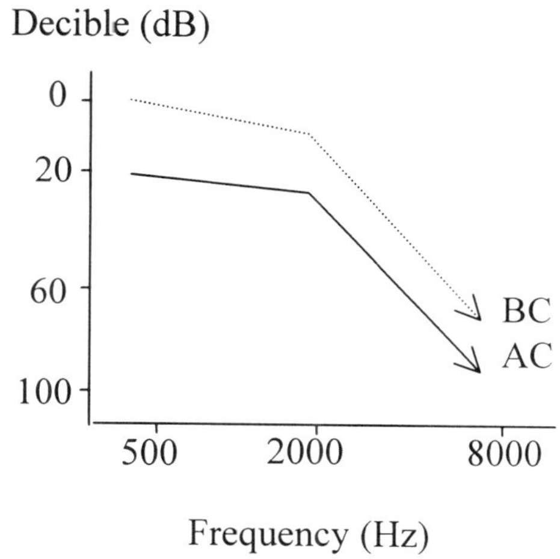

(A) **Normal:** No hearing loss, hearing close to 'zero' decibel, AC (air conduction) > BC (bone conduction)
(B) **Conductive hearing loss:** Mild hearing loss, BC at least 15 decibels better than AC, usually less than 20 decibels. It is found in otitis media, cerumen occluding ear canal, perforated ear drum, fluid in middle ear or effusion, patent ventilating tube in ear drum.
(C) **Sensorineural hearing loss:** Severe hearing loss, precipitous drop of both AC and BC, usually more than 60 decibels. It is found in otosclerosis, acoustic neuroma, presbycusis, excessive exposure to loud noise, and Meniere's disease.
(D) **Mixed (conductive plus sensorineural) hearing loss:** This graph in low frequency appears as a conductive loss but with a high frequency, sensorineural type.

9. Brain stem auditory evoked potential (BAEP) and different diseases:
   (A) **Normal:** Different waves represent different anatomical location:
   Wave I = Auditory nerve
   Wave II = Cochlear nucleus
   Wave III = Superior olivary complex (lower pons)
   Wave IV = Lateral lemniscus
   Wave V = Inferior colliculus
   Wave VI = Thalamus
   Wave VII= Thalamic radiations

Diagram **96**

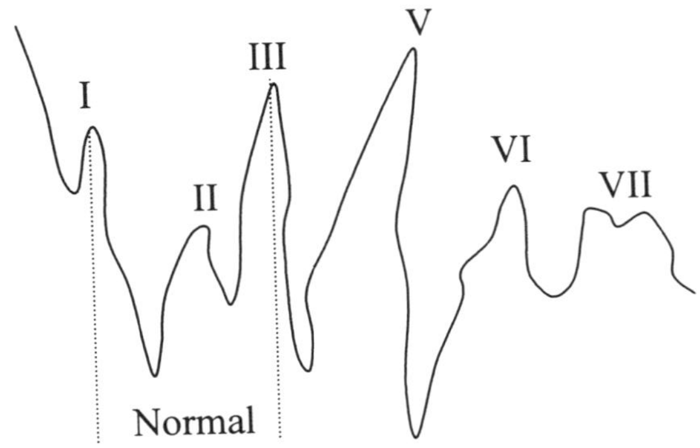

It is the electrical response generated within the auditory pathways from the VIII th cranial nerve to diencephalon. Seven different waves are produced form outside (VIII cranial nerve) to inside (thalamic radiations). **Normal conduction** means high altitude and short interwaves distance. **Abnormal conduction** means low altitude and prolong interwaves distance.

It can differentiate middle ear, cochlear and retrocochlear disorders.

(i) **Middle ear disorder:** Delayed responses but good morphology and normal interwave intervals.

(ii) **Cochlear disorders**: Well formed responses at normal absolute latencies and interwave intervals.

(iii) **Retrocochlear disorders:** Poor morphology and prolonged interwave intervals.

(iv) **VIII cranial nerve or lower auditory brain stem disorder:** Prolongation occurs between wave I and III.

(v) **Upper brain stem disorder:** Prolongation occurs between wave III and V.

(B) **Patients with intracanalicular acoustic neuroma right ear:** Normal BAEP study in left ear but in right ear, prolongation occurs in interpeak latency between wave I and III and it indicates delayed conduction between distal eighth cranial nerve and lower pons. It is also found in other cerebellopontine angle tumors.

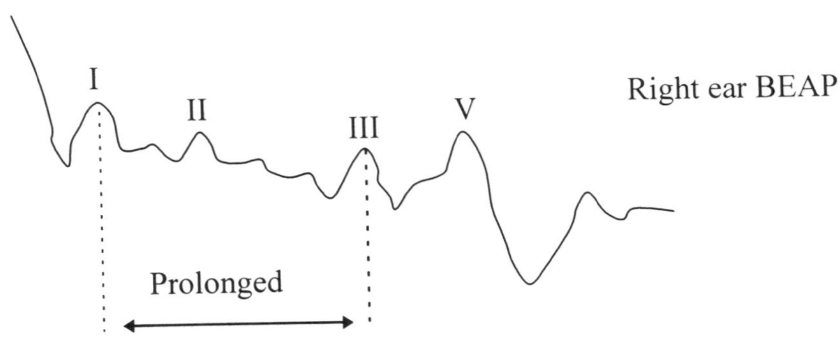

(C) **Patients with brain stem hemorrhage except the lower third of the pons:** Wave I,II, and III are normal but IV and V are lost.

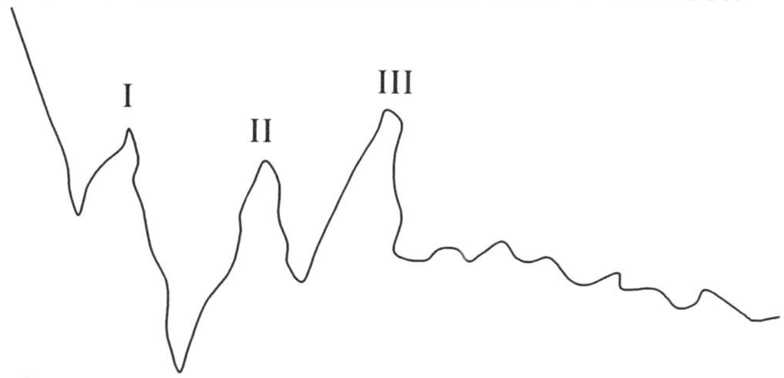

BAEP is also abnormal in brain stem gliomas.

(D) BAEP is not altered with high barbiturate levels (or other medications) or metabolic disorders.

(E) Normal BAEP in brain stem lesions when it does not involve the auditory pathways: Ventral pontine infarcts producing the **locked-in syndrome or lateral medullary infarcts.**

10. **Patients with different hearing problems**.

(A) **Meniere's disease**: A 60 year old man with Meniere's disease in left ear.

(i) Tympanometry: Normal in both ears.
(ii) Audiometry: Sensorineural hearing loss in (L) ear
(iii) Acoustic reflexes: Normal in both ears.
(iv) BAEP study: No evidence of retrocochlear disorder in either ear.

(B) **Presbycusis**: A 80 year old man with bilateral hearing difficulties.

(i) Tympanometry: Normal in both ears.
(ii) Audiometry: Moderate to severe sensorineural hearing loss bilaterally.
(iii) Acoustic reflexes: Absent ipsilaterally, which may normally be present in elderly patients.

Treatment: Hearing aid may be helpful plus counseling for realistic expectations.

(C) **Acoustic neuromas**: A 45 year old man with left ear acoustic neuroma.

(i) Tympanometry: Normal in both ears
(ii) Audiometry: Sensorineural hearing loss in (L) ear only, right ear is normal.
(iii) **BAEP study**: Prolongation occurs in interpeak latency between wave I and III in left ear, and normal study in (R) ear. **This is characteristic finding.**
(iv) Acoustic reflexes: Absent in (L) ear

(D) Otosclerosis: A 35 years old man with otosclerosis in (R) ear

(i) Tympanometry: Abnormal in (R) ear, normal (L) ear.
(ii) Audiometry: Mixed loss in (R) ear, normal (L) ear.

(E) Exposure to loud noise: A 37 year old man works in the factory.
(i) Tympanometry: Normal in both ears
(ii) Audiometry: Sensorineural loss in both ears

(F) Otitis media: A 20 year old with (L) otitis media
(i) Tympanometry: Abnormal in (L) ear, normal (R) ear
(ii) Audiometry: Conductive hearing loss (L) ear, normal (R) ear.
(iii) Acoustic reflexes: Absent (L) ear, normal (R) ear.

11. **Flowmetry or urodynamic studies and diseases:**

(a) Normal

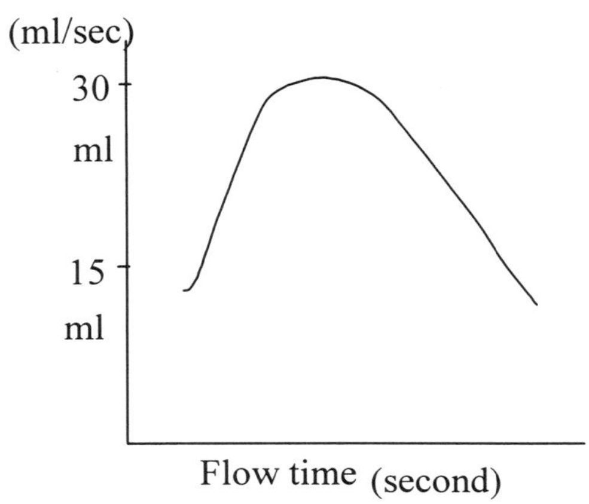

(b) Obstruction

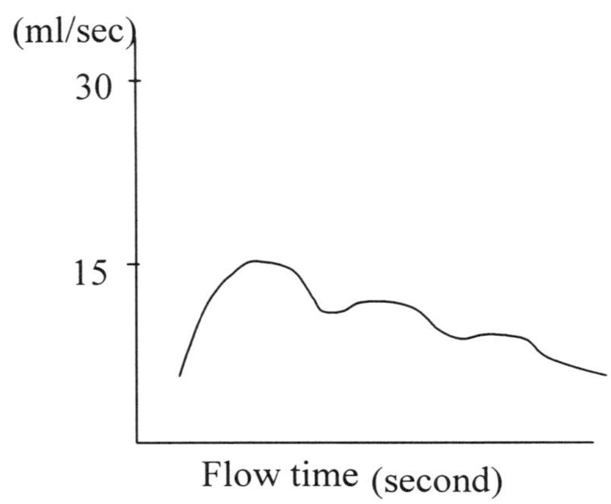

(c) Hypocontractile detressur

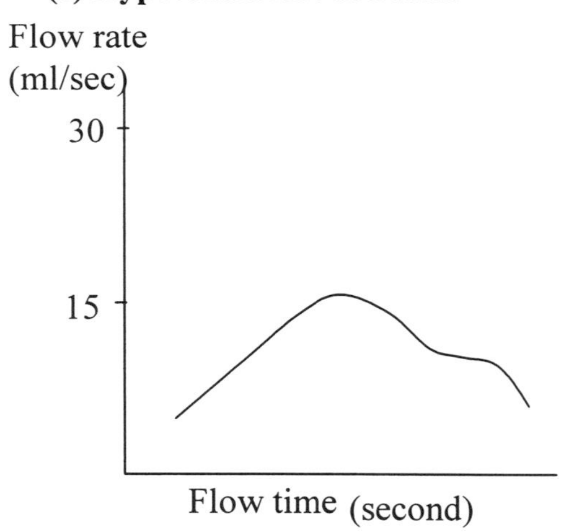

(d) Abdominal straining

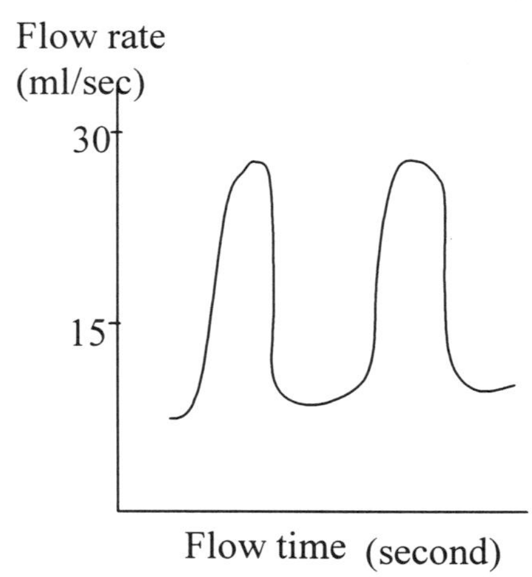

(e) Low amplitude fluctuating Detrusor contraction

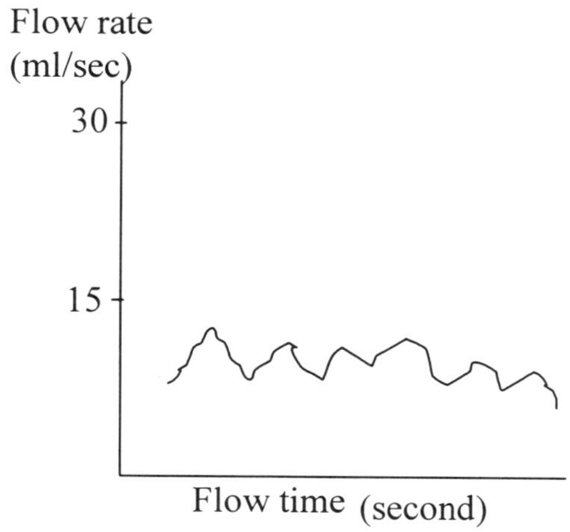

(f) Sphincter dyssynergia

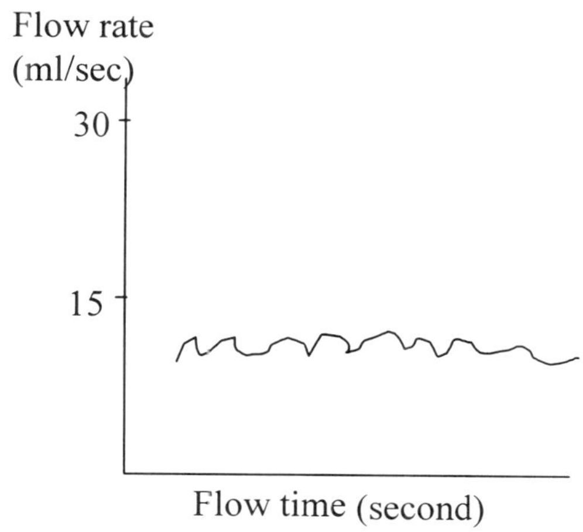

Normal urinary flow rate:

Male age 18-55 is 21 ml/sec.
Male age 56-80 is 9 ml/sec.
Female age 18-55 is 15 to 18 ml/sec.
Female age 56-80 is 10 ml/sec.

Normal detrusor pressure: It should be <15 cm H_2O.

Decreased bladder compliance: Pressure rises rapidly with filling.

(A) **Normal bell-shaped curve: Normal flow rate.**

(B) **Bladder outlet obstruction with normal detrusor function:** Maximum flow is achieved **soon after the onset** of voiding, peak and mean flow are decreased and prolonged flow rate.

(C) **Hypocontractile detrusor muscles:** Maximum flow is achieved **near the middle of the voiding**, peak and mean flow are decreased and prolonged flow time.

(D) **Intermittent flow due to abdominal straining:** Patients with **decreased outflow resistance** the peak flow rate may be normal or above normal.

(E) **Intermittent flow due** to low amplitude fluctuating detrusor contraction: This condition is **rare,** rule out suprasacral neurologic disease or idiopathic detrusor instability.

(F) **Intermittent flow due to sphincter dyssynergia**: It is **more common and faster** in changes of urine flow, than in low amplitude fluctuating detrusor contraction.

12. Cystograms in different disease conditions:

Diagram **100**

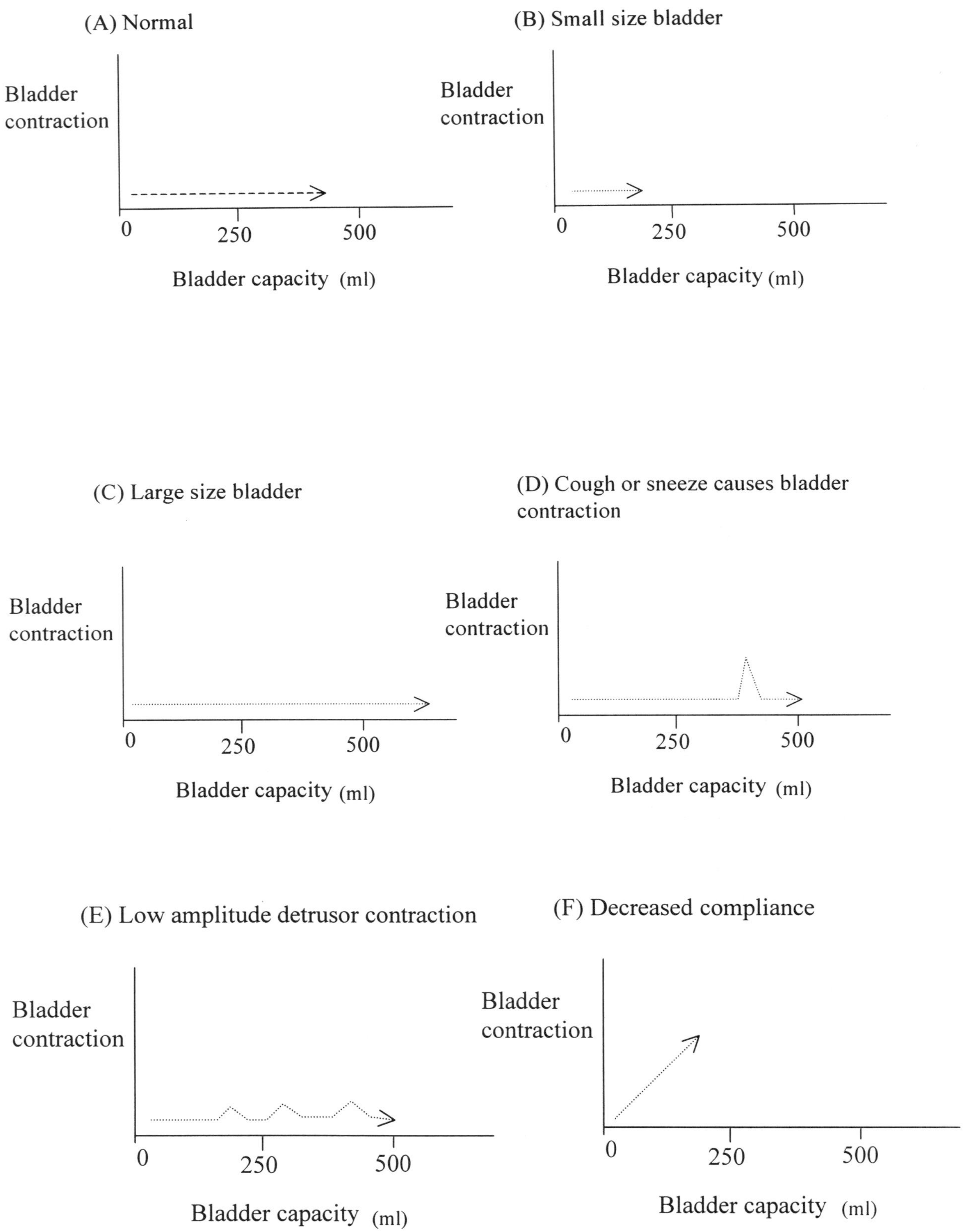
(A) Normal
Bladder contraction
0
250
500
Bladder capacity (ml)
(B) Small size bladder
Bladder contraction
0
250
500
Bladder capacity (ml)
(C) Large size bladder
Bladder contraction
0
250
500
Bladder capacity (ml)
(D) Cough or sneeze causes bladder contraction
Bladder contraction
0
250
500
Bladder capacity (ml)
(E) Low amplitude detrusor contraction
Bladder contraction
0
250
500
Bladder capacity (ml)
(F) Decreased compliance
Bladder contraction
0
250
500
Bladder capacity (ml)

Diagram**101**

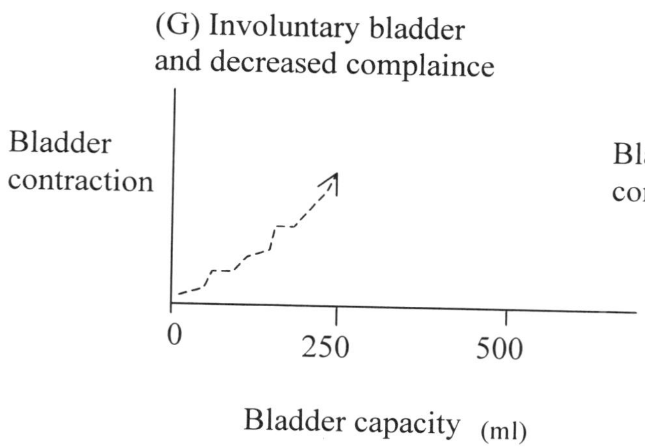

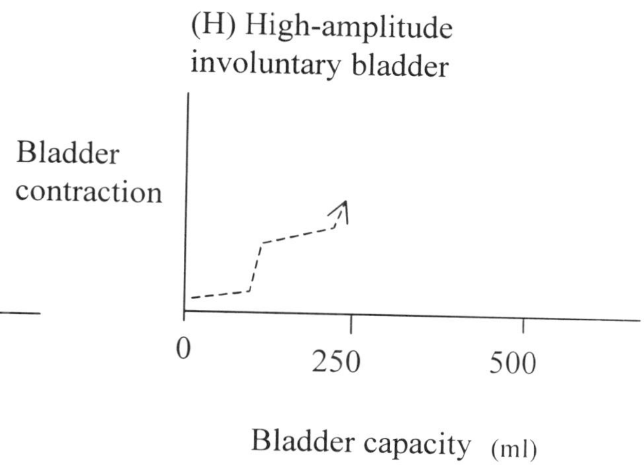

(A) Normal filling curve, normal compliance, and no involuntary bladder contraction. The bladder capacity is 450 ml.

(B) Small bladder capacity due to hypersensitivity, normal compliance and no involuntary bladder contraction.

(C) Large bladder capacity, increased compliance, and it is characteristic of patients with decreased sensation and bladder decompensation. Most patients will have absence or poor detrusor function but it is not correct to make that diagnosis from this curve.

(D) Bladder contraction is due to cough or sneeze and this curve represents total bladder pressure. To make this diagnosis additional recording of intravesical and intraabdominal (or intrarectal) pressure are necessary.

(E) Low amplitude detrusor contraction. This is a characteristic of **patients with suprasacral neurologic disease or idiopathic detrusor instability.**

(F) Decreased compliance.

(G) Decreased compliance and involuntary bladder contraction.

(H) High amplitude early involuntary bladder contracton.

13. Normal combined pressure-flow curve representing pressure of the abdomen, inside the bladder, detrusor muscles and urinary flow of the bladder.

Diagram **102**

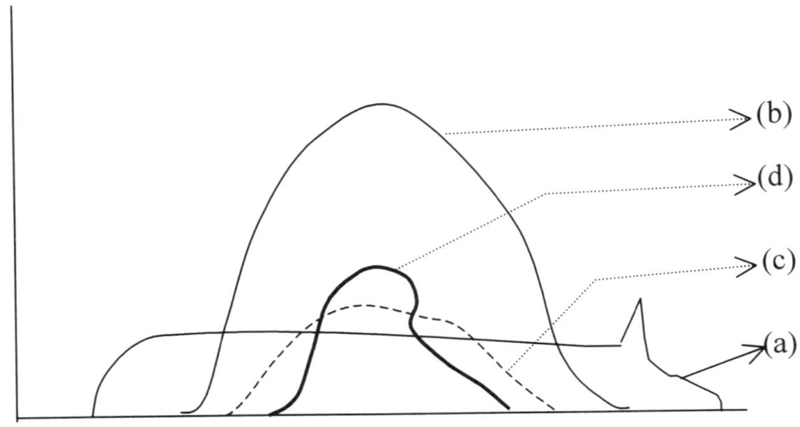

(a) Abdominal pressure (cm H_2O)
(b) Intravesical pressure (cm H_2O)
(c) Detrusor muscles pressure (cm H_2O)
(d) Urinary flow rate (ml/second)

(i) A patient appears with very high intravesical (250 cm H_2O) pressure and detrusor (150 cm H_2O) pressure, but decreased urinary flow rate (5 ml/sec) and normal intraabdominal pressure:
Most likely diagnosis: **Bladder outlet obstruction but normal neurological function .**

(ii) A patient appears with normal intravesical (40 cm H_2) pressure and detrusor (40 cm H_2O) pressure, but decreased (5 ml/sec) urinary flow rate and normal intraabdominal pressure:
Most likely diagnosis: Hypocontractile detrusor but normal neurological function.

(iii) A patient appears with high intravesical (150 cm H_2O) pressure and detrusor (150 cm H_2O) pressure, but severely decreased (1 ml/sec.) flow rate and normal intraabdominal pressure:
Most likely diagnosis: **Dyssynergic bladder sphincter, detrusor hyperreflexia and synergic bladder neck. This indicates neurologic dysfunction of the sphincter.**

(iv) A patient appears with normal intravesical (40 cm H_2O) pressure and detresor (40 cm H_2), but absence of urinary flow and normal intraabdominal pressure (20 cm H_2O):
Most likely diagnosis: Low compliance, incompetent bladder neck, distal bladder sphincter did not open. All these are due to the injury of sacral spinal cord, efferent nerve root, or disease (diabetes).

14. **Oxygen saturation and pressure gradient in normal heart:**

Normal left atrial (LA) saturation = 95-100%
Mean pressure = 8 (range 2-12) mm Hg
Normal left ventricle (LV) saturation = 95-100%
Mean pressure = 130/8 mm Hg
Normal aortic (A) saturation = 95-100%
Mean pressure = 130/70 mm Hg
Normal right atrial (RA) saturation = 75%
Mean pressure = 3 (range 1-5) mm Hg
Normal right ventricle (RV) saturation = 75%
Mean pressure = 25/4 mm Hg
Normal pulmonary artery (PA) saturation=75%
Mean pressure=25/9 mm Hg
Normal pulmonary capillary wedge pressure = 9 mm Hg

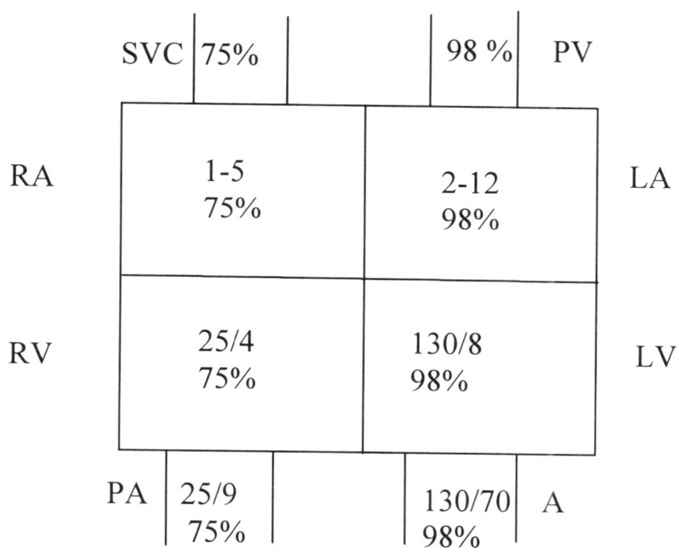

15. **A patient with VSD (left to right shunt)**:
(↑RV pressure and saturation, ↑PA pressure and saturation).

Diagram **104**

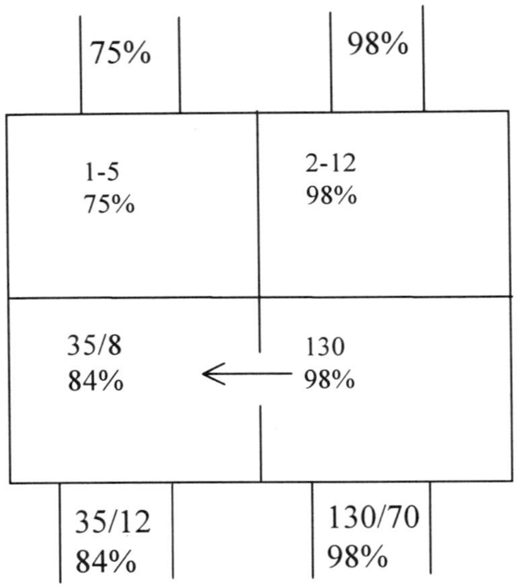

16. **A patient with ASD (left to right shunt):**
(↑RA pressure and saturation, ↑RV pressure and saturation, ↑PA pressure and saturation).

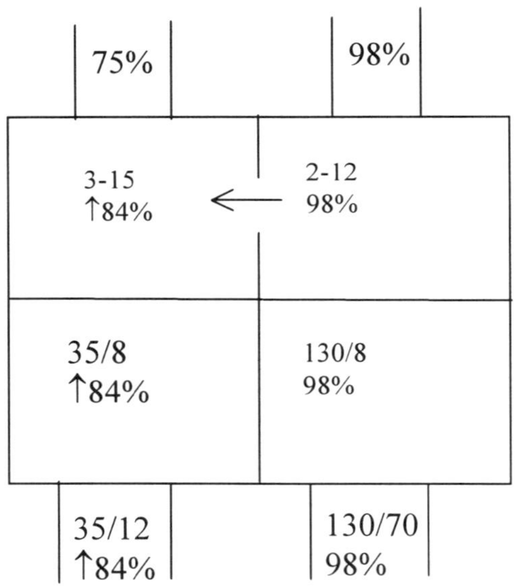

17. A patient with TOF (Tetralogy of Fallot, right to left shunt)
(↑RV pressure, ↓PA pressure, ↓LV saturation, ↓aortic saturation)

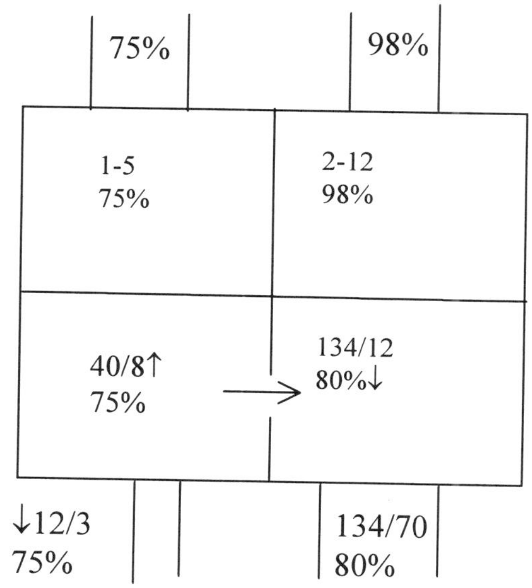

18. **Calculation of cardiac output (CO) and shunt:**
The following parameters are provided:
O_2 consumption = 240 ml/minute
Systemic artery O_2 content = 190 ml/L
Systemic venous O_2 content = 150 ml/L
Pulmonary artery O_2 content = 160 ml/L
Pulmonary venous O_2 content = 190 ml/L
Oxygen Capacity = 200 ml/L

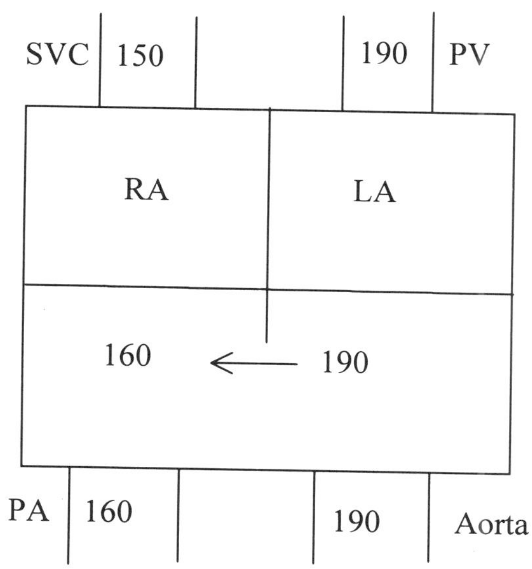

Diagram **106**

(a) Systemic cardiac output

$$\text{(or systemic blood flow SBF)} = \frac{O_2 \text{ consumption}}{\text{Systemic A - V } O_2 \text{ content difference}}$$

$$= \frac{240}{190 - 150} = 6L / \text{minute}$$

(b) Pulmonary cardiac output

$$\text{(or pulmonary blood flow PBF)} = \frac{O_2 \text{ consumption}}{\text{Pulmonary V - A } O_2 \text{ content difference}}$$

$$= \frac{240}{190 - 160} = 8 \text{ L / minute}$$

(c) Left - to - right shunt = 8 - 6 = 2 L / min due to VSD.

(d) $$\text{Effective blood flow(EBF)} = \frac{O_2 \text{ consumption}}{\text{Pulmonary venous } O_2 \text{ - Mixed venous } O_2 \text{ content differe}}$$

$$= \frac{240}{190 - 150} = 6 \text{ L / min}$$

EBF is the fraction of the mixed venous return received by the lungs without contamination by the shunt flow.

(e) **Normal or without any shunt** = SBF, PBF and EBF should be all equal.

(f) The size of a left-to-right, when there is no associated right-to-left shunt = PBF-SBF.

(g) The presence of a left-to-right shunt in addition to a right-to-left shunt then,
left-to-right shunt = PBF-EBF
right-to-left shunt = SBF-EFB

(h) The significance of the shunt is determined by the ratio of PBF/SBF (or QP/QS).

(i) A ratio of <1.5 = Small L to R shunt
(ii) A ratio of 2 or more = Large L to R shunt
(iii) A ratio of < 1.0 = R to L shunt
(iv) When O_2 consumption is not measured, then **ratio of PBF/SBF is measured**

$$= \frac{\text{Systemic arterial } O_2 \text{ saturation - Mixed venous } O_2 \text{ saturation}}{\text{Pulmonary venous } O_2 \text{ saturation - Pulmonary arterial } O_2 \text{ saturation}}$$

$$= \frac{190 - 150}{190 - 160} = \frac{40}{30} = 1.3 \text{ (small L to R shunt)}$$

19. **ECG diagnosis in different arrythmias:**

(A) Ventricular tachycardia: (VPC's in succession at a rate 100 per minute or more)

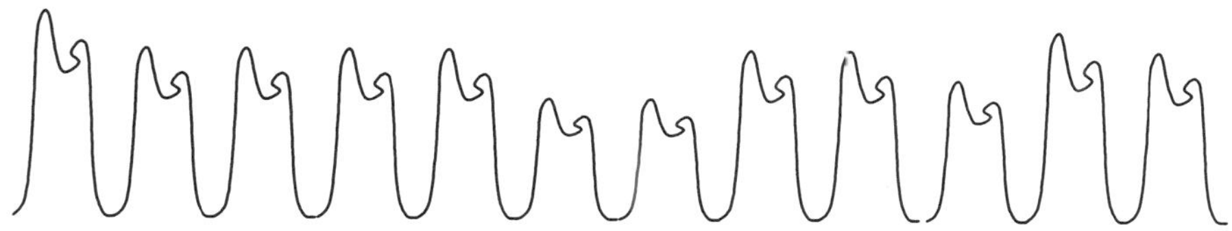

(B) Ventricular fibrillation: (Absence of QRS complex and T waves, presence of low-amplitude baseline undulations which are variable in amplitude and periodicity.

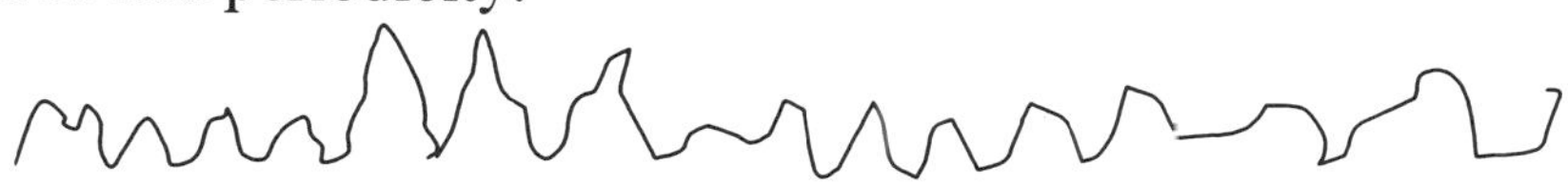

(C) Ventricular flutter: (Ventricular tachyarrythmia has sinusoidal or zigzag QRS's at the rate 240 to 280 per minute)

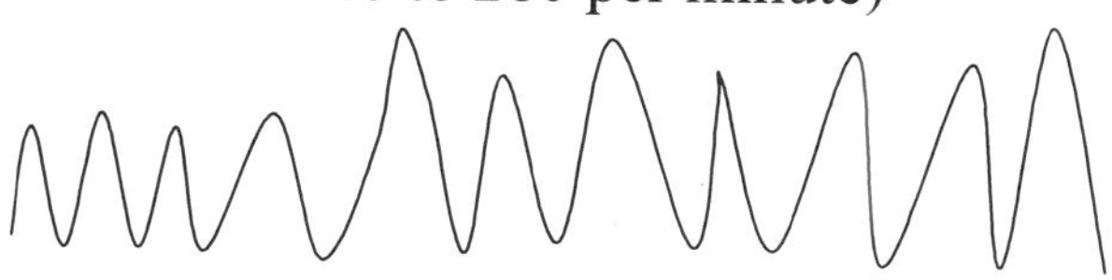

(D) Accelerated idioventricular rhythm (AIVR): (Three or more consecutive QRS complexes of ventricular origin at a rate between 50 to 100 per minute)

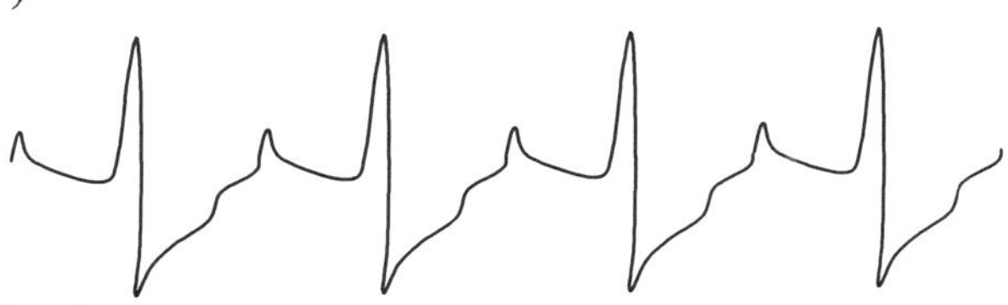

(E) **Ventricular premature complexes (VPC's):** (The QRS is wide, premature, the ST segment and T wave are opposite in direction of the QRS complex ; no premature P wave precedes the premature QRS Complex).

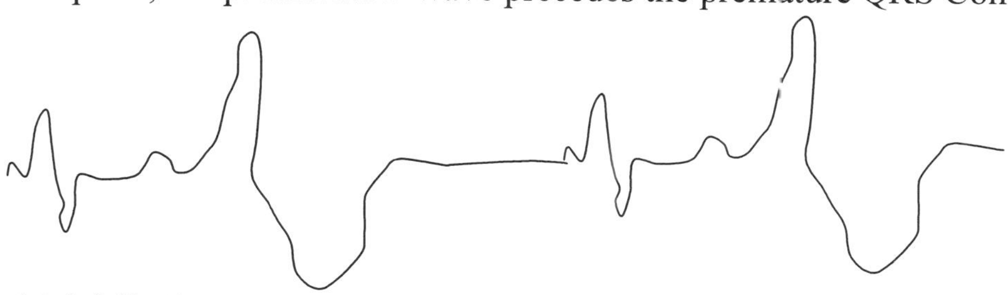

(F) **Atrial flutter:**

(i) (Atrial rate 250 to 350 beats per minute, narrow QRS, ventricular rate 125 to 175 / minute or low, AV conduction ratio is 2:1 or variable. The characteristic saw tooth appearance of P waves.)

Diagram **108**

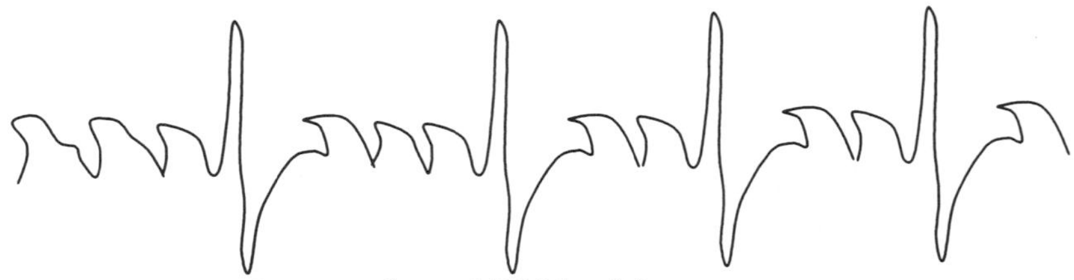

(ii) (Atrial flutter with complete AV block)

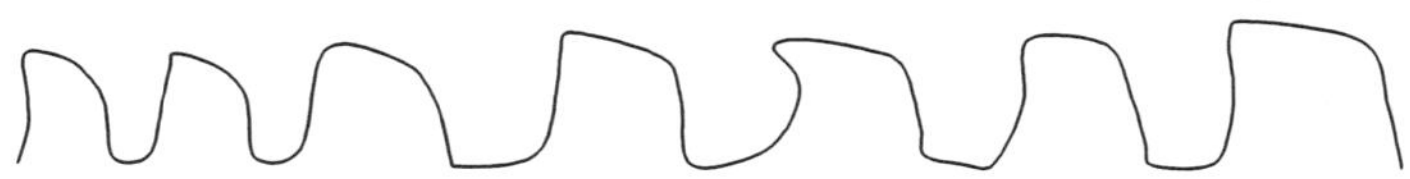

(G) **Atrial fibrillation:**

(i) Absence of P waves, irregular atrial rate of 350 to 600 / minute, rapid irregular ventricular rate 150 to 200 / minute

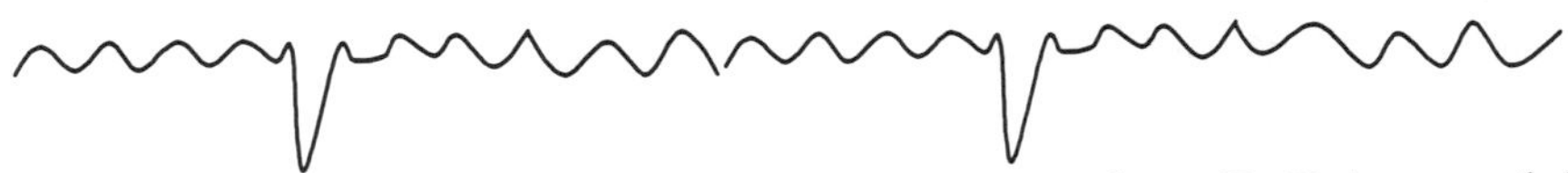

(ii) Ashman phenomenon : (In atrial fibrillation, short R-R interval follows a long R-R interval results in aberrant conduction, 5th QRS complex right bundle branch)

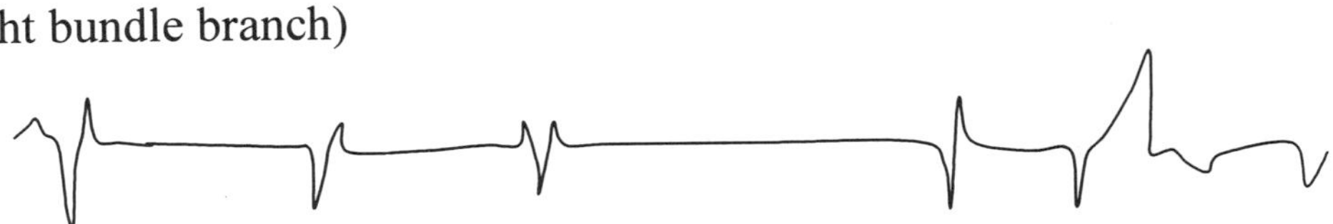

(H) **Atrial premature complexes (APC's):** (Abnormal, inverted, premature P waves, and prolonged PR interval, normal QRS complex)

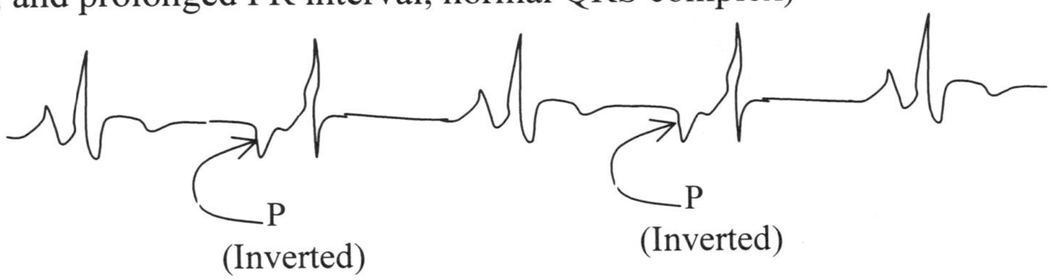

(I) **Sinoatrial block (SA block):**

(i) **First-degree**: Conduction delay from sinus node to the atrium, it is **not** detected in standard ECG but can be diagnosed in electrophysiologic studies (EPS)

(ii) **Second-degree SA block type I (Wenckebach)**: (PP interval is constant and PR interval is progressively increases until a P wave is not conducted).

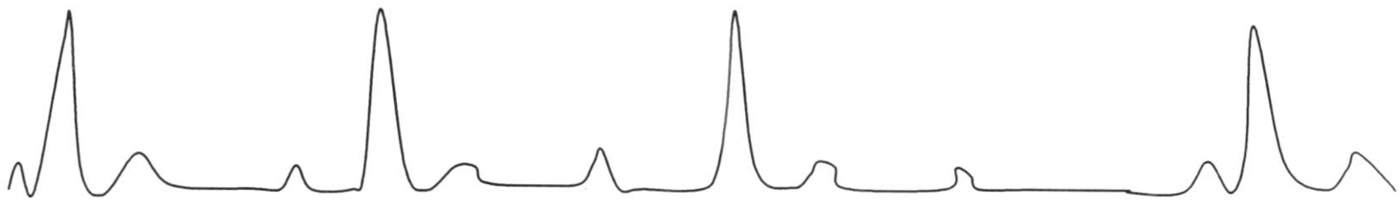

(iii) **Second-degree SA block type II:** (PP interval is double, absence of P wave due to intermittent failure of conduction of sinus impulses to the surrounding atrial tissues)

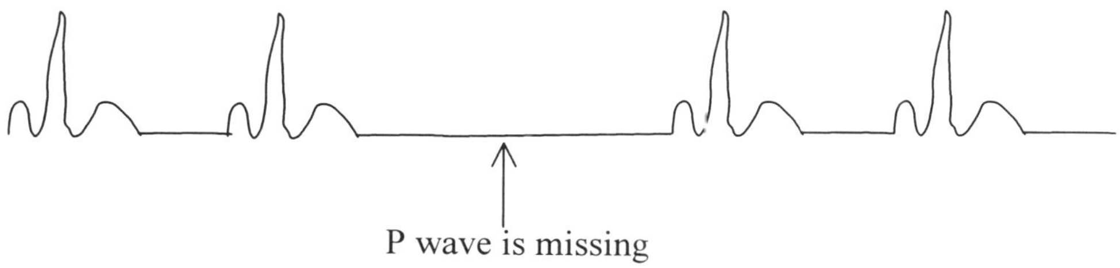

(iv) **Third-degree SA block or atrial arrest:** (Lack of atrial activity means complete absence of P waves or presence of ectopic subsidiary atrial pacemaker)

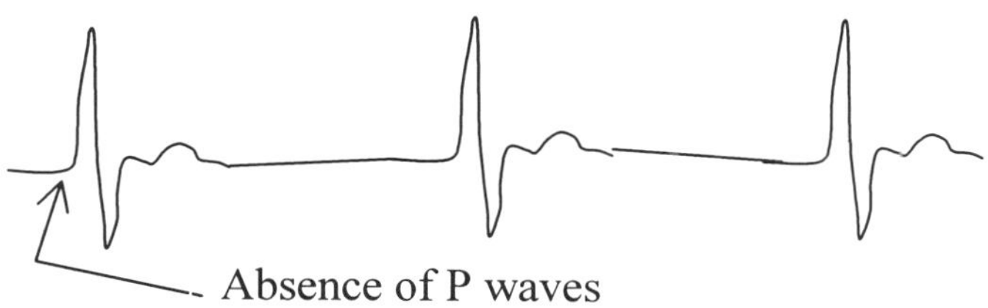

20. **Wandering atrial pacemaker:** (When heart rate slows down, the P wave become inverted, then it gradually becomes normal as the heart rate speeds up again, cyclical increase in R-R interval, and PR interval shortens with inverted P waves)

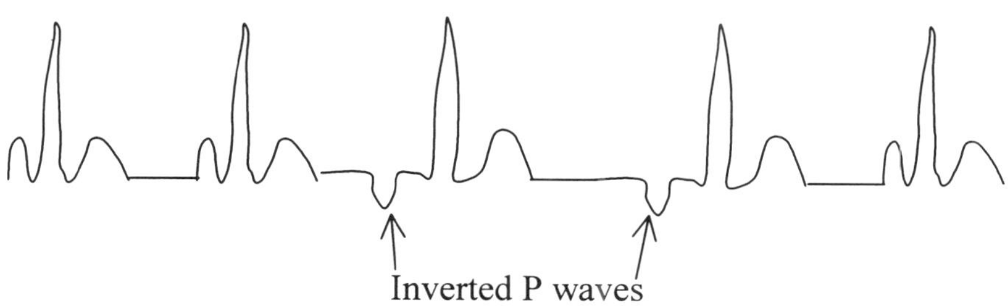

21. **Sick sinus syndrome or tachycardia-bradycardia syndrome:** (Tachyarrythmias are mostly due to atrial flutter, fibrillation, or any tachycardias with retrograde conduction to the atria can cause override suppression of the sinus node)

Diagram **110**

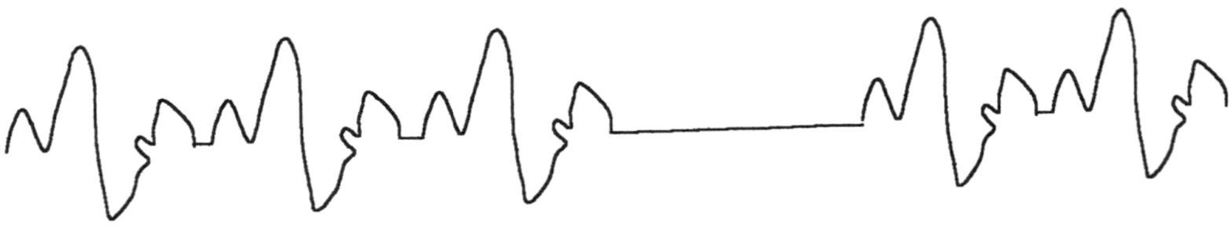

22. **Paroxysmal Supraventricular tachycardia or atrial tachycardia (PAT) :** (Atrial rate is 150 to 200 beats per minute, P waves are different then sinus P waves P waves overlaps on QRS complex)

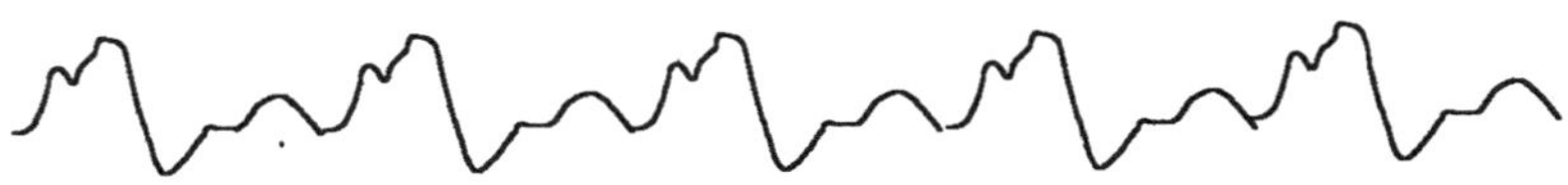

23. **Wolff-Parkinson-White (WPW) Syndrome:** (Triad of wide QRS complex, short P-R interval and slurring or delta wave in the ascending part of QRS Complex)

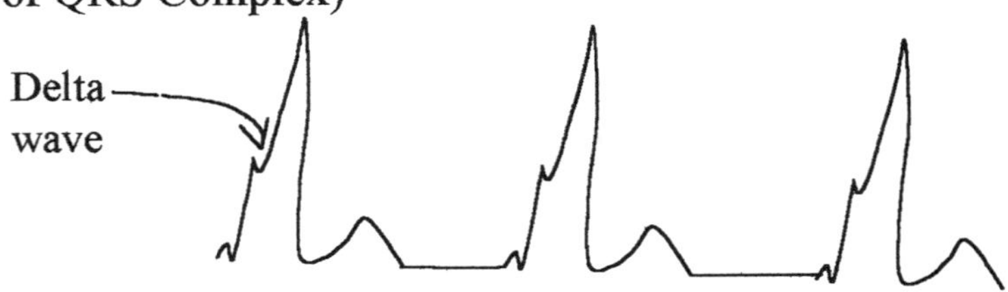

24. **Severe anterior wall ischemia with or without infarction:** (Prominent inverted T waves in precordial leads and patients may have stenosis of the left anterior descending coronary artery).

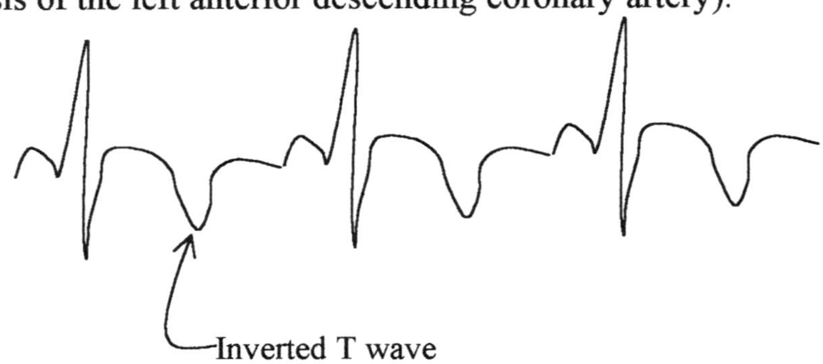

25. **Anteroseptal myocardial infarction (hypercute phase)**: (Tall positive T wave in V2 to V3 plus ST-segment elevations and Q waves in V1 to V3).

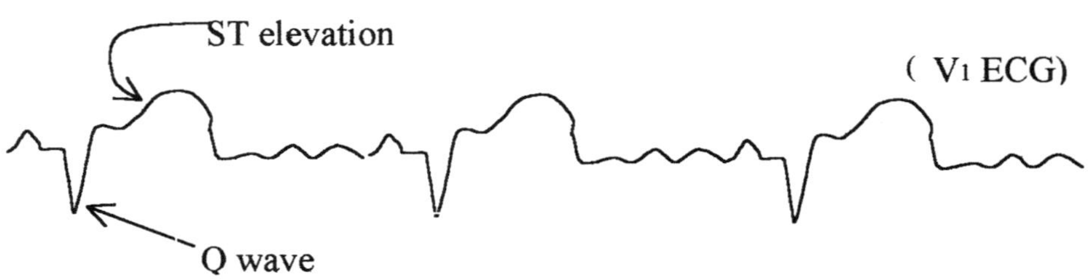

26. Acute anterior infarction: (ST elevation in lead I, aVL and precordial leads and may have reciprocal ST depression in leads II, III, and aVF)

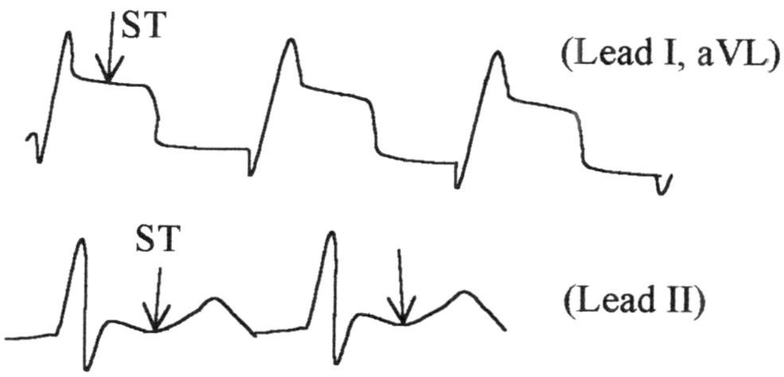

27. **Acute inferior or posterior infarction**: **(Reciprocal ST depression in leads V1 and V3).**

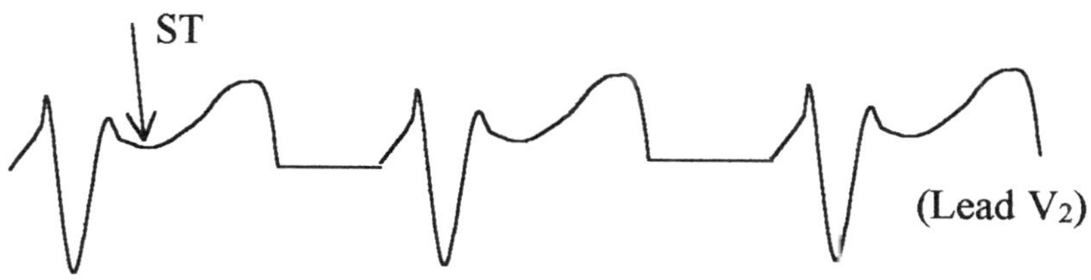

28. **Acute pericarditis:** (ST elevations in Leads I,II, aVF,V2,V6 due to ventricular injury and PR-segment deviation opposite to the ST-segment due to atrial injury)

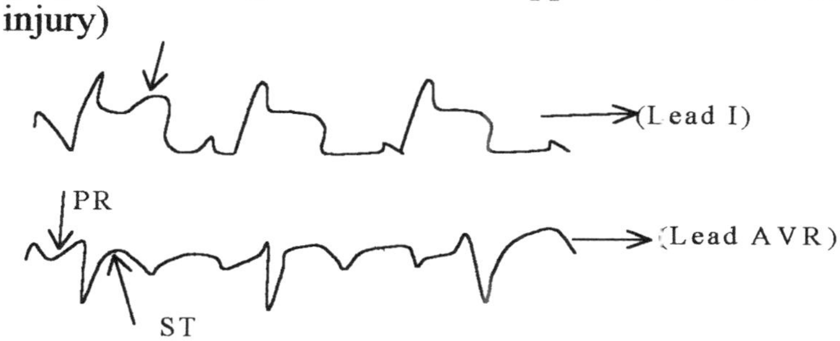

29. **Pericardial effusion with cardiac tamponade:** (Beat-to-beat variation in QRS axis or amplitude with sinus tachycardia)

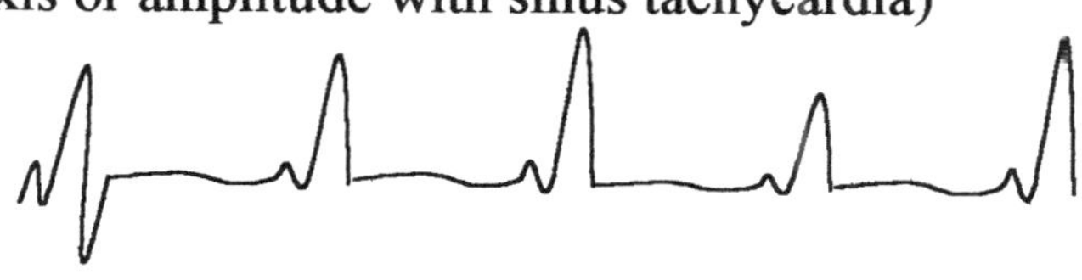

30. **Hypothermia**: (Convex hump at the J point)

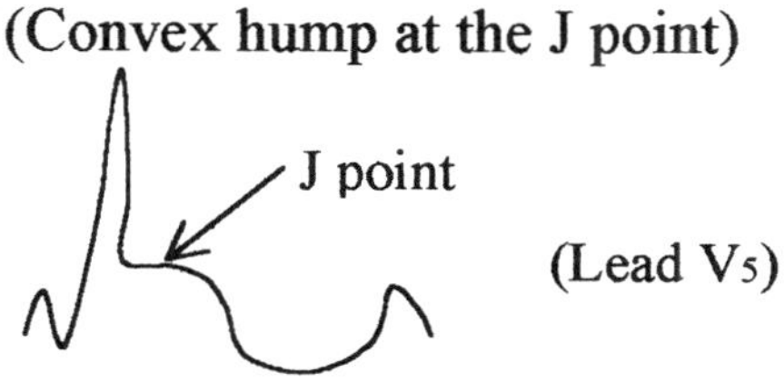

31. **Hypokalemia**: (Prominent U wave)

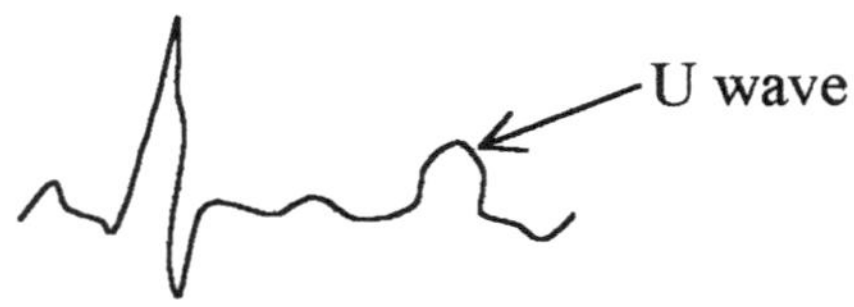

32. **Overdose of TCA (Tricyclic antidepressants):** (Prolongation of QRS and QT with sinus tachycardia)

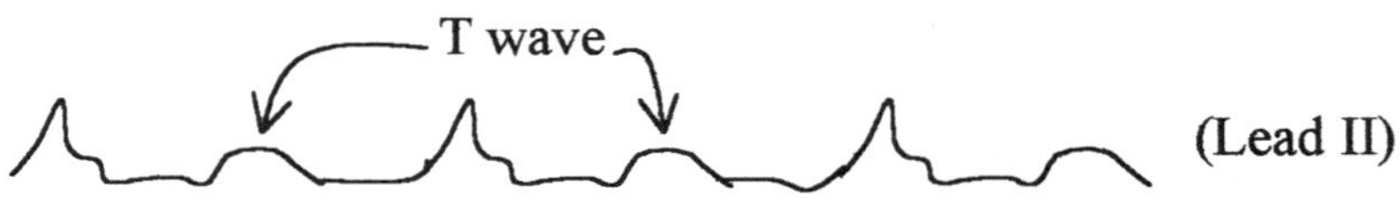

33. **Hypocalcemia:** (Prolongation of QT interval, ST segment only)

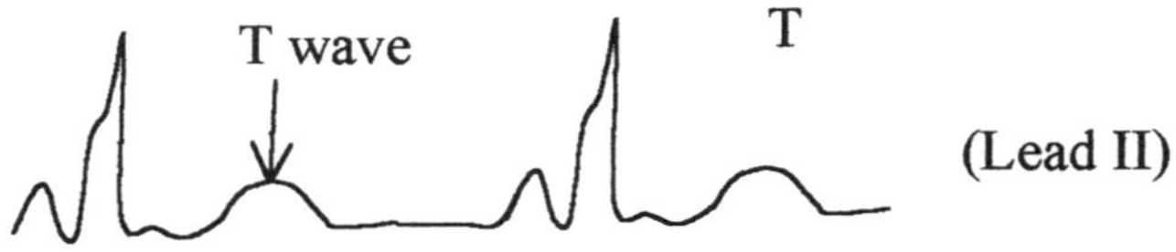

34. **Hypercalcemia:** (Short ST segment and QT interval)

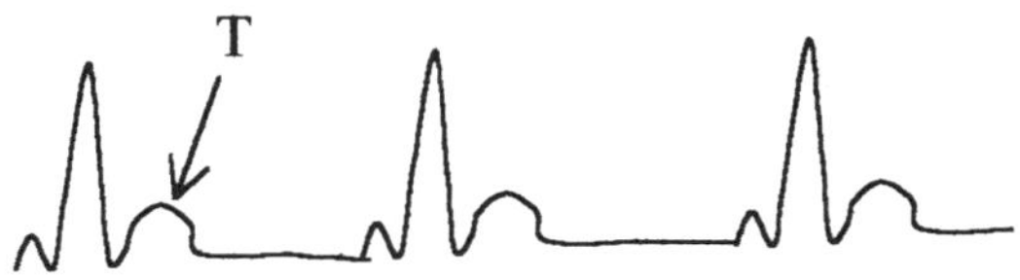

35. **Hyperkalemia:** (Narrow and peaking of the T wave)

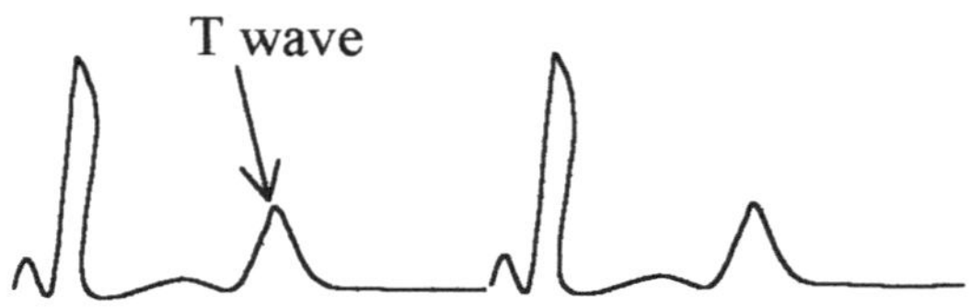

36. **Antiarrythmic drugs:** (Quinidine, TCA, procainamide, disopyramide, phenothiazines, sotalol, amiodarone): Prolongation of the QT interval

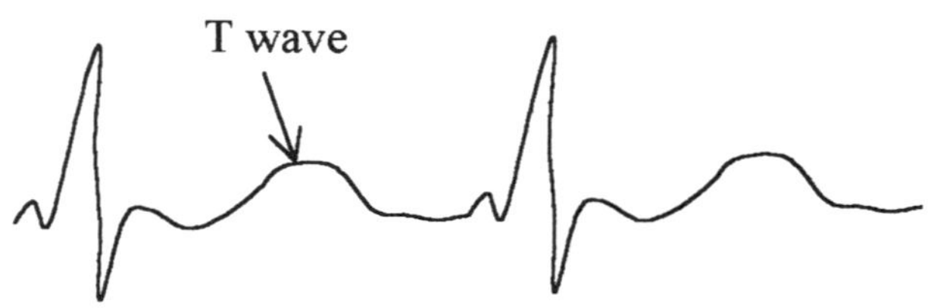

37. **Digitalis toxicity:** (Prolongation of the PR interval is the first sign ; atria fibrillation with AV block or atrial tachycardia with AV block)

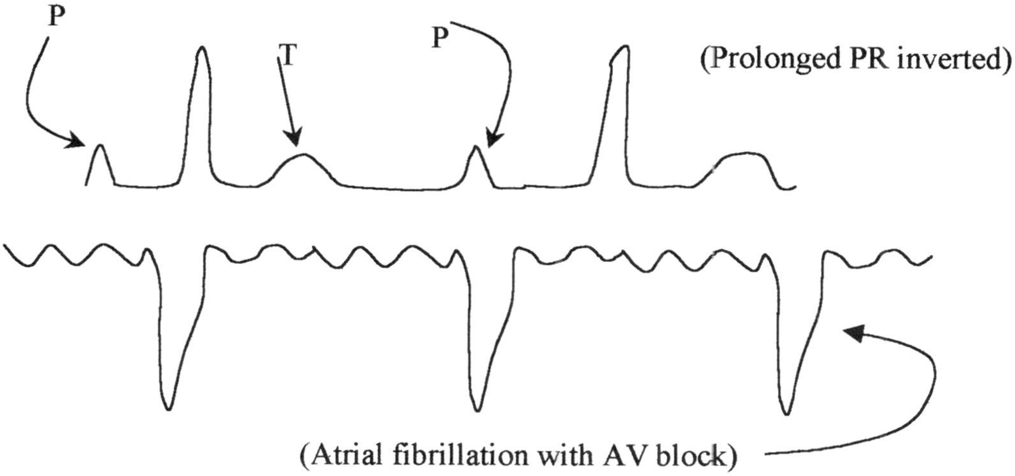

38. **Subarachnoid hemorrhage or other intracranial bleed:**
(prolongation of QT interval sometimes deep, inverted T wave).

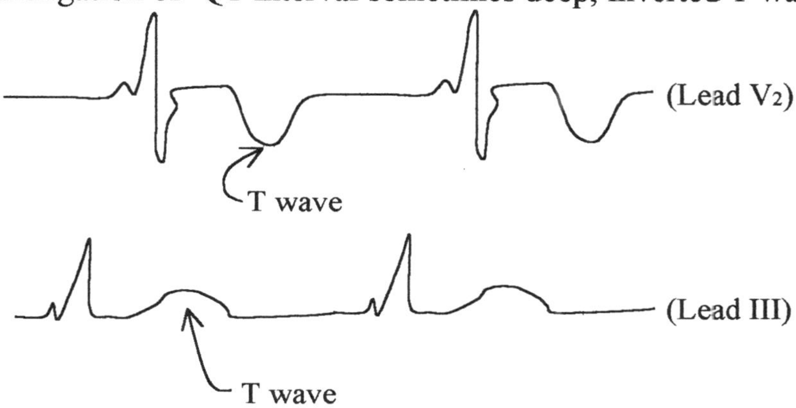

39. **Left ventricular function curves**:

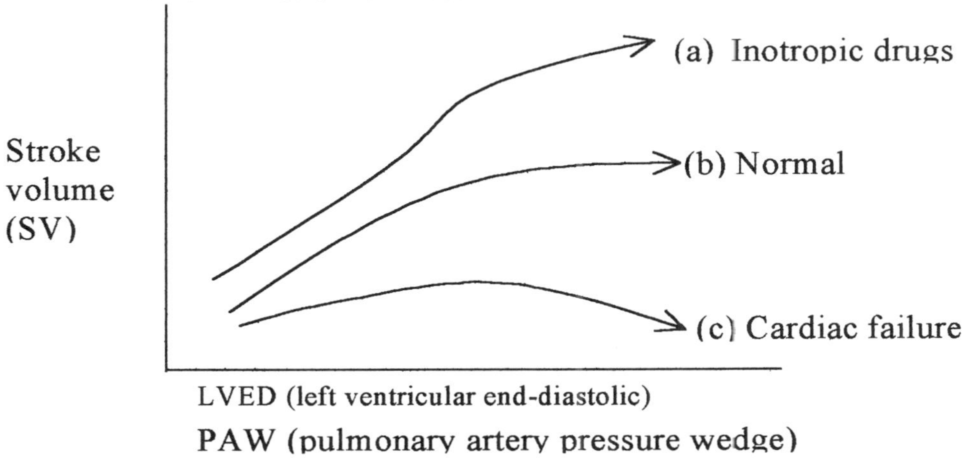

Diagram **114**

(a) Increased contractility and SV due to use of inotropic drugs.
(b) Normal cardiac function and SV.
(c) Cardiac failure and decreased SV.

40. **Relationship between RA (right atrial) pressure and CO (Cardiac output) or VR (Venous return).**

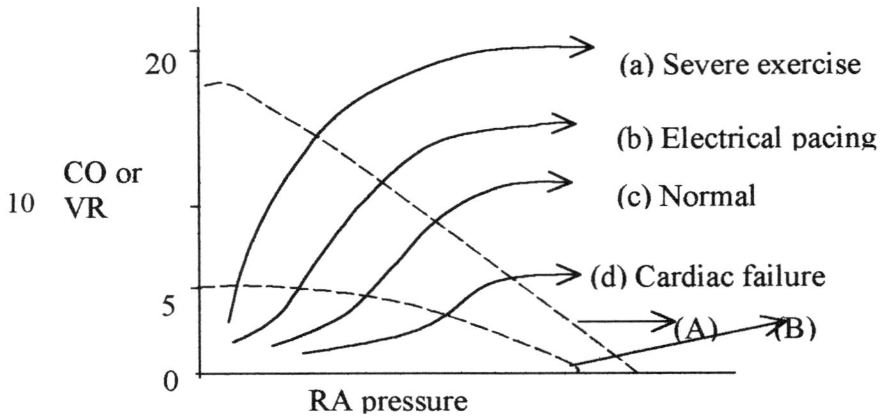

(A) and (B) represents the inverse relationship between RA pressure and CO or VR.
B represents normal physiologic condition.
A represents increased sympathetic stimulation.
a = Severe exercise
b = Electrical pacing
c = Normal
d = Cardiac failure

41. Water deprivation and urinary osmolality

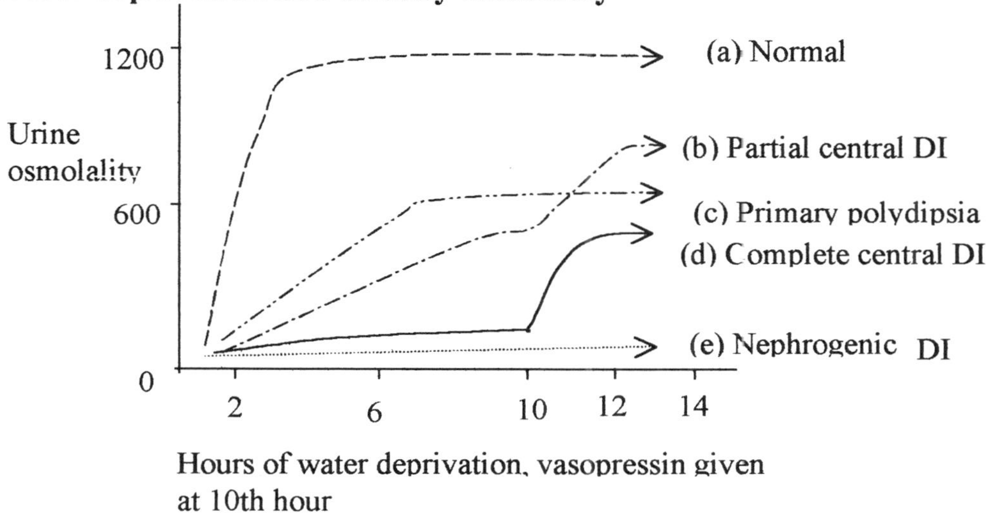

(a) **Normal response curve** (increased urine osmolality with water deprivation and no change with vasopressin)
(b) **Partial central D1** (diabetes insipidius) (partially increased urine osmolality with water deprivation and significant increased after vasopressin)
(c) **Primary polydipsia** (Partially increased urine osmolality with water deprivation but no increase in osmolality with vasopressin)
(d) **Complete central DI**: (no change in urine osmolality with water deprivation but increase osmolality with vasopressin)
(e) **Nephrogenic DI** (no increase in urine osmolality with water deprivation and vasopressin).

RESPIRATORY SYSTEM

1. **Most common lethal genetic disease in U.S.A**: Cystic fibrosis. Frequency in Caucasians is 1 in 2000 and carriers of defective gene is 1 in 20. Gene is located on the long arm of chromosome 7. The mutation at amino acid 508 position results in pancreatic insufficiency but not on the lung.

2. **Excessive electrolyte levels in the sweat in cystic fibrosis is due to**: Impermeability of the sweat duct epithelium to chloride. In a normal person, chlorides are located on the luminal membranes of the epithelial cells. The chlorides go into the lumen and draw water. In cystic fibrosis, there is inadequate amount of water in secretion.

3. **Important points to remember in cystic fibrosis**:
   (a) Most common cause of death is either respiratory failure or pulmonary complication.
   (b) Infertility in males are due to azoospermia and in females, anovulation.
   (c) Most common organism causing infection is **Staphylococcus aureus**.
   (d) Pseudomonas infection indicates poor prognosis. **P.cepacia** is resistant to multiple antibiotics resulting fatal pneumonia.
   (e) NaCl concentration, 70 mEq per liter in sweat is the most probable diagnostic test.
   (f) cDNA probes also give correct diagnosis.
   (g) History of cough, recurrent respiratory infections, viscous, and purulent sputum; signs of poor nutritional status, malabsorption, clubbing, and recurrent pneumothorax.
   (h) Rusty brown sputum is suggestive of **Aspergillus fumigatus** infection.
   (i) Hypertrophic osteoarthropathy may cause severe and continuous pain.
   (j) For **S.aureus** infection, use dicloxacillin or cephalosporin, and for Pseudomonas infection, use a combination of gentamicin/carbenicillin and tobramycin/ticarcillin.
   (k) Experimental therapies: Aerosolized human recombinant DNase and gene therapy.
   (l) Lung function: Obstructive lung disease. $\downarrow O_2$, $\uparrow CO_2$ $\uparrow FEV_1$(forced expiratory volume in 1 second <30% indicates end stage pulmonary disease).

4. **Most common presentation of sarcoidosis**: Asymptomatic, next is fatigue but CXR findings of bilateral hilar, paratracheal adenopathy, and reticulonodular infiltrates.

5. **Acute sarcoidosis or Löffgren's syndrome**: Erythema nodosum, arthritis, uveitis and/or fever along with mediastinal adenopathies and pulmonary reticulonodular infiltrates. This is symptomatic sarcoidosis. Other diseases should be considered when there is fever, anorexia, and weight loss.

6. **Most commonly involved organ in sarcoidosis**: Lungs.(Other involved organs are skin, CNS, eyes, kidneys, heart, and musculoskeletal).

7. **Most commonly involved cranial nerve**: VII or facial. (II, VIII, IX, X cranial nerves are also involved causing papilledema (II), deafness, vertigo (VIII), dysphagia, absent gag reflex (IX), and vocal cord paralysis (X).

8. **Lupus pernio**: Skin manifestations in sarcoidosis of violaceous plaques over the nose, cheeks, and ears.

9. **Heerfordt's syndrome in sarcoidosis**: Anterior uveitis with parotitis and facial nerve palsy.

10. **Most common eye manifestation in sarcoidosis**: **Uveitis**.(Other involved parts are retina, conjunctiva, and lacrimal glands).

11. **Most frequently involved bones in sarcoidosis**: Phalanges, metacarpals, and metatarsals. (Osteoporotic, cystic, and reticulated changes).

12. An asymptomatic patient, 28 years of age, with bilateral symmetric hilar and paratracheal lymphadenopathy or with arthralgia, erythema nodosum, and uveitis (typical presentation of sarcoidosis).
MOST LIKELY DIAGNOSIS: Sarcoidosis.
CHEST X-RAY: (B/L) symmetric hilar and paratracheal lymph nodes enlargement. CT scan can demonstrate lymphadenopathy better than CXR.
DIAGNOSIS CONFIRMED By: Biopsy of the lung is most specific but it **is only needed when clinical & radiological findings are suspicious**. Biopsy shows granulomas but absence of mycobacteria, fungi or refractile material.
TREATMENT: **Spontaneous total remission** occurs in 80 to 90 % of patients within 3 years without treatment. **Prednisone** is the drug of choice only when the function of a vital organ deteriorates or in hypercalcemia. Topical steroids are used on the skin and for eye conditions. For skin lesions, methotrexate and chloroquin have been used. Dietary restriction of calcium in hypercalcemia.

13. **'Activity' of sarcoidosis means**:
    (a) **Worsening of clinical conditions.**

(b) **Worsening of CXR and pulmonary functions.**
(c) ↑Serum calcium level.
(d) ↑Serum angiotensin 1-converting enzyme level.
(e) Experimental: Positive gallium lung scan and alveolitis in bronchial lavage.

14. **Management of a sarcoidosis patient, exposed to tuberculosis, has positive PPD**: Appropriate prophylaxis or treatment should be given.

15. **Neurologic complications of sarcoidosis**: Diabetes insipidus is due to involvement of hypothalamus and posterior pituitary. Manifestations of space occupying lesions (focal seizure, headache) are due to granulomas of the brain.

16. **Pulmonary functions in sarcoidosis**: ↓Po_2, →Pco_2, ↓vital capacity, ↓diffusion. Pulmonary functions may be abnormal with normal CXR and vice versa.

17. **Complication of discontinuation of steroid therapy in sarcoidosis**: Recurrence of the disease. So, alternate day therapy of prednisone with lower dosage (10 to 15 mg) will reduce the recurrence and complications of prolonged steroid therapy (↑weight,↑fluid retention, diabetes mellitus).

18. **Radiological grading of sarcoidosis**:
(a) Grade 0: normal CXR.
(b) Grade 1: only lymph node enlargement.
(c) Grade 2A: combination of lymph node enlargement and diffuse pulmonary parenchymal disease.
(d) Grade 2B: diffuse pulmonary disease and normal lymph node.
(e) Grade 3: pulmonary fibrosis (honeycombing or hilar retraction).
Most common CXR finding is reticulonodular pattern with nodules of 3 to 5 mm in diameter.

19. **Most common type and source of pulmonary emboli: Thromboemboli** (blood clots) come from the thrombi in **proximal deep veins of the lower extremities and pelvis**. (Superficial veins of lowers extremities do **not** cause pulmonary thromboembolism). **Rare** sources of emboli are fat droplets, neoplastic cells, air bubbles, exogenous materials (talc and cornstarch materials in IV drug abusers), accidental intravenous catheters, and catheter introducers.

20. **Risk of pulmonary embolism**: **After surgery for hip fracture is 5-10%.** After abdominal and thoracic surgery over the age 40 years is 1%.

21. **Most important factor for venous thrombosis after surgery: Immobilization.**

22. **Cancer increases thromboembolisms due to: Factors released from tumors** (↑coagulability, ↓fibrinolysis, alter endothelial cells).

23. **Most common cause of acute pulmonary hypertension: Pulmonary thromboembolism.**

24. **Relation between mean pulmonary artery pressure (MAP) and pulmonary vascular obstruction** (PVO):
<50% PVO =<20 mm Hg of MAP.
50-75% PVO = 20-40 mm Hg of MAP.
(* Normal right ventricle cannot generate > 40mm Hg pressure except in chronic right ventricular hypertrophy).

25. **Characteristic of acute pulmonary emboli: Multiple**, involves both lungs but more in **right** than left, **involve lower lobe vessels** more than the upper ones.

26. **Most common arterial blood gas (ABG) changes in acute pulmonary embolism: Hypoxia**; other changes are ↓Pco_2 due to ↑RR (respiratory rate), ↑MV (minute ventilation).

27. A 50 year old man appears with H/O dyspnea, pleuritic pain, cough, leg pain, and swelling. On physical examination the patient has tachypnea (≥20/min), rales, tachycardia (>100/min), deep vein thrombosis, and fourth heart sound.
Pulmonary angiogram: Filling defect of vessels of at least 2 to 3 mm. in diameter **(most confirmatory test).**
ABG: Nonspecific findings, ↓O_2, ↓CO_2.
CXR: Nonspecific findings, basillar atelactasis, elevation of hemidiaphragms, unilateral pleural effusion, and increased parenchymal densities - these are typical findings.
EKG: Sinus tachycardia. R/O myocardial infarction and pericarditis.
Thoracocentesis: Exudate.
Ventilation- Perfusion Scan: Abnormal perfusion scan but normal ventilation scan.
Most likely diagnosis: **Pulmonary embolism.**
Treatment:
(a) Hemodynamically stable: IV heparin and oral anticoagulation for 5-7 days, then oral anticoagulation for at least 3 months.

(b) Above condition + anticoagulant contraindicated: Interrupt inferior vena cava (IVC).
(c) Hemodynamically unstable: Thrombolytic therapy + same as treatment in (a).
(d) Above condition in c + anticoagulation contraindicated: Pulmonary embolectomy + interrupt IVC. Primary goal of therapy is to prevent a fatal recurrence. Supportive treatments are oxygen, analgesic, and cardiorespiratory management.

28. **Mechanism of action of heparin**: Inhibitory effect of antithrombin III upon the coagulation enzymes, Factors IXa, Xa, XIa, XIIa, and thrombin. During heparin therapy, try to maintain the activated partial thromboplastin time (aPTT) at 1.5 to 2.5 times of control.

29. **Most common and most serious complication of heparin**: Bleeding which is due to increase dose and effect of heparin on clotting factors. Thrombocytopenia appears after few days of therapy.

30. **Action of warfarin: Site of action: Liver**.
Mechanism: Inhibit the γ-carboxylation of specific glutamic acid residues in vitamin K dependent factors II, VII, IX, and X.

31. **Thrombolytic agents**: Streptokinase (SK), urokinase (UK), and tissue-type plasminogen activator (t-PA).
Mechanism of action: Converting plasminogen to plasmin.(Plasminogen is an inactive proenzyme, and palsmin is fibrinolytic proteinase. Plasmin causes breakdown of thrombus in pulmonary and deep veins. SK and UK form a complex with plasminogen but t-PA acts on plasminogen which is associated with fibrin unlike SK and UK.
Contraindications:
Definite: Recent or active internal bleeding, head injury, intracranial surgery, and hemorrhagic stroke. **Relative**: Uncontrolled severe hypertension; within 10 days of major surgery, trauma, and internal organ biopsies; within 1 year of nonhemorrhagic stroke.

32. **Prophylaxis for deep vein thrombosis:**
(1) **Low dose heparin**: Medical patients with risk factors for deep vein thrombosis. Surgical patients over age 40 recommended for abdominal or thoracic surgery. Medication given preoperatively.

(2) Intermittent pneumatic compression of the calves or thighs– Eye or neurologic surgery in which bleeding could be dangerous, open prostatectomy, and gynecologic cancer.
(3) Warfarin: Hip fracture, hip replacement **(or low molecular weight heparin), and knee replacement (and intermittent pneumatic compression).**

33. **Most death due to pulmonary embolism**:
(a) Patients deteriorate very rapidly.
(b) Inadequate therapeutic level of anticoagulant because of low dosages given.
(c) Misdiagnosis.

34. **Causes of death within 1 year despite adequate treatment with anticoagulant**:
(a) Cancer.
(b) Chronic lung disease.
(c) Left sided congestive heart failure.
* Long term survival inversely proportional to age.

35. A 40 year old man appears in the emergency room with respiratory failure and multiple fractures of long bones and pelvis, secondary to recent automobile accident. Physical examination shows petechiae over the upper half of the body including axilla, conjunctiva, oral mucosa, and cyanosis. No apparent head injury was noted.
CXR: Diffuse alveolar infiltrate but no fracture of ribs.
Most likely diagnosis: **Fat embolism syndrome**.
Diagnosis confirmed: By physical findings & history, dyspnea, tachypnea, and hypoxemia within 72 hours after injury &/or cerebral confusion or dysfunction, and petechiae are diagnostic. No laboratory tests are diagnostic. Presence of fat globules in the pulmonary capillary blood sample, support the diagnosis.
Pathogenesis: Endothelial injury, caused by fatty acids which produce from fat droplets by lipoprotein lipase, causes increased microvascular permeability and interstitial edema. It is **not** due to mechanical obstruction by fat droplets. Cerebral symptoms are due to direct brain injury by emboli with hemorrhage and necrosis but rarely by hypoxia. The reason for petechiae is unknown but petechiae from thrombocytopenia may be due to DIC (disseminated intravascular coagulation).
Treatment:
(a) Supportive: Oxygen, ventilator management, ↑PEEP may reduce high oxygen requirement, fluid restriction, and diuretics.
(b) Long bone fractures: Stabilization of the fracture, maintain systemic perfusion.

* Corticosteriod may prevent the development of this syndrome but there are no effects once the syndrome has developed.

Prognosis: Good, mortality <10%.

36. **Most common organism for lung abscess**: Anaerobic bacteria which produces necrotizing pulmonary infections. It is a normal flora of the oropharynx. (Nosocomial infection is caused by **S.aureus** or Gram-negative bacilli).

37. **Septic pulmonary emboli are most commonly caused by**: S.aureus. It is mostly found in intravenous drug users with tricuspid valve endocarditis.

38. **Most common site of aspiration pneumonia**:
    (a) Recumbent position: Superior segments of the lower lobes or posterior segments of the upper lobes.
    (b) Upright or semiupright position: Basillar segments of the lower lobes.

39. **Most likely source of the anaerobic lung abscess:**
    (a) Periodontal infection (pyorrhea, gingivitis).
    (b) Aspiration (found in complication of general anesthesia; drug addict, alcoholic, seizure, and patients with neurologic disorders).

40. A 50 year old woman appears with 3 weeks H/O cough, fever, recent onset of putrid sputum which has a very noxious taste. She had H/O dental infection 4 weeks ago. (*Putrid sputum mostly indicates anaerobic infection).
    CXR: Cavity containing air-fluid level with parenchymal infiltrate: **Most diagnostic study is CXR.**
    Most likely diagnosis: Anaerobic lung abscess.
    Treatment:
    (a) Appropriate antibiotics: Clindamycin, penicillin, or penicillin plus metronidazole.
    (b) Physiotherapy with postural drainage: It should be done carefully to avoid spillage of purulent material into the noninfected portion of the lungs.

41. **Indications for surgery (lobectomy) in the lung**:
    (a) Lung abscess unresponsive to medical treatment.
    (b) Lung cancer.
    (c) Life threatening hemorrhage.
    (d) Bronchial obstruction.

42. **Indications for bronchoscopy in lung abscess patient**:

(a) Atypical clinical presentation.
(b) Unresponsive to antibiotics.
Bronchoscopy is done to diagnose neoplasm, foreign body, and bronchostenosis.

43. **Antibiotics used in different organisms causing lung abcesses**: Sensitivity is the best way to select antibiotics.
    (a) **S.aureus**: Vancomycin.
    (b) **Group A beta-hemolytic streptococci**: Penicillin G.
    (c) **Gram-negative bacilli (P.aeruginosa):** Ticarcillin plus aminoglycoside or ceftazidime.
    (d) **Nocardia**: Sulfonamides.

44. **Poor prognosis in lung abscesses**:
    (a) Aerobic bacteria, **S.aureus**, Gram-negative bacilli.
    (b) Lung cavity > 6 cm in diameter.
    (c) Symptoms > 6 weeks.
    (d) Abscess with bronchial obstruction.
    (e) Multiple small abscesses.
    (f) Immunologically compromised.
    (g) Elderly, debilitated patients.

45. **Kartagener's syndrome**: Subset of immotile cilia syndrome, situs inversus, and bronchiectasis. Immotile cilia is due to absent or aberrant of dynein arms which make them immotile. Situs inversus is due to abnormal embryonic migration of the viscera (not due to cilia). Bronchiectasis is due to recurrent infections.

46. **Immotile cilia syndrome**: Autosomal recessive, males infertility are due to immotile sperm, females have decreased fertility, associated with sinusitis, **and bronchiectasis**.

47. **Most common cause of bronchiectasis in children and young adults: Cystic fibrosis**.

48. **Important factors causing bronchiectasis**:
    (a) Bronchopulmonary infection & obstruction.
    (b) Immune deficiency states.
    (c) Hereditary diseases.
    (d) Congenital anatomical defects.

(e) Young's syndrome, aspiration, inhalation of irritant, and after heart-lung transplantation.

49. **Young's syndrome**: Bronchiectasis, chronic sinopulmonary infections, and obstructive azoospermia.

50. **Yellow nail syndrome**: (very rare) Yellow nails, bronchiectasis, lymphedema of the feet, recurrent pneumonia.

51. **Most common site of bronchiectasis**: Left lung, lower lobes, medium- sized bronchi.

52. A 60 year old man appears with H/O chronic cough, purulent sputum which may contain intermittent blood streaking.
    CXR: Increased bronchovascular markings, atelactasis and cavities. Tram tracks, tram line of tubular shadows or gloved finger shadows are significant. **It is the most diagnostic study.**
    Lung function: ↑Residual volume (RV), ↓Forced expiratory volume in one second (FEV_1),↓Forced vital Capacity,↓FEV_1/FVC,↓Forced expiratory flow (FEF 25-75%)↓O_2,→CO_2,↓ventilation-perfusion & ratio.
    Bronchography: Not done.
    Chest CT scan: Can replace bronchography.
    Sinus radiography: R/O sinus infection.
    Sputum culture: To identify the organism.
    Most likely diagnosis: **Bronchiectasis**.
    Treatment:
    (a) Antibiotics: Initially start ampicillin, then switch to appropriate antibiotics after culture and sensitivity results. Penicillin allergic patients should receive initially either tetracycline or trimethoprim- sulfamethoxazole.
    (b) Chest physiotherapy & postural drainage.
    (c) Hydration; bronchodilators are used in bronchospasms, oxygen is used in hypoxia.
    (d) Treatment for sinusitis, if necessary.
    (e) Prophylaxis: Annual influenza vaccines.
    (f) Rarely, surgery for massive hemoptysis.
    (g) If unfit for surgery, then bronchial artery embolization.
    (h) Lung transplantation for end-stage disease.

53. **Most common malignant lung tumor**: **Brochogenic carcinoma**.
    Two subgroups are –**Non-small cell lung cancer (NSCLC, most common type-75%),** small cell lung cancer (SCLC,20%). **NSCLC includes**

adenocarcinoma (35%), squamous cell carcinoma (30%), and large cell carcinoma (10%).

54. **Most common cause of cancer death in both males and females**: **Lung cancer** (28% of all cancers).

55. **Most common type of lung cancer with tobacco smoking**: **SCLC**.

56. **Mechanism of producing cancer by the tobacco smoking**:
    (a) It contains active carcinogens.
    (b) It contains procarcinogens.
    (c) Mutations (transversions versus transitions) in oncogenes and tumor suppressor genes.*Passive smoke exposure also increases lung cancer.

57. **Genetic susceptibility to lung cancer**:
    (a) Major antosomal gene has been indentified. It is inversely correlated with age of lung cancer patients.
    (b) Proto-oncogenes.
    (c) Tumor suppressor genes.
    (d) Genes encoding enzymes.
    (e) Two P-450 isoenzyme are CYP2D6 & CYP1A1.

58. **Environmental carcinogens causing lung cancer**:
    (a) Asbestos.
    (b) Radon.
    Others are chromium, arsenic, nickel, etc.

59. **Protection of lung cancers by the following**:
    (a) 13-cis-retinoic acid.
    (b) Vitamin A.
    (c) β-carotene.
    (d) Vitamin C.
    (e) Vitamin E.
    (f) Selenium.
    Vitamin A and its derivatives have effects on differentiation of respiratory epithelium.

60. **Risk of lung cancer in chronic obstructive pulmonary disease (COPD):** Increases even without smoking.

61. **Sex and lung cancer**: Male > Female, black males have the highest incidence of lung cancer.

62. **Genetic abnormalities with lung cancer**:
    (a) Rb and p53 genes mutaion: Tumors suppressor genes found in both SCLC and NSCLC.
    (b) Chromosome 3p, 5q, 9p, 11p, 13q, 17p deletions; p53 overexpression has poor prognosis.

63. **Type of cells and lungs cancer**:
    Type II cell is the stem cell of alveolar epithelium. It proliferates and causes lung cancer.

64. **Increase of bioactive peptides directly, increases lung cancer**: Bioactive peptides are derived from pulmonary neuroendocrine cells. **Bioactive peptides are bombesin-like peptides and calcitonin gene-related peptides are growth factors for bronchial epithelial cells**. Tobacco smoke may increase bombesin like peptides. Other growth factors are derived from inflammatory and epithelial cells may increase in tobacco smoking.

65. A 50 year old male smoker appears with **H/O** new productive cough with thin secretion and hemoptysis. Occasionally, secretion has a **salty flavor (classical presentation of bronchoalveolar carcinoma).**
    Physican examination: Unilateral wheezing.
    CXR: Mass, atelactasis, or cavity.
    Most likely diagnosis: **Local lung cancer**.
    A 55 year old male smoker appears with **H/O** chest pain, dyspnea, and irregular heart beat.
    Physical examination: Cardiac tamponade.
    CXR: Pleural effusion.
    Diagnosis confirmed: Fiberoptic bronchoscopic biopsy.
    Most likely diagnosis: Local invasion of lung cancer.
    Superior vena cava (SVC) syndrome: Blockage of SVC, either by tumor or thrombus, causes facial suffusion & swelling.
    Horner's syndrome: Unilateral facial anhidrosis, ptosis, and miosis due to disruption of cervical sympathetic nerves.
    Pancoast syndrome: Shoulder and arm pain with or without Horner's syndrome due to tumor in apex and superior sulcus of the lung.
    Hoarseness: Due to recurrent laryngeal nerve involvement either directly or through the malignant lymph nodes.

66. A 60 year old male smoker can appear with signs and symptoms of metastasis of lung cancer to the brain, adrenal, liver, bone, skin and cervical - supraclavicular lymph nodes.
Rarely, patient appears with paraneoplastic syndromes which has six categories: Systemic, neurologic, endocrine, renal, cutaneous, and hematologic.

67. A large number of patients, with H/O tobacco smoking appears completely asymptomatic.
CXR: Solitary pulmonary nodule < 6 cm in diameter. Rest of the lungs are normal.
Most likely diagnosis: Lung cancer.
Diagnosis: Flexible fiberoptic bronchoscopic biopsy.
Treatment: It should begin as soon as possible because the cure rate is high in this presentation.

68. **Most important radiologic study in lung cancer**: **CXR**. Try to compare with the old chest X-ray. If the lesion doubles < 6 weeks or > 18 months time, then it strongly suggest a benign condition. Heavy calcifications particularly in popcorn, solid, or concentric pattern also suggests a benign condition but carcinoma can present adjacent to calcified granuloma.
CT scan of lungs, liver and adrenal: To look for sites of metastasis and enlarged lumph nodes in the lungs.
MRI: It is useful to detect the matastasis in the mediastinum, spinal cord, and vertebrae.

69. **Pathological diagnosis of lung cancer**:
Least invasive: Sputum cytology, good for central pulmonary lesions only.
Noninvasive: Pleural fluid cytology, skin and lymph nodes (cervical & supraclavicular) biopsies.
Invasive:
(a) **Flexible fiberoptic bronchoscopy is widely practiced because** it allows visualization of all the central, lobar, segmental, & subsegmental airways. It is done in awake patients with sedation, has low morbidity, and mortality. Sensitivity of the test is approximately 95% but for peripheral lesions, 60-70%.
(b) **Needle biopsy under fluoroscopic or CT guidance**: Sensitivity of the test is 90-95%. It is good for the lesions that lie close to visceral pleura.
(c) **Cervical medinoscopy**: Appropriate for the patients with mediastinal **lymph nodes** enlargement.

(d) **Thoracotomy with biopsy**: Appropriate for the patients with strong suspicion of malignancy.

70. **Preoperative pulmonary function tests in patients with lung cancer**: **FEV_1< 800 to 1000 ml** indicates poor postoperative outcome. Loss of lung tissues are directly proportional to loss of FEV_1(forced expiratory volume in 1 second). **High CO_2 indicates** bad prognosis but low O_2 is not a strong indicator for poor outcome.

71. **NSCLC staging**:

Tumor

TO	No Tumor.
TX	No tumor, positive cytology.
TIS	Carcinoma in situ.
T1	Tumor < 3 cm diameter, no visceral pleural, or lobar bronchial involvement.
T2	Tumor < 3 cm diameter, visceral pleural, or > 2 cm from carina.
T3	Direct extension to pleura, chest wall, or < 2 cm from carina.
T4	Invades great vessels, heart, trachea, esophagus, vertebrae, or malignant pleural effusion.

Nodes

N0	No involvement.
N1	Ipsilateral hilar or peribronchial.
N2	Ipsilateral mediastinal or subcarinal nodes.
N3	Contralateral mediastinal or hilar nodes;any supraclavicular or scalene nodes.

Metastasis

N0	None.
M1	Any.

72. **SCLC staging**:
   (a) Limited: Tumor confined to chest plus supraclavicular nodes, but excluding cervical and axillary nodes.
   (b) Extensive: Tumor beyond the above confines.

73. **Most important preventing measure against lung cancer**:
   (a) To avoid smoking actively and passively.
   (b) Chemoprevention with retinoic acid derivatives, carotenoids, vitamin E, vitamin C, and selenium **are experimental**.

74. **Treatment for lung cancer**: **(chemotherapy: CT, radiotherapy: RT)**.

(A) **Small cell lung cancer.**

(a) Limited stage (good performance status): Combination CT + Chest RT.

(b) Extensive stage (good performance status): Combination CT.

(c) Complete tumor responders (all stages): Prophylactic cranial RT.

(d) Poor-performance-status patients (all stages): Modified-dose combination CT, palliative RT.

(B) **Non-small cell lung cancer.**

(a) **Resectable (stages I, II, IIIa, and selected T3, N2 lesions):** Surgery, postoperative radiotherapy for N_2 disease. Radiotherapy for nonoperable patients.

(b) **Nonresectable (N2 and M1).**

(i) Confined to chest: High dose chest RT.

(ii) Outside the chest: RT to symptomatic local sites; CT for good-performance-status patients, with evaluable lesions.

(C) **All patients**.

(a) To stop smoking tobacco.

(b) To treat other medical problems.

(c) RT for CNS metastasis, weight-bearing bony lesions, symptomatic local lesions such as obstructed airways, nerve paralysis, and hemoptysis in non-small cell lung cancer. **Small cell cancers are unresponsive to CT**.

75. **Prognosis for lung cancer:** Depends on the staging but overall prognosis is poor.

76. **Most common etiology of asthma**: **Unknown**. It is an inflammatory condition that includes a number of distinct disease entities. It shows hyperresponsiveness to foreign stimuli.

77. **Pathogenesis of asthma**:

(a) **Airway smooth muscles constriction** due to local release of bioactive mediators or neurotransmitter is **the most accepted phenomenon.**

(b) Thickening of the airway epithelium.

(c) Presence of free liquids within the bronchial lumen.

78. **Acute asthmatic response is due to**:

(a) Acetylcholine (airway constrictor): It constricts airway smooth muscles by **directly stimulating muscarinic receptors of the M3 subtype**. It is **released from intrapulmonary motor nerves.**

(b) Leukotrienes (airway constrictor) LTB4, produced by polymorphonuclear leukocytes, is a chemoattractant molecule. **LTC4 and LTD4, contractile**

agonists, cause bronchial constrictions. LTC4, LTD4, LTE4, and LTB4 are derived from arachidonic acid by lipooxygenation. Arachidonic acid is produced from epithelial cell membrane phospholipids during cellular activation. Mast cells, alveolar macrophages, and eosinophils have the capacity to produce leukotrienes. Leukotrienes synthesis inhibitors or receptor antagonists are effective in exercise & aspirin induced asthma.

(c) Neuropeptides (airway constrictor): When the nerves are excited neuropeptides, substance P and neurokinin A (substance K) are released from secretary nerves. They induce constriction of airways through NK1 and NK2 receptors respectively.

(d) Nitric oxide (airway dilator): It is produced by airway epithelial cells and inflammatory cells in asthma. Paradoxically high level of free nitric oxide ($NO^{\bullet}$) forms toxic oxidation product ($OONO^{-}$) which damages the airway epitheliums.

(e) Histamine, kinins, and platelet activating factor (PAF): Unimportant in asthma.

79. **Response of airways in asthma:**In the beginning of an asthma attack, all airways constrict but during reversal, larger airways dilate before the smaller airways.

80. **Pathological responses in asthma:** Mucosal changes include **edema, hyperemia**, infiltration of mast cells, eosinophils, and lymphocytes bearing TH_2 phenotype. Those cells produce **IL-3, IL-4, IL-5, and granulocyte-macrophage colony stimulating factor**, thereby increase the production of **IgE**. Deposition of type III & type V collagen in the lamina propria of the airway wall.

81. **Tachypnea in asthma is due to:** Stimulation of intrapulmonary receptors causing stimulation of central respiratory centers. It is **not** due to changes in ABG (arterial blood gas).

82. **Different types of asthma:**
Intrinsic asthma: Unknown cause.
Exercise-induced asthma: It is caused by exercise.
Aspirin-induced asthma: It is caused by aspirin.
Occupational asthma: It is caused by an offending environment. Elimination of an offending environment does not reduce the asthma attack immediately. Sometimes it takes years to get better or remain asthmatic forever.

83. **ABG in asthma:**

↓O_2 ↓CO_2. In asthma patients, when **CO_2 is normal with moderate to severe airflow obstruction** that indicates mechanical load on the respiratory system and subsequent respiratory failure. ABG is **not** done in mild asthma attacks.

84. **Lung function tests in asthma**:
All ↓[peak expiratory flow rate (PEFR), forced expiratory volume in the first second (FEV_1), maximal midexpiratory flow rate (MMEFR)] **except** ↑total lung-capacity (TLC) and ↑residual volume (RV).

85. **CXR in asthma**: In **mild to moderate** asthma, CXR is **not** needed unless there are adventitious sounds in addition to wheezing. In **severe asthma, CXR is needed** to R/O any other complication like pneumothorax and pneumomediastinum.

86. **Sputum findings in asthma**: Colored sputum does **not** always mean infection. Asthma patients may have clear or opaque sputum with a green or yellow tinge. So Gram-stain or Wrigt-stain should be done. Colored sputum could be due to eosinophil, Charcot-Leyden crystals (crystalized eosinophil, lysophospholipase), Curschmann's spirals (bronchiolar casts contain mucous and cells), or Creola bodies (airway epitheliums with cilia).

87. A 50 year old man appears with H/O dyspnea and tachypnea. Physical examination shows bilateral wheezing which is polyphonic (more than one pitch sound) in nature.
Diagnosis is made by: Rapid response to bronchodilator therapy.
Treatment for asthma in general:
(a) **Bronchodilators**:
   (i) Inhaled β-adrenergic agents are the principal therapy.
   (ii) Theophylline: It is used **only** in patients using inhaled steroids in order to prevent future use of oral steroids.
(b) Anti-inflammatory agents:
   (i) **Systemic corticosteroids**: Steroid "pulse" with prednisone; methylprednisolone in life-threatening condition.
   (ii) **Inhaled corticosteroids**: Oral thrush is a major complication. It is used in moderate to severe asthma along with bronchodilators.
   (iii) **Disodium chromoglycate**: It is a mast cell membrane-stabilizing agent which is used in prophylaxis for asthma.

88. A 60 year old man using consistently four or more treatments of β- adrenergic agent per day.
Diagnosis: Moderate asthma.

Treatment: Add inhaled steriod.

89. **Treatment for asthma in the emergency room**:
   (a) PEFR or FEV_1 is <40% + clinical condition is **not** life threatening: Inhaled β_2 agonist and IV aminophylline (dosage should be determined by previous treatment status): If no improvement, then give IV steriod + repeat inhalation treatment in 20 minutes until PEFR or FEV_1 is >40% of the predicted value. If no improvement, then admit the patient for further treatment.
   (b) PEFR or FEV_1 is >60%: Only inhaled β_2 agonist in the ER (emergency room) then advise the patient to take β_2 agonist + inhaled steriod as an outpatient.
   (c) PEFR or FEV_1 is between 40-60%: Inhaled β_2 agonist +IV aminophylline initially, further treatment will depend upon the patients response of the therapy.

90. **Treatment for status asthmaticus**:
   (a) Oxygen (to acheive oxygen saturation values between 92-94%).
   (b) Inhaled β_2 agonist.
   (c) IV aminophylline (monitor the serum level).
   (d) IV steriod (high-dose).
   (e) If no improvement and $\uparrow CO_2$ then: Intubation and mechanical ventilation to achieve normal ABG ($Paco_2$ of 50 to 60 is acceptable in asthma).

91. A 50 year old women appear with respiratory distress which gets worse during supine position. Physical examination shows cyanosis and paradoxical movement of the abdomen.
   Diagnosis confirmed by: Measurement of **transdiaphragmatic pressure** with or without electromyographic recording. Fluroscopy is less reliable.
   Most likely diagnosis: Bilateral diaphragmatic paralysis.
   Treatment:
   (a) Ventilatory support.
   (b) In permanent paralysis: Diaphragmatic pacing.

92. **Most common cause of diaphragmatic paralysis in postoperative cardiac patients**: Phrenic nerve cooling.

93. **Diaphragmatic hernia**:
   (a) Traumatic: H/O injury, **CXR shows abdominal contents inside the chest which is confirmed by CT scan**. Treatment: Surgical repair.

(b) Weakness or impaired development of diaphragmatic muscles:Usually formed in middle-aged obese patients.
Treatment: Conservative.
(c) Congenital: Found in children.

94. **Most important muscle of respiration: Diaphragm.**

95. **Most important cause of diaphragmatic dysfunction**: Lung hyperinflation (asthma and COPD).

96. **Hoover's sign in COPD** (chronic obstructive pulmonary disease): **Inward deformities of the lower rib cage** in COPD is due to shortening of horizontal fibers of the diaphragm.

97. **Most common tumor causing unilateral diaphragmatic paralysis**: Bronchogenic carcinoma involves the phrenic nerve.

98. **Confirmatory study for unilateral diaphragmatic paralysis**: **Fluoroscopic findings** of paradoxical diaphragmatic movement on cough and sniff. Initial CXR shows elevation of diaphragm in one side. Patients are asymptomatic.

99. **Causes for bilateral diaphragmatic paralysis**:
(a) Cervical trauma (C3 to C5).
(b) Myopathies:
(i) Limited (localized to diaphragm): Due to collagen vascular disorder, acid maltase deficiency.
(ii) Generalized: Hypothyroidism, muscular dystrophy and polymyositis.
(c) Unknown.

100. Most common site of scoliosis causing chest wall **deformities**: **Dorsolumbar.** Scoliosis is a lateral angulation and rotation of the spine. It is more common in **right** than left.

101. **Cobb's angle in scoliosis**: Angle between upper and lower portion of the spinal curves which is found in X-ray.
<70^0 angle: **No** respiratory function difficulty is noted.
70-120^0 angle: May be **mild** difficulty in pulmonary function.
>120^0 angle: **Dyspnea and respiratory failure.**

102. **Kyphosis**: Anteroposterior angulation of the spine. It is a less serious condition.

103. **Treatment for Kyphoscoliosis**:

(a) Oxygen: If patient is hypoxic.
(b) Surgery: Traction, plasters, and rods.
(c) Ventilator management in respiratory failure.
(d) Bronchodilator for bronchospasms.
(e) Antibiotics for infections.
(f) Weight loss for obese.
(g) Stop smoking for tobacco smoker.

104. **Association between ankylosing spondylitis and respiratory condition**: **Upper lobe fibrosis** may develop in some patients. It is an inflammatory disease, result in fusion of vertebral and costotransverse joints, occasionally involves clavicular and sternomanubrial joints. Unlike kyphoscoliosis, **it does not cause corpulmonale and respiratory failure.**

105. **Cardiac abnormality in pectus excavatum**: **Mitral valve prolapse.** Pectus excavatum patients are usually asymptomatic but in some patients, cardiac output may not increase appropriately during exercise. Treatment is cosmetic surgery.

106. **Fibrothorax**: It may be a primary disease of the chest wall resulting from pulmonary diseases (hemothorax or asbestosis).
Treatment: Same as kyphoscoliosis. Sometimes pleurectomy is needed.

107. **Most frequent cause of 'Flail chest'**: **Accidental trauma in the chest** and/or after CPR (cardiopulmonary resuscitation) Flail chest is due to double fractures of three or more adjacent ribs or combined sternal and rib fractures.
Treatment for flail chest.

(a) Oxygen for hypoxia, clear airways.
(b) Ventilator for respiratory failure.
(c) Antibiotic for infection.
(d) Chest fixation for **large** flail chest.

108. **Frictions between the lung and chest wall are reduced by**: Glycoprotein rich in hyaluronic acid is secreted by mesothelial cells of the pleura.

109. **Hydrostatic pressures in pleuras**:
Visceral pleura: 10 cm H_2O (depends on pulmonary circulation).
Parietal pleura: 30 cm H_2O (depends on systemic circulation).
Oncotic pressures in both pleurae are the same (25 cm H_2O).

110. **Pleural effusion and CXR view: Lateral decubitus film is the best way**. It can detect as little as 150 cc of pleural fluid. Posteroanterior view **can miss** up to 300 cc of pleural fluid.

111. **Radiologic appearance of pseudotumor in pleural effusion**: **It is due to loculation of pleural fluid in the interlober fissure, mostly in the minor fissure.**

112. Preferred investigative procedures in order to know the pulmonary abnormalities in pleural effusion: **Ultrasonography or CT scan**.

113. **Criteria for exudative pleural fluid**: (At least one of three criteria)-
   (a) Pleural fluid/serum protein ratio > 0. 5
   (b) Pleural fluid/serum LDH ratio < 0.6
   (c) Pleural fluid LDH greater than two thirds of serum LDH.

114. **Criteria of transudative pleural fluid**:
   (a) Pleural fluid/serum protein ratio < 0.5
   (b) Pleural fluid/serum LDH ratio < 0.6
   (c) Pleural fluid/serum glucose ratio 1.0

115. **Absolute values of pleural fluid**:

	Transudate	Exudate
Protein	<3 gm/dl	>3 gm/dl
LDH	<200 IU/L	>200 IU/L
WBC count	<1000	>1000
Glucose	>60 mg/dL	<60 mg/dL.

116. **Therapeutic thoracocentesis and hypoxia**: 50% of the patients will have lower Pao_2 up to 20 mm Hg. Other complications are pain, infection, pneumothorax, bleeding, and puncture of the liver and spleen.

117. **Thoracocentesis in pleural effusion**:
   (a) Diagnostic: 30 to 50 ml of fluids are needed.
   (b) Therapeutic: Up to 1000 to 1500 ml of fluids can be removed.
   Newly discovered pleural effusion should be tapped. A thoracocentesis is diagnostic in 75% of patients and it is an extremely helpful procedure to exclude empyema.

118. **Pleural fluids and different diagnosis**:
   (a) Bloody **fluids** (without trauma): Malignancy, pulmonary embolism causing infarction.
   (b) White **fluids**: Chyle, cholesterol, lymphoma.
   (c) Black **fluids**: Aspergillosis.
   (d) Yellow-green **fluids**: Rheumatoid pleurisy.
   (e) Putrid odor: Anaerobic empyema.
   (f) Ammonia odor: Urinothorax.
   (g) ↑Polymorph WBC: Bacterial infection.
   (h) ↑Lymphocyte: Lymphoma, leukemic effusion.
   (i) ↑Lymphocyte but ↓mesothelial cells: TB (tuberculosis).
   (j) ↑Eosinophil: Nonspecific, long standing fluid.

119. **Indication for percutaneous pleural biopsy**: To differentiate between malignancy and TB in a patient whose exudative pleural fluid shows ↑lymphocytes.

120. **Most common cause of transudative pleural effusion**: **Congestive heart failure is** due to biventricular failure with venous hypertension. In chronic heart failure for months may increase the total protein >3 gm/dl.

121. **Pleural fluid accumulates by different mechanisms in the different disease condition**:
   (a) Pneumonia: Increased permeability of the microvascular circulation.
   (b) Congestive heart failure: Increased hydrostatic pressure in microvascular circulation.
   (c) Hypoalbuminemia: Decreased oncotic pressure in microvascular circulation.
   (d) Lung collapse: Decreased pressure in the pleural cavity.
   (e) Cancer and trauma: Decreased lymphatic drainage from the pleural cavity.
   (f) Ascites: Migration of fluids from peritoneal cavity.

122. Most common cause of exudative pleural effusion: Pneumonia or lung abscess.

123. **Types of exudative pleural effusion: Two**

Complicated	Uncomplicated
(a) ph <7.20	>7.30
(b) Polymorph >100,000 per cubic (severely increased) millimeter	Moderately increased
(c) LDH >1000	<500

(d) Glucose <40 g/dl	same as blood
Positive Gram-stain & culture	Negative

124. **Complication of poorly treated empyema**: Bronchopleural and bronchopleurocutaneous fistulas.
Treatment: Surgery (open drainage, resection of ribs, decortication, and reconstruction).

125. **Most common location of the upper abdominal abscess: Subphrenic**.

126. Boerhaave's syndrome: It is due to **spontaneous** esophageal rupture. **Most common cause of esophageal rupture** is **due to endoscopy or esophageal dilatation.** Esophageal rupture can occur with foreign body or trauma.

127. **Esophageal rupture**: Patients appear with fever, dyspnea, chest pain, and dysphagia.
Physical examination: Subcutaneous emphysema.
Diagnosis confirmed: Barium sulfate or water soluble compound.
Study of exudate:
(a) Early:↑polymorph, then ↑salivary amylase.
(b) Late: pH 6.0, presence of anaerobic mouth organisms.
Treatment:
(a) Surgery: Repair.
(b) Medical: Antibiotics to cover anaerobe, parenteral nutrition, drainage of mediastinum and pleura.

128. **Serous pleural effusion in primary pulmonary tuberculosis (TB) is due to: Hypersensitivity** phenomenon. It occurs in 66% of patients within 5 years.

129. **Second form of pleural effusion in subpleural TB ruptures into pleural space**:
Pleural fluids consist of **protein >4 gm/dl**, **low** glucose (rarely lower than 20 mg/dL), pH, between 7.00 and 7.30(**pH >7.40 excludes the TB**), increase leukocytes 5000 cells (90-95% **lymphocytes;** in the beginning, there is increase in polymorph), adenosine deaminases and lysozymes are present.
Signs & symptoms: **Fever, non-productive cough, chest pain, and tachypnea.**
Diagnosis of TB:
(a) Multiple samples from a closed pleural biopsy: (+) in 50 to 80%.
(b) Positive culture: 30% to70%.
(c) Positive acid fast stain: <10%.

(d) ELISA or PCR: To detect the mycobacterial antigen.
(e) Positive PPD (intermediate-strength): 70%.

Treatment:
(a) Antituberculous medications.
(b) Short-term corticosteriod may be used in seriously ill patients.

130. **Response to antituberculous treatment**: Fever disappears in 2 weeks (maximum 8 weeks). Effusion disappears in 6 weeks (maximum 16 weeks).

131. **Most common cause of chylothorax**: **Throracic duct lymph (chyle) leakages are** due to **mediastinal lymphoma (50%). Others are** thoracic surgery (20%) and truama (5%).

132. **Best way to diagnose chyle:** Triglyceride >110 mg/dL (rarely between 50-110 mg/dL).

133. **Yellow-nail syndrome-triad of lymphatic drainage abnormalities**: Lymphedema, slowly growing yellow nails, and pleural effusion. It is due to either hypoplasia or dilation of lymphatics.

134. **Meig's syndrome: Triad**.
Benign fibroma (or other ovarian tumor), right sided pleural effusion, and ascites. It is found mostly in postmenopausal women with H/O increased abdominal circumference & chest pain. Fluids move from abdomen into the chest through small diaphragmatic defects or lymphatics.
Diagnosis by: CT scan.
Treatment: Removal of the tumor resolves the effusion within 2-3 weeks.

135. **Pleural effusion in uremia: Bloody exudate.**

136. **Most frequent cause of exudative pleural effusion after 60 years of age**: Invasion of lung cancer.

137. **Most frequent mechanism of pleural effusion in breast cancer**: Breast cancer metastasis to liver then spreads further or the invasion of lymphatics in the chest wall.

138. **Composition of exudative pleural fluid due to cancer:**

RBC:	30,000 to 50,000/ml
Lymphocytes:	>50%
pH:	<7.30

Glucose: <60mg/dL
Positive cytology: 60%
Positive biopsy: 70%(only)

139. **Prognosis for malignant pleural effusion**: Poor except in breast cancer and small cell cancer of the lung.

140. **Most common cause of malignant mesothelioma**: Asbestos (80 to 90% cases).

141. A 50 year old man, with H/O exposure to asbestos, appears with dyspnea, weight loss, cough, and chest pain.
CXR: Pleural effusion.
Pleural fluid: Bloody, pH <7.30.
Diagnosis: ↑Level of hyaluronic acid in pleural fluid; special stain, and electronmicroscopic study of biopsy tissue.
Most likely diagnosis: Malignant mesothelioma.
Differential diagnosis: Benign mesothelioma is large, pedunculated and has histology of fibroma.
Treatment: Surgical removal of the mass.
Prognosis: Poor.
Associated findings are: Clubbing and pulmonary osteoarthropathy.

142. A 25 year old man, appears with H/O right sided chest pain, cough, and difficulty in breathing. Patient denies H/O trauma.
CXR: Right sided pneumothorax with expiratory or lateral decubitus film (viseral pleural line is noted).
Diagnosis: Simple pneumothorax.
Treatment: Right sided chest tube.

143. **Recurrence rate of simple pneumothorax**: **30% in the same side** and 10% in the opposite side.

144. **Tension pneumothorax**: It is due to increased positive pressure through a "ball-valve" mechanism.
Small size (<20%): Only observation, resolves within 1 to 2 weeks.
Large pneumothorax: Chest tube; air aspiration.
Recurrent pneumothorax: Chemical pleurodesis or surgical repairs may be needed.

145. **Most common cause of secondary pneumothorax**: Emphysema. Other causes are trauma, pulmonary diseases, insertion of central lines, barotrauma, and rarely Ehlers-Danlos syndrome and Marfan syndrome.

146. **Most common presentation for mediastinal masses**: Asymptomatic. Other symptoms are chest pain, cough, dyspnea, & hoarseness.

147. **Investigation for mediastinal masses**:
CXR: Initially detect the masses.
CT scan: Initial procedure of choice.
Mediastinoscopy or mediastinotomy: It is performed for anterior and middle compartment lesions.
Thoracotomy: May be necessary for middle and posterior compartment lesions. It is also therapeutic for surgical removal of the mass.

148. **Different specific presentations in different mediastinal masses:**
(a) Myasthenia gravis: Thymoma.
(b) Hypercalcemia: Parathyroid tumors.
(c) Hypoglycemia: Mesotheliomas, teratomas, fibrosarcomas.
(d) Neurologic symptoms: Neurogenic tumors.

149. **Most common cause of mediastinal masses in young adults**:
(a) Anterior: Thymoma (20% of all mediastinal tumors).
(b) Middle: Lymphoma (Hodgkin).
(c) Posterior: Benign neurogenic tumors (**neurilemoma, neurofibroma, and ganglioneuroma**).

150. **Most common cause of mediastinal mass in older patients**: Metastatic bronchogenic carcinoma.

151. **Treatment for neurogenic mediastinal tumors**:
(a) Removal of the masses.
(b) Postoperative radiation for neuroblastomas.

152. **Treatment for thymoma**: (66% of all thymomas are malignant).
(a) Surgical resection.
(b) Followed by radiotherapy.

153. **Most common presentation for thymoma**: Myasthenia gravis (40%).

154. **Prognosis for lymphatic tumors**:

(a) Best prognosis: Hodgkin lymphomas.
(b) Worse prognosis: Non-Hodgkin lymphomas, angiomatous lymphoid hamartomas, plasmacytomas.

155. **Teratomas:**
(a) Found in anterior mediastinum.
(b) 33% are malignant.
(c) Cystic teratomas are frequently found.

156. **Most common type of diaphragmatic hernia**: **Through the esophageal hiatus**. Others are through the foramen of Bochdalek (posterolateral) and formen of Morgagni (retrosternal).

157. **Most common cause of superior vena cava (SVC) syndrome**: Bronchogenic carcinoma.

158. **SVC syndrome**: Symptoms: Dyspnea, dysphagia, wheezes, and headache.
Signs: Edema and congestion of the face; dilatation of collateral veins in the upper chest and neck.

159. **Benign causes of SVC syndrome**:
(a) Aortic aneurysm.
(b) Retrosternal thyroid (enlarged).

160. **Diagnosis of SVC syndrome**: Chest CT scan/MRI. **No invasive procedures are allowed because of dilated blood vessels**.

161. **Treatment for SVC syndrome with malignancy**: Irradiation and chemotherapy should be started before mediastinal tissue biopsy. Attempt should be made to get tissues from somewhere else.

162. **Causes of pneumomediastinum:**
(a) Patients are on ventilator: Alveolar rupture.
(b) Trauma: Rupture of esophagus or tracheobronchial tree.

163. **Pneumomediastinum**: Symptoms: Chest pain and dyspnea.
Signs: Subcutaneous emphysema with crepitus.
Hamman's sign: Crunching sound synchronus with heart beat on auscultation. Normal cardiac activity.
Diagnosis: Lateral CXR.
Treatment:

(a) Simple or mild: Resolves spontaneously.
(b) Traumatic or severe: Surgical repair and drainage.

164. **Nasal polyps are associated with**:
(a) Cystic fibrosis.
(b) Aspirin-sensitive asthma.

165. **Most common organisms for acute otitis media**:
(a) Streptococcus pneumoniae.
(b) Hemophilus influenzae.
Treatment: Antibiotics.

166. **Most common cause for serous otitis media**: Failure to clear fluid from middle clear.
Treatment: Antihistamines and decongestants.

167. **Most common cause for chronic otitis media**: Eustachian tube obstruction.
Treatment: Drainage of the tube, antibiotics for infections, antihistamines, & decongestants, if needed.

168. **Complications of otitis media**:
(a) Mastoiditis, osteomyelitis, basal skull structure's infection, brain abscess, meningitis,& dural abscess.
(b) Facial palsy.
Treatment: Antibiotics, drainage of abscess, surgery for inner-ear problems.
(c) Fungal infections for immunocompromised hosts (aspergillus and candida).
Treatment: Antifungal medication.

169. **Otitis externa**:
Symptoms: Severe pain and discharge from the external ear canal.
Signs: Ear and tragus are painful to touch.
Most common organism: Pseudomonas.
Diagnosis: By clinical findings, **no culture is needed.**
Treatment:
(a) Topical antibiotics + topical corticosteriods.
(b) Oral antibiotics are used in cellulitis, erythema, or lymphadenitis.

170. **Malignant otitis externa**: It is a serious otitis externa infections found in diabetes and immunocompromised host. It can involve the following cranial

nerves, VII, IX, X, XI; can infect the jugular vein, middle ear, mastoid, and temporobandibular joint.

Treatment.

(a) IV antibiotics (**broadspectrum**).

(b) Surgery.

171. **Swimmer's ear**: Otitis externa occurs after swimming due to **exposure to water.**

Treatment: Ear drops containing alcohol + glycerine mixture.

172. **Most common cause of acute rhinitis**: Common cold.

173. **Most common cause of sinusitis**: Complication from common cold or other URI (upper respiratory infections) or from periodontal infections below the maxillary sinus.

Most common organism: Streptococcus pneumoniae and hemophilus influenzae.

Treatment:

(a) Acute: Antibiotics, antihistamines, & decongestants.

(b) Chronic and unresponsive to above treatment: Surgery.

174. **Most common organism in fungal sinusitis which occurs rarely: Aspergillus**. Other funguses are Candida, Penicillium, and Mucor.

175. **Most common nonmalignant tumor of the jaw**: Epulis (granulomatous and fibrous tissue growth).

176. **Ludwig's angina**: It is a bacterial infection causing painful swelling of the anterior floor of the mouth, dysphagia, and drooling.

Treatment: IV antibiotics, corticosteriod, surgery.

Complications: Respiratory obstruction is due to rapid progression.

177. **Complication from periodontal abscess**: Infections can spread along the tissue planes to the neck, mediastinum, and basal structure of the skull. Abscess is formed due to poor dental status, diabetes, trauma, immunocompromised hosts and the elders.

178. **A 57 year old man appears with jaw swelling:**

(a) **Swelling with H/O trauma:** R/O fracture.

(b) **Swelling without H/O trauma but no pain:** R/O bony or soft tissues tumor (epulis, cyst, osteoma, ameloblastoma,& malignant epithelioma).

(c) **Swelling (bilateral) of the mandible**: R/O Paget's disease, osteitis fibrosa due to hyperparathyroidism, leontiasis ossea (rare condition with enlargement of the jaw with **normal** hands & feet).

(d) **Swelling without H/O trauma with pain and fever:**
  (i) Ludwig's angina.
  (ii) Infections of the salivary glands.
  (iii) Infections of the lymph nodes.

179. **Pain in the lower jaw without swelling:**
  (a) Dental caries, periodontal disease, or otomandibular syndrome (temporomandibular dysfunction).
  (b) **Cardiac angina is the most important** in differential diagnosis.

180. **Pain along the distribution of VII cranial nerve**:
  (a) Herpes zoster involves **division I** of VII cranial nerve.
  (b) Trigeminal neuralgia involves **division II** more than I or III.

181. **Most common cause of acute onset of hoarseness**: Bacterial or viral infection. Other causes are overuse and irritants (smoke or fumes).
  Treatment:
  (a) Treat the infection with antibiotics.
  (b) Avoid the irritants.
  (c) Do **not** use corticosteriod: It can enhance irritation and infection.

182. A 50 year old man appears with **H/O** hoarseness for 2 to 3 weeks; initial investigation of choice: Direct examination of the laryngeal structures.

183. A 40 year old woman appears with **H/O** hoarseness. She had thyroid/parathyroid surgery done few years ago.
  Most likely diagnosis: Recurrent laryngeal nerve paralysis.

184. **Associated medical conditions with snoring**: Apnea, hypertension, myocardial infarction, and stroke.

185. **Snoring**: It occurs in deep sleep. It is produced by vibrations of the soft tissues of the nasopharynx due to turbulant flow of air through the narrowed airway.
  Diagnosis: By history.
  Treatment.
  (a) Symptomatic for the bed partner.
  (b) Medical: Weight loss, nasal decongestants medication to reduce upper airway inflammation.

(c) Surgery: Uvulopalatopharyngoplasty.

186. A 36 year old woman appears with H/O recent onset of snoring with or without dry skin and sleepiness:
Mostly likely diagnosis: **Hypothyroidism.**
Hypothyroidism should be ruled out with anybody with recent onset of snoring.

187. **Most common cause of death in pneumonia and COPD: Respiratory failure.**

188. **Types of acute and chronic respiratory failure**:
(a) Hypoxic respiratory failure (HRF).
(b) Hypercapnic-hypoxic respiratory failure (HHRF).

189. **Hypoxic respiratory failure (HRF):** It is defined as severe arterial hypoxemia (Pao_2 <50 mm Hg) that cannot be corrected by increasing the inspired oxygen concentration to >50%(FIO_2 >0.5). Hypoxemia is due to the large right-to-left intrapulmonary shunt which is approximately between 25 to 50%. At a Pao_2 level of 50 mm Hg, hemoglobin is 80% saturated and a further **small reduction Pao_2 will significantly reduce oxygen content**.

190. **Hypercapnic-hypoxic respiratory failure (HHRF):** It is defined as a life-threatening condition with inadequate CO_2 excretion (↑$Paco_2$) is due to hypoventilation. (Examples are COPD, drug overdose, neuromuscular weakness).

191. **Mechanisms of hypercapnia in different conditions:**
(a) Airflow obstruction: COPD, asthma.
(b) Normal lungs: Overdose of sedative drugs, neuromuscular weakness.

192. **In HHRF, what values of $Paco_2$ defined as respiratory failure?:** It depends on the precipitating condition and previous condition of the patient.
(a) Asthma, drug overdose, or neuromuscular weakness: $Paco_2$ >45 mm Hg is considered significant.
(b) COPD with previous normal $Paco_2$ values: $Paco_2$>55 mm Hg is considered as respiratory failure.

193. **Mechanisms of hypoxemia in HHRF**:
(a) COPD, asthma: Perfusion of poorly ventilated lungs. There is a mismatch of ventilation-perfusion (V/P). $Paco_2$ 58+Pao_2 42=100 mm Hg.

194. **Alveolar-arterial O_2 gradient in pure hypoventilation**: A-a O_2 gradient is not increased in hypoxemia due to pure hypoventilation. So, hypoxemia is corrected by modestly increasing FIO_2 which displaces nitrogen.

195. Depressed mental status in acute hypercapnea (↑$Paco_2$) is due to: Low CSF (cerebrospinal fluid) pH (**not** due to ↑CO_2 level). CO_2 diffuses rapidly through blood-brain barrier. (**Important for board exam**).

196. **Causes of hypoxic respiratory failure**: ARDS, pneumonia, atelactasis, pulmonary emboli, pulmonary hemorrhage, and cardiogenic pulmonary edema.
Important points to remember in respiratory failure:
In **elderly patients the most common cause of respiratory failure is cardiogenic pulmonary edema** (mortality is 40%). Respiratory failure due to cardiopulmonary arrest has the **highest mortality** (80%). Respiratory failure **due to drug overdose** has the **best prognosis (survival 95%)** or **least mortality**. Least common cause of respiratory failure in elderly is **asthma** (<1%). More than one condition may be present simultaneously in respiratory failure in a large number of patients.

197. **Important points to remember for hypoxic respiratory failure:**
    (a) At any age, past history of normal physical condition, hypertension, or **heart disease**.
    (b) H/O acute difficulty in breathing with present H/O accidental injury, sepsis, or chest pain.
    (c) Physical examination: Tachypnea (>35), tachycardia,↓BP, and diffuse crackles in the chest.
    (d) CXR: Small, white lungs; infiltrates, atelactasis, or consolidation.
    (e) ABG: **Respiratory alkalosis, metabolic acidosis.**
    (f) BUN: **Increased** but **normal** potassium.
    (g) EKG: Sinus tachycardia, LVH, or myocardial infarction.
    (h) **Hyperventilation** and increased right-to-left intrapulmonary shunt.

198. **Important points to remember for hypercapnic-hypoxic respiratory failure (e.g. COPD, drug overdose, neuromuscular weakness)**:
    (a) At any age, past H/O emphysema and bronchitis in elderly patients.
    (b) Past history of difficulty in breathing, wheezing or depression; recent H/O URI, drug overdose, or muscle weakness.
    (c) Physical examination: Tachypnea (>30); **tachycardia; decreased** breath sound; lower extremities edema; and altered level of consciousness.
    (d) CXR:

(i) COPD or asthma: Hyperinflated, large, black lungs with increased bronchovascular markings.
(ii) Drug overdose or neuromuscular weakness: Hypoinflated small black lungs.

(e) ABG: **Respiratory acidosis, mixed metabolic and respiratory acidosis.**
(f) BUN: **Normal** but **low potassium.**
(g) EKG: RVH, "P" pulmonale, normal, or low voltage.
(h) (i) COPD: Hypoventilation, ↑**A-a gradient,** V/P imbalance, normal, or increased minute ventilation.
(ii) Drug overdose or neuromuscular weakness: Hypoventilation,→**A-a gradient,↓minute ventilation (→ means normal, ↓ means decreased).**

199. In ARDS, relation between CXR findings and Pao_2 levels: **Very poor correlation** betwen Pao_2 levels, extravascular lung water, & radiographic densities.

200. **ARDS** (adult respiratory distress syndrome): This is due to acute lung injury in healthy people. Patients appear with tachypnea, profound shortness of breath, unresponsiveness with supplemental oxygen which result in severe hypoxemia (Pao_2/FIO_2 <200). ARDS has low pulmonary compliance (<40 ml of air/cm of H_2O; normal is 100 ml/cm of H_2O), and low thoracic gas volume suggests small functioning lungs.

201. **ARDS is mostly (80%) associated with**: Systemic infections, pulmonary infections, aspiration of gastric contents, or severe trauma. **ARDS is maximum in patients with septic shock or severe sepsis** (Important for board exam.).

202. **Most import pathogenetic mechanism in ARDS**: **Inflammatory response** to distant or local tissue injury (**Important for board exam**).

203. **First sign of hypoxia: Tachycardia** then tachypnea, anxiety, increased sweating, confusion, cyanosis,↑BP, then ↓BP,↓HR (heart rate), seizure, and lactic acidosis develop in order of progression.

204. **First sign of hypercapnea: Somnolence,** then lethargy, irritability, tremor, slurred speech, headache, asterixis, papilledema, and coma develop in order of progression.

205. **ARDS resolves rapidly in the following conditions**: Postictal, heroin overdose.

206. **Most likely mechanism of pulmomary endothelial damage in acute lung injury**: **Unknown.** It may be due to various cytokines. Initial damage of pulmonary epithelium then release of cytokines, arachidonic acid, and PAF (platelet activating factor). Then activation of complement, coagulation, and kinin. Neutrophils adhere to endothelial cells and then release free oxygen radicals and protease which damage the **endothelial cells** as well.

207. **Treatment for hypoxic respiratory failure**:
   - (a) **Not** effective: Corticosteroids, surfactants, and nonsteroidal anti-inflammatory agents.
   - (b) Free radical scavenger (experimental): Shows improvement in sepsis-induced ARDS.
   - (c) Most important management is supportive care: To maintain adequate Pao_2 and to avoid oxygen toxicity, barotrauma, fluid overload, infection, GI bleeding, thromboembolism, and malnutrition.
   - (d) Ventilator management:
     - (i) Physicians should use the ventilator settings with which they are comfortable with.
     - (ii) Ventilator settings are: $FIO_2 < 0.5$, respiratory rate 10-15/min (assist-control), PEEP <10 cm H_2O, tidal volume 6-8 ml/kg, flow rate >70 L/min, plateau pressure <35 cm H_2O end inspiration,& sensitivity: -0.5 to -1.5 cm H_2O. **It should be adjusted with ABG values**.
     - (iii) ABG does **not** have to be within the normal range, Pao_2 close to 55 mm Hg and $Paco_2$ 60-70 may be accepted if we can avoid lung over distension, oxygen toxicity, **air trapping, and circulatory compromise**.
     - (iv) **↑PEEP may improve oxygenation but excessive increase of PEEP decreases cardiac output due** to increase of intrathoracic pressure which results in hypoxia.
     - (v) Tidal volume should be low in ARDS because functioning lung volume is low.

208. **Prognosis of ARDS**:
   - (a) Survival is the lowest with MSOF (multi system organ failure, 30%).
   - (b) Survival is highest (85%) when ARDS is an isolated problem.

209. **Most common pulmonary outcome in postextubation patients of ARDS**: **Normal pulmonary functions**. Only few patients will have abnormal pulmonary functions.

210. **Measurement of lung overdistension in ICU (intensive care unit):** To measure end-inspiratory pressure. Lung overdistension damages the capillary wall causing pulmonary edema and also damages the alveoli causing pneumothorax & mediastinal emphysema.

211. A 70 year old man appears with chest pain, palpitation, & hypertension. He had a H/O heart attack in the past.
Physical examination: Elevated neck veins, peripheral edema, 3rd and 4th heart sounds, left ventricular enlargement, lift & heave.
CXR: Cardiomegaly, vascular pedicle (>53 mm), peribronchial and vascular congestion, Kerley lines (septal lines), and pleural effusion.
EKG: LVH, past and ongoing ischemic cardiac changes.
Pulmonary artery wedge pressure: >18 mm Hg.
Cardiac index: <3.5 L/min/m^2.
Most likely diagnosis: Cardiogenic pulmonary edema.

212. A 50 year old woman appears with shock or trauma. She has an unremarkable past medical history.
Physical examination: Hyperdynamic pulses, physiologic gallop, normal neck veins, & no edema.
CXR: Air bronchogram (80%), normal heart size, vascular pedicle<48 mm, and peripheral infiltrates.
EKG: Sinus tachycardia.
Pulmonary artery wedge pressure: <15 mm Hg. Cardiac index: >3.5 L/min/m^2.
Most likely diagnosis: Noncardiogenic pulmonary edema (ARDS).

213. Most common clinical presentations hypercapnic-hypoxic respiratory failure (HHRF): Lower respiratory disease (COPD, asthma). Both of them have severe ventilation-perfusion mismatch.

214. **Acute HHRF may be divided into the following categories**:
   (a) Ventilation-perfusion mismatch: COPD, asthma.
   (b) ↓Minute ventilation and ↑wasted ventilation: Ankylosing spondylitis, kyphoscoliosis, and obesity-hypoventilation syndrome.
   Clinical presentations in (a) and (b) are both similar.
   (c) ↓Minute ventilation (↑$Paco_2$): Upper airway diseases; metabolic disorders (↓pH, ↑pH, ↓p, ↓Mg, ↓k); neuromuscular diseases (trauma, tumor, myasthenia gravis, polyneuritis, polymyositis, **dermatomyositis, and Parkinson diseases**); and alteration of mental status (brain tumor, brain hemorrages with or without trauma, drug overdose, poison, and central hypoventilation).

215. Barbiturate and morphine overdoses: Barbiturate causes coma with normal $Paco_2$.Morphine causes moderate unconsciousness with increased $Paco_2\uparrow$.

216. **Most common precipitating event in COPD patients result in HHRF: Bronchospasm**. It is due to a change in weather, infection, or failure to take medications.

217. **Indication for assisted ventilation in HHRF**: When patients deteriorate with supplemental oxygen, brochodilators, antibiotics, appropriate fluids, and electrolytes. ABG values are **not** very important to make that decision. Patients with minor alteration of mental status, exhaustion, tachypnea (>36/minute), paradoxical thoracoabdominal respiratory movement, and excessive use of accessory muscles may require intubation.
Most patients improve with conservative therapy without ventilator support.

218. **Most important indication for early (<2 weeks) tracheostomy**:
Inadequate removal of copious and tenacious secretions through ET (endotracheal) tube. When patients require ET intubation more than 2 weeks, then tracheostomy is indicated.

219. **Ventilator management in HHRF**: Similar as discussed in HRF. Additional recommendation are as follows:
   (a) Correct respiratory acidosis by removal of $Paco_2$.
   (b) Stabilize alveolar ventilation once $Paco_2$ is normal.
   (c) Patients with known baseline elevated $Paco_2$, do not attempt to reduce the $Paco_2$.
   (d) Keep end-inspiratory plateau pressure <35 cm H_2O.
   (e) Measure end-expiratory alveolar pressure and to avoid air trapping, use lowest minute ventilation and longest expiratory to inspiratory time.

220. Therapy for acute HHRF with airway obstruction:
Drug of choice:
   (a) Albuterol which improves FEV_1 or peak flow.
   (b) Ipratropium: Drug of choice with cardiac arrythmias, slower onset of action than albuterol & no toxicity.
   (c) Theophylline: If patients do not improve with other drugs then use theophylline, keep serum level <15 mg/L.

221. **Therapy for acute HHRF with arrythmias:**

(a) Treat the respiratory failure.
(b) Correct alkalosis, k and Mg.
(c) Reduce theophylline or β_2-agonist.
(d) In SVT (supraventricular tachycardia): Cardizem, adenosine, or digoxin.
(e) Do **not** use β-blocker in asthma because it causes bronchospasm.

222. **Therapy for acute HHRF with thick secretion.**
(a) Treat infection with second-generation cephalosporin to kill **Streptococcus pneumoniae** and **Hemophilus influenzae**.
(b) Correct dehydration with 0.45 normal saline.
(c) Postural drainage, vibration, and percussion.

223. Therapy for acute HHRF in different conditions:
(a) Volume overload: Diuretics.
(b) Hypoxia: Oxygen to keep Pao_2>55 mm Hg.
(c) GI bledding: H_2 blocker.
(d) Prevention of deep venous thrombosis: Heparin.
(e) Hypokalemia: Kcl.
(f) Anti-inflammatory: Methylprednisone which also improves FEV_1.
(g) Agitation: Lorazepam is used only when a patient is on ventilator.

224. **Management of hypoxia in ARDS:**
(a) Keep the Pao_2 60 mm Hg and saturation 90%: Initially give 100% oxygen.
(b) In young patients, acceptable Pao_2 <60 mm Hg: Usually requires intubation.
(c) To prevent oxygen toxicity, try to keep FIO_2 <0.6 but increase the PEEP to recruit lung units.
(d) **Assisted ventilation to allow $Paco_2$ 60-70 mm Hg, sedation, rarely paralysis.**

225. **Management of ARDS in different conditions**:
(a) Hypotension: Fluid, vasoactive medications to keep the BP normal.
(b) Keep the cardiac index >3.5 $L/min/m^2$.
(c) Keep the hemoglobin >10 gm/dl.
(d) Fluid overload: Diuretics, keep dry.
(e) Respiratory infection:
  (i) Prevention: Hand washing, elevate bed 30°, good respiratory therapy, jejunal enteral feeding, & mechanical turning.
  (ii) Antibiotics.
(f) Nutrition: 25-30 kcal/kg protein, 1.5 gm/kg, try enteral feeding first, if failed then TPN (total parenteral nutrition).
(g) Weaning and extubation: As soon as possible, first reduce the PEEP.

226. **Most common indication for single lung transplantation (SLT): COPD.**

227. **Most common indication for double lung transplantation (DLT): Cystic fibrosis.**

228. **Most common indication for heart-lung transplantation (HLT): Eisenmenger's/congenital heart disease.**

229. **Most common immediate complication after lung transplantation: Pulmonary edema**.

230. **Most common becterial infection within 30 days of lung transplantation: Staphylococcus aureus**. Then, organisms of the Enterobacteriaceae family.

231. **Most common bacteria colonize the airway after lung transplantation: Pseudomonas**. It can cause chronic purulent bronchitis in patients with chronic rejection.

232. Prophylaxis in lung transplantation patients inorder to avoid pneumocystis carinii infection: Trimethoprim-sulfamethoxazole is given three times a week. This infection occurs after three to six months postoperatively.

233. **Most common non-bacterial infection after lung transplantation**:
CMV (cytomegalo virus). It appears 4 to 8 weeks postoperatively. CMV causes pneumonia first and eventually, spreads further.
Treatment: Ganciclovir.

234. **Most common fungal infection after lung transplantation: Candida albicans**.

235. A 40 year old man appears with fever, dyspnea, & cyanosis. He had lung transplantation surgery done 25 days ago and **presently receiving immunosuppressive medications**.
CXR: Infiltrate.
Most likely diagnosis: Acute rejection of **lung transplantation**.
Treatment: Methylprednisolone.

236. Immunosuppressive medications used after lung transplantation: Cyclosporine, azathioprine, methylprednisolone, & antilymphocyte agents (OKT3, RATG).

237. **Most common cause of hemoptysis: Pneumonia or lung infection**;other causes are lung tumor, pulmonary TB, bronchiectasis, bronchitis, cystic fibrosis, ruptured blood vessels in the bronchial mucosa, & pulmonary infarction.
Investigations: CXR, chest CT scan,& bronchoscopy.

238. **Different types of chest pain**:
(a) Pleuritic: Sharp, severe, enhanced by breathing +pleural friction rub.
(b) Pericarditis: Pain has no relation with breathing, relieved by leaning forward+pericardial friction rub.
(c) Pulmonary embolism: Feeling anterior chest pressure which may persist for hours.
(d) Myocardial ischemia: Pressure-type anterior chest pain, often with radiation to left (rarely, right) shoulder, arm, neck, or jaw; history of physical exertion may be present.

239. **Lymphatics are present throughout the lungs except:** Alveoli.

240. **Lung and systemic blood pressure**: Angiotensin-converting enzyme, produced by pulmonary endothelial cells, maintains the systemic blood pressure by converting angiotensin I to angiotensin II, and by metabolizing bradykinin.

241. **Most common type of alveolar epithelial cells: type I (98%);** type II is only 2%. Human lungs contains 500 million alveoli.

242. **Most commonly used test to measure pulmonary function tests: Spirometry**. It measures the airway movements into and out of the lungs during controlled ventilatory maneuvers. It measures the following parameters:
(a) FEV_1: Forced expiratory volume in 1 second.
(b) FVC: Forced vital capacity.
(c) FEV_1%: FEV_1/VC ratio (VC-vital capacity). Most commonly helpful pulmonary function parameters are ABG and carbon monoxide (CO) diffusing capacity.

243. **Lung volume is measured by: Plethysmography.**
Lung volume includes the following parameters:
(a) TLC: Total lung capacity.
(b) FRC: Functional residual capacity.
(c) RV: Residual volume.
(d) ERV: Expiratory reserve volume.

Plethysmography is done by placing the person in an air-tight box and allowing the person to breathe through a mouth piece connected outside.
Boyle's law=Pressure x volume of a gas is constant at a constant temperature.

244. Calculation of alveolar oxygen tension (P_{AO_2}):
$P_{AO_2} = P_{IO_2} - P_{ACO_2} [F_{IO_2}+(1-F_{IO_2})/R]$.
$P_{IO_2} = P_{O_2}$ of the expired gas.
P_{ACO_2}= Alveolar P_{CO_2} (or arterial P_{CO_2}).
F_{IO_2}=Fractional concentration of O_2 in the inspired gas.
R=Respiratory exchange ratio (0.8).
Simplified equation:
Alveolar P_{O_2}=150 - Pa_{CO_2} X 1.2

245. A-a gradient (alveolar-arterial oxygen gradient):
(a) **Simplified equation**: $(A\text{-}a)D_{O_2}=(P_{ATM}-P_{H_2O})-(Pa_{O_2}-Pa_{CO_2})$.
(b) Mostly used equation:
(i) $(A\text{-}a)\ D_{O_2}=P_{AO_2}-PaO_2$.
(ii) $P_{AO_2}=P_{IO_2}-P_{ACO_2}/R + Pa_{CO_2} \times F_{IO_2}(I-R)/R$.
P_{ATM}=Atmospheric pressure, P_{H_2O} =partial pressure of H_2O vapor.
P_{AO_2}=Alveolar oxygen tension, PaO_2=Arterial oxygen tension.
P_{ACO_2}=Alveolar CO_2 tension, Pa_{CO_2}=Arterial CO_2 tension.
$P_{IO_2}=F_{IO_2}(P_{ATM}-P_{H_2O})$.
R=Respiratory exchange ratio
In 100% oxygen, F_{IO_2}=1, P_{ACO_2} and Pa_{CO_2} is equal,.
R=1, simplified formula can be used.
(c) **Normal** A-a gradient= Normal lung function;**up to 5 to 15 mm Hg** is normal or mild gradient is due to nonuniform distribution of ventilation &/or small right-to-left shunt.
(d) Hypoxia with **normal** A-a gradient= Drug overdose, neuromuscular weakness.
(e) Hypoxia with **increased** A-a gradient=Lung dysfunction (COPD, pneumonia etc).

246. Lung function test:
(a) Obstructive: $\downarrow FEV_1/VC\%$,$\rightarrow\uparrow$TLC,$\downarrow FEV_1$,$\uparrow$RV,$\uparrow$FRC, $\downarrow$ERV, $\downarrow$VC, $\uparrow$RV /TLC.
The hallmarks are $\downarrow$ **FEV_1/VC%**, $\downarrow FEV_1$,$\rightarrow\uparrow$TLC.
Examples: Emphysema, Chronic bronchitis, mucous gland hyperplasia;asthma (reversible pulmonary disease).
In clinical practice, FEV_1 is used more commonly because it is easy to measure.

(b) Restrictive: ↓**TLC,** ↓**VC**;↑ FEV_1/VC%,↓ERA.

The hallmarks are ↓**TLC,**↓**VC,** ↓**ERV.**

Examples: Diseases of the chest wall (e.g. kyphoscoliosis, obesity), neuromuscular diseases (e.g. Guillain-Barre syndrome, myasthenia gravis), space-occupying lesions (e.g. pleural effusions, tumors, cardiomegaly), pulmonary fibrosis, pleural thickening, pneumonia, collapse, tuberculosis, pneumothorax, and surgical removal of portion of a lung.

Pulmonary fibrosis= ↓**TLC,** ↓**ERV**, ↓FRC, ↓**RV**, collapse points **is zero.**

Chest wall restriction= ↓**TLC,** ↓**ERV**, ↓FRC, →**RV**, collapse points **is RV.**

Neuromuscular weakness= ↓**TLC,** ↓**ERV**, →FRC, ↓**RV**, collapse points **is FRC.**

247. **Chronic obstruction in airways is mostly due to: Obstruction in the peripheral airways (not central)**.

248. (A)**Simple chronic bronchitis**: This includes:
   - (a) Enhanced mucous secretion.
   - (b) H/O cough on most days for at least 3 months in a year for at least 2 years.
   - (c) Ruled out tuberculosis, bronchiectasis, and other lung diseases.
   - (d) **H/O** exposure to bronchial irritants like smoking tobacco. It is commonly found in men over the age of 40.

(B) **Chronic obstructive bronchitis (or small airways diseases):** A small number of patients, with simple chronic bronchitis, result in **irreversible obstruction** in bronchioles and bronchi less than 2 mm in diameter.

(C) **Asthmatic bronchitis**: Bronchitis patients with **bronchospasms**.

(D) **Chronic asthmatic bronchitis**: Patients with chronic airway obstruction, productive cough, and episodic **bronchospasms**. It is commonly found in elderly smokers.

(E) **Emphysema**: Permanent abnormal enlargement of airways distal to terminal bronchioles due to noxious stimuli. Airways are damaged without fibrosis.

The term COPD has been used broadly in all of the above conditions.

249. **Relationship of cigarette smoking with simple chronic bronchitis and asthmatic bronchitis**:
   - (a) Cigarette smoking is the most important cause for above mentioned bronchitis.
   - (b) Only 15 to 20 % smokers develop airway obstruction.
   - (c) Mucous hypersecretion is not always present in smokers.

250. Mucous gland **hyperplasias in** simple chronic bronchitis and asthmatic bronchitis: Mucous gland hyperplasias (**not** hypertrophy) in the larger airways are the **most characteristic abnormality.**

251. **Most common bacterial organisms** causing infection in simple chronic bronchitis and asthmatic bronchitis: **Hemophilus influenzae** and **Streptococcus pneumoniae**. Patients receiving multiple antibiotics may develop psuedomonas infection which is rare.

252. **Hemoptysis in asthmatic bronchitis**: **Blood streaked sputum and eosinophils** containing sputum are occasionally found during bronchospasm. Severe hemoptysis indicates serious conditions like neoplasms.

253. **Most important method to clear bronchial secretions**: Deep breathing followed by deliberate coughing.

254. **Major causes of chronic disabilities in older patients in order:**
   (a) First: Heart diseases.
   (b) Second: Schizophrenia.
   (c) Third: Chronic obstructive bronchitis and emphysema (COPD).

255. **Alveolar destruction in COPD is due to**: Imbalance of proteases (proteolytic enzymes) and antiproteases in the lower respiratory tract. Proteases (elastase & elastases) are produced by polymorphs and macrophages in the lungs;cigarette smoking enhances these enzyme secretions causing alveolar destruction.

256. **Smokers-nonsmokers, FEV_1 and alpha 1- antitrypsin deficiency:**
   (a) Heavy smokers with normal enzymes: ↓ FEV_1 38 to 59 ml/year.
   (b) Nonsmokers with normal enzymes: ↓ FEV_1 29 to 37 ml/year.
   (c) Nonsmokers with decreased enzymes: ↓ FEV_1 to 80ml/year.
   (d) **Heavy smokers** with decreased enzymes: ↓ FEV_1 to 150 ml/year.

257. **COPD and alpha-1- antitrypsin deficiency**:
   (a) In a normal person, PiMM (Pi is protease inhibitor, two M genes) are present.
   (b) In symptomatic alpha-1-antitrypsin deficiency, PiZZ (two Z genes) are present. **Only Z gene leads to COPD.**
   (c) PiMZ phenotype (heterozygous) are mostly asymptomatic.

258. **Types of emphysema in different diseases**:
   (a) Panacinar emphysema-Alpha-1-antitrypsin deficiency.

(b) Centrilobular emphysema: Chronic airway obstruction due to smoking.
Panacinar type: Defects are present throughout the acini.
Centrilobular type: Defects are mostly in the central portion of the lobule.
Both types may be found in the same lung.

259. **A 60 year old man appears with H/O weight loss, dyspnea, and cough with mucoid scanty sputum.**
Physical examination: Mild end expiratory wheezes, marked hyperinflation, & quiet lungs.
CXR: Bilateral hyperlucent, overinflated lungs.
ABG: Mild hypoxic with normal or low P_{CO_2}.
Lung function tests:↓ FEV_1,↑TLC, ↑↑RV.
Pulmonary artery pressure: Normal or slightly increased.
Cardiac output: Low.
Most likely diagnosis: **Emphysematous type of COPD**. It is called "**pink puffers**"because patients can maintain normal or nearly normal arterial oxygen tension by hyperventilation.

260. A 64 year old man appears with H/O cough with copious mucopurulent sputum with recent onset of dyspnea. Patient denies H/O weight loss.
Physical examination: Rhonchi with noisy breathing and rales are noted.
CBC: **Normal;increased eosinophil count is found in asthmatic bronchitis**.
CXR: Old infiltrates bilateral.
ABG: Hypoxia with chronic retention of P_{CO_2}.
Lung function tests: **↓ FEV_1, →↓TLC, ↑RV.**
Pulmonary artery pressure: Markedly increased.
Cardiac output: Almost normal.
Most likely dlagnosis: Bronchial type of COPD. It is called "**blue bloaters**"because patients have low arterial oxygen tension, cyanosis, and right-sided congestive heart failure.

261. **Management of patients with COPD:**
- (a) All patients should be treated as **having reversible** pulmonary diseases.
- (b) **Bronchodilators** therapy for asthma and asthmatic bronchitis.
- (c) **Prophylaxis.**
  - (i) **Avoid** active and passive smoking.
  - (ii) **Pneumococcal vaccine and yearly influenza vaccine.**
- (d) **Antibiotics** for bacterial infections.
- (e) **Corticosteriods are helpful in the following conditions:**
  - (i) Wheezes or noisy breathing on auscultation.
  - (ii) Presence of nasal polyps or vasomotors rhinitis.

(iii) Increased eosinophil count in sputum or blood.
(iv) Evidence of atopy (↑IgE, positive allergic skin test, and H/O hay fever).
(v) When there is 20% improvement in FEV_1, after acute inhalation bronchodilator or few days to weeks of bronchodilator treatment.

(f) Discontinue postural drainage, if it is not helpful to patients.
(g) Monitor clinical conditions and lung functions.
(h) Oxygen therapy to keep the oxygen saturation >90%.
(i) Pedal edema: Diuretics.
(j) Avoid high altitude (<4000 feet).
(k) **Single lung transplantation**: **End-stage emphysema is the most common indication.**

262. **Treatment for alpha1-antitrypsin deficiency emphysema**: Intravenous alpha 1- antitrypsin concentrate. It is used in patient who are nonsmokers and have fixed airflow obstruction.

263. **Most common side effects after intravenous alpha-1-antitrypsin infusion**: **Fever**. It is found in <1% of all patients.

264. **Physical therapy in COPD patients**:
(a) It does **not** improve pulmonary functions but it increases cardiovascular and skeletal muscles activities. It should be done under guidance of physician or physical therapist.
(b) Patients should be asked to do "**slow, deep breathing**"rather than rapid, shallow, panicky breathing. **Breathing exercises encourage diaphragmatic breathing** but do not change usual breathing pattern of COPD patients.

265. **Flow volume curve in airways obstruction**:
(a) **Fixed (intrathoracic or extrathoracic)**: Both inspiratory and expiratory flows are **decreased.**

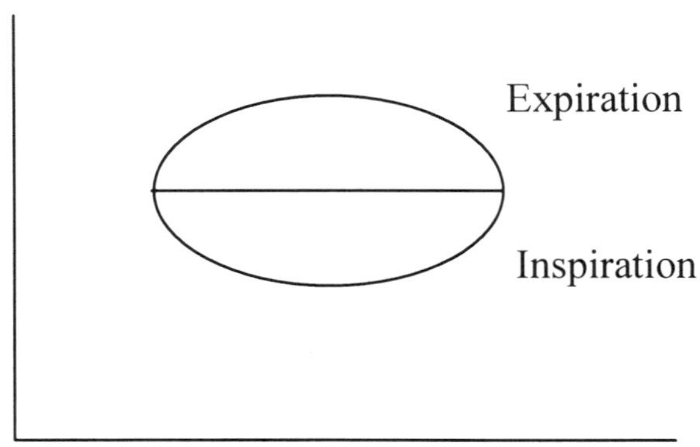

(b) **Extrathoracic variable obstruction**: Severely **diminished inspiratory flow** and mildly decreased expiratory flow.

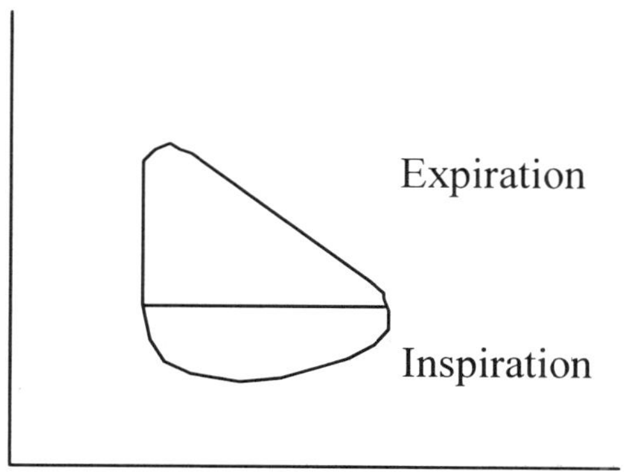

(c) **Intrathoracic variable obstruction: Severely diminished expiratory flow** and mildly decreased inspiratory flow.

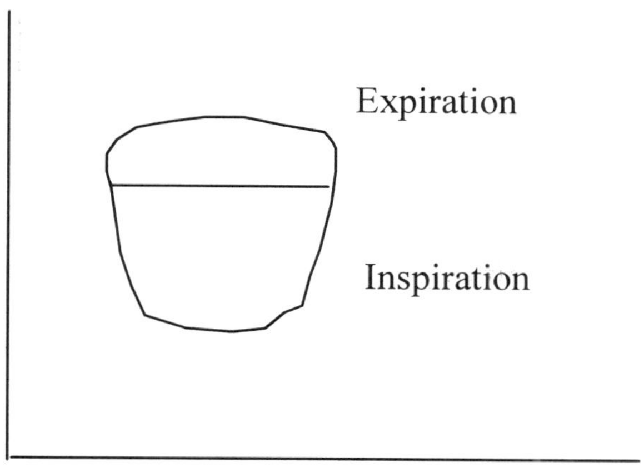

266. **The Most common cause of obstruction below the tracheal bifurcation:** A **primary neoplasm** within or outside of the airways. Other causes are enlarged lymph nodes, foreign bodies and inflammatory changes.
Physical examination: Unilateral expiratory wheezes.
CXR: Unilateral hyperinflated lung distal to obstruction.
Spirometry: Nonspecific, may be normal or abnormal.
Definitive diagnosis: **Bronchoscopy.**
Treatment: According to the respective disease condition. Partial obstruction may progress to complete obstruction of the bronchus and "obstructive atelactasis".

267. **Obstruction above the tracheal bifurcation**: Two types: partial and complete.

(A) **Partial obstruction**: **Most common clinical presentation is stridor** which is also associated with intercostal retractions.
   (a) **Intrinsic** airways obstructions are due to tracheal stenosis, bilateral vocal cords paralysis, neoplasms or granulomas (sarcoidosis or fungi) of the upper respiratory tract and hypopharynx, vasculitis (Wegener's granulomatosis), laryngeal edema, or spasm.
   (b) Extrinsic airways obstruction are due to enlargement of thyriod, mediastinal infection, and paratracheal neoplasm.

Treatment:
   (i) To treat the underlying cause.
   (ii) Tracheostomy, intubation, or surgical repair, if obstruction persist.

(B) **Complete obstruction**: Most common cause is aspiration of poorly chewed food ("**cafe coronary**"), patients apear with acute asphyxia.

Treatment: **Heimlich maneuver** is to apply sharp blow to the back or forced pressure applied to the epigastrium.

268. **Most common complication of high inspired oxygen used in obstructive atelactasis distal to tracheal bifurcation:**
Pulmonary atelactasis because oxygen is rapidly absored in the bloodstream unlike nitrogen which is poorly soluble. Lungs filled with high oxygen are more likely to collapse than that filled with nitrogen.

269. A 50 year old man went for a routine yearly physical examination. He has a history of **only mild cough** for the last few months.
CXR: Atelactasis of the partial right lung.
Most likely diagnosis: **Bronchogenic carcinoma**. It should be considered when there is obstructive atelactasis in an asymptomatic or mildly ill patient.

270. **Middle lobe syndrome**: The middle lobe bronchus in the right lung is compressed by enlarged hilar lymph nodes due to tuberculosis or granulomatous lung diseases.

271. A 65 year old man appears with severe dyspnea.
Physical examination: Tympanic percussion sound and reduced breath sounds in right-side.
CXR: Large trabeculated bullae are occupying most of the right hemithorax.
Bullae have irregular thin margins (lung cysts have regular margins; bullae **that occuping less than 50%** of the hemithorax do **not** cause symptoms unless associated with obstructive airways disease. Bullae do **not** have endothelial lining like cysts. Ventilation-perfusion scan, chest CT, or pulmonary

angiogram may be necessary: To exclude emphysema and to **evaluate the normal lung.**

Mostly likely diagnosis: Symptomatic bullae in right hemithorax.

Treatment:

(a) Asymptomatic: Conservative.

(b) Symptomatic: Surgery is indicated when there is no emphysema and the other lung is normal.

Complication: Pneumothorax is due to rupture of bullae.

272. **Most common sites of bronchogenic cysts**: **Subcarinal and paratracheal regions** in **the lower lobes parenchyma**. Patients are usually asymptomatic. Bronchogenic cysts are detected by routine CXR.

CXR: Air-fluid level, regular margins, lack of trabeculations.

Diagnosis is confirmed by: Thoracotomy and resection; chest CT with needle aspiration which may help in diagnosis and drainages of cysts.

Complication: Rarely infections occur. Infection may not be resolved with antibiotics.

Treatment:

(a) Surgical resection.

(b) Antibiotics for infections.

273. **Treatment for bronchopulmonary sequestrations**: Surgical resection only. Bronchopulmonary sequestrations are formed in early gestation by **abnormal budding** in the tracheobronchial tree. It is **non** functional, found **most commonly in the bases of the lungs posteriorly**. Patients are **asymptomatic** except when there are secondary infections.

CXR: Opacity in the lung.

MRI:(to avoid angiography of the aorta): To detect an abnormal vascular supply from aorta to sequestration which is not found in cysts.

274. **Pathogenesis in ILD (interstitial lung diseases):**

(a) **Intra-alveolar inflammation: First detectable** lesion in ILD is the **lower respiratory tract inflammatory exudates.** Macrophages, lymphocytes, and neutrophils are all present in the alveoli. Inflammatory cells migration depends on cytokines and chemokines.

(b) **Injury**: **The most important finding is the epithelial cell injury** due to free radicals (oxidants), immune cells, inflammatory cells, proteases, and viral infections. After the epithelial cells injury, there is **exudation of the plasma** and formation of **fibrin-rich exudates.** Alveolar basal laminas are also destroyed.

(c) F**ibrosis of the alveoli or its collapse**: Either the lungs are repaired completely or become fibrotic. Major factors are the **macrophages and alveolar epithelial cells** which control the formation and clearance of the **intra-alveolar** fibrins.

275. **Most useful investigation to detect physiologic abnormalities in interstitial lung diseases** (ILD): **Pulmonary function tests**;CXR is nonspecfic but is very helpful to include or exclude the different cateogories of ILD.

276. A 60 year old man, who has ILD, **recently develops clubbing in the fingers**.
Most likely diagnosis: Lung cancer should be ruled out.
Physical examination: **Basilar, crepitant"Velcro-like"rales are found in both lungs of ILD.**
Diagnosis is confirmed by: Fiberoptic bronchoscopy and lung biospy.

277. **ILD patients with pneumothorax which is found in CXR:** R/O tuberous sclerosis, neurofibromatosis, histiocytosis X, and lymphangioleiomyomatosis.

278. **ILD patients with enlarged hilar or mediastinal lymph nodes**: R/O Gaucher's disease, sarcoidosis, LIP (lymphocytic interstitial pneumonia), amyloidosis, and silicosis (**egg shell** calcification).

279. **Most common symptom in ILD: Breathlessness.** Other symptoms are cough, dyspnea etc.
   (a) Cough: It is found in BOOP (bronchiolitis obliterans organizing pneumonia), IPF (idiopathic pulmonary fibrosis), and eosinophilic pneumonia.
   (b) Pleuritic chest pain in ILD: R/O systemic rheumatoid disease and some drug induced diseases.
   (c) Hemoptysis in ILD: R/O alveolar hemorrahage syndrome or lymphangioleiomyomatosis.
   (d) Sudden onset of acute dyspnea and pleuritic chest pain: R/O pneumothorax.

280. **Smoking and ILD**:
   (a) Goodpasture's syndrome without smoking: 20% patients have pulmonary involvements.
   (b) Goodpasture's syndrome with smoking: 100% patients have pulmonary involvements.
   (c) Histiocytosis X: 90% patients are active smokers.

281. **Genetic patterns and ILD**:

(a) Autosomal recessive: It is found in Gaucher's disease, Niemann- Pick disease, and Hermansky- Pudlak syndrome.
(b) Autosomal dominant: It is found in tuberous sclerosis, neurofibromatosis, and familiar IPF (interstitial pulmonary fibrosis).

282. **CXR and ILD**: Important points to remember.
(a) **Normal CXR can be present** in 5 to 10% of patients with biopsy confirmed diseases.
(b) **Honeycomb (cystic)** pattern appears in the **later part** of the diseases.
(c) **Diffuse ground glass pattern** appears in the **early part** of the diseases.
(d) **Typical presentations** are the following:
(i) Nodular infiltrates.
(ii) Reticular infiltrates.
(iii) Reticulonodular infiltrates (combination of **i & ii**).

283. **HRCT (high-resolution computed tomography) and ILD:** Important points to remember.
(a) HRCT may be **normal in biopsy-confirmed diseases.**
(b) **HRCT can detect lung abnormalities before** CXR becomes positive in the following diseases: Sarcoidosis, silicosis, scleroderma, and asbestosis.
(c) **Normal** HRCT cannot exclude ILD.
(d) Advantages of HRCT are the following: Quantify the extent of involvement in ILD, may detect early ILD, and may diagnose specific ILD.
(e) HRCT can detect the appropriate sites for lung biopsies.

284. **Classic findings of PFT (pulmonary function tests) in ILD**:
(a) Decreased lung volumes (↓VC, **↓TLC, normal or supernormal ratio of FEV_1/FVC**, ↓diffusing capacity or DLco.
(b) Decreased static lung compliance.
(c) Increased transpulmonary pressure.

↑TLC is the classic finding in ILD. (Dlco means diffusing lung capacity of carbon monoxide).

285. **↓TLC is found in the following diseases**: These are **exceptions** to classic findings.
(a) Sarcoidosis.
(b) Tuberous sclerosis.
(c) Histiocytosis.
(d) Neurofibromatosis.
(e) Lymphangioleiomyomatosis.

286. **Most confirmatory procedures for diagnosis of ILD: Thoracoscopic or open lung biopsy.**

287. **Therapy in ILD patients:**
   (a) **Corticosteroids are the main treatment.** It is continued until the pulmonary functions are normal for one year. Anti-inflammatory effect of corticosteroids prevent further damages of the lungs.
   (b) **Cyclophosphamide** is an immunosuppressive agent. It is used when patients get worse with corticosteroids (prednisone), or cannot tolerate steroid therapy.
   (c) Azathioprine can be used as an alternative to cyclophosphamide.
   (d) Supportive therapies include oxygen and antibiotics.
   (e) Single lung transplantation may be indicated in unresponsive patients.

288. **Prophylactic vaccinations in ILD patients**: Pneumococcal vaccine and yearly influenza vaccines should be given.

289. **Most common symptom in drug-induced ILD**: Nonproductive cough with mild degree.

290. **Drug-induced ILD**: (Important points to remember).
   (a) **Nitrofurantoin-induced ILD is most common. It is not dose related. Acute ILD appears 2 hours to 10 days after the onset of therapy.**
   (b) ILD can present in acute, subacute, or chronic conditions.
   (c) **False diagnosis of pneumonia** is common when cough and fever are presenting symptoms.
   (d) Blood smear shows **increased eosinophil count.**
   (e) ABG shows **hypoxemia and hypocarbia.**
   (f) Pulmonary function tests show restrictive lung diseases.
   (g) CXR: Reticulonodular or alveolar infiltrate.
   (h) Treatment: Discontinue the drug causing ILD.

291. **Most common antineoplastic drug causing ILD:**
   Bleomycin. Other antineoplastic drugs causing ILD are the following.
   (a) Methotrexate: ILD appears with cough, fever, and dyspnea within a few days to weeks after the onset of therapy. Increased eosinophil count in peripheral blood smear but it is absent in the lungs.
   (b) Cyclophosphamide: ILD appears within few weeks to 6 years after the onset of therapy.
   (c) Nitrosourea (BCNU and methyl-CCNU): ILD appears in **more than 50% of patients** when doses of >1500 mg per square meter have been used.

292. **Most common cardiovascular drug causing ILD: Amiodarone** is an antiarrhythmic drug used in refractory ventricular dysrhythmias. ILD is **less if the maintenance dose is <400 mg/day.** ILD can present either an acute onset which mimic ARDS/infectious pneumonia or gradual onset with fever, cough, & dyspnea.
Treatment: **Discontinue the drug**; for some reason, if the drug is to be continued, then use corticosteroid therapy.

293. **Most effective treatment for chronic eosinophilic pneumonia (CEP): Corticosteroids. It is extermely effective**. Patients **improve within 2 to 4 days after the onset of therapy** CEP patients usually appear with fever, cough, night sweat, dyspnea, and weight loss.
CBC: **Shows increased eosinophil count** (10 to 40 % of the total cells count).
CXR: Peripheral, nonsegmental alveolar infiltrates.
BAL: Increased eosinophil count (>40%).
Recurrence would show same CXR findings as the initial one.

294. A 20 year old man appears with **hemoptysis, dyspnea, gross hematuria, and fatigue. Major findings are pulmonary hemorrhage and progressive glomerulonephritis.**
CBC: Hypochromic microcytic anemia.
CXR: Bilateral symmetrical alveolar infiltrates.
DLco: Increase (≥30%) which is suggestive of intrapulmonary hemorrhage due to CO uptake by the intraalveolar RBC's.
Anti-glomerular basement membrane antibody (anti-GBM): **Positive in 95% of patients**.
Anti-alveolar basement membrane antibody (anti-ABM): Positive.
Diagnosis is confirmed: By immunoflurescent studies of **kidney tissues**.
Most likely diagnosis: Goodpasture's syndrome.
Treatment:
(a) Symptomatic pulmonary therapy: Oxygen, respiratory supports.
(b) Corticosteroids, cytotoxic medicines with plasmapheresis until circulating anti-GBM antibodies were removed.

295. **The most common opportunistic infection in pulmonary alveolar proteinosis: Nocardia**. In pulmonary alveolar proteinosis, the following points are important.
(a) H/O exposure to asbestos, silica, or cement dust; patients appear with dyspnea and cough.

(b) It is associated with Fanconi's anemia, myeloblastic leukemia, and chronic myelocytic leukemia.
(c) It is due to **intraalveolar accummulation of an acellular periodic acid-Schiff positive, lipoproteinacious material.**
(d) **Diagnosis is confirmed** by bronchoscopic lung biopsy.
(e) **Treatment of choice** is the whole lung lavage with 40 to 60 litres of fluids under general anesthesia, through double-lumen ET tube.

296. **Chronic silicosis and mycobacterium TB**: There are higher incidences of TB in pulmonary silicosis patients. So, yearly PPD test should be done, and appropriate prophylaxis with INH should be given if PPD is positive.

297. **Lung cancer and asbestosis**: Incidences of lung cancer are higher in pulmonary asbestosis patients.

298. **Caplan's syndrome**: It is an uncommon syndrome found in coal mine workers with multiple peripheral nodules. It may develop in miners with rheumatoid arthritis or without arthritis with positive circulating rheumatoid factors.

299. **Most ominous sign in smoke inhalations: Stridor**. Other signs are dyspnea, wheezing, tachynea, and cyanosis.

300. **Leading cause of accidental poisoning in USA**: Carbon monoxide (CO).

301. **Carbon monoxide poisoning is confirmed by**: **Blood HbCO level (not by pulse-oximetry) which is elevated.** (HbCO is carboxy-hemoglobin).

302. **Severity of CO poisoning and HbCO level**: Patients clinical presentations depend on **duration and extent of exposure to smoke, rather than HbCO level.**

303. **Most commonly involved organ in CO poisoning**: CNS. In a nonsmoker, symptoms appear when HbCO **levels reach 10%;** smokers tolerate slightly higher levels.

304. **Classical clinical findings of cherry red lips and nail beds** in CO poisoning: It is **rarely** found. Patients usually appear with a headache, nausea, vomiting; seizures and unconsciousness are found in severe poisoning which may also manifest with **rhabdomyolysis, pulmonary edema**, and **metabolic acidosis**.

305. **Treatment for CO poisoning:**

(a) Mild: No treatment is needed.
(b) Moderate: 100% oxygen which displaces CO from Hb.
(c) When HbCO is >25%, neurological or cardiac symptons: Hyperbaric oxygen at 2.5 atmosphere absolute (ATA).

306. **Halftime for elimination of CO:**
(a) Without oxygen therapy: 240 minutes.
(b) With 100% oxygen therapy: 60 minutes.
(c) With hyperbaric (2.5ATA) oxygen: 20 minutes.

307. **Silo-filler's disease**: It is a racheobronchitis due to nitrogen dioxide. Patients appear with dyspnea, cough, and bilateral rales due to pulmonary edema.
Treatment:
(a) Acute: **Crticosteroids are highly effective**; bronchoditators, oxygen, and mechanical ventilation if needed.

308. **Most common site of oxygen toxicity**: Pulmonary capillary endothelium.

309. A 50 year old man was treated with 100% oxygen for over 6 hours due to smoke inhalations. After 6 hours of oxygen therapy, he complains of **substernal pain with dry cough.**
Most likely diagnosis: Oxygen toxicity.
Treatment: To avoid the excessive use oxygen, probably 40 to 50 % oxygen is safe. Remember, do **not** use corticosteroids which can damage the lungs further.

310. **Total radiation doses and lung injuries:**
(a) <2000 GY=Safe, do **not** cause radiation pneumonitis.
(b) >4000 GY=Dangerous,100% of patients develop radiation pneumonitis.
Radiation pneumonitis depends on the doses, duration, and number of fractions.

311. **Treatment for radiation pneumonitis**:
(a) Supportive care: Antitussive for cough, oxygen for hypoxia, and antipyretics for fever.
(b) Severe pneumonitis: Corticosteroids may be helpful but it should not be used as prophylaxis.

312. **Most common cause of chemical aspiration**: Aspiration of gastric acid.

313. **Most important factor causing lung injury during chemical aspiration**: **The pH of** the material (pH ≤2.5 usually causes severe pneumonitis). Other factors are volume of the aspirate >0.4 ml/kg body weight can cause pneumonitis.

314. **Treatment for aspiration pneumonia**:
   (a) Remember, do **not** use prophylactic antibiotics because it enhances infections with resistant organisms.
   (b) **First, to establish the airways.**
   (c) Suction the airways.
   (d) Oxygen for hypoxia.
   (e) Bronchodilators for bronchospasms.
   (f) Do **not** use corticosteroids.
   (g) Severe aspiration–Ventilator management. **To improve oxygenation in gastric acid aspiration, PEEP is commonly used.**

315. **Preventions of pre-intra-postoperative aspiration**: **(Important for board exam)**.
   (a) NPO for at least 12 hours before general anesthesia.
   (b) Use H_2 blocker (single dose) or an antacid (single dose 10 ml per oral) preoperatively 2 hours before surgery in order to increase the gastric pH.

316. **Hydrocarbon pneumonia**: **It is not an important for the board examination** becuase it is **rare** in adults.

317. **Most common agent casuing lipoid pneumonia**: **Mineral oil** which is used as laxative, nasal drops for congestion of the nose, and for dysphagia.
   Most common clinical presentation is asymptomatic with positive lipoid pneumonia in CXR. Symptomatic patients mostly appear with cough and exertional dyspnea;sometimes with fever, chest pain, and hemoptysis.
   Diagnosis is confirmed by: Lipid-laden macrophages in the sputum.
   Treatment.
   (a) To stop using mineral oil.
   (b) Corticosteroid may be used briefly, only in severely affected patients.

318. **Most important complication in near-drowning**: **Asphyxia**. It leads to hypoxemia, metabolic acidosis, and hypercarbia.

319. A 20 year old man was brought to the emergency room by EMS with H/O drowning in a swimming pool for an unknown peroid of time. Patient required

intubation, CPR (**cardiopulmonary resuscitation**) and placed on mechanical ventilator. **The patient has smell of alcohol in his breath**.

Physical examination: Cyanosis, pink frothy endotracheal secretions in an agitated patient.

ABG:↓Pao_2, ↓pH,↑$Paco_2$.

SMA6:↑Na, ↑Cl, ↓K.

CBC: Initially normal Hb (hemoglobin) and hct (hematocrit), after 12 hours hct falls slightly due to hemolysis.

EKG: Initial sinus tachycardia with nonspecfic ST segment and T wave changes are the most common presentation. Subsequently, it becomes normal.

CXR: Pulmonary edema.

Treatment:

(a) Ventilator management, oxygen for hypoxia.
(b) Cerebral edema: Mannitol, minimum PEEP.
(c) Corticosteroids.
(d) Bronchodilators for bronchospasms.
(e) Do **not** give prophylactic antibiotics.

320. **Drowning**: Two types.

(a) **"Wet"**drowning: Most common, large amount of water was aspirated due to laryngeal relaxation after brief initial spasms.
(b) **"Dry"**drowning: Little or no water was aspirated due to severe laryngospasm.

321. **Immediate cause of death in drowning: Cardiac arrythmia**.

322. **Prognosis** for drowning depends upon: Presence or absence of coma. The prognosis is directly proportional between the interval of drowning and first gasping breathing. The shorter the interval is, the better the prognosis.

323. **High-altitude pulmonary edema (HAPE) is due to: Pulmonary hypertension** increases pulmonary capillary leak which results in pulmonary edema.(No cardiac causes).

HAPE: Patients appear with dyspnea, tachypnea, and crackles in the bases of the lungs. It is found above 9500 feet altitude.

324. **High-altitude cerebral edema (HACE) is due to: Hypoxemia** increases cerebral blood flow, which results in cerebral edema.

HACE: **Very rare**, patients appear with headache, confusion, ataxia, papilledema, and coma.

325. **Acute mountain sickness (AMS) is due to**: **Hypoxemia but exact mechanism is uncertain.** Patients appear with headaches, anorexia, and disturbed sleep. It is a self-limited condition and usually found above 8000 feet altitude.

326. **Most common symptom in high-altitude retinal hemorrhages (HARH)**: **Asymptomatic**. Patients rarely present with visual symptoms. Eye examination shows **dilated retinal vessels and peripheral hemorrhages**.

327. **Definitive treatment for HARH, HACE, and HAPE**:
   (a) Immediately give oxygen.
   (b) Bring the patients back to lower altitudes.
   (c) Give PEEP or CPAP (continuous positive airway pressure), or place the patient in a pressurized bag, if the procedure of descent is delayed.

   Symptomatic treatment is the following: Rest, hydration, analgesics, avoid achohol use.

   Prophylactic treatment is the following:
   (a) **Slowly climb up the mountain** (1000 feet/day between 7000 to 10,000 feet altitudes, above that altitude is only 500 feet/day).
   (b) **Acetazolamide** which reduces respiratory alkalosis due to increase of renal bicarbonates excretion.

   Do **not use other diuretics and corticosteroids.**
   (c) Bring the patient back to lower altitudes when symptomatic.

328. A 70 year old man lived in very high altitude (over 14,000 feet) for several years. He has a long term history of cough, dyspnea, palpitation, muscular weakness, cyanosis, and rarely stupor.
   CBC: High hct (70).
   ABG:$\downarrow Pao_2$,$\uparrow Paco_2$.
   Most likely diagnosis: Monge's disease (chronic mountain sickness).
   Treatment: Move the patient to a lower altitude.

329. **Most important treatment in decompression illness (DCI) or Caisson's** disease: Maximum concentration of oxygen is given by face mask. Then recompression treatment is done in hyperbaric chamber with 100% oxygen. DCI can occur during decompression in the divers those who went 25 feet below the seawater or rapid ascent from sea level to 18,000 feet. Patients appears with mild symptoms (joint pains, numbness, pruritis) or severe symptoms (unconsciousness, vertigo, nystagmus, substernal pain, tachypnea, or hypovolemic shock). In DCI, inert gas (mostly nitrogen) dissolved in the tissues and venous blood causes above mentioned clinical manifectations

which are also partly due to release of vasoactive mediators, platelet aggregations, and activation of complements.

330. **Signs and symptoms in arterial gas embolism (AGE) are due to**: **Distribution of gases in the carotid arteries** result in **acute cerebral dysfunctions** which includes blindness, unconsciousness, paralysis, or seizures. AGE can occur when divers ascend to the surface after deep diving, in blast injury, or during decompression at high altitude.
Treatment: Same as DCI and should begin as soon as possible. Maximum concentration of oxygen by face mask. Then, recompression treatment in a hyperbaric chamber with 100% oxygen.

331. **Most common ways the bacteria gets into the lungs:**
   (a) **First**: **Aspiration of oropharyngeal secretions** which are responsible for most bacterial infection and anaerobic infections. **Most common cause of pneumonias**.
   (b) **Second**: Inhalation of airborne microorganisms which are responsible for TB, legionella, and viruses.
   (c) **Third**: Bacteremia.
   (d) **Fourth**: Extension of infections directly to the lungs from the adjacent organs (e.g.,liver, chest wall, diaphragms). **Least common cause of pneumonias.**

INFECTIOUS DISEASES

1. **Most common etiologic agent of community acquired pneumonia (outpatient, hospitalized ICU, and non-ICU patients): Streptococcus pneumoniae (pneumococcal pneumoniae). It is the most common bacterial pneumonia in the world.**

2. **Blood cultures and pneumonias: It is positive only in 30% of all pneumonias. Remember, positive blood and pleural fluid cultures in pneumonias are highly specific.**

3. **Sputum specimens and pneumonia**: Purulent sputum should have **>25 leukocytes and <10 squamous cells** per low-power field in microscopic examination.

4. **Most important factor causing virulency in S.pneumoniae:** S.pneumoniae have **polysaccharide capsules** which inhibit phagocytosis by the neutrophils.

5. **S.pneumoniae and toxins**: S.pneumoniae do **not** produce any major tissue destructive toxins. All of them contain **pneumolysin** and some strains release **hyaluronidase** enzyme. Pneumolysins are released during bacterial destruction, and also causes disruption of respiratory epitheliums.

6. Most common cause of **S.pneumoniae pneumonia**: Patients aspirate **oropharyngeal secretions** which contains encapsulated pneumococci.

7. **Most frequent site of spread from pneumoccocal pneumonia: Subarachnoid space.** Patients develop meningitis. S.pneumoniae can also spread by **bacteremia** to other organs, resulting in endocarditis, pericarditis, septic arthritis, and peritonitis. S.pneumoniae can also spread locally to other organs, result in sinusitis, mastoiditis, otitis media, conjunctivitis, and rarely the soft tissues of the neck or retropharyngeal space **(Ludwig's angina).**

8. A 50 year old man appears with a sudden onset of **high fever (up to39.5^0),** chill, **rigor**, **diaphoresis, tachypnea**, cough, **productive sputum**, and **pleuritic right sided chest pain**. Few days ago, the patient had H/O URI symptoms.
   Physical examination: Bronchovascular breath sounds and wet rales in (R) side of the chest, increased vocal or tactile fremitus which is diminished if ipsilateral pleural effusion or empyema is present. Reflex splinting of the (R) sided chest is noted due to the pain.

CBC: Leukocytosis (22000 to 33000↑) with shift to the left (↑polymorphs 80%). (Normal or decreased WBC count may be present in alcoholics or immunosuppressed patients).

ABG:↓Pao_2,↓$Paco_2$,→pH (7.45),(↓**$Paco_2$, pH is <7.40 means metabolic acidosis which indicates shock**; acidosis should be corrected as soon as possible.).

CXR: Lobar consolidation of the (R) upper lobe.(It may be **absent** in patients with dehydration or immunosuppression or severely neutropenic, but after rehydration therapy consolidation would be visible).

sputum Gram stain: Gram positive diplococci (50 bacterial cells per 100 x field), polymorphs (26 cells per 100 x field), Squamous cells (9 cells per 100 x field).

Sputum cultures: S.pneumoniae.

Blood cultures: S.pneumoniae.

Most likely diagnosis: Pneumococcal pneumonia in the (R) upper lobe.

Treatment: **It should be started immediately.**

(a) Penicillin G is the medicine of choice.
(b) Penicillin allergic patients: Cephalosporin because cross-allergenicity is low.
(c) Severe Penicillin allergic patients: Try erythromycin but organism may be resistant. Do **not** give tetracycline which is **not** effective.
(d) **Highly resistant organisms**: Vancomycin, clindamycin,(antibiotics should be adjusted after the sensivity results), cefotaxime, or ceftriaxone etc.

9. A patient with the diagnosis of pneumococcal pneumonia is being treated with penicillin. After 24 hours, the patient still has high fever with the worsening of symptoms and signs of pneumonia.
   Most likely diagnosis: **Penicillin resistant** pneumococcal pneumonia because fever should be reduced or normal within 24 hours.
   Treatment.
   Cefotaxime, ceftriaxone, vancomycin, clindamycin, etc. Antibiotics should be adjusted after the sensitivity results.

10. Any suspected bacterial pneumonias with pleural effusions when organisms are not known: Pleural tap should be done to examine the fluid to identify the microorganism and fluid cultures should be done.

11. Patients diagnosed to have pneumococcal pneumonia, appears with cardiac failure, heart murmurs, and enlarged spleen.
    Most likely associated diagnosis: Endocarditis.

12. Major complication due to sepsis of inadequately or untreated pneumococcal pneumonia patient.
    (a) Meningitis: Positive kernig's or Brudzinski's sign.
    (b) Endocarditis.
    (c) Purpura fulminans: Symmetric purpura and gangrene of extremities (fingers or toes).
    (d) DIC.

13. Detection of **pneumococcal capsular antigen** is extremely important:
    (a) In patients those are **partially treated.**
    (b) Gram stain is negative.
    (c) Sputum culture is negative.
    Problems of this study:
    (a) False negative results are common.
    (b) Cross-reactivity with antigens of other bacterias.

14. **Important guidelines to identify and treat in any acute bacterial pneumonias:**
    (a) Try to make every effort to make the correct diagnosis as soon as possible but the treatments should **not** be delayed which could be life-threatening in seriously ill patients.
    (b) Satisfactory (not contaminated with oropharyngeal secretions) sputum specimen is important, once it is collected. To obtain pus from the pulmonary tissues may be postponed or not necessary.
    (c) First procedure should be **least traumatic** to make the diagnosis. If it fails, then go for the next less traumatic procedure.

15. **Problems to identify the real organisms causing bacterial pneumonias by Gram stain of the sputum specimens:**
    (a) Gram stain may **show more than one organism** which may be contaminated with oropharyngeal secretions, to identify the real organism is difficult.
    (b) If the blood or pleural fluid culture shows **one organism**, then **that organism is the right organism. More than one organism can be present in the lungs**.

16. **Recommendations to give pneumococcal vaccines**:
    (a) Functional or anatomic **asplenia.**
    (b) Chronic pulmonary diseases.
    (c) Healthy adults 65 years or over.
    (d) Chronic liver diseases.

(e) Chronic cardiac diseases.
(f) Diabetes, alcoholics, and chronic CSF leaks.

17. **Pneumococcal vaccine**:
   (a) It has 23 antigenic capsular polysaccharides which are responsible for 90% of all infections.
   (b) Protective effect is 79% in healthy adults.
   (c) It does not produce pneumococcal infections.
   (d) After vaccination, patients may develop fever, swelling, and pain at the site of an injection.

18. **Most bacterias have an outer cell wall except**: **Mycoplasma** Cell wall contains muramic acid.

19. **Major virulence factors in bacterias which prevent phagocytosis: Capsules** (pneumococcus and H.influenzae). Other factors are exotoxins (tetanus and cholera).

20. **Most common organism and sites of acute hematogenous osteomyelitis**: **S.aureus** infection in the **lumbar or thoracic vertebral spine**. Patients appear with fever, back pain, and symptoms of cord compression. S.aureus first appear in the intervertebral discs. Then spread to the adjacent vertebrae.
   X-ray: Narrowing of the intervertebral discs.
   CT scan: It can detect small bony changes.
   Bone scan: Not diagnostic;there is increased uptake of radionuclide.
   MRI: **Confirms the diagnosis** and **extent of the diseases**. MRI detects osteomyelitis earlier than X-ray and CT.
   Treatment: Antistaphylococcal antibiotics for 4 to 6 weeks + surgical debridement to drain abscesses, to **remove necrotic tissues and foreign bodies, if present**. Hematogenous osteomyelitis is most common in **spine** because vertebrae are **more vascular than other skeletal tissues.**

21. **S.aureus septic arthritis in sternoclavicular joint are typically found in.**
   (a) IV drug users.
   (b) Patient with subclavian IV catheters.

22. **S.aureus septic arthritis mostly occurs**: In **damaged** joints (s/p arthritis, surgery, prosthetic devices, injections, or aspirations). It **rarely** affects the normal joints either by hematogenous or spreads from adjacent **infected areas.**
   Diagnosis: **Arthrocentesis should be done before** the antibiotics treatment.

23. **S.aureus and (R) sided endocarditis**: It involves mostly the **tricuspid valve**. It is found in **IV drug users**. They are usually young and without previous cardiac problems.
    Presenting symptoms: Fever, acute onset of chest pain, and hemoptysis due to septic pulmonary emboli. No cardiac failure is noted.
    CXR: Multiple nodular infiltrates (bilateral) with or without cavity.
    Treatment: Appropriate antibiotics for 2 to 3 weeks (Nafcillin or vancomycin, plus gentamicin). Recurrence: Commonly occurs.
    Mortality: Low.

24. **S.aureus and (L) sided endocarditis:** It involves mostly the mitral valve. It may be found in elderly patients with existing cardiac valvular diseases in 75 % cases. Almost half of the patients will have either S.aureus skin infections or central venous catheters.
    Presenting symptoms: Fever, fatigue for couple of weeks followed most commonly with (L) **sided heart failure** (dyspnea, pulmonary edema, cyanosis) **in 50% cases** or CNS symptoms in other half.
    CXR: Pulmonary edema.
    Treatment: Antibiotics for 4 to 6 weeks (**nafcillin or vancomycin; add gentamicin for first 7 days**).
    Mortality: High.

25. **Most common cause for hospital acquired bacteremia**: Coagulase-negative staphylococci is **S.epidermidis**; **second** common organism is **S.aureus**. **Most common source for S.epidermidis infection is infected central venous catheters**;other sources are infected vascular grafts, prosthetic heart valves, and joints.

26. **S.aureus and bacteremia:** Two types.
    (a) **Nosocomial bacteremia**:
    Source: IV catheters:
    Symptoms & signs: Fever, sepsis, may include metastatic abscesses, endocarditis, and osteomyelitis.
    Treatment: Prolonged IV antibiotics and removal of sources (e.g., catheter).
    (b) **Community acquired bacteremia:**
    Source: skin infections, IV drug use, infected focuses (heart or peripheral tissues).
    Symptoms & signs: Same as nosocomial bacteremia.
    Treatment: Same as nosocomial bacteremia; Stop IV drug use.
    In all patients, source of infections should be found. If not found, then patients should be treated as they have endocarditis.

27. **Most common organism which is responsible for paraspinous or epidural abscess: S.aureus**. It is secondary to vertebral osteomyelitis.

28. **Most common toxin causing toxic shock syndrome (TSS)**: **Enterotoxin** rather than TSST-1(toxic shock syndrome toxin-1). **TSS is most commonly due to infected skin or other areas** rather than tampon. **Most common organism is S.aureus**.
Symptoms and signs: Fever, rashses (macular or scarlet fever-like), desquamation of skin in palms and soles (1 to 2 weeks after the onset of symptoms).

29. **Most common organism for skin cellulitis: Streptococcus pyogens;next is S.aureus**.

30. **Most common organism for furuncle, boil, or folliculitis in the skin: S.aureus.**

31. **Most common cause for toxic epidermal necrolysis**: Drug hypersensitivity reactions.
Signs and symptoms: Ulcerations of the skin and mucous membranes (absence Nikolsky's sign, which means easy separation of skin with minimal pressure).
Pathology: Epidermis is infiltrated with inflammatory cells.
Morality: High.

32. **Antibiotics for S.aureus bacteremic infections**:
    (a) **Community acquired (nosocomial): Vancomycin;** for metastatic infections or no source for bacteremia, all should be treated as endocarditis.
    (b) Hospital acquired (mostly resistant to drugs) should be guided by susceptibility testing or vancomycin.
        (i) Catheter related, after removal of the catheter fever and bacteremia disappears within 72 hours, **no** endocarditis, and **no** metastatic lesions: Antibiotics should be given for 2 weeks.
        (ii) Catheter related, persistent fever, endocarditis, or metastatic lesions: Antibiotics should be continued as in endocarditis.
    (c) Nosocomial S.epidermidis infection: Vancomycin.

33. **Prevention for hospital-acquired S.aureus infections**:
    (a) Strict hand washing technique.
    (b) Use separate gloves for each patients.

(c) Prophylactic antibiotics before and during the procedures for potential wound infections and implanted device infections.
(d) Patients with recurrent infections in the catheters, skin, or dialysis shunts: Do nares culture.
  (i) **Positive nares culture** for S.aureus: Use **topical mupirocin** ointment, then repeat the culture for effectiveness.
  (ii) If topical therapy is **ineffective**: **Use together rifampin + trimethoprim-sulfamethoxazole orally**, minocycline, ofloxacin, or ciprofloxacin.

34. **Most common organism causing both hematogenous and contiguous osteomyelitis: S.aureus**. When patients have **prosthetic materials** inside the body joints (metallic rod in bones) then S.epidermidis is the most common organism.

35. **Diabetes, foot ulcers, and osteomyelitis**: Diabetic patients mostly stay in the hospital for foot infections than for any other complication. Osteomyelitis develops from foot ulcers/infections by contiguous spread.

36. **Earliest bony changes in hematogenous osteomyelitis**: **Osteopenic or lytic lesions**. It takes **2 to 4 weeks** to develop. Subsequently new bone formations with sequestra and sclerotic changes occur.

37. A 19 year old female, who lives in a college dormitory, appears with **H/O** tracheobronchitis URI symptoms, fever, sore throat, nonproductive cough, **chills, but no rigors**. Her roommate had the similar symptoms 2 to 3 weeks ago.
Physical examination: Mildly injected throat with **enlarged cervical lymph nodes.**
Diagnosis:
(a) Serologic test: Compliment fixation (CF) titer ≥1:32. **Four fold rise of CF titer usually confirms the diagnosis.**
(b) Bed side cold agglutination test which represent agglutinations of RBC. Titer of cold agglutinin >1:64.
Most likely diagnosis: **Mycoplasma pneumoniae infection.**
Treatment:
(a) Mycoplasma pneumoniae: **Erythromycin, tetracycline**, or **doxycycline.**
(b) M.fermentans: **Doxycycline/or quinolone** or clindamcycin or tetracycline.
(c) M.hominis: Clindamycin or tetracycline.
(d) Ureaplasma urealyticum: Erythromycin or tetracycline.
Complications:

Mycoplasma pneumonia: Most patients have CXR finding of lower lobe segmental collapse (R)side or interstitial infiltrates.

38. **Most common cause for rash and pneumonia together**: **Mycoplasma pneumoniae**. Other causes are herpes simplex, Epstein-Barr virus, chlamydia, TB, meningococci, and fungus.

39. **Most frequent extrapulmonary complication of mycoplasma infections**: CNS (peripheral neuropathy, cranial nerves involvement, and Guillain-Barre syndrome may be present).

40. **Different mycoplasma infections:**
    (a) **M.hominis:** It should be suspected in purulent **surgical wounds which is negative in Gram stain and culture**, or in **immunocompromised patients after genitourinary manipulations**. It also causes PID (pelvic inflammatory diseases).
    (b) **Ureaplasma urealyticum:** It may cause nongonococcal urethritis, PID, and salpingitis.
    (c) **M.fermentans:** It may affect normal or immunocompromised patients (AIDS, leukemia, and chemotherapy). Patients appear with respiratory distress, fever, vomiting, and diarrhea.

41. **Relation between mycoplasma and HIV**: Patients with infection due to HIV-1 and simultaneous infection with mycoplasma which may enhance HIV replication or cytopathic effect, results in accelerated HIV infections.

42. **Causes for aspiration pneumonia:**
    (a) Obstruction of esophagus: Cancer or TE fistula secondary to treatment for cancer.
    (b) Neurogenic diseases affecting deglutition: Strokes are the most common cause.

    Obstruction of the esophagus: It causes aspiration of the oropharyngeal secretions proximal to obstruction. **Most common organism are aerobic bacterias which are normal floras**. **Most pathogenic organisms are Streptococcus pneumoniae**, S.aureus, and H.influenzae. Remember, normal people can aspirate small volumes during sleep but do **not** develop pneumonias.

43. **Aspiration pneumonias**: **Signs & Symptoms**: Fever, dyspnea, and purulent sputums.

    Physical examination: Coarse rhonchi in the dependent part of the lungs.

CXR: Infiltrates in the posterior aspects of the lower lobes and posterior parts of the upper lobes (dependent parts of the lungs).

Diagnosis confirmed:

(a) Presence of **food particles** in tracheal secretions: The **most definitive** findings.
(b) Presence of glucose (normally absent) in the oropharyngeal secretions.
(c) When diagnosis is **not** confirmed, then swallowing of the thin water-soluble contrast materials may be diagnostic.
(d) Patients with reflux: pH study of the lower esophagus which is acidic due to acidic gastric secretions.

Treatment for aspiration pneumonias:

(a) Intravenous penicillin or clindamycin + an aminoglycosides; alternate therapy is cephalosporins (2nd or 3rd generation).
(b) Tracheobronchial toileting.
(c) Nutrition: Enteral or TPN.
(d) Surgical repair for reflux.

44. **Most virulent type and factors of H.influenzae is**: **Type b because it is an extremely resistant to clearance**. The most virulent factors are the **capsules** which inhibits opsonization, intracellular killing and clearance; other factors are **fimbriae** which **increase adherence** of the H.influenzae to mucosal surfaces.

45. **Most common type of H.influenzae infection in HIV (human immunodeficiency virus) patients: Nontypable H.influenzae**;another study shows type b is the most common.

46. **Most common organisms of acute purulent sinusitis: Nontypable H.influenzae and staphylococcus pneumoniae.**

47. **H.influenzae pneumonia**: Patients appear with fever and cough.
CXR: **Lobar** consolidation.
Positive sputum Gram stain: Suggest the diagnosis.
Positive sputum culture: **Not** diagnostic because it colonizes in the respiratory tract.
Diagnosis is confirmed by: **Positive blood culture.**
Treatment: Ceftraixone or cefotaxime is the medicine of choice. Adults with **H/O** CSF leak or head trauma can develop **H.influenzae meningitis** which appears as high CSF WBC count (>1000 per cubic ml), low glucose, and nonspecific Gram stain. **PRP capsular antigens in CSF are also diagnositic**

even when the patient was treated with antibiotics before spinal tap was done. Positive CSF culture is most diagnostic for meningitis.

48. **Most common Hemophilus species causing endocarditis**: **H.parainfluenzae.** It can cause arterial embolization from endocarditis.

49. **Antibiotics prophylaxis for H.influenzae infections: Rifampin** is the medicine of choice.

50. **American Heart Association (AHA) recommendation of preventive antibiotic therapy for patients with postoperative cardiac prosthetic devices:** AHA **does** not recommend to continue antibiotics for 6 months or more.

51. **Most common cause of infective endocarditis:** Infection; most commonly is due to **bacteria**, other organisms are fungi, chlamydia, and rickettsia.

52. **Most common bacterias in different endocarditis:**
    (a) Previously normal valves: **Streptococci (alpha-hemolytic).**
    (b) Prosthetic valves (PVE): **Staph.epidermidis.**
    (c) IVDU (intravenous drug users): **Staph.aureus.**
    (d) Patients with GI (gastrointestinal, particularly colonic) problems: **Streptococcus bovis.**
    (e) Trauma to skin and mucous membranes: **Staphylococci, diptheroids.**
    (f) PVE after 1 year of surgery: **Streptococci (alpha hemolytic).**
    (g) **Rarely** occurs in **Non** IVDU: **Pseudomonas and fungi.**
    (h) Minor trauma to gum and teeth: **Strep. viridans.**
    (i) Endocarditis of the left side of the heart: **Streptococci.**
    (j) Endocarditis of the right side of the heart: **Staph.aureus.**
    (k) Acute endocarditis with sepsis: **S.aureus.**
    (l) Subacute endocarditis: **Streptococci, enterococci.**

53. **Most common risk factors for endocarditis:**
    (a) Prosthetic valves.
    (b) Degenerative cardiac diseases in elderly patients 65 or over.
    (c) Patients with a bicuspid aortic valve (males > females).
    (d) Conditions lead to bacteremia such as.
        (i) IV catheters.
        (ii) Noninvasive dental & gum procedures.
        (iii) Invasive urologic procedures (cystoscopy).

(iv) Surgical procedures of prostate, gallbladder, respiratory, intestinal mucosa, esophagus (dilatation), and skin (abscesses).

54. Large friable vegetations and emboli are due to **H.parainfluenzae,** candida albicans.

55. **Libman-Sacks endocarditis**: It is a nonbacterial thrombotic endocarditis (NBTE) found in SLE (systemic lupus erythematosus).
Marantic endocarditis: It is a NBTE found in chronic wasting diseases.
NBTE: There are depositions of **fibrins and platelets** in **the damaged endothelial cells** of the heart, results in vegetations which are sterile initially. Subsequently over vegetations, bacterias proliferate which also stimulate further depositions of fibrins and platelets over the bacterial layers. Majority of the bacterias are inactive so bactericidal effects of antibiotics are **not** very effective. Bacteremia from vegetations are cleared by RE system (reticuloendothelial) in the liver, spleen, and bone marrow. When there is **less clearance,** then **bacteremia persists**.

56. **In non-IVDU endocarditis, most commonly involved valve:** Aortic valve.

57. **Most common complication of endocarditis**: CHF (congestive heart failure).

58. **CHF most commonly occurs in:** Left sided endocarditis with aortic valve involvements.

59. **Endocarditis with cerebral abscess, most common organism**: S.aureus.

60. **Endocarditis**:
Signs & symptoms: **Most common is fever which is low grade (<39.4^0),** joint pain, muscle pain in lower back and thighs, and severe night sweats.
Cardiac:
(a) **Endocardial:** Heart murmurs of valvular insufficiencies due to destruction of the valves or valvular stenosis due to large vegetations.
(b) Myocardial: Myocarditis, infarctions, or abscesses.
Extracardiac: Infarctions of brain, kidneys, or spleen from left sided endocarditis, pulmonary infarctions from right sided endocarditis; vascular reaction includes petechiae, Roth spot (retinal hemorrhages), Osler's nodes, splinter hemorrhages; abscess formations, and infected mycotic aneurysms.
Endocarditis in IVDU: Most common presentations are fever and septic pulmonary embolisms/infarctions in younger patients. S.aureus is the most common organism. Heart murmurs and cardiac failure **are absent. Tricuspid**

valves are mostly involved because **right sided cardiac involvements are predominant**. The clinical presentations in left sided endocarditis mimic non-IVDU cases.

61. **Absent heart murmur in endocarditis are due to:**
    (a) Tricuspid valve endocarditis.
    (b) When patients are examined initially; murmurs appear subsequently.

62. Endocarditis patients with persistent fever despite appropriate antibiotics is due to: Valve ring abscesses.

63. Diffuse myocarditis in endocarditis is due to: Immune complex vasculitis.

64. **A 60 year old man appears with severe headache and difficulty in vision for the last few days. He was treated appropriately for endocarditis almost an year ago. Physical examination:** Cranial nerve paralysis.
    Most likely diagnosis: **Cerebral mycotic aneurysm which is about to rupture**. (Aneurysm more than 1 cm usually ruptures).
    Diagnosis is confirmed by: MRI, angiography (cerebral).
    Treatment: Surgery is needed if enlarging or bleeding. Cerebral aneurysms may heal with only medical treatment. **Intrathoracic, intraabdominal, or peripheral mycotic, aneurysms are required surgical treatment.**

65. **Nosocomial endocarditis**: Patients develop symptoms of endocarditis within 4 weeks of procedures done in the hospital. **Elderly patients** appear with **left sided heart failure and heart murmur**. Almost 50% of patients have **prosthetic valves**. Most common reason to develop bacteremia is **central venous catheter. The aortic valve is most commonly involved.**

66. **Diagnosis in infective endocarditis**:
    (a) Definitive diagnosis:
        (i) Postoperative cardiac patients and dead patients: Histologic examination of vegetations and cultures.
        (ii) Other conditions: **Positive blood cultures**+echocardiographic findings of vegetations, valve ring abscess, or dehiscence of newly placed prosthetic valves.
        (iii) Two major criteria.
        (iv) One major and three minor criteria.
        (v) Five minor criteria.

67. **Major criteria for infective endocarditis are the following:**

(A) **Blood cultures**:
  (a) Two separate cultures positive for the following organisms:
    (i) **Strep. viridans, S.bovis, HACEK (Hemophilus, Actinobacillus, Cardiobacterium, Eikenella, and Kingella).**
    (ii) **Community-acquired S.aureus or enterococci without primary focus.**
  (b) Positive blood cultures more than 12 hours apart.
  (c) Positive blood cultures: 3 out of 3, majority of ≥4 with first and last ≥1 hour apart.

(B) Echocardiography: Vegetations, valvular ring abscesses, new valvular regurgitations, or new prosthetic valve dehiscence.

68. **Minor criteria for infective endocarditis are the following:**
  (A) IVDU or predisposing cardiac conditions.
  (B) Fever 38^{0}c or more.
  (C) Systemic or pulmonary emboli, mycotic aneurysms.
  (D) Immunologic conditions: Rheumatoid factors, glomerulonephritis, Osler's nodes, Roth's spots in retina, and Janeway lesions.
  (E) Echocardiographic findings are suggestive of endocarditis but not definitive.
  (F) Microbiologic findings or serologic findings are consistent with endocarditis but **not** definitive.

69. A 40 year old man who is IVDU is admitted with **H/O** fever.
Physical examination: No sources of infections are found.
First investigation of choice: Blood cultures. Blood cultures are usually positive within one week. **(Important for Board examination).**
Management of patients in different conditions:
  (a) Positive blood cultures, positive clinical signs with positive endocarditis by echocardiography: **Treat as endocarditis.**
  (b) Positive blood cultures with positive clinical signs but negative TTE echocardiography: **Treat as endocarditis** and do TEE echocardiography if (-) ve repeat the test after one week.
  (c) Positive blood cultures with negative clinical signs and positive echocardiography: **Treat as endocarditis.**
  (d) Positive blood cultures with negative clinical signs and negative TTE echocardiography: Do TEE echocardiography, if (-) ve repeat the test after 1 week and look for any other source of infections; if there are no other sources, treat the **patients as endocarditis.**
  (e) Negative blood cultures, no sign of endocarditis, and patients are doing well, **discharge the patients home.**

(f) If the blood cultures are negative but the signs of endocarditis are present, patients should be **treated as endocarditis.**

70. **Management of nosocomial and prosthetic valves endocarditis:**

(a) IV catheters with S.aureus endocarditis: **Removal of the catheter+antibiotics** for endocarditis.

(b) Intravascular devices+bacteremia+endocarditis: **Removal of the intravascular devices** such as arterio-venous fistula, pacemaker wire, graft for hemodialysis, and cardiac assist balloon pump +antibiotics for endocarditis.

(c) IV catheters with S.epidermidis bacteremia without prosthetic valve: Removal of the catheter may **not** be necessary+antibiotics. No echocardiography is needed because **S.epidermidis** rarely causes native valve endocarditis (NAV).

(d) IV catheters with S.epidermidis bacteremia with prosthetic valves: Removal of the catheter, antibiotics, and echocardiography should be done.

(e) IV catheters with fungi positive blood cultures but no clinical signs of endocarditis and no prosthetic valves: Removal of the catheter, antifungal therapy, and echocardiography should be done.

(f) IV catheter with fungi positive blood cultures and clinical signs of endocarditis with or without prosthetic valves: Removal of the catheter+antifungal therapy+echocardiography should be done.

(g) Patients with prosthetic valves, fever, and positive bacterial cultures: Most likely have endocarditis and should be treated appropriately.

(h) Patients with prosthetic valves with fever: **First do 3 to 4 sets of blood cultures,** start antibiotics empirically. If blood cultures are positive then repeat the cultures to make sure that those become negative.

71. **Antibiotic therapy for infective endocarditis:**

(A) **Streptococcal infections**:

(a) Penicillin-responsive: Penicillin, or penicillin+streptomycin or gentamicin; or ceftraixone.

(b) Penicillin-responsive with **H/O** penicillin allergy: Cefazolin, ceftriaxone, or vancomycin.

(c) Relatively resistant to penicillin: Penicillin (higher dosages) + streptomycin or gentamicin.

(d) Enterococci or other streptococci: Penicillin or ampicillin + gentamicin; or streptomycin.

(e) Enterococci or other streptococci with **H/O** penicillin allergy: Vancomycin+gentamicin; or streptomycin.

(B) **Staphylococcal infections:**

(a) Methicillin-responsive: Nafcillin or oxacillin.
(b) Methicillin-responsive with **H/O** penicillin allergy: Cefazolin with or without gentamicin;or vancomycin.
(c) **Methicillin-resistant: Vancomycin.**
(d) Methicillin-resistant with prosthetic device: Vancomycin + rifampin + gentamicin.
(e) Methicillin-responsive with prosthetic device: Nafcillin or oxacillin+gentamicin with or without rifampin.

72. **Most common cause of death in infective endocarditis**: **Cardiac failure**. It is shifting towards **neurologic complications** (emboli, infections, or aneurysms) because cardiac valves are replaced by surgery with prosthetic valves in critically ill-patients.

73. Duration of antibiotics required before the repeat of blood cultures become negative in patients with infective endocarditis.
(a) **S.aureus**: 3 to 5 days after the onset of therapy.
(b) **S.aureus treated with vancomycin**: 10 to 14 days after the onset of therapy.
(c) **Streptococci and enterococci**: 1 to 2 days after the onset of therapy.
Blood cultures should be repeated daily until the cultures become negative.

74. **Best outcome in infective endocarditis**: Streptococcus viridans infection in non-IVDU patients.

75. **Worst outcome in infective endocarditis**: Early onset of prosthetic valve endocarditis.

76. **Prevention of bacterial endocarditis (AHA recommendation)**:
(A) Procedures for urogenital and gastrointestinal tract:
(a) Penicillin non-allergic patients: Ampicillin, gentamicin, and amoxicillin.
(b) Penicillin allergic patients: Vancomycin+gentamicin.
(c) Alternate low risk patients: Amoxicillin.
(B) Procedures for oral, dental, or upper respiratory tract:
(a) Penicillin non-allergic patints: PO Amoxicillin or IV ampicillin.
(b) Penicillin allergic patients: PO Erythromycin or IV clindamycin.
(c) High-risk patients: with or without prosthetic heart valve and penicillin non-allergic patients Ampicillin, gentamicin, and amoxicillin.
(d) High-risk patients with or without prosthetic heart valve and penicillin-allergic patients:Vancomycin.

77. **Pneumonias with cavities-most common organisms**: **Klebsiella**, **then pseudomonas.**
Lung gangrene: Extensive lung necrosis is found in Gram negative infections with systemic toxicities. Lung necrosis is due to extracellular products produced by these organisms. Pseudomonas produces virulent factors such as exotoxin A, exoenzyme S, neural protease, and elastase. **K. pneumoniae** do not produce any of those virulent factors so mechanisms are unknown.

78. **Aerobic Gram negative bacterial infections (GNB)**: Two types:
(a) Hospital acquired (nosocomial).
(b) Community acquired.
Hospital acquired GNB pneumonias are most commonly found in:
(i) Postoperative patients.
(ii) Severely ill ICU (intensive care unit) patients on mechanical ventilator, may **not** have underlying chronic lung disease.

79. **Poor prognostic sign in GNB pneumonias**: Leukopenia.

80. **Diagnosis of GNB pneumonias**: It is difficult because GNB are present in the oropharyngeal secretions in **normal** persons. Blood cultures are positive in nosocomial GNB infections=8% only.
Blood cultures are positive in community acquired GNB infections =20 to 30 % only.
Pleural fluid cultures are positive in effusion =30% only. BAL (bronchoalveolar lavage) or PSB (protected specimen brush) may be helpful, BAL is more helpful in immunocompromised hosts because specimens can be examined for special staining and cytology.

81. **Treatment for GNB pneumonia**:
(a) **Pseudomonas**: **Ceftazidime + amikacin**, ticarcillin+amikacin, or imipenem/cilastin+amikacin. (Monitor renal functions closely).
(b) Combination therapies for normal renal functions: **Cefuroxime + gentamicin,** Cefotaxime + gentamicin, or pipercillin+gentamicin.
Single therapy for abnormal renal functions: Cefotaxime or ticarcillin/clavulanate.
Remember, **if patients are improving, continue the same treatment despite culture results which may be confusing.**

82. **Most important complications of GNB pneumonias**: **Empyema**;other complications are superinfections, metastatic infections, lung necrosis, and

multiple organ failure. Empyema pleural fluids consist of pH ≤7.2, **positive Gram stain, WBC count >30,000/dl.**

83. **Therapies for extensive lung necrosis depends on potential complications**:
    (a) Definitive therapy: Surgical resection.
    (b) Pneumothorax: Chest tube.
    (c) Antibiotics.
    (d) Supportive therapies.

84. **Risk factors for Legionellae infections**:
    (a) Glucocorticoid administration or its endogenous production.
    (b) OKT3 therapy.
    (c) Chronic cardiac or pulmonary patients.
    (d) Elderly patients over 50 years of age.
    (e) Hairy cell leukemia.
    (f) AIDS patients.
    Factors that do **not** cause any risks are: Cyclosporine, cytotoxic medications, neutropenia, or hematologic cancers except hairy cell leukemias.

85. **Most important nutritional element for Legionellae**: **L-cysteine** in growth media.

86. **Most common subgroup of Legionellae causing infections: L.pneumophila subgroup 1.**

87. **"Typical" presentations of Legionnaires' disease**: It is found in few patients. Patients appear with fever, mild GI symptoms (vomiting, abdominal pain, or diarrhea without dehydrations);respiratory symptoms & signs (sputum with rarely blood stained, rales, or effusion) appear later.

88. **Most definite diagnostic test for Legionellae infections**: **Culture of the respiratory tract secretions such as sputum**.

89. **Treatment of choice for Legionellae infections**: **Erythromycin.** Experimental medications which are more effective than erythromycin are the quinolone antimicrobials (ciprofloxacin) and macrolide antimicrobials (azithromycin, clarithromycin).
    (a) Severe infections: Add rifampin.
    (b) Organ transplantation in patients: Use quinolone medicines because they do not interfere with cyclosporine levels.

90. **Sites of extrapulmonary infections caused by Legionella**: **Dialysis shunts**, sinuses, peritoneum, prosthetic valves, pericardium, or different organ abscesses (e.g.,brain, kidneys, bowel).

91. **Pontiac fever:** Patients appear with fever, myalgia, and headache (flue-like symptoms). It is a self-limited, (unproven) legionellae infection, mostly epidemic in origin; found in Jacuzzi-type bath or spa, factories, and offices.
Diagnosis:
(a) Isolation of legionellae from water.
(b) Increase antibody titer.
(c) Very difficult to diagnose non-epidemic infections.

92. **Most common organism causing cellulitis: Group A streptococcus;2nd is S.aureus**.
Cellulitis: Gr.A streptococci spread into the subcutaneous tissues and epidermis, result in **pain, erythema, and swelling.**
Treatment: Penicillin, dicloxacillin.
Patients are susceptible to develop cellulitis in the following conditions:
(a) Chronic lymphatic stasis or lymphedema (lymphoma, lymph nodes resection during mastectomy or prostatectomy due to cancer and filariasis).
(b) Recurrent saphenous vein donor-site cellulitis caused by streptococci (group A, C, or G).

93. **Most common organism for necrotizing fascitis (Important for Board examination)**: **Group A streptococci.** Necrotizing fascitis is a progressive infection of the subcutaneous tissues which damage the fascia and fat (but skin may be spared).
Progressive local infections (first to last):
(a) **Within day 1**: Pain, erythema, heat, swelling, and tenderness.
(b) **Day 1 to 2**: Skin color changes from red to purple then to blue. Blisters or bullae form with yellow clear fluid.
(c) **Day 4 to 5**: Skin becomes gangrenous.
(d) **Day 7 to 10**: Clear line of demarcation between dead skin and healthy skin, extensive necrosis of the subcutaneous tissues under the dead skin. Patients are very sick, unresponsive, and emaciated.
Treatment:
(a) **"Bearclaw fasciotomy"** which is an aggressive fasciotomy and debridement; irrigation with Dakan's solution. **This is the most important treatment.**
(b) Appropriate antibiotics: Clindamycin, penicillin.

94. A 40 year old man appears with **H/O** sudden onset of pain in the right lower extremity, fever, and mild confusion. Patient had **H/O** minor surgery or trauma recently.
Physical examination: Hypotension, tachycardia, right lower extremity redness, tenderness, and swelling.
CBC: Thrombocytopenia, mild leukocytosis with shift to left.
SMA_8:↓Ca, ↑creatine phosphokinase, ↑BUN; U/A-hematuria. (U/A = Urinalysis).
ABG:↓pH, ↓Pao_2.
Most likely clinical diagnosis: **Streptococcal toxic shock syndrome.**
Diagnosis is confirmed by:
(a) Isolation of the organism from the deep tissue specimens (95%).
(b) Positive blood cultures (60% only).
Treatment: **Clindamycin is the drug of choice;** or penicillin.
Most common strains isolated: **M types 1,3,12, and 28.**
Toxin: Pyrogenic **exotoxins A** and/ or **B** are noted.

95. **Prophylaxis in Military service**: Monthly injection of benzathine penicillin reduces the incidence of pharyngitis and rheumatic fever caused by Streptococci.

96. **Mechanism of action of clindamycin in streptococcal infections**: Clindamycin suppresses M protein synthesis. It has a longer postantibiotic effect.

97. **Non-group A streptococcal infections:**
(a) **S.bovis:** Patients with GI cancer with bacteremia and subacute bacterial endocarditis.
Treatment: Penicillin.
(b) **Streptococci group C and G**: Patients with coronary artery bypass develop cellulitis of the donor site of saphenous vein.
Treatment: Penicillin, vancomycin, clindamycin, and erythromycin.
(c) S.milleri: Patients develop contiguous abscesses formations such as tooth abscess and periappendiceal abscess etc.
Treatment: Penicillin.
(d) S.agalactiae: Patients develop postpartum sepsis, soft tissue infections, septic arthritis, and osteomyelitis.
Treatment: Penicillin, vancomycin, or 1st generation cephalosporin.
(e) Enterococcus faecalis: Patients develop endocarditis, UTI, and bacteremia. It **causes nosocomial infections due to antibiotic resistance** but **is not due to** virulence.

Treatment: Ampicillin or vancomycin+aminoglycoside.

98. **Most common organism for acute bacterial meningitis**: **S.pneumoniae.** Next common organism is N.meningitidis and then **L.monocytogenes**. In large urban hospitals like Massachusetts General Hospital most common cause of bacterial meningitis is **nosocomial** and most common organisms are **E.coli (1st) and Klebsiella (2nd)** which are Gram-negative bacilli.

99. **Most common predisposing factors causing pneumococcal meningitis**: **Acute otitis media with or without mastoiditis;** (20% other factors are pneumonia, sinusitis, recent or remote head injury, CSF rhinorrhea, and alcoholism).

100. **Most common bacterial organism causing meningitis after complications of neurosurgical procedures: S.aureus.** It also occurs after penetrating skull injury, staphylococcal bacteremia, and endocarditis.

101. **Most common organism causing Gram-negative bacillary meningitis**: **E.coli.**

102. **Most common bacterial meningitis in cancer**: **Pseudomonas aeruginosa (1st), then E.coli (2nd).**

103. A 45 year old man appears with signs of meningitis (stiff neck, positive Kernig's and Brudzinski's signs). Patient has been suffering from URI symptoms with fever for the last few days.
Physical examination: Petechial, purpuric, or ecchymotic rash over the body.
Mostly likely diagnosis: **Meningococcal meningitis**. Other organisms causing **petechiae** with meningitis are:
    (a) Viral aseptic meningitis: It occurs in the summer months. Patients appear with meningeal signs plus macular and petechial rashes. Spinal tap shows several hundreds WBC with increased polymorphs in early stage.
    (b) **Very rarely, S.pneumonae, H.influenzae, and S.aureus.**

104. **Sensorineural deafness in bacterial meningitis is due to:**
    (a) **Inner ear infection or toxic products** spread from subarachnoid space along the cochlear aqueduct.
    (b) **Acoustic nerve involvement.**

105. **Neurologic complications of bacterial meningitis**:
    (a) Seizures with meningitis: **S.pneumoniae is the most common organism.**

(b) Focal cerebral signs (hemiparesis, visual field defects, dysphagia, and gaze preference): It is due to **decreased blood flow** secondary to increased intracranial pressure.
(c) **Todd's paralysis**: Postictal lateralizing findings which last only few hours.
(d) Cerebral edema and subsequent temporal lobe herniation.
(e) Residual neurologic damage after recovery.
(f) Temporary cranial nerves (3rd,4th,6th, or 7th) involved.

106. **CSF examination in bacterial meningitis**:
(a) **Pressure**: Increased (200 to 300 mm H_2O; >450 mm H_2O means acute cerebral edema).
(b) **Most confirmatory test**: **Positive CSF culture.**
(c) **Gram-stain**: Positive in 60 to 80% cases. It gives morphologic diagnosis.
(d) Cell count: **WBC count 100 to 10,000 per cubic millimeter with polymorphs ≥80%,** cell count**>50,000 may indicate cerebral abscess,** lowest cell count 10 to 20 may by found in **N.meningitidis, and H.influenzae**. Increased lymphocytes count is usually due to TB and syphilis.
(e) Protein: **Increased, >100 mg/dL**; >1000 mg/dL or more indicates subarachnoid obstruction is due to meningitis.
(f) Glucose: Decreased,40 mg/dL or less (or less than 50% of simultaneous blood level). Remember, normal glucose does **not** exclude meningitis.
(g) C-reactive protein: Increased. It is normal in viral meningitis.
(h) **Rapid diagnosis of bacterial antigens by latex agglutination (LA)**: It is helpful when Gram stain is negative. The following bacterias are indentified by LA technique-H.influenzae type b, pneumococci, meningococci (group A, B, C, and Y), group B streptococci, and E.coli K1. It **cannot** diagnose gonococcous and nontypable H.influenzea. E.coli K1 and group B meningococci have common antigenic determinant, may show false positivity.

107. **Hypoglycorrhachia (low CSF glucose) in pyogenic bacterial meningitis is due to**:
(a) **Decreased carrier- facilitated diffusion** of glucose in CSF from blood.
(b) **Increased utilization of glucose by host cells.**

108. **Blood cultures in bacterial meningitis**:
(a) **H.influenzae**: 80% have positive blood cultures.
(b) **Pneumococci**: 50% have positive blood cultures.
(c) **Meningococci**: 30 to 40% have positive blood cultures.

109. **Indications of head CT scan in bacterial meningitis**: (Do **not** delay the treatment of meningitis in order to obtain CT scan).
   (a) Focal cerebral signs and papilledema.
   (b) Mass lesion (cerebral abscess, subdural, and empyema).
   (c) When patients are **not** improving with medical therapy such as subdural empyema, complicating hydrocephalus, cerebral infarctions, ventricular empyema, or persistent basillar meningitis.
   (d) Parameningeal accumulations (epidural and subdural infections are due to otitis, mastoiditis, or lung abscess).

110. **The syndrome after antibiotic therapy for meningococcal meningitis-(Important)**: It is a syndrome which includes **fever, arthritis, and pericarditis.** It is found after 3 to 6 days of antibiotics therapy only in 10% of patients.

111. **Persistence or recurrence of fever in bacterial meningitis**: (Important).
   (a) Patients are improving clinically: Drug fever.
   (b) Patients are getting worse clinically:
      (i) Inadequate antibiotic therapy.
      (ii) Neurologic complications (subdural empyema, ventriculitis, or cortical vein thrombophlebitis): **Do head CT scan.**
      (iii) Metastatic complications (septic arthritis, endocarditis, pericarditis, or empyema in the thoracic cavity).
      (iv) Post meningococcal therapy syndrome.

   Diagnosis:
   (a) Repeat CSF examinations.
   (b) Appropriate investigations for different presentations.

   Treatment: According to the underlying problems.

112. **Most common organism causing recurrent bacterial meningitis**:
   (a) Community acquired: **S.pneumoniae**.
   (b) Nosocomial (or hospital) acquired: **S.aureus**.

113. **Recurrent bacterial meningitis (Important points to remember)**:
   (a) H/O head trauma is very common.
   (b) **Most common organisms** enter the subarachnoid space through **a defect in the cribiform plate.**
   (c) Skull fracture at the base or erosive mastoiditis can cause recurrent meningitis.
   (d) Neurosurgical procedures are the most important causes of recurrent meningitis.

(e) CSF rhinorrhea or otorrhea.
(f) Immunologic deficiencies can cause recurrent bacterial meningitis.
(g) Rarely, nonbacterial causes mimic bacterial meningitis:
  (i) **Behcet's syndrome**: Relapsing oral and genital ulcers with meningitis.
  (ii) **Mollaret's meningitis**: Repeated fever with mild **meningitis** without neurological involvement. Initially CSF contains endothelial cells and polymorphs, later replaced with lymphocytes.

114. A 35 year old man appears with **H/O** persistent rhinorrhea for 4 to 6 weeks after a head injury.
Treatment:
(a) Surgical repair is indicated when CSF leak is more than 4 to 6 weeks.
(b) Do **not** give prophylactic penicillin therapy for long time to prevent pneumococcal infections. It enhances infections with drug-resistant organisms.

115. Treatment for bacterial meningitis: **Best way to select antibiotics after the sensitivity tests.**
(a) **S.aureus**: **Nafcillin or vancomycin.**
(b) **S.pneumoniae**: **Penicillin.** or ampicillin; cefotaxime; ceftriaxone or vancomycin.
(c) **H.influenzae**: **Cefotaxime.**
(d) **Pseudomonas**: Ceftazidime plus tobramycin or gentamicin.
(e) **Listeria**: **Penicillin or ampicillin.**
(f) **Enterobacteriaceae**: Cefotaxime or ceftazidime (E.coli, Klebsiella, Proteus). Cefuroxime causes sensorineural hearing loss and slower sterilization of CSF.

116. **Repeat CSF examination in bacterial meningitis**: (Important) **It should be done in the following conditions:**
(a) Patients are not improving within 1-2 days after therapy.
(b) Pneumococcal meningitis.
(c) Gram-negative meningitis particularly postoperative neurosurgical patients.
It should **not** be done:
(a) Routinely.
(b) When patients are improving clinically.
(c) Meningococci and H.influenzae meningitis patients are improving clinically.

117. **Important management of bacterial meningitis in different conditions**:
(a) Brain swelling: Use **corticosteroid** after the onset of antibiotics therapy.

(b) Increased intracranial pressure: Mannitol can be used.
(c) Normal blood pressure: Fluid restrictions (1200 to 1500 ml/day) to avoid brain edema due to ↑ADH secretions in meningitis.
(d) Hypotension: First fluid resuscitations until the BP is normal then fluid restrictions.
(e) Acute convulsion: Diazepam.
(f) Maintenance therapy for convulsion: Dilantin.

118. **Pyogenic focus (mastoid abscess) with bacterial meningitis and surgery**: Treatment:
(a) Surgery is indicated after the antibiotics to **control and complete recovery from meningitis**. Antibiotics should be continued during and after surgery.
(b) **Bezold abscess** (hyperacute mastoid infection): Surgery is required **after 2 days of antibiotics therapy.**

119. **Isolation of patients with meningococcal infections**: **Respiratory isolation which is discontinued after 24 hours** of appropriate antibiotics treatment.

120. **People susceptible to acquire infection when exposed to meningococcal infections**:
(a) College roommates.
(b) Close family members.
(c) Nursery school occupants.
(d) Mouth to mouth resuscitations and needle stick with contaminated fluid in hospital personnel. Remember the hospital personnel who are responsible for taking care of patients with meningococcal infections are **not** at risk for acquiring the infections.

121. A 35 year old female was brought to the emergency room in the month of February. She told the doctor, this is the sickest illness she ever experienced. She appears with acute onset fever, headache, vomiting, myalgia, and diaphoresis for the last 24 hours.
Physical examination: BP ↓,↑HR, meningeal signs (Kernig's and Brudzinski's signs) are present with petechiae over the skin, mucous membrane, or conjunctiva.
CBC: Leukocytosis with a shift to the left, thrombocytopenia, or leukopenia.
PTT:> 50 seconds.
Fibrinogen: >150 microgram/dl.
CSF Gram-stain: Positive **N.meningitidis**.
CSF culture: **Confirmatory test.**
Blood culture: Highly suggestive.

PCR (polymerase chain reaction): Rapid method of diagnosing infections in CSF and blood. Rapid detection of capsular polysaccharides antigen: Most commonly positive in type A and C.

Diagnosis: Meningococcal meningitis.

Treatment: Penicillin, ampicillin, or ceftriaxone; chloramphenicol for penicillin allergic patients.

122. **Treatment for other meningococcal infections**:
   (a) Pericarditis: Antibiotics and removal of pericardial fluid.
   (b) Cardiac failure: Treat the heart failure.
   (c) Pneumonia: Antibiotics.
   (d) Urethritis (due to orogential sex): Penicillin and/or tetracycline.
   (e) Chronic meningococcemia (painful skin lesions, migratory polyarthritis, and tenosynovitis): Antibiotics.

   It is difficult to distinguish from gonococcal dermatitis- arthritis syndrome.

123. **Prophylaxis for meningococcal infections**: **(Important for Board examination).**
   (a) **Rifampin**: **It is the drug of choice.** PO 600 mg every 12 hours for 2 days.
   (b) Ceftriaxone: It is used when rifampin is contraindicated. Single dose of 250 mg should be given.
   (c) Meningococcal vaccine has been used in the U.S. military effectively due to crowdedness.

124. **Traveler's diarrhea and recommendations**:
   (a) **Cook it, boil it, or peel it.**
   (b) If diarrhea develops use oral rehydrating solutions containing glucose and electrolytes.
   (c) Antibiotic: Ciprofloxacin for infectious diarrhea.
   (d) Antimotility drug: Loperamide which reduces the duration of secretary diarrhea. It is contraindicated in bloody diarrhea, inflammatory colitis, or high fever.

125. **Prophylaxis for malaria infections**: Plasmodium falciparum is the most common type.
   (a) Apply insect repellents.
   (b) Long-sleeved clothing.
   (c) Use mosquito net.
   (d) Put permethrin in clothing and mosquito netting.
   (e) **Medications: Chloroquine phosphate;** in case of drug resistence use mefloquine or doxycycline.

(f) Late relapses with P.vivax and P.ovale: Primaquine phosphate.

126. **Advice to travelers:**

(a) Jet lag: Short acting benzodiazepines; avoid alcohol and excessive food during flight.
(b) Altitude sickness: Acetazolamide (diuretics).
(c) STD (sexually transmitted diseases): Latex condom.
(d) Motion sickness:
  (i) Short travel: Diphenhydramine.
  (ii) Long travel or cruise: Sustained- release transdermal scopolamine.

127. **Immunizations to adults international travelers- traveling to developing countries**:

(a) Hepatitis A-Immunoglobulin (2 ml, for less than 3 months visit and 5 ml, for 3 to 5 months visit). It is not needed when patients have anti-hepatitis A IgG antibodies.
(b) Yellow fever vaccine: Live, attenuated vaccine. It **cannot** be used in HIV-infected travelers.
(c) Typhoid vaccine: Oral live vaccine **cannot** be used in HIV-infected travelers, persons receiving antibiotics or mefloquine.
(d) Meningococcal, rabies, and Japanese B encephalitis.
(e) **No need for cholera vaccine, only food and water precautions.**

128. **Immunizations recommeded for all adult travelers**:

MMR (measles, mumps, rubella), hepatitis B, DT (diptheria, tetanus), and poliomyelitis.

129. **Most common nosocomial infection (hospital acquired): UTI** (urinary tract infection). Most frequent cause of UTI is frerquent use of **Foley catheters.**

E.coli is the most common organism. Patients are mostly asymptomatic or mildly symptomatic. Infecting bacterias colonize at the tip of the urethral meatus, enter and infect the bladder urine during catheterization.

Treatment: Removal of the catheter and antibiotics for UTI.

Prophylaxis:

(a) Use Foley catheter only when it is absolutely necessary.
(b) Remove the catheter as soon as possible.
(c) No need to do routine catheter tip culture.
(d) No routine urine culture is needed.
(e) No need to use antibiotic containing cream in the perinium or in the catheter tip.
(f) Use of systemic prophylactic antibiotics is unsettled while catheter is inside.

(g) Bladder irrigation with antibiotic is **not** helpful.
(h) **Closed drainage system is very helpful**. It means catheter should **not** be disconnected from the urine bag to empty the bag.

130. **Most common organism causing intravenous catheter related infections**: **S.aureus** and **S.epidermidis**; other organisms are Gram-negative bacilli and candida.
Treatment: Removal of the catheter, antibiotics, or antifungal medication.

131. **Surgical wound infections**: Most common organisms are **S.aureus and S.epidermidis.**
Prophylaxis: Antibiotics are used **no** more than 24 hours after postoperative course.
Treatment: Appropriate use of antibiotics.

132. **Different nosocomial infections:**
(a) Patients with renal transplantation: **Cryptococcus and Listeria** are the most important organisms.
(b) Ventricular shunt infections: **S.epidermidis** is the most common organism.
(c) Infectious diarrhea after antibiotic therapy: **Clostridium difficile** is the most common organism.
(d) Epidemic keratoconjunctivitis: **Adenovirus** can spread from the contaminated tonometers and hands of opthalmologist.

133. **Prevention of tuberculosis: (Important)**.
(a) Yearly PPD testing, early testing for high risk patients.
(b) PPD positive: Do CXR.
(c) PPD positive, CXR negative: Only INH.
(d) PPD positive, CXR positive: Antituberculous medications.
Remember, **annual CXR** is **not recommended**.

134. **Prophylaxis for hepatitis B:**
(a) Hepatitis B vaccine should be given to all health care workers (doctors, nurses, medical students, laboratory workers, and all other workers with potential risks).
(b) Reduce the injury through education, proper handling, and disposal of the sharps.

135. **Most important risk factor for immunocompromised host**: **Granulocytopenia**. It is defined as a count of $\leq$500 polymorphs and band forms per microliter.

136. **Most important cause for granulocytopenia**: **Malignancy**; other causes are cytotoxic medications used for cancer.

137. **Granulocytopenia associated with:**
   (a) AML (acute myelogenous leukemia): Quickly develops bacterial (Gram-negative, anaerobes, or alpha-streptococci) infections because of damaged mucosal defense barrier.
   (b) Aplastic anemia without steroid: Bacterial infections are not developed as quickly as AML due to of the intact mucosal defense barrier.
   (c) Aplastic anemia with steroid or cyclosporine therapy: Increases risk for viral or fungal infection.

138. **Most common types of infections in granulocytopenic patients**: **E.coli;** K.pneumoniae, and P.aeruginosa (Gram-negative organisms). **E.coli** is the most common; **P.aeruginosa is the most virulent organism.** Most common Gram-positive organisms are **S.epidermidis** and S.aureus.

139. **Infections associated with GI injuries (abscess, peritonitis)**: Anaerobic bacterias are common with granulocytopenia.

140. **Most common candida infections with granulocytopenia**: C.albicans.

141. **Most common organism causes pseudomembranous colitis (PMC)**: Clostridium difficile.

142. **Most frequent cause for PMC:** Antibiotics (ampicillin, clindamycin, and cephalosporins).

143. C.difficile **colitis** is due to: **Toxins are attached to the colonic mucosa and cause colitis**; it is **not** due to the bacterial invasions into the colonic mucosa. **Toxin A (enterotoxin) is the most commonly responsible**. **Toxin B (cytotoxin)** does **not** attach to the mucosa, it causes additional damage in severe cases.

144. A 50 year old man appears with H/O **acute abdominal pain, mild fever, and severe diarrhea**. The patient was taking ampicillin for last 5 days.
Physical examination: Abdominal tenderness and mild dehydration.
CBC: **Leukocytosis** (up to 50,000 per cubic millimeter).
Most likely diagnosis: Pseudomembranous colitis.
Diagnosis:

(a) Endoscopy is the best and most rapid way to make a diagnosis.
(b) Stool culture: **Not diagnostic** because 10 to 25 % of patients in the hospital may carry this organism and only 75% of isolates release toxins.
(c) Abdominal CT scan: May be helpful in patients with acute abdominal symptoms.

Treatment:
(a) Discontinue the antibiotics.
(b) **PO vancomycin is the drug of choice** or metronidazole.
(c) **To prevent relapse or recurrence** weeks or months after discontinuation of antibiotics: Try to restore normal fecal flora by giving lactobacilli or live yeast **(Saccharomyces boulardii)** for few weeks.

145. **Most frequent source of botulism in the USA: Home-canned food. Type A and B of Clostridium botulinum are the most common in USA.**

146. A 35 year old woman appears with H/O sudden onset of diplopia, nausea, vomiting, and abdominal pain for the last 12 hours. She ate canned food last night.
Physical examination: Paralysis of VI cranial nerve, ptosis, and dilated both pupil.
Most likely diagnosis: Foodborne botulism.
Diagnosis is confirmed by:
(a) Botulinum toxins are found in food, serum, gastric contents, or stool (in diarrhea).
(b) C.botulinum organisms are found in food and/or stool.

Treatment:
(a) Antitoxin is the treatment of choice.
(b) Penicillin is used to eradicate the organism.
(c) Gastric lavage, cathartics, and enema to remove toxins from the GI tract.
(d) Ventilatory support: **Respiratory failure is a most serious complication of botulism.**

Prevention: Botulism is due to germination of spores and toxins released by vegetative forms.
(a) To destroy spores: Use heat or irradiation of the food.
(b) To inactivate toxins: Terminal heating of food before eating.
(c) To inhibit germination of spores: Reduce pH, sodium nitrate, refrigerating, freezing, drying, salt, or sugar.

147. **Most common type of tetanus in USA: Generalized**. Other types are **localized and cephalic**. Tetanus is due to neurotoxin released by Clostridium tetani at the site of injury. Patients are moslty over 60, unimmunized, H/O

injury, appear with **trismus (most common presentation),** diaphoresis, irritability, drooling, and hydrophobia.
Diagnosis: Clinical presentation.
Treatment: Penicillin. Human tetanus immunoglobulin (TIG) (Tetanus is rare in USA, and is not important for an examination).

148. **Most common organism in community acquired aspiration pneumonias**: **Anaerobes (90% cases)**. Most common anaerobes is **Bacteroides fragilis**.

149. **Transient anaerobic bacterimia is found in 85% of the cases:** After dental procedures or cleaning.

150. **Most common cause of vaginitis**: Bacterial vaginosis (45% of all cases) is due to anaerobes. Patients appear with foul vaginal discharge. Presence of "clue cells" and a vaginal pH > 4.5 are important findings. It also causes PID (pelvic inflammatory diseases), endometritis, and tubo-ovarian abscess.

151. **Anaerobes are the most common organisms causing following infections**:
   (a) Animal and human bites.
   (b) Intraabdominal abscess.
   (c) PID.
   (d) Skin and soft tissue infections particularly in diabetes (uncontrolled).
   (e) Gas gangrene, necrotizing cellulitis, and **Fournier's gangrene** which **is a serious infection and subsequent gangrene of the scrotum or perinium**. It is **found in diabetes or trauma**.

152. **Enteric infections and presentations:**
   (a) **S.aureus food poisoning**: Symptoms are acute onset of vomiting which begins <**4 hours** after the intake of contaminated foods.
   (b) **Bacillus cereus** enterotoxin food poisoning: Symptoms & signs of food poisoning appear >8 hours after the intake of contaminated foods.
   (c) **Giardia lamblia** infection: It occurs in **mountainous regions of the USA. Treatment: Metronidazole.**
   (d) **Enterotoxigenic E.coli, salmonella, or shigella infection**: It occurs in the developing countries from the contaminated water and food.
   (e) **Cryptosporidium**, microsporidium, CMV, C.jejuni, C.difficile, and Mycobacterium avium-intracellulare infections: They are found in homosexual males with diarrhea.

153. A 30 year old woman appears in the emergency room with H/O fever, chills, mild abdominal pain, and diarrhea. She went to a developing country for vacation 2 weeks ago.

Physical examination: The patient looks acutely ill and appears with rose spots (rashes over the chest and abdomen), abdominal mild tenderness, and mild hepatosplenomegaly.

Diagnosis is made by:

Blood cultures: Positive for Salmonella typhi is the most definitive test.

Bone marrow culture: It is the most sensitive test. It is helpful when a patient received antibiotic before a blood culture was done.

Stool culture: May be positive for S.typhi.

CBC: Leukopenia, thrombocytopenia, and anemia.

The Widal test: An O agglutination titer (1:80 or four fold increase support the diagnosis.

Diagnosis: Typhoid fever.

Treatment: **Chloramphenicol is the drug of choice**; trimethoprim-sulfamethoxazole or ampicillin. Some are resistant to all of the above mentioned medications. **The drug of choice is ciprofloxacin.**

Complications: Intestinal bleeding and perforation.

Prevention:

(a) Cook it, boil it, or peel it to avoid contaminated food and water.
(b) Typhoid vaccine or live oral vaccine Ty21a: It is partially protective.

154. **Most common form of salmonella infections**: Inapparent infections which may lead to chronic carrier states.

Most common clinical manifestation in Salmonella infections: Enterocolitis with diarrhea.

Enteric typhoid fever: **S.typhi**. **It is found only in humans**.

Enteric paratyphoid fever: **S.paratyphi A, B, and C**; **most common is type A.**

Chronic carrier of typhoid: Infection in the gall bladder more than one year duration.

Transient carrier of typhoid: Self-limited. The carrier state disappears in several weeks to months.

155. **Clinical presentations of salmonella infections:**

(a) **Paratyphoid fever or enteric fever**: It is caused by **S.paratyphi A (most common), B, and C.** Patients appear with fever, relative bradycardia, rose spots, leukopenia, and enlarged spleen. Enteric fever without S.typhi is a mild variety.
(b) **Salmonella bacteremia**: Most **common type is S.choleraesuis.** Patients appear with fever, chills, metastatic infections to bones, heart, brain and

abdominal aortic mycotic aneurysm. Patients have no GI symptoms and have negative stool cultures.

(c) **Salmonella enterocolitis:** Patients appear with fever, chills, abdominal pain, and diarrhea. Fever disappears in 3 days and diarrhea disappears in 7 days. Reactive arthritis is a complication when patients have HLA-B27 phenotype.

(d) **Asymptomatic intestinal carrier of Salmonella:** It is either due to inapparent infection or sequelae of clinical disease (convalescent carrier).

156. **Relationship between Schistosoma haematobium infections and Salmonella**: Patients with S.haematobium infection may become a chronic carrier of Salmonella in the urinary tract.

157. **Diagnosis of different Salmonellae infections:**
   (a) Enterocolitis: Positive stool culture is diagnostic.
   (b) Bacteremia: Positive blood culture is diagnostic.
   (c) Enteric fever: Positive blood and stool cultures are diagnostic.

158. **Treatment for different Salmonellae infections**:
   (a) Carriers:
      (i) Transient: No treatment is needed.
      (ii) Chronic (over 1 year): **Ampicillin and probenecid** together for 6 weeks or **fluroquniolones.**
      (iii) **With gall stones or chronic cholecystitis and patients have relapses**: Antibiotics and cholecystectomy.
   (b) **Enterocolitis:** It is **self-limited** and the **majority of the patients do not require antibiotics.**
      (i) Fluid and electrolytes replacement therapies.
      (ii) Antibiotics are used in the following clinical conditions such as elderly patients, leukemia, lymphoma, sickle cell diseases, or very sick patients. **Fluroquinolones** (e.g., ciprofloxacin, norfloxacin) are the most effective drugs; other drugs are ampicillin, amoxicillin, or trimethoprim-sulfamethoxazole.
      (iii) Antispasmodic (e.g., loperamide or diphenoxylate with atropine) May be used for spasm but it prolongs diarrhea.

159. **Most common shigella infection in the USA are caused by: S.sonnei.**

160. A 80 year old man appears with H/O fever, chills, abdominal pain, & initial watery diarrhea followed by blood and mucous about 30 times per day for last few days.

Physical examination: Dehydration, tachycardia; presence of blood and **mucous in the stool.**
Most likely diagnosis: **Shigellosis (Bacillary dysentery)**.
Definitive diagnosis: Stool cultures should be done for 3 consecutive days, usually **positive** within 24 hours.
Stool microscopic examinations: **Presence of polymorphs** which are absent in diarrhea caused by enterotoxigenic bacteria and viruses. **Polymorphs are present** in Salmonella (nontyphoidal), yersinia, and campylobacter.
Treatment:

(a) **Ciprofloxacin** is the drug of choice.
(b) Fluid and electrolytes for dehydration.
(c) Do **not** use antimotility agents (e.g., loperamide etc.) which inhibit intestinal clearance of the Shigellae.

161. **Fluroquinolones (e.g., ciprofloxacin, norfloxacin, ofloxacin) are the drug of choice in the following infectious diarrhea: (Important)** Salmonella, Shigella, Campylobacter, and most of the organisms causing diarrhea. **They are not effective in diarrhea caused by C.difficile**.

162. **Complication of Shigellosis: Arthritis or Reiter's syndrome** may develop (only in 2% cases) after weeks or months of recovery from shigella infection.

163. **Prevention of shigellae infections:**
(a) Avoid contaminated food and water.
(b) Proper hand washing technique.
(c) **No** chemoprophylaxis is effective.

164. **Most common campylobacter organism causing enteritis: C.jejuni or C.coli**.

165. A 30 year old man appears with H/O fever, myalgia, abdominal pain, and bloody diarrhea for the last 24 hours. He has passed stool 10-12 times. He ate improperly cooked chicken or turkey sandwiches about 3 days ago.
Physical examination: Diffusely tender abdomen. It mimics appendicitis.
Most likely diagnosis: **Campylobacter enteritis**.
Diagnosis: **Clinical presentation; positive stool culture confirms the diagnosis**.
Treatment:
(a) Fluid and electrolytes for dehydration.
(b) Erythromycin, tetracycline, clindamycin, or quinolones.

Prevention: **To avoid** improperly cooked food, unpasturized milk, and contaminated (nonchlorinated) water. To stay away from sick pet puppies or kittens which may harbor C.jejuni.

166. **Complications of Campylobacter enteritis**:
(a) Guillain-Barre syndrome (GBS).
(b) Hemolytic-uremic syndrome (HUS).
(c) Toxic megacolon.
(d) Colonic hemorrhage.
(e) Pseudomembranous colitis (PMS).
(f) Reiter's syndrome.

167. **Most common type of E.coli causing traveler's diarrhea**: **Enterotoxigenic E.coli (ETEC).**
ETEC patients appear with **abdominal** pain and watery diarrhea while visiting in developing countries. It is self-limited to 1 to 5 days but sometimes it continues longer period of time. ETEC is **severe** when it produces both ST (heat -stable) and LT (heat-labile) toxins or only ST toxin, rather than LT alone.
Other types are the following:
(a) Enteroinvasive E.coli (EIEC): Patients appear with signs and symptoms of **inflammatory colitis** that includes **high fever, abdominal pain, bloody or dysenteric diarrhea** which mimic Shigellae infections. It is self-limited to 1 to 3 days.
(b) Enterohemorrhagic E.coli (EHEC): EHEC patients appear with **gross bloody** diarrhea with very low fever or little inflammatory exudates in the stool. It is self-limited to 5 to 12 days and is associated with Shiga-like toxin producing E.coli O157: H7 or O26: H11.
Hemolytic-uremic syndrome is an important complication.
Definitive diagnosis: To detect specific types is very expensive and is not needed routinely. ELISA and gene probe in ETEC; sereny test and gene probe in EIEC; and serotype and **gene probe in EHEC are the specific tests**.
Treatment:
(i) **Fluid and electrolytes are the main treatment in all E.coli infections.**
(ii) It is a self-limited disease, so routine antibiotics should not be used except in ETEC.
(iii) ETEC: Quinolones, trimethoprim-sulfamethoxazole, or tetracycline which reduces the duration of illness.
(iv) Bismuth subsalicylate: It may be used in **traveler's diarrhea with caution due to salicylate toxicity**. It reduces the symptoms.

(v) EHEC: Use of antibiotics is controversial.
(vi) Hemolytic-uremic syndrome: Plasma exchange may be needed.

168. **Prevention of E.coli enteritis: Cook it, boil it or peel it is to avoid food and water contaminations.**

169. **Most common organism for traveler's diarrhea: Enterotoxigenic E.coli (30-70%);** next common cause is unknown; Shigella, Salmonella, and Campylobacter may be the infecting organisms.
Traveler's diarrhea: It is due to food and water contaminations.
Preventions:
(a) cook it, boil it, or peel it.
(b) Ciprofloxacin 500 mg once daily, begin medication one day before reaching the destination and one day after leaving that place. It is helpful in short-term travelling (less than 3 weeks, upto 90% protection).
(c) Bismuth sub-salicylate (BSS): It is also helpful (60% protection).
Treatment:
(a) Advice should be given by the traveler's primary care physician to avoid consultation with the local physicians and laboratories.
(b) Fluid and electrolytes are given to avoid dehydration.
(c) Ciprofloxacin 500 mg bid for 3 days.
(d) Loperamide with antibiotics are more effective than antibiotics alone.
(e) BSS may be helful.
(f) Do not use kaolin/pectin preparation.

170. A 30 year old man appears with H/O fever, abdominal pain, and diarrhea with occasional blood for 7 days. He went to Belgium recently and ate improperly cooked pork meat. The patient also noticed some arthritis like pain in the joints for last 12 hours.
Physical examination: Abdominal tenderness which may mimic appendicitis.
Most likely diagnosis: **Yersinia enterocolitica infection**.
Diagnosis is confirmed by: Detection of yersinia from stool or blood.
Treatment: Fluroquinolones may be the drug of choice.
Complications:Erythema nodosum and reactive polyarthritis are present in HLA -B27-positive patients.

171. A 22 year old Native American appears with H/O fever, chills, and painful swelling of the lymph nodes of the groin or neck. He takes care of different animals, particularly dog.
Physical examination: Swelling is tender, hot, oval shaped, approximately 5 to 7 cm in length, and nonfluctuant.

Most likely diagnosis: **Bubonic plague**.
Diagnosis is made by: Detection of Yersinia pestis in blood or aspirate from swelling (bubo).
Treatment: **Streptomycin is the drug of choice**, tetracycline, or chloramphenicol.
Complication:
Pneumonias: H/O cough, chest pain, and hemoptysis.
CXR shows patchy bronchopneumonia.
Isolation:
(a) Without pneumonia: Drainage and secretion precautions.
(b) With pneumonia: Strict isolation for 3 days after starting antibiotic therapy to avoid airborne spread.

172. **Most common organism causing ecthyma gangrenosum**: **Pseudomonas aeruginosa**. **P.aeruginosa infections are also found in**:
(a) Extensive third-degree burn.
(b) Cancer patients receiving chemotherapy.
(c) Patients with urinary tract catheterization.
(d) Patient with neutropenia: Bacteremia in neutropenic patients arise from lower intestinal tract.

173. **Most common clinical presentation in Listeria infections: Meningitis (50 to 60%),** next common is bacteremia only, CNS parenchymal diseases, or endocarditis.

174. **Listeria meningitis patients and associated diseases**:
(a) 25 % have cancer.
(b) 25 % have received organs (Patients with transplantations).
(c) 30 % are normal.
(d) 20 % have diabetes mellitus, cirrhosis, or under glucocorticoid treatment.

175. **Listeria meningitis**: **There is no special or characteristic features.** Patients appear with high fever, headache, signs of meningeal irritations, or seizure.
Physical examination: Focal neurologic deficit.
CSF:
WBC count 100 to 10,000 with increased polymorphs.
Protein: 50 to 300 mg/dL.
Glucose: less than 50 mg/dL.
Gram stain: Gram positive bacilli are present in 25 % cases.
Culture: Positive is diagnostic.
Blood culture: Positive only in 60 % of meningitis.

Diagnosis is confirmed by: Positive CSF or blood culture.

176. **Listeria related CNS parenchymal diseases**: A previously healthy patient appears with H/O fever, headache, and vomiting for 5 days followed by decreased consciousness, hemiparesis (50% of cases), seizures, and cranial nerve paralysis (33% of cases; includes V, VI, VII, IX or X cranial nerves).
Diagnosis is confirmed by: Positive blood culture with clinical findings; CSF culture and Gram stain **are** negative in most of the cases.
CSF: **Normal** or mildy increased protein and cell count.

177. **Treatment for all Listeria infections:**
   (a) Ampicillin is the drug of choice.
   (b) Ampicillin plus gentamicin for severely ill or immunocompromised patients.
   (c) Trimethoprim-sulfamethoxazole for patients allergic to penicillin.
   (d) Do **not** use cephalosporins, quinolones, or imipenem.

178. **Prevention for Listeria infections:**
   (a) Hospitalized patients with listeria infection should be isolated from other immunocompromised patients.
   (b) To avoid improperly cooked meat, raw milk, or raw vegetables.

179. A 40 year old fisherman appears with H/O painful, throbbing, and burning sensation in the middle of the index finger of the right hand for the last 2 days. He had a minor cut in that area 7 days ago.
Physical examination: Tender, well-defined, elevated, violaceous lesion in the middle of the index finger.
Most likely diagnosis: **Erysipeloid (E.rhusiopathiae is the organism)**.
Preferred diagnostic method: Skin biopsy.
Treatment: Penicillin, cephalosporin, clindamycin, imipenem, and ciprofloxacin.

180. **Complications of erysipeloid infections:**
   (a) Sterile arthritis of the adjacent joint.
   (b) Systemic infections and bacteremia **are very rare**. The majority of bacteremic patients develop endocarditis (mostly on the native valve).

181. **Most common clinical presentation of actinomycosis:** Cervicofacial lesions. Patients appear with subacute or chronic swelling in the submandibular region.
Physical examination: Very poor oral and dental hygiene. **Pus containing sulfur granules is a characteristic** finding.

Most likely diagnosis: Actinomycosis.
Preferred diagnostic test: Presence of the **Actinomyces organisms in the pus or tissue.**
Treatment: **Penicillin is the drug of choice**, other medications are tetracycline, clindamycin, imipenem, and cephalosporins.

182. **Abdominal-pelvic actinomycosis occurs due to**:
(a) Postoperative acute appendicitis with perforation.
(b) Perforated colonic diverticulitis.
(c) Postoperative patients after acute lower intestinal trauma.
(d) IUCD (intrauterine contraceptive device) can cause pelvic actinomycosis.

183. **Most common clinical manifestation of nocardiosis**: **Pneumonia**. It is found in immunocompromised patients such as AIDS and organ recipient patients. Patients appear with nonspecific signs and symptoms like any other pneumonia patients. The head CT scan should be done because lung infection can spread to the CNS.
CXR: Infiltrates or cavitary lesions.
Head CT: Cavitary brain lesions.
Preferred diagnostic test: **Culture of sputum, BAL, lung aspirate, or lung biopsy. Patients with AIDS, pulmonary nocardiosis, and brain mass should undergo** needle biopsy for definitive diagnosis.
Treatment: Trimethoprim-sulfamethoxazole is the drug of choice.

184. A 40 year old man appears with H/O fever (103°-104°F), chills, sweats, weakness, weight loss, joints pain, testicular pain, and difficulty in urination. He works in a slaughter house with sheeps and goats.
Physical examination: Pulse did not increase with the rise of temperature; enlarged spleen and lymph nodes are occasionally present.
Most likely diagnosis: **Brucellosis**.
Preferred diagnostic test: **Culture positive body fluid or tissues.**
CBC: Neutropenia, thrombocytopenia.
Blood culture: May or may not be positive for **B.melitensis.**
Treatment: Doxycycline, tetracycline, rifampin, fluroquinolones; **in CNS disease use ceftriaxone with rifampin**; localized drainage of abscess (if any).

185. **Localized brucellosis is due to: B.suis** is the most common organism in USA. B.suis can affect the CNS, bones, joints, heart, lungs, testes, prostate, kidneys, liver, spleen, and skin.

186. A 35 year old immunocompromised man appears with H/O painful single axillary lymph node enlargement in right hand for last 2 days. He has few cats in his house. Almost 3 weeks ago, one of the cats scratched his hand. Seven days later, he developed erythematous papules which were crusted subsequently.

Physical examination: Tender, enlarged lymph node in the right axillary region; mild splenomegaly.

Most likely diagnosis: **Cat scratch disease. Bartonella henselae is the most common organism**.

Diagnosis is made: Examination of the tissues (lymph node).

Treatment: Trimethoprim- sulfamethoxazole, rifampin, or ciprofloxacin.

Bacillary angiomatosis: H/O cat scratch; infection caused by **B.henselae**; patients appear with H/O single or multiple, red or purple cutaneous, or subcutaneous nodules. Liver, spleen, or internal lymph nodes may be involved.

Preferred diagnostic study: Examination of the tissue particulary Warthin-Starry stain confirms the diagnosis.

Treatment: Erythromycin, doxycycline, or azithromycin.

187. **Most common complications of bartonellosis:**

(a) **Acute hemolytic anemia**. Patients quickly develop anemia and jaundice.
(b) Secondary salmonella infections.

In bartonellosis, patients appear with H/O tick bite (sandfly) 2 to 3 weeks before the onset of Oroya fever which includes fever, muscle pain, and joint pain, and tender lymph nodes.

Preferred diagnostic test: Peripheral blood smear reveals bacilli within RBC.

Treatment: Chloramphenicol (because this disease is associated with salmonella), penicillin.

Prevention: Insecticide to kill the sandfly (vector).

188. Increased number of tuberculosis (TB) patients for the last 12 years in USA is due to: **HIV epidemic**. Approximately 11 % of U.S.- borne tuberculosis patients are HIV positive.

189. **Mechanism of spreading tuberculosis in HIV infections and AIDS patients**:

(a) Reactivation of latent tuberculosis in a newly infected HIV patients.
(b) Higher risk of acquiring new infections from the surrounding environment.
(c) Spreading infections to other individuals live or stay around HIV positive active tuberculosis patients.

190. **Most commonly involved organ in tuberculosis**:

Pulmonary (85%); extrapulmonary (15%).

191. **Active tuberculosis patients (non-HIV) may appear with two very important negative findings**:
   (a) Patients feel 'feverish' but absence of fever during measurement.
   (b) Negative TST (tuberculin skin tests) are found in 20 to 25% of all patients with active tuberculosis.

192. **Pulmonary tuberculosis**: Patient appears with H/O night sweat, weight loss, and cough with bloody sputum.
   Physical examination: Rales noted initially in the right upper lobe of the lung. Rhonchi appears when secretions become voluminous and sticky.
   CXR: Fibronodular shadows in the right or left upper lobe of the lungs.
   Preferred diagnostic study: **Sputum culture is the confirmatory test**.
   AFB (acid-fast bacilli) stain of sputum and respiratory secretions are suggestive but **not** diagnostic. Diagnosis can be made by the clinical presentations and the radiological findings.
   Treatment: **HIV infected patients should receive 12 months of therapy and non-HIV should receive therapy for 6 months**. INH and rifampin are given daily for six months. In addition to that pyrazinamide (PZA), streptomycin (SM), or ethambutol (EMB) daily for the first two months. Physician should decide how may **antituberculous** drugs patients need. It depends upon the patients history of IVDU, HIV positivity, degree of exposure in the surroundings, or number of previous hospital admissions.

193. **Most commonly involved part of the lungs in reactivated adult tuberculosis**:
   (a) First: The posterior and apical segments of the right upper lobe.
   (b) Second: The apical and posterior segments of the left upper lobe.
   (c) Third: The superior segments of the lower lobes of the both lungs.

194. **Multidrug treatment in active tuberculosis is due to**:
   (a) Enhance bacterial clearance.
   (b) Prevent the emergence of drug-resistant mutants as dominant strains.
   (c) Shorten the duration of treatment.

195. **Mechanism of action of different antituberculous drug**:
   (a) INH and rifampin: Superior bactericidal effects.
   (b) Ethambutol: Prevent emergence of drug resistance.
   (c) Pyrazinamide: Early and rapid reduction of tuberculous bacilli.

(d) Streptomycin: Enhances initial bactericidal activity. It is used only in severely ill patients with extensive tuberculosis because IM (intramuscular) injections are inconvenient.

196. **Side effects of antituberculous drugs**:
(a) INH: Lupus reaction, hepatitis, neuritis.
(b) Rifampin: Flu syndrome, hepatitis, nephritis, low platelets count.
(c) Ethambutol: Optic neuritis (retrobulbar).
(d) Pyrazinamide: Hepatitis, arthralgia, and arthritis due to increased urates level, rash, and GI symptoms.
(e) Streptomycin: Vestibular and auditory damage.

197. **Problems of antituberculous drugs in AIDS patients**:
(a) Reduced serum level of the drugs are due to AIDS enteropathies.
(b) Increased drug resistance.
(c) Increased treatment failure.
(d) Rifampin induced hepatic catabolism of other drugs, so monitor drug level.s
Management:
(i) Give maximum therapeutic dosages.
(ii) Monitor serum drugs level.
(iii) Watch for patients therapeutic response.

198. **CNS penetration of antituberculous medications**:
(a) Well penetration through blood-brain barrier: INH and PZA.
(b) Less well penetration: RIF.
(c) Very poor penetration: EMB, SM, and other aminoglycosides.

199. **Complications of antituberculous drugs**:
(a) RIF: Urine and fluids **turn red**, monitor other drug levels for hepatic catabolism.
(b) INH: **Monitor LFT's** (liver function tests); drug interactions with dilantin and antifungal medications.
(c) EMB: **Watch for visual acuity and color vision.**
(d) SM: **Audiometry to monitor hearing loss**, adjust the dose in renal diseases.
(e) PZA: **Gout due to increased urate levels.**

200. **Important points to remember while managing patients with tuberculosis**:
(a) Physicians mistake to recognize high risk patients, deal with nonadherence patients, and fail to give effective antituberculous treatment from the onset, might result in emergence of **multidrug** resistance.

(b) Directly observed therapy is **not** necessary for all patients but it is important to avoid multidrug resistance and rising prevalence of tuberculosis.
(c) Instead of daily therapy, twice or thrice weekly therapy may be effective in certain nonadherence patients.
(d) Counseling and educating patients about the disease are important.
(e) To avoid GI symptoms, medications should **not** be taken with foods, antacids, or an **H_2-blocker** which inhibit the absorption of antituberculous drugs.
(f) Patients who develop serious hepatitis: First, discontinue the hepatotoxic drugs and monitor LFT's. When it becomes normal resume the medication one at a time in a 3 to 4 day interval.

201. **Prolonged duration of antituberculous therapy is indicated in the following conditions**:
(a) Cavitary tuberculosis with delayed sputum conversion or clinical response.
(b) HIV-infections and AIDS patients.
(c) Meningeal tuberculosis.
(d) Miliary tuberculosis.
(e) Uncooperative patients with irregular or interrupted therapy.
(f) If patients sputum culture **remains** positive after **3 months of treatment, they need another 3 months of treatment after the sputum culture becomes negative.**

202. **Sputum culture becomes negative after antituberculous treatment**: Within 3 months (95% of cases).

203. **Post antituberculous treatment, advice to patients**:
Return to the physician when clinical condition is not normal. Routine surveillance is **not** recommended after treatment.

204. **Patients with borderline functions of the adrenal and rifampin therapy**: Rifampin enhances **hypocortisolism** by catabolizing the endogenous steroids. An addition of a steriod may by helpful.

205. **Indication for steriod therapy in tuberculous patients**: It is helpful in meningitis and pericarditis. Low dose of prednisone is used to reduce inflammation and fibrotic changes.

206. **Multidrug- resistance tuberculosis means (MDR- tuberculosis)**: Resistance to INH and RIF.
Important points in MDR- tuberculosis patients:

(a) Treatment duration is doubled.
(b) Low cure rate.
(c) Preventive treatments for infected contact persons are compromised.
(d) MDR- tuberculosis proven or suspected patients should be managed in a special facility.

207. **Extrapulmonary tuberculosis:** Most common sites of involvement are **lymphatic and pleural**. It is only 16% of all non-HIV tuberculosis pleural. Patients appear with weight loss and fever in severe disease conditions.

(a) **Lymphatic tuberculosis**: Painless cervical lymph nodes enlarge with sinus tract formations.

Diagnosis: **Excisional biopsy with positive culture**, PPD positive.

(b) **Pleural tuberculosis**: Patients may be asymptomatic or symptomatic with pleural effusion.

Diagnosis: Biopsy and positive culture.

(c) **CNS-meningeal tuberculosis:** Patients appear with fever, confusion, seizures, and coma.

Diagnosis: Due to lack of AFB in CSF, **useful diagnostic tests are PCR, antibody measurements, or tuberculostearic acid levels**.

LP shows ↑protein, ↓glucose, ↑cells (initial polymorphs then lymphocytes).

(d) **Bones-joints tuberculosis**: Patients appear with pain in the lumbar and lower thoracic vertabrae or in weight bearing joints.

Diagnosis: Needle biospy, culture of spinal lesions, synovial biopsy, and culture of joints.

(e) **Pericardial tuberculosis**: Patients appear with cough and dyspnea. Physical examination shows decreased heart sounds.

Diagnosis: CXR shows enlarged heart and EKG shows low voltage.

(f) Disseminated tuberculosis: Patients appear with fever and weight loss. **CXR may be normal or lagging. PPD is positive only in 50% of cases.**

Diagnosis: Culture of fluids obtained from different organs.

(g) **GI-peritoneal tuberculosis**: Patients appear with mild abdominal pain and distension. Most common site is ileum.

Diagnosis: **Laparascopic ileal biopsy, culture of peritoneal fluids,** or stool cultures.

(h) **Genitourinary tuberculosis**: Patients appear with hematuria, weight loss, or other symptoms of different organs (e.g., kidneys, bladder, ureters, testis, and uterus).

Diagnosis: Urine cultures, tissue biopsy, and cultures.

208. **HIV infection and AIDS patients with tuberculosis**:

(a) In early HIV infections with tuberculosis, the patients clinical presentations are the same as a non-HIV with tuberculosis.
(b) The chances of extrapulmonary tuberculosis is very high (60 to 80 % of cases) in patients with CD4 counts < 50.
(c) TST (tuberculin skin tests) is positive only 10 to 20% of cases in advanced AIDS patients.
(d) CXR shows interstitial or miliary pattern, hilar adenopathy, and pleural effusions.

209. **Most common cause of tuberculosis in USA**: Endogenous reactivation of latent infection is the most common cause. Most important example is **HIV infected individuals.**

210. **Prevention of tuberculosis:**
(a) In USA, most effective therapy is IPT (**I**NH **p**reventive **t**herapy).
(b) In the rest of the world, the most effective therapy is BCG (bacille Calmette-Guerin).
(c) IPT is the most important in HIV infected patients.
(d) INH resistant organism: Give rifampin prophylaxis.
(e) INH and RIF resistant organism: Ofloxacin and ethambutol, or ofloxacin and PZA may be effective. **Consultations with the experts are indicated.**

211. A 40 year old man is receiving INH prophylaxis. The patient is **asymptomatic** but the routine LFT's **reveals a fourfold increase of transaminases from his baseline values.**
Management:
(a) **Do not discontinue INH** because about 20% of patients over the age of 35 may have benign increase of LFT's.
(b) Monitor LFT's very closely. If patients become symptomatic or progressively rising LFT's, discontinue the INH. **Expert consultations are indicated** to resume INH or other antituberculous drugs.

212. **CDC (Center for Disease Control) guidelines to prevent nosocomial (hospital) tuberculosis transmission**:
(a) **Administrative measures**: Teach the staff to recognize and isolate active cases early. Tuberculin testing should be done for all hospital workers.
(b) **Engineering or environmental measures**: Isolation of proven or suspected cases in negative-pressure rooms.
(c) **Personal respiratory protection by**: Respirator or masks that can filter out the infectious 'droplet nuclei', e.g., HEPA filtration respirators.

213. **Most common cause for NTM (nontuberculous mycobacteria) lymphadenitis: MAC (M.avium complex includes M.avium and M.intracellulare).** NTM can affect the lung, lymph nodes, skin, or present as disseminated diseases. Advanced HIV patients can appear with extrapulmonary or disseminated diseases, which appear as fever, weight loss, diarrhea, abdominal pain, hepatosplenomegaly, or lymphadenopathy.

Diagnosis of disseminated diseases: Positive cultures of the organism from blood, stool, bone marrow, or tissue biopsy.

Prophylaxis: **Rifabutin** is recommended for patients with CD4 + T lymphocyte counts <100 cells per microliter.

Treatment: Azithromycin or clarithromycin must be given, 2nd drug should be added (e.g., ethambutol and/or rifabutin, clofazimine, rifampin, or ciprofloxacin). AIDS patients should receive treatment for at least 18 to 24 months or life time if clinical and microbiological improvements occur.

214. A 25 year old man appears in the emergency room in the month of July with H/O fever, headache, retro-orbital pain, photophobia, and myalgia. He had visited the Rocky Mountains 3 days ago when he was exposed to a tick.

Physical examination: Mild conjunctivitis and rashes all over the body. Patients may appear with fever and headaches for 2 to 3 days. **After those symptoms relieve for 1 or 2 days**, then a relapse of fever, myalgia, and headache occur which lasts for 3 to 4 days. **This is a typical presentation. Typical presentation is absent in the Rocky Mountain spotted fever**.

Most likely diagnosis: **Colorado tick fever (CTF).**

Preferred diagnostic method:

(a) Isolation of the virus (D.andersoni) from serum or whole blood is the definitive test.
(b) Detection of virus on the RBC by immunofluorescent stain is the rapid diagnostic method.
(c) ELISA method to detect antibody titer.

Treatment: Only supportive therapy.

Prevention: To wear protective clothing, use tick repellents, and rapidly remove the tick.

Differential diagnosis:

Rocky Mountain spotted fever: Pink, macular rash over the wrist and ankle appear within a 4 day onset of fever. Patients do **not** feel normal between the illness.

215. A 28 year old man appears in the emergency room in the month of June, with H/O fever, headache, myalgia, retro-orbital pain, photophobia, and conjunctival injections for the last 4 days. Yesterday, the patient develops macular rashes

over the wrist and ankle which subsequently spread all over the body. Recently, he visited wooded areas in North Carolina and was **exposed to a tick**.
Physical examination: Rashes all over the body including palms and soles.
Most likely diagnosis: **Rocky Mountain spotted fever (RMSF).**
Preferred diagnositc method:
(a) Clinical: Detection of the tick on the scalp or groin.
(b) Rapid diagnosis: Detection of R.rickettsiae in skin or rash biopsy with immunofluorescence stain.
Treatment:
(a) Tetracycline, doxycycline, chloramphenicol, or quinolones.
(b) Remove the tick as soon as possible, if present.
Prevention: To avoid the tick.
Differential diagnosis:
RMSF is **less** in Rocky Mountain areas and there are maximum reported cases in North Carolina. To differentiate from Meningococcemia with meningitis, patients appear with purpura and petechiae in the early phases of the disease which is absent in RMSF.

216. **Most common reported sexually transmitted disease (STD) infection in the USA**: **Gonorrhea**. Chlamydia, herpes simplex virus (HSV), and human papilloma virus (HPV) are more commonly unreported infections. Chlamydia is the most common unreported infection.

217. **Most common type of male urethritis**: Nongonococcal urethritis (NGU). Most common organism is **Chlamydia**. Next common is **Ureaplasma** urealyticum.

218. **Postgonococcal urethritis syndrome is due to:** Simultaneous untreated **chlamydia infection**. Patients complain of urethritis even after appropriate therapy for gonococcus infection with β-lactam antibiotics.
Treatment: Ceftriaxone should be followed by oral tetracycline.

219. **Most common ulcerative genital lesions in USA**: **HSV (herpes simplex virus)**.

220. A young woman with dysuria, pyuria, and urinary frequency:
(a) **Bacterial cystitis**: Urine has more than 10^5 bacterias/ml of urine.
(b) Urethral syndrome or Urethritis: Urine has less than 10^4 bacterias/ml of urine. Most common organism in urethritis is **Chlamydia.**

221. **Most common sign of vaginitis**: Increased vaginal discharge, types of discharges in different vaginitis:
   (a) Candida: Curdlike, white discharges.
   (b) Bacterial vaginosis: Gray, malodorous discharges.
   (c) Trichomonas vaginalis: Profuse, frothy discharges.

222. **Candida vaginitis**: Most common organism is **C.albicans.** Vaginal discharges: pH <4.5, no bad odor.
Diagnosis: Culture is more reliable than microscopic examination of yeast or pseudohyphae, but culture is positive in asymptomatic women.
Treatment: Most effective treatment is **vaginal application of clotrimazole or miconazole**. No need to treat sexual partners and asymptomatic carrier. Increased candida infections are due to: Diabetes, antibiotics, or oral anovulatory steroids.

223. **Trichomonas vaginitis is due to T.vaginalis**: **Vaginal discharges** – pH >5.0, fishlike odor in KOH preparation.
Diagnosis: Culture is more diagnostic than microscopic examination.
Treatment: Metronidazole. Male partners should be treated with metronidazole.

224. **Bacterial vaginosis (BV) is due to Gardnerella vaginalis**: It is a gram-variable coccobacillus.
Viginal discharges: pH >5.0, fishlike odor in KOH preparation.
Diagnosis: By **exclusion** of trichomonas, candida, and purulent cervicitis. Sometimes clue cells (vaginal epithelial cells containing G.vaginalis) are present.
Treatment: Metronidazole 500 mg BID for 7 days is effective. This indicates that the principle cause of the patients symptoms are due to anaerobes. Clindamycin is also effective. Male partners should be treated.

225. Most characteristic clinical manifestation in gonococcal (GC) urethritis in male: Dysuria with yellowish, purulent urethral discharge. Fifty percent of infected males are **asymptomatic**. The principal complication is disseminated gonoccal infection (1% cases). **GC infections in pharynx and rectum:** Most of the patients are **asymptomatic.** Pharyngeal infections appear as exudative pharyngitis with cervical lymph nodes enlargement. Rectal infections appear as proctitis with mucopurulent bloody discharges.
Epididymitis under 35 years: Coliform bacteria is the most common organism.
Epididymitis over 35 year: Chlamydia and GC.

Most common site of GC infections in female: Endocervix (80 to 90%), most of the patients are asymptomatic, most important complication is salpingitis.

226. **DGI (disseminated gonococcal infections):** Patients appear with migratory polyarthralgias which are asymmetric, associated with finger or toe skin lesions which include papules, pustules, or bullae on erythematous bases. Urethral symptoms are absent.

227. **Diagnosis of GC infections**:
   (a) **In females**: **GC cultures are diagnostic**. Gram stain of normal vaginal flora may give false positivity for GC.
   (b) In males:
      (i) Untreated symptomatic (urethral discharges) patients: Gram stain has a specificity of 95 to 98 % and a sensitivity of 90 to 98%. So urethral cultures are not routinely indicated.
      (ii) Asymptomatic patients: **Culture of the** anterior urethra is diagnostic. Gram stain is less sensitive.
   (c) Pharyngeal and rectal GC infection: The culture is diagnositic. In throat cultures, confusion between GC and meningococci may occur because GC is less frequent.

228. **Treatment for GC infections**:
   (a) Uncomplicated genital, pharyngeal, or rectal infections in both men and women: Ceftraixone once plus doxycycline for 7 days are the drugs of choice.
   (b) Disseminated GC infections: Ceftriaxone or spectinomycin.

229. **Most common cause of 'typical chancre' in North America**: Genital herpes.
Primary syphilis: Painless, cleanbased, single, and indurated ulcer is a **chancre**.
Chancroid: Painful, exudative, multiple, and nonindurated.
Secondary syphilis: It appears 4 to 8 weeks after the primary syphilis. Most common clinical presentations (80%) are skin rashes which are pink, macular, symmetrical, nonitchy, nonvesicular, or nonbullous. Rashes first appear on the margins of the ribs or the sides of the chest. Later on, it spreads all over the body, particularly on the palms and soles.
Relapsing syphilis: Approximately one third of the patients of primary or secondary syphilis have **recurrences of skin lesions** after the resolutions of initial skin lesions. These lesions are fewer, more indurated than initial lesions. They are also infectious.

Latent syphilis: No signs of syphlis and CSF are normal.
Two types:
(a) **Early latency**: First year after the resolution of the primary or secondary lesions or newly reactive positive serologic test which was negative for the last one year in an asymptomatic patient. It is infectious.
(b) **Late latency**: It means after one year of duration and it is **noninfectious except in pregnant women.**

Late syphilis: It is **noninfectious**, slow progressing, appears as late benign (gummatous), cardiovascular, or neurosyphilis.

230. **Syphilis and HIV infections**: (Important).
(a) Syphilitic skin lesions can enhance the spreading of HIV infections.
(b) Most common clinical presentation is secondary syphilis.
(c) Chancre is more likely present in HIV- positive than HIV- negative individuals.
(d) Higher incidence of therapeutic failure whicn may lead to neurosyphilis.
(e) In an **early stages** of HIV-infection, titer may be higher than non-HIV but in the **advanced stages**, titer may be low or absent.

231. Diagnostic tests for syphilis:
(a) Specific, confirmatory, and treponemal antibodies: FTA-ABS, MHA-TP. They are positive in yaws, pinta, endemic syphilis (bejel).
(b) Nonspecific, nonconfirmatory, and nontreponemal antibodies: VDRL, RPR. These are screening tests.

VDRL: Most patients with secondary syphilis have titer at least 1:16. False positive tests have titer less than 1:8.
VDRL is positive in only 70% of cases of cardiovascular or neurosyphilis, so FTA-ABS is the only test positive in some of those patients. MHA-TP is **less** sensitive in primary syphilis only, otherwise as good as FTA-ABS.

232. **False-positive serologic test:** VDRL or RPR is positive (less than 1:8), FTA-ABS or MHA-TP is negative, and patients do **not** have the disease.
Two types:
(a) Acute (<6 months duration): Bacterial, viral, atypical pneumonias, or malaria.
(b) Chronic (>6 months duration): SLE, HIV infections, narcotic addicts, elderly patients (over the age 70, >1% positive; over the age 80, 10% positive), or leprosy.

233. **False-positive VDRL or RPR and high titer**: In lymphoma and other diseases titer is more than 1:8.

234. **A 19 year old woman has H/O chronic false-positive VDRL titer**: Rule out autoimmune diseases e.g., SLE, thyroiditis, or others.

235. **False-positive FTA-ABS are found**: SLE, rheumatoid arthritis, biliary cirrhosis, or other chronic inflammatory diseases with hyperglobulinemia.

236. **Treatment for syphilis:**
   (a) **Primary, secondary, and early latent (<1 year):** Benzathine penicillin G 2.4 million units IM. In penicillin allergic patients, use doxycycline 100 mg twice daily for 10 days.
   (b) Late latent (>1 year duration), cardiovascular syphilis, or **late benign (bone, skin, visceral gumma):** Benzathine penicillin G 2.4 million units IM weekly x 3 dosages.
   (c) **Neurosyphilis (symptomatic or asymptomatic**) Aqueous penicillin G IV 2 to 4 million units every 4 hours for 10 days.

237. **Follow-up for all syphilis patients after treatment:**
   (a) **HIV-negative patients**: VDRL titer and clinical examinations at 3, 6, and 12 months after therapy.
   (b) **HIV-positive patients:** VDRL titer and clinical examinations at 1,2,3,6,9, and 12 months.
   (c) **Late-latent syphilis**: Examination at 24 months after therapy. Spinal tap is needed, if it was not done before therapy in order to diagnose inadequately treated asymptomatic neurosyphilis.

   HIV-positive patients and treatment for syphilis:
   (a) Treatment failure is usual.
   (b) More aggressive follow-up is needed.
   (c) More aggressive treatment is usually not needed.

238. **VDRL titer after therapy for early (primary, secondary, or early latent) syphilis:** VDRL should be **nonreactive** after 12 to 24 months.

239. VDRL titer remains **positive after 24 months due to the following reasons**:
   (a) Very high initial VDRL titer.
   (b) Repeated infections.
   (c) Advanced stages of syphilis.
   (d) Prolonged infections.
   (e) In early syphilis, a small percentage of patients may have very low titer. Do **not** miss recurrent infections.

(f) In late syphilis, the presence of low titer for a long period of time is not alarming.

240. Indications for **retreatment of syphilis** after **initial therapy**:
(a) Rising VDRL titers (four folds or higher).
(b) Clinically symptomatic patients.
(c) In neurosyphilis, when a repeated follow up spinal tap shows increasing cell counts, protein, and VDRL titer than before.

241. **CSF results become negative after therapy for neurosyphilis:** First CSF cells disappear, 2nd is protein, and last CSF- VDRL which would take years to become negative.

242. Treatment for asymptomatic patients have sexual contact with people of symptomatic **syphilis**: All asymptomatic people should be treated for syphilis who came in sexual contact with a person who has syphilis within 90 days. Most of the syphilis develops within 60 days. Thirty percent of contacts would develop syphlis within 30 days of contact, if untreated.

243. A 40 year old man diagnosed to have early syphilis was treated with a first injection of penicillin. Two hours later he develops low grade fever, myalgia, and headache. The patient became more symptomatic after 8 hours. The physician advised him to take some salicylates. Patient becomes completely asymptomatic within 24 hours of penicillin therapy.
Most likely diagnosis: **Jarisch- Herxheimer reaction (JHR)**.
Treatment: Salicylates.
Local complications: Patients with syphilis of the coronary ostium or optic nerve, may develop inflammation in this JHR which has less clinical importance. These inflammatory changes may be benefitted by corticosteroids.

244. **Mechanism of Jarisch-Herxheimer reactions: Unknown.**
The following mechanism have been proposed:
(a) Antigens release from spirochetes.
(b) Activation of complement cascade.
(c) Transient consumption of C3, C4, C6, and C7.
(d) Transient reduction of treponemal antibodies.
(e) Endotoxemia but T.pallidum does not contain biologically active endotoxin.

245. A 25 year old man appears in the emergency room with H/O fever, shaking chills, vomiting, and nose bleeding. He recently visited the Rocky Mountains and slept one night in a rodent-infected cabin in a western National Park. **H/O**

fever usually lasts for 4 days, then disappears for 10 days without treatment but reappears again.
Physical examination: Tachycardia, conjunctival injections.
Most likely diagnosis: **Tick-borne relapsing fever due to O.hermsii which is a night feeder, so patient doesn't recall a tick bite.**
Diagnosis: Identification of spirochetes in peripheral blood smear.
Treatment: Tetracycline is the drug of choice.
Louse-borne relapsing fever appears with hepatosplenomegaly and jaundice. The fever lasted for 6 days. Then, it disappeared for 9 days but reappeared again once. **The Jarisch-Herxheimer reaction (JHR)** is common in louse-borne relapsing fever. This reaction begins 2 to 3 hours after the treatment with tetracycline. Patient appears with fever (1^0 above the normal), rigors, initial slight fall of BP followed by rise in BP, and transient leukopenia. JHR is associated with increased phagocytosis of spirochetes by polymorphs and a temporary rise of TNF (tumor necrosis factor), IL-6, and IL-8 (IL-interleukin).

246. **Most characteristic clinical presentation of Lyme disease:** Erythema chronicum migrans (ECM).

247. **Most common cardiac abnormalities in Lyme disease**: Variable degrees of atrioventicular block (first degree, Wenckebach, or complete heart block). Cardiac involvement is usually a short duration (3 days to 6 weeks) and heart murmur is absent.

248. **Lyme disease**: It is caused by spirochete, **Borrelia burgdorferi and ixodid ticks** are the primary vector. Patient appears initially with a characteristic of ECM (erythema chronicum migrans) which is followed by neurologic, joints, or cardiac abnormalities within weeks or months.
Early presentations: It appears initially with red maculopapular rashes at the site of a tick bite. It expands up to 15 cm with partial central clearing. The outer borders of the rash are red, flat, and nonscaling. It is associated with the malaise, fatigue, lethargy, fever, chills, myalgia, and arthralgia. Some patients appear with mild transient encephalopathy (severe headache, neck pain, and stiffness) but CSF is normal.
Late presentations:
(a) Neurologic: Patients appear with meningitis, encephalitis, chorea, cranial nerve paralysis (**particularly bilateral facial nerve involvement** which may be the only finding). Patients with meningitic symptoms have no meningeal signs (absence of Kernig's and Brudzinski's signs). CSF shows increased lymphocytes (approximately 100 cells/cubic millimeter) and

sometimes EEG (electroencephalogram) shows diffuse slowing. Neurologic manifestations last for several months but usually resolve completely.

(b) **Arthritis**: Arthritis symptoms may appear as early as few weeks or as late as 2 years. It involves usually larger joints, particularly knee joints. Joints appear swollen, hot, less tender, and rarely red. Baker's cysts may form and rupture within a short period of time. Fever is absent but fatigue is common. Analysis of joint fluid shows **polymorphonuclear leukocytosis** (ranges from 500 to 100,000 cells per cubic millimeter, with an average of 25,000), **glucose levels are more than two-third** of the serum, **C3 and C4 levels are more than one-third**, protein levels are 3 to 8 gm/dl, and **absence** of rheumatoid factor and ANA (antinuclear antibodies).

(c) **Cardiac**: Variable degree of atrioventricular block.

(d) **Late important findings**: Acrodermatitis chronica atrophicans (rare in USA).

249. **Diagnosis of Lyme disease:**

(a) Most of the diagnosis is made clinically with H/O exposure of the tick.

(b) **Definitive diagnosis**: Culture of B.burgdorferi from skin biopsy specimen.

(c) Increase of IgM specific antibody by ELISA method (the peak is 3 to 6 weeks after onset of the diseases).

(d) Most common nonspecific laboratory findings ↑ESR,↑IgM (nonspecific), or ↑AST (asparate transaminase).

250. **Treatment for lyme disease:**

(a) **Early disease: Amoxicillin and add probenecid** (some experts recommendation), doxycycline.

(b) **Arthritis**: **Amoxicillin plus probenecid, doxycycline.**

(c) Carditis: **Ceftriaxone**, penicillin.

(d) **Bell's palsy only (no other neurologic abnormalities)**: Same as item number (a).

(e) Meningitis: **Ceftriaxone**, penicillin.

(f) Pregnancy:

(i) Early disease: Amoxicillin.

(ii) Asymptomatic seropositive patients: No medication.

(iii) Disseminated diseases: Penicillin.

251. **Jarisch-Herxheimer reactions are found after treatment in the following diseases**:

(a) Syphilis.

(b) Relapsing fever.

(c) Lyme disease.

252. **Prophylaxis for lyme disease.**
   (a) Prophylactic antibiotic is **not** recommended.
   (b) In a very early stage of development of the ECM and documented tick bites, use of antibiotic is effective.

253. A 35 year old man appears with H/O **fever, conjunctivitis, hepatosplenomegaly, jaundice,** abdominal pain, trunchal rash, and pretibial, raised, erythematous lesions are called 'Fort Bragg fever'. A patient may appear with **biphasic illness** such as initial fever which resolves, after that **headache and meningeal signs appear**.
   Most likely diagnosis: Leptospirosis.
   Diagnosis:
   (a) **Blood and CSF cultures**: Identification of Leptospira confirms the diagnosis.
   (b) Rising agglutinating antibody titer (four fold rise).
   Treatment: Doxycycline, penicillin.

254. **Conjunctivitis with preauricular lymphadenopathy**: Most commonly due to **adenovirus infections.**

255. **Most common sexually transmitted bacterial infection in USA: Chlamydia trachomatis.**

256. **Clinical characteristics of trachoma**: It is an eye infection caused by C.trachomatis. Clinical diagnosis can be made if any two of the following findings are present:
   (a) Lymphoid follicles in the upper tarsal plate.
   (b) Herbert's pits (lymphoid follicles) along the corneal limbus.
   (c) Pannus formations in cornea.
   (d) Scarring formations in conjunctiva.

257. **Diagnosis of chlamydia infections:**
   Definitive diagnosis:
   (a) **By identification of the organism in cell culture** but it is **rarely** positive **in an adult with a late scarring disease**.
   (b) Other methods that make the diagnosis:
      (i) PCR: To detect chlamydial DNA.
      (ii) ELISA: To detect chlamydia antigen.
      (iii) Immunoflourescent study: To detect elementary bodies with monoclonal antibodies.

258. **Treatment for chlamydia infections.**
   (a) Eye infections only: Azithromycin by mouth.
   (b) Uncomplicated urethritis, cervicitis: **Doxycycline (7 days), azithromycin (single dose).**
   (c) Epididymitis, salpingitis, endometritis: Doxycycline (10 to 14 days).
   (d) LGV (lymphogranuloma venerium): Doxycycline for 21 days.
   (e) Sexual partners should be treated.
   (f) All sexual contacts within 60 days should be treated.

259. **Most common organism in epididymitis with urethritis**: C.trachomatis or N.gonorrhoea.

260. **Most common organism in epididymitis.**
   (a) <35 years: C.trachomatis.
   (b) >35 years: Uropathogens causing complicated UTI.

261. **Most common organism in NGU (nongonococcal urethritis)**: C.trachomatis.

262. **Chlamydia pneumonia**: An elderly patient appears with (afebrile pneumonia) nonproductive cough, sore throat, and hoarseness.
   Physical examination: Auscultation reveals localized crackles in the chest.
   CXR: Subsegmental pneumonia (unilateral).
   Treatment: Tetracycline or erythromycin.

263. A patient is complaining of **unremitting pain and a splitting headache. He was treated with narcotic analgesics:** R/O rickettsial infection.

264. **Rickettsial infections**: It is caused by R.prowazokii. Body lice can get infection from an infected individual. Infected body lice can cause infection to normal individuals.
   Signs & symptoms of typhus fever: Patients appear with **severe headache,** fever, chills, and myalgia. On the 5th day of illness, patients develop reddish-pink macular rashes over the trunk and axilla. Patients progressively develop altered mental status.
   Physical examination: Relative bradycardia with the rise of temperature, photophobia, conjunctivitis, mildly inflammed pharynx, and no rales.
   Treatment: Doxycycline is the treatment of choice, or tetracycline.
   Prevention:
   (a) To destroy body lice and its feces.

(b) Prophylactic doxycycline use in weekly dosages is effective for 2 to 3 weeks only.

265. **Interferons (IFN):** They are glycoprotein cytokines which have antineoplastic, antiviral, and immunomodulating properties.
Mechanism of action: IFN binds with intact cell membrane.
Toxicity: Frequent use of IFN can cause influenza-like symptoms (fever, chills, malaise, and headache).
Uses:
(a) Hepatitis.
(b) Respiratory papillomatosis.
(c) Respiratory infections.
(d) Condylomata acuminata.

266. **Acyclovir**: Acyclovir is an acyclic analogue of guanosine.
Mechanism of action: Viruses release **thymidine kinase** which phosphorylates acyclovir to acyclovir monophosphate which is further phosphorylated to form **triphosphate** which binds **with viral DNA.** Acyclovir is not effective on the viruses which does not release thymidine kinase such as EBV (Epstein-Barr virus) and CMV (cytomegalo virus).
Toxicity: Acute tubular necrosis, reversible elevation of serum creatinine.
Uses:
(a) Herpes encephalitis.
(b) Herpes lesions in the genitalia.
(c) Mucocutaneous herpes infections in the immunocompromised hosts.

267. **Ganciclovir:**
Ganciclovir is an acyclic nucleoside analogue of acyclovir.
Mechanism of action: Same as acyclovir but it is effective against all herpes viruses, CMV, and EBV. The mechanism of action against CMV and EBV is not entirely clear but viruses may stimulate cellular thymidine kinsase (TK) or viral kinase activities which initiate phosphorylation of ganciclovir to monophosphate, ultimate triphosphate which binds with viral DNA.
Toxicity: Neutropenia, thrombocytopenia.
Uses:
(a) CMV retinitis.
(b) Life threatening CMV infections in AIDS or other immunocompromised patients.
(c) It can prevent the reactivation of CMV infections in **organ transplantation recipients**.

268. **Most common cause of absenteeism from work**: Common cold. Most common organism for common cold is **rhinovirus**.

269. **Most common complication of viral cold**: Secondary bacterial infections. Sinusitis (fever and/or facial pain) is common in adults.

270. **Most common types of viruses responsible for pharyngitis, bronchitis, croup, and laryngitis**: **Myxoviruses** (Influenza, parainfluenza, and RSV). Influenza (types A, B) parainfluenza (types 1, 2, 3), and RSV (A, B1, B2) are most common.

271. **Antiviral drugs used in different viral infections**:
    (a) Ribavirin: RSV.
    (b) Acyclovir: Herpes simplex.
    (c) Amantadine: Influenza A.

272. **Elderly patients and RSV infecitons**: Type A is the most common and most dangerous type.
    Diagnosis of RSV: Confirmed by positive RSV culture of respiratory secretions.
    Treatment of RSV: Hydration, oxygen, bronchodilators, and ribavirin (inhalation).

273. **Most common bacterial superinfections after influenza viral pneumonia: Streptococcus pneumoniae, S.aureus, or H.influenzae.**

274. **Nonpulmonic complications of influenza virus**:
    (a) Aseptic meningitis, myelitis, and encephalopathy are found during acute illness. Encephalitis is found after an acute illness.
    (b) Rarely complications are adults, Reye's syndrome, Guillain-Barre syndrome, DIC, myoglobinuria, myocarditis, or pericarditis.
    (c) Associated bacterial infections are **meningococcal, or S.aureus (toxic shock syndrome).**

275. **Treatment for infuenza virus infections**:
    (a) Rimantadine or amantadine is effective only in type A infection. Amantadine has CNS toxicity and it is excreted unchanged in the urine.
    (b) Symptomatic treatments are antipyretics and cough suppressants. Do **not** use aspirin under the age of sixteen to avoid Reye's syndrome.
    (c) Use antibiotics to cover S.aureus secondary bacterial infections.

276. **Indications for using influenza vaccine:**
 (a) Elderly patients (65 and over).
 (b) Elderly patients in the nursing home or chronic care facilities (50 to 60% effective in reducing hospitalization and pneumonia).
 (c) Patients with chronic pulmonary, cardiac, metabolic, renal, immunodeficient diseases, and hemoglobinopathies.
 (d) All health care workers in any facilities.
 (e) It can be used on anybody who wants to avoid influenza.

277. **Adenoviruses causing the following complications in transplantation recipients:**
 (a) Bone marrow recipient: Hemorrhagic cystitis. Patients receiving cyclophosphamide without infection can manifest with hemorrhagic cystitis.
 (b) Renal transplantation recipients: Hemorrhagic cystitis but the problem is less severe.
 (c) Liver transplantation recipients: Disseminated liver disease and failure of transplantation.

278. **Adenoviruses causing the following diseases**:
 (a) Most common respiratory infection is **acute pharyngitis.**
 (b) Most important urinary complication is **acute hemorrhagic cystitis**. Patients appear with hematuria and dysuria. It is a self-limited disease. Patient has normal BP, temperature, and renal function tests.
 (c) **Pharyngoconjunctival fever (PCF):** Patients appear with **nonexudative pharyngitis, bilateral contagious conjunctivitis** (itchy, painless, hypermic conjunctiva, and watery discharge) and fever. It is a self-limited disease and no specific treatment is available.
 (d) Epidemic keratoconjunctivitis (EKC): Patients appear with unilateral keratoconjunctivitis, preauricular lymphadenopathy, no fever, and no pharyngitis, EKC is a contagious illness.

279. **Most common infectious cause of blindness in USA**: **Herpes keratitis**. It is caused by HSV-1.

280. **Most common cause of genital herpes**: HSV-2. Men appear with ulcerative lesions over the genitalia. Women appear with dysuria, urinary retention, and ulcerative lesion over the genitalia.

281. **Most common cause of focal, sporadic encephalitis in USA**: Herpes simplex encephalitis. It is mostly caused by HSV-1. It causes hemorrhagic necrosis of

the temporal lobe. HSV travel along the olfactory or trigeminal nerve to the temporal lobe of the brain.
CSF:↑protein,→glucose.
Preferred diagnostic method: Cultures to isolate the viruses, PCR study of CSF.
Treatment: **Acyclovir is the treatment of choice,** or vidarabine may be used. Rapid infusion of acyclovir can crystalize in the renal tubules particularly in dehydrated patients.

282. **Most common cause of HSV infections in immunocompromised patients**: **Reactivation of latent infection**. Patients appear with severe infections, such as esophagitis, dermatitis (orofacial and perineal), colitis, and hepatitis.

283. **Most common infection after allograft transplantation**: Human **cytomegalovirus (HCMV)**.

284. **Most common cause of HCMV infection in allograft patients**: HCMV-seropositive donar. Other causes are reactivated infection of the HCMV-seropositive recipient and exogenous blood products given after transplantation surgery.

285. **Clinical manifestations of HCMV infections**:
   (a) Immunocompetent person: Either asymptomatic or mononucleosis- like syndrome. Nonspecific symptoms are low grade fever, malaise, or loss of appetite. Laboratory tests may show atypical lymphocytosis, ↑LFT's, Cholestasis, or rarely ↓platelets.
   (b) AIDS patients: **Most common is HCMV retinitis.**
      (i) Eye: Retinitis.
      (ii) CNS: Encephalopathies, neuropathies, and myelopathies.
      (iii) GI: Colitis, esophagitis, or rarely gastritis.
   (c) Allograft transplantation patients: Symptoms develop after 4 to 6 weeks of transplantation.
      (i) **HCMV mononucleosis**: This is a most common complication. Patients appear with fever, hepatitis, ↓WBC, ↓platelets.
      (ii) Liver: Hepatitis.
      (iii) Lungs: Pneumonitis (diffuse interstitial infiltrates).

286. **Diagnosis of HCMV infections**:
   (a) Preferred diagnostic method: Isolation of the virus from urine, blood, saliva, or tissue biopsy specimens.

(b) PCR (polymerase chain reaction) study of the body fluids and biopsy specimens.

287. **Treatment for HCMV infections**:
(a) Ganciclovir: Dose-related neutropenia is the most common side-effect.
(b) Foscarnet: Most common side effect is nephrotoxicity.
(c) Prophylaxis: Most important prophylactic use of ganciclovir or foscarnet in both solid organ and bone marrow transplantation recipients.

288. A 19 year old man appears with H/O sore throat, fever, headache, or malaise for the last 5 days. Patient was seen by a private doctor 2 days ago. The doctor prescribed ampicillin. Since then, the patient developed rashes all over the body.
Physical examination: Tender cervical lymph nodes, mild jaundice, palpable spleen.
CBC: Atypical lymphocytosis.
Urinalysis: Albuminuria.
Most likely diagnosis: Infectious mononucleosis due to EBV (Epstein-Barr virus).
Diagnosis: Clinical presentations plus atypical lymphocytosis. Diagnosis is confirmed by a positive heterophil test.
Treatment:
(a) No treatment is necessary in most of the patients.
(b) Discontinue ampicillin or penicillin.
(c) Acetaminophen or aspirin is used as symptomatic treatment for patients with normal or mildly abnormal LFT's.
(d) Glucocorticoid may be helpful in patients with acute tonsillar obstruction.
(e) Intravenous immunoglobulin therapy may be helpful in patients with severe hemorrhagic thrombocytopenia refractory to glucocorticoid therapy.
(f) Acyclovir may be used in AIDS patients with progressive EBV infection or oral hairy leukoplakia.
(g) Interferon may be helpful in patients with X-linked lymphoproliferative diseases.

289. **EBV may be an etiologic agent for the following diseases**:
(a) Anaplastic nasopharyngeal carcinomas: Patients have high levels of IgA antibodies to EBV.
(b) Hodgkin diseases: EBV DNA may be present.

290. **Most common malignancy caused by HTLV-I**: ATL (adult T-cell leukemia/lymphoma). **Acute form** for ATL appears with high WBC counts,

hypercalcemia, and skin manifestations. It is an aggressive mature T-cell lymphoma. Most patients with acute and lymphoma-type ATL die within 6 months due to rapid growth of tumor cells, opportunistic infections (Pneumocystic carinii), and hypercalcemia.

291. **Breast and bottle feeding in HTLV-I infected mother:** Transmission of HTLV-I from infected mother to newborn is much higher in breast-feeding (20%) than in utero or perinatal transmission (1 to 2 % in bottle-feeding infants). HTLV-II is probably transmitted via breast milk but it does not go through the placenta.

292. **Breast and bottle feedings in HIV-1 infected mother**: In the USA, breast feeding is **not** recommended, so transmissions of HIV-1 from infected mothers to the newborn are almost all of them in utero or perinatal transmission. In case of breast feeding rate of transissions is 15%.

293. **Risk factors for transmission of HTLV**:
    (a) Intravenous drug abuse.
    (b) Sexual contacts.
    (c) Birthplace in a viral endemic area.
    (d) Simultaneous infections with HTLV-I and HIV-1 appear to progress the disease process rapidly, probably due to cell proliferative effects of HTLV-I upon HIV-1- infected T cells. It is not found in HTLV-II. **HIV-1 is more infectious than HTLV-I**.

294. **A little or no risk for infection of HTLV**:
    (a) Health care workers who experience a needle stick.
    (b) Health care workers whose skin or mucous membrane was exposed directly without protective devices.

295. **No risk for infection of HTLV**:
    (a) Casual contacts.
    (b) Mosquito bites.

296. An effect of transfusion of blood infected with HTLV-I or II - It is rare in USA.
    CNS: Chronic progressive demyelination of the long motor tracks of the spinal cord.

297. **Transmission of HTLV-I or II**:

(a) **Sexual**: Male to female and female to male transmissions are found in both HTLV I and II. Male to male transmission occurs only in HLTV I. No heterosexual transmission is found in type II.
(b) **Parenteral**: Intravenous drug use and infected blood transfusions can cause either I or II.
(c) Ulcerative genital lesions or elevated virus loads (mother to infant or heterosexual): Both transmit only HTLV-I.
(d) Cellular transfusion products: Both I and II can be transmitted.
(e) Sharing of 'works': Both I and II can be transmitted.

298. **Do not breast-feed if mother has**: CMV, AIDS, DIC, active TB, postpartum psychosis, neurosis, nephritis, eclampsia, or **herpetic lesions in the breasts**. Hepatitis is **not** a contraindication of breast-feeding unless there is crack in the nipple through which contaminated blood can infect the baby.

299. **Allowed breast-feeding if mother has:** Hepatitis, mastitis (give antibiotic and local care) or, inverted nipple (with difficulty).

300. **HTLV-I is causing TSP/HAM (tropical spastic paraparesis/HTLV-I-associated myelopathy)**: It is a neurologic syndrome characterized by a **chronic, slowly progressive appearance** of spastic paraparesis. It is due to demyelination of the long motor neurons of the spinal cord. Patients appear with stiff-gait, followed by spasticity, impotence, and incontinence. It has **no** waxing and waning unlike multiple sclerosis.
Diagnosis: HTLV-I antibodies and clinical presentations.
Treatment:
(a) Corticosteroids: May help in rapidly progressive diseases.
(b) Danazol (androgenic steroid): Improves urinary and fecal incontinence.

301. HTLV-II can cause the following diseases:
(a) Hairy T-cell leukemia.
(b) TSP/HAM may occur with HTLV-II viruses.
(c) B-cell cancer.
(d) LGL (large granulocytic cell leukemia).
(e) Cancer with NK (natural killer) cell phenotype.

302. **CDC (Center for Disease Control and Prevention) guidelines for prevention and counseling for HTLV-I and II**:
(a) Blood should be screened before transfusion.
(b) Positive donors should not be allowed to donate blood.
(c) Use of condoms can prevent the transmission of the viruses.

303. A practicing physician should mention the following facts when talking to a person who is HTLV+:
   (a) The complications are rare in HTLV-I diseases.
   (b) No specific disease is caused by HTLV-II viruses.
   (c) Both the viruses are **not** transmitted easily.
   (d) HTLV and HIV viruses are **not** the same.

304. **Coxsackieviruses**: Two groups; A and B.
   (a) **Group A**: Generalized myositis of skeletal muscles with flaccid paralysis.
   (b) **Group B**: Focal myositis, encephalitis causing spastic paralysis, generalized infections causing **myocarditis**, **pancreatitis,** and infections in the brown fat.

305. **Most common presentation of nonpolio enterovirus infections**: **Asymptomatic**. Most common symptomatic infection includes undifferentiated febrile illness (summer grippe) which is associated with upper respiratory symptoms. Aseptic meningitis, pleurodynia, and hand-foot-mouth disease comprises characteristic enterovirus syndrome.

306. **Most common causes for aseptic meningitis**: **Nonpolio enteroviruses**. It is most frequently caused by the following enteroviruses:
coxsackieviruses A (2, 4, 7, 9, 10), B (1 to 5).
echoviruses (3, 4, 6, 9, 11, 14, 16-19, 25, 30, 33), and enteroviruses (70, 71).
Patients appear initially with undifferentiated febrile illness (fever, headache, sorethroat, and myalgias) followed by symptoms and signs of meningitis (severe headache, vomiting, stiffness of the neck, and photophobia).
CSF:
   (a) Cell count:<10 to >3000 per cubic millimeter (average 50 to 500), initially increased polymorphs (<90%) which is quickly replaced by monocytes.
   (b) Protein: Normal (<40 mg/dL) or mildly elevated (rarely exceed 100 mg/dL).

Other CNS diseases caused by **enteroviruses are:**
   (a) Paralytic disease: Muscle weakness is more usual than paralysis and recovery is mostly complete except for the few cases which are fatal, and have bulbar paralysis.
   (b) Encephalitis: Enteroviruses only responsible for 10 to 20% of all cases. Most commonly involved enteroviruses are coxsackieviruses (A9, B2, B5), echoviruses (4,6,9,11,30), and enterovirus (71).

307. **Most common causes of epidemic pleurodynia (Bornholm disease): Group B coxsackieviruses (B3 and B5).** Patients appear with sudden onset of fever and sharp intermittent localized unilateral pain over the intercostal muscles of the lower chest wall. Presence of sweating, tachypnea, and grunting indicates pneumonia or pleural inflammation. The presentation may be **biphasic** that means initially symptomatic phase(2 to 7 days) followed by asymptomatic phase (1 or 2 days) then a recurrence of the symptoms again.
Physical examination: Muscle tenderness and sometimes swellings are noted.
Serum: Elevated CPK (creatine phosphokinase).
Treatment:
(a) Symptomatic: Analgesics (salicylates or others).
(b) Application of heat to the affected muscles.
Prognosis: Excellent.

308. **Most common cause of myocarditis and pericarditis:**
Group B coxsackieviruses.
Patients are predominantly males, **most common clinical diagnosis is pericarditis (60%) than myocarditis (40%).**
Treatment:
(a) Supportive such as analgesics, treatment for arrythmias, cardiac failure, and hemodynamic complications.
(b) Bed rest is an important treatment because exercise increases myocardial necrosis in mice.
(c) Do **not** use corticosteroids.
Prognosis: Good.

309. **Most common organism causing AHC (acute homorrhagic conjunctivitis)**: **Enterovirus 70**. Other organism is coxsackievirus A24. Patients appear with **H/O** foreign body sensations, pain in the eye, conjunctivitis, photophobia, and lacrimation.
Physical examination: **Most important finding is subconjunctival hemorrhage**. In addition to that, edema and swelling of the conjunctiva are present.
Treatment:
(a) **Symptomatic**: Cold compress, topical use of antihistamine/decongestant eye drops.
(b) Do **not** use corticosteroids.
Prevention: Hand washing, avoid contaminated clothing and towel, and sterilization of instruments are mandatory.
Prognosis: Good. Rarely, AHC caused by enterovirus 70 (**not** coxsackievirus 24) can cause motor paralysis like poliomyelitis.

310. **Major etiologic agent causing acute nonbacterial gastroentertitis**: **Norwalk virus group**. It is most commonly transmitted by fecal-oral route. **Adult patients appear with more diarrhea** than vomiting, along with abdominal discomfort. **Stools are loose, watery**, but **no** blood, WBC, or mucus.

311. **Acute nonbacterial gastroenteritis**:
Diagnosis: **Detection of virus in the stool** or antigenic responses to viral-specific antigen by ELISA or radioimmunoassay.
Treatment:
(a) **Dehydration**: Fluids and electrolytes in order to hydrate the patients.
(b) **To reduce the GI symptoms**: **Bismuth subsalicylate may reduce abdominal cramps and duration of the GI symptoms** but it does **not** reduce the viral excretion, and number, weight, or water contents of the stools.
Prevention: Avoid contaminated food and water, careful handwashing, and proper disposal of contaminated materials.

312. **Yellow fever vaccine**: This attenuated vaccine cause protective antibody for at least 10 years or a lifetime. It should be given at least 10 days before the arrival to the endemic area.
Contraindications:
(a) People with H/O allergy to egg.
(b) Pregnant women, unless the risk of exposure is very high. No birth defects have been reported from yellow fever vaccine.
Indications:
(a) HIV patients can receive this vaccine if needed.
(b) Travelers visiting to yellow fever endemic areas.

313. **Most common site of GI bleeding in yellow fever: Stomach.** Patients appear with very mild, mild, moderately severe, or malignant form.
(a) **Very mild**: Fever and headache are the symptoms which disappear within 2 days.
(b) **Mild**: Sudden onset of fever, headache, epistaxis, bleeding from the gums, bradycardia, or albuminuria. Patients improve within 3 days.
(c) **Moderately severe**: Bleeding, jaundice, vomiting, bradycardia in relation with fever, and marked albuminuria. Patients improve within 4 days or get worse with hemorrhagic manifestations from upper and lower GI tracts.
(d) **Malignant form**: It has three periods.
(i) **Period of infections** (0-3 days): Fever, initial tachycardia **followed by bradycardia despite rise of temperature (Faget's sign)**, bleeding from

the gums followed by bleeding from the stomach, and strawberry tongue.

(ii) Period of remission (beginning on day 4): No fever, nausea, and headache. Patients feel better and it lasts for a few hours to 2 days.

(iii) **Period of intoxication (beginning on day 4 to 6 and lasts for 2 weeks):** Fever, epigastric pain/ tenderness, blood vomiting, nose bleeding, albuminuria followed by oliguria or anuria, hypotension, coma, or death. Patients may appear lucid until the terminal phase.

314. **Diagnosis of yellow fever:**

(a) **Definitive diagnosis:**

(i) Alive patients: Isolation of the virus from blood.

(ii) Dead patients: Isolation of the virus from liver or other tissues.

Liver biopsy should not be attempted because it can cause uncontrolled bleeding.

(b) **Most rapid diagnostic test**: Detection of specific IgM by ELISA method.

(c) Routine CBC: Low WBC, neutrophils, and platelets count.

(d) Serum bilirubin: Elevated (9 to 20 mg/dL).

(e) PT and PTT: Prolonged.

(f) Coagulation Factors II, V, VII, IX, and X: Decreased.

(g) AST and ALT: Elevated.

(h) BUN/creatinine: 108/5.9 (elevated).

(i) CSF: Elevated proteins with normal cell counts.

315. **Treatment of yellow fever:**

(a) Bed rest, fluids and electrolytes therapy.

(b) Blood transfusions.

(c) Analgesics (except aspirin) and antiemetics.

(d) In DIC patients, heparin may be used cautiously.

(e) In renal failure, dialysis may help.

(f) Patients should be inside the bed nets to avoid mosquito transmission to other patients and hospital workers.

316. **Hantavirus pulmonary syndrome (HPS)**: It is a North American disease. HPS caused by hantavirus which is transmitted through rodent-feces either by inhalation or percutaneous contamination. Patients appears with fever, muscle pain, vomiting, abdominal pain for 3 to 6 days, followed by cardiopulmonary symptoms such as dyspnea, cough, noncardiogenic pulmonary edema, and hypoxia.

CBC: Low platelets, high leukocytes with atypical lymphocytes and band counts, and high hematocrits.

PT and PTT: Prolonged.

Urinalysis: Proteinuria and high creatinine.

Preferred diagnostic method: Detection of IgM (specific) antibody of the virus by ELISA method.

Treatment:

(a) Oxygen for hypoxia.

(b) Crystalloids are recommended as fluids because colloids enhances pulmonary edema due to increased pulmonary capillary permeabilities.

(c) Avoid overhydration because it increases pulmonary edema.

Prognosis: Half of the patients have fatal outcome. HPS syndrome also caused by Muerto canyon virus which is a hantavirus. Patients appear with fever, muscle pain, vomiting (influenza like symptoms), followed by dyspnea, acute pulmonary edema, hypotension, and death in 75% of patients. Diagnostic tests, laboratory tests, and treatment are the same as above.

317. A group of mentally retarded young adults were brought to **the park for recreational activities**. Inside the park, there were **many birds** and **full of bird feces** all around the area. Few days later, most of them developed flulike symptoms such as fever, chills, nonproductive cough, and muscles pain. Only few of them were complaining of substernal or pleuritic chest pain.

CXR: Most of them have **normal CXR** except a **few of them show patchy infiltrates with hilar adenopathies.** Only one person has miliary infiltrates which subsequently healed with 'buckshot' calcifications. No pleural effusions are noted.

Most likely diagnosis: **Histoplasmosis**. It is due to H.capsulatum. It causes acute pulmonary infection. Histoplasmosis is due to respiratory inhalations of spores present in bird and bat feces.

H.capsulatum causing **chronic pulmonary** infections: Patients symptom mimic pulmonary tuberculosis but histoplasmosis is milder and more indolent than TB. Patients initially appear with fever, night sweats followed by dyspnea and hemoptysis (indicates cavitary disease).

CXR: Initially interstitial infiltrates followed by cavity formations and fibrosis.

An AIDS patient went to the same park. The patient appears with fever, weight loss, and chills.

Physical examination: Hepatosplenomegaly, lymphadenopathies, oropharyngeal ulcerations, and hypotension.

CBC: Leukopenia, thrombocytopenia.

SMA6: Low Na, High k.

ESR: Elevated.

LFT: Elevated alkaline phosphatase.

CXR: Interstitial infiltrates (bilateral).

Most likely diagnosis: Disseminated histoplasmosis with adrenal insufficiency. In some AIDS patients, infections are due to reactivation of dormant infections. Rare complications of disseminated disease: Meningitis, endocarditis, and GI bleeding which is due to mucosal ulcerations.

318. **POHS (presumed ocular histoplasmosis syndrome):** Patients appear with loss of vision and three characteristic findings:
(a) Spots or punched-out lesions in the choroid.
(b) Neovascular membrane in the macula.
(c) Pericapillary scars or atrophy.
(d) Absence of inflammatory changes in anterior chamber or vitreous.
Patients are young adults and without any pulmonary or disseminated infections.
Treatment:
(a) Laser photocoagulation is the treatment of choice.
(b) No antifungal therapy is indicated.

319. **Diagnosis in different types of histoplasmosis**:
(a) **Definitive diagnosis**: Identification of H.capsulatum by culture of the sputum or histopathologic study of involved organs (e.g.,lungs, lymph nodes, liver etc.).
(b) Primary pulmonary histoplasmosis: Sputum cultures are **rarely** positive, so diagnosis is made by **clinical, radiological, and H/O exposure to birds or bats.**
(c) Chronic pulmonary histoplasmosis: Definitive diagnosis by **positive sputum cultures** or histopathologic study and special stains of the lung tissues obtained by flexible fiberoptic bronchoscopy.
(d) Disseminated histoplasmosis:
(i) Histopathologic study: Shows intracellular yeast forms.
(ii) Positive cultures of blood, bone marrow, liver, lungs, and lymph nodes.

320. **Treatment for histoplasmosis**: Itraconazole is the drug of choice for most patients.
(a) Primary pulmonary histoplasmosis: No antifungal therapy is needed.
(b) Progressive or severe lung infections(chronic and disseminated): Amphotericin, itraconazole, or ketoconazole.
(c) Immunocompromised patients (AIDS, patients with organ transplantation, cancers, corticosteroids therapy, rarely CNS and cardiac histoplasmosis): **Amphotericin is the drug** of choice or **itraconazole is an effective alternative therapy.**

(d) AIDS patients with milder disease: **Itraconazole is the drug of choice** or fluconazole can be used as an alternative. Life long therapy is needed to prevent the relapse.
(e) Mediastinal fibrosis due to histoplasma infections: Antifungal therapy is not effective. It is not recommended. Surgical treatment may be helpful in entrapment or obstructive syndromes.

321. **Coccidioidomycosis:** It is commonly found in desert areas (Arizona, California, Texas, New Mexico), and is caused by **Coccidioides** immitis. Infections begin in the **lungs** by inhalation of arthroconidia. Patients appear with dry cough, fever, chest pain, weight loss, arthralgia (no effusion), and rashes (maculopapular, erythema multiforme, or erythema nodosum).
CXR: Mostly normal except in a few cases interstitial infiltrates are found. **Hilar lymph nodes enlargement are the characteristic findings**.
Definitive diagnosis: Identification of C.immitis from pulmonary secretions and other clinical specimens.
Treatment:
(a) Immunocompetent patients with or without pnuemonia: No antifungal therapy is needed.
(b) Immunocompromised patients with pulmonary diseases: Amphotericin is the drug of choice.
(c) **Extrapulmonary diseases**: Fluconazole or itraconazole is the drug of choice. None of them suppress steroid synthesis unlike ketoconazole. Fluconazole is effective in meningitis.
Complications:
(a) **Pulmonary**: Lung nodule formations. It is a **benign mass** but it mimics malignancy, so percutaneous needle aspiration or resection is necessary.
(b) Extrapulmonary dissemination in immunocompromised patients:
(i) Skin: Cutaneous or subcutaneous nodules.
(ii) CNS: Involves basilar meninges.
(iii) Joints (particularly knee) and vertebrae.

322. **Most common candida infections in human: Candida albicans.**
Clinical manifestations of candida infections:
(a) **Mucocutaneous infections**: Pseudomembrane formations over the oropharyngeal areas. It also extends in the esophagus and stomach. **Gastrointestinal candida infection are common in cancer patients. HIV infections should be suspected** when there are no predisposing factors.
(b) **Systemic candidiasis:**

(i) **Candida positive blood culture**: It is common in burn, AIDS, cancer patients, and patients with central catheters. Mortality rate ranges from 40 to 80% except in catheter related infections which are lower.
(ii) **Liver and spleen**: 'Bulls eye' lesions are diagnosed by sonogram or CT scan. Diagnosis is confirmed by positive biopsy.
(iii) **Kidney**: Most common mode of spread is by **hematogenous route**. It produces '**fungus balls'** in the kidneys and ureters. It is also due to ascending infections from the urinary bladder. Upper urinary tract involvements are diagnosed by **triad: Candiduria, candida organisms within urinary casts, and candidemia.**
(iv) **Eye**: It can affect any structures, **Endopthalmitis is the most serious complication**. It is either due to hematogenous or **direct spread from postoperative complications**.
(v) **Heart**: **Candida is the most common cause of fungal endocarditis**. One of the most common complication of disseminated candida infection is candida myocarditis.
(vi) CNS: Intracerebral abscesses and meningitis.

323. **Diagnosis of fungal infections:**
(a) **Mucocutaneous lesions**: Clinical diagnosis; KOH preparation which shows spherical budding yeasts form and pseudohyphae.
(b) Esophageal candidiasis: Endoscopic biopsy.
(c) Remember, **blood cultures may be negative** in 50% of cases of disseminated candidiasis.
(d) Positive cultures and heavy growth of candidas in urine, sputum, tracheal aspirate, or wounds do **not** always means disseminated infections.
(e) **Definitive diagnosis** is made by positive histopathology and culture of the tissue specimens obtained by biopsy.
(f) **Newer genotypic methods** (DNA probes, electrophoretic **karyotyping, and** restriction fragment length polymorphism) are the most important and sensitive way of identifying different strains of candida.

324. **Treatment recommedations for disseminated candida infections:**
(a) Remove the catheter, if it is present. Remember, **catheter removal plus antifungal therapy should be given to all patients with catheters**.
(b) Surgical segmental venous resection in suppurative peripheral thrombophlebitis.
(c) Candidemia: Amphotericin and fluconazole.
(d) Non-neutropenic patients with catheter related candidemia: Remove the catheter plus fluconazole.

(e) Documented disseminated infections (CNS, cardiac, liver, and spleen) or multiorgan diseases: Amphotericin plus flucytosine.
(f) Hepatosplenic candidiasis: Fluconazole alone may be used or associated with initial treatment with amphotericin, with or without flucytosine.
(g) **Candida peritonitis**: It is due to complication of CAPD (continuous ambulatory peritoneal dialysis). First remove the catheter, then treat with amphotericin or fluconazole. If catheter cannot be removed, give amphotericin or fluconazole in the dialysate fluids.
(h) **Candida endocarditis:** Remove the valve and antifungal therapy.
(i) **Candida eye infections**: Amphotericin with or without flucytosine plus vitrectomy to remove vitreous abscesses.
(j) **Candida cystitis**: Most of the patients improve with removal of the catheter. Fluconazole (less toxic) or flucytosine may be used in persistent candiduria. If patients need the catheter, rinse the bladder with amphotericin or miconazole.

325. **Treatment for localized candida infections:**
(a) **Mucocutaneous:** Use topical preparation of clotrimazole, nystatin, miconazole, or ketoconazole.
(b) **Vulvovaginitis:** Single dose therapy with clotrimazole, miconazole, or fluconazole.
(c) **AIDS patients with oropharyngeal or esophageal lesions:** Fluconazole is more effective than ketoconazole but **fluconazole resistant diseases should be treated with either low-dose amphotericin or itraconazole (cross-resistance may develop).**

326. **Aspergillosis**: Most common organism is Aspergillus fumigatus. Invasive form of the diseases are found mostly in **immunocompromised patients** such as AIDS and cancer patients on chemotherapy (particularly acute leukemia). It is also found patients with in heart transplantation and diabetes.
(a) **Lungs**: The primary site of infection in the lungs include **infiltrates, nodules**, 'target lesions' (necrotic center surrounded by pulmonary hemorrhage due to pulmonary emboli), or **fungus balls (matted hyphae and debris) in a cavity.**
(b) **CNS**: **Abscesses are characteristic.** CSF glucose is normal and cultures are negative.
(c) **Heart**: Endocarditis is found in intravenous drug abusers or patients with prosthetic valves. Blood **cultures are negative**. Patients with postoperative endocarditis and negative blood **cultures,** always rule out aspergillus infections.

327. A 40 year old male farmer who is immunocompromised and chronic asthmatic, appears in the winter with H/O fever and grossly visible brown flecks in the sputum which are hyphae.
CXR: 'Tram-line'or ring markings (thickened bronchi) and upper lobe fibrotic changes are present.
Blood: Eosinophilia, elevated IgA and IgE.
Sputum: Eosinophilia.
Most likely diagnosis: Allergic bronchopulmonary aspergillosis.

328. **Treatment for aspergillosis**: **Amphotericin, itraconazole**.

329. **Most common presentation in mucormycosis**: **Rhinocerebral mucormycosis**. It is found in patients with diabetic ketoacidosis, other acidotic conditions, immunocompromised patients (hematologic malignancy with neutropenia, immunosuppressive therapy, or on prolonged broad-spectrum antibiotics therapy). Infections spread from oronasal cavity to sinuses (particularly ethmoidal), then from sinuses to retroorbital region and CNS.
Physical examination: **Black necrotic turbinates** with nasal septum perforation, proptosis, periorbital edema, and decreased vision. Paralysis of 3rd, 4th, 6th, and opthalmic branch of 5th cranial nerves are known as "**orbital apex syndrome**".
Treatment:
(a) **Amphotericin is the drug of choice.**
(b) Surgical debridement of necrotic tissues.

330. **Black necrotic tissue lesions are found in**:
(a) Mucormycosis.
(b) Pseudomonas aeruginosa.
(c) Pseudallescheria boydii.

331. **Cavernous sinus thrombosis are found in**:
(a) S.aureus.
(b) Fungal infections.
(c) Rhinoscleromas.
(d) Midline granulomas.
(e) Aggressive orbital tumors.

332. **Most common mycetoma infection in USA**: **Pseudallescheria boydii**. Other organism is A.madurae. Patients usually work in the field with barefeet in swampy soil and H/O repeated trauma to the feet. Patients appear with painless

nodules (in the feet) with or without rupture yielding granulation tissues or pus. Finally, sinus tract formations with release of fungal granulation tissues.

Diagnosis: Identification of mycetoma in the tissue specimens.

Treatment:

(a) Eumycetoma (P.boydii): Itraconazole plus surgical debridement.

(b) Actinomycetoma (A.madurae): Trimethoprim-sulfamethoxazole plus surgical debridement.

333. **Most important complication of group A streptococcal throat or upper respiratory infection**: Rheumatic fever (RF). It is a delayed nonsuppurative complication of group A streptococcal infection. RF is a self limited diseases.

334. **Most important complication of RF**: Damaged heart valves.

335. **Group A streptococcal skin infections can cause**: Poststreptococcal acute glomerulonephritis. It never causes rheumatic fever.

336. **The mechanism by which group A streptococci produces connective tissue inflammatory changes:**

(a) Unknown.

(b) Autoimmune phenomenon: Tissue damages are due to host's own immunologic responses to streptococcal infections.

(c) Toxin: Streptolysins S and O, both can damage the tissues.

(d) Antigen-antibody complexes localized to the sites of injury (heart valves).

337. **Jones criteria and acute rheumatic fever (ARF)**: In order to diagnosis ARF, patients should have two majors or one major and two minor manifestations along with evidence of preceding group A streptococcal infections.

(A) **Major manifestations are the following:**

(a) Polyarthritis (larger joints, mostly knee or ankle).

(b) Carditis (apical systolic or middiastolic **heart murmur,** pericarditis, and CHF).

(c) Chorea (Sydenham's type indicate rapid, purposeless involuntary movements mostly in face & upper extremities.

(d) Subcutaneous nodules.

(e) Erythema marginatum.

(B) **Minor manifestations are the following:**

(a) Clinical presentations:

(i) Fever.

(ii) Arthralgia.

(b) Laboratory findings: Elevated ESR and CRP (C-reactive protein).

(c) EKG: Prolonged PR intervals.

(C) Evidence of group A streptococcal infections:

(a) Positive throat cultures.

(b) Positive rapid streptococcal antigens test.

(c) Rising or elevated streptococcal antibody titers (more than 240 Todd units/ml).

338. **Most common clinical presentation in first attack of ARF**: **Arthritis** (75% of cases), next is carditis (40 to 50% of cases), chorea (15%), subcutaneous nodules and erythema marginatum (less than 10%). (You have to remember arthritis only).

339. **Joints fluid composition of arthritis in ARF:**

(a) Negative bacterial cultures.

(b) Cell counts: Thousands of WBC with predominant of polymorphs.

340. **Treatment for ARF:**

(a) Mild cases or equivocal cases: No treatment is needed.

(b) Arthritis with or without mild carditis: Aspirin. Do **not** use aspirin in moderate to severe carditis.

(c) Severe carditis with CHF: Corticosteroid is usually helpful.

(d) Group A streptococcal throat infections: Benzathine penicillin G.

Remember, **antiinflammatory** agents (aspirin, corticosteroids) **do not 'cure'** the disease, **nor do they prevent the subsequent development of rheumatic heart disease**. **Antibiotics** neither prevent the subsequent development of carditis, nor they can modify the course of rheumatic attack.

341. **Prevention of ARF:**

(a) Most effective management is the 1M injection of benzathine penicillin G every 4 weeks. It may be given every 3 weeks in high risk areas of the world.

(b) Patients with any **organic heart diseases** particulary rheumatic valvular disease, must receive the antibiotic prophylaxis before any dental or surgical procedures. **This recommendation is extremely important to avoid baceterial endocarditis.**

(c) Duration of rheumatic fever prophylaxis by 1M or PO is not settled, but life long prophylaxis are needed for patients with significant rheumatic heart diseases.

(d) Patients with **functional heart murmur** should **not** receive antibiotic prophylaxis before any dental or surgical procedures.

GASTROINTESTINAL DISEASES

1. **Most common sites of mild to moderate upper gastrointestinal hemorrhage**: **Duodenum** (41%), next is stomach (35%) which is followed by esophagus (24%).

2. **Most common sites of severe upper GI hemorrahges: Esophagus (59%);** stomach (24%); duodenum (17%).

3. **Most common cause of hematochezia (bright red blood in the stool which indicates distal or colonic bleeding)**: **Diverticula (23% of all cases),** next is unidentified locations (15%) which is followed by hemorrhoids (12%) In most of the cases of hematochezia (90%) bleeding is distal to the ileocecal valve. Brisk hemorrhages from the proximal GI tract can cause hematochezia in 10% cases.

4. **Most common sites of 'coffee grounds' vomiting**: Bleeding occurs **proximal to duodenojejunal junction**. It could be due to bleeding from nasopharynx, liver, pancreas, or respiratory tract.

5. **Most common sites of bleeding in melena: Upper GI tract** but sometimes bleeding occurs from mid-or distal small intestine or proximal colon can cause melena.

6. **Clinical presentation in patients with GI hemorrhage**: Patients appear with signs & symptoms of GI bleeding plus pallor, dizziness, diaphoresis, dyspnea, or syncope. **Initial immediate noninvasive assessment** should include:
   (a) **Presence of shock**: It indicates more than 15 to 20% of the acute loss of blood volume.
   (b) **Change of postural vital signs**: Systolic hypotension, tachycardia, or widening of pulse pressure in the upright position, indicates more than 10 to 15% of the acute loss of blood volume. If patients have no acute blood loss and they are clinically stable blood pressure and pulse should be recorded in sitting and standing position.
   (c) In acute bleeding, hemoglobin and hematocrit levels are **unreliable**. Patients may have severe blood loss with normal hematocrit.
   (d) It will be highly inaccurate estimate the amount of bleeding by **measuring nasogastric lavage** which is otherwise helpful. In duodenal ulcer, there will be small amount of blood in the nasogastric lavage because it mostly passes to the distal intestine.

(e) Presence of **large blood clots and bright red blood** in the stomach indicate **severe** upper GI bleeding.
(f) Severe upper GI bleeding may be associated with increased frequency of stool.The color of the stool may vary from dark black to dark red and increased bowel sounds.

7. **Initial emergency management of patients with severe acute GI bleeding**:
(a) **Fluid**: Saline or other standard electrolyte solutions should be started immediately. Fluids cannot replace the blood.
(b) **Oxygen**: To improve oxygen carrying capacity to the tissues.
(c) **Pulmonary artery and peripheral arterial catheters:** To monitor the adequacy of resuscitation and severity of the hemorrhage. It is needed only in severe bleeding.
(d) Try to obtain the **pertinent history** such as previous bleeding, GI ulcers, cancer, alcohol use, vascular anomalies (Osler-Weber-Rendu syndrome), and forceful vomiting before bleeding (Mallory-Weiss syndrome).
(e) **Physical examination** reveals abdominal tenderness (in ulcers), palpable mass (in cancer), and other pertinent findings. A rectal examination should be done to feel the mass and to look at the color of blood.
(f) **Nasogastric tube lavage** with room temperature water should be done after adequate resuscitation, history, and physical examination. It should be done in both upper and lower GI bleeding. It causes vasoconstriction of smaller gastric vessels. **(Never use ice cold water which causes gastric mucosal necrosis)**.
(g) After initial evaluation, blood should be sent for type & cross matching, CBC, PT, PTT and SMA6. **Blood transfusion should be given as soon as the blood is available in severe bleeding**.

8. **Patients with severe GI bleeding with disproportionate rise of BUN: creatinine ratio**: Indicates **proximal** GI bleeding.

9. **Most common cause of upper GI bleeding**: **Peptic ulcer disease**. It is usually but **not** always associated with epigastric pain or heart burn, particularly in elderly patients. Bleeding from the **varices** (esophageal or gastric) is usually but **not** always associated with chronic liver disease. **Gastritis caused by alcohol or nonsteroidal antiinflammatory agents**, appear with abdominal discomfort which is not relieved by food or antacids.

10. In patients with severe GI bleeding with shock and did receive multiple units of blood, preferred diagnostic procedure is: **Endoscopy**. It should be done **after** appropriate resuscitation and clinical examination of the patients. By this

procedure, physicians can diagnose the **site of bleeding in more than 95% of patients and treatment to stop the bleeding can be done immediately**. **Patients with severe GI bleeding and unstable condition**: Patients should be transferred to an intensive care unit or in the operating room for adequate monitoring and resuscitation. Endoscopy should be done by an expert.

11. **Indications for urgent endoscopy in upper GI bleeding**:
    (a) Shock or changes of postural vital signs.
    (b) Patients have received multiple transfusions.
    (c) Hematocrit is less than 30.
    (d) Recurrent bleeding from an unknown origin.
    (e) Prior to surgery.

12. **Indications for nonurgent endoscopy in upper GI bleeding**: **All patients** with acute GI bleeding should be investigated by endoscopy.

13. **Contraindications to endoscopy:**
    (a) Acute myocardial infarction.
    (b) Hemodynamically unstable patients.
    (c) Severe chronic lung disease.
    (d) Terminal cancer patients.
    (e) Agitated patients.

14. Definitive therapy can be done by endoscopy in the following upper GI bleeding.
    (a) Acute bleeding form varices (esophagus or stomach) can be controlled by sclerotherapy or varix band ligation in 90% of patients.
    (b) Active bleeding from ulcers can be stopped by endoscopic multipolar electrocoagulation, heater probe coagulation, or injection of dilute epinephrine.

15. **Benifits of endoscopy**:
    (a) It controls acute bleeding.
    (b) Reduces blood transfusions.
    (c) Decreases surgical procedures.
    (d) Reduces duration of stay and cost of hospitalizations.

16. **Indications of barium radiographic study in upper GI bleeding**:
    (a) Patients are not bleeding excessively.
    (b) Patients do not need endoscopic hemostasis.
    (c) Patients do not have chronic liver disease.

17. **Contraindications of barium radiographic study in upper GI bleeding**:
    (a) Patients are bleeding excessively.
    (b) Patients need endoscopic hemostasis.
    (c) Patients have chronic liver diseases.

18. **Problems of barium radiographic study in upper GI bleeding**:
    (a) It **cannot detect actual site of bleeding** when there are multiple sites of lesions.
    (b) Large amounts of retained blood in the upper GI tract prevent to detect ulcers by barium.

19. **Indications of angiography in upper and lower GI bleeding**:
    (a) Failure of endoscopic detection of **active brisk bleeding.**
    (b) Therapeutic indications **to stop the active bleeding** by infusion of vasopression or coil embolization.

20. **Contraindications of angiography in upper and lower GI bleeding**: Patients do **not** have active bleeding.

21. **Problems of angiography in upper and lower GI bleeding**:
    (a) It can detect the sites of bleeding but may **not** diagnose the etiology of bleeding.
    (b) It needs a specialized unit.
    (c) It is an expensive and an invasive procedure.

22. **Diagnostic steps** in patients with hematochezia.
    (a) First step: Proctoscopy to detect bleeding in anorectal junction, rectum, and anus.
    (b) Second step: Sigmoidoscopy can detect polyps, lacerations, cancers, and other conditions.
    (c) Third step depends upon the patients condition:
        (i) Patients with modest blood loss, normal hematocrit, and normal vital signs: Double contrast barium radiography can detect smaller polyps and superficial mucosal laceration in colitis.
        (ii) Patients present with lower GI tract blood loss and anemia: Colonscopy is the next step. It is done after cleansing the colon with oral nonabsorbable electrolyte solutions.
        (iii) Patients present with continuous brisk bleeding, the following steps should be considered:
        -Upper endoscopic evaluation to rule out upper GI bleeding.

-Angiography if bleeding is more than 30 to 50 ml/hour.
-Technetium RBC scintigraphy if bleeding is more than 3 to 10 ml/hour.
-Surgical resection of the sites of bleeding. Angiography or scintigraphy is helpful before surgery to localize the sites of surgery.

23. **Advantages of colonoscopy in lower GI bleeding**:
 (a) To stop bleeding immediately by coagulation methods.
 (b) To remove the polyps.
 (c) To take biopsy of mass lesions.

24. **Indications of surgery in GI bleeding**:
 (a) Failure of endoscopic injections and coagulation therapies.
 (b) Failure of two endoscopic therapeutic attempts.
 (c) Patients have received more than 6 to 8 units of blood.
 Only 10% of patients need surgery.

25. **Most common location of bleeding of unknown origin that means both upper GI endoscopy and pancolonoscopy failed to detect the sites of bleeding**: Lesions located **anywhere between** distal to the inferior duodenal angle to proximal to the ileocecal valve. Unknown sites are in the small intestine.
 Most helpful diagnostic procedures:
 (a) Technetium scintigraphy is the most helpful procedure.
 (b) In addition to that, angiography can also detect the sites of bleeding.
 (c) Rarely used methods are small bowel enteroclysis or enemas to detect polyps, cancers, or diverticula (Meckel's) and small bowel enteroscopy can detect vascular ectasia particularly jejunum.

26. **Most common site of GI bleeding in cancer patients with iron-deficiency anemia**: Colon cancer.

27. **Most common site of GI bleeding in noncancer patients with iron-deficiency anemia**: Small intestine, **most common cause is duodenal ulcers.**

28. **Step by step approach to patients with GI bleeding (first to last)**:
 (a) Quick recognition and **assessment of the bleeding.**
 (b) Resuscitation should be started immediately.
 (c) Differentiation from upper to lower GI bleeding.
 (d) Empiric treatment for upper GI bleeding.
 (e) Appropriate diagnosis.
 (f) Proper treatment.

29. **In HIV positive patients, white plaques on the lateral surface of the tongue, most likely clinical diagnosis**:
Hairy leukoplakia. It contains large numbers of Epstein-Barr viruses. Candida may be present on the superficial layers and antifungal treatment may not be very effective. A patient with hairy leukoplakia, HIV testing must be done.

30. **Blue or purple color macular lesions over the palate in HIV positive patients, most likely clinical diagnosis**: **Kaposi's sarcoma**. Diagnosis is confirmed by biopsy.

31. **Oral mucosal lesions of lupus may be present in the following condition**:
(a) Patients have the lupus.
(b) Patients will develop the lupus.
(c) Patients will never develop the lupus.
It appears with reticular solitary or bilaterally asymmetric hyperkeratotic lesions which resemble atrophic lichen planus.
Treatment:
(a) Topical fluocinonide.
(b) Intralesional application of triamcinolone.

32. **The following medications can cause mucosal hyperpigmentations, if used for prolonged period of time**:
(a) Cyclophosphamide.
(b) Minocycline.
(c) Nystatin.
(d) Chloroquine.
Differential diagnosis of **malignant melanoma** can be ruled out by biopsy of hyperpigmented lesions.

33. **Most common oral soft tissue tumor**: Small, pedunculated, hyperplastic fibrous connective tissue masses which are covered with normal- appearing mucosa. It could be due to irritation, dentures, drug induced (cyclosporin, phenytoin, nifedipine), or palatal papillomatosis.

34. **Treatment of mucous retention cysts or mucoceles in the oral cavity**: Conservative surgical excision. It is due to the injury of minor salivary glands. It is a small recurring nodule which is found inside the cheeks, lips, floor of the mouth, or on the posterior palate.

35. Patients appear with painful swelling of the salivary glands.

Physical examination: Mild purulent or no exudate is expressible from the duct.
Diagnosis is confirmed by: Bacterial cultures.
Most likely diagnosis: Bacterial sialadenitis.
Treatment: Cephalexin or dicloxacillin.

36. **Rarely, mumps like illness occur in adults in the following disease conditions**:
    (a) CMV.
    (b) Coxackie A virus.
    (c) Influenza.

37. **Few common causes of xerostomia (decreased salivary secretion)**:
    (a) Chronically used the following drugs: MAO inhibitors, antidepressants, neuroleptics, and parasympatholytics.
    (b) Systemic disease: Sjogren's syndrome, sarcoidosis, HIV infection, and irradiation to the head or neck in malignancy.
    (c) Temporary: Antihistamines, fear, depression, and dehydrations.
    Treatment for xerostomia:
    (i) Mild or moderate xerostomia: Frequent sips of water, sugarless hard candies, chewing gum, or saliva substitute at night.
    (ii) Severe xerostomia (following irradiation): Pilocarpine.

38. Most common causes of 'transfer dysphagia' (when the bolus of food cannot be propelled from the mouth to esophagus): Neurologic diseases or pharyngeal muscles weakness.

39. **Odynophagia (pain while swallowing) is most commonly seen in**:
    Patients with reflux, other causes are viral, fungal infections or radiation to the esophageal mucosa. It indicates esophageal diseases.

40. **Most common symptoms of esophageal diseases**: Heartburn (pyrosis). It is also present in 20% of normal individuals.

41. **Most common symptom of GERD (gastroesophageal reflux disease)**: Heartburn, other symptoms are dysphagia, regurgitation, or iron deficiency anemia mostly due to chronic blood loss.

42. **Most important diagnostic aids in GERD**: History and physical examination.

43. **Approach to diagnosis and treatment in GERD patients**:

(A) Patients with symptoms of short duration and no other complications: Empiric treatment for GERD.
   (i) Well response: Patients may need prolonged maintenance therapy.
   (ii) Poor response: Endoscopy with esophageal biopsy.
(B) Patients with dysphagia only: Patients need barium swallow study.
   (i) Normal: Empiric treatment for GERD.
   (ii) Abnormal: Endoscopy with esophageal biopsy.
(C) Patients with chronic history, weight loss, anemia, hematemesis, and heme-positive stool: Endoscopy with esophageal biopsy.
(D) Patients have required endoscopy with esophageal biopsy:
   (i) Endoscopy and biopsy reveal reflux esophagitis: Patients may need prolonged maintenance therapy.
   (ii) Endoscopy and biopsy reveal normal esophagus, but patients are very symptomatic, no response to empiric therapy: Patients need esophageal manometry with Bernstein test (catheter is placed in midesophagus, normal saline is infused for 5 minutes followed by infusion of 0.1N hydrochloric acid for 5 minutes, patients develop symptoms which disappear with infusion of normal saline) and 24-hours esophageal pH monitoring.

44. **Most important clinical significance of Barrett's esophagus (columnar epithelium)**: It is a precursor of **adenocarcinoma** and also **indicates severe reflux**. Normal squamous epitheliums of esophagus are replaced by columner epitheliums due to severe reflux.

45. **Most common clinical symptom of esophageal stricture**: Dysphagia.
Initial diagnostic study: Barium swallow shows esophageal stricture.
Final diagnostic study: Endoscopy with biopsy and /or brush cytology must be done if stricture is present to rule out cancer.

46. **Complications of GERD**:
   (a) Esophageal ulcers.
   (b) Esophageal strictures.
   (c) Barrett's esophagus.
   (d) Pulmonary aspiration.

47. **Treatment of GERD**:
First step: Changes of lifestyle and nonsystemic therapies.
   (a) Elevate the head portion of the bed (**not** the chest portion) by 6 to 8 inches.
   (b) Avoid food and fluids at least 3 hours before bed time.

(c) Avoid fatty food, chocolate, peppermint, onion, coffee, cigarette, and alcohol.
(d) Take antacids 1 hour after meals, bedtime and prn.
(e) Advice to lose weight.

Second step: Systemic treatment when the first step was not effective.
(a) H_2- receptor antagonists: Cimetidine, ranitidine, famotidine, or nizatidine.
(b) Prokinetic agents used in addition to gastric acid suppressants: Metoclopramide (CNS side effects), cisapride (used in nocturnal GERD), or bethanechol.

Third step: Patients who did not respond to H_2- receptors antagonist.
(a) Proton pump inhibitor: Omeprazole.

Fourth step: Patients who did **not** respond to previous treatment or required long-term maintenance therapy: Surgical fundoplication.

48. **Indications of surgical fundoplication in GERD**:
(a) Medical managements have failed despite 6 months of adequate therapies.
(b) Patients have good evidence of reflux.
(c) Patients require long term medical therapies.

49. **Most effective surgical procedure in GERD**:
Nissen fundoplication: It is a most effective procedure which surrounds the lower end of the esophagus with a cuff of gastric fundal muscles to maintain the sphincter competence. It is a **complete** procedure. Other **partial** procedures are Belsey and Hill repair.

50. **Treatment for complications of GERD**:
(A) Esophageal ulcers: H_2-receptor antagonist or proton pump inhibitor.
(B) Esophageal strictures:
  (a) Midly symptomatic patients: Advice on diet, dentition, and appropriate medical therapy.
  (b) Moderate to severely symptomatic patients: Dilatation of the esophagus. Most patients become asymptomatic if the lumen is kept 13 to 15 mm in diameter.
  (c) Patients need dilatation every 4 to 6 months and stricture is stable: No other intervention is necessary.
  (d) Patients need dilatation every 3 to 4 weeks but are not tolerating dilatation well:
    (i) Surgical fundoplication to prevent the reflux.
    (ii) Esophageal replacement by the colon, jejunum, or stomach is the last resort. It has high morbidity and mortality.

(iii) Repeated dilatation may be reduced by using high-dose of H_2-antagonists or preferably omeprazole along with dilatations.

(C) **Barrett's esophagus (premalignant condition, columner epitheliums)**.

(i) **Medical**: To prevent the reflux use high-dose of H_2-antagonists or proton pump inhibitor. It may cause regression of the columner epithelium, which are premalignant, in some patients.

(ii) **Periodic endoscopic biopsies**: To look for dysplastic changes for adenocarcinoma. Dysplasia could be mild, moderate or severe.

(iii) **Esophagectomy**: It is needed when patients have confirmed high-grade dyplasia.

(D) **Pulmonary aspiration**:

(a) Elevate the head portion of the bed at night or while sleeping.

(b) Gastric acid suppressants.

(c) Prokinetic agents.

(d) Do **not** advice antireflux surgery when patients have primary pulmonary problems with documented reflux because there is no direct relationship between the reflux and primary pulmonary diseases.

51. **Most important clinical presentation of esophageal motor disorders**: Chest pain or esophageal colic. Patients complain of mild or severe pain which mimics myocardial infarction or dissecting aortic aneurysm. The pain is usually substernal which can radiate to the neck, jaw, or arms. It is impossible to differentiate between the esophageal chest pain and the anginal attack because both are identical and may respond to nitroglycerin.

52. **Clinical presentation in scleroderma achalasia, and transfer dysphagia**:
Scleroderma: Patients appear with GERD due to primary failure of sphincter muscles.
Achalasia: Patients appear with dysphagia, esophageal retention, regurgitation, and aspiration of the food materials into the tracheobronchial tree due to failure of the lower esophageal sphincter to relax and loss of peristolsis of the esophagus.
Transfer dysphagia: Patients are unable to transfer both solid or liquid foods from the pharnyx to the esophagus. It is found in upper esophageal sphincter (UES) malfunction or oropharyngeal mascular weakness.

53. **Radiological studies in different esophageal motor disorders**:

(a) LES (lower esophageal sphincter) dysfunction: Manometric examination directly determines the LES function.

(b) UES (upper esophageal sphincter) and oropharyngeal dysfunctions: Videoesophagogram is the best diagnostic study.

(c) Achalasia: Barium study shows dilated esophagus with smooth tapering beak which is diagnostic (irregular tapering beak may suggest malignancy).
(d) Scleroderma: Barium study shows that barium is retained in the esophagus for longer period of time in supine position.

54. **Treatment of the different motor disorders**:
   (A) Achalasia: (Aim is to relax LES and relieve the obstruction).
      (a) Isosorbide dinitrate, long-acting nitrate, or nifedipine (calcium channel blocker).
      (b) Pneumatic bag dilatation: Perforation is the complication, it should be done by an expert.
      (c) **Heller esophagomyotomy**: Direct section of lower esophageal muscles, sparing some gastric muscle fibers to prevent reflux. It is done when dilatation fails or to avoid perforation due to dilatation. Laparoscopic surgery can be done.
   (B) Diffuse spasm:
      (a) Nitroglycerin, anticholinergics, or nifedipine.
      (b) Balloon dilatation of LES: It is helpful in patients with abnormal LES functions and high basal tone with difficult relaxation.
   (C) Nutcracker esophagus: Sublingual nitroglycerin, anticholinergics, or nifedipine. (They reduce the force of esophageal contractions and relieve the pain).
   (D) Scleroderma:
      (a) Treat the reflux medically.
      (b) Do **not** recommend antireflux surgery because it can lead to dysphagia, muscle atrophy, or collagen deposition.

55. **Cause of chest pain in nutcracker esophagus**: It is due to microvascular coronary artery disease.

56. **Most common tumors of the esophagus**: **Squamous cell carcinoma and adenocarcinoma of the esophagus**. Rarely found benign tumors are leiomyomas, polyps, or papillomas.

57. **Squamous cell cancers are associated with the following conditions**:
   (a) Squamous cancers of the head and neck.
   (b) Improperly or untreated achalasia.
   (c) Patients with history of alcohol or tobacco intake.

58. **Most common clinical symptoms of esophageal cancer**: **Progressive dysphagia**. Initially dysphagia occurs with solid food for several months

before dysphagia occurs with liquid. Other symptoms are steady, boring pain (which means mediastinal involvement and inoperability), halitosis, hoarseness (involvements of recurrent laryngeal nerve), weight loss, coughing after drinking fluids (means complete obstruction and aspiration or tracheoesophageal fistulas) and clubbing which is found in benign and malignant tumors.

59. **Diagnostic studies of suspected esophageal carcinomas**:
   (a) First investigation of choice is barium esophagogram with double contrast technique. It may be normal or abnormal (irregularity and narrowing of the lumen).
   (b) If esophagograms are normal and patients are symptomatic: Endoscopy with biopsies and brushing should be done. Adenocarcinomas of the gastroesophageal junction should be ruled out by the careful retroflexed view of the cardia from below during endoscopy.
   (c) If esophagograms are abnormal: Endoscopic biopsies and brushing should be done.
   (d) Esophageal cancer is confirmed and to rule out any metastasis to the mediastinal lymph nodes and liver, the following investigations are necessary: CXR, liver function tests, CT scan, endoscopic ultrasound (it detects the level of involvement and mediastinal lymph nodes abnormalities).

60. **Indications of bronchoscopy in esophageal cancers**: Bronchoscopy is indicated in patients with upper and midesophageal cancers to rule out asymptomatic invasions of tracheobronchial tree.

61. **Treatment of esophageal cancers (squamous cells and adenocarcinomas)**:
   (a) Involvement of **lower third** of the esophagus without widespread metastasis: Surgical resection of the cancers with restoration of gastroesophageal continuity.
   (b) Radiotherapy is effective mostly in the **upper third**, and is also in the middle third of the esophageal cancers. Adenocarcinomas are **not** radiosensitive tumors unlike squamous cells carcinomas.
   (c) **Combinations** of chemotherapy (cisplatin and flurouracil) and radiotherapy **are superior** than radiotherapy alone.
   (d) Extraesophageal spreads of cancers:
      (i) To maintain the esophageal lumen by dilatation, silastic tube, or metal stent.
      (ii) To destroy the tumor and maintain the esophageal lumen by **endoscopic laser** therapy or **intraluminal heat-coagulating probe.**

62. **Most common cause of acquired postcricoid web of esophagus**: Iron deficiency anemia (Plummer-Vinson syndrome).
Treatment: Iron therapy.

63. A 30 year old man appears with H/O dysphagia of solid or liquid food every 3 to 4 months. He was unable to swallow a bolus of meat or bread which was regurgitated, after that patient was able to eat without any problem for 3 months.
Preferred diagnostic method: Video study of the lower esophageal ring.
Most likely diagnosis: **Schatzki's ring (lower esophageal ring)**.
Treatment: Dilatation of lower esophageal ring by endoscopic balloon or a bougie.

64. **Patients with H/O dysphagia and barium study reveals diverticulum**: Dysphagia may be due to diverticulm or associated motor disorders.

65. **Zenker's diverticulum of the pharynx**: A patient appears with characteristic H/O retaining food or saliva which needs post prandial throat clearing by pressing on the neck and empty the diverticulum.
Complication: Perforation during endoscopy or passing tubes in the esophagus.
Treatment:
(a) Small diverticulum: It improves with the section of cricopharyngeus muscles.
(b) Large diverticulum: Diverticulectomy or diverticulopexy with section of cricopharyngeus muscles.
Other diverticulums are:
Traction diverticulum: Located at the level of carina but scar tissue traction is not found.
Epiphrenic diverticulum: Located in the right side of esophagus just above the LES.
Treatment: No treatment is necessary.

66. **Most important method of confirming the infectious diseases of the esophageal mucosa**:
Endoscopic biopsy. Organisms causing the infections are candida, CMV, HSV in immunocompromised hosts.
Treatment:
(a) Candida: Nystatin, clotrimazole, fluconazole, or low-dose IV amphotericin depends on the severity of the lesions.

(b) HSV: Acyclovir.
(c) CMV: Ganciclovir.

67. **Most common reason of caustic injury to the esophagus in adults**: Suicide attempt. Most common materials are lye crystals and liquid lye preparations for drain cleaning. Esophageal injuries are possible without injuries to the oral cavities.
Preferred diagnostic method: History is important and degree of esophageal injuries are confirmed by emergency endoscopy.
Treatment: Definitive therapies have not been established.
(a) Liquid lye burns: Emergency esophagogastrectomy.
(b) Solid lye burns: Corticosteroids, broad-spectrum antibiotics.

68. **Most common complication of esophageal perforations**:
Mediastinitis.
Esophageal perforation could be due to blunt trauma, penetrating injuries (knifes, gunshot) or vomiting.
Mallory- Weiss syndrome: Esophageal mucosal tear is located just below the gastroesophageal junction due to vomiting.
Preferred diagnostic method: Endoscopy.
Treatment.
(a) Conservative therapy: Majority of the patients improve with this therapy.
(b) Surgical repair is needed in <5% of patients.
(c) To stop bleeding: Endoscopic electrocoagulation is needed.
Boerhaave's syndrome: Complete esophageal rupture is located **above** the gastroesophageal junction on the left side due to vomiting, weight lifting, or straining during defecation.
Preferred diagnostic method: Radiologic study with water soluble contrast material should be done carefully.
Treatment:
(a) Emergency surgical repair is the best treatment of choice.
(b) Patients are unstable for surgery: Nasogastric suction, antibiotics, and mediastinal drainage prn.

69. **Most common cause of gastritis**: Helicobacter pylori (HP).
HP is present in all patients with superficial gastritis which usually resolves once the HP infection is controlled. Patients appear with epigastric pain, nausea, and vomiting. HP could be superficial, type B is antral predominant, or type AB causes pangastritis.

70. **Most common type of peptic ulcer causing gastric cancer**: Gastric ulcer. It causes low acid secretions, more severe antral gastritis and superficial fundic glands gastritis. Duodenal ulcer causes high acid secretion and lowers the risk of gastric cancer.

71. **Diagnostic methods for HP**:
    (a) Most important is noninvasive methods:
        (i) Serology with an ELISA method to detect IgG or IgA antibodies.
        (ii) ^{13}C or ^{14}C-urea breath tests after an oral urea load.
    (b) Invasive methods: Antral biopsy and culture. These procedures are not done routinely. False-negative result can occur because the organism is suppressed by the antibiotic, bismuth, or omeprazole.

72. **Dyspepsia in a HP infection is due to**: Functional disorder which is independent of HP infection. So in some patients dyspepsia may persist, even when HP infections are in control.

73. **Absence of immune markers in HP infections**: **HP pangastritis.** Antibodies fall within months after the organisms have been killed.

74. **HP infection and vitamin deficiency**: Vitamin B_{12} deficiencies are found in some patients of HP infections by nonimmunologic mechanisms unlike pernicious anemia which has immunologic mechanisms. Approximately 90% of patients with **pernicious anemia have antibodies against parietal cells** which block the vitamin B_{12} binding sites, react with parietal cell H^+-K^+-ATPase and intrinsic factors. Genetic factors are also important in pernicious anemia.

75. **Causes of atrophic gastritis**:
    (a) HP.
    (b) Pernicious anemia.

76. **Pernicious anemia and gastric cancer**: **Gastric adenocarcinomas** have increased frequencies in prenicious anemias. Pernicious anemias are diagnosed by **multiple biopsies**. Dysplastic changes in the epithelial cells warrant close follow-up and /or surgical therapy. The ratio of pepsinogen I to pepsinogen II **falls** in proportion to glandular atrophy.
    Treatment for pernicious anemia: Vitamin B_{12}.

77. **Endoscopic findings in different disease conditions**:

(a) Watermelon stomach (gastric antral vascular ectasia): Erythematous folds or linear vascular streaks are converging at the pylorus. Biopsy confirms the diagnosis. It is found in nongastric conditions, chronic iron deficiency anemia, or acute GI bleeding.
Treatment:
(a) Repeated coagulations with endoscopic laser or heater probe.
(b) Antrectomy.

Relation: It is **not** found in HP infection.

(b) Phlegmonous gastritis: Pus formations within the gastric mucosa and walls. It is due to alpha-hemolytic streptococci, E.coli, proteus, or S.aureus.

Treatment: Surgery because medical treatment is not effective.

(c) Blood under a plastic wrap (subepithelial, intramucosal bleed or hemorrhagic gastritis). It is found in patients with **alcohol abuse**.

(d) Chronic erosive gastritis (varioliform gastritis): Gastric erosions are found on top of gastric nodules. It is found in HP infections.

(e) Eosinophilic gastritis: Infiltration of eosinophils within mucosal and muscular layers of the stomach particularly antrum, with peripheral high eosinophil counts.
Treatment.
(i) Glucocorticoids.
(ii) Surgery is performed only for obstruction.

(f) Granulomatous gastritis: Granulomas are found in the gastric mucosa particularly antrum. It is found in sarcoidosis, Crohn's disease, TB, histoplasmosis, and syphilis.
Treatment:
(i) Treat the underlying disease conditions.
(ii) Spontaneous resolutions may occur in some patients.

78. **Menetrier's disease**:
These are the following features:
(a) Gaint folds in the stomatch fundus and body.
(b) Protein- losing gastropathy causing low albumin in the serum.
(c) Decreased stomach acid secretions.
(d) Foveolar hyperplasia, mucosal thickening, glandular hypertrophy.

Preferred diagnostic method: Biopsy.
Relationship: No risk of cancer but HP infections may present.
Treatment:
(a) Treat the underlying HP infections, if present.
(b) Antiulcer therapy.

79. **Most common causes of peptic ulcers**:

HP infection is the most common infection in the World. More than 90% of duodenal ulcers (DU) and 75% of gastrointestinal ulcers (GU) are associated with HP infections. Approximately 10 to 20% of patients infected with HP develop peptic ulcers.
Next common cause is nonsteroidal anti-inflammatory drugs (NSAID's) which is followed by stress ulcers.

80. **A 50 year old woman who is taking NSAID has occult blood in the stool**: **Most likely diagnosis:** Drug related ulcers or colonic cancer. **Recommendations**: Thorough investigations (endoscopic biopsy) should be done to rule out cancer.

81. **Mechanism of action of NSAID's causing ulcers**: They inhibit **the enzyme** cyclo-oxygenase. This enzyme catalyzes the formation of prostaglandins (PG) precursor endoperoxide from arachidonic acid which is produced by cell membrane phospholipids. There are decreased mucosal PG production which usually protects the cell membranes.

82. **Important points to remember in NSAID's causing peptic ulcers**:
    (a) Three types of ulcers are produced: Superficial, endoscopic, and clinical ulcers.
    (b) The risks of ulcer and bleeding are maximum within first 3 months of treatment but both can begin within few days.
    (c) All aspirin dosages including baby aspirin can reduce mucosal PG (prostaglandins) production.
    (d) All aspirin dosages except baby aspirin can cause ulcers.
    (e) Elderly women have increased incidence of ulcers because of increased consumption and poor tolerance.
    (f) Diagnosis is made by endoscopy.

83. **Antral G cell hypersecretion of gastrin in duodenal ulcer (DU) disease**: It is a rare form of DU which is found in both HP dependent and independent ulcers. Fasting gastrin levels are modestly elevated and after meals gastrin levels are highly elevated.

84. **NSAID's causing peptic ulcer is most commonly seen in**: Elderly patients with degenerative joint diseases.

85. **Recurrence rate in petic ulcer diseases**: Most common in peptic ulcers which are not related to NSAID's. NSAID's causing peptic ulcers usually improve with the discontinuation of the medications.

86. **Genetic factors in peptic ulcer diseases**:
   (a) First-degree relatives of ulcer patients have three fold increase of developing ulcers.
   (b) DU patients families do **not** have high incidence of GU ulcers and vice-versa.
   (c) DU patients families have high incidence of DU; GU patients families have high incidence of GU.
   (d) Genetic families with ulcers may have been exposed to early HP infections.

87. **Most common cause of delayed gastric emptying**: Functional bowel disorders. It is also found in drugs, diabetic neuropathy, or connective tissue diseases.

88. **Most common presentation of peptic ulcers**: **Epigastric pain which is burning in nature**. Majority of the patients(70%) with dyspepsia (epigastric distress) do **not** have ulcer diseases due to high visceral sensations. Approximately 40% patients with documented ulcers do **not** have abdominal pain due to **low visceral sensations**. Abdominal tenderness in physical examination may be present in **ulcer or nonulcer diseases**. Epigastric abdominal pain does not necessarily means ulcer disease.

89. A patient had surgery for an ulcer, appears again with symptoms of ulcer.
   Endoscopy: No ulcer has been found.
   Most likely diagnosis: Visceral hyperalgesia.

90. **Important points in endoscopy**:
   (a) It is the best method to diagnose peptic ulcer disease.
   (b) Biopsy is **not** indicated in DU ulcer disease because it is always benign.
   (c) Biopsy is indicated in GU ulcer disease becasue it can cause cancer.
   (d) Repeat endoscopy in GU ulcer disease is important to confirm healing after 8 to 12 weeks of medical therapy except in young patients with GU are due to NSAID and appear benign.

91. **American College of Physician recommends in patients with epigastric discomfort or pain**:
   (a) Patients with uncomplicated dyspepsia: Empiric therapy should be given with antiulcer medications. Further investigations (endoscopy and radiographic studies) are **not** needed if patients are under the age of 40 and responsive to medical therapy.

(b) Patients with complicated dyspepsia (weight loss, back pain, and loss of appetite) in any age or older than 50, require NSAID on a regular basis, and **unresponsive** to medical therapy: Endoscopy should be done to confirm the diagnosis and obtain biopsy to rule out malignancy.

92. **NIH recommedations of HP diseases**:
   (a) Patients with HP infections and H/O taking NSAID should be treated for HP.
   (b) Patients with confirmed HP diseases should be treated for HP infections to eradicate the microorganism.
   (c) Patients with GU diseases should have endoscopy done and HP status should be obtained because 70% of GU diseases are due to HP and 30% of GU diseases are due to NSAID.
   (d) Patients with nonulcer dyspepsia unresponsive to medical therapy should be tested for HP infections.

93. **Diagnostic testing for HP infections**:
   (a) Most sensitive and specific serologic test- **^{14}C- or ^{14}C- urea breath test** because HP produces urease. **It is good for both diagnosis and follow-up**. Other serologic tests are ELISA which is **not** suitable for follow-up and quick office test which is rapid and inexpensive.
   (b) Test which requires endoscopy: **Most specific test is culture (up to 100%) and most sensitive test is histology** (up to 99%). Other test is rapid urease test which is also highly sensitive and specific (up to 98 %).

94. **Drug that prevents both GU and DU in NSAID users**: Misoprostol is the only drug which can prevent both ulcers. It is the only synthetic PG available in the USA.

95. **Most effective antisecretary agents are**: Acid-pump inhibitors. They are expensive and lack of long term usage.

96. **Treatment of NSAID ulcers**:
   (a) Stop the NSAID medications.
   (b) Osteoarthritis with pain: Use acetaminophen, low dose ibuprofen, or naproxen sodium.
   (c) Rheumatoid arthritis: Use low dose prednisone which has no adverse effect on ulcers. After the ulcer heals, use antiinflammatory medications with misoprostol therapy.

97. **Treatment of HP ulcers**:

(a) Tripple therapy combinations have success rate >90%.
   (i) Tetracycline + clarithromycin + bismuth subsalicylate + antisecretary drug.
   (ii) Tetracycline + metronidazole + bismuth subsalicylate + antisecretary drug.
   (iii) Amoxicillin + clarithromycin + bismuth subsalicylate.

(b) Double threrapy combinations are the following:
   Best success rate (>90%) in double threrapy:
   (i) Amoxicillin + clarithromycin + antisecretary drug.
   (ii) Amoxicillin + metronidazole + antisecretary drug.
   (iii) Clarithromycin+omeprazole.

98. **Prevention of ulcers**:
   (a) Patients with cured HP infections: No maintenance anti-secretary threapy is needed.
   (b) Patients with resistant HP infections: Half of the healing dose of anti-secretary therapy is recommended.
   (c) Patients with ulcers caused recent bleeding or potential for bleeding: Continuation of anti-secretary therapy is recommended.
   (d) Very sick patients with ulcers, secondary ulcers due to balloon dilatation, or large ulcers: Use acid pump inhibitors (omeprazole).

99. **Indications for emergency surgery for peptic ulcers**:
   (a) Perforation.
   (b) Bleeding.
      (i) Severe hemorrhage.
      (ii) Bleeding >6 units of blood.
      (iii) Active bleeding in visible vessels.
      (iv) Slow, persistent bleeding.
      (v) Recurrent bleeding on medical therapy.
   (c) Fixed gastric outlet obstruction.

100. **Treatment for gastric outlet obstruction**:
   (a) First conservative management with nasogastric tube for 8 to 10 days.It relieves most of the inflammatory obstruction.
   (b) Surgery is indicated when conservative management fails.

101. **Elective procedure of choice in DU patients**: Highly selective vagotomy (HSV).

102. **Procedure of choice in perforation of GU**: To close the perforation, HSV, and antibiotic to prevent infection. HSV should not be done if perforation is more than 24 hours old, possibility of peritonitis, or a very sick patient.

103. **Operative procedures of gastric ulcer patients**:
   (A) Elective operations:
      (i) Ulcer in the body of the stomach (highest incidence): Billroth I (antrectomy).
      (ii) GU with DU (2nd most common incidence): Vagotomy + antrectomy.
      (iii) Prepyloric: Vagotomy+antrectomy.
   (B) Emergency operations:
      (i) Bleeding and stable patients: Distal gastrectomy which removes the ulcer +Billroth I anastomosis.
      (ii) Bleeding and unstable patients: Excision of the ulcer alone, or with vagotomy and pyloroplasty. If ulcer cannot be excised, bleeding should be stopped by sutures with or without biopsy.
      (iii) Perforation: Procedure of choice is distal gastrectomy + Billroth I anastomosis. These procedures are contraindicated if patients are very sick, possibilities of peritonitis, or perforations of more than 24 hours. In those patients procedures of choice are excision of the ulcer + closure of perforation + vagotomy + pyloroplasty. In severely ill patients, ulcers are patched with omentum after the biopsies were taken from each quadrant.

104. **Postoperative vagotomy patients with recurrent ulcers**: Treatment of choice is cimetidine (H_2- receptor antagonist). Most common presentation is recurrence of ulcer pain (95%), other presentations are bleeding, obstruction, or perforation.
   Preferred diagnostic method: Endoscopy.

105. Gastrinoma with recurrent ulcers.
   (a) First localization of the tumor and removal of the tumor.
   (b) When tumor cannot be localized even after laparotomy (no tumor is found in pancreas, duodenum, or retroperitoneal areas): Treatment of choice is omeprazole. If that fails, total gastrectomy is the treatment of choice.

106. **Most common cause of postoperative recurrent peptic ulcer**: **HSV** (highly selective vagotomy), next common is truncal vagotomy and drainage, ZES (zollinger-Ellison syndrome) should be ruled out.

107. **Zollinger-Ellison syndrome (ZES):** ZES is very common in postoperative recurrent DU. ZES should be suspected in preoperative DU patients who have the following features like multiple ulcers, ulcers in the distal duodenum or jejunum, family history of (MEN I) multiple endocrine neoplasia syndrome, hypercalcemia, or renal stones.

Preferred diagnostic method:

(a) Elevated plasma gastrin levels which are also found in other condition like vagotomy.

(b) **Characteristic of ZES**: **Paradoxical rise of plasma gastrin after secretin which** is **not** found after vagotomy or retained antrum syndrome.

(c) Post meal elevation of gastrin is modest in ZES, no change in retained antrum syndrome, and highly elevated gastrin levels in G cell hyperplasias are due to either primary or post vagotomy.

108. A 50 year old man appears with H/O upper abdominal pain, borborygmi, diarrhea, sweating, tachycardia, or palpitation within 1 hour after feeding. Patient develops hypoglycemic symptoms in the second hour after feeding due to hyperinsulinemia secondary to initial hyperglycemia. Patient had recent H/O gastrojejunostomy or pyloroplasty operation.

Most likely diagnosis: Dumping syndrome or postgastrectomy syndrome.

Pathogenesis: It is due to destruction of antropyloric mechanism (gastric resection pyloroplasty), bypass operation (gastrojejunostomy), or hyperosmolar food is 'dumped' into the upper small intestine.

Treatment:

(a) **Dietary management is the most important: Low carbohydrate** which has low osmolarity, **delayed liquid intake for 30 minutes after food** prevents rapid passage of hyperosmolar food from stomach to intestine, and **reclining for 30 minutes** to prevent rapid passage of food from stomach to intestine by gravitational force.

(b) **Medical therapy**: Pectin, ephedrine, and the long acting somatostatin. Somatostatin prevents the release and action of vasoactive peptides from the intestine and also prevents hypoglycemia by inhibiting the secretion of insulin. It prevents the late dumping syndrome which is due to hypoglycemia.

(c) **Surgical therapy**: It is used only in patients with failure of dietary management and medical treatment. The procedures are the following:

(i) Construction of a Roux-en-Y gastrojejunostomy.

(ii) Conversion of Billroth I to Billroth II.

109. **Postvagotomy diarrhea**: Patients appear with episodic loose bowel movement 1 to 2 hours after the intake of foods.

Treatment:

(a) Diet: Avoid milk, juice, carbonated liquids, and banana.

(b) Medical: Cholestyramine and broad-spectrum antibiotics are not very useful.

(c) Surgical: None.

110. **Postgastrectomy anemia**: It is due to deficiencies of iron, folate, and vitamin B12. **Iron deficiency is the major factor** because gastric acids are necessary to absorb ferric iron from the diet. Iron deficiency is more with gastrectomy than vagotomy.

111. **Most common cause of upper GI bleeding**: Peptic ulcler.

112. **Most common presentation in upper GI bleeding**: Hematemesis, melena, or both.

113. **Management of upper GI bleeding:**

(a) Best outcome is expected when patients are managed in ICU (intensive care unit) by an expert in this field.

(b) First step is to restore intravascular volume by giving 0.9% saline solution and to maitain oxygen-carrying capacity to the tissues. Systolic BP<100 mm Hg or heart rate >100/minute indicates volume loss more than 20 %. A positive Tilt test (drop of systolic BP >10 mm Hg or increase of heart rate >20/minute upon sitting or standing) indicates acute blood loss more than 1 liter.

(c) Blood should be drawn for CBC, SMA6, coagulation profile, and typing-crossmatch.

(d) Hematocrit is not a reliable indicator in actue blood loss. It should be maintained around 10 grams/dl.

(e) **Elevated BUN, normal creatinine,** and **presence of melena indicates significant upper GI bleeding**. Adequate replacement of volumes can be assesd by the normalization of BUN.

(f) Insert nasogastric tube to asses the blood clots or fresh blood.

(g) **Therapeutic endoscopy is extermely important.** Diagnostic endoscopy is **not** recommended in actue bleeders.

(h) Surgical consultations should be obtained early. It is **not** the first-line of therapy.

114. **Most of the recurrent bleeding of peptic ulcers occurs**: Within first 48 hours of initial bleeding.

Management:

(a) Same as above in severe bleeding.
(b) In stable patients: Endoscopy is recommended.
(c) Continuous infusion of H_2-receptor antagonist for ulcer therapy.

115. **Post bleeding management**:
(a) Rule out HP infections: Treat the HP infections if positive.
(b) Rule out NSAID use: Discontinuation of the drug is the best, if not possible add prostagladin misoprostol with NSAID, or use with minimum doses. Maintenance therapy with H_2-receptor antagonist is recommended when patients cannot tolerate misoprostol or ulcer is in duodenum.
(c) Medical treatment is the first-line of therapy.
(d) Try to avoid surgery, if necessary to control bleeding do simple suturing of the ulcer or HSV.

116. **Indication of medical treatment failure in perforation of peptic ulcers**: After 6 hours of medical therapy if signs & symptoms of peritonitis get worse that indicates medical failure. Surgical procedure of simple closure of perforation with proximal selective vagotomy is indicated.

117. **Most common presentation of perforation of peptic ulcer**: Sudden onset of acute abdominal pain. Other signs and symptoms are grunting, abdominal tenderness, and boardlike rigidity.
CBC: Leukocytosis.
Serum amylase: Elevated.
Preferred diagnostic method: Left decubitus film or erect posture CXR shows free intraperitoneal air in majority of the cases. When X-ray is negative then upper GI series with gastrograffin along with CT scan can confirm the diagnosis.
Treatment:
(a) **Medical**:
  (i) Resuscitation with fluid and electrolytes.
  (ii) Continuous NG suction from dependent part of the stomach.
  (iii) Antibiotics (ampicillin-sulbactam and gentamicin).
  (iv) Recognition of HP infections and treatment.
  (v) Perforation due to NSAID: Discontinue the drug, reduce the doses, or add misoprostol.
(b) **Surgical**: Closure of the perforation plus proximal selective vagotomy.

118. **Most common associated finding in gastric outlet obstruction**: Previous or coexistent DU or GU.

Preferred diagnostic method: Endoscopy and biopsy to rule out cancer or HP infection.

Treatment for obstruction:

(a) Decompression of the stomach.
(b) Fluid and electrolytes.
(c) H_2-receptor antagonist.
(d) Treat the HP infection.
(e) Endoscopic dilatation with balloon.

119. **Most common site of ulcer in Zollinger- Ellison syndrome (ZES)**: Duodenum.

120. **Most common clinical presentation in ZES**: **Patients appear with abdominal pain due to peptic ulcer**. It is mostly found in male patients between the ages 35 and 65. Diarrhea is the next common presentation, sometimes it is present before abdominal pain. Patients with ZES do **not** respond well to H_2-receptor antagonist, treatment of HP infections, or surgical therapy.

121. **Most common presentation of ZES when it is a part of MEN I which is autosomal dominant**: **Renal stones are** due to hypercalcemia secondary to hyperparathyroidism (parathyroid hyperplasia). Other findings are pancreatic and pituitary tumors.

122. **Cause of hypergastrinemia**: (normal gastrin level is <100 pg/ml).

(a) ZES: This is the only nonphysiologic type.
(b) HP infection.
(c) Pernicious anemia.
(d) Atrophic gastritis.
(e) Renal failure.

123. **How to distinguish elevated gastrin level in ZES from other physiologic condition?**:

(a) Fasting serum gastrin level >1000 pg/ml (normal is <100) and fasting gastric pH <2.5 **are diagnostic of ZES which** is found in 40% patients.
(b) Fasting gastrin level <1000 pg/ml, pH <2.5, and increased basal acid output (>10.6 mEq/hour in males and >5.6 mEq/hour in females) are also diagnostic.
(c) Gastrin level after intravenous secretin: Normal individual gastrin level is <200 pg/ml and in ZES it is elevated >1000 pg/ml.

124. **Treatment of ZES:**
   (a) The H^+-K^+-ATPase inhibitor, **omeprazole is the drug of choice**. It inhibitis gastric acid hypersecretion. Medicine should be given for long period of time.
   (b) Surgery is **only** indicated to those who cannot or would not tolerate omeprazole: **Total gastrectomy is the surgical treatment of choice**, selective vagotomy which reduces the acid secretion plus low dose of omeprazole can be used.
   (c) Parathyroidectomy in hyperparathroidism, MEN I. It reduces the acid secretion and increases the sensitivity of omeprazole.
   (d) Identification of metastatic tumor by CT scan; MRI is the best for liver metastasis; selective angiography is the best for primary disease. Treatment for metastasis is surgical resection if feasible and chemotherapy (streptozotocin,5-FU, doxorubicin). The patient who did not respond to chemotherapy may respond to alpha-interferon or octreotide.

125. **Can gastric ulcer turn into gastric cancer?**: No.
Gasrtic cancer focus may be present along with gastric ulcer which apparently may look benign by endoscopy or radiography. **All gastric ulcers should be examined for biopsy and cytology to rule out gastric cancer**.

126. **Few important etiologic factors may cause stomach cancer**.
   (a) Blood group A.
   (b) Genetic factors (three-fold increase in first-degree relatives).
   (c) HP infection (gastric adenocarcinoma, lymphoma, DU).
   (d) Food (salted fish, smoked fish, salty food, starchy food, animal fat, cabbage, potato, pickled vegetables, cooked cereal, and bacon).
   (e) Progressively reduced incidence of cancer in pernicious anemia.
   (f) Deficiencies of magnesium and vitamin A (unproven).
   (g) Nitrosamines are carcinogenic.
   (h) Achlorhydria of the stomach which increases nitrosamines synthesis.
   (i) Adenomatous polyp >2 cm in size (most of the polyps are benign).

127. **Factors prevent stomach cancer**:
   (a) Refrigeration of food.
   (b) Increased intake of vitamin C blocks the nitrosamines synthesis unlike achlorhydria of the stomach.

128. **Most common presentation of early stomach cancer**: **Asymptomatic with normal physical examination**. Stomach cancer patients appear with epigastric pain after eating food, epigasrtic distress, dysphagia in proximal lesions,

anorexia, weight loss (non-specific), anemia due to occult blood loss in stool, vomiting due to pyloric obstruction which is a late finding, and boring pain radiating to the back indicates penetration of the tumor into the pancreas.

129. **Angina pectoris, CHF in gastric cancer patients are due to**: **Anemia**.

130. **Signs and symptoms of stomach cancer**: First is asymptomatic with normal physical examination.
    (a) Liver metastasis: Hepatomegaly, jaundice, and ascitis.
    (b) Spleenic or portal vein involvement: Splenomegaly.
    (c) Rare metastasis: Virchow's node (left supraclavicular adenopathy), Blumer's shelf (nodules in perirectal wall).
    (d) Extragastric presentation: **Trousseau's syndrome** (recurrent thrombophlebitis); hyperpigmented, verrucous, and elevated skin lesions on flexor surface of the body; acanthosis nigricans, CNS (ataxia, loss of memory, hostility), and localized neuropathy (sensory, motor).

131. **Laboratory findings in gastric cancer**:
    (a) Remember, elevated carcinoembroynic antigen is usually found in metastatic disease. It is a **late** finding.
    (b) Iron deficiency anemia, microangiopathic hemolytic anemia, or megaloblastic anemia in pernicious anemia patients.
    (c) Stool containing occult blood in <50% patients.
    (d) Presence of acid secretion does **not** exclude stomach cancer. **Most of them have reduced gastric acid secretions**, few have absence, or increased secretions (antral cancer).
    (e) Increased LFT's particulary alkaline phosphatase, and 5' necleotidase indicate metastasis to the liver.

132. **Most of the tumor in GI tract are malignant except**: Colonic tumor which is mostly benign. Most common gastric cancer is **adenocarcinoma**. Most common type is bulky mass with deep central ulceration projecting into the lumen and invading the wall.

133. **Diagnostic studies of gastric cancer**:
    (a) Initial barium study can detect even a very small lesion.
    (b) Diagnosis is confirmed by endoscopy, biopsy, and cytological examination.

    Please remember that **location of the ulcers have nothing to do with the cancers. Cancer can occur in any part of the stomach.**

(c) **Endoscopic ultrasonographic probes** are very important to detect the invasion of the cancer through the stomach wall and lymph nodes. CT scan and abdominal sonogram are useful to detect the metastasis.

134. **Treatment of choice in stomach cancer**: **Surgical resection is the most curative therapy**. Micrometastasis can be present frequently, so additional **postsurgical combined chemotherapy** with 5 FU, doxorubicin, and methotrexate (FAMTX) is needed. It is **radioresistant**.

135. **Poor prognosis of gasrtic cancer depends on**:
   (a) Involvement of perigastric lymph nodes.
   (b) Linitis plastica (diffusely infiltrating cancer) and infiltrating lesions have very poor prognosis.

136. **Most common type of lymphoma (5% of all cancers) of the stomach**: **Non-Hodgkin lymphoma**. Patients appear with **pain** which is the most frequent symptom. **Palpable mass** is the most frequent physical finding. **Mild anemia due to occult blood in the stool**.
   Diagnosis: Gastroscopy, biopsy, and cytology.
   Treatment: Surgical resection followed by radiotherapy and /or chemotherapy. It is highly radiosensitive tumor.

137. **Management of the gastric polyp**: It depends on the size of the polyp in diameter.
   (a) **<2 cm**: No malignancy.
   (b) **>2 cm or polyp of any size causing symptoms**: Polyp should be removed because >2 cm in size may change to cancer.
   (c) **Pedunculated polyp**: Removed by cautery-snare technique by fiberoptic endoscopy.
   (d) **Sessile polyp >2 cm**: Segmental gastric resection may be needed.

138. **(A) Gastric emptying time**:
      (a) Liquid: $T_{1/2}$ is 6 to 12 minutes.
      (b) Solid: $T_{1/2}$ is 45 to 70 minutes.
   (B) Duodenum to cecum emptying time of chyme (food, water, and electrolytes): 40 to 180 minutes.
   (C) Colonic emptying time of digested food: 40 to 60 hours.

139. **Treatment for delayed gastric emptying**:
   (a) Metoclopramide (side effects are anxiety, sedation, or fatigue).
   (b) Domperidone (less CNS side effects).

(c) Cisapride (releases acetylcholine, useful in gastroparesis).
(d) Erythromycin (macrolide antibiotic, useful in gastroparesis by initiating phase 3 in the stomach).

140. **Delayed gastric emptying is found in**:
(a) Anorexia nervosa (delayed with solid food only, **not** with liquid; no delayed activity in bulimia).
(b) Parvovirus like agents (Norwalk or Hawaii viruses) causes tachygastria (unknown etiology, intractable vomiting, and slow antral muscle activites).
(c) Postgastretomy.
(d) Diabetic gastroparesis (delayed gastric emptying) in DKA.

141. **Rapid gastric emptying are noted in**:
(a) Dumping syndrome.
(b) ZES (Zollinger-Ellison syndrome).
(c) DU (Duodenal ulcer).
(d) Pancreatic insufficiency.

142. **Most common collagen vascular disease causing delayed intestinal motility**: Progressive systemic sclerosis. Other conditions are hypothyroidism, amyloidosis, muscular dystrophy, or jejunal diverticulosis.

143. **Treatment of diabetic mellitus with diarrhea**:
(a) To control the diabetes.
(b) Clonidine (alpha-2-adrenergic drug) may be effective. Diabetes causes increased motility of the small intestine which is also found in hyperthyroidism, carcinoid syndrome with increased 5-hydroxytryptamine production, or infectious diarrhea **(E.coli or Shigella)**.

144. **What is the hallmark of the irritable bowel syndrome? Colonic cramping abdominal pain** and an altered bowel habits.

145. **Important points to remember in irritable bowel syndrome**:
(a) The symptoms are **intermittent** with variable periods of **asymptomatic phases.**
(b) Most common **bowel** habit is **constipation aternating with increased frequency of low volume stool**, some patients may have only constipation or only loose stools at the onset.
(c) Most **commonly found in yound adult women.** Always rule out other diseases (colonic cancer, **diverticulitis) when it occurs after age 40.**
(d) It is also present in 25% of otherwise healthy individuals.

(e) Preferred diagnostic methods are colonoscopy and barium enema.
(f) Patients with no organic diseases, therapies includes reassurance, low fat, and high fiber diet those decreases colonic intraluminal pressure. If there is no improvement, the following medications may be added such as anticholenergic drugs, low dose TCA (tricyclic antidepressants), octreotide, specific 5-HT_3 antagonists (ganisetron).
(g) Patients with documented psychoneurosis, **use anxiolytic or antidepressants.**

146. **Most common site of colonic involvement in painful colonic diverticular disease**: **Left colon.**
Patients appear with symptoms similar to irritable bowel syndrome but problem mostly in left lower quadrant. Symptomatic patients with complication may have left lower abdomal mass, increased WBC counts, and occult blood in the stools. **Asymptomatic patients may have gross hematochezia**.
Preferred diagnostic method: Barium enema or colonscopy.
Treatment: Low fat and high fiber diet which reduces colonic intraluminal pressure.

147. **Ogilvie's syndrome**: It is a form of **primary colonic pseudo-obstruction**, commonly **paraneoplastic**. There is decreased postprandial colonic motility results in abdominal distension.

148. **Psychiatric patients with diarrhea**: It may be due to overuse of laxatives (oxyphenisatin and bisacodyl). It is very important to **make the correct diagnosis.**

149. **Treatment for functional diarrhea**: Loperamide, diphenoxylate, or opioid analogues. Patients appear with functional diarrhea with normal anatomic and histological findings. It is due to increased prostaglandin E_2 production in the colon by the specific food or increased concentration of fecal bile salts. Cholestyramine is useful to decrease the diarrhea when it is caused by increased bile salts.

150. **Microscopic or collagenous colitis**: Patients appear with functional diarrheal symptoms with no anatomic abnormalities.
Preferred diagnostic method: **Rectal biopsy**.

151. Mechanism of action of the following drugs:
(a) Dopamine antagonist.
(i) Peripheral: Domperidone.

  (ii) Peripheral and central: Metoclopramide.
- (b) Agonist of muscarinic receptors on muscle wall: Acetylcholine analogues.
- (c) 5-HT_4 agonist: Cisapride.
- (d) Binds to motilin receptors: Erythromycin.
- (e) Blocking inhibitory neurons: Octreotide.
- (f) Reduce progesterone and relaxin (smooth muscle inhibitory hormones): Leuprolide.

152. **Diarrhea**: Presence of liquid stools more than 200 grams per day.

153. **Osmotic diarrhea**: It is due to accumulation of nonabsorbed solutes in the gut lumen. **Diarrhea stops when patients fast or stop taking poorly absorbable solute**. Fecal fluid has solute gap.
Solute gap = Osmolality–2[(Na^+)+(K^+)]. Solute gap must be associated with **large stool volume** loss in osmotic diarrhea.

154. **Secretary diarrhea**: It is due to secretary stimulus on intestinal mucosa. Stools are large in volume and watery (more than 1 liter per day). Diarrhea persists with fasting.

155. **Different causes of secretary diarrhea**:
- (a) Enterotoxin-induced diarrhea: Asiatic cholera, **E.coli, Campylobacter, Salmonella, Shigella, Clostridium difficile**.
- (b) Carcinoid syndrome casuing diarrhea is due to serotonin & subance P.
- (c) Medullary carcinoma of the thyroid causing diarrhea is due to increased calcitonin.
- (d) Pancreatic islet cells tumor causing diarrhea is due to high circulating level of VIP (vasoactive intestinal peptide).
- (e) Bile acid diarrhea is due to secretary effects of bile acids on colonic mucosa. Type I is most common.
  Type I: Ileal disease or resection of ileum.
  Type II: Ileal transport defects of bile acid.
  Type III: Postcholecystectomy, postvagotomy.
  Treatment: Cholestyramine for type I and II. Type III rarely responds to this treatment.

156. **Treatment for radiation enteritis**:
- (a) **Medical**: Antidiarrheal drugs, broad-spectrum antibiotics for bacterial infections, and prednisone.
- (b) **Surgical**: Segmental resection or fistula closure is needed in 15% of patients. Patients with radiation enteritis appear with abdominal cramping

pain, diarrhea, and vomiting within the first few weeks of initial radiation. Patients appear asymptomatic **between symptomatic phases**.

157. **Examination of the stool**:
   (a) **Stool containing WBC**: Presence of **scattered WBC is normal**. Presence of WBC means inflammation.
   (b) **Stool containing pus**: **Shigella, invasive E.coli**, idiopathic ulcerative colitis have maximum pus cells. Salmonella, **Entamoeba histolytica, Gonococci, and Campylobacter also have pus cells**. It is also found in Crohn's disease, ischemic colitis, TB colitis, and antibiotics causing colitis. Absence of pus in single stool examination does **not** exclude these diseases.
   (c) **Stool does not contain pus**: **Toxigenic E.coli,** viruses, Giardia, microscopic colitis, IBS (irritable bowel syndrome), laxative overuse, and malabsorption snyndrome.
   (d) **Stool may or may not contain pus**: Radiation enteritis to both small and large intestines.
   (e) Stool contains **both pus and occult blood**: Inflammatory bowel disease.
   (f) Stool contains **only occult blood and no pus**: Rule out cancer, ischemic damage of the gut, or heavy metal poisoning.
   (g) **Stool or urine turns pink with alkali**: Phenolphthalein ingestion.
   (h) **Stool contain fat**: Giardiasis, malabsorption syndrome.

158. **Proctosigmoidoscopic findings in different diarrheal conditions**:
   (a) Pseudomembrane: Antibiotics-associated diarrhea.
   (b) Solid stool: IBS, fecal impaction, or psychiatric illusion disorder.

   This procedure should be performed **without** laxatives, suppositories, or enemas because they can induce trauma which can give **false positive** finding or wash away exudate which can give **false negative finding**.

159. **Rectal biopsy** should be done from the posterior wall of the rectum on a valve. The following diseases are diagnosed by rectal biopsy because stool examinations may be normal in microscopic colitis, melanosis coli, amyloidosis, granulomatous inflammation, and Whipple's disease.

160. **Fecal water containing more sodium than plasma**: Stool is contaminated with urine. Recollection of the stool is indicated.

161. **Treatment of diarrhea**:
   (a) Most important is to treat the underlying disease. The symptomatic and supportive therapy for undiagnosed conditions.

(b) Prevention or correction of fluid and electrolytes: Oral intake of fluids and salty foods, oral glucose-saline solutions, or intravenous fluid therapy when patients are unable to tolerate oral therapy or very severe dehydration.
(c) Opiates: Loperamide, codeine, or lomotil (diphenoxylate with atropine) may be used.
(d) Antibiotics: Used in severely ill patients with blood or pus in the stool. Do **not** use in mild diarrhea.
(e) Antisecretory durgs: Phenothiazines, aspirin, indocin, motrin, glucocorticoids, or somatostain analogues.
(f) Bismuth subsalicylates: Prevents enterotoxigenic E.coli infection, and to treat acute infectious diarrhea by bacteria or virus.

162. **Treatment causes worsening of diarrhea:**
(a) Oral glucose-saline solution or liquids **plus salty food** may increase the stool volume.
(b) Gatorade (23 mEq of Nacl per liter), other soft drinks, tea, and citrus juices have low or absence of sodium.

163. **WHO (World Health Organization) recommended the following oral rehydrating solution (ORS) in millimoles (grams) per liter**: Glucose, 111 (20); Nacl, 60(4); Kcl, 20(2); $NaHCO_3$, 30(2); osmolality is 331 mOsm per kilogram. Glucose is given as polymer to prevent hypertonicity. High sodium may be required in short-bowel syndrome.

164. **Sites of absorption of different nutrients**:
(a) Proximal small intestine: Fat, calcium, and iron. Iron is mostly absorbed in duodenum.
(b) Mid small intestine: Protein.
(c) Proximal and mid small intestines: Carbohydrate, folic acid, and water-soluble vitamins except B_{12}.
(d) Distal small intestine (ileum): Vitamins B_{12}, bile salts.
(e) Small intestine and colon: Water, electrlytes.

165. **Triglycerides require bile salts for absorption except**: MCT (medium chain triglycerides) can be absorbed directly into the portal vein. More than 93% of dietary fats are absorbed and less than 7% are excreted in the stool in normal individuals.

166. **Mode of absorption**:
(a) Active absorption: Glucose, galactose, L forms of amino acids, sodium, calcium, and folic acid.

(b) Passive diffusion: Water, potassium.
(c) Facilitated diffusion: Fructose.
(d) Endocytosis: Nutrients are absorbed by cell membrane.

167. **Most important transport protein for vitamin B_{12}**: Transcobalamin II.

168. **Steatorrheal stools float in the water are due to**: **High gas content** (**not** due to high fat content).

169. A patient appears with H/O weight loss, diarrhea which consists of bulky, greasy, and malodorous stool. Patient also stated the difficulty in flushing the toilet.
Most likely diagnosis: **Malabsorption syndrome.**
Preferred diagnostic method:
(a) **Screening test**: Serum carotene level <0.06 mg/dL with adequate oral intake.
(b) Specific test:
   (i) **Urinary D-xylose**: <5 grams/5 hour indicates small **intestinal disease, or bacterial overgrowth**. It is normal (>5 grams/5 hour) in pancreatic disease.
   (ii) **Bentiromide test**: Arylamine excretion <50% in 6 hours is diagnostic of pancreatic insufficiency.
   (iii) **Breath tests:** ^{14}C-xylose breath test: Elevated in small intestinal (SI) bacterial overgrowth. Lactose-H_2 breath test: Elevated in lactase deficiency.

170. **Small intestinal biopsies are abnormal and diagnostic in the following malabsorptive diseases:**
(a) Immunedeficiency syndrome.
(b) Abetalipoproteinemia.
(c) Whipple's disease.

171. **Small intestinal biopsies are normal and nondiagnostic in the following malabsorptive diseases**:
(a) Ulcerative colitis.
(b) Functional bowel disease.
(c) Liver and pancreatic diseases.
(d) Primary disaccharidase deficiency.

172. **Treatment for pancreatic exocrine insufficiency**: Large doses of **pancreatic extract** (Viokase, Cotazyme, Creon, Pancrease MT) **with each meal**. Adjuvent

therapy with sodium bicarbonate and and H_2-receptor antagonist provide the best results by raising duodenal pH.

173. **Preferred diagnostic method of diagnosing bacterial overgrowth causing malabsorption**: Noninvasive breath test. It is found in SI stasis, blind-loop syndrome, or elderly patients with decreased acid secretion and abnormalities in SI motility.
Treatment: Cephalosporin (Keflex) plus metronidazole, or augmentin.

174. **Intestinal resection and steatorrhea**:
(a) <100 cm ileal resection, proximal to ileocecal valve: **Mild steatorrhea** and chloretic diarrhea are the frequent problems.
(b) >100 cm ileal resection: **Large steatorrhea** is due to loss of ileal absorptive surface, reduced bile acids, and overgrowth of the bacteria when ileocecal valve is damaged or removed.

175. **Most common disaccharide deficiency**: **Lactase deficiency**. **Primary** lactase deficiency: Patients appear with symptoms in adulthood and the reasons for delayed symptoms are not clear.
Diagnosis: History and confirmed by lactose-H_2 breath test.
Treatment:
(a) Avoid the milk or milk products.
(b) Use lactase (derived from Aspergillus oryzea) with milk or milk products.
Secondary lactase deficiency: It is due to the damage of enterocytes by any disease condition.
Sucrase deficiency: Rare, patients appear with diarrhea.
Treatment: Avoid sucrose, starch, and dextrin from diet.
Glucose- galactose malabsorption: Rare, use fructose, and avoid glucose-galactose.

176. **Important points to remember in nontropical sprue (gluten- sensitive enteropathy, adult celiac disease):**
(a) Etiology is unknown. Gluten (protein found in wheat, barley, oats, and rye) can damage the enterocytes by an immunologic mechanism.
(b) Patients with abdominal pain and sprue, always **rule out lymphoma** of the small intestine (SI).
(c) HLA-B8 and HLA-DRw3 are present in up to 90% of patients (normally is found up to 30% of individuals).
(d) Most severely damaged portion is proximal part of SI.
(e) **Preferred diagnostic method is SI biopsy.**

(f) Treatment: Gluten-free diet (avoid all grains except rice and corn) relieves the symptoms fast or delayed for months.
(g) Patients with dermatitis herpetiformis, always rule out **sprue.**
(h) Associated complications include jejunum and ileum ulcers, bleeding or perforation, which are not responsive to treatment.

177. **Treatment for short bowel syndrome**:
(a) Parenteral hyperalimentation for weeks or months.
(b) Slow introduction of oral feeding (high proteins, vitamins, minerals, and MCT).
(c) Antidiarrheal drugs, cholestyramine.
(d) Steroids may help in water absorption.
(e) Rarely, H_2-receptor antagonists and pancreatic extracts are used.
(f) Diarrhea unresponsive to above therapies may respond to somatostatin analogues (sandostatin).

178. **Relationship of smoking with ulcerative colitis (UC) and Crohn's disease (CD)**: **(Important)**.
UC: Cigarette smoking protects UC. It may begin after stops smoking in susceptible individuals. Most of the UC **patients are nonsmoker.**
CD: It is strongly associated with smoking; 80% of patients are smoker in CD.

179. **Relationship of inflammatory bowel disease (IBD) with UC or CD in family history**: 20% patients of IBD have relatives with UC or CD.

180. **Most common sites of CD and UC**:
CD: Distal ileum and right colon.
UC: Rectum and sigmoid colon.

181. **Most definitive diagnostic test of iron deficiency anemia in UC**: Low serum ferritin level (not serum iron or TIBC). Serum ferritin also reflects the iron storage. TIBC is total iron binding capacity.

182. **Long term compliction of UC and cancer**: **Colonic adenocarcinoma**. It is more common in pancolitis than left-sided colitis. Cancer is directly proportional to the duration of the UC.
Please remember that the cancer is **not** related to the severity of the initial attack, course of the disease, or medical therapies.

183. **Long term complication of CD and cancer**: Intestinal adenocarcinoma. It also depends on extent and duration of the diseases, but the relationship is not clear unlike UC.

184. **Long term complication of IBD and cancer**: Slightly increased risk of leukemia, lymphoma, or bile duct cancer.

185. **Precursor of cancer in UC**: **Intestinal mucosal dysplasia** which is diagnosed by colonoscopic biopsy. **Indications of colonoscopy and biopsies** throughout the length of the colon:
   (a) After 8 to 10 years of UC.
   (b) Repeat every 1 to 2 years after the initial examination.
   Indications for surgery in UC:
   (a) Confirmed dysplasias of the intestine.
   (b) DALM (dysplasia-associated lesion or mass).
   Management of patients with indefinite dysplasias:
   (a) Follow-up examination after 3 to 6 months.
   (b) Confirmed by an experienced pathologist as soon as possible.

186. **Extraintestinal manifestations of IBD associated with HLA-B27**: Uveitis, sacroiliitis, and ankylosing spondylitis.

187. **Pregnant and lactating women with IBD on medications**:
   (a) Corticosteroids and sulfasalazine can be continued in pregnancy and lactation as long as the mothers symptoms improve.
   (b) Avoid metronidazole in the first trimester.
   (c) Use of 6-mercaptopurine or azathioprine is controversial.

188. **Postpartum complication of asymptomatic IBD**: Patients become symptomatic.

189. **Most common clinical presentations in UC and Crohn's colitis (CC)**:
   (a) UC: Rectal bleeding.
   (b) CC: Perianal diseases, abdominal pain and tenderness.

190. **Most common endoscopic findings in UC and CC**:
   (a) UC: Rectal diseases, diffuse symmetric mucosal involvement.
   (b) CC: Apthous or linear ulcer.

191. **Most common radiological findings in UC and CC**:
   (a) UC: Continuous disease.

(b) CC: Asymmetric noncontinuous disease, stricture, and fistula.

192. **Most common pathological findings in UC and CC**:
(a) UC: Crypt abscesses.
(b) CC: Crypt abscesses plus sinus tract/fistula, transmural disease, and lymphoid aggregation.

193. **Presentations of IBD**:
(a) **Mild**: Blood in the stool may or may not be present, <4 stools/day, ESR <30 mm/hour. Normal vital signs, hemoglobin, clinical signs, and radiological findings.
(b) **Severe**: Blood is present in the stool, >6 stools/day, ESR >30 mm/hour. Patients have fever, tachycardia, decreased hemoglobin, abdominal tenderness, radiological findings of colonic edema, thumbprinting, air-fluid levels.
(c) **Fulminant or toxic**: Blood is continuously present in the stool, >10 stools/day, ESR>30 mm/hour. Patients have all the findings of severe disease. In addition to that, severe anemia, abdominal distension, radiological findings of dilated colon or small intestine are present.

194. **Treatment of UC**:
(a) **Mild to moderate diseases**:
   (i) **Oral anti-inflammatory drugs**: Sulfasalazine, olsalazine, or mesalamine.
   (ii) **Systemic anti-inflammatory drugs**: Predinsone. It is also used in CD.
   (iii) **Topical anti-inflammatory drugs**: Mesalamine enema or suppository, corticosteroid enema or foam.
   (iv) No antibiotics, no surgical consultation.
(b) **Severe disease**:
   (i) Oral anti-inflammatory drugs: Same as above.
   (ii) Systemic anti-inflammatory drugs: Prednisone, ACTH.
   (iii) Topical anti-inflammatory drugs: Corticosteroid enema or foam.
   (iv) Surgical consultation, no antibiotics.
(c) **Fulminant disease**:
   (i) Systemic anti-inflammatory drugs: Prednisone, ACTH.
   (ii) No oral or topical therapy.
   (iii) Antibiotics: **Metronidazole, sulfasalazine.** Both are used in CD.
   (iv) Surgical therapy: UC can be cured by colectomy.
(d) **Maintenance treatment**: Sulfasalazine, olsalazine, or mesalamine only. Do **not** use corticosteroids.

195. **Complications of steroid therapy**:
   (a) Early: Elevated blood pressure, acne, facial hair, and Cushingoid features.
   (b) Late: Cataract, aseptic necrosis, and osteoporosis.

196. **Common complications of drugs used in UC and CD**:
   (a) **Metronidazole**: Peripheral neuropathy can be diagnsoed in neurologically asymptomatic patients by clinical examination and nerve conduction studies.
   (b) **Sulfasalazine**: Folic acid deficiency, sperm motility, and morphology (in 80% male patients) can be reversible with mesalamine treatment.
   (c) Olsalazine: Diarrhea which can be reduced by adjusting the doses.
   (d) Mesalamine: Less side effects than sulfasalazine.

197. **Indications for immunosuppressive therapies (6-mercaptopurine, azathioprine) in long term UC and CD patients**:
   (a) Patients unresponsive to medical treatment.
   (b) Patients who are steroid-dependents.
   (c) Some patients with fistulas.
   (d) Patients unresponsive to maintenance therapy.
   (e) Patients cannot tolerate mesalamine.

   Other chemotherapeutic drugs recently used in UC and CD patients:
   (a) Intravenous cyclosporin plus steroids used in UC.
   (b) Intravenous methotrexate plus steroids used in CD.

198. **Treatment for toxic megacolon (severe colitis):**
   (a) Fluid and electrolytes resuscitation.
   (b) Blood transfusion in severe anemia.
   (c) Patients who never received steroids: Parenteral ACTH or corticosteroids.
   (d) Patients with severe tenesmus: Steroid enemas or foam inside the rectum may provide rapid relief along with systemic steroids.
   (e) **Patients with fever, leukocytosis, and abdominal tenderness**: Metronidazole plus an aminoglycoside.
   (f) **Patients with perforations**: Surgical therapy.
   (g) **Nutrition**: Parenteral nutrition is for severely ill patients. Oral therapy is for less severely ill patients.

199. **Treatment of Crohn's disease (CD)**:
   (a) **Nutrition**: It is very important in CD unlike UC.
      (i) Iron, water- soluble vitamins, folic acid, calcium, and magnesium.
      (ii) Excess protein is needed for loss of protein.
      (iii) Avoid lactose in lactose intolerance.

(iv) Avoid fat in fat malabsorption.
(v) Add fiber in constipation.
(vi) Avoid fiber in diarrhea or intestinal narrowing.
(vii) TPN (total parenteral nutrition) is useful in failure of oral nutrition, short bowel syndrome, or failure of medical therapies.

Dietary management is equally effective as corticosteroid therapy.

(b) **Drugs**: Metronidazole, sulfasalazine, or mesalamine. Corticosteroid should be discontinued with clinical improvement.

(c) Surgical therapy is indicated to manage the complications only: It does **not** cure CD.
(i) Intestinal obstruction.
(ii) Uncontrollable bleeding.
(iii) Complicated fistulas.
(iv) Resistant to medical therapies.
(v) Unable to discontine corticosteroid.

(d) Gastroduodenal CD: Corticosteroid with H_2-receptor antagonist or omeprazole.

(e) Jejunoileitis due to CD:
(i) **Mild**: Oral mesalamine or alternating antibiotics.
(ii) **Moderate to severe**: Elemental diet or conticosteroid is equally effective.
(iii) **Corticosteroid resistant**: Immunosuppressive threapies.

200. **Most common causes of death** in UC and CD.
(a) UC: Colonic perforation, cancer, or postcolectomy complications.
(b) CD: Postsurgical complications (pulmonary emboli and sepsis).

201. **Most common type of intestinal ischemia**: Colonic (60% of cases), next common is acute mesenteric (30%), chronic mesenteric, or focal segmental. Ischemic injury to the bowel is due to anatomical obstruction (occlusive) or nonocclusive vasoconstriction.

202. **Normal oxygen consumption of the intestine can be maintained even with reduced blood flow**: Blood flow can be reduced up to 20 to 25 % of normal but normal oxygen consumption can be maintained because 20% of mesenteric capillaries open at one time.

203. Most common **cause of acute mesenteric ischemia: Superior mesenteric artery emboli (SAME-50%)** which originates mostly from left atrial or ventricular thrombus. Other causes are nonocclusive mesenteric ischemia (NOMI) and superior mesenteric artery thrombus (SMAT).

204. A 60 year old man appears with acute abdominal pain in the emergency room. He had H/O CHF, arrythmias, and recent myocardial infarction.

Physical examination:

(i) Initial: Normal abdomen.

(ii) Several hours later: Abdominal tenderness and guarding are noted. Patient also become hypotensive. While waiting in the emergency room, patient did pass **maroon or bright red bloody stools.**

Laboratory findings:

(a) CBC: Leukocytosis.

(b) ABG: Metabolic acidosis.

(c) Elevated serum phosphate, LDH, amylase, intestinal alkaline phosphatase, and CPK (creatine phosphokinase).

(d) Abdominal X-ray (plain film): Initially was normal, subsequently developed ileus, formless loops of small bowel or 'thumbprinting' signs are due to submucosal hemorrhages of small intestine or right colon.

(e) **Preferred diagnostic test**: **Selective mesenteric angiography is the best diagnostic test for both occlusive and nonocclusive types.**

Most likely diagnosis: **Acute mesenteric ischemia (AMI)**. In AMI, initial symptom (abdominal pain) is out of proportion than physical findings. **Please remember that diagnosis should be made before intestinal infarction which is manifested by maroon or bright red bloody stools, abdominal tenderness, rigidity, abnormal abdominal x-ray, and laboratory findings**. **Normal abdominal x-ray cannot exclude acute mesenteric ischemia**.

Treatment:

(A) First resuscitations:

- (a) Treat the congestive heart failure, arrythmias, myocardial infarction, and hypotension. **Improve cardiac output would improve the intestinal blood flow.**
- (b) Fluid and electrolytes are used for hypovolemia.

(B) Broad spectrum antibiotics STAT.

(C) Plain film of the abdomen to exclude other diagnosis (**not** to diagnose AMI). When other diagnosis are excluded then confirm the diagnosis by superior mesenteric artery (AMA) angiography.

(D) Infusion of papaverine through SMA angiography catheter.

(E) **Surgical therapy**: To restore intestinal blood supply or remove the dead intestine. Postoperative heparin anticoagulant therpay for 2 days to avoid late thrombus formation.

205. **Most common associated finding in mesenteric vein thrombosis (MVT)**: Almost 60% of patients with MVT have history of **peripheral venous thrombosis (PVT)**.

206. **Few important points in MVT (It only represents 5 to 10% of AMI)**:
   (a) MVT is due to deficiencies of antithrombin III, protein S, protein C, myeloproliferative disorders, hypercoagulable states, or oral contraceptives.
   (b) **Preferred diagnostic studies**: **Ultrasound, CT, or MRI of the abdomen**. Selective mesenteric angiography can be diagnostic but is not done routinely.
   (c) **Acute MVT resembles arterial form of AMI**. Patients symptoms, signs abdominal x-ray, medical, and surgical managements are same in both the conditions.
   (d) Other forms are subacute (weeks to months) or chronic.

   Subacute: Patients appear with nonspecific abdominal pain, normal physical examination, and laboratory findings.

   Chronic: Patients are **mostly asymptomatic** or may develop bleeding from esophageal varices, enlarged spleen, pancytopenia, thrombocytopenia. No treatment is needed for asymptomatic patients. To control the bleeding is very important.

207. **Most common site of ischemic injury to the intestines**: Colon.

208. **Most common type of colonic ischemia**: **Reversible colopathy (submucosal or intramural hemorrhage)**. Other type are chronic ulcerating colitis, transient colitis, gangrene, stricture, or fulminant colitis.

209. **Important complication of postoperative ruptured aortic aneurysm**: Colonic ichemia (CI) is noted up to 60% of patients.

210. Most common cause of CI: Unknown. The predisposing factors are the following: Over age 60, cocaine abuse, long distance run, coagulopathies, drugs (e.g., estrogens, vasopressin, danazol, and psychotropic drugs), or SLE (systemic lupus erythematosus).

211. **Important points to remember in colonic ischemia**:
   (a) Unlike AMI, CI is not associated with major vascular occlusion or low cardiac output.
   (b) Patients appear with crampy, left lower abdominal pain, passage of mild bright red or maroon blood mixed with stool. Symptoms subside within 24 to 48 hours, and mucosal healing is noted within 2 weeks.

(c) Most common sites of involvement are in the left colon (**splenic flexure, descending colon, and sigmoid colon). 'Watershed' areas** (splenic flexure and rectosigmoid) are involved in local nonocclusive ischemic injuries. Remember, systemic hypoperfusion usually involves the right colon.

(d) **Colonoscopy is the best method to make the diagnosis. It should be done on the unprepared bowel within 48 hours of the onset of symptoms** because thumbprinting (submucosal hemorrhage) sign may disappear after that. Combination of barium enema and sigmoidoscopy are also helpful.

(e) Mesenteric angiography is useless because colonic blood flow becomes normal when the symptoms appear. It is only indicated when clinical manifestation suggests AMI because AMI has mortality up to 90% when diagnosis is made after intestinal infarctions.

(f) Uncomplicated (no gangrene or perforation) patients are treated with bowel rest, broad spectrum antibiotics, and maintain normal cardiac function. Discontinue mesenteric vasoconstrictors (digitoxin vasopressing agents).

(g) Complicated (gangrene or perforation): Laparatomy and resection of the colon.

(h) Asymptomatic stricture: Only observation because it might disappear within 2 years.

(i) Symptomatic (obstruction) stricture: Surgical resection of the colon.

212. **'Small meal syndrome'in chronic mesenteric ischemia (CMI):** Patients appear with the symptoms of dull or crampy, periumbilical or epigastric pain which begins 10 to 30 minutes after eating and disappears within 1 to 3 hours. Patients progressively reduce the meal size because of the pain.

Physical examination: Nonspecific systolic bruit in upper abdomen may be found.

Diagnostis test: No specfic test is available. Diagnosis is made by physical examination, **exclusion of other diseases, and angiography.** Stenosis or occlusion of vessels in angiography does **not** confirm the diagnosis. Tonometric determination of decreased **small bowel pH after meal** due to decreased blood flow to the intestine and increased blood flow to the stomach.

Treatment: Surgical revascularization is needed in patients with weight loss, vascular obstruction, and typical pain.

213. Most common **vascular abnormality of the GI tract**: **Vascular ectasia (VE) of the right colon** which includes angiodysplasia or arteriovenous malformation (AVM). Most common sites of VE is cecum or ascending colon because of increased tension (T) = DP (D= diameter, P= intramural pressure).

214. **Most common cause of lower GI bleeding in the elderly patients: Vascular ectasia.**
Patients appear with bright red blood, maroon-colored stools, or melena which stops spontaneously in majority of the patients.
Preferred diagnostic study: Angiography or colonscopy. Biopsy is **not** done because it can cause bleeding.
Treatment:
(a) **Heater probe and bipolar coagulation** are the **most commonly used treatment**. Other treatments are laser therapy and sclerosis.
(b) Patients with **active** bleeding: Superior mesenteric artery vasopressin infusion, right hemicolectomy, or subtotal colectomy only as a last resort.

215. **Most common associated findings in VE**: **Cardiac disease** (50% of patients), next common is **aortic stenosis** (25% of patients).

216. **Blue rubber bleb nevus syndrome is mostly associated with**: Intestinal lesion and GI bleeding. Characateristic cutaneous lesions which are blue, raised, up to 5 cm in size, found in trunk, face, and extremities (**not** in mucous membrane).
Diagnosis: Endoscopy, barium, or angiography.
Treatment:
(a) Resection of the involved segment of the bowel in recurrent bleeding.
(b) Endoscopic laser surgery **could be dangerous** because it may involve full thickness.

217. **Watermelon stomach**:
Etiology: Unknown.
Lesion: Tortous dilated vessels radiating outward from the pylorus like a waterlemon.
Most commonly found in: **Women**, achlorhydria, atrophic gastritis, or cirrhosis. Patients appear with acute or chronic occult bleeding.
Diagnosis: Endoscopy.
Treatment: Endoscopic therapy or antrectomy.

218. **Most common presentation of the hemangiomas of the colon**: Occult blood loss in the stool. Most of the lesions are small, reddish purple in color, polyp like appearance.
Diagnosis: Endoscopy.
Treatment:
(a) Small or few hemangiomas: Endoscopic local ablation.

(b) Large or multiple hemangiomas: Resection of the hemangiomas or involved portion of the colon.

219. **Most common site of Dieulafoy's ulcer**: **Stomach**. Patients are mostly men and have a mean age of 52. Patients appear with sudden onset of severe hematemesis or melena due to eroding arteries in the submucosa. **Most common site of ulcer is 6 cm distal to the cardioesophageal junction.**
Diagnosis: Endoscopy.
Treatment: Endoscopic therapy to treat bleeding.

220. **Frequency of cancer in adenomatous polyps of the colon depends on**:
(a) Size of the polyps: **More than 2 cm in** size have a rate of cancer 40%, smaller than 2 cm have lesser chances of cancer.
(b) Cancer is directly proportional to the degree of dysplasia.

221. **Most common symptom of adenomatous polyps**: **Asymptomatic**. Patients may appear with hematochezia or occult blood in asymptomatic patients.
Preferred diagnosis: Double contrast barium enema, fiberoptic sigmoidoscopy, or colonoscopy.
Treatment:
(a) **Pedunculated polyps**: Electrocautery snare. No biopsy is necessary in benign lesions.
(b) **Small (1 to 8 mm in size) sessile polyps**: Biopsy of the polyp should be done and destroyed with 'hot biopsy' forcep.
(c) **Large (>8 mm in size) sessile polyps**: Several electrocautery sessions may be needed for complete removal and biopsy should be done.
(d) **Very large (>3 cm in size) sessile polyps**: Endoscopic removal is neither possible nor safe.

222. **Follow-up recommendations after colonoscopic polypectomy**: Follow-up colonoscopy after 3 years of initial procedure to look for any new or missed lesion. If the examination shows no polyp, then repeat examination after 3 years is recommended. When polyps are found then appropriate management should be done.

223. **Risk of colorectal cancer in inherited polyposis syndrome:**
(a) Inherited polyposis: Risk of cancer is 1%.
(b) Inherited nonpolyposis: Risk of cancer is 6%.

224. **Two types of adenomatous polyposis syndrome**:
(a) Gardner syndrome: **Extraintestinal benign growth.**

(b) Familial adenomatous polyposis: **No** extraintestinal growth.

Both are inherited as an **autosomal dominant**, mutant gene is present **on 5q**, **highly malignant**, and most commonly appear with **upper GI polyps.** Polyps appearing distal to duodenum are mostly benign. Familial adenomatous polyposis may occur without a family history due to spontaneous mutations.

225. **Most common extraintestinal manifestations of Gardner syndrome**: **Benign osteomas (particularly mandibular)**, soft tissue tumors (lipomas, fibrosarcomas, and sebaceous cysts). Other associated findings are supernumerary teeth, mesenteric fibromatosis, and desmoid tumors. **The triad of Gardner syndrome are colonic polyposis, bone and soft tissue tumors.**

226. **Screening recommendations for adenomatous polyposis syndrome**:
   (a) Flexible proctosigmoidoscopy should be done every year in all first-degree relatives between 12 to 40 years of age.
   (b) After 40 years of age, it should be done every 3 years.
   (c) Above recommendations are most appropriate for patients with **mutant gene**. It should also be done in patients without **mutant gene** because genetic markers are **not** 100% specific and sensitive.
   (d) **Endoscopic diagnosis of stomach and duodenal polyps** are important in patients with colonic polyps. It should be done soon and then every 2 to 3 years interval.

227. **Mode of inheritance of Lynch syndrome I and II (hereditary nonpolyposis colorectal cancer, HNPCC)**: Autosomal dominant.

Lynch syndrome I: Site-specific colon cancer.

Lynch syndrome II: Cancer family syndrome.

In both syndromes, patients appear in mid 40's with colon cancer proximal to the splenic flexure.

228. **Recommendations for the family members of both Lynch syndromes**: **Colonoscopy should begin 5 year earlier** than the age of youngest member of the family diagnosed to have cancer. It should be done every two years.

229. **Most common associated cancer in Lynch syndrome II**:
   (a) Female genital cancer (ovarian, uterine): Ultrasonography of ovary and uterus are recommended.
   (b) Breast cancer: Mammography should be done earlier than general population.

230. **Most common CNS tumors in Turcot's syndrome (hereditary adenomatous polyposis)**: Medulloblastoma, ependymoma, and glioblastoma.

231. **Most common associated abnormalities in juvenile polyposis**: Pulmonary AVM (arteriovenous malformation). Patients with juvenile polyposis appear with abdominal pain, rectal bleeding, and subsequently anemia.

232. **Syndrome associated with protein-losing enteropathy**: **Cronkite-Canada syndrome**. It does **not** run in the family. Patients appear with GI polyposis, skin hyperpigmentation, alopecia, and nails dystrophy. Polyps may turns into malignancy.

233. **Most common associated cancer in Cowden's syndrome (multiple hamartoma syndrome)**: **Thyroid and breast cancers**. Patients with this syndrome appear with keratosis of the hands and feet, facial tricholemmomas, and oral papillomas. Mode of inheritnce is an **autosomal dominant.**

234. **Relationship of food and colorectal cancers**.
    (a) Saturated fat: High incidence of colon cancer.
    (b) Monosaturated fatty acids: Protect from colon cancer.
    (c) Aspirin, NSAID's: Protect from colon cancer.
    (d) Dietary fibres: May protect from colon cancer.
    (e) Low calcium and vitamin D: Increase colon cancer.
    (f) Obesity and excess caloric intake: Increase colon cancer.

235. **Most common type of colorectal cancers**: Adenocarcinomas.
    Polypoid lesions: Mostly found in right side.
    Annular constricting lesions: Mostly found in left side.

236. **Most common sites of colorectal cancers**: **First is sigmoid colon**, next is rectum.

237. **Colorectal cancers and other diseases**:
    (a) Chronic ulcerative colitis: Approximetely **10 to 20 times higher** incidence of colorectal cancers than general populations.
    (b) Crohn's disease: **Approximately 4 to 7 times higher** incidence of colorectal cancer than general populations.
    (c) Family history of the following diasease have higher incidence of colorectal cancers: Familial polyposis syndrome, Lynch syndrome I and II, and sporadic colorectal cancer.

238. **Risk of colon cancer in a first-degree relatives of a person with colon cancer**: Two to threefold higher incidence of colon cancer.

239. **Risk of adenomatous polyps in a first-degree relatives of a person with adenomatous polyps**: Two to threefold higher incidence of adenomatous polyps.

240. **Chromosomes and colorectal cancers**: Chromosomes **5, 17 (p53 gene), 18(**DCC gene means deleted colon cancer tumor suppressor gene) and overexpression of the **c-myc genes.**

241. Molecular changes in colorectal cancers:
   (a) **Normal cells to enhance growth**: Due to APC (adenomatous polyposis coli tumor suppressor gene) loss.
   (b) **From enhanced growth to formation of adenomas**: Due to **DNA demethylation**, ras mutation, MCC (mutated colon cancer tumor suppressor gene) loss, or DCC loss in order of sequence from first to last.
   (c) **From adenomas to carcinomas**: Due to p53 loss (in chromosome 17) which is tumor suppressor gene.
   (d) **From carcinomas to metastasis**: Due to **nm23 loss** which is metastasis suppressor gene.

242. A 55 year old man appears with history of **rectal bleeding, decrease in stool caliber, change in bowel habits**, abdominal pain, and iron deficiency anemia.
   Preferred diagnostic method: Best method is **colonoscopic biopsy;** double-contrast baruim enema after sigmoidoscopy. Endoscopic ultrasonography is done for staging of rectal cancer.
   Initial digital rectal examination is important to rule out distal lesions. **A complete pelvic examination is important.**
   Most likely diagnosis: **Colorectal cancer.**
   Treatment.
   (a) **Surgical management**:
      (i) Primary cancer of the colon and rectum: Complete surgical removal of the affected portion of the intestine, including omentum, and lymph nodes.
      (ii) Cancer of the right and left colon: Hemicolectomies.
      (iii) Cancer of the sigmoid and upper part of the rectum above 6 cm from anal verge: Anterior resection and removal of margin of the normal colon above and below the cancer areas.
      (iv) Cancer within 5 cm of the anal verge: Combined abdominoperineal resection and permanent colostomy. Small, early rectal cancer may be

treated with local excision with or without radiation to the pelvis. Combined radiation and chemotherapy before surgery may be helpful.

(v) Cancer of the anus: **Combined radiation and chemotherapy**: Surgery is indicated when lesions do not respond to the above therapy and for recurrence of lesions.

(b) **Radiation therapy**: Combined radiation (50 Gy) and chemotherapy (5-flurouracil), are standard therapy. Preoperative radiation decreases postoperative recurrence.

(c) **Chemotherapy**: Combined therapy with 5-FU and levamisole or 5-FU and leucovorin are effective. Later therapy is useful for metastasis. Topoisomerase I inhibitors such as camptothecins are also effective.

243. **Postoperative follow up in colorectal cancer**:

(a) First colonoscopy after one year of surgery. Subsequent colonoscopy every three years because small adenomas require 3 years to become large adenomas which are premalignant.

(b) Carcinoembryonic antigen (CEA): It may be **elevated** before any clinical symptoms or other laboratory tests abnormalities. Early detection of recurrence is possible.

(c) CT scan or MRI: To look for metastasis.

244. **Most common sites of metastasis of colon cancer and presentation:**

(a) Rectal: Hepatomegaly.

(b) Abdominal metastasis: SI and LI obstructions, ascitis.

(c) Pelvic metastasis: Urinary bladder functional abnormalites, sacral nerve pain, sciatic nerve pain, in women vaginal bleeding or discharges.

(d) Lungs metastasis: Asymptomatic until advanced stages.

(e) Bones metastasis: Asymptomatic until advanced stages.

Please remember that intestinal recurrence is very rare (Important for the examination).

245. **National Cancer Institute's dietary guideline for prevention of colorectal cancer**:

(a) Increase dietary fibers to 20 to 30 grams/day.

(b) Reduce intake of fat to <30% of calories.

(c) Increase vegetables and fruits in diet.

(d) Avoid cigarettes and tobacco.

(e) Avoid obesity.

(f) Avoid alcohol or consume in moderation.

246. **Guidelines for screening patients to detect colorectal cancer**:

(a) Digital rectal examination annually after age 40.
(b) Fecal occult blood testing annually after age 50.
(c) Flexible sigmoidoscopy every 3 to 5 years after age 50.

247. **Most common malignant neoplasms of the small intestine (SI)**:
(a) Proximal SI: Adenocarcinomas. Most common site is duodenum.
(b) Distal SI: Lymphomas, carcinoids.

248. **Risk factors for SI neoplasms:**
(a) Patients with regional enteritis especially after surgical bypass of a segment of SI.
(b) Patients with AIDS, immunodeficiencies, long standing celiac disease: Intestinal lymphomas.
(c) Peutz-Jeghers syndrome: Intestinal adenocarcinomas.
(d) Gardner syndrome: Intestinal periampulary adenocarcinomas.

249. **Most common clinical presentations of SI neoplasm**: **Asymptomatic**.
Large tumors (benign and malignant) appear as **intestinal obstructions**. Signs and symptoms of intestinal obstructions are vomiting, abdominal mass and distension, visible presistolsis.
Signs and symptoms of metastasis: Severe weight loss, hepatomegaly, jaundice, and ascites.

250. **Diagnostic studies for SI neoplasms:**
(a) Upper GI series with barium is the most important.
(b) Fiberoptic endoscopic biopsy and brushed are most diagnostic.
(c) Ultrasonography and CT scan to look for extent of the disease and metastasis.
(d) Peroral intestinal biopsy for intestinal lymphomas.
(e) Dysproteinemia is a typical finding of Mediterranean lymphomas and manifested by the presence of abnormal fragments of IgA (devoid of light chains) in the serum and urine.
(f) Elevated serum serotonin or urinary 5-hydroxy-indoleacetic acid in carcinoid syndrome.
(g) Nonspecific finding is hypochromic, microcytic anemia.

251. **Treatment for SI neoplasms**:
(a) Surgical management of the mass.
(b) Whipple procedure (pancreaticoduodenal resection): Duodenal cancer or large villous adenomas.
(c) Surgical excision for stage I lymphomas.

(d) Combined chemotherapy and surgical management for extensive lymphomas.
(e) Radiation therapy for localized recurrences or bulky tumors.

252. **Most common causes of acute pancreatitis**: Choledocholithiasis, next is ethanol abuse.
Most common cause of acute pancreatitis during pregnancy:
Gallstones. It occurs mostly in third trimester.

253. **Most common drugs causing pancreatitis in AIDS patients**: Sulfur-containing diuretics, pentamidine, and ddI. Pancreatitis is usually mild. It occurs within 2 months of treatment and is **not** dose related.

254. **Highest mortality (up to 50%) in pancreatitis**: **Postoperative pancreatitis** after intra-and extra-abdominal operations.
Other causes of pancreatitis.
(a) Lipemia with **serum triglyceride levels >1000 mg/dL**. High triglyceride levels may be due to alcohol abuse, estrogen therapies, parenteral lipid infusions, and primary hyperlipidemias.
(b) Gallstones and stones in the bile ducts.
(c) Drug induced pancreatitis.
(d) ERCP (endoscopic retrograde cholangiopancreatography).
(e) Acute hypercalcemia.
(f) Pancreatic divisun (anomaly) may cause pancreatitis.
Please remember that **pancreatic infection** is an **extremely rare** or **poorly proven cause** of pancreatitis. Increased triglycerides level is **not an effect** of pancreatitis.

255. A 60 year old chronic alcoholic man appears with history of mid-epigastric pain which is radiating straight to the **back in the midline** at the level of lower thoracic vertebral region. The pain is chracterised by **steady, dull, or boring**, gets **worse in supine position,** reaches peak intensity **from 15 to 60 minutes** after the onset.
Physical examination: Mild fever, tachycardia, **borderline hypotension, and** upper abdominal tenderness. **Absence of abdominal rebound tenderness and rigidity which are present in perforation.**
Laboratory examination: CBC: Leukocytosis.
Hematocrit: **Elevated** due to hemoconcentration.
SMA8: **Elevated** BUN and glucose; **low** total clacium and normal ionized calcium.
Serum amylase: **Elevated (more than 5 times of normal)**.

Serum lipase: **Elevated**.

Plain X-ray of abdomen: Localized ileus of loop of jejunum ('sentinel loop`), generalized paralytic ileus, absence of colonic gas shadow ('colon cut-off' sign), or calcification over the pancreatic area.

Abdominal sonogram: Absence of gallstone and acute cholecystitis, normal size of common bile duct.

Abdominal CT scan: Mild ascitis, pancreatic inflammatory and necrotic changes, and absence of spleenic vein thrombosis.

Most likely diagnosis: Acute pancreatitis.

Treatment:

(a) Mild pancreatitis:

- (i) NPO (nothing per mouth).
- (ii) Nasogastric aspiration for paralytic ileus and vomiting.
- (iii) Analgesics: Meperidine.
- (iv) Fluid and electrolytes for volume depletion.

Please remember, do **not** give prophylactic antibiotics or TPN (total parenteral nutrition).

(b) Systemic complications:

- (i) Circulatory failure or shock: Admission to 1CU, adequate fluid replacement, and vasopressor medications.
- (ii) Sepsis: Antibiotics.
- (iii) ARDS (adult respiratory distress syndrome): Patients should be managed appropriately.
- (iv) ARE (acute renal failure): Patients should be treated accordingly.

(c) Local complications:

- (i) Gram-negative sepsis in ascending cholangitis and biliary pancreatitis: Appropriate antibiotics (gentamicin, ampicillin, and metronidazole) should be given as soon as possible.
- (ii) Pancreatic necrosis diagnosed by CT scan: Fine-needle aspiration under CT guidance should be done immediately. Gram-stain of the aspirate is accurate in >95% patients.

Patients with positive Gram-stain: Antibiotics (fluroquinolones, imipen/cilastatin, and metronidazole) and immediate surgery (necrosectomy to remove necrotic, tissues and continued lavage of the necrotic space).

Patients with negative Gram-stain: The Management is controversial. Repeat CT scan and fine needle aspiration are recommended. Initial negative Gram-stain becomes positive in many patients.

256. Patients appear with **Grey turner's sign** (large ecchymosis in the flanks) or **Cullen's sign** (large ecchymosis in the umbilical area) **after one to two weeks**

from the onset of pancreatitis: It represents **blood dissecting from the pancreas along the fascial planes.**

257. **ACR (amylase-creatinine) ratio**: The ratio of **amylase concentration** in urine over plasma, **divided** by the creatinine concentration in urine over plasma. It is helpful in diagnosing asymptomatic macroamylasemia.

258. **Liver function tests in different pancreatitis**:
   (a) Elevated AST (aspartate aminotransferase): Pancreatic inflammation or alcoholic liver disease.
   (b) Elevated ALT (alanine aminotransferase) and alkaline phosphatase: Gallstones associated pancreatitis.

259. **Preferred diagnostic methods in different conditions of pancreatitis**:
   (a) Pancreatic necrosis: It can be identified and quantitated by lack of contrast enhancement after bolus injection.
   (b) Cholelithiasis or dilated bile ducts: Ultrasonography is the best method.
   (c) Local complications and extent of pancreatitis: CT scan.

260. **Accurate predictors in the development of pancreatic necrosis**:
   (a) Elevation of serum C-reactive protein to >120 mg/liter.
   (b) Elevation of polymorphonuclear elastase.

261. **Prognosis of acute pancreatitis can be estimated by the Glasgow and Ranson's criteria which are measurements of clinical and laboratory findings during the first 48 hours after admission**: **Three or more positive** criteria indicate **complicated pancreatitis; four or more indicate higher mortality**. Remember **they cannot replace clinical observation of individual patients.**
   Glasgow criteria for all pancreatitis (within 48 hours):
   (a) Age >55.
   (b) WBC >15,000/cu mm.
   (c) Arterial Po_2 <60 mm Hg.
   (d) Glucose >180 mg/dL (no pre-existing hyperglycemia).
   (e) BUN >45mg/dL.
   (f) LDH >600 IU/L.
   (g) Calcium <8 mg/dL.
   (h) Albumin >3.2 gm/dl.
   Ranson's criteria for mainly ethanol-induced pancreatitis: At the time of admission:
   (a) Age >55.

(b) WBC >16,000/cu mm.
(c) Glucose >200 mg/dL (no pre-existing hyperglycemia).
(d) AST >250 IU/L.
(e) LDH >350 IU/L.
Within 48 hours of admisssion:
(a) Arterial Po_2 <60 mmHg.
(b) BUN rise >5 mg/dL.
(c) Hematocrit decrease >10 %.
(d) Base deficit >4 mEq/L.
(e) Fluid deficit >6 L.
(f) Calcium <8 mg/dL.

262. **Most common type of chronic pancreatitis**: **Chronic calcifying pancreatitis**, other type is chronic obstructive pancreatitis.

263. **Most common cause of chronic calcifying pancreatitis**: **Alcohol (70 to 80% of cases).** Alcoholic pancreatitis is a **chronic progressive** disease. Alcohol abuse **initially causes pancreatitis at ages 35 to 45;** 5 to 10 years **later** develops **alcoholic liver disease. This is very important to remember that alcohol abstinence may relief abdominal pain and future development of diabetes mellitus but does not prevent progressive pancreatic fibrosis and exocrine malfunction. Other causese of chronic pancreatitis:**
(a) Idiopathic.
(b) Hereditary pancreatitis: Autosomal dominant, symptoms begin at age 10, **higher incidence of adenocarcinoma.**
(c) Metabolic: **Primary heperparathyroidism**, patients are clinically **asymptomatic.**
(d) Obstruction: **Tumors**, stones, post-traumatic strictures. Removal of causes prevent progression of the disease.
(e) Senile or atrophic pancreatitis (**benign, nonprogressive**): **Absence of pain is characteristic. Absence of alcohol abuse** but presence of **smoking and obesity**. Patients appear with malabsorption symptoms.
(f) Tropical pancreatitis: No relation with alcohol, no definite relation with malnutrition.

264. **Does gallstone-associated acute pancreatitis develop chroinic pancreatitis?**: No.

265. **Most common cause of chronic obstructive pancreatitis**: Tumors.

266. **Most sensitive pancreatic function tests for chronic pancreatitis**: **Secretin test (decreased pancreatic output** of bicarbonate and enzymes in duodenal contents, after intravenous injection of secretin (cholelcystokinin or cerulein). Other test is Lundth test (determination of trypsin concentration in proximal jejunum after liquid test meal). **None** of those tests are used widely because of time consumption. Diagnosis of chronic pancreatitis depends on the following:

(a) Symptoms & signs: Pain mimics **acute** pancreatitis or **gradual onset** of pain (intermittent or chronic, epigastric and/or right or left subcostal region, radiates straight through the back) which may be aggravated by the **food or alcohol**. **Pancreatic calcification, malabsorption, and diabetes mellitus appear when the patient's pain started to reduce usually 6 to 9 years after the onset of symptoms (This is important)**.

(b) Radiologic studies:

(i) PA/oblique abdominal X-ray: Calcifications of the pancreas.

(ii) CT scan: May detect **small calcifications** which may be missed by plain X-ray.

(iii) ERCP: To rule out strictures, large ductal stones, or pseudocysts.

(c) Pancreatic funtion tests: Already discussed.

(d) Abnormal Schilling test of vitamin B_{12} absorption: It is a **specific** test, but not sensitive. Remember, clinical vitamin B_{12} deficiency does not occur frequently.

267. **Treatment for chronic pancreatitis**:

(a) **Pain**: **The most important management is to control the pain. Narcotics** should be used in acute pain even in alcoholics.

(b) Acute attacks in chronic pancreatitis: Patients should be admitted to the hospital, NPO, and intravenous hydration.

(c) Pancreatic enzymes (pancrelipase): Viokase, Cotazyme, or Ilozyme.

(d) H_2-receptor blocker.

(e) Somatostatin analogue: Octreotide (Sandostatin).

(f) Severe pain: ERCP or CT scan of the duct should be done.

(i) Dilated (≥8 mm in diameter) duct: Duct decompression by endoscopically introducing a stent acorss the ampulla of Vater, or permanent duct decompression by longitudinal pancreaticojejunostomy.

(ii) Normal or nondilated pancreatic duct: Partial pancreatectomy, such as Whipple operation (pancreaticoduodenectomy).

(g) Malabsorption: Most common malabsorption is fat malabsorption which is due to lipase deficiency. Pancreatic enzymes (Viokase, Cotazyme, or Ilozyme) or enteric-coated enzymes (pancrease or creon) are used.

268. **Complications of chronic pancreatitis**: Pseudocysts, pancreatic ascites, obstruction of common bile duct and gastric oulet, and compression/thrombosis of splenic vein.

269. **Life threatening complications of pancreatic pseudocysts**: Infections, hemorrhages into the cyst, or ruptures. These are rare but should be treated adequately.

270. **Diagnosis and treatment for pancreatic pseudocysts**:
   (a) Diagnosis: Ultrasonograpy, CT scan, or endoscopic ultrasonography.
   (b) Treatment:
      (i) Asymptomatic small cysts: No treatment is needed.
      (ii) Large (>5 cm in diameter): **Internal drainage into stomach, duodenum, or jejunum is the best surgical method**. Excision is **rarely** possible. Alternative method is percutaneous or endoscopic aspiration and drainage for several weeks are also helpful.

271. **Treatment for pancreatic ascites**: Surgical correction of the leaking pancreatic duct by providing drainage into the loop of jejunum or by partial removal of the pancreas.

272. **Treatment for obstructive complication of chronic pancreatitis**:
   (a) Common bile duct obstruction: Drainage of bile into the intestine surgically.
   (b) **Gastric outlet obstruction**: Gastrojejunostomy plus vagotomy are performed because of increased DU in chronic pancreatitis.
   (c) Compression thrombosis of splenic vein leads to gastric fundic varices: **Splenectomy.**

273. **Most common cancer of the pancreas**: **Ductal adenocarcinomas.**

274. **Molecular abnormalities in pancreatic cancer**:
   (a) Deletion and mutations of the p53 gene: Most common molecular abnormalities.
   (b) **Mutation in the codon** 12 of the K-ras gene.
   (c) Altered EGF and erb B-2 receptor pathways.

275. **Definitive risk factors for pancreatic cancer:**
   (a) Chronic pancreatitis (No relation with cholecystectomy or gastrectomy).
   (b) Nonpolyposis colon cancer syndrome.
   (c) Cigarette smoking (No relation with alcohol or coffee).

(d) Male over age 60 (**Please remember that diabetes mellitus is not a risk factor for pancreatic cancer**).

276. **Incidence of pancreatic cancer can be reduced by:**
   (a) Consumption of low cholesterol diet with olive oil and fish.
   (b) Avoid smoking.
   (c) Avoid chemical exposures (coal tar derivatives, coke, benzidine, beta-naphthylamine).
   (d) Avoid high cholesterol and high fat diet with high linoleic acid content.

277. **Most common clinical presentations of pancreatic cancer**: **Abdominal pain** (90% of patients) which is nonspecific, aggravated by lying supine or eating food, relieved by bending forward, lying on the side, drawing the knees to the chest, or crouching forward in all four extremities.
   Other presentations are the folllowing:
   (a) Jaundice: Due to obstruction of CBD.
   (b) Light colored stools: Due to obstruction of CBD.
   (c) Weight loss: Due to malabsorption (mostly fat, then protein) and poor food intake.
   (d) Emotional lability: In pancreatic tail cancer.
   (e) Mostly mild diabetes: Due to insulin resistance caused by increased plasma of IAPP (islet amyloid polypeptide).
   (f) Depression, vomiting.
   (g) **Courvoisier's sign**: Palpable gallbladder in cancer of the pancreatic head.
   (h) Enlarged Liver: In cancer of the pancreatic head.
   (i) **Trousseau's syndrome**: Superficial thrombophlebitis, rarely present.

278. **A known pancreatic cancer patient appears with the following symptoms**:
   (a) Severe hearing loss: Due to temporal bone metastasis.
   (b) Dysphagia: Due to esophageal metastasis.
   (c) Painful, swollen testis: Due to testicular metastasis.

279. **Most specific and sensitive tests** to diagnose pancreatic cancer: ERCP.
   (a) **Endoscopic retrograde cholangiopancreatography (ERCP):** It has the **highest positive and negative predictive values** in comparison to **ultrasonography and CT scan**.
   (b) Remember pancreatic function tests are **not** necessary to diagnose cancer.
   (c) **Endoscopic ultrasonography is nore sensitive** then ultrasonography, CT scan, and angiography to diagnose **portal vein involvement and lymph node metastasis.**

(d) CT scan is needed for staging of the tumor. It is done **in absence** of metastasis or in absence of pancreatitis.

(e) Aspiration cytology under ultrasound or CT guidance should **not** be done in a resectable cancer mass, because it can cause intra-abdominal seeding to the tumor cells. It can be done only in a nonresectable mass.

(f) **Nospecific routine battery of tests are** done in suspected pancreatic cancer patients:

  (i) Serum lipase, amylase, and glucose: Elevated. They are also elevated in **chronic pancreatitis**.

  (ii) Bilirubin, AST, and alkaline phosphatase: Elevated, They are also elevated in hepatic disorders.

  (iii) Calcification in abdominal X-ray.

  (iv) Symptomatic patients with bony or pulmonary metastasis: No need for further diagnostic studies.

(g) Serologic studies such as CEA, monoclonal antibodies, and galactosyltransferase: Nonspecific and less sensitive.

280. **Abdominal X-ray or CT scan shows pancreatic calcifications in the following conditions**:

(a) Chronic pancreatitis.

(b) Primary ductal cancer.

(c) Pancreatic mucosal cancer (mucinous cystadenocarcinomas appear as curvilinear calcification).

(d) Solid and papillary epithelial cancers.

281. **Treatment of choice in pancreatic cancer**.

(a) **Surgical resection. Pancreaticoduodenectomy is the procedure of choice**. Only 10% of all pancreatic cancers are resectable.

(b) Palliative porcedures:

  (i) To relieve biliary obstruction: Cholecystojejunostomy or choledochojejunostomy.

  (ii) To decompress biliary trees: Endoscopic stenting is better than percutaneous stenting. It is useful in patients who have high surgical risks and few months of life expectancy.

  (iii) Unresectable tumor is found during surgery or a patient has life expectancy of 6 to 7 months: Double bypass surgery should be done.

  (iv) Incomplete on functional obstruction (up to 60% of patients): To enhance gastric emptying or to relieve gastric stasis symptoms, a **combination** of bethanechol (cholinergic drug) **and metaclopramide or cisapride** (prokinetic durg) are used.

(v) Combination of chemotherapy 5-FU or SMF (streptozotocin, mitomycin-C and 5-FU) and external-beam radiation **are more effective** than isolated chemo or radiotherapy).

282. **In food poisoning, intervals between the time of ingestion of contaminated food and onset of symptoms is very important (Important for the Board examination)**:
(a) Staphylococcus aureus: 2 to 6 hours.
(b) Clostridium organisms: 8 to 24 hours.
(c) Vibrio vulnificus: 24 to 48 hours.
(d) Salmonella organisms: 12 to 48 hours.
(e) Bacillus cereus heat-stable toxin (nausea, vomiting): 6 hours.
(f) Bacillus cereus heat-labile toxin (diarrhea): 12 hours.
(g) Mushroom poisoning (Amanita phalloides): 8 hours.
(h) Parasites (Anisakis simplex): 1 to 12 hours.

283. **Characteristics in different food poisoning (Important for Board examination)**:
(a) **S.aureus**: Patients appear with vomiting, crampy abdominal pain, and **diarrhea for 2 to 6 hours** after eating food contaminated by enterotoxin. It is due to contamination of food by the carrier, food which is uncooked, improperly cooked, or unrefrigerated.
(b) **Clostridium organisms (C.perfringens type A is a common cause of foods poisoning in USA)**: Patients appear with diarrhea and crampy abdominal pain 8 to 24 hours after eating food contaminated by vegetative forms of bacterium. It is **rarely fatal** except in elderly, debilitated individuals. Food is mostly unrefrigerated. Enterotoxins are producing the symptoms. C. botulinum toxin caused food-borne botulism due to ingestion of contaminated food.
(c) **Vibrio organism:**
(i) **V.vulnificus (100% mortality)**: Patients appear with a sudden onset of fever, chills 24 to 48 hours after **eating raw seafood (usually oysters).** Patients subsequently manifest bullous hemorrhagic rashes, low BP, renal failures, and death. Most of the patients had **H/O** chronic underlying diseases such as diabetes mellitus, cirrhosis, or hemochromatosis.
(ii) **V.parahaemolyticus**: It is also due to uncooked seafood particularly oysters.
(iii) **V.cholerae**: It causes cholera due to contaminated **water**. **Food-borne cholera** caused by V.cholerae 01, El Tor biotype are due to raw or

incompletely cooked food. **Non-01 V.cholerae** are found in raw oysters cause milder symptoms than 01 type.

(d) **Salmonella organisms (nontyphoidal S.enteritidis and S. typhimurium)**: Patients appear with **diarrhea, vomiting, fever, myalgias, and abdominal cramps 12 to 48 hours after eating contaminated food**. The symptoms are **usually mild** except in elderly persons and immunocomprised patients. It is due to unrefrigerated food, inadequate cooking, or unhygienic condition.

(e) **Bacillus cereus**:
  - (i) Heat-stable enterotoxins: Patients appear with nausea, vomiting **6 hours after eating** contaminated foods.
  - (ii) Heat-labile enterotoxins: Patients appear with diarrhea 12 hours after eating contaminated foods.

(f) **Escherichia coli O157: H7**: It is mostly found in **incompletely cooked contaminated hamburgers**.
  - (i) **Uncomplicated infections**: Patients appear with diarrhea (frequently bloody), vomiting, fever, and abdominal cramps.
  - (ii) **Complicated infections**: Patients appear with hemorrhagic colitis and hemolytic uremic syndrome which includes hemolytic anemia, low platelet counts, and acute renal failure. It is a fatal condition.

(g) **Listeria infections**: It is found in contaminated uncooked meat, poultry food (soft cheese), and milk. It usually affects the elderly individuals, diabetes, immunocompromised individuals, and pregnant women.

(h) **Yersinia enterocolitica**: Patients appear with **diarrhea with or without blood, vomiting,** fever, and **pain in the right lower quardrant** of the abdomen due to mesenteric adenitis. It is found in contaminated incompletely cooked meat specially pork and is also found in contaminated **milk.**

(i) **Campylobacter organisms**: **C.jejuni** infections occur due to ingestion of incompletely cooked poultry foods, meat, and raw milk. Patients appear with febrile prodrome, vomiting, **bloody diarrhea**, and abdominal pain. **C.coli** also appears with similar clinical manifestation.

(j) **Shigella infections**: It is due to fecal-oral transmission of the organism results from poor hand washing technique of food handlers and crowded living environment. Patients appear with bloody diarrhea and abdominal pain.

284. **Contaminated food and bacterial infectious diarrhea**:
  - (a) V.vulnificus: **Raw seafood (oysters).**
  - (b) E.coli: Incompletely cooked **hamburgers or ground beef.**
  - (c) Campylobacter: Poultry foods, meat, and milk.

(d) Bacillus cereus: **Fried rice** (heat-stable toxins), meat products (enterotoxins).
(e) Yersinia enterocolitica: **Pork**, milk.
(f) Shigella: Poor hygiene of food handlers, fecal-oral transmission.
(g) Listeria: Raw meat, poultry, and milk.
(h) V.cholerae: Water, raw seafood.
(i) V.parahaemolyticus: Raw seafood.
(j) Salmonella: Raw eggs, mayonnaise, meat, and poultry.
(k) S.aureus: Meat, cheese, cream buns, pasta, and custard pies.
(l) C.perfringens A: Meat, vegetable soup.
(m) C.botulinum: Uneviscerated cured fish, meat, home presservative vegetables.

285. **Bloody diarrheas are found in different infectious diarrheas**:
(a) E.coli.
(b) Yersinia enterololitica.
(c) Campylobacter (C.jejuni and C.coli).
(d) Shigella.

286. **Contaminated food and non bacterial diarrheas**:
(a) Food-borne Norwalk virus and hepatitis A virus: Raw shellfish (clams and oysters).
(b) Giardia intestinalis (G.lamblia): Salads, fruits, and foods.
(c) **Parasites (Anisakis simplex)**: Raw fish (Patients appear with abdominal pain 1 to 12 hours after ingestion of fish. Treatment is to remove the worm by endoscopy).

287. **Poisoning by food-borne toxins, plants, and mushrooms**:
(a) Amnesic shellfish poisoning (ASP): Patients appear with vomiting, diarrhea, abdominal cramps, disorientation, confusion, and persistent or permanent loss of shor-term memory.
(b) Ergot alkaloids (mycotoxins): Patients appear with arterial spasm, thrombosis, and ischemic necrosis of the extremities.
(c) Mushroom poisoning (A. phalloides): Patients appear with vomiting, watery diarrhea approximately 8 hours after ingestion of mushroom, subsequently develop **acute liver failure, hepatocellular necrosis, and death. Treatment is liver transplantation.**

288. **Most common symptoms of internal hemorrhoids**: **Bleeding and prolapse.**

Patients appear with painless, bright-red anal bleeding. Presence of pain indicates anal fissure or abscess. Acute prolapse or thrombosis of hemorrhoids are severely painful.

Treatment:

(a) Initially, high-bulk diet.
(b) Avoid prolong sitting at stool.
(c) Injection of sclerosing agent (5% phenol in oil) into the submucosa of hemorrhoids.
(d) Rubber-band ligation.
(e) Photocoagulation with infrared device.
(f) Electrocoagulation with bipolar electrode.
(g) Thermocoagulation with heater probe.
(h) **Surgical excision** is the best method in **fourth-degree hemorrhoids.**
(i) **Thrombosed external hemorrhoid** appears as painful bluish mass present at the anal verge: Excision of the hemorrhoid if the pain persists more than 48 hours.

289. **Most common sites of anal fissure**: **Posterior midline (over 90% of cases),** rest are in the anterior midline.

290. **Patients appear with fissure off the midline indicates**: Cancer, sexually transmitted disease, or Crohn's disease.

291. Patients appear with painful defecation and spots of blood on toilet tissue. Diagnosis is confirmed by **inspection**. Rectal examination is very painful, so it is **not** necessary.

Most likely diagnosis: **Anal fissure**.

Treatment:

(a) Stool should be bulk and soft.
(b) Sitz bath.
(c) Acute fissure: Heals spontaneously.
(d) Chronic fissure: Lateral subcutaneous internal anal sphincterotomy.

292. **Presentation of anorectal abscesses**:

(a) Deeper abscesses: Gradual symptoms with abdominal pain.
(b) Superficial abscesses near the skin: Throbbing pain.
(c) Larger abscesses: Patients also develop fever along with pain.

Preferred diagnositc method: Indurated tender mass palpable in rectal examination.

Treatment:

(a) Prompt surgical incision and drainage.

(b) Standard therapy for immunocompromised hosts may **not** be adequate.

293. Patients appear with **H/O** perianal **pus, blood, mucus, and discomfort**.
Preferred diagnostic method:
(a) **Anoscopy** to detect primary opening **which is at the dentate line** where the infections were originated. Hooked probe confirms the patency. Secondary opening is outside over the skin.
(b) Proctosigmoidoscopy is done routinely.
Treatment: Surgical correction.
Goodsall's rule: It indicates usual relationship of primary and secondary fistulas orifices except the long anterior fistula.

294. **Most common sexually transmitted disease (STD) in USA**: **Chlamydia trachomatis infections.**
Treatment: **Tetracycline is the drug of choice**. Other STD's are the following:
(a) Gonococcal proctitis: Patients appear with purulent bloody discharge, pain, and frequent defecation.
Diagnosis is confirmed by positive culture.
(b) **Syphilis**: Patients appear with mucosal ulcers. Primary lesions heal spontaneously. Secondary lesions are multiple plaques with a white odorous discharge.
(c) **Condylomata acuminata induced warts**: It is due to human papillomavirus, usually types 6 and 11. Patients appear with small discrete excrescences (or warts) around the perianal areas, pruritus, and bleeding.
Treatment:
(i) Local application of 25% podophyllin in tincture of benzoin.
(ii) Fluguration with electrocautery.
(iii) Surgical excision.

295. A yound woman appears with **H/O** anal pain, mucous discharge, bleeding, and obsessive straining to defecate.
Examination shows indurated, ulcerated lesions in anterior rectal mucosa 8 to 10 cm above the anal verge.
Most likely diagnosis: **Solitary rectal ulcer syndrome**.
Preferred diagnostic method: Biopsy.
Treatment:
(a) Avoid straining during defecation because straining causes ulcers.
(b) Use bulk agents.
(c) Surgical treatment is not satisfactory unless the patients have true rectal prolapse.

296. A multiparous woman appears with **H/O** a sense of incomplete evacuation and a constant desire to defecate. Examination reveals perineum balloons downward during straining.
Most likely diagnosis: **Descending perineum syndrome**.
Treatment:
(a) Education, not to strain.
(b) Bulk agents.
(c) Rarely local surgical therapies are needed.

297. **Rectal prolapse and procidentia**:
(a) Rectal prolapse: Protrusion of rectal mucosa.
(b) Rectal procidentia: Protrusion of entire thickness of the rectum.
Treatment:
(a) Prolapse: Fixation procedure or excision.
(b) Procidentia: Surgical repair through perineum or abdomen.

298. **Human papillomavirus is etiologically linked to**: **Anal carcinoma (epidermoid)**. Patients appear with pain, bleeding, and mass.
Preferred diagnosis: Biopsy.
Treatment:
(a) Combined radiation and chemotherapy are the treatment of choice.
(b) It is followed by local or radical surgical excision.
Bowen's disease: Chronic squamous cell cancer in situ.
Treatment: Local excision.
Paget's disease: Intraepithelial mucinous adenocarcinoma.
Treatment: Local excision.

299. **Most common cause of ascites**: Portal hypertension (90% of cases) is due to cirrhosis.

300. **Most common clinical presentation of ascites**: Increased abdominal girth and rapid weight gain.
Physical examination: Dullness in flanks in supine position and shifting dullness. Less than 1500 ml of ascitic fluid cannot be detected by clinical examination.
Preferred diagnostic test: Ultrasonography or abdominal CT scan.
Ascitic fluid examination for cytology and culture–**Exudate**: Protein content ≥ 2.5 gm/dl.
Transudate: Protein content <2.5 gm/dl.
Portal hypertension: Serum-ascites albumin gradient >1.1 gm/dl.

Peritoneal inflammation or cancer: Serum-ascites albumin gradient <1.1 gm/dl.
Malignant chylous ascites: WBC>300 mm^3, triglycerides>200 mg/dL.
TB peritonitis: WBC>500, mostly lymphocytes;ascitic adenosine deaminase ≥32.3 U/L.
Cirrhosis: Polymorphs<250, protein <2.5 gm/dl.
SBP: Polymorphs>250, albumin <1 gm/dl.
Cardiac ascites: Polymorphs<250, protein>2.5gm/dl.
Hepatic metastasis: Serum alkaline phophastase ≥350 mU/ml.
Hepatoma plus ascites: Elevated serum alpha-fetoprotein.

301. **Most common cause of malignant ascites**: **Peritoneal carcinomatosis**. It arise from primary peritoneal disease such as mesothelioma or from metastatic spread.

302. **Most common cause of chylous ascites**: **Malignancy, especially lymphoma**. Other rare causes are trauma, peritonitis, and intra-abdominal operation.
Ascitic fluids: Do **not** contain any malignant cells, serum-ascites albumin gradient <1.1 gm/dl, WBC 300 to 1000, triglycerides>200 mg/dL.
Other diagnostic methods: CT scan, bone-marrow aspiration.
Treatment:
(a) Treat the underlying lymphomas is most important.
(b) Give MCT (medium-chain triglycerides) instead of fat, because MCT can absorb directly into portal bloodstream bypassing the lymphatics.
(c) Sometimes, TPN to reduce chylous ascites.
(d) Both benign and malignant ascites do **not** respond well to diuretics or salt restrictions.

303. **Most common causes of pancreatic ascites**: Ruptured pancreatic pseudocyst sencondary to pancreatitis. **Alcohol is a common cause of pancreatitis and the most common cause of chronic liver failure**. To distinguish the two different types of **pancreatic ascites:**
(a) Pancreatic ascites **without** cirrhosis: Low (<1.1 gm/dl) serum-ascites albumin concentration gradient. Elevated amylase level in ascitic fluid.
(b) Pancreatic ascites **with** cirrhosis: High (>1.1 gm/dl) serum-ascites albumin concentration gradient. Elevated amylase level in ascitic fluid.
(c) Pancreatic ascites **due to trauma**: ERCP (endoscopic retrograde cholangiopancreatography) is helpful.
Treatment of different causes of ascites:
(a) Alcoholic pancreatitis: Conservative therapy.
(b) Nontraumatic pancreatitis: Conservative therapy.

(c) Pseudocyst pancreatitis: Surgery to drain the cyst.
(d) Traumatic pancreatitis: Repair of the pancreatic duct.

304. **Most common cause of ascites in HIV-infected patients**: Portal hypertension due to alcoholism or chronic viral hepatitis. Other cause are abdominal lymphomas, peritoneal infections (cryptococcosis, coccidioidomycosis, or TB).

305. **Other rare causes of ascites**:
(a) Renal: When serum albumin falls below 2.0 gm/dl, always rule out associated hepatic causes.
(b) Connective tissue disorder: SLE.
(c) Endocrine ascites: Myxedema, struma ovarii, **Meig's syndrome (ascities, pleural effusion, and benign ovarian tumors)**, and ovarian overstimulation syndrome.

306. **High (>1.1 gm/dl) serum-ascites albumin concentration gradient is found in the following liver & other diseases**:
(a) Cirrhosis.
(b) Alcoholic hepatitis.
(c) Hepatic metastasis.
(d) Fulminant hepatic failure.
(e) Acute fatty liver of pregnancy.
(f) Congestive/restrictive cardiac failure.
(g) Myxedema.
(h) Budd-chiari syndrome.
Please remember that **bile leak has low** (<1.1 gm/dl) gradient.

307. **Low (<1.1 gm/dl) serum-ascites albumin concentration gradient is found in the following diseases(except cirrhosis)**:
(a) Pancreatic cancer.
(b) Pancreatic ascites.
(c) TB peritonitis.
(d) SLE, nephrotic syndrome.
(e) Bowel obstruction or infarction.
(f) Bile leak.

308. **Types of acute peritonitis**:
(a) Primary: Without a recognizable cause e.g., spontaneous bacterial peritionitis.
(b) Secondary: With recognizable causes e.g., perforation, surgery.

(c) Tertiary: Peristence of intra-abdominal sepsis without a recognizable focus of infection e.g., following surgery of peritonitis, immunocompromised patients, or patients with transplantation.

309. A 50 year old man appears with sudden onset of acute pain in the abdomen and vomiting.
Physical examination: Abdominal rigidity, tenderness, and rebound ternerness all over the abdomen.
Most likely diagnosis: **Acute peritonitis.**
Preferred diagnostic method:
(a) Initial: Plain abdominal X-ray ot rule out free air or any other causes.
(b) Ultrasonography and CT scan: Very important to make the diagnosis.
(c) Abdominal paracentesis: It is mandatory when ascites is associated with peritonitis. Definitive diagnosis can be made from ascitic fluid analysis.
Treatment:
(a) Resuscitation: Intravenous fluid and electrolytes.
(b) Laparotomy: It is the treatment of choice for secondary or tertiary peritonitis.
(c) Antibiotic plus antifungal therapies: Broad spectrum antibiotics (to cover enterococci, S.epidermidis, enterobacter) plus amphotericin or fluconazole (to cover candida which is common in secondary or tertiary peritonitis).

310. **Most common organisms causing SBP (spontaneous bacterial peritonitis)**:
(a) Enteric gram-negative aerobes **(E.coli, Klebsiella pneumoniae)**.
(b) Enteric gram-positive aerobes **(Streptococcus pneumoniae)**.
Please remember that anaerobes rarely cause SBP.

311. **Most common cause of SBP**: **Cirrhosis**. Remember, SBP is a marker of severe hepatic failure. Most important predictor of the first-episode of SBP:
(a) Low ascitic fluid portein content.
(b) Elevated serum bilirubin.
Future predictor of SBP:
(a) Patients with ascitic fluid total protein content of <1 gm/dl develop SBP within 3 years in approximately 1/4th of patients.

312. Patients appear with **H/O** cirrhosis, develop fever and abdominal pain due to acute peritonitis;**or** patients appear with **H/O** liver disease, develop sepsis, deterioration of liver function but absence of clinical ascites; or patients appear with H/O cirrhosis with ascites, develop acute deterioration in liver or kidney function, encephalopathy, or unexplained leukocytosis.
Most likely diagnosis: **SBP (spontaneous bacterial peritonitis)**.

Preferred diagnostic method: **Abdominal paracentesis.**
Paracentesis findings of the peritoneal fluids:
(a) SBP:≥250 polymorphs/cubic millimeter.
(b) Intra-abdominal abscess or secondary peritonitis:>500 polymorphs/cubic millimeter.
(c) Culture: It may be **negative up to 50% of cases**. It is **not** required to make the diagnosis. Presence of multiple organisms indicate perforated viscus. To indentify the **source** of peritoneal infections the **following investigations are mandatory**:
  (a) Blood culture.
  (b) CXR.
  (c) Urinalysis.
  (d) Urine culture.
  (e) To look for any other sources of infections.

Treatment for SBP:
(a) **SBP with cirrhosis: Cefotaxime is the drug of choice.**
(b) **Please remember that laparatomy should not be done.**
(c) **Prophylactic antibiotics: Quinolone e.g., norfloxacin**. It cleanses the gut flora.

313. **Poor prognostic indicators of SBP patients**:
(a) Presence of renal failure.
(b) Elevated serum aminotransferases.
(c) Onset of SBP in the hospital or hospital acquiring infections.

314. **Risk of recurrence of SBP patients**:
(a) Patients are **not** on prophylactic antibiotics.
(b) Low total protein content in ascitic fluid.
(c) Inadequate liver functions.

315. **Most common type of the TB infection HIV positive patients**:
(a) **Newly acquired infection.**
(b) Rapidly progressive disease which results in extrapulmonary TB.
(c) Patients are mostly symptomatic.
(d) Emergence of resistant strains of TB.

316. **Most common signs & symptoms of peritoneal TB**: **Ascites**, next common is abdominal pain and swelling. Other findings are fever, positive PPD, weight loss, and abdominal tenderness.

317. **Definitive diagnostic test for TB peritonitis**:

(a) Laparascopy with direct peritoneal biopsy is the best diagnostic method.
(b) Other diagnostic test is elevated (≥32.3 U/L) ascitic concentration of ADA (adenosine deaminase) which is a marker of T lymphocyte and macrophage activation.

318. **Contraindication of laparascopic biopsy in TB peritonitis**: Fibroadhesive tubercular peritonitis.

319. **Treatment of TB peritonitis**: Two or three anti-tuberculous drugs for 9 months.

320. **Important risk factors for intra-abdominal TB**:
(a) **HIV infection.**
(b) **Patients receiving immunosuppressive treatment.**
(c) Peritoneal dialysis.
(d) Intravenous drug abuse/alcohol abuse/cirrhosis.
(e) Elderly patients.

321. **Most common organism causing peritonitis in CAPD (continuous ambulatory peritoneal dialysis) S.epidermidis,** next is S.aureus, Streptococci.

322. **Diagnosis and treatment of CAPD**: Diagnosis is made by **cytology of infected dialysate which has high WBC counts** and cloudy fluids.
Treatment:
(a) Infusion of **broad-spectrum antibiotic** into the peritoneum (to cover both gram-positive and Gram-negative organisms) through dialysis catheter.
(b) Do **not** remove dialysis catheter.
(c) To continue the dialysis.
Patients did not respond to the above mentioned therapy should be treated as follows:
(a) Admission to hospital, if OPD management fails.
(b) Removal of catheter.
(c) Intravenous antibiotics.

323. **Most common presentation in familial Mediterranean fever**: Peritonitis. Patients appear with abdominal pain and fever.
Treatment: Colchicine.

324. **Etiology of mesenteric panniculitis and retractile mesenteritis**: Idiopathic. Patients may be asymptomatic or appear with abdominal pain, swelling, and mass. Diagnosis is made by laparatomy.
Treatment:
(a) Surgical resection should **not** be done unless there is intestinal obstruction.

325. **Most common etiology of acute appendicitis**: **Fecolith**.

326. **Most common presentation of acute appendicitis**: **Abdominal pain in the right lower quadrant**. Pain may begin in the periumbilical or epigastric region, initially colicky then steady. Pain increases in severity with progression of the disease. Please remember that vomiting is **not** a common sympton.
Physical examination: Tenderness in the right lower quadrant at McBurney's point. **Obturator sign**: Presence of pain when rotating a flexed hip in supine position.
Psoas sign: Presence of pain when raising a straightened leg against resistance.

327. **Diagnosis and treatment of acute appendicitis**:
Diagnosis:
(a) Initial CBC: Polymorphonuclear leukocytosis.
(b) Urinalysis: To rule out UTI.
(c) Serum amylase: To rule out pancreatitis.
(d) SMA-6: To rule out electrolyte abnormalities and dehydration.
(e) Abdominal X-ray: Appendicolith may or may not be present, presence of free air indicates perforation.
(f) Ultrasonography: Sensitivity and specificity of the test are more than 90%. **It is a confirmatory test.**

Remember, when a patient appears with typical history, physical examination is characteristic, then **no confirmatory test is necessary**. When the diagnosis is in doubt, don't give any antibiotics, **only careful observation for 6 to 12 hours may be diagnostic**. Patients with appendicitis usually get worse with observation. To expedite the process, ultrasonography or CT scan can be done.
Treatment:
(a) Surgical appendectomy is curative.
(b) Broad-spectrum antibiotics to cover Gram-negative rods and anaerobes before and after surgery.

328. A 55 year old man appears with history of subacute and constant pain in the **left lower quadrant with fever**. Patients may have either constipation or loose stools. **There is no blood in the stool (please remember this point)**.
Most likely diagnosis: Colonic diverticulitis.

Most commonly involved site is **sigmoid colon.**

Preferred diagnostic test:

(a) **Abdominal CT scan**: It shows bowel wall thickening, diverticuli, and abscess formation.

(b) Previously most commonly performed test was barium enema: It may show spiculation, spasm, abscess, or perforations.

(c) Do **not** perform endoscopy because it can cause perforation.

Treatmetnt:

(a) **Initial therapy**: Third generation cephalosporin plus metronidazole (to cover anaerobes).

(b) **Mildly symptomatic patients:** Bowel rest plus oral antibiotics (outpatient therapy).

(c) **Acute abdomen or severe pain**: Early surgical consultation.

(d) **Abscess formation:** Initial percutaneous catheter drainage is followed by definitive surgical management.

329. **Complications of colonic diverticulitis**:

(a) Stricture formation.

(b) Hemorrhage.

(c) Fistula formation to small intestine, bladder, colon, or vagina.

330. **Amount of radiation is needed to cause radiation enterocolitis**: **More than 5000 rads**. Patients appear with **H/O** nausea, vomiting, and diarrhea with or without blood during the initial radiation therapy. The complications of high dose radiation includes fibrosis, strictures, fistulas, abscess, and hemorrhages from the intestine.

Preferred diagnostic method:(History is very important).

(a) **Endoscopy**: Initial findings are mucosal edema and ulceration, late findings are vascular dilatations and strictures.

(b) Nonspecfic test is barium enema.

Treatment:

(a) Iron therapy: For anemia.

(b) Initial dilatation is followed by surgery: For strictures.

(c) Surgical management: For fistula and abscess.

(d) Antimotility drugs: For diarrhea.

331. **Most common cause of isolated proximal small intestinal ulceration**:

(a) NSAID's (nonsteroidal anti-inflammatory drugs).

(b) Slow-release potassium pills.

Please remember that NSAID's can cause ulcereation in the right colon.

Diagnostic study for small ulcerations:

(a) Enteroclysis is better than barium enema which can miss small size ulcers.
(b) Small intestinal enteroscopy: It is the best method to visualize the ulcer directly but is **not** widely available.

Treatment: Discontinue the medications or reduce the doses if it is mandatory.

Liver+Gallbladder+Bile ducts

1. **Alcoholic hypoglycemia is due to**:
   (a) Ethanol is not converted to glucose.
   (b) Ethanol may inhibit gluconeogenesis.

2. **Most important organ of chemical modification of exogenous drugs and toxins, or endogenous hormones**: **Liver**. It mostly involves the cytochrome P-450-dependent microsomal mixed function oxidase system.

3. **Most important source of bilirubin: Heme** moiety of hemoglobin in senescent or old RBC's that are sequestered and degraded in the mononuclear phagocytic cells of the spleen, liver, or bone marrow.

4. **The following informations are important**:
   (a) Daily bilirubin production is about **4 mg/kg body weight.**
   (b) **Unconjugated** bilirubin is about 95% of circulationg bilirubins and it is water soluble.
   (c) Unconjugated bilirubin is bound reversibly to **albumin** (affinity site 10^8 M^{-1}) in the plasma.
   (d) Inside liver cells, bilirubin and other organic anions bind with **ligandin** (2% of total cytoplasmic proteins).
   (e) Bilirubin **diglucuronide** predominates in human bile (up to 80%), a small amount is monoglucuronides.
   (f) **Most urobilinogens are** absorbed from the intestines (mostly terminal ileum and colon), re-excreted in bile into stool, and a small amount appear in urine.

5. A 30 year old man is completely asymptomatic, appears with **H/O** mild scleral icterus.
   Phyical examination: Unremarkable except mild scleral icterus.
   Plasma sulfobromophthalein disappearance rate: Mildly abnormal in some patients.
   CBC: No hemolysis.
   LFT's: Normal **except** elevation of the unconjugated bilirubin.
   Most likely diagnosis: Gilbert's syndrome.
   Pathogenesis: Due to inadequate conjugation process in the liver (less than 3 mg/dL).
   Treatment: None.
   Important points to remember:
   (a) Liver biopsy is **not** needed. It is usually normal.

(b) Diagnosis is made by the following: An asymptomatic patient with mild jaundice, normal physical examination, elevated unconjugated bilirubin, and no signs of hemolysis.
(c) Phenobarbital reduces the plasma bilirubin level.

6. **Fasting increases the unconjugated bilirubin in the following diseases**:
(a) Gilbert's syndrome.
(b) Crigler-Najjar syndrome (type II).
Pathogenesis in both the disease: Unknown.
A slight elevation of bilirubin production may be a contributing factor.

7. **Crigler-Najjar syndrome**: (Type I is **not** important for the examination. Most of the patients die due to kernicterus in infancy).
Type II: Autosomal dominant, patients appear with severe asymptomatic unconjugated hyperbilirubinemia but rarely develop kernicterus.
Physical examination: Unremarkable except moderate to severe jaundice.
Laboratory studies: Elevated unconjugated bilirubin (6 to 45 mg/dL), rest are normal.
Plasma sulfobromophthalein disappearance rate: Normal.
Cholecystography and histology: Normal.
Diagnosis is made by the following: Clinical manifestation (asymptomatic jaundice), elevated unconjugated bilirubin, and reduction of plasma bilirubin by phenobarbital.
Pathogenesis: Severely decreased glucuronyltransferase enzyme activities.
Treatment: Phenobarbital.

8. An adult woman appears with **H/O** jaundice, otherwise asymptomatic. She is receiving **estrogen therapy recently for menstrual problem**. The degree of icterus **increases** with estrogen therapy.
Physical examination: Unremarkable except jaundice.
Laboratory studies: Elevated both unconjugated (40%) and **conjugated (60%)** bilirubins (1 to 25 mg/dL).
Plasma sulfobromopthalein disappearance rate: **Slow initially** with secondary rise.
Oral cholecystography: **Nonvisualization of gallbladder.**
Urinary coproporphyrin: **Positive.**
Most likely diagnosis: **Dubin-Johnson syndrome (D-J syndorme is an autosomal recessive)**.
Diagnosis is made by the following: Clinical manifestation (asymptomatic jaundice), elevated both **unconjugated and conjugated** bilirubins, slow disappearance of sulforbromophthalein, nonvisualization in cholecystography,

and positive urinary coproporphyrin excretion. Liver biopsy is **not** needed but it reveals pigmentations in centrolobular cells.
Treatment: None is available.
(a) Avoid estrogen.
(b) Minimal reduction of plasma bilirubin with phenobarbital.

9. **Rotor's syndrome**: Autosomal recessive, asymptomatic patients appear with jaundice.
Physical examination: Unremarkable except jaundice.
Laboratory studies: Elevated both unconjugated (40%) and conjugated (60%) bilirubins (1 to 20 mg/dL).
Plasma sulfobromopthalein disappearnce rate: Markedly slowed without secondary rise (unlike Dubin-Johnson syndrome).
Cholecystography and histology: Normal (unlike D-J syndrome).
Urinary coproporphyrin: Positive (like Dubin-Johnson syndrome).
Diagnosis is made by following: Clinical manifestations (asymptomatic jaundice), elevated both unconjugated and conjugated bilirubins, markedly slowed plasma sulfobromopthalein disappearance rate, positive urinary coproporphyrin excretion, and normal cholecystography.
Treatment: None is available.

10. **Most common causes of postoperative jaundice**: **Multifactorial.** It is due to increased bilirubin production (e.g., reabsorption of hematomas, hemolysis of transfused RBC) and reduced hepatic clearance (e.g, bacteremia, hypoxia, and TPN). It resolves spontaneously in 1or 2 weeks.

11. **Most important laboratory findings in postoperative jaundice**: **Elevated serum bilirubin**, other findings are **elevation** of alkaline phosphatase or GGTP (gamma-glutamyl transpeptidase), normal synthetic function and mildly elevated transaminases (AST and ALT).

12. A patient appears with **H/O** intermittent and recurrent jaundice which lasted from few days to few months separated by normal hepatic functions and asymptomatic conditions.
Most likely diagnosis: **Benign recurrent cholestasis** It is a familiar syndrome of unknown etiology.
Treatment: None.

13. **Abnormal liver function tests in different diseases**:
(a) Isolated disorder of bilirubin metabolism: Elevated bilirubin but other hepatic tests are normal.

(b) Biliary obstruction: Elevated GGTP and alkaline phosphatase.
(c) Bony diseases: Elevated alkaline phophatase and normal GGTP.
(d) Drug (e.g., phenytoin) or alcohol use: Elevated GGTP and normal alkaline phosphatase.
(e) Liver diseases (e.g. hepatitis): Elevated (AST and ALT) transaminases.

14. **Clinical presentations in biliary obstruction and liver diseases**:
   (a) **Biliary obstruction**: Patients appear with **H/O** fever, upper abdominal pain, rigors, or previous surgery to biliary system.
   Physical examination: High fever, abdominal tenderness, or mass.
   (b) Liver diseases: Patients appear with **H/O** viral prodrome, alcohol use, hepatitis exposure, transfusion, intravenous drug use, or exposure to hepatotoxins.
   Physical examination: Ascites, breasts enlargement, spider angiomata, dilated periumbilical veins, encephalopathy, or asterixis.

15. **Diagnostic studies in biliary obstruction and liver diseases**:
   (a) **Initial studies should include**: CBC, serum bilirubin, AST, ALT, alkaline phosphatase, and PT (prothrombin time).
   (b) Noninvasive studies are:(Two).
      (i) **Ultrasonography:** It is a **first procedure** of choice in obstructive diseases.
      (ii) **Abdominal CT scan**: It may be the procedure of choice in order to know the **level of obstruction** and **exact anatomical structures.**
   (c) Invasive studies are indicated when **dilated ducts are identified** and to visualize the biliary tree directly.
   Invasive studies are:(Two).
      (i) ERCP (endoscopic retrograde cholangiopancreatography): Direct visualization, examination, biopsy, and therapy (e.g. stenting of distal lesions, papillotomy for removal of stone).
      (ii) PTC (percutaneous cholangiography): Direct visualization and therapy (e.g., stenting of proximal lesions).

16. **Presence of dilated ducts in a patient who had cholecystectomy in the past**: It does not indicate obstruction.

17. **Imaging studies of choice in biliary obstructions**:
   (a) Negligible obstruction: No studies are needed.
   (b) Possible obstruction: Ultrasonography or CT scan.
   (c) Most likely obstruction: Direct cholangiography.

18. **Treatment of hyperbilirubinemia in different conditions**: It depends upon the causes.
    (a) Type I Crigler-Najjar syndrome: Liver transplantation.
    (b) Type II Crigler-Najjar syndrome: Phenobarbital.
    (c) Hepatic parenchymal diseases causing cholestasis: Few specific therapy.
    (d) Progressive cholestasis due to cirrhosis or other conditons: Liver transplantation, avoid alcohol, or drugs.
    (e) Cholestasis causing fat malabsorption: Fat soluble vitamins, MCT.
    (f) Pruritus: Less frequent bathing, skin softeners, cholestyramine. Ursodeoxycholic acid (chloretic bile acid) may be effective in primary biliary cirrhosis and primary sclerosing cholangitis.

19. Important points to remember for hepatic transaminases (normal 40 IU/L).
    (a) AST or SGOT is present mostly in **mitochondria,** less in cytoplasm.
    (b) ALTor SGPT is present mostly in **cytoplasm.**
    (c) AST and ALT are elevated in hepatic diseases.
    (d) **Remember this point** that transaminases levels do **not** correlate with diseases severity and prognosis.
    (e) Serum transaminases levels may **fall in** massive hepatic necrosis (Important).
    (f) Serum transaminases levels do **not** increase above 300 IU/L in severe alcoholic hepatitis.
    (g) Elevated transaminases levels are more than 15 times of normal (40 IU/L) in chronic bile duct obstruction indicate associated cholangitis.
    (h) Serum transaminases levels **are helpful** in monitoring the course of and chronic parenchymal liver diseases **except** in massive heptic necrosis and severe alcoholic hepatitis.
    (i) The high ratio of AST (mitochondria) to ALT (cytoplasm) indicates hepatocellular necrosis (e.g. alcoholic hepatitis).
    (j) AST levels are less than **10 times of normal** in myocardial and skeletal muscles diseases.

20. Different diseases and liver enzymes.
    (a) **Liver disease**: Elevated serum levels of 5'-nucleotidase (5'-NT), leucine aminopeptidase (LAP), or gamma-glutamyl transpeptidase (GGTP). Elevated alkaline phosphatase levels are found in both liver and bone diseases.
    (b) **Bone disease**: Elevated alkaline phosphatase (3 to 10 times normal) but **normal 5'-NT, LAP, and GGPT.**
    (c) **Liver and bone diseases**: Elevated alkaline phosphatase (3 to 10 times normal).

(d) **Extrahepatic bile duct obstruction: Highest level** (more than 10 times normal) of alkaline phosphatase (Important).
(e) **Intrahepatic cholestasis, primary or metastatic cancer, leukemia, lymphoma, or sarcoidosis: Very high levels** (3 to 10 times normal) of alkaline phosphatase.
(f) **Hepatitis, cirrhosis: Mild to moderate** (up to twice normal) increase of alkaline phosphatase.
(g) **No hepatobiliary disease**: Approximately 1/3rd of patients with **mildly elevated** alkaline phosphatase have no hepatobiliary disease (Important).

21. **How to distinguish the origin (liver or bone) of elevated serum alkaline phosphatase? (Normal 25 to 85 IU/L)**.
   (a) **Liver disease**:
      (i) Elevated alkaline phosphatase, 5'-NT, LAP, and GGTP. Elevated 5'-NT and LAP are found in normal pregnant patients.
      (ii) Elevated alkaline phosphatase and GGTP, but normal 5'-NT and LAP.
   (b) **Bone disease**:
      (i) Elevated alkaline phosphatase and normal 5'-NT, LAP, and GGTP.
   (c) **Pregnant patients**:
      (i) Elevated alkaline phosphatase and GGTP: Liver disease.
      (ii) Elevated alkaline phosphatase and **normal** GGTP: Bone disease.

22. **How to monitor abstinence from alcohol ?**: Serum GGTP levels should decrease in abstinence from ethanol.

23. **Elevated GGTP can be found in the following conditions**:
   (a) Hepatobiliary use.
   (b) Alcohol use.
   (c) Diabetes.
   (d) Myocardial infarction (Impotant).
   (e) Pancreatic disease.
   (f) Pulmonary disease.

24. **Regan isoenzymes are found in the following conditions**:
   (a) Hepatoma.
   (b) Lung cancer.

25. **Elevated alkaline phosphatase levels are found in following conditions**:
   (a) Hepatobiliary disease.
   (b) Bone disease.
   (c) Intestinal disease.

(d) Placenta.
(e) Kidney disease.
(f) Leukocytes.

26. **Most common type of mitochondrial antibody is found in primary biliary cirrhosis**: M_2 Presence of mitochondrial antibody indicates parenchymal liver disease but its absence does **not** exclude that disease. **It is rarely found in obstructive liver disease.**

27. **Most common associated finding in primary biliary cirrhosis**: Gallstones.

28. **Urine and bilirubin**:
    (a) Clinical jaundice and presence of bilirubin (conjugated) in urine: Hepatobiliary disease.
    (b) Clinical jaundice and absence of bilirubin (unconjugated) in urine: Hemolysis, inffective erythropoiesis, or inherited bilirubin conjugation defect.

    Remember, presence of urobilinogen in urine or stool is not helpful to make the diagnosis.

29. **Presence of spur cells (acanthocytes) in advanced alcoholic cirrhosis indicates**: Increase of cholesterol in the membrane.

30. **Normalization of laboratory tests occur in acute viral hepatitis**: **Within 4 to 6 months**. Acute infection become chronic if laboratory abnormalities persist beyond 6 to 12 months. Chronic **hepatitis is found only in hepatitis B, C, or D** and absent in hepatitis A, E.

31. Patients appear with mild fever, malaise, anorexia, nausea, vomiting, arthralgias, or **'flu' like symptoms** and characteristic **loss of taste for coffee or cigarettes**. Subsequently develop jaundice and pruritus.

    Physical examination: Enlarged, tender liver is noted. Enlarged spleen is found in 20% of patients. Jaundice is present.

    Laboratory findings:
    (a) **Elevated** AST, ALT, total and direct bilirubins, alkaline phosphatase, globulin, and PT (prothrombin time).
    (b) Decreased albumin and glucose.
    (c) **CBC:** Normal or decreased with atypical lymphocytosis, but increased in severe case.

    Most likely diagnosis: **Acute viral hepatitis.**

32. **Most common complications of acute viral hepatitis**:
    (a) Severe hepatic necrosis and failure are found in hepatitis **D and E, rare in** B, C, and A.
    (b) Chronic hepatitis is present in B, C, and D (absent in A and E).
    Remember, hepatitis A has better prognosis than B, C, and D.
    (c) Cholestatic hepatitis is found in hepatitis A. Cholestasis causes dark color urine, light color stools, pruritus; elevated direct bilirubin and alkaline phosphatase levels.
    (d) Rarely, aplastic anemia may be present in icteric or convalescent phase: Treatment is bone marrow transplantation.

33. **Extrahepatic manifestations found in prodromal phase of acute viral hepatitis are the following**:
    (a) Arthralgias, arthritis.
    (b) Urticaria.
    (c) Cutaneous vasculitis.
    (d) Pancreatitis.
    (e) Other vasculitis manifestations: Polyarteritits nodosa, glomerulonephritis, and cryoglubulinemia are found in chronic hepatitis B and C.

34. **Diagnostic significance of serologic tests in viral hepatitis**:
    (a) Anti-hepatitis A (HAV) IgM positive: Current or recent infection or convalescence. **It indicates active infection.**
    (b) Anti-hepatitis A (HAV) IgG positive: Current or past infection. It indicates **protective immunity.**
    (c) Hepatitis B (HBV) surface antigen (HBsAg) positive: Acute or chronic infection. It indicates infection.
    (d) Hepatitis-e antigen (HBeAg) positive: Acute or chronic infection. It is transiently positive during viral replication. **It indicates infectivity.**
    (e) Hepatitis core antigen (HBcAg): Not tested.
    (f) Anti-hepatitis core (HBcAb) IgM or IgG positive: Acute, or chronic infection; or carriers. Remember it is **not** protective. IgM positive means active virus replication.
    (g) Anti-hepatitis e (HBeAb) positive: During convalescence, in some chronic cases and carriers.
    Remember it is **not** protective. It indicates **low** infectivity.
    (h) Anti-hepatitis B-surface (HBsAb) positive: In late convalescence period. It is **protective.**
    (i) Antibody to hepatitis C virus (HCV) positive: Patients are **infectious**. It is **not** protective. Usually positive 5 to 6 weeks after the onset of clinical infection.

(j) Antibody to hepatitis D virus (HDV) positive: Patients are infectious. It is **not** protective.
(k) Antibody to hepatitis E virus (HEV) positive IgM: Current or recent infection;or convalescence. It indicates **infection.**
(l) Antibody to hepatitis E virus (HEV) positive IgG: Current or previous infection. It indicates immunity.

35. **Hepatitis antibodies with or without protective effects**:
   (a) protective effects:
      (i) Anti-hepatitis A IgG antibodies.
      (ii) Anti-hepatitis B IgG antibodies.
      (iii) Antibody (IgG) to hepatitis E virus (HEV).
   (b) No protective effects:
      (i) Anti-hepatitis core antibodies.
      (ii) Anti-hepatitis e antibodies.
      (iii) Antibody to hepatitis C virus (HCV).
      (iv) Antibody to hepatitis D virus (HDV).

36. **Few important points in hepatitis A infection:**
   (a) It is tansmitted through **contaminated food and water,** person-to-person, and promiscuous homosexual. It is a RNA virus.
   (b) There is no chronic form or carrier state.
   (c) Patients appear with 'flue' syndrome and self-limitted mild jaundice; rarely with acute cholestatic hepatitis for several months which is diagnosed by HAV in the stool and HAV RNA in the serum.
   (d) Fecal shedding of the virus is **brief** between 2 to 5 weeks after exposure, it **stops with the appearance of anti-HAV** (IgG + IgM) **in the serum around 4 to 5 weeks.**
   (e) Serum anti-HAV (IgM) is usually present up to 4 to 5 months or may persist up to 1 year or longer.

37. **Few important points in hepatitis B infections:**
   (a) It is transmitted mainly via parenteral route (transfusions or injections), contaminated body fluids and secretions (sexual partners), from infected mothers to newborn infants. Unlike hepatitis A, fecal oral transmission is **not** important because large doses of viruses are needed. It is common in workers and patients in clinical laboratories, dialysis and oncology units, drug users who shares needles, male homosexuals, and handlers of primates. It is a DNA virus.
   (b) Unlike hepatitis A, it has a chronic form, carrier state, and extrahepatic manifestations.

(c) Remember, it is **more common in Down syndrome,** lymphoproliferative diseases, and leprosy due to increased exposure and /or impaired immunity.
(d) Patients appear with jaundice and extrahepatic manifestations (urticaria, other rashes, arthritis, rarely vasculitis, glomerulonephritis). Remember, up to 33% of patients with **polyarteritis nodosa** may have HBV infections. Patients manifestations are more **prolonged and variable** than hepatitis A.
(e) Intitial manifestation is HBs Ag-emia.
(f) HBeAg and HBV DNA are present **before** the transient rise of ALT.
(g) Anti-HBc (first IgM, then IgG) appears during the acute clinical presentation.
(h) There is a **window period** between the disappearance of HBsAg and appearance of HBsAb; **anti-HBc is the only marker of hepatitis B infection during the window period.**
(i) Approximately 95% of HBsAg positive patients become negative and have normal outcome.
(j) Less than 1% develop severe hepatic necrosis.
(k) Approximately 5% of patients develop chronic hepatitis.

38. **Few important points is hepatitis D infections (HDV or Delta-agent)**:
(a) It is a **complication of hepatitis B infection.** Approximately 5% of hepatitis B patients have HDV infection. HDV is an incomplete RNA virus (HBV is a DNA virus).
(b) In USA, it is transmitted mostly by **blood products or contaminated needles,** but in high prevalence areas by person-to-person contact.
(c) Unlike HBV, incidence is **very low** in dialysis patients, institutional patients, and male homosexuals.
(d) Perinatal transmission is **not** important.
(e) Remember **fulminant hepatic failure is more in HBV and HDV together** than HBV alone, but the possibilities of chronic hepatitis are the **same.**
(f) Recent evidence suggests that HDV is associated with hepatocellular cancer.
(g) **Anti-HDV IgM** is detected in acute and **IgG** in chronic infections or HDV-RNA in the serum. Remember patients also have **positive** HBsAg, anti-HBc, and predominantly anti-HBe.

39. **Few important points in hepatitis C virus (HCV) infections**:
(a) It includes all **non-A, non- B** viruses except for the enterically transmitted disease which is called hepatitis E. It is a RNA virus.
(b) HCV infection does **not** give immunity due to genomic variability, so multiple infections are possible.

(c) HCV is a major cause of **post-transfusion** hepatitis but incidence has declined significantly.
(d) **Detection of HCV- RNA in the serum** by EIA-2 (enzyme linked immunoassay and RIBA (recombinant immunoblot assay) or PCR study (less sensitive) are **the best methods** to diagnose HCV infections.
(e) HCV infections are **found in** drug abusers sharing needles, dialysis patients, clotting factor recipients, and recipients of organ transplantation.
(f) HCV is **less** likely transmitted sexually and perinatally.
(g) Patients clinical manifestations are **same as** other acute hepatitis.
(h) **Liver biopsy in HCV** infection shows **lymphoid aggregates, microvesicular fat in hepatocytes, or injury to the bile duct.**
(i) HCV **causes more chronic hepatitis** than HBV but **rarely causes severe hepatic failure** unlike HBV.

40. **Few important points in hepatitis E infections (HEV)**:
(a) It is a **form of non-A, non-B** which is enterically transmitted.
(b) HEV is exclusively transmitted via the **fecal-oral route.** Acute HEV infection gives **lifelong immunity.**
(c) Patients appear with **acute hepatitis** and **predominantly janudice** (may be cholestatic). Skin rash and arthralgias may be present.
(d) HEV is a **self-limitted disease** and does **not** become chronic.
(e) HEV has **higher** case fatality rate than other acute hepatitis, especially in third trimester pregnancy.
(f) HEV infections can be diagnosed by detecting anti-HEV IgM and/or IgG by EIA method.

41. **Liver biopsy and diagnosis of viral hepatitis**:
(a) It is **nonspecific** and **not indicated** to diagnose viral hepatitis.
(b) It is **contraindicated** in severly ill patients due to coagulation defect.
(c) It is **indicated** when diagnosis is uncertain or deteriorating clinical condition or biopsy report might change the management or concern over chronic hepatic changes.

42. **Treatment for viral hepatitis:**
(a) **Nonspecific symptomatic and supportive care.**
(b) Most patients can be treated at home with adequate rest (but **not** confined to bed).
(c) **Nonspecific diet** but most patients prefer low-fat and high-carbohydrate diet which are palatable.
(d) Small doses of **antinausea drugs** (hydroxyzine, trimethobenzamide) may be helpful.

(e) Avoid alcohol.
(f) Patients plan to return to work or school depend upon the patients symptoms, strenuousness of the job, and transmission of diseases to others.
(g) Hospitalization is necessary in severely ill patients (encephalopathy, prolonged PT, and persistent vomiting).
(h) Liver transplantation is the ultimate therapy.
(i) Corticosteroids are **not** helpful **except** in rare condition of prolonged cholestasis in hepatitis A.

43. **Prevention of viral hepatitis**:
(A) Hepatitis A:
(i) Strict hand washing, wearing gloves, personal hygiene, boiling, or ultraviolet radiation.
(ii) Passive immunization **with immune serum globulin should be given** to immediate family members, individuals with close contacts, and sexual contacts. It is **not** indicated for causal contacts in work place or school unless someone sharing food, beverage, or contaminated items (Important).
(B) Hepatitis B:
(i) Hepatitis B vaccine should be given initially, then at 1 month and 6 month (total 3 doses).
(ii) Hepatitis B vaccine should be given to all newborn infants and high-risk adolescents (intramuscularly into the deltoid muscle is most effective).
(iii) **Hepatitis B immunoglobulin plus vaccine** should be given to health professionals after needle stick and to infants born to HBsAg-positive mothers.
(iv) Postexposure prophylaxis and management:
(a) Blood should be obtained immediately from the donor and recipient for viral serologic studies.
(b) Exposed person (recipient) should receive HBIG plus vaccine pending serologic results.
(c) If the exposed person already has positive HBsAg or anti-HBs, then HBIG and vaccine will **not** be helpful.
(d) HBIG is effective up to 14 days after exposure.
(e) Sexual contacts with acute hepatitis B person, exposed person should receive HBIG plus vaccine.
(f) Family members of acute hepatitis B do **not** need prophylaxis but **do need in chronic hepatitis B (Important).**
(g) Infants under 12 months should receive HBIG plus vaccine if primary caregiver has acute hepatitis B.
(C) **Hepatitis C:**

(i) Avoid contaminated blood transfusions.
(ii) Immune serum globulin is **not** recommended pretransfusion or after needle stick infected with HCV only because there is no evidence of neutralizing (protective) antibody to HCV.
(iii) Prophylaxis resembles hepatitis B.

(D) Hepatitis D:
(i) Prevention of **hepatitis B by vaccine also protect hepatitis D because** HDV infection occurs simultaneously or preceeding HBV infection.
(ii) Avoid HBV-positive serum and secretions.

(E) Hepatitis E: No active or passive immunization is available at this time.

44. **Liver damage caused by drugs and toxic agents are mostly due to**: **Metabolites** of the drugs and toxic agents (rarely due to parent drugs and toxic agents). Liver damages are done by two pathogenetic mechanisms:
(a) Intrinsic hepatotoxins (few days of latent period, dose-dependent, and predictable fashion): Examples are **acetaminophen, mushroom,** industrial chemicals. Toxic metabolites are formed by the cytochrome P-450 from parent compounds.
(b) Idiosyncratic hepatotoxins (variable latent period up to few months, less frequent, and unpredictable fashion): Examples are **isoniazid, phenytoin,** chlorpromazine, and halothane. Patients appear with fever, rash, arthralgias, and eosinophilia.

45. A 19 year old female appears in the emergency room with H/O nausea, vomiting, diarrhea, and ingestion of unknown quantities of over the counter medications. Patient becomes asymptomatic for short period of time, subsequently develops hypoglycemia, lactic acidosis, coagulation abnormalities, and encephalopathy.
Liver aminotransferase: More than 5000 U/L.
Most likely diagnosis: Acetaminophen toxicity.
Preferred diagnostic test: Serum acetaminophen levels are elevated.
Liver damage: Zonal necrosis.
Treatment:
(i) N-acetylcysteine is the most specific treatment of choice.
(ii) Charcoal by mouth.
Prognosis: Depends upon serum acetaminophen levels.

46. **Different medications and hepatotoxicities**:
Amoxicillin- clavulanic acid: Cholestatic jaundice. Resolves completely within 4 to 6 months.

(a) **Erythromycin (mostly estolate):** Cholestatic jaundice, mimic acute cholecystitis or cholangitis. Excellent prognosis.

(b) **Isoniazid (INH)**:
   - (i) INH is converted to acetylhydrazine (hepatotoxic) through cytochrome P-450.
   - (ii) INH toxicities in **younger** patients are **self-limited,** so routine monitoring of LFT's are **not** recommended.
   - (iii) **Several-fold elevation of aminotransferase** over **the age of 35,** even in an asymptomatic patient **is very serious and INH should be discontinued (Important).**

(c) **Oral contraceptives**:
   - (i) **Cholestatic jaundice is due to estrogen** component which has **direct** hepatoxic effects.
   - (ii) It also causes hepatic neoplasms (adenomas), hepatic vein thrombosis **(Budd-chiari syndrome)**, and cholesterol gallstone.
   - (iii) Treatment: To discontinue the medication and cholestyramine for pruritus.
   - (iv) Cholestasis resolves completely within 3 months.

(d) **Amiodarone**:
   - (i) It produces **pseudoalcoholic lesion** (mimic acute alcoholic hepatitis).
   - (ii) Remember, it **rarely causes jaundice** but hepatomegaly may be present.
   - (iii) Abrupt withdrawal of the amiodarone can cause cardiac arrythmias and sudden death.

(e) **Methyldopa**:
   - (i) It mimics acute viral hepatitis, chronic active hepatitis, or INH induced hepatitis.
   - (ii) It causes positive Combs' test which has **no** relation to hepatic damage.
   - (iii) Complete recovery is expected.

(f) **Phenytoin**:
   - (i) Patients symptoms (fever, rash, and enlarged lymph nodes) begin within 6 weeks of therapy.
   - (ii) Leukocytosis with atypical lymphocytosis and eosinophilia are present.
   - (iii) It is converted to **arene oxides** which are hepatotoxic. Genetic abnormalities to detoxify arene oxides may be present.

(g) **Flucloxacillin**: Vanishing bile duct syndrome or ductal lesion.

(h) **Tetracycline, corticosteroids, valproic acid, and alcohol**: Fatty liver.

(i) **Methotrexate, hypervitaminosis A**: Hepatic fibrosis.

(j) **Allopurinol, FUDR (chemotherapy)**: Hepatic arteritis.

(k) **FUDR**: Sclerosing cholangitis.

(l) **Aspirin, oxacillin**: Nonspecific hepatitis.

(m) Anticancer drugs, azathioprine: Veno-occlusive disease, nodular hyperplasias.
(n) Vinyl chloride: Angiosarcoma.

47. A 70 year old elderly obese woman appears in the emergency room with H/O fever, chills, sweating for few days, followed by jaundice and rashes. She had surgery under general anesthesia about 10 days prior to these symptoms.
Physical examination: Jaundice and rashes.
CBC: Mildly elevated eosinophils.
Most likely diagnosis: Halothane induced hepatotoxicities.
Mechanism of halothane hepatotoxicities:
(i) Halothane metabolites are directly hepatotoxic.
(ii) Immune-mediate reaction on the liver by forming haptens with cell membrane proteins.

48. **Most common form of chronic hepatitis**: **Chronic persistent hepatitis (CPH).** It is an inflammatory process mostly confined to **portal areas**, but absence of fibrosis and cirrhosis.

49. **Few important points in CPH (chronic persistent hepatitis):**
(a) Patients appear with **mild nonspecific symptoms** (Jaundice, anorexia, and abdominal discomfort).
(b) Extrahepatic manifestations (arthritis, vasculitis, and glomerulonephritis) are **less than CAH** (chronic active hepatitis).
(c) Hepatomegaly, palmer erythema, and spider telangiectasias are present.
(d) **Absence** of ascites, encephalopathy, and portal hypertension.
(e) Elevated bilirubin, AST, ALT, and globulins.
(f) Normal albumin and PT (prothrombin time).
(g) Biopsy is **not** indicated but continued observation is important.
(h) Rarely, it can progress to CAH, cirrhosis, or liver failure.
(i) Treatment includes symptomatic, nutritional support, avoid hepatotoxins. Small amount of alcohol may be allowed if it is not an etiologic factor.

50. **Few important points in CAH (chronic active hepatitis)**:
(a) Most common cause of CAH is post-transfusion or community acquired hepatitis C (50%), next common (20%) is chronic HBV infection with or without associated HDV.
(b) Patients may be **asymptomatic** or **symptoms** of liver disease (jaundice, anorexia, fever, or ascites) or **extrahepatic manifestations** (rash, glomerulonephritis, vasculitis, thyroiditis, pneumonitis, ulcerative colitis, Sjogren's syndrome, or amenorrhea).

(c) Physical examination shows hepatomegaly or splenomegaly, spider telangiectasias, with or without jaundice; in advanced stages patients appear with cirrhosis, ascites, and encephalopathy.
(d) Serum aminotransferase is **elevated** mildly to severely more than 1000 IU/L, serum globulin is **elevated.**
(e) Low serum albumin level.
(f) Treatment: Orthotopic liver transplantation in severe cases.

51. **Few important points in autoimmune hepatitis**:
   (a) It is characterized by **sever hyperglobulinemia.**
   (b) **Young women** are mostly affected with **extrahepatic manifestations.**
   (c) Presence of **smooth muscle antibodies (66%),** antinuclear antibodies (50%), antimitochondrial, and anti- double stranded DNA.
   (d) Associated with HLA-A1, B8, DR3, and DR4.
   (e) Presence of anti-liver/kidney microsomal (anti-LKM1) anti-body, anti-LKM2, anti-LKM3 are directed against cytochrome P-450 2 D6, P-450 2C9, and UDP-glucoronyltransferase respectively.
   (f) Treatment: Corticosteroid with or without low-dose azathioprine.

52. **Few important points in chronic hepatitis B**:
   (a) Most common (66%) presentation is CPH and rest (33%) is CAH.
   (b) 2 to 10% of acute hepatitis B patients become chronic.
   (c) Disease progress to liver failure, cirrhosis, and hepatocellular carcinoma.
   (d) Treatment:
      (i) **Recombinant interferon- alpha 2b** with or without brief antecedent dose of corticosteroids (which does **not** work alone).
      (ii) Liver transplantation in end-stage liver disease.

53. **Few important points in hepatitis and liver transplantation**:
   (a) Posttransplantation patients for chronic hepatitis B **always get reinfected** due to viremia during the time of surgery or extrahepatic viral replication.
   (b) Reinfection is **less** in fulminant hepatic failure, combined HBV and HDV infections, or posttransplant treatment with high-dose of HBIG.
   (c) Posttransplant reinfection may cause **fibrosing cholestatic hepatitis syndrome and liver failure.**
   (d) Liver transplantation is **contraindicated** in liver failure due to chronic hepatitis B with active viral replication.

54. **Few important points in chronic hepatitis D**:
   (a) Simultaneous infections of HBV and HDV cause more **fulminant hepatic failure but** do **not** increase chronic disease.

(b) **High-dose of interferon-alpha** may be effective in chronic HBV and HDV infections.
(c) **Liver transplantation is more effective in combined HBV and HDV infections** than HBV infection alone because HDV inhibits HBV viral replications.

55. **Few important points in chronic hepatitis C:**
    (a) It represents most cases of non-A, non-B, or posttransfusion hepatitis.
    (b) Most patients remain **asymptomatic without any liver disease** for many years.
    (c) Patients may be symptomatic with abnormal liver function tests and may be **asymptomatic** between symptomatic phases.
    (d) Chronic HCV infection is present in type II cryoglobulinemia and some cases of type III.
    (e) Treatment:
        (i) Interferon-alpha in high dose is effective.
        (ii) Orthoptic liver transplantation in hepatic failure.

56. **Post liver transplantation complication in chronic hepatitis C**: (Important). **Recurrence of hepatitis C.** It is usually mild and easily managed, only few cases lead to chronic active hepatitis, cirrhosis, or hepatic failure.

57. **Diagnosis and management of asymptomatic patients with elevated serum aminotransferase:** (Important).
    (A) Diagnosis: Rule out liver, muscle, or other extrahepatic diseases. Liver disease is either subclinical presentation of acute viral hepatitis, chronic toxic/viral hepatitis, or alcohol steatohepatitis.
    (B) Management:
        (a) First observation, follow up studies, and hepatitis serology should be done.
        (b) Avoid alcohol or hepatotoxic drugs.
        (c) **Persistence of abnormal liver function beyond 6 to 12 months indicates chronic hepatitis, so biopsy is indicated.**

58. **Diagnosis and management of asymptomatic patients with positive HBsAg and/or anti-HCV**: (Important).
    (A) Diagnosis:
        (i) Healthy carrier state.
        (ii) Subclinical acute viral hepatitis.
        (iii) Chronic hepatitis or early cirrhosis.

    Liver biopsy can differentiate these three conditions.

(B) Management:

(i) **HBsAg positive persons with normal clinical findings and liver function tests:** Biopsy findings are normal. Observation and follow up liver function tests and hepatitis profile are indicated.

(ii) **Anti-HCV positive persons with normal clinical findings and liver function tests:** May be **false positive** anti-HCV which is confirmed by negative antibody (RIBA-2) testing.

(iii) **HBsAg or anti-HCV positive persons with abnormal clinical findings and liver function tests:** Management depends upon the duration and severity of disease. **Liver biopsy is** indicated in persistence of abnormal liver function tests beyond 6 months. Interferon therapy may be helpful.

59. **Most common organisms in pyogenic liver abscess: Gram negative enteric bacteria (E.coli,** Klebsiella pneumoniae, Streptococcus fecalis, and Proteus vulgaris), next is anaerobes (bacteroides).

Signs and symptoms: Patients appear with right upper quadrant pain, tenderness, fever, and leukocytosis.

Preferred diagnostic method:

(a) **Ultrasonography or CT scan** to diagnose liver abscess.

(b) **Direct aspiration of the abscess, culture, and cytology to identify the organism.**

Treatment:

(a) Antibiotics to cover gram negative and anaerobes.

(b) Drainage of the abscess.

(c) In multiple abscesses larger accessible abscess should be drained.

(d) Metronidazole in amebic abscess.

(e) Underlying obstruction: Endoscopic or surgical approach to relieve obstruction.

60. **Most common causes of hepatic granulomas**:

(a) Sarcoidosis is the most common cause.

(b) Coccidioidomycosis: In western USA.

(c) Mycobacterium avium- intracellulare: In AIDS patient.

Most common presentation in hepatic granulomas:

Asymtomatic, rarely causes CAH and cirrhosis.

Diagnosis: Biopsy and look for generalized underlying disease.

Treatment: Appropriate to underlying conditions.

61. **Most common worldwide cause of liver abscess**: **Amebic liver abscess is** due to Entamoeba histolytica. Patients appears with fever, right upper quadrant

abdominal pain, sometimes referred to right shoulder due to involvement of hemidiaphragm. Only few patients have amebic colitis or cysts in the stool.

Diagnosis: History of endemic region, ultrasonography, indirect hemagglutination is indicative but **not** diagnostic. Aspiration is **not** needed for diagnosis.

Treatment:

(a) **Metronidazole** is the drug of choice.
(b) **Oral diiodoquine** may be added.
(c) Aspiration is needed when abscess is about to rupture or not responsive to metronidazole.

62. **Few important points of alpha$_1$-antitrypsin (A_1AT) deficiency in adults**:
   (a) PiZZ homozygotes who did **not** have liver disease in childhood, **develop cirrhosis in adults only in 10% cases.**
   (b) PiZZ patients with liver disease have a high incidence of **liver cancer.**
   (c) PiZZ is more common in **males** than females.
   (d) Adults with cirrhosis of unknown etiology, **A_1AT deficiency should be suspected.**
   (e) Diagnosis of A_1AT deficiency is made by measuring **enzyme in the serum or directly analyzing protease inhibitor phenotype.**
   (f) **Remember,** emphysema need **not** be present to make diagnosis.
   (g) Treatment for cirrhosis with A_1AT deficiency is **liver transplantation.**
   (h) Gene therapy may correct enzyme deficiency but cannot suppress overproduction of abnormal Z protein (normal is M protein). **Z protien provokes injury to the liver.**

63. **Few important points of Wilson disease**:
   (a) **Autosomal recessive,** molecular defect on **chromosome 13.**
   (b) **Excess accumulation of copper** in liver, brain, cornea, and kidneys.
   (c) Most commonly involved organ is **liver.**
   (d) **In liver, most common syndrome** is postnecrotic cirrhosis, liver dysfunction, and portal hypertension.
   (e) Diagnosis is confirmed by **low serum ceruloplasmin (<20 mg/dL) plus Kayser-Fleischer rings.** Wilson disease patients may have **normal** serum ceruloplasmin level (15% cases) or **absence** of Kayser- Feleischer rings, in those cases liver biopsy to quantify total hepatic **copper (>250 microgram per gram of dry liver tissues) is diagnostic.**
   (f) Treatment:
      (i) Lifelong chelation therapy.
      (ii) Liver transplantation.

64. **Most common cause of death in hereditary hemochromatosis: Hepatocellular cancer. Other features of hemochromatosis:**
   (a) **Autosomal recessive,** genetic defect on **chromosome 6** near the human leukocyte antigen A (HLA-A) allele.
   (b) **Excessive absorptions of iron** from the intestine and deposits in many organs particularly liver. Only homozygotes have liver injury and heterozygotes have increased iron stores but no liver injuries.
   (c) Patients appear with **abdominal pain and hepatomegaly** after the age of 40.
   (d) Initial laboratory studies reveal **elevation** of **transferrin saturation and ferritin.**
   (e) Definitive diagnosis is made by **liver biopsy to quantify the iron** (>10,000 microgram per gram of dry liver tissues, >20,000 in cirrhosis).
   (f) Treatment: **Phlebotomy** can prevent or reverse hepatic fibrosis but cannot reverse advanced cirrhosis.
   (g) **Family member** should be screened by **HLA typing** and serial measurement of **transferrin saturation and ferritin levels.**
   (h) Remember, HLA type is **not** helpful in general population screening.

65. **Most common hepatobiliary complication of TPN (total parenteral nutrition): (Important)**.
   Hepatic steatosis.
   Few important points in TPN **induced hepatic steatosis:**
   (a) Enzymes (AST, ALT) peak **around 2** weeks after onset of TPN and **then decline despite continuation of TPN without any changes.**
   (b) It is **completely reversible** with discontinuation of TPN.
   (c) **Biliary sludge and gallstones** are formed when TPN is used for 4 weeks or more, 50% of cases after 6 weeks, and 100% after 12 weeks. It is due to gallbladder stasis and decreased bile flow.
   (d) **Bile stasis** can be **reduced** by cholecystokinin, enteral feeding, or pulsed infusion of amino acids.
   (e) Long term use of TPN most commonly causes **steatohepatitis, cholestasis, and hepatic fibrosis.** The management is to discontinue the TPN, avoid caloric excess, cyclical infusion of TPN, and enteral feeding.

66. **Treatment of protoporphyria with liver disease**: Aim is to reduce production and increased excretion of protoporphyrin by the following:
   (a) **Hematin:** Reduces protoporphyrin production.
   (b) **Cholestyramine and activated charcoal:** Both bind protoporphyrin in intestine, promote excretion, and reduce enterohepatic circulation.
   (c) **Liver transplantation:** For severe liver disease and jaundice.

Few important points in protoporphyria:

(a) Presence of **jaundice** means very severe illness.

(b) Patients appear with skin photosensitivity, scarring **sun-exposed skin, and pigmented gallstones.**

(c) Diagnosis is made by the elevated protoporphyrin levels in RBC or feces. Liver is involved when RBC protoporphyrin levlels are >1000 microgram/DL, so liver biopsy is indicated.

67. **Most commonly involved organ in sarcoidosis**: **Liver (granulomatous disease),** next is lung, or lymph nodes.
    Physical examination: Hepatomegaly.
    LFT: Elevated alkaline phosphatase.
    Liver biopsy: Granulomas are diagnostic.
    Treatment:
    Corticosteroid is used in symptomatic patients because it can reduce the symptoms but cannot change the liver disease (Important).

68. **HELLP syndrome:** It is found in severe preeclampsia and eclampsia second or third trimester, or postpartum period.
    H: Hemolysis.
    EL: Elevated liver enzymes.
    LP: Low platelets.
    Patients also have anemia, elevated LDH, but normal PT, PTT, and fibrinogen.
    Treatment:
    (a) Prompt delivery which resolves the symptoms.
    (b) Plasmapheresis is used in patients with persistent thrombocytopenia.

69. Most common **non-neoplastic cause of death** in hepatobiliary and digestive disease: **Cirrhosis.**

70. **Most common cause of cirrhosis in USA and Europe: Alcoholic liver disease** which includes fatty liver, a reversible consequence of acute alcohol ingestion, to reversible cirrhosis **(Laennec's cirrhosis)**.

71. Risk factors for developing cirrhosis:
    (a) Duration and amount of alcohol ingestion: **The significant amount is eighty grams of ethanol per day for 20 years.** Remember, **progression depends upon the total dose,** not the type of alcohol beverage, or pattern of intake. (Eighty grams of ethanol is present in eight 12-oz beers, a liter of wine, or a half-pint of spirits).
    (b) Hepatitis B or C infection.

(c) Genetic factors.
(d) Gender: Females have higher incidence.
(e) Nutritional status: Poor nutrition (poor intake or abnormal metabolism) causes liver disease but adequate nutrition does **not** prevent it.

72. **Types of alcoholic liver injury**:
(a) Fatty liver (severe hepatomegaly, no fever, and no jaundice).
(b) Alcoholic hepatitis (hepatomegaly, fever, and jaundice).
(a) Fatty liver:
(i) It can develop even after single binge of alcohol, unlike hepatitis.
(ii) Patients apper with moderate to severe hepatomegaly, **rarely** right upper quardrant tenderness and epigastric discomfort.
(iii) Liver function tests are normal or moderately elevated, but **absence of jaundice.**
(iv) **It resolves completely within 6 weeks** of discontinuation of alcohol.
(b) Alcoholic hepatitis:
(i) It usually develops **after several weeks to months of alcohol ingestion.**
(ii) Patients appear with **jaundice, mild fever, and hepatomegaly.**
(iii) Presence of spider angiomas, ascites, and palmer erythemas suggest associated **cirrhosis.**
(iv) Patients appear with fever, always rule out bacterial peritonitis, pneumonia, or UTI.
(v) Elevated both AST and ALT (<500), AST >ALT.
(vi) AST or ALT >500 indicates additional hepatic injury (HCV or drugs such as acetaminophen).
(vii) AST or ALT values **become normal within few days,** followed by **elevation of bilirubin up to 20 times normal.**
(viii) Patients poor prognosis are directly proportional to amount of drinking, degree of inflammation (leukocytosis), perivenular fibrosis, and indices of liver failure (coagulopathy, encephalopathy, ascites, or hepatorenal syndrome).

73. **Treatment of alcoholic liver injury**:
(a) **Abstinence is the most improtant** management.
(b) Family and social support.
(c) Alcoholics Anonymous (12-step programs).
(d) **Disulfiram** which inhibits acetaldehyde metabolism.
(e) Patients with withdrawal symptoms (tachycardia, high BP, and agitation): Use benzodiazepines.
(f) Multivitamins including thiamine, pyridoxine, vitamin K, and folate.

(g) Fluids and minerals (phosphate, magnesium).
(h) **Methylprednisolone** is used in severe hepatitis only. It should **not** be used in mild hepatitis, GI bleeding, or bacterial infections.
(i) **Future** therapies include androgenic steroids, propylthiouracil (PTU), invasive nutritional management.
(j) **Liver transplantation.**

74. **Important points in postviral cirrhosis:**
(a) Chronic hepatitis B virus (HBV) and hepatitis C virus (HCV) are the **second leading cause of cirrhosis in USA.**
(b) HBV infection induced cirrhosis depends upon the HDV infection, HBeAg, and alcohol use.
(c) HCV infection induced cirrhosis depends upon the age of exposure, duration of infection, and degree of liver injury.
(d) **This is very important to remember** that in chronic HCV infection patients may have **mild or moderate elevation of AST or ALT with severe liver damage (fibrosis) in biopsy. Liver biopsy is very important.**
(e) **The response of treatment with inferferon** (reduced fibrosis and tissue mRNA levels) can be detected by biopsy.

75. **Cryptogenic cirrhosis:**
(a) It is a progressive liver disease **without viral infections, cholestasis, or genetic causes.**
(b) Cryptogenic cirrhosis with autoimmune hepatitis (75%) **have better survival** than non-autoimmune group (25%).

76. **Genetic disease causing cirrhosis**:
(a) Hemochromatosis is the most common cause.
(b) Wilson's disease.
(c) $Alpha_1$-antitrypsin deficiency.

77. **Important points in primary biliary cirrhosis:**
(a) Immune-mediated, unknown etiology.
(b) Presence of antimitochondrial antibodies and progressive destruction of intraheptic bile ducts in **biopsy is diagnostic.**
(c) It may be associated with other autoimmune diseases **(CREST syndrome**, rheumatoid arthritis, thyroiditis, pernicious anemia, renal tubular acidosis, or sicca complex).
(d) Middle-aged females appear characteristically with **gradual onset of pruritus. Other presentations are malabsorption of fat- soluble vitamins (A, D, E, K),** hepatosplenomegaly, jaundice, and dry skin.

(e) **Treatment:**
  (i) Ursodeoxycholic acid (UDCA) reduces the concentration of toxic bile acids in the liver.
  (ii) Immunosuppressive drugs may be helpful: Azathioprine, methotrexate, chlorambucil, and prednisone.
  (iii) Cholestyramine reduces pruritus.
  (iv) Vitamins A, D, E, K.
  (v) Liver transplantation.
  (vi) Experimental drug: Cyclosporine.

78. **Important points in secondary biliary cirrhosis**:
  (a) It is due to chronic biliary intrahepatic or extrahepatic obstruction for 6 months.
  (b) Intrahepatic cholestasis is **most commoly due to primary sclerosing cholangitis** other than PBC, next is cystic fibrosis.
  (c) Extrahepatic obstruction is motly due to **Choledocholithiasis,** biliary cancer, pancreatic cancer, chronic pancreatitis, or iatrogenic.
  (d) Patients clinical presentations depend upon the underlying primary diesase, usual presentations are pruritus, jaundice, and deficiencies of vitamins A, D, E, K.
  (e) **Severely elevated (fivefold) alkaline phosphatase,** mild elevation of AST or ALT, with hypercholesterolemia are characteristic.
  (f) Treatment:
    (i) Surgery or biliary stent: For extrahepatic obstruction.
    (ii) Cholestyramine for pruritus.
    (iii) Vitamins A, D, E, K.
    (iv) Ursodeoxycholic acid.
    (v) Liver transplantation.
    (vi) Future therapy: Ursodeoxycholic acid plus methotrexate.

79. **Liver function tests abnormalities in chronic right sided heart failure**: Hepatic congestion (nutmeg liver) causes **severe elevation of bilirubin (up to 10 folds),** PT (2 to 6 seconds prolonged), but modest elevation of AST and ALT (<3 folds). Patients appear with cardiac and pulmonary symptoms.

80. **Complication of bone marrow transplantation and/or pyrrolizidine alkaloid therapy**: **The syndrome of hepatic veno-occlusive disease** which is characterized by rapid onset of enlarged liver, ascites, and weight gain. It is **not** a true cirrhosis.
Liver function tests: Elevated bilirubin, AST, and ALT.

81. **Budd-chiari syndrome:** It is due to **acute or subacute obstruction to hepatic venous outflow.** It is **not** a true cirrhosis.

82. Complication of **nonalcoholic steatonecrosis- Cirrhosis (33 % of cases)** if the underlying causes are **not** removed. The underlying causes are the following:
   (a) Diabetes mellitus.
   (b) Jejunoileal bypass surgery.
   (c) Abetalipoproteinemia.
   (d) Weber Christian disease.
   (e) TPN.
   (f) Synthetic estrogen, diethylstilbestrol.
   (g) Amiodarone.

83. **Drug induced hepatic fibrosis is due to**:
   (a) INH.
   (b) Antimetabolites (methotrexate). It is dose-dependent and intermittent therapy causes less fibrosis than continuous therapy.

84. **Most common cause of portal hypertension**: **Cirrhosis.**

85. **Most common site of lesion in portal hypertension**: **Sinusoidal and intrahepatic.** It may be presinusoidal obstruction (portal vein thrombosis, schistosomiasis), or post sinusoidal obstruction (e.g., veno-occlusive disease, right-sided cardiac failure, and Budd-Chiari syndrome).

86. **Portal venous pressure**:
   (a) Normal condition: <10 mm Hg.
   (b) Portal hypertension: Portal venous pressure at least **5 mm Hg more than nonportal abdominal veins (inferior vena cava).**

87. **Most common presentation of cirrhosis with portal hypertension**: **Bleeding from varices** in esophagus/stomach.

88. A patient appears with ascites, enlarged spleen, gastroesophageal varices (painless bleeding), encephalopathy, distended abdominal wall veins (caput medusae), and abnormal liver functions (coagulopathy or infection).
   Most likely diagnosis: Portal hypertension is due to cirrhosis. (In **noncirrhotic portal hypertension,** liver functions are **normal.** In **presinusoidal lesions** such as portal vein thrombosis or schistosomiasis, **most common** clinical presentations are **enlarged spleen and variceal bleeding.** In **postsinusoidal obstruction,** most common clinical presentations are **weight**

gain, enlarged spleen, also rapid onset of ascites. In **portal hypertension which is due to neoplasm or infection,** patients appear with anemia, heart **failure, or hypercoagulable state).**

Diagnostic studies are the following:

(a) Serum: AST, ALT, bilirubin, albumin, and PT.

(b) Abdominal ultrasonography with doppler probe: To look for hepatic parenchyma, blood flow to hepatic and portal veins, or varices.

(c) Abdominal CT or upper endoscopy: Varices are present in **both intrahepatic and extrahepatic lesions.**

(d) Direct measurement of portal hemodynamics by hepatic vein catheterization (it is **invasive and only indicated when ultrasound and doppler** studies are **not** conclusive): **Normal wedged hepatic venous pressure gradient (WHPG) is < 5 mm Hg, it is the difference between (wedge hepatic venous pressure) WHVP and 1VC (inferior vena cava). When it (WHPG) exceeds 12 mm Hg** then **hemorrhage from varices can occur** but it does **not** corelate with extent of elevation above 12 mm Hg.

89. **Risk factors for variceal bleeding:** (Remember that gastrin has **very little role** in this bleeding).
   (a) WHPG is >12 mm Hg.
   (b) Large variceal size.
   (c) Endoscopy shows red wales or cherry red spots over the varix, that means hemorrhages within the vessels.
   (d) Jaundice and poor liver functions.

90. **Diagnosis of variceal bleeding:** Vigorous gastric lavage followed by emergency endoscopy should be done when a patient is stabilized by fluid, blood, and appropriate respiratory care.

91. **Treatment of variceal bleeding**:
   (a) **Hemodynamic stabilization:** Fluid, electrolytes, and blood in hypotensive patients.
   (b) **Endotracheal intubation:** For ventilation and to avoid aspiration of blood.
   (c) **Emergency endoscopy:** To look for and stop acute bleeding and recurrence of bleeding.
   (d) **To control bleeding:**
      (i) Endoscopic direct or paravariceal injection with sclerosant.
      (ii) Endoscopic band ligation.
      (iii) **Drugs:** Intravenous vasopression and nitroglycerin; or octreotide (experimental).

(iv) **Minnesota or Sengstaken- Blakemore tube for** balloon tamponade of blood vessels at the gastroesophageal junction: It is **done only when endoscopy and medications fail.**
(v) Patients with persistent bleeding: Surgical portal decompression is performed on an emergency basis.
(vi) TIPS (Transjugular intrȧhepatic portasystemic shunt): It is an alnertative to surgery. It decompresses portal circulation and stops bleeding in up to 95% of patients. It is good for patients waiting **for liver transplantation**.

92. **Prevention of initial or recurrent variceal bleeding**:
   (a) **Beta-blocker (propranolol or nadolol):**
      (i) **Prophylactic use in patients with moderate to large varices with normal liver functions.**
      (ii) It **also reduces the bleeding in congestive gastropathy (or portal hypertensive gastropathy)** which is a bleeding from submucosal veins in the proximal stomach due to portal hypertension.
      (iii) It **also reduces the rebleeding.**
      (iv) It reduces **bleeding by reducing the heart rate.**
   (b) **Sclerosant therapy.**
      (i) Prophylactic use is **not** effective.
      (ii) Endoscopic sclerotherapy: It is done only when beta-blocker is ineffective or cannot be used. It needs follow up every 3 to 6 months.
   (c) **No** synergistic effect of beta-blocker and sclerotherapy.
   (d) Portacaval shunt surgery.
   (e) Liver transplantation.

93. **Side effects of beta- blocker**:
   (a) Bronchospasms.
   (b) Heart failure.
   (c) Impotence.
   (d) Lethargy.

94. **Long-term use of TIPS and its complications:**
   (a) Shunt occlusion.
   (b) Encephalopathy.

95. **Most common cause of ascites**: Cirrhosis.

96. **Most accurate method to classify ascites**: **Serum-ascites albumin gradient (SAAG)** is the difference between serum albumin and ascitic fluid albumin.

(a) SAAG value ≥1.1 gram/dl: Portal hypertension.
(b) SAAG value <1.1 gram/dl: Rule out neoplasms, tuberculosis, bile leak, or pancreatitis by analyzing amylase, triglycerides, mycobacterial cultures, or cytology.

97. **Diagnostic methods of ascites**:
   (a) Paracentesis:
      (i) SAAG value.
      (ii) Cell count, Gram stain, albumin.
      (iii) Ascitic fluid culture in blood culture media.
   (b) Abdominal sonogram with doppler flow study:
      (i) To asses structure and blood flow in the portal, hepatic, and splenic veins.
      (ii) To asses parenchyma of the liver and spleen.
      (iii) To asses size of the biliary tree.
      (iv) To rule out neoplasms.
      (v) To rule out any peritoneal diseases.

98. **Treatment for ascites:**
   (a) **Restriction of sodium (40 ot 60 mEq/day).**
   (b) **Diuretics:** Spironolactone, lasix, or both. (Lasix causes more azotemia than spironolactone).
   (c) **Patients with pedal edema:** Therapeutic paracentesis.
   (d) Patients without pedal edema: Paracentesis should be associated with infusion of albumin or dextran.
   (e) **Refractory ascites:** Peritoneovenous shunting or TIPS.
   (f) **Most definitive treatment: Liver transplantation.**

99. **Complications of peritoneovenous shunting**:
   (a) Catheter infections.
   (b) Shunt occlusion.
   (c) Mild DIC (disseminated intravascular coagulation).

100. **Most common complication of ascites: SBP (spontaneous bacterial peritonitis) is most common and serious** complication, other complications are hepatic hydrothorax, tense ascites with leakage, and abdominal wall hernias.

101. **Few important points in SBP**:
   (a) Most common organisms are E.coli, Pneumococcus, Klebsiella, and anaerobes.

(b) Patients appear with **either subtle presentation** (mild abdominal pain/tenderness) or **serious presentation (**fever, severe abdominal pain, encephalopathy, azotemia, or abnormal liver function tests).

(c) **Presumptive diagnosis:** Ascitic fluid has PMN count (250 per cubic millimeter. **Remember, Gram stain and culture are mostly negative despite infections.**

(d) **Treatment of choice:** Cefotaxime or ceftriaxone.

(e) **Response to antibiotics should be documented by reexamination of ascitic fluid:** fluid shows 50% reduction of WBC counts.

(f) **Prophylaxis:** Norfloxacin is used in patients with history of SBP to prevent recurrence, susceptible to develop SBP (low-protein ascites or GI bleeding), or candidates for liver transplantation.

102. **Hepatopulmonary syndrome:** It is a triad which includes the following:

(a) **Liver diseases:** Chronic liver disease or severe liver disease.

(b) **Pulmonary vessels:** Right to left shunt through pulmonary A-V fistulas, bronchial varices, and pulmonary hypertension.

(c) Reduced arterial oxygenation.

Lung function tests: Normal lung volumes but reduced diffusing capacity.

Treatment:

(a) **Oxygen:** It reduces the symptoms but cannot help the diseases process.

(b) **Liver transplantation:** It helps in resolution of the syndrome in most patients.

103. **Hepatorenal syndrome (or functional renal failure):** It includes **severe liver disease and ascites which are associated with functional renal failure without intrinsic abnormalities of the kidneys.**

Etiology: Unknown, but reduced renal blood flow, cortical perfusion, glomerular filtration, and increased endothelin-1(vasoconstrictor).

Diagnosis: Low urine sodium (<10 mEq/L), oliguria, and normal intravascular volume in patients with cirrhosis.

Treatment:

(a) **Liver transplantation:** It is **most effective treatment.**

(b) Antibiotics for infections.

(c) Fluids to maintain adequate volume.

(d) **Avoid NSAID's**: It inhibits renal vasodilatation.

Prognosis: poor.

104. **All clotting factors are synthesized in the liver except:** Factor VIII. In severe liver disease, all factors will be reduced except Factor VIII.

105. **Feminization of men with end-stage liver diasease (ESLD) is due to**: Increased estrogen and diminished testosterone. Other complications of **ESLD are thinning and spontaneous fractures of bone** due to osteoporosis, osteomalacia, or both.

106. **Most common benign hepatic tumor**: Cavernous hemangioma.
Most common clinical presentation: Asymptomatic.
Diagnosis: MRI, CT with bolus contrast.
Treatment.
(a) Asymptomatic patients: None.
(b) Symptomatic patients: Resection; rarely required radiotherapy or hepatic artery ligation.

107. **Most common predisposing factors in hepatocellular adenomas**: **Oral contraceptives;** next is glycogen storage disease type I.
Patients appear with abdominal mass, tumor infarctions, intratumor hemorrhage (fever, pain, and increased WBC counts), or intraperitoneal hemorrhage.
Diagnosis: Ultrasonography, CT, or MRI.
Treatment:
(a) Discontinue oral contraceptives.
(b) Asymptomatic patients: Observation.
(c) Symptomatic patients: Tumor resection.
Prognosis: Rarely, change to malignancy.

108. **Hepatic malignant tumor in adults:**
(a) **Most common tumors are metastatic tumors, most commonly arise from stomach, colon, and pancreas.** Other metastatic tumors are melanoma tumors of the oropharynx, lungs, and bladder.
(b) Non-metastatic tumors of the liver:
(i) Hepatocellular carcinoma (hepatoma): **It is not common in USA** and Western Europe. It is found in male patients with cirrhosis, hepatitis B and C, and hemochromatosis. It **may be associated** with aflatoxins, mycotoxins, estrogenic and androgenic steroids, thorotrast, alpha-1-antitrypsin deficiencies, or glycogen storage diesases I and II.
Signs and symptoms: Patients appear with **weight loss, abdominal pain and mass (most common presentations);** obstructive jaundice or paraneoplastic syndromes (fever, erythrocytosis, hypercalcemia, and hypoglycemia).
Diagnosis:

(a) **Elevated serum alpha-fetoprotein level (>1000 ng/ml) or progressively rising levels.**
(b) **Ultrasonography, CT, or MRI.**
(c) **Biopsy.**

Treatment:
(a) **Surgical resection: Treatment of choice in USA.**
(b) **Chemotherapy:** Adriamycin or combination with other antineoplastic drugs.
(c) Radiotherapy: Not effective.
(d) Liver transplantation: It is curative only in few patients with **unresectable tumors.**

Prognosis: Bad.

(ii) Fibrolamelar carcinoma: It is a variant of hepatocellular carcinoma. It is found in both sexes, noncirrhotic young patients, and has longer survival.

Treatment: Surgery.

(iii) Cholangiocarcinoma and angiosarcoma.

109. Most common extranodal sites of involvement in Hodgekin, non-Hodgkins, and malignant histiocytosis: **First is spleen and second is liver.**

110. **Most common presentation of hepatic tumors**: Right upper quardrant or epigastric mass.

111. **Most common diagnostic imaging studies are done in hepatic tumors**: Ultrasonography, CT, or MRI.

112. **Diagnostic studies for metastatic tumors in liver**:
(a) **Initial screening study**: Ultrasonography.
(b) **Percutaneous biopsy: Two biopies from** same skin site have higher yeilds and lower risk of bleeding.

113. Diagnostic studies for primary tumors of the liver:
(a) Initial diagnosis is made by: Ultrasonography, CT or MRI.
(b) When diagnosis is certain and preoperative patients: No preoperative biopsy is needed.
(c) When diagnosis is **not** certain: Biopsy is indicated for appropriate diagnosis and management.
(d) **Contraindications of needle biopsy: Hemangioma, angiosarcoma, and hepatocellular adenoma** may cause bleeding; echinococcal cyst may spread further.

(e) **Difficulty in diagnosis** by needle biopsy: Hepatocellular adenoma, focal nodular hyperplasia.
(f) Laparascopic direct biopsy of visible tumor is helpful.
(g) **CT or ultrasound guided fine-needle percutaneous aspiration biopsy (best method).** It has the **best result and** less bleeding than standard biopsy.

114. Most common cause of **fulminant liver failure: Viral hepatitis.** Other causes are medication (acetaminophen), toxins (Amanita phalloides), or metabolic (Wilson's diseases).

115. **Complication of fulminant hepatic failure before transplantation: Cerabral edema and herniation.**
Management before transplantation:
(a) Elevation of head, monitor intracranial pressure (ICP).
(b) Hyperventilation to reduce cerabral edema and ICP.
(c) Mannitol (diuretics), barbiturate coma to reduce ICP.

116. **Most common cause for liver transplantation**: **Chronic active hepatitis/crytogenic cirrhosis.** Other important causes are alcoholic liver disease, fulminant hepatic failure, and primary biliary cirrhosis.

117. **Donor selection for liver transplantation**: ABO blood type and body size compatibility.

118. **Posttransplantation complications and management**:
(a) Vascular (thrombosis of the anastomosed hepatic artery or portal vein): Retransplantation for early hepatic artery thrombosis.
(b) Infection: It **is very common due to immunosuppression.**
   (i) Bacterial: Prophylactic antibiotics plus treat the underlying infections.
   (ii) Fungal: Amphotericin.
   (iii) Herpes virus: Acyclovir.
   (iv) CMV: Ganciclovir, acyclovir.
   (v) Pneumocystis carinii: Prophylactic trimethoprim- sulfamethoxazole can prevent infection.
(c) Biliary tract leak and strictures.
(d) Renal failure.
(e) Rejection: It is very common.

119. **Posttransplantation (liver) immunosuppressive therapy:**
(a) Cyclosporine: Its absorption **depends upon bile.**

(b) FK 506 (tacrolimus): Its absorption does **not** depend upon bile.
(c) Prednisone is used in combination with cyclosporine or FK506.
(d) Azathioprine.

120. Side effects of immunosuppressive drugs:
(a) **Cyclosporine and FK506:**
(i) Neurotoxicity: Headache and tremor.
(ii) **Nephrotoxicity:** Increased BUN, creatinine, and potassium; glucose intolerance.
(iii) Post-transplantation lymphoproliferative disorders.
(b) **Prednisone:**
(i) Increased pretransplantation bone loss.
(ii) Increased cholestatic liver disease.
(c) **Azathioprine:**
(i) Bone marrow suppression.

121. **Rejection after liver transplantation:** It is very important to make diagnosis and treat promptly.
(a) Diagnosis: Histologic findings in rejection: Periportal infiltrate, bile duct epithelial damage, and endothelitis.
(b) Treatment:
(i) Additional steroids or antilymphocyte drugs.
(ii) Switch to FK506 from cyclosporine.

122. Most common causes of fulminant hepatic **failure (hepatic failure with encephalopathy less than 8 weeks)**: Acute hepatitis B (with or without hepatitis D), hepatitis A, acetaminophen. (Remember, hepatitis C and E **rarely** cause fulminant hepatic failure).
(A) **Dignosis:** Encephalopathy with liver failure must be present.
(i) **PT: Elevated (Important finding).**
(ii) Serum bilirubin: **Less helpful** because patients may be in coma without significant elevaton of bilirubin.
(iii) AST or ALT: Elevated **but cannot distinguish between** this and acute hepatitis without encephalopathy.
(B) **Treatment: First start supprotive measure,** if no improvement **then immediately contact liver transplant center (Important).**
(i) **Supportive therapies.**
(a) **Endotracheal intubation** if patients are unable to protect airways.
(b) **Lactulose** (enema or nasogastric tube):
(c) **Cerebral edema** (CT scan is **not** reliable, invasive monitoring of ICP should be done): Mannitol, barbiturates.

(d) **Coagulation abnormalities:** It should be corrected with FFP (fresh frozen plasma) before ICP monitoring.
(e) **Antibiotics:** It should be started after appropriate cultures (blood, urine, and others) were obtained. Remember, it can control the infection but **cannot** change the survival.

(ii) **Liver transplantation:** It is the best treatment of choice.
(iii) Experimental therapy: (These are not effective) Corticosteroids, PGE (prostaglandins), L-dopa, hyperimmune globulin (hepatitis B), exchange transfusion, plasmapheresis, and extracorporeal circulation (**No need to rember experimental therapies).**

123. **Adverse prognostic factor in fulminant hepatic failure with or without acetaminophen**:
(a) PT: Elevated (international normalized ratio > 6.5 in acetaminophen and >3.5 in non-acetaminophen cases).
Other factors are:
(i) Acetaminophen: Elevated creatinine >3.4 mg/dL.
(ii) Non-acetaminophen: Elevated bilirubin >18 mg/dL, **more than 1 week duration from jaundice to encephalopathy**, age over 40 years.

124. Most common cause of encephalopathy due to chronic liver disease: Cirrhosis with portal- systemic shunting (spontaneous, TIPS, or surgically created).
Diagnosis is made by the: Presence of encephalopathy with chronic liver disease.
LFT's: Not helpful, mildly elevated.
PT: Severely elevated or progressively rising means acute hepatocellular necrosis.
Patients with chronic alcoholic liver disease: It is extermely important to **rule out other causes of metabolic encephalopathies** (Wernicke- Korsakoff syndrome, hypoglycemia, acute alcoholic intoxication), or CNS lesions (subdural hematoma, meningitis).
Treatment:
(a) **Supportive measures:**
(i) Improve liver function, stop toxic agents, use lactulose or neomycin.
(ii) Treat the underlying reversible precipitating factors (sedatives, hepatotoxic agents, hypoxia, hypokalemia, constipation, infection, GI bleed, diuretics, and azotemia) unlike fulminant heptic failure.

(b) **Liver transplantation:** It is the **best** treatment of choice. **Remember, prompt referral to liver transplant center is very important.**

Prognosis.
(a) Encephalopathy with chronic liver disease: Bad.

(b) Encephalopathy is due to reversible precipitating factors: Good.

125. **Complications of prolinged use of neomycin in hepatic encephalopathy**: Ototoxicity and malabsorption.
Treatment:
(a) Discontinue neomycin.
(b) Give lactulose.

126. **Most common cause of hepatic encephalopathy: Multifactorial.**
Important causes the following:
(a) Toxins (ammonia and marcaptans).
(b) Elevated GABA (gamma-aminobutyric acid): It is produced by the intestine and it inhibits the brain.
(c) Increased concentration of aromatic amino acid and decreased concentration of branched-chain amino acids in brain and serum.

127. **Signs and symptoms of hepatic encephalopathy**:
(a) **Subclinical encephalopathy:** Patients appear with H/O impaired work performance or driving ability. Psychomotor tests and bedside tests (drawing or number connection) are abnormal.
(b) **Clinical encephalopathy:** (Stage I to IV) Patients appear with mild confusion, asterixis, tremor, sleep disorder, and restlessness (stage I); disorientation, lethargy, primitive reflexes (suck), and dysarthria (stage II); somnolence, speech disorder, hyperreflexia, and hyperventilation (stage III); or coma, decerebrate posturing, and flaccidity (stage IV).

Few important presentations to remember:
(i) No seizure.
(ii) **EEG changes are non-specific** but is a sensitive indicator for hepatic encephalopathy: Symmetrical slowing initially in frontal areas.
(iii) **Brain stem reflexes are preserved** such as pupillary light reflex, oculocephalic, and oculovestibular.

Diagnosis: It is made by **neurologic signs and symptoms with advanced liver disease but other diseases should be excluded.**
(a) To exclude other diseases: Routine LFT's, BUN, creatinine, **calcium, and electrolytes**.
(b) Toxicologic screen.
(c) Serum ammonia and CSF glutamine: Limited values.
(d) CT scan of head: To exclude subdural lesions.

128. **Treatment for heptic encephalopathy**: Most important is supportive measures:

(i) Improvement of hepatic functions.
(ii) Prevention or correction of factors which enhance encephalopathy.
(iii) Stop all hepatotoxic drugs.
(iv) Decrease production and absorption of enteric toxins: **Lactulose (orally or enema) or neomycin.**
(v) Vegetable protein is helpful for long term management: It is less likely to produce encephalopathy than animal protein.

129. **Most predominant organic solute of hepatic bile**: **Bile salts,** other constituents of bile are electrolytes (same as plasma), phospholipids (most common is phosphotidylcholine or lecithin), proteins, cholesterol (unesterified form), and bilirubin.

130. **Methods of diagnosis in patients with suspected cholestasis**:
(a) **Initial studies:** LFT's show **disproportionate** elevation of GGTP, alkaline phosphatase, and 5'-nucleotidase; increased conjugated bilirubin, cholesterol and PT (due to malabsorption of vitamin K).
(b) **Next investigation of choice is ultrasonography**: It can distinguish the site (extrahepatic or intrahepatic), nature (gallstones, mass, or stricture) of obstruction. Remember, CT or MRI has no advantage over ultrasonography in **large duct obstruction.**
(c) **When cancer is suspected** to look into entire abdomen including retroperitoneum and pancreas: **Investigation of choice is CT or MRI.**
(d) **Cholestatic patients with normal bile duct by ultrasonography:** Liver biopsy is performed to look for parenchymal diseases.

131. **Methods of treatment in patients with cholestasis**:
(a) Specific treatment to cure or control specific problems:
(i) Cholecystectomy: Gallstones.
(ii) Withdrawal of drugs and immunosuppressive medications which are responsible for cholestasis.
(iii) Resection: Neoplasms.
(b) Procedures to relief obstruction of the bile duct: Roux-en-Y choledochojejunostomy.
(c) Medications:
(i) Rifampin and phenobarbital reduce cholestasis.
(ii) Cholestyramine reduces pruritus. It is also reduced by naloxone.
(iii) Fat soluble vitamins (A, D, E, K), calcium, and low-fat diet.
(iv) Ursodeoxycholic acid reduces cholestasis.
(d) **Liver transplantation:** It is the procedure of choice in end-stage liver disease.

132. **Intrahepatic cholestasis is caused by the following drugs**:
   (a) **Cyclosporine or steroids**: Metabolic effects at the level of hepatocytes, little or no hepatic inflammation.
   (b) **Chlorpromazine:** Hypersensitivity reaction causing fever, elevated AST, ALT, and alkaline phosphatase.
   (c) Captopril, benoxaprofen, and sulindac.

   Treatment for drug induced cholestasis: Stop the drugs.

133. **Most common cause of extrahepatic biliary obstruction: Neoplasms** (cancer of the liver, gallbladder, and bile duct cause proximal bile duct obstruction; cancer of the pancreas and ampulla cause distal obstruction) **Other causes are the following:**
   (a) Metastatic tumors: It can cause **both extra or intrahepatic biliary obstruction.**
   (b) Benign tumors: Pancreatic cystadenoma and villous adenoma of the papilla of Vater cause **distal bile duct obstruction (extrahepatic).**
   (c) Nonobstructive metabolic cholestasis (paraneoplastic syndrome): It is due to complication of extrahepatic malignancies such as lymphoma or renal cell cancer **(Stauffer's syndrome).**
   (d) Cholangiocarcinoma.
   (e) Rarely, gallbladder adenocarcinoma.

134. **Most common cause of death in cholangiocarcinoma**: **Local hepatic invasion rather than distant metastases.**

135. **Few important points in cholangiocarcinoma:**
   (a) **Extrahepatic biliary obstruction** is more common than intraheptic obstruction.
   (b) **Klatskin tumors:** It is a tumor at bifurcation of the common hepatic duct which can directly invade the liver.
   (c) Patients appear with **progressive obstructive jaundice, vague abdominal pain, and severely elevated alkaline phosphatase.**
   (d) It is more common in patients with **primary sclerosing cholangitis or choledochal cysts.**
   (e) **Initial diagnostic studies**: Ultrasonography or CT.
   Most useful study: Cholangiography.
   Diagnosis is confirmed by: Endoscopic **brush cytology,** needle aspiration, or laparatomy.
   (f) Treatment:

(i) **Intraductal radiation (brachytherapy): It is the best treatment of choice.**
(ii) **Not effective:** Surgery, chemotherapy, and radiotherapy.

136. **Gallbladder adenocarcinoma is most commonly associated with**: Gallstones.

137. **Few important points in gallbladder adenocarcinoma:**
   (a) It is **mostly associated with large stones** (>3 cm in diameter) or **calcification** of gallbladder wall (porcelain gallbladder).
   (b) Remember, cholecystectomy is **not** an indication in patients with asymptomatic gallstone because incidence of cancer is < 0.1 %.
   (c) Patients are mostly asymptomatic initially, symptoms of abdominal pain and progerssive jaundice indicate advanced stage.
   (d) Preoperative investigations are ultrasonography, CT, or cholangiography.
   (e) More than 80% of gallbladder cancers are **not diagnosed before surgery.**
   (f) Treatment:
      (i) Cancer restricted to gallbladder: Cholecystectomy.
      (ii) Advanced stages (jaundice): Chemotherapy and radiotherapy have little benefits.

138. **Best method to diagnose choledochal cyst in adult**: ERCP. Other methods are ultrasonography and CT.

139. **Few important points of choledochal cyst in adults**:
   (a) Patients appear with jaundice, abdominal pain, and palpable mass. Fever is present in associated cholangitis.
   (b) Treatment: Surgery (complete excision of cyst).
   (c) **Complications:** Cholangiocarcinoma, brown pigment gallstones, and liver abscess.

140. **Patients with chronic pancreatitis and elevated serum alkaline phosphatase**. Ultrasonography: Dilated common bile duct.
   (a) **Next recommended diagnostic study of choice: Periodic liver biopsies are needed to detect progressive hepatic fibrosis**.
   (b) **Treatment:** Choledochojejunostomy to relieve ductal obstruction.

141. **AIDS cholangiopathy:**
   (a) Patients with **advance immunodeficiency** may appear with acalculous cholecystitis, stenosis of the papilla of Vater, or multifocal stenosis of the biliary tree.

(b) Pathogenesis: **Unknown,** but colonization of bile with cryptosporidia and microsporidia.
(c) Diagnostic studies:
(i) Initial: Ultrasonography.
(ii) **Final: ERCP is most diagnostic.**
(d) Treatment: No specific treatment.
Remember, **it is a late complication of AIDS, rarely fatal, but poor prognosis.**

142. Patients with PSC (primary sclerosing cholangitis) suddenly **develop increased cholestasis, Cholangiography:** Single stricture is found.
Most likely diagnosis: Cholangiocarcinoma.

143. **Few important points in PSC (primary sclerosing cholangitis)**:
(a) It is an obliterative inflammatory fibrosis of the large bile ducts.
(b) Most commonly associated with idiopathic inflammatory bowel diseases (ulcerative colitis or Crohn's disease) but **PSC has no relation with severity of bowel disease.**
(c) Etiology: Unknown, but associated with HLA B8 and DR3.
(d) Most definitive diagnostic study: ERCP. It shows **multiple irregular strictures and dilatations** of intra and extrahepatic bile ducts. **Liver biopsy** can detect the stage and rate of disease progression.
(e) Patients appear with gradual onset of chronic cholestasis (jaundice), **pruritus, and elevated alkaline phophatase**. Presence of fever, chills, night sweats, and abdominal pain **indicate bacterial cholangitis.**
(f) Treatment: Nonspecific therapy.
(i) Ursodeoxycholic acid: It reduces symptoms, improves LFT's, but **cannot** stop pregression of disease.
(ii) Antibiotics: For infections.
(iii) Endoscopic stenting or balloon dilation of focal strictures: It reduces cholestasis, replaces surgery, but has little long term benefit.
(iv) Liver transplantation in end-stage liver disease.

144. **Most common type of gallstones in USA: Cholesterol gallstones (80%),** pigment (calcium) stones (20%).

145. **Most common cause of recurrent acute pancreatitis: Small gallstones.**

146. **Most common cause of nonalcoholic pancreatitis**: **Gallstones.**

147. **Four stages of gallstones diasease:**

(a) **Stage I (lithogenic stage):** Stones have **not** formed yet but on the process of formation (because bile is supersaturated with cholesterol, mucus, galbladder stasis, rapid nucleation, and crystal growth).
(b) Stage II (asymptomatic gallstones): Gallstones have formed but patients are asymptomatic.
(c) Stage III (symptomatic gallstones): Patients appear with **biliary colic** (continuous severe pain in the epigastirc or right upper quadrant, sometime radiating to the back or scapula, lasting more than half hour) but absence of fever and peritonitis. There is **transient elevation** of AST, ALT, alkaline-phophatase, and bilirubin.
(d) Stage IV (complication of gallstones):
   (i) **Acute: (Two).**
      (A) Acute cholecystitis.
      (B) Choledocholithiasis.
   (ii) **Chronic:** (Three).
      (A) Chronic cholecystitis.
      (B) Adenocarcinoma of the gallbladder.
      (C) Choledochoduodenal fistula with gallstone ileus.

148. **Diagnostic studies of gallstones**:
(a) **Ultrasonography: It is the best diagnostic procedure of choice and accuracy rate is up to 95%. Problems are the following:** It **cannot detect the number and type** of gallstones, **cystic duct obstruction, and common bile duct (CBD) stones but provides clue to CBD stones because of dilatation of CBD.**
(b) **Plain X-ray of the abdomen:** It can detect only pigmented (calcium) stones. Calcification indicates chronic cholecystitis.
(c) **Oral cholecystogram (OCG):** It can detect the **size and type of stones** (cholesterol stones are radiolucent and float).
Failure to visualize the gallbladder is due to following:
   (i) Acute and chronic liver diseases.
   (ii) Chronic cholecystitis with loss of gallbladder mucosal function.
   (iii) Cystic duct obstruction.
(d) **Hepatobiliary radionuclide scan (DISIDA, HIDA, or PIPIDA):** It can asses **patency** of the **cystic duct and common bile duct,** failure of the radionuclide material enter in the gallbladder and the intestine indicates obstruction of the cystic duct and CBD respectively. **It is the investigation of choice in patients with cholecystitis with cystic duct obstruction.**
(e) Direct injection of contrast material into the biliary tree either by PTC **(percutaneous fluroscopy guided) or ERCP: It is the investigation of**

choice when CBD stones or (narrowing) stricture cannot be diagnosed by any other methods.

149. **Treatment for gallstones and other biliary conditions:**
   (a) **Asymptomatic small gallstones (< 3 cm in diameter):** No treatment is needed.
   (b) **Asymptomatic large gallstones (> 3 cm in diameter):** Cholecystectomy (because it can turn into cancer).
   (c) **Asymptomatic porcelain gallbladder: Cholecystectomy** (because it can turn into cancer).
   (d) **Symptomatic gallstones:** Cholecystectomy is the curative therapy.
   (e) **Acute cholecystitis:** Cholecystectomy.
   (f) **Symptomatic patients with nonvisualized gallbladder by OCG. (chronic cholecytitis):** Cholecystectomy.
   (g) **CBD stones:** Direct choledochoscopy and stone extraction during cholecystectomy.
   (h) **Ascending cholangitis:** Antibiotic plus endoscopic sphincterotomy which which can remove the stone.
   (i) **Ursodeoxycholic acid can dissolve cholesterol gallstones.** It is used in **midly symptomatic, high risk, and for patients who do not want surgery.** Prophylactic use in severely obese patients can reduce gallstones by 80%.
   (j) Experimental: Lithotripsy.

   Remember, **laparoscopic cholecystectomy and removal of CBD stones are the best treatment of choice.**

150. **Complications after cholecystectomy**:
   (a) **Diarrhea:** It is due to increased delivery of bile salts into the colon. Treatment: Cholestyramine.
   (b) **Recurrent upper abdominal pain is due to:**
      (i) Retained CBD stones, abscess, or surgical complications.
      (ii) **Postcholecystectomy syndrome: Patients symptoms persist because the gallbladder was removed due to misdiagnosis.** Actually patients have peptic ulcer, irritable bowel syndrome, pancreatitis, or biliary dyskinesia.

151. **Biliary dyskinesia:** It is a functional biliary obstruction due to spasm of sphincter of Oddi (or motor dysfunction).

   Diagnosis is made by following criteria:
   (i) Patients appear with right upper quadrant pain with transient elevation of LTF's.

(ii) Elevated basal sphincter of Oddi pressure.
(iii) Dilated (>11 mm) CBD by ultrasonography.
(iv) Delayed emptying of CBD (>45 minutes) after ERCP.

Treatment: Endoscopy sphincterotomy is the treatment of choice.

CRITICAL CARE MEDICINE

1. **Diagnosis of respiratory failure:** It is done through **systemic ABG** (arterial blood gas) analysis only.

2. **Diagnostic of criterion hypercapnic respiratory failure or ventilatory failure**: **High $Paco_2$.**

3. **The ratio of respiratory rate (F) and tidal volume (V_T) 100 or more indicates (F/V_T)**: To **start or continue mechanical** ventilation.

4. **Few important points when managing patients on the mechanical ventilator**:
   (a) Maximum inspiratory pressure (**MIP) is more than 20 cm H_2O indicates need for ventilatory support,** less than 20 cm H_2O indicates wean off from ventilatory support.
   (b) **Vital capacity (VC) less than 10 ml/Kg body weight indicates need for ventilatory support (**normal is 50 ml/Kg body weight).
   (c) Forced expiratory volume (FEV_1) in 1 second **less than 75% of forced VC is** found in airway obstructions (e.g.,asthma and COPD), normal value is 75 to 80% of forced VC.

5. **Most important approach to the critically ill patients**: **Quick initial clinical assesment and intervention**. The subsequent steps are the following:
   (a) Broader and comprehensive diagnostic and treatment plans depend upon the physiology and pathophysiology.
   (b) Appreciation of organ system independence.
   (c) Directed and dynamic management plans.

   Remember, physicians **must avoid to collect data for their own interest** and **must concentrate in clinical assesment.**

6. **Diagnosis of failure of arterial oxygenation**: **Low $Paco_2$.**

7. Alveolar- arterial oxygen tension difference (PAo_2 - Pao_2):
   $PAo_2 = PIo_2 - (Paco_2/RQ)$.
   PAo_2= Alveolar oxygen tension.
   PIo_2 = Inspired oxygen tension (oxygen delivered to the patient).
   $Paco_2$= Arterial carbon dioxide (from ABG).
   RQ= Respiratory quotient (0.8).
   Pao_2= Arterial oxygen (from ABG).

8. **Pulse oximetry:** It measures **systemic arterial saturation (Sao_2) by** differential absorption of certain wavelength of light (with hemoglobin) that passes through fingers or other parts of the body where it is applied. These lights only detect hemoglobin that is **saturated by oxygen (not carbon monoxide).**

9. **Best method** to asses tissue oxygenation of different organs: To **analyze the respective organ system functions by simple biochemical tests.** Other methods are to measure intragastric pH and Pco_2 by tonometer.

10. **Ventilatory failure, causes and management:**
    (a) Narcotics overdose: Use naloxone.
    (b) Benzodiazepines overdose: Use flumazenil.
    (c) Ventilatory failure due to COPD, anesthesia, or other drugs: Use doxapram.
    (d) Some COPD patients: Theophylline may be helpful.
    (e) Some drugs overdose: Hemodialysis or charcoal hemoperfusion.
    (f) Pneumothorax, hemothorax, empyema: Thoracostomy tube is helpful.
    (g) Thick respiratory secretions: **Removal of the secretions by chest physiotherapy and gentle endotracheal suction.** Additional help in COPD patients with **iodinated glycerol** which helps in secretion clearance.

11. **Arterial hypoxemia, causes and management**:
    (a) **Pneumonia or infections:** Patients should lie **down on the side of normal or nondiseased lung** in order to improve Pao_2.
    (b) **Plumonary edema: Pao_2 improves in prone position** than supine.
    (c) **Lung atelactasis: Pao_2 improves in upright position** than supine, and also improves **with sedative** if patients have pain.
    (d) **Hypoventilation (narcotic overdose) causing hypoxia:** Naloxone.
    (e) **Hypoxia due to high altitude, carbon monoxide, asthma, and COPD:** Supplemental oxygen.

12. **Indications for mechanical ventilation:**
    (a) **Ventilatory failure (acute hypercapnia), acute hypoxemia are the most common indications** (Pao_2 <50-60 mm Hg in inspired oxygen fraction ≥0.4 or P $(A\text{-}a)o_2$ >300 mm Hg on inspired oxygen (F_{IO_2} of 1.0 or 100%).
    (b) Patients need hyperventilations (head trauma, cerebral edema).
    (c) MIP (maximum inspiratory pressure) more than 20 cm H_2O.
    (d) Minute ventilation (V_E) >10 L /minute.
    (e) Vital capacity (V_C) < 10-15 ml/Kg body weight.
    (f) Ratio of respiratory rate (F) and tidal volume (V_T) ≥100.
    (g) Dead space (V_D) to tidal volume (V_T) fraction ≥0.06.

13. **Indications for weaning from mechanical ventilation:**
    - (a) When the reason for mechanical ventilation is **no longer present: Most important indication.**
    - (b) Pao_2 >50 to 100 mm Hg on an FIO_2 of 0.4.
    - (c) $P(A\text{-}a)o_2 < 300$ mm Hg on an FIO_2 of 1.0.
    - (d) MIP less than 20 cm H_2O.
    - (e) Minute ventilation (V_E) < 10 L/minute.
    - (f) Vital capacity (V_C) between 10 to 15 ml/ Kg body weight.
    - (g) Ratio of $F/V_T \leq 100$.
    - (h) Ratio of $V_D/V_T < 0.6$.

14. **Complications of positive pressure ventilation:**
    - (a) Volutrauma (or barotrauma).
    - (b) Pneumothorax.
    - (c) Mediastinal emphysema.
    - (d) Systemic air embolism.
    - (e) Lung cyst.
    - (f) **Decreased cardiac output is** due to decreased peripheral venous return, **results in hypotension.**

15. Indications for PEEP (positive end-expiratory pressure, PEEP), increases arterial oxygenation by increasing lung volume:
    - (a) It prevents or reverses atelactasis.
    - (b) It helps in weaning from mechanical ventilation.
    - (c) It improves arterial oxygenation at a low inspired oxygen fraction.

    Please remember that PEEP does not improve ventilation and $Paco_2$ may be elevated due to **elevated V_D/V_T.**

16. **Complications of PEEP (it is found in high levels):**
    - (a) Volutrauma (or barotrauma).
    - (b) Decreased cardiac output is due to decreased **pheripheral venous retrun, results in hypotension.**

17. **Methods of weaning from mechanical ventilator:**
    - (a) **From AMV (assisted mechanical ventilation) and other modes of PPV** (positive-pressure ventilation):
        - (i) ET tube should be connected to a **T- piece tubing** which is connected with desired oxygen.
        - (ii) Switch to SIMV without using T-piece.

(b) **From SIMV (synchronized intermittent mandatory ventilation),** here ventilator breaths are delivered to the patients only at the end of **spontaneous expiration to avoid hyperinflation.** Both SIMV and IMV are PPV mode):

   (i) **Progressively reduce the ventiltor respiratory rate (F) until** patients can maintain normal minute ventilation (V_E) by spontaneous breathing.

   (ii) SIMV and PSV (pressure-support ventilation) may be combined for weaning. PSV helps spontaneous breathing with a preset positive airway pressure to achieve a desired tidal volume (V_T).

Remember PSV should be used only in stable patients during the process of weaning. PSV can be reduced as long as the V_T is normal, begin SIMV in an intermediate rate, and reduce ventilator rate slowly to avoid collapse.

18. **Method of weaning from PEEP**.
    (a) Patients is on **low level of PEEP** for collapse: They can be weaned without trouble.
    (b) Patients with **diffuse parenchymal lung problems:** They should be weaned from PEEP slowly (2 to 5 cm H_2O), monitor Pao_2 and Sao_2 very closely. Pao_2 more than 80 mm Hg on an FIO_2 ≤ 0.4 is considered adequate level for weaning.

19. **Relationship between airway pressure (Pa) and pleural pressure (Ppl) in different types of ventilation (spontaneous, IPPV, CPAP, and CPPV)**:
    (a) Pressure **gradient between Pa and Ppl is increased in CPAP and CPPV** than in IPPV and spontaneous breathing **(Important).**
    (b) Ppl is negative in spontaneous breathing and CPAP; Ppl is positive in CPAP; Ppl is **negative** in IPPV except in end of inspiration and beginning of expiration when **it is positive.**

20. **Blood gas and oxygen content in CO poisoning: Pao_2 is normal, low Sao_2 and Cao_2 (arterial blood oxygen content).**
    Treatment:
    (a) Supplemental oxygen at an FIO_2 of 1.0(100%).
    (b) Hyperbaric oxygenation.

21. **Effect of dopamine in different doses:**
    (a) 2 to 5 microgram/kg/min: Increases renal and mesenteric vasodilatation (dopaminergic effect).
    (b) 5 to 10 microgram/kg/min: Improves cardiac output (beta-1 effect).
    (c) >10 microgram/kg/min: Increases peripheral vasoconstriction (alpha-1 effect).

22. **Effects of dobutamine:**
    (a) **Please remember that it does not raise the blood pressure (BP)** because its alpha-1 actions are balanced by its beta-1 actions.
    (b) It may **reduce the BP** in some unstable patients due to predominant beta-2 actions.
    (c) It does **improve cardiac output** (beta-1 actions).
    (d) It has **no** effect on renal and mesenteric blood flow.
    (e) It **can be used in hypotensive patients along with high dose of dopamine.**

23. **Hypoxia is due to shunting of blood (cardiac output):** Hypoxia (Pao_2) is directely proportional to the amount of shunting of cardiac output. **Pao_2 improves with high inspired oxygen if shunting is less than 30% of cardiac output,** above that level there **is very little increase** of Pao_2 even with FIO_2 0.8 to 1.0.

24. **Treatment of cyanide poisoning causing hypoxia.**
    (a) Amyl nitrate (inhalations), sodium nitrite (IV): They produces **methemoglobin which binds free cyanide ions.** Sodium nitrite is used only in critical cases because it causes hypotension and methemoglobinemia.
    (b) Sodium thiosulfate (IV): It **converts cyanide to thiosulfate** which is less toxic and is quickly excreted from the body.
    (c) New antidote is hydroxocobalamine.

25. **Neuromuscular diseases with respiratory failures (mostly hypercapnic) and management**:
    (a) Guillain-Barre syndrome: Plasmapheresis.
    (b) Myasthenia gravis: Pyridostigmine, corticosteroids, plasmapheresis, and thymectomy.
    (c) Botulism: Enema and lavage, penicillin, antitoxin, and surgical debridement of contaminated wounds.
    (d) Bulbar paralysis may cause aspiration and respiratory obstruction: Treat accordingly (ET tube intubation, suction, and ventilator management).
    (e) Generalized weakness with atelactasis or pneumonia: Treat appropriately (oxygen and antibiotics).
    (f) Kyphoscoliosis with chronic hypoxia causing right heart failure and pulmonary hypertension: Treat appropriately (oxygen, respiratory and cardiac managements).

(g) **Patients with paralysis or severe weakness: Initially managed with CMV or AMV.**
After improvement, SIMV may be used if there is no fatigue, if patients show improvement in MIP (maximum inspiratory pressure) and V_C (Vital capacity) then **PSV or T- piece should be attempted.**

(h) Hypertension, diaphoresis, and tachycardia in neuromuscular disease: Use esmolol.

(i) Hypotension in spinal cord injury or other conditions: Intravenous fluids, high-dose of dopamine, or alpha-1 agonist (phenylephrine).

(j) Patients with bradycardia: Atropine.

(k) Patients with asystole: Cardiac pacing.

26. **ABG changes is asthma and COPD: (Important).**
   (a) **First is hypoxia** due to mismatch of ventilation and perfusion.
   (b) Next is **hypercapnia** due to airway obstruction plus fatigue of the respiratory muscles and **FEV_1 is reduced to 750 ml or 25% of the predicted value.** (Remember, **increased $Paco_2$** and **normal FEV_1 is found in narcotic or sedative overdose or in inhalation of high oxygen).**
   (c) **Metabolic acidosis is more serious** than respiratory acidosis in obstructive lung disease.

27. **Management of patients in asthma and COPD:**
   (a) **Acute hypoventilation should be managed immediately** than chronic hypoventilation.
   (b) **Treatment:** Beta-2-adrenergic agonists, theophylline, anticholinergic drugs, and corticosteroids. **The drug of choice is beta-2-agonists (metaproterenol and albuterol).** The side effects of beta-2-agonist (tremor and tachycardia) can be reduced in **aerosol form.** Epinephrine and isoproterenol are **not** used because of both beta-1 and beta-2 effects.
   (c) **Hypoxic patients without ventilator: Use low oxygen** to keep Pao_2 60 mm Hg to avoid respiratory depression.
   (d) **Hypoxic patients on ventilator or pneumonia: Use high oxygen.**
   (e) **Indications for intubation:**
      (i) Acute respiratory acidosis with or without metabolic acidosis.
      (ii) Patients are **responsive to maximal therapy.**
      (iii) **Progressive deterioration of ABG** despite maximal therapy.
      (iv) Patients become confused, uncooperative, or somnolent.

28. **Ventilator management in asthma and COPD:**
   (a) The goal in severe obstructive lung diseases is to **maintain adequate expiratory time to avoid auto- PEEP (or $Paco_2$ retention)** and **slow**

inspiratory flow to optimize the distribution of ventilation and **to reduce the airway pressure to achieve preset tidal volume (V_T).**

(b) To achieve above mentioned goal, patients need to **be sedated** during CMV or AMV to **give slow ventilator rate (F)** and **small I: E ratio. Tidal volume should** be between 7 to 10 ml/Kg body weight **and an adequate FIO_2 to achieve normal Pao_2.**

(c) Patients with chronic hypoventilation and $Paco_2$ retention: (Important): **Do not reduce the $Paco_2$ rapidly** which results in **uncompensated metabolic alkalosis.**

(d) **Patients with severe drops in pH, elevated $Paco_2$ due to low ventilator rate (F) and tidal volume (V_T):** Sodium bicarbonate may be given PRN but be careful about the $Paco_2$ elevation.

(e) **PEEP is contraindicated** in asthma and COPD because lung **volumes are already increased.** Remember, **high PEEP is dangerous, PEEP of 5 cm H_2O does not cause hyperinflation, low PEEP may prevent airway atelactasis during expiration.**

29. **Weaning from mechanical ventilator in asthma and COPD (obstructive lung diseases)**:
   (a) **Asthma patients:** Weaned and extubated quickly if respond to therapy.
   (b) **COPD patients (marginal pulmonary function and $Paco_2$ rentention):** Patients should be weaned slowly and ABG in **normal condition should match with the ABG on the ventilator. Use SIMV or T-piece with or without PSV and little PEEP.**
   (c) COPD patients **unable to meet objective criteria for extubation:**
      (i) Decision of extubation would depend on subjective criteria (alertness, cooperation, and prognosis).
      (ii) When the patients can maintain desired **minute ventilation (V_E) spontaneously for 30 to 60 minute: Patients can be extubated.**

30. Ventilator management of pneumonia:
   (a) Most commonly used types of ventilation are **CMV, AMV, and SIMV** modes of PPV (positive pressure ventilation).
   (b) **PEEP is needed** for **diffuse bilateral pneumonias** like in other forms of ARDS.
   (c) **PEEP should be used carefully in unilateral pneumonia** because it can overdistend the normal lung, may worsen arterial oxygenation.
   (d) The goal is to achieve normal ABG.

31. Most common gas exchange abnormality in ARDS (**reduced lung volume, most common cause is sepsis): Hypoxemia.** Other findings are elevated $Paco_2$

and V_D/V_T. Remember, respiratory presentation of MOSF is ARDS, **sepsis is the most common cause in both conditions.**

32. **Ventilator management of ARDS and MOSF**: Most patients are ventilated and oxygenated adequately by CMV, AMV, and SIMV with low V_T (10 to 15 ml/kg body weight) Pmax less than 35 cm H_2O, lowest **possible level of PEEP to reduce an F_{IO_2} of ≤ 0.6.** When Pmax is needed more than 35 cm H_2O, PCV may be added with or without IRV. **I:E ratio** can be used **1:3 or greater.**

33. **Most common finding in all forms of shock: Microcirculatory insufficiency.** The ultimate findings are cell membrane dysfunction, abnormal cell metabolism, and cellular death.

34. **Most common finding in** cardiogenic shock: **Severely reduced tissue perfusion is** due to primary myocardial dysfunction, results in hypoxia and metabolic acidosis.

35. **Most important factor in pulmonary edema: Increased capillary permeability, other factors are low oncotic** pressure and **increased left atrial pressure.**

36. Most important factor in **preload** (presystole): **Total circulating blood volume,** other factors are atrial contraction and distribution of blood volume. Important factors in afterload: Aortic root diastolic pressure, **ventricular size, and impedance**. Afterload mimic and calculated by measuring:
    systemic vascular resistance = (Mean arterial pressure - Mean RAP) / systemic cardiac output.
    (RAP= right atrial pressure).

37. **Conversion of angiotensin I to angiotensin II occurs in the: Lungs. Inactive angiotensinogen** is converted to **active angiotensin I in the Kidneys.**

38. **Degrees of hypovolemic shock:**
    (a) Mild (10% loss of blood volume): Mild reduction of BP and moderate reduction of cardiac output (CO).
    (b) Moderate (20% loss of blood volume): Moderate reduction of BP and moderately severe reduction of CO.
    (c) Severe (40% loss of blood volume): Severe reduction of BP and CO.

39. Most common organisms **cause septic shock:**

(a) **Gram-negative organisms** are **E.coli,** Klebsiella, Enterobacter, and Pseudomonas. **Most important sources of** infections are **GU and GI tracts,** then respiratory tract, wound, and intravascular catheter.
(b) Gram positive organisms are Staphylococcus, Streptococcus.
(c) Fungal: Candida.

40. **Most common cause of cardiogenic shock: Acute myocardial infarctions. Anterior infarction causes more shock** than inferior infarction (**Important**).

41. **Most important example of shock due to acute vascular obstruction: Acute cardiac tamponade** causes decreased diastolic ventricular filling. It is **due to trauma, cardiac rupture,** neoplasms, or infections. **Remember,** symptoms depend upon **the rapidity of accumulation rather than amount. Rapid accumulation of 100 to 200 ml can cause symptoms.**
Treatment: Percutaneous pericardiocentesis, removal of only **50 to 100 ml** is adequate for normal cardiac function.

42. **Complications of shock.**
(a) DIC: Most common cause is sepsis.
(b) ARDS: Most common cause is sepsis.
(c) ARF (acute renal failure): Most common cause is **decreased renal perfusion results in ATN (acute tubular necrosis).**

43. **Clinical presentations of cardiogenic shock:** Patients appear with **hypotension** (systolic arterial pressure < 90 mm Hg or > 60 mm Hg below baseline), **tachycardia, and hyperventilation.**
Physical examination shows **cold clammy extremities, thready pulse, and altered sensorium.**
Special clinical presentations in different causes of cardiogenic shock:
(i) Critical AS (aortic stenosis) or MS (mitral stenosis): Tachyarrythmias (atrial fibrillation).
(ii) Rupture myxomatous mitral valve: Sudden onset of shock and pulmonary edema in asymptomatic patients.
(iii) Viral myocarditis: H/O mild viral symptoms followed by slow onset (weeks to months) of low output cardiac failure.
(iv) Myocardial infarctions: (Three types of presentations).
  (a) **Massive infarction or rupture ventricle: Acute** onset of shock, severely low BP, and pulmonary edema.
  (b) **Ruputre of interventricular septum, mitral valve rupture/dysfunction: Nonacute onset** of shock, pulmonary edema **within several days, and new systolic murmur.**

(c) **Recurrent infarctions: Gradual onset** of low cardiac output shock after several days of infarctions.

44. **Management of cardiogenic shock (five important points):**
(a) **First and most important is the rapid recognition of the shock.**
(b) **Second is to correct the initial problems.**
(c) Maintain the functions of the vital organs.
(d) To correct the secondary consequences of the shock.
(e) To identify and correct the aggravating causes.

Approach and set up for patients care:
(i) **Critical care team: Experienced physicians and appropriate set up are the most important** in the management.
(ii) **Past and present medical history:** It should be obtained very quickly and appropriately.
(iii) **Physical examination:**
(a) Most important is patency of the airway: Intubation, if necessary.
(b) Breathing should be established.
(c) Circulatory assement (low BP, rapid and slow pulse, bradycardia, and narrow pulse pressure).
(d) Differential diagnosis of **sinus tachycardia (seven H's):** Hypovolemia, hypotension, hypoxia, heart failure, hyperthermia, hyperadrenergic states (reflex tachycardia in anterior MI) and hyperthyroidism.
(iv) **Intravenous access and fluids:** Two rapid IV accesses; blood is obtained for hematologic, chemical, type and cross-matching; **isotonic solutions (**normal saline or Ringer's lactate) should **be infused immediately.**
(v) **Blood analysis also includes:** ABG, blood culture, cardiac enzyme panels, and toxicology screen.
(vi) Monitoring of the patients:
(a) EKG: Serial standard 12-leads.
(b) Arterial pressure: More severe the shock the more central should be the arterial catheter which has **higher complications than peripheral catheters (**femoral or radial.) Complications include **bleeding, thrombosis, infection, embolism, aneurysm, and vasospasms.**
(c) Assesment of **cardiac filling pressures:** Swan-Ganz catheter (pulmonary artery balloon catheter) is important in cardiogenic shock. **Right ventricular preload** is measured by right atrial pressure (**normal 2-10 mm Hg)** and right ventricular end-diastolic pressure (**normal 2 to 8 mm Hg, normal systolic pressure 15 to 30); left ventricular preload** is measured by pulmonary artery diastolic pressure (**normal 4 to 12, normal systolic pressure 15-30) and pulmonary capillary**

wedge pressure (**normal 3-15)** provided there is **no obstruction between pulmonary artery and left ventricle.**

Few important points to remember:

(i) **Increase of oxygen saturation from SVC (superior vena cava) to pulmonary artery more than 7% indicates left-to right shunt.**

(ii) **Left ventricular volume** is very important determinant of the preload, the relation **between volume and pressure of left ventricle** depends on distensibility (or compliance) of the ventricle.

(d) Urinary catheter to measure urine output: Urine output **less than 20 ml/hour indicates inadequate renal perfusion which is most commonly due to hypovolemia.**

45. Therapy of patients with cardiogenic shock:

(a) **Oxygen:** Try to keep the oxygen saturation ≥90%; to avoid pulmonary oxygen toxicity in ventilator patients try to keep the $FIO_2 \leq 0.6$.

(b) **Hypovolemia causing hypotension without pulmonary edema:** IV normal saline should improve the BP. Do **not** give excessive fluid which can cause pulmonary edema.

(c) If **patients do not improve with the volume or progerssively getting worse:** Immediate invasive monitoring of hemodynamics to measure RA, RV, PA, and pulmonary capillary wedge pressures; cardiac index (normal 2.6-4.2 L/min/m^2) and arterial-mixed venous oxygen contents difference (normal 3-5 ml/dl) to measure the cardiac output.

(d) **Metabolic acidosis:** Sodium bicarbonate should be given when pH < 7.0 and $Paco_2$ is normal. **Try to keep the pH ≥7.30.** Do **not** overcorrect metabolic acidosis, it causes CNS acidosis (because co_2 can diffuse quickly through blood-brain barrier than HCO_3), hypokalemia, sodium and water overload.

(e) **Arrythmias: (**Not all arrythmias need treatment).

(i) Arrythmias should be treated when it alters the hemodynamic status.

(ii) PVC on the monitor in clinically stable patients: **No need for treatment.**

(iii) Ventricular tachycardia: Electrical countershock, of no response use lidocaine.

(iv) Ventricluar fibrillation: Electrical countershock therapy.

(v) Atrial flutter, fibrillation, and tachycardias with hemodynamic compromise: Electrical cardioversion therapy, digoxin (Do **not** use beta-blocker and calcium-channel blocker in patients with shock because **death** can occur).

(vi) Sinus bradycardia: Atropine is useful.

(vii) A-V block with inferior wall MI (myocardial infarction): **It responds to atropine** because A-V block is neurologically mediated.

(viii) **A-V block with anterial wall MI: It does not respond to** atropine because A-V block is due to ischemia of A-V node or bundle of His. Treatment of choice is **external (transthoracic) or internal (transvenous) electrical pacing.**

(f) **Sympathomimetic amines: Dopamine, dobutamine, epinephrine, and norepinephrine** are used to improve cardiac output, increased arterial BP (try to keep systolic 100 to 130 mm Hg and diastolic 60 to 80 mm Hg), and increased blood flow to vital organs (e.g., CNS, heart, and alrenals).

Please remember that isoproterenol is not recommended for cardiogenic shock because it increases myocardial oxygen demand, although **it dilates** coronary arteries but ischemic portion of the heart **is hypoperfused which is documented by increased lactate production.** It can be used **temporarily** in A-V block unresponsive to atropine before **the pacemaker is available.**

(g) **Amrinone (predominant inotropic and less chronotropic action)**: It can be used as an **alternative to dobutamine** in severe low-output cardiogenic shock or in combination with dopamine or dobutamine.

Side-effects: Low plateletes count and elevated liver enzymes.

(h) **Digoxin:** Remember, **it is not used in cardiogenic shock (**because of narrow therapeutic-to- toxic ratio and splanchnic ischemia) **except in atrial flutter unresponsive to electric cardioversion to** control the heart rate.

(i) **Nitroglycerin**: It is a **vasodilator (**mostly **effective on venous vessels** than arteriolar vessels) which is used in **acute pulmonary edema with MI.**

Side effects: Hypotension and headache.

(j) **Nitroprusside:** It is a **vasodilator (both venous and arteriolar vessels)** which is used in MI with power failure provided the **patients have indweling systemic and pulmonary catheter to monitor the hemodynamics.**

(k) **Vasodilators:** They reduce the cardiac preload and afterload. They are useful in **severe heart failure and/or shock** with adequate cardiac filling pressure and **ability of ventricle to adjust** in preload or afterload (**not** effective in obstructive heart disease).

(l) **Pain with shock:** IV morphine can be used very cautiously.

Side effects of morphine: Hypotension, bradycardia, respiratory depression, and biliary spasm.

Treatment: Naloxone.

(m) **Thrombolytic agents:** Streptokinase and TPA (tissue plasminogen activator) should be used **in MI as early as possible (Important).**

(n) **IABP (Intra-aortic balloon counterpulsation):** It is used in **cardiogenic shock due to acute ventricular septal rupture or acute papillary muscle**

rupture/dysfunction causing mitral insufficiency. It is only used temporarily before patients go for major surgery (cardiac).
Side effects: Limb ischemia, vascular damage, and infections.

(o) **Nutritional therapy in shock**: (Important) Initially, unstable patients should receive NPO plus parenteral nutritions. Enteral feeding should be started in stable patients.

46. **Most common cause of death in ICU**: **Septic shock (**sepsis is manifested with fever, tachycardia, tachypnea, leukocytosis; shock is manifested with hypotension and MOSF).
SIRS (systemic inflammatory response syndrome): It is the most recent definition of sepsis which is body's inflammatory response in infections and noninfections (trauma, pancreatitis).

47. **Few important definitions of sepsis**:
    (a) **Sepsis:** The systemic response to infection which is manifested by the temperature (<36° or >38°), respiratory rate (>20 breaths/min. or $Paco_2$ <32 mm Hg), WBC (< 4000 or >12000 cells per cubic millimeter, or >10% band forms).
    (b) **Severe sepsis:** Sepsis plus organ dysfunction, hypotension, or hypoperfusion. It may be associated with lactic acidosis, alteration in mental status, or oliguria.
    (c) **Septic shock: Sepsis plus hypotension** despite adequate fluid therapies and hypoperfusion. It may include lactic acidosis, alteration of mental status, or oliguria.
    (d) **Hypotension:** Systolic BP<90 mm Hg or reduction >40 mm Hg from the baseline.
    (e) **MOSF (multiple organ system failure):** Actuely ill patients with altered organ function, **intervention is absolutely needed to maintain the homeostasis.**

48. **Important structural component of different organisms causing sepsis**:
    (a) Staphylococci: Teichoic acid antigens, TSST-1 (toxic shock syndrome toxin-1).
    (b) Gram-negative organisms: Endotoxins (lipopolysaccharides **LPS initiates the septic** shock pathogenetic cascade).
    (c) Pseudomonas aeruginosa: Toxin A.
    (d) Streptococcus pneumoniae: Polysaccharide capsule.
    (e) Candida albicans: Polysaccharides are present on surface.

49. **The following endogenous mediators are released by the monocytes, macrophages, neutrophils, endothelial cells, and plasma in sepsis**:
   (a) Cytokines (TNF, IL 1,2,6,8).
   (b) PAF (platelet activating factor).
   (c) EDRF (endothelial-derived ralaxing factor, N_2O).
   (d) Endorphins.
   (e) MDS (myocardial depressant substance).
   (f) Arachidonic acid metabolites (prostaglandins, leukotriens); **elevated thromboxane B_2, 6-keto PGF_1-alpha in sepsis.**
   (g) Complement (C_{5a}, C_{3a}).
   (h) Kinin.
   (i) Coagulation (Factor XII or Hageman factor).

50. **Acute phase of septic shock, the following parameters:**
   (a) **Decreased:** BP, CVP, SVR (systemic vascular resistance), EF (ejection fraction).
   (b) **Increased:** Left ventricular systolic and diastolic volume, heart rate, CO (cardiac output).
   (c) **No change**: Stroke volume.

51. **Calculation of ejection fraction (%)**: (LV- left ventricle).

$$\frac{\text{LV diastolic volume (ml)} - \text{LV systolic volume (ml)}}{\text{LV diastolic volume}}$$

Normal = (130-50)/130 = 80/130 = 60%.
Shock = 200-140/200 = 60/200 = 30% (decreased).

52. **Clinical presentation of septic shock**:
   (a) **First:** Signs and symptoms of primary focus of infection (UTI or pneumonia).
   (b) **Second:** sings and symptoms of systemic inflammatory response (**fever is the most common presentation with or without shaking chills,** remember that immunocompromised, elderly, or debilitated patients may be **hypothermic or normothermic);** ederly patients may present with altered mental status, tachypnea, and respiratory alkalosis in sepsis.
   (c) **Third:** Signs and symptoms of shock (low BP, MOSF, and lactic acidemia).

53. **Diagnosis and treatment for septic shock.**
   (A) **Diagnosis:**

(i) **Blood culture or culture from the site of infection:** It is the **most definitive diagnositc method,** but it is positive up to 60% cases due to intermittent bacteremia and prior antibiotic therapy.
(ii) Gram-stain of fluids (CSF), pus: It is extremely valuable for **early diagnosis and management.**

(B) **Treatment:**
(i) Infection: Appropriate antibiotics.
(ii) Abscess or empyema: Surgical drainage.
(iii) Hypotension: IV fluids and vasopressor drugs (to keep the mean arterial pressure 60 mm Hg and more, pulmonary artery wedge pressure 14-18 mm Hg).
(iv) Inadequate tissue perfusion: IV fluids, inotropic, and vasopressor durgs (to keep the cardiac index >2.2 L/min/m^2 in nonseptic shock and >4.0L/min/m^2 in septic shock, and normal lactate level).
(v) Hypoxemia: Oxygen to keep saturation >92%.
(vi) Anemia: Blood transfusion to keep hemoglobin level >10 g/dl.
(vii) Respiratory failure: Mechanical ventilator to keep normal ABG.
(viii) CNS, renal, and hepatic: Try to keep their functions normal.

54. Hyperthermic syndromes: Hyperthermia is T >37.2°C, heat injury syndromes begin when the T > 40°C (104°F).

(a) **Heat cramps:**
Signs and symptoms: Nausea, vomiting, fatigue, and muscle cramps.
Effects and Causes: Excessive losses of Nacl and H_2O are due to exposure and exertion in hot weather.

(b) **Heat exhaustion: It is the most common head injury syndrome found in athlets.**
Signs and symptoms: Same as heat cramps plus pallor, excessive sweating, postural hypotension, incoordination, and core temperatures of 37.5 to 39°c (99.5 to 102.2°F).
Effects and causes: Severe losses of Nacl and H_2O are due to exposure and exertion in hot humid weather. It may be preceeded by the heat cramps. In the elderly patients, it is due to inadequate cardiovascular response to heat.

(c) **Heat stroke** (Two types).
(i) **Exertional:** It is caused by working or exercising in warm environment due to disruption of thermoregulatory mechanism results in CNS depression, hypohydrosis, core T ≥41°c and severe physiologic and biochemical changes.
(ii) **Nonexertional:** It is mostly found in elderly, debilitated, intoxicated, paralyzed, or schizophrenic individuals due to impaired CNS and

peripheral thermoregulatory mechanisms, impaired awareness, or acclimatization, and poor cardiac output.

Signs and symptoms in both types: Rhabdomyolysis, acute renal failure, hypotension, vasodilatation, cardiac failure, arrythmias, ARDS, acute hepatic failure, and GI bleeding.

Laboratory findings:

(a) **Elevated:** K, phosphate, creatinine, WBC, hct (hemoconcentration), lactic acids, proteinuria, and urinary sediment.
(b) **Decreased:** Phosphate, platelets, glucose, and fluids.

Treatment for hyperthermic syndromes:

(a) **Most important is active cooling,** next is to remove from hot environment, and inhibition of thermogenesis.
(b) **In the emergency room: Continuous core temperature and ECG monitoring.**
(c) Airway, IV glucose, saline, or colloid solutions.
(d) **Hypotension: Fluids, small dose of isoproterenol in emergency situation;** if hypotension persists then put arterial and pulmonary catheters. Do **not** give alpha-agonist which impedes heat loss.
(e) Metabolic acidosis (pH <7.30): Sodium bicarbonate to keep the pH 7.30 and above.
(f) SVT is due to severe hyperthermia: **Cooling** can reverse SVT to normal sinus rhythm. **Do not give digoxin because high k causes heart block (Important).**
(g) **Phosphate: It should be given when** level is around 1 mg/dL.
(h) Do **not** use corticosteroids and antibiotics.

55. **Complications of neuroleptic medications: NMS (neuroleptic malignant syndrome)**. Patients appear with high core temperature, altered level of consciousness, elevated serum creatine kinase, and extrapyramidal muscular rigidity.

56. **Milignant hyperthermia: Signs and symptoms:** Abrupt rise in core temperature, metabolic and respiratory acidosis, ventricular arrythmias, and vigorous musle contractions.

    Cause and effects: Anesthesia. It is chemically or stress induced hypermetabolic myopathic syndrome.

57. Hypothermic syndromes: **Two types.**

    Hypothermia is T <35°C (95°F).

    (a) **Primary or accidental:** Due to cold environment.
    (b) **Secondary:** Dysfunction of hypothalamic thermoregulations.

Sings and symptoms:

(i) **Initial:** Tachypnea, tachycardia, increased BP, and increased cardiac output are due to increased catecholamine secretion.

(ii) **Subsequent:** Respiratory depression, bradycardia, decreased BP, decreased cardiac output, and hypoxia.

EKG findings: Sinus bradycardia, A-V block, prolonged QT interval, wide QRS, and inverted T-wave.

Laboratory findings: Metabolic acidosis (↓pH), low Na, high k, glucose, and phosphate.

Treatment:

(A) **Mild (34-36°C).**

- (i) **Prevent further heat loss (remove wet/cold clothing), increase core temperature (blankets), and prevent complications.**
- (ii) CPR in patients without vital signs.
- (iii) **Warm oxygen for hypoxia.**
- (iv) **Warm IV dextrose and saline.**
- (v) **Warm environment (overhead lights, thermostat).**

(B) **Moderate to severe (≤ 33°C):**

- (i) **Admit to ICU.**
- (ii) **Peripheral rewarming:** Heating blankets and pads, hot water bottles, and heated lights.
- (iii) **Central core rewarming:** Inhalation of heated, humidified oxygen, warmed IV fluids, gastic lavage, and colonic irrigations.
- (iv) Avoid pressure necrosis by providing special beds.
- (v) **Tempereture should rise 0.5 to 1.0°C/hour,** if **not** then may consider pertoneal dialysis, hemodialysis, bypass, or bladder lavage.
- (vi) **Antibiotics: For secondary infection which is a common complication.**
- (vii) **MOSF:** Treat accordingly.

58. **Complications of hypothermia.**

- (i) **Infections.**
- (ii) **Rhabdomyolysis.**
- (iii) GI: Upper GI bleeding, gastric dilatations, and ileus.
- (iv) Liver: Severe hepatic dysfunctions.
- (v) Pancreas: Acute pancreatitis.
- (vi) Hematologic: Low WBC and platelets, hemoconcentrations, and increased blood viscosity.

59. **Most common cause of death due to poisoning in USA: Carbon monoxide,** other important causes are analgesics, cocaine, and TCA (tricyclic antidepressants).

60. **Most common causes of death from cardiovascular drug in USA.** **Calcium channel blocker,** next is digitalis.

61. **Most barbiturates are metabolized by the liver except:** Phenobarbital is excreted unchanged by the **kidneys.**

62. **Characteristic of barbiturate poisoning: Bullous skin lesions and persistence of pupillary light reflex even in stage IV coma.**

63. **Characteristic of anticholinergic poisoning: Psychosis, seizures, hyperpyrexia, dilated pupils,** dry skin, dry mucous membrance, flushing, and urinary retention.
    Treatment: Physostigmine is used in only severe case of pure anticholnergic poisoning. Remember, it should **not** be used in poisoning of cyclic antidepressants because of their anticholenergic properties.

64. **Characteristics of poisoning with calcium channel blocker** (e.g., nifedipine, diltiazem, verapamil, and amlodipine): Hypotension, bradycardia, pulmonary edema, cardiac arrest, A-V block (mostly in verapamil), and coma.
    Treatment:
    (i) **IV calcium is the drug of choice.**
    (ii) If no response, use dopamine, dobutamine, amrinone, and epinephrine.
    (iii) **Pacing** may be used in verapamil overdose.
    (iv) **Glucagon** is used for associated beta-blocker overdose.

65. **Characteristics of carbon monoxide poisoning:**
    (a) CNS: Headache, altered mental status, and convulsion.
    (b) Cardiac: Arrythmia, myocardial infarctions, and chest pain.
    Treatment:
    (i) Oxygen (100%).
    (ii) Hyperbaric oxygen.
    Detection of extent of poisoning:
    (i) Carboxyhemoglobin is **unreliable** because most patients receive oxygen on the way to ER.
    (ii) Level of coma indicates neurophychiatric outcome.

66. **Most common cause of insecticide poisoning: Organophosphate.** It is a irreversible acetylcholinesterase inhibitor.
Signs and symptoms:
(i) **Initial: Flulike syndrome (abdominal pain, vomiting, headache, dizziness).**
(ii) **Around 24 hours after poisoning:**
CNS: Confusion, convulsion, psychosis, coma, fasciculation, weakness, or paralysis of the muscles.
Lungs: Dyspnea, pulmonary edema, and cyanosis.
Pancreas: Sometime pancreatitis.
Heart: Ventricular tachycardia (outside USA).
Treatment:
(a) **IV pralidoxime: Specific antidote, it is the treatment of choice.**
(b) Atropine: Physiologic antidote, it reverses muscarinic effect and reduces pulmonary secretion.
(c) Establish airway, breathing, and ventilatory support PRN.
(d) Removal of clothes.
(e) Decontamination of skin prn.

67. **Treatment of choice for carbamate insecticides**: **Atropine.**
Signs and symptoms: It is **benign and mimic milder form of** organophosphate poisoning but **no** CNS effects.

68. **Most commonly involved organ in paraquat toxicity: Lungs.**
Signs and symptoms:
(i) Lungs: Pulmonary edema, fibrosis, and **hypoxia (which causes death)** because it **reduces O_2 to Superoxide free radicals.**
(ii) Esophagus: Perforation and esophagitis after ingestion.
Treatment:
(a) Do **not** give oxygen unless absolutely needed.
(b) Gastric lavage as soon as possible.
(c) Fuller's earth (15% solution) or bentonite (7% solution) is to absorb paraquat (soil or clay with water at home).
(d) Activated charcoal or kayexalate may be used.

69. **Most common cause of death from prescription drug in USA: TCA (tricyclic antidepressant)**.

70. **TCA toxicities:**
(a) Signs and symptoms:

(i) **CVS: Cardiac arrythmias (most common is ventricular tachycardia), hypotension.**
(ii) **CNS:** Seizures, coma.
(iii) **EKG: Prolonged QRS complex is the most characteristic in TCA toxicities.**

(b) Treatment:
(i) **IV $NaHCO_3$: Treatment of choice.** It reduces cardiac arrythmias and hypotension by keeping blood pH 7.50.
(ii) Airway, breathing, ventilation, and oxygen.
(iii) IV fluids (must avoid pulmonary edema).
(iv) **Phenytoin:** It can **reverse** prolonged QRS complex but **it is used for convulsion.** It can be used **prophylactically in amoxapine overdose to avoid seizures.**
(v) **Seizures:** Diazepam, pentobarbital, pancuronium bromide, and phenytoin.
(vi) Remember, do **not** use physostigmine.

71. **Theophylline toxicities**:
First sign: Tachycardia.
First symptom: Vomiting.
Other signs and symptoms:
(i) CNS: Seizures.
(ii) Heart: Arrythmias, CVS Collapse.
(iii) Lungs: Respiratory arrest.
Loboratory findings: Metabolic acidosis, low k, and high glucose.
Treatment.
(i) **In severe toxicity: Chracoal or hemoperfusion is the treatment of choice.**
(ii) Discontinue theophylline, supportive care, and cardiac monitoring.
(iii) Propranolol: For cardiac arrythmias.
(iv) Diazepam: To control seizures.
(v) Give k, $NaHCO_3$, and fluids: To correct the imbalance of fluids and electrolytes.

72. **Ethylene glycol toxicites:** It causes metabolic acidosis due to aldehyde, glycolate, and lactate formations and deposition of oxalate crystals into heart, lungs, and kidneys.
(i) Early: Seizure, altered mental status, low calcium.
(ii) 12 hours after ingestion: Congestive cardiac failure.
(iii) 24 - 72 hours after ingestion: Renal failure.
Treatment:

(a) Gastric lavage STAT, ethonol infusion.
(b) Sodium bicarbonate, $cacl_2$.
(c) Hemodialysis.

73. **Methanol toxicities**:
Signs and symptoms:
(i) Eye: Diplopia, photophobia, blurred vision, sensation of "in a snowstorm" blindness.
(ii) CNS: Altered mental status, seizure, coma.
(iii) GI: Abdominal pain, pancreatitis.
Treatment:
(a) IV ethanol infusion.
(b) $NaHCO_3$ for metabolic acidosis.
(c) Hemodialysis: It is indicated when serum methanol level >50 mg/dL, severe metabolic acidosis, or visual disturbance. It removes methanol and its metabolites (formaldehyde, formic acids).

74. **Isopropanol or rubbing alcohol toxicities:**
Signs and symptoms: Same as ethanol ingestion.
Treatment: Supportive management only; rarely hemodialysis is needed.
Metabolism: Partly metabolized to acetone.

75. **Lithium toxicities.**
Signs and symptoms:
(i) CNS: Ataxia, altered mental status, parkinsonism.
(ii) CVS: Low BP, myocarditis, arrythmias.
(iii) Renal: Nephrogenic diabetes insipidus, renal failure.
Treatment:
(a) **Hemodialysis: It is the treatment of choice because** it is highly dialyzable toxin.
(b) Stop lithium, do gastric lavage.
(c) IV fluids and electrolytes.

76. **Iron toxicities.**
Signs and symptoms.
(i) GI bleeding, vomiting, abdominal pain.
(ii) After that a **quiescent phase is noted.**
(iii) Then progress to metabolic acidosis, shock, liver failure, and death.
Laboratory findings: High glucose and WBC counts.
Abdominal X-ray: Radiopaque tablets are visible.
Treatment:

(a) **Deferoxamine: It is the treatment of choice.**
(b) Gastric lavage and $NaHCO_3$.

77. **Most common cause of death from illicit drug abuse in USA: Cocaine.**
Signs and symptoms:
(i) CVS: Chest pain, palpitation, arrythmia, high BP, myocardial infarction, cardiac arrest.
(ii) CNS: Altered mental status, ischemic stroke, focal neurologic signs.
Seizures which progress to status epilepticus.
(iii) Psychophysiologic: Violent behavior, suicide attempt.
Urine metabolites: Benzoylecgonine, ecgonine methyl ester.
Treatment:
(a) Supprotive care, cardiac monitoring.
(b) IV labetalol (alpha and beta-blocker) for CVS presentations.
(c) **Nitrates and/or calcium channel blockers** are used for angina.
(d) **Thrombolytic therapy for acute MI.**
(e) **Grandmal seizures may progress to status** epilepticus: Anticonvulsants (e.g., benzodiazepines, phenytoin, phenobarbital) may **not** control the seizures. **It is better to treat with pancuronium bromide and pentobarbital or thiopental to produce coma.**
(f) $NaHCO_3$ for metabolic acidosis.
(g) Treat rhabdomyolysis if present.

78. **Benodiazepines toxicities**:
Signs and symptoms: Ataxia, coma.
Treatment: Flumazenil: It is used **only in hospital overdose cases.** Remember it can cause **seizures** in patients coingested TCA with benzodiazepines, or **increased ICP** in head-injury patients.

79. **Most leading analgesic drug overdose in USA**: **Salicylates (aspirin), next is acetaminophen** (e.g., tylenol, tempra, panadol).

80. **Acetaminophen toxicities (toxic dose is about 10 grams in adult):**
Signs and symptoms.
(i) 12 to 24 hours after ingestion: Nausea, vomiting.
(ii) 48 to 96 hours after ingestion: Coagulopathy, hepatic coma.
Treatment:
(i) Mucomyst or N- Acetylcysteine is the drug of choice.

81. Salicylates toxicities: (Mild toxic level is >30 mg/dL, severe toxic level is 80 to 100 mg/dL).

Signs and symptoms:

(i) **Mild to moderate: Hearing loss, hyperpyrexia, hyperventilation, diaphoresis, facial flushing.**

(ii) **Severe toxicity: GI bleeding, purpura, hypernatremia, dehydration, pulmonary edema, death.**

Treatment.

(a) **Forced alkaline diuresis with $NaHCO_3$.**

(b) IV fluids and electrolytes.

(c) Vitamin K.

(d) **Hemodialysis:** It is done in critical patients, serum level >100 mg/dL, unresponsive to $NaHCO_3$ therapy.

82. **Ibuprofen toxicities**:

Signs and symptoms: Mild gastroenteritis.

Treatment: Stop the drug and supportive care only.

83. **Emergency management in the patients with coma due to drug overdose**:

(a) Airway, ventilation, perfusion.

(b) Continue cardiac and pulse oximetry monitoring.

(c) **IV Naloxome 2 mg, thiamine 100 mg, and 50% glucose 50cc (in hypoglycemic patients**) should be given after the insertion of IV and drawing of the blood samples.

(d) Volume replacement, correct metabolic acidosis.

(e) Antidotal therapies.

(f) Treat seizures and cardiac arrythmias.

84. **Caustic alkali, acids, and other chemicals are exposed to the eyes and management**:

(a) Irrigation **with normal saline** (at least 30 min for alkali exposure).

(b) Opthalmologic consult STAT.

85. **Few important physical examination findings in drug abuse**:

(a) Cocaine: Destruction of nasal mucosa and cartilage.

(b) Heroin: Pulmonary edema.

(c) IV drug abuse: Needle tracks.

(d) Organophosphate: Changes in neurologic status.

(e) Gasoline: Odor of gasoline in breath.

(f) Spider bite (black widow): Boardlike abdomen.

86. **Most common cause of cyanide poisoning: Smoke inhalations.**

Signs and symptoms: seizures, shock, lactic acidosis due to hypoxia, cardiorespiratory failure.
Treatment: Specific antidote **amyl nitrate then sodium nitrite.**

87. **Digitalis toxicities:**
Signs and symptoms: Sinus bradycardia, yellow or blurred vision, vomiting.
Treatment: Digibind (digoxin-specific FAB antibodies) is a specific antidote.

88. **Hallucinogens (LSD, PCP, mushroom, mescaline) toxicities:** LSD is **not** addictive and it causes "**flashbacks**". PCP (**phencyclidine)** is known as '**Angel dust'**. **PCP overdose: Hypertensive crisis, nystagmus, heperpyrexia, sensory anesthesia,** seizures and respiratory arrest.
Treatment of hallucinogens overdose:
(a) Quiet room, talking down the patients.
(b) Sedation: Benzodiazepines.
(c) Prolonged toxic psychosis: Haloperidol.
(d) **Do not give** ascorbic acid to enhance PCP excretion because it can cause renal failure when rhabdomyolsis is present.

89. **Few important antidotes in toxicities.**
(a) Digitalis: Digibind FAB antibodies.
(b) TCA: $NaHCO_3$.
(c) Organophosphate: Pralidoxime, atropine.
(d) Opiates, darvon, lomotil: Naloxone.
(e) Carbon monoxide: Oxygen.
(f) Atropine: Physostigmine.
(g) Acetaminophen: N- Acetylcysteine.
(h) Calcium channel blockers: Calcium chloride.
(i) Benzodiazepines: Flumazenil.
(j) Beta-blocker: Glucagon.
(k) Cyanide: Amyl nitrate, then sodium nitrite.
(l) Methyl or ethyl alcohol: Ethyl alcohol with dialysis.
(m) Nitrites: Methylene blue.

NEUROLOGY

1. **Contraindications of lumbar puncture**:
   (a) Increased intracranial pressure (mass or obstructive hydrocephalus).
   (b) Bleeding disorders.
   (c) Localized skin or epidural infections.

2. **Preferred investigations of choice in different CNS disease**:
   (A) **MRI plus Gd (gadolinium enhancement).**
      (i) **Spine:** Postoperative disc diseases, **AVM of the spinal cord (or MRI alone).**
      (ii) **Brain.**
         (a) Posterior fossa: Meningioma.
         (b) Tumors: **Gliomas, lymphomas, meaningiomas, metastases.**
         (c) Others: Abscess, empyema, acute and chronic meningitis, sarcoidosis, multiple sclerosis (or MRI only), AIDS, postoperative and radiation treatment.
   (B) **MRI only:**
      (i) **Spine: Degenerative disc disease, metastatic diseases in spine, AVM of the spinal cord (or MRI plus Gd), trauma (or CT scan).**
      (ii) Brain:
         (a) **Posterior fossa**: Acoustic neurinoma, cholesterol granuloma, intra-axial gliomas, epidermoids, craniovertebral junction, and basilar artery aneurysm.
         (b) **Tumors:** Hamatomas, sellar tumors.
         (c) **Others: AVM, aneurysm, infarction, head trauma (or CT only), multiple sclerosis (or MRI plus Gd), congenital anomalies, hydrocephalus, and cerebral atrophy.**
   (C) **CT plus C (contrast enhancement):**
      (i) Spine: None. It is a second choice in postoperative disc disease when MRI is **not** available.
      (ii) **Brain.**
         (a) **Posterior fossa: None.** It is a second choice in meningioma when MRI is **not** available.
         (b) **Tumor:** None. It is the **second choice** in gliomas, lymphomas, meningiomsa, and metastases when MRI is **not** available.
         (c) **Others:** None. It is the second choice in AIDS when MRI is **not** available So, it is **not** the best diagnostic method when MRI is available or **only CT scan should be done.**
   (D) **CT scan only:**

(i) **Spine: Trauma (or MRI only).** It is the **second** choice in degenerative disc disease when MRI is **not** available.

(ii) Brain:

(a) Posterior fossa: None.

(b) Tumors: None. It is the second choice in hematomas when MRI is not available.

(c) **Others: It is the best diagnostic method in subarachnoid hemorrhages and acute stroke or infarction. It is also the best diagnositc method in head trauma or parenchymal intracranial injury (or MRI only).**

3. **Best diagnostic methods for head trauma:**

(a) First 48 hours: CT scan.

(b) After 48 hours: **MRI is superior** than CT scan to detect cerebral contusions, axonal shearing injuries, and small bleeding.

4. **Best diagnostic methods for stroke or cerebral infarcts**:

(a) **First 24 hours:** CT scan may remain **normal** but **MRI shows hyperintensity in the infarct area. MRI is the best method but CT scan is the most frequently used study.**

(b) **Old infarcts: MRI and CT scan are equally good.**

(c) Elderly patients with high BP, atherosclerosis: MRI shows hyperintensities when CT is normal.

(d) Patients with vasculitis or SLE: **MRI shows hyperintensities** when CT is normal.

5. **Best diagnostic method in AVM and aneurysms**:

(a) **MRI is superior to CT because MRI can** detect **aneurysm as small as 3 mm** and surrounding bleeding.

(b) Subarachniod hemorrhage: CT scan is the best method. Remember, in suspicious cases subarachnoid hemorrhage **should not be excluded unless CSF is normal.**

6. **Best diagnostic methods for metastases, gliomas, lymphomas, and meningiomas.**

MRI plus Gd.

7. Patients with AIDS may have brain lymphoma and toxoplasma granulomas simultaneously, MRI **cannot** distinguish those two lesions but it can be distinguished by:

(a) Rising toxoplasma IgG progressively in toxoplasmosis.

(b) Response of the lesions with anti-Toxoplasma therapy.

8. **Best diagnostic postoperative follow-up studies for evaluation of tumor recurrence or radiation necrosis:**
   (a) **MRI plus Gd or CT plus C.**
   (b) Chronic postradiation **demyelenation of the white mater: MRI plus Gd is better** than CT plus C.
   (c) To distinguish radiation necrosis from tumor recurrence:
   PET (positron emission tomography) to measure metabolic rate.
   (i) Hypoactivity: Radiation necrosis.
   (ii) Hyperactivity: Recurrent tumors.

9. **Best diagnositc study in multiple sclerosis and white mater disease: MRI. MRI plus Gd can differentiate from active lesions from old healed lesions**.

10. **Best diagnostic method for hydrocephalus, cerebral atrophy, sellar tumors, congenital** anomalies of CNS, **posterior fossa lesions and tumors: MRI.**

11. **Best diagnostic method** for acoustic neurinoma, cholesterol granuloma, intra-axial gliomas, epidermoids, craniovertebral junction, basilar artery aneurysms, arachnoid cyst: **MRI**.

12. **Best diagnostic method for trauma to the spine.**
    (a) **First conventional X-ray to rule out fractures or dislocations.**
    (b) **CT scan** can detect fractures of the neural arch, articular facets, transverse fracture of the vertebral bodies, and post traumatic herniated disc.
    (c) **Patients with clinical evidence of spinal cord injury: MRI is done** tc detect hematomyelia or epidural hematoma.

13. **Best diagnostic method for degenerative disc disease, demyelenating disorder, hydromyelia, and primary tumors of the spinal cord: MRI.**

14. **Best diagnostic study to distinguish between postoperative scarring and recurrent disc prolapse in degenerative disc dieases: MRI plus Gd.**

15. **Best diagnostic study is to distinguish between** intramedullary cyst (gliomas, ependymomas) and hyromyelia:
    MRI plus Gd because MRI may look identical.

16. **Best diagnostic method for AVM:**

(a) Large size: MRI or MRA.
(b) Small size: Myelography may be needed.

17. **Complication of very rapid correction of hyponatremia in patients with coma**:
Central pontine myelinolysis.

18. **Complication of using naloxone in coma patients of unknown cause**:
Withdrawal symptoms if the patients are drug addict.

19. **Position of the patients in coma**: **Semiprone in the drainage position and change side to side. Never put them in fully supine position which can cause aspiration.**

20. **Best outcome in coma patients are due to**: **Depressant drug poisoning.** Patients usually recover completely with appropriate medical care.

21. **Pupillary reactions in different causes of coma**:
(a) **Metabolic: Normal and symmetric pupillary response to light except** in rare cases of poisoning with drugs having anticholinergic effects which can transiently paralyze the puplis.
(b) **Structural brain disease:** Pupil are **mostly asymmetric**, sometimes fixed to light response.

22. **Few important points in outcome of patients with coma**:
(a) **Persistence of coma more than 4 weeks almost never associated with complete recovery.**
(b) Duration of coma is **directly proportional** to the permanent disability.
(c) **Coma due to trauma have better outcome than coma due to medical illness (but 50%** patients die with traumatic coma due to head injury).
(d) Younger patients have better prognosis than older patients in traumatic coma.
(e) **Drugs induced coma have the best prognosis and complete recovery.**
(f) Medical illness causing coma **lasting more than few hours** have the poor prognosis, only 15% regain the pre-illness health status.
(g) **Earliest accurate prediction of neurological recovery can be made in 66% of patients by the end of the first day (24 hours).** Patients who are awake, normal neuro-opthalmologic examinations, and speaking few words. They have 70% chances of good outcome.
(h) **On day three:** Patients with normal corneal reflex, speak few words, and move. They have 74% chances of good outcome.

(i) **On day seven:** Patients with open eyes, speak words, and make localized motor response. They have 99% chances of good outcome.

23. **Six-hour observation of absence of brain function is sufficient to declare brain death except**:
Drug or alcohol which needs 12 hour absence of brain function and negative drug or alcohol screen.

24. **Most common cause of BLOC (brief loss of consciousness)**: **Syncope** which is defined as temporary reduction of cerebral blood flow. **It is due to brief dysfunction of vasodepressor cardiovascular reflexes** in majority of the cases.

25. **Most common cause of BLOC in patients over age 50 without any cardiac, neurologic, or systemic illness**: **Benign syncope.** Remember that **24 hours ECG monitoring is recommended** in those cases, because 20% patients may have undiagnosed underlying cardiac disorders.

26. **Most common causes in different brain tumors:**
    (a) **Metastatic: Most common primary site of origin are lungs;** other sources are breast, melanoma, colorectal, and kidneys.
    (b) **Primary extra-axial (not originates from brain but from meninges, cranial nerves, and surrounding structures): Most common is meningioma, other tumors are acoustic neuroma and pituitary adenoma.**
    (c) Primary intra-axial: (**Originate from the brain): Most common is glioblastoma;** other tumor are anaplastic astrocytoma and astrocytoma.

27. **Symptoms and signs of brain tumors:**
    (a) **Increased intracranial pressures:** Headaches, vomiting, lethargy, and confusion.
    (b) **Focal brain dysfunction:** Focal seizures, cranial nerve palsies, hemianopia, and hemiparesis.

28. **Diagnosis and treatment of brain tumors**.
Diagnosis:
    (a) **MRI is the best method,** next is CT scan. **MRI plus Gd (T_1) is the most precise method to diagnose brain tumors.** Remember Gd (T_2) images are useful to detect the extent of edema and post radiation demyelenation of the white matter.

(b) **MR-guided stereotaxic biposy is the best method, bleeding is the complication (2% of cases). Open brain biopsy should not be done.**

Treatment:

(a) **First consideration is surgical removal of the tumor except multiple metastases. Single metastatic lesion can be removed surgically, it is the best treatment choice.**

(b) Small meningiomas or acoustic neuromas: No treatment is needed to reduce ICP. **Surgery is the treatment of choice.**

(c) **Dexamethasone:** It reduces the ICP and edema of the brain tissue. It is the steroid of choice.

(d) **Mannitol:** It is used in severe elevation of ICP to reduces the pressure rapidly.

(e) Intubated patients with high ICP: Try to keep **$Paco_2$ around 25 mm Hg to** reduce cerebral circulation and edema.

(f) **Seizures** (20% of all cases of tumors): **Phenytoin is the drug of choice** because it can be given IV or orally (carbamazepine or valproic acid is given only orally).

(g) **All supratentorial tumors should be treated with anticonvulsant before surgery even in patients without seizures (Important).** It is **not** needed in posterior fossa tumors or acoustic neuromas because of **low probability of seizures.**

(h) Surgical managements are the following:

(i) **The complete excision is the ultimate goal of treatment. The combination** of neurosurgical anesthesia, the capacity to control ICP, and **laser surgery helps in radial resection.**

(ii) **No surgery:** Please remember that intra-axial tumors (gliomas) **cannot** be even resected partially because they invade **indispensable** areas of the brain. **Radiotherapy is the best treatment of choice.**

(iii) **Dexamethasone** should be given for at least 5 days after surgery to reduce cerebral edema.

(iv) Anticonvulsant (phenytoin): Monitor blood level to avoid postoperative convulsions.

29. **The greatest surgical risk of brain tumors**:

(a) Impaired neurologic function and postoperative neurological deficit.

(b) Deep leg vein thrombophlebitis leading to pulmonary embolisms: Avoided by the use of compression boots and early passive exercises.

(c) Seizures: Maintain phenytoin serum levels.

30. **Radiation therapies of brain tumors**:

(a) External beam radiation: It is used in malignant gliomas and metastatic brain tumors. It is **not curative in multiple metastatic brain tumors but it is the treatment of choice.**
(b) Radiotherapy is **not** effective: Recurrent meningiomas and acoustic meuromas. Reoperation is the best therapy.
(c) **Primary brain lymphomas:** It is highly responsive to radiotherapy, combination with chemotherapy are the best treatment of choice.

31. **Most common complication of radiotherapy in brain tumors**:
(a) Dementia: It is less in localized radiation than whole brain radiation.
(b) Impaired mobility.
Remember, most patients with brain tumors on radiotherapy **die before the presentation of brain injury.**

32. **Chemotherapy of brain tumors:**
(a) **It is not very effective in brain tumors** because of inadequate delivery of drugs, inherent resistence, and heterogeneity of the tumor cells.
(b) **Primary brain lymphomas: The best treatment of choice are the chemotherapy plus radiotherapy** than radiotherapy alone.
(c) **Malignant astrocytomas:** The best and most effective treatment of choice are the **combination** of procarbazine, vincristine, and CCNU (cyclohexylchloroethylnitrosourea). They are probably better than BCNU (biscloroethylnitrosurea) alone. **BCNU is the best single drug of choice and most frequently used.**
(d) **Rarely,** chemotherapy is effective in **gliomas (primary brain tumors): The best treatment of choice is radiotherapy.**

33. **Single or multiple brain metastases**:
(a) **Single metastasis:** Non-small cell carcinoma of the lung and renal cancer.
(b) **Multiple metastases:** Small cell carcinoma of the lung, breast cancer, and melanomas.
Remember, multiple metastases are more common than single metastasis.

34. **Most common cause of death in patients with** systemic illness and brain metastases: **Systemic illness is the most common cause of death (not** the brain metastases).

35. **The treatment for different types of brain tumors:**
(a) Single metastasis: Surgery.
(b) Multiple metastases: Radiation therapy.
(c) Few metastases and stable patients: Surgery may be attmpted.

(d) Meningeal carcinomatosis: **Radiation therapy to the brain and spinal cord. It rarely** gives long remission. Patients with limited systemic metastases, **intrathecal chemotherapy with methotrexate** through an Ommaya reservior may be appropriate.

Future therapy: Isotope emitting radionuclides coupled to monoclonal antibodies.

(e) Pituitary adenomas:
  (i) Surgical removal is the best treatment.
  (ii) Inadequate surgical removal or large tumor: Radiotherapy.
  (iii) Medical: Bromocriptine life long therapy is **not** very effective.

(f) Adult craniopharyngioma (benign): Surgical removal.

(g) Small meningiomas and acoustic neuromas: Surgery.

(h) Arachnoid cyst (slow growing, asymptomatic patients): No treatment is needed.

(i) Oligodendrogliomas:
  (i) **Complete surgical excision** is the treatment of choice.
  (ii) Chemotherapy: Combination of procarbazine, vincristine, and CCNU.

(j) Medulloblastomas:
  (i) Surgery and radiation therapy.
  (ii) Chemotherapy: Cyclophosphamide and vincristine.

(k) Primary brain lymphomas: **(Unresectable tumor).**
  (i) Dexamethasone.
  (ii) Multidrugs chemotherapy, radiotherapy.

36. Meningiomas and chromosomal association: Loss of a portion of chromosome 22 (same as neurofibromatosis type 2).

37. All patients who **develop hearing loss in the** middle years of life, most likely diagnosis: **Acoustic neuromas.**

Best diagnostic physiologic method:

(a) Auditory evoked response (remember, audiometry is **not** diagnostic and caloric test of labyrinthine function is always abnormal).

(b) MRI can detect even a very small tumor.

Treatment: Microsurgery.

38. **Few important points in acoustic neuroma.**

(a) It is a growth of Schwann cells of the VIII cranial nerve, **unilateral, not familial.**

(b) **Bilateral acoustic neuromas is diagnostic of neurofibromatosis type 2.** It is **rare, familial, autosomal dominant, gene deletion on chromosome 22, and almost 100% penetrance in successive generations (Important).**

39. **Early symptoms of pituitary adenomas: Nonspecific headache,** other presentations are hypothyroidisms, infertility, acromegaly, amenorrhea, galactorrhea, or Cushing's syndorme.
   Remember, it produces **bitemporal visual field defects** due to compression on the optic nerve.
   (a) **Preferred diagnostic methods:** MRI plus hormonal studies.
   (b) **Treatment**: Surgical removal is the best therapy; bromocriptine is less effective occasional radiotherapy for large or incompletely removed tumor.

40. **Pituitary apoplexy:** It is due to hemorrhage in the large pituitary tumor.
   Sings and symptoms: Sudden onset of headache, unilateral blindness, and partial opthalmoplegia.
   Preferred diagnostic method: MRI.
   Treatment: Emergency surgical decompression.

41. **Presentations of pineal tumors (true- pineocytomas, pineoblastomas; or teratomas, germinomas)**: Patients appear with increased ICP, pupillary dysfunction, paresis of upward gaze, convergence nystagmus, and hydrocephalus. **Germinomas cause precocious puberty in male** due to destruction of pineal glands. **True pineal tumors cause delayed puberty.**
   Treatment: Surgery but still difficult to control.

42. **Most common gliomas of the brain**: **Astrocytomas.**
   Remember, it **can occur as a late result of radiation to the head or skull.**

43. **Most malignant form of astrocytomas: Glioblastoma multiforme (or astrocytoma type IV). It is the most common form of primary brain tumor (>50 % of cases).** Astrocytoma type III or anaplastic astrocytoma is **less** malignant variety.
   Treatment of glioblastoma: Surgery, radiation, and chemotherapy.

44. **Signs and symptoms of glioblastomas and anaplastic astrocytomas**: Both have **similar clinical presentations** which includes **seizures, focal neurologic deficitis, and headaches.**
   Diagnostic study: CT and MRI studies are alike in those two conditions. Chromosomal relation with glioblastomas and anaplastic astrocytomas.
   (a) Glioblastoma: **Chromosome 10 is characteristic, rarely 17.**
   (b) Anaplastic astrocytomas: **Chromosome 17 (mutation of tumor suppressor gene, p53).**

45. **Most benign tumor of all the gliomas: Oligodendrogliomas.**
Signs and symptoms: Same as low-grade astrocytomas, seizures are the early symptoms.
Location: Cerebral hemispheres especially in the **frontal lobe.**
Diagnosis: MRI or CT scan, many have flecks of calcium.
Treatment:
(a) **Complete surgical excision is the treatment of choice.**
(b) Chemotherapy: Combination of procarbazine, vincristine, and CCNU is better than radiotherapy alone.
Complications:
(a) It can **bleed spontaneously.**
(b) Anaplastic oligodendrogliomas can spread **through spinal fluid to the meninges.**

46. **Chromosomal abnormality and medulloblastoma: Chromosome 17.** It occurs in 4th ventricle, **mostly in young adults.**
Signs and symptoms: Cerebellar and brain stem dysfunctions.
Treatment:
(i) Surgery and radiation therapy.
(ii) Chemotherapy: Cyclophosphamide and vincristine.

47. **Brain tumor is associated with tuberous sclerosis**: **Gangliogliomas.** It is a **slow growing tumor,** found in young adults, and occurs in **temporal lobe.**
Prognosis: Good even when it is untreated.

48. **Most common extranodal site of involvement in primary brain lymphomas**: **Eye.** Lymphomas are found in both AIDS and non-AIDS patients. It diffusely affects the brain and **rarely develops systemic lymphomas.**
Treatment: (This tumor cannot be resected).
(i) Dexamethasone.
(ii) Multidrugs chemotherapy, radiotherapy.

49. **To differentiate between abscesses and granulomas of the brain**:
(a) Remember, CT or MRI **cannot** differentiate these two conditions.
(b) Clinical presentation may differentiate the conditions.
(c) **Biopsy should be done** when clinical presentation **cannot** distinguish. **It is the most confirmatory diagnostic procedure because mistake could be detrimental in patients management.**

50. **Most common presentation of vascular malformations**: **Seizures**.

Diagnosis.

(a) Large-caliber vessels: CT or MRI.

(b) Small-caliber vessels: **Angiography** because CT or MRI findings may look like tumor, so an **attempt to do biopsy will be devastating.**

(c) Some capillary variety: May be missed even by angiography.

51. **Brain tumor produces erythropoietin and may cause polycythemia**: **Capillary hemangioblastomas.** It may be associated with retinal angiomatosis and cyst or tumors of kidneys, pancreas, and adrenals (von Hippel syndrome).

52. **Lumber CSF pressure may be normal or low with elevated ICP (CSF presssure >250 mm indicates serious neurologic disease)**: **Brain herniation and intracranial mass lesions.** (Lumbar pressure does **not** always accurately reflect ICP).

53. **Most common signs and symptoms of elevated ICP**:

(a) Symptoms: Most common headache, others are vomiting, diplopia, and tinnitus.

(b) Signs: **Papilledema** (it may be **absent** in the elderly) **is most common,** others are loss of vision, psychomotor retardation.

Remember, patients may be **asymptomatic in elevated ICP without shift.**

Treatment:

(i) Initial (impending herniation, to reduce the intracranial volume): Hyperventilation (keep $Paco_2$ 25 to 30 mm Hg) STAT then mannitol, and dexamethasone.

(ii) Definitive: To treat the underlying pathological conditions.

54. **Pseudopapilledema (anomalous elevation of the optic disc due to hyaline bodies)**: It is found in **retinitis pigmentosa.**

55. An elderly obese woman came to the ER with H/O headaches, vomiting, diplopia, visual loss, vertigo, and tinnitus for last few days.

Physical examination: It shows **bilateral papilledema (always present),** mild retinal hemorrhage plus exudate, diplopia (VI cranial nerve palsy, **false localizing sign).** The rest of the neurological examinations are normal.

Investigations:

(a) CT or MRI: Normal (abnormal in tumor, abscesses).

(b) MRA: Normal (abnormal in dural sinus thrombosis).

(c) Lumber CSF: Pressure is elevated (>300 mm) but **cell counts, glucose, and protein are normal**.

Most likely diagnosis: **Benign intracranial hypertension.**

Etiology: Unknown in most of the cases.

Treatment:

(i) **Medical:** Corticosteroids and diuretics are the mainstay of therapy.

(ii) Large volume lumbar tap (alternate day) may be effective.

(iii) **Papilledema: Incision of the optic nerve sheath is the treatment of choice.**

Remember, **high rate of spontaneous remission** also occurs without treatment.

56. **Drugs causing benign intracranial hypertension.**
    (a) Vitamin A.
    (b) Oral contraceptives.
    (c) Steroid therapy/ withdrawal.
    (d) Phenytoin.
    (e) Tetracycline, sulfonamides.
    (f) Nalidixic acid.
    (g) Nitrofurantoin.

57. **CSF pressure and hyrocephalus**:
    (a) Acute hydrocephalus: Increased.
    (b) Chronic hydrocephalus: Normal or low.
58. **Most common cause of acute and chronic hydrocephalus**:
    (a) **Acute:** Ventricular outflow obstruction (hemorrhage/infarction, trauma, tumor, subarachnoid bleeding, meningitis, encephalitis).
    (b) **Chronic: Aqueductal stenosis is the most common** complication of subarachnoid bleeding.

59. **Presentation, diagnosis, and treatment of hydrocephalus**:
    (a) Clinical presentations:
        (i) **Acute: Severe headaches, vomiting, lethargy, papilledema, VI cranial nerve palsy,** bilateral extensor planter response, hyperactive reflexes, and **elevated** ventricular CSF pressure.
        (ii) **Chronic: Dementia, unsteady gait,** urinary incontinence, psychomotor retardation, bilateral pyramidal and extrapyramidal signs, and **normal** CSF pressure.
    (b) **Best diagnostic study: MRI**.
    (c) **Treatment**:
        (i) Acute: To treat the **primary lesion is the treatment of** choice; ventricular drainage and CSF diversion are very improtant.
        (ii) **Chronic: Ventricular shunting.**

60. Patients appear with H/O severe throbbing, frontal, and occipital headaches **in erect posture but resolves completeley when lying flat. Patients also complain of photophobia, stiffneck, and dizziness.**
Most likely diagnosis: Intracranial hypotension (0 to 55 mm; normal CSF pressure 70 to 200 mm).
Treatment: **Symptomatic.**
(i) Post-lumber puncture: Epidural blood patch (injection of 10 ml of patient's own blood into the epidural space to seal a dural leak) is rarely needed in persistently symtomatic patients.
(ii) Hypovolema: IV fluids.
Complication: Subdural effusion. It resolves when intracranial hypotension disappear.

61. **Most common type of head injury**: **Nonpenetrating.** It is a **diffuse axonal injury (DAI)** in which axons are either sheared at the time of impact or degenerate later due to traumatic/ ischemic damage. Brain injury could be due to **brain contusion and intracranial hematoma.**

62. **Clinical presentations of epidural hematoma due to head injury**:
Epidural: H/O head injury (baseball or fall from a horse), **lucid interval is the most characteristic** (brief loss of consciousness, then period of lucidity, followed by acute clinical deterioration), **laceration of the middle meningeal artery and fracture of temporal bone.**
Diagnosis: CT scan is the best procedure of choice because it can detect both skull bones **and brain tissue** injury (MRI is good for soft tissues only); skull x-ray is done when CT is **not** available.
Treatment:
(a) **Surgery** is to stop the bleeding and remove the blood.
(b) ICU management for severe head injury and intracranial hypertension.

63. **ICU management for severe head injury and intracranial hypertension**:
(a) Intubation and ventilation: To keep arterial $Paco_2$ 30-35 mm Hg.
(b) Maintain systolic BP between 100 and 160 mm Hg.
(c) Maintain CPP >70 mm Hg (CPP = MAP-ICP).
(d) Adequate sedation (with morphine) but muscle relaxants (vacuronium) as needed.
(e) Anticonvulsant therapy (phenytoin).
(f) Ventricular drainage for increased ICP, if fail use mannitol.
(g) Head elevated 30 degree and in neutral position.
(h) IV fluids with 0.5 normal saline (do **not use dextrose and water).**

64. **Clinical presentation of subdural hematomas**: **Three subgroups** (acute, subacute, and chronic).

   (A) **Acute:** H/O severe head injury (motor vehicle accident, assaults, fall in alcoholic or elderly); clinical manifestation progressively deteriorates, laceration of the bridging veins (drains blood from the surface of the brain to major sinuses) or cortical veins in Sylvian fissure.

   Best diagnostic study: CT scan.

   Treatment:

   (a) Early surgical intervention may improve the outcome.

   (b) ICU management for severe head injury.

   (B) **Subacute:** H/O minor head injury, usually older than 50, may be on anticoagulants, symptoms **usally begins after 2 to 7 days of injury.**

   Diagnosis: CT scan.

   Treatment: Surgery + medical management.

   Prognosis: Good, if diagnosed early and managed properly.

   (C) **Chronic:** H/O **very minor head injury** (striking head on a door) or may forget about the injury; **no loss of consciousness; symptoms begin 1 to 6 weeks after the injury,** usually occurs in elderly, alcoholic, dementia, or chronic illnesses. The symptoms include worsening headache in the morning, unsteady gait, confusion, focal weakness, and difficulty in writing.

   Best diagnostic method: CT scan.

   Treatment:

   (a) Some resolves spontaneously.

   (b) Surgery: Evacuate the clots by twist drill hole and puncture of the dura with or without subdural drain (**avoid craniotomy).**

65. **Intraparenchymal bleeding**: H/O head injury, progressive deterioration of symptoms depend upon the amount of bleeding (1 to 100 ml).

   Best diagnostic method: CT or MRI.

   Treatment:

   (a) More than 15 to 20 ml blood: Surgical evacuation.

   (b) Medical management (ICU) for severe head injury.

66. **Indication for intubation in head injury patients**: Glasgow coma scale **score of 8 or less** (patients who are unable to follow commands, do **not** open eyes to noxious stimuli, fail to utter words or comprehensive sounds are considered in coma).

67. **Glasgow coma scale (GCS)**: (The lowest score is 3, highest is 15, need intubation **8 or less means severe injury, or 9 to 12 is moderate,** and **13 to 15 is mild injury.**

(A) Eye open:

(i) Spontaneously	4
(ii) To speech	3
(iii) To pain	2
(iv) Never	1

(B) Best verbal response.

(i) Oriented	5
(ii) Confused speech	4
(iii) Inappropriate	3
(iv) Incomprehensible sound	2
(v) None	1

(C) Best motor response:

(i) Obeys commands	6
(ii) Localizes pain	5
(iii) Withdrawl from the stimulus	4
(iv) Decortication	3
(v) Decerebration	2
(vi) None or flaccidity	1

68. **Signs of increased ICP and possible intracranial disaster in adults**:
   (a) Respiratory rate >20.
   (b) Heart rate < 60 or change >10/minute.
   (c) BP: Increased systolic >15 mm Hg and/ or widening of pulse pressure.
   (d) **Pupillary changes:** Dilated, asymmetric, decreased response to light, and irregular shape.
   (e) Decreased level of consciousness.
   (f) One point decrease in GCS score.

69. **Post-traumatic or postconcussive syndrome after minor head injury (GCS score 13 to 15)**: Patients appear with loss of recent memory, lack of concentration, abstract thinking. Most of the symptoms subside within first 3 months after injury but **symptoms of permanent cognitive deficits** may persist, chronic dizziness, and disequlibrium may persist. Some patients suffer **transiently** from headaches, insomnia, and depression.
   Treatment for headaches persist more than 60 to 90 days: Propranolol.

70. **Problems of patients with moderate head injury (GCS score is 9 to 12):** Depression, behavioral and cognitive problems, increased irritability, social disruption, and traits of impetuousness (violence in action).
   Treatment:
   (a) Antidepressants for depression.

(b) Psychological intervention: Social workers and psychiatrist.

71. **Most common site and type of injury to the spinal cord**: (Remember, most injuries to spinal column do **not** traumatize the spinal cord). **Cervical (50%);** approximately 50% of such patients become **quadreplegic. The spinal cord damage is due to** direct trauma, **compression** by the displaced or broken bones, and **ischemia** due to compression or laceration of spinal arteries.
Two types of injuries:
(A) Acute complete or spinal shock: Patients appear with loss of all sensorimotor functions (**flaccidity** and **loss of reflexes at and below the level of injury),** and occasional **priapism.**
(B) **Incomplete spinal cord injury.**
  (i) Central cord syndrome (less severe injury): It is due to **ischemia or hematomas** of the spinal cord, result in **syrinogomyelia-like clinical** syndrome (**weakness in distal portion of the upper extremities associated with lost or decreased pain and temperature sensations in the arms but sparing the touch and mostly all functions below the cervical cord level).** The upper extremity weakness generally improves.
  (ii) Partial hemisection or anterior spinal artery syndrome: Ipsilateral loss of proprioceptive sensation, distal weakness, contralateral impairment of pain and temperature.

72. **Treatment of spinal cord injury**:
(a) Management in first few hours after injury (most important).
  (i) Airway and ventilation.
  (ii) Neck immobilization.
  (iii) Protection against shock.
(b) Neurosurgery or orthopedic treatment.
(c) **Large dose of methylprednisolone within 8 hours: It reduces the neurological dysfunction in acute traumatic paraplegia.**
(d) Hypotension (low BP, low heart rate): Leg elevation to improve venous return plus IV fluids.
(e) **To prevent deep vein thrombosis:** Vigorous fluid replacement, antiembolism stockings, and early mobilization.
(f) **To prevent UTI:** Intermittent catheterization at 4 to 6 hour interval, acidification of urine with vitamin C and cranberry juice reduces the incidence of UTI.
(g) Nutrition: Early heavy nutrition (enteral or parenteral) with vitamins for rapid wound healing and rehabilitation.
(h) To prevent decubitus ulcers: Rotating beds.

(i) Reflex spasms (or autonomic dysfucntion of the bladder) causing bladder distension and UTI: **Diazepam (small doses)** and baclofen.
(j) Physical, occupational, and rehabilitation therapies: For long term skin care, prevention of UTI, management of bladder dysfunction, sexual problems, and emotional- vocational therapies.

73. **Compression on the spinal cord:**
(a) Lesion compressing **lateral side (unilateral) of the spinal cord:**
Brown-Sequard syndrome: Ipsilateral hemiparesis, loss of vibration and position senses with **contralateral loss** of pain and temperature. It is due to compression on the lateral side of the spinal cord.
(b) Lesion compressing **posterior portion** of the spinal cord.
Bilateral loss of position and vibratory sensations, **with preservation of** pain and temperature sensations and motor power.
(c) **Earliest signs** of spinal cord compression: Weakness, hyperreflexibility, and spasticity. Loss of vibratory and position senses, and followed by paresthesias.
(d) **Late signs of** spinal cord compression: Loss of pain, temperature sensation, bladder, and bowel functions.
(e) Cervical lesions: Quadriplegia.
(f) Thoracic lesions: Paraplegia.
(g) **Upper lumbar lesions:** Bladder and bowel dysfunctions, extensor planter (conus medullaris syndrome) **but normal motor functions.**
(h) **Lesions below the first lumbar vertebral body (cauda equina)**: Loss of bladder and bowel functions, lower motor neurone findings in leg, and normal planter reflexes.

74. **History and physical examination in patients with neck pain and back pain:**
(A) History:
(i) **First symptom is the pain** which may be followed by neurologic dysfunction.
(ii) **Radicular pain indicates nerve root compression (herniated disc).** It is enhanced by straining, coughing, and sneezing.
(iii) **Funicular pain indicates compression of the long tracts of the spinal cord.** It is more diffuse, less sharp, enhanced by **stretch of the cord (neck flexion, straight leg raising),** and increased intraspinal pressure (coughing, straining, and sneezing).
(iv) Most spine pain begins **acutely or subacutely** with or without H/O strenuous activities. It is a **dull aching pain** exaggerated by movement

and relieved by rest. The pain persists during rest indicates serious illnesses (tumors or herniated disc).

(B) Physical examination:

(i) Movement of the spines and paravertebral structures should be **done very carefully.**

(ii) **Spinal cord compression** should be suspected if patients have the following signs.

(a) Lhermitte's sign: Parasthesias radiating into the arms, legs, or back during neck flexion.

(b) Referred pain to the thoracic or lumbar area during neck flexion.

(c) Severe pain in gradual movement of the cervical spine.

(iii) **Non-herniated disc pain is** relieved by lying down and exaggerated by flexion **(Important).**

(iv) **Stright leg raising sign:** It is positive in any severe pain particularly which radiates to the lower extremities.

(v) **Crossed straight leg raising sign (**referred pain to the opposite leg or back when nonpainful leg is eleveted): It indicates root compression.

(vi) Pain during forced extension of the hip: L4 and above lumber roots diseases.

(vii) Point tenderness indicates tumor infection.

(viii) Remember, any inconsistencies during examination **indicate psychological abnormalities.**

75. **Investigations and management of the patients with neck and back pain:**

(A) **Investigations:**

(i) **Best diagnostic test is MRI except subluxation** of the vertebral bodies which is diagnosed by **flexion and extension plain radiographs of the neck or back.**

(ii) Remember, most patients do **not** need any investigations.

(iii) Plain x-ray is helpful in fracture, dislocation, or subluxation; otherwise it is **not** helpful.

(B) Treatment:

(i) Patients without any serious structural diseases: Treat the neck or back pain without further investigations.

(ii) **Severe pain:** Bed rest on a firmly support mattress in the most comfortable position for 2 to 3 days plus analgesics (aspirin or acetaminophen) and local heat application.

(iii) Low back pain: Semi-Fowler's position (slightly elevated head with pillow under the knees).

(iv) Neck pain: Cervical pillow and soft neck collar.

(v) **Remember these points:** Most patients (up to 80 %) improve completely within 4 weeks; **don't allow neurological examination during rest;** only patients with serious diseases need further investigations.

76. **Most common structural lesion causing low back pain**: **Herniated disc (lateral is more common than medial)**. Most common sites are **between L4 and L5 or L5 and S1 compressing the L5 or S1 root respectively.** In the cervical region most common sites are C6 and C7 (C7 root) or C5 and C6 (C6 root). Most common symptom is the **pain** (dull aching) **which is exaggerated by activity and relieved by rest. Patients may have no or little pain or pain in a bilateral radicular distribution in medial herniation.**

Best diagnostic study: MRI.

Treatment:

(a) Bed rest.

(b) Indications for surgery.

(i) Severe persistent pain unresponsive to bed rest and analgesics.

(ii) Foot drop.

(iii) Myelopathy.

(iv) Urinary dysfunction due to compression on the cauda equina.

Operative procedure: Removal of the involved disc and leave as much bone as possible; **rarely** fusion of the lumber spines.

77. **Spondylosis:** Two types are cervical and lumbar. It is **chronic degenerative disease** of the intervertebral discs plus reactive changes of the adjacent vertebrae, mostly found in the **ederly** patients.

(A) **Cervical:** Two types of presentations are **radiculopathy or myelopathy** but both are not present at the same time.

(i) **Radiculopathy:** Less acute pain, slow onset, and no muscle spasms.

(ii) **Myelopathy: Little or no pain;** weakness, atrophy, and fasciculations in **the upper extremities (**mostly involves small muscles of the hand), associated with spastic paraparesis and reduced proprioception **in the legs. (Remember, in amyotrophic lateral sclerosis** fasciculations are noted **outside of cervical segments).**

Best diagnostic method: MRI.

Treatment:

(a) **Conservative:** Brief period of bed rest plus cervical traction and stabilization of the neck with a soft collar.

(b) **Surgery**: It is indicated in progressive neurologic signs with conservative treatment.

(i) **Up to 2 segments fusion: Anterior removal of the disc** material with spinal fusion.

(ii) **More than 2 segments fusion:** Laminectomy with foraminotomy.

(B) **Lumbar:** It is differentiated from herinated disc by the **characteristic pseudoclaudication from cauda equina compression** which is manifested by pain, weakness, and paresthesias of the **lower extremities.** The symptoms are **exaggerated by the walking** and ceases by the standing, sitting, or lying down. (Remember, to differentiate from **vascular claudication** which is manifested by reduced or absent pulses in lower extremities and the patient knows **exactly how much** he/she can walk before symptoms begin unlike pseudoclaudication in which some days a patient can walk longer than otherdays).

Best diagnostic method: MRI.

Treatment:

(a) Mild stenosis: Conservative therapy.

(b) Severe stenosis: **Decompressive laminectomy is the treatment of choice.**

78. **Facet syndrome:** It is due to osteoarthritis or trauma of the zygapophyseal joints and synovial membranes. Patients appear **with pain in the back, thigh, and buttock.** The pain relieved by flexion movement, and **exaggerated by the extension of the vertebrae or rest.**

Treatment: Conservative or anesthetic block of the joints.

79. **Most common neoplastic growth causing spinal cord compression**: **Extradural** and **metastatic.** Other types are paravertebral (primary or metastatic), intradural (mostly benign), and intramedullary.

(A) **Extradural: Most extradural tumors are metastatic which arise from the breast, lung, prostate, or kidney;** primary malignant vertebral body tumors are chordoma and osteogenic sarcoma.

Signs and symptoms: First symptom is localized pain followed by symptoms of spinal cord compression (weakness, numbness, paraplegia in the **legs** before trunk and upper extremities).

Best diagnostic study: MRI, but remember plain x-ray can detect bone lesions (85% of cases).

Treatment:

(a) Metastatic tumors: **Corticosteroids** (to reduce spinal cord edema) **plus radiotherapy; chemotherapy** may be added.

(b) Primary tumors (Diagnosis is confirmed by biopsy):

(i) **Malignant tumors:** Corticosteriods plus surgery followed by radiation therapy; if unresponsive to radiation and chemotherapy,

resection of the vertebral bodies may prevent or delay the paraplegia.

(ii) Benign tumors: Surgery.

(B) **Paravertebral tumors** (Primary neoplasms or metastatic lesions).

Signs and symptoms: Gradual onset of severe, unremitting pain, sometimes burning in quality localized to the spine and radiating along the dermatome, **anhydrosis, hyperhydrosis, Horner's syndrome, or diaphragmatic paralysis.**

Best diagnostic method: MRI.

Treatment:

(a) Metastatic tumors: **Radiation therapy,** if available chemotherapy.

(b) Undiagnosed tumors (first biopsy should be done to confirm the diagnosis): If malignant, then radiotherapy and chemotherapy should be given.

(C) **Intradural extramedullary tumors:**

Most tumors are **benign.** Most common type is **meningiomas, next is neurofibromas.**

(i) **Meningiomas:**

Signs and symptoms: First symptom is the pain. It is present in 75% patients of meningiomas; In remaining patients (25%) appear with painless spinal cord compression symptoms like degenerative or demyelenating diseases.

Best diagnotic method: MRI plus Gd.

Treatment: Surgical removal is the treatment of choice.

(ii) Neurofibromas:

Signs and symptoms: Radicular pain is the first symptom, followed by signs of spinal cord compression after months or years. Positive family history of cutaneous stigmata is present.

Laboratory investigation: Elevated CSF protein.

Best diagnostic study: MRI.

Treatment: Surgical extirpation of the lesion.

(D) **Intramedullary tumors:** Most common is **low grade astrocytomas,** next is ependymomas.

Signs and symptoms: First symptom is the **pain** which is followed by signs of spinal cord dysfunction. The characteristic of intramedullary lesions (early onset of bladder or bowel dysfunction, and dissociated sensory loss except sacral areas) **cannot** distinguish definitely from extramedullary lesions.

Best diagnostic study: MRI (It can distinguish from extramedullary lesions).

Biopsy can distinguish from abscess and syringomyelia.

Treatment:

(i) Surgical removal of the tumor.
(ii) Partially resectable tumor: **Surgery followed by radiotherapy.**
Ependymoma syndrome: Hydrocephalus, enlarged ventricles, headaches, and papilledema are present due to tumor's protein exudate blockage.

80. **Investigation of choice in spinal arachnoiditis: Myelography.** CSF may have high protein, high cells, and low glucose (although depends upon the underlying diseases such as TB or bacterial infections).
Signs and symptoms: Patients appear with characteristic pain in the neck and back or radicular pain, **rarely** spinal cord dysfunction leads to paraplegia.
Treatment:
(i) Nonspecific treatment.
(ii) Treat the underlying diseases.

81. Most common and serious vascular disorder compressing the spinal cord: **Spinal epidural hematoma.** It is due to spontaneous, trauma, bleeding disorders, anticoagulant, or vascular malformations.
Sings and symptoms: Sudden, severe localized back pain followed by rapid spinal cord dysfunction leads to paraplegia.
Best diagnostic method: MRI.
Treatment: Emergency surgical evacuation.
Other vascular disorders are intradural or intramedullary. **Remember,** Symptoms of AVM compressing spinal cord are **exaggerated during menstruation or pregnancy.**
Best diagnostic methods: MRI, angiography.
Treatment:
(i) Microsurgery is the treatment of choice.
(ii) If surgery is **not possible,** then embolization of malformation and ligation of the feeding arteries should be performed.

82. Arnold-chiari malformation (adult form): Patients remain asymptomatic until adult age.
Signs and symptoms: Dysfunction of the cerebellum, pyramidal tracts, posterior columns, and lower cranial nerves; signs of hydrocephalus (due to obstruction or coexisting syringomyelia of the cervical spinal cord and medulla).
Best diagnostic study: MRI.
Treatment:
Surgical enlargement of foramen magnum and decompression of the cervicomedullary junction may be helpful.

83. Most common cause of **acute flaccid paralysis:** Guillain-Barre syndrome (GBS). It has two types: Acute inflammatory demyelinating polyneuropathy (AIDP) and axonal GBS.

84. **Etilogy, clinical presentation, and treatment of GBS(Guillain-Barre syndrome)**:
   (A) **Etiology:** Immune-mediated disorder, 60% of cases have underlying infections **(Campylobacter jejuni, mycoplasma, and herpes virus; C.jejuni is mostly associated with severe axonal GBS)**.
   (B) **Clinical presentations: Most important finding is early loss of tendon reflexes.** Patients appear with tingling, pins-and- needles sensation in the lower extremities, dull low back pain followed by weakness, a**scending paralysis, respiratory and swallowing difficulties** within few hours or days from the initial symptoms.

   Best diagnostic test: None.
   CSF protein- Elevated after the first week only (characteristic finding).
   Electrodiagnostic study: Mild abnormalities in early stages may be helpful.
   Treatment:
   (i) Best effective therapy: Plasmapheresis (when patients have good veins), intravenous immunoglobulin (when patients don't have good veins). Remember, corticosteroid is **not** effective alone. Plasmaphereisis or IVIg may **not** be effective in axonal GBS. **Plasmapheresis means exchange of patient's plasma for albumin**.
   (ii) For respiratory failure: Intubation and ventilator management.

85. **Chronic inflammatory demyelinating neuropathy (CIDP) of chronic GBS:** It mimic GBS but **slower onset of signs and symptoms.**
   Physical examination: Weakness, areflexia in the legs.
   Laboratory findings: Elevated CSF protein, prominent demyelenating features in NCV (nerve conduction velocity).
   Treatment:
   Best treatment of choice: **Corticosteroids,** next is plasmapheresis or IVIg.

86. A patients appear in the ER with H/O unilateral wrist drop (radial nerve palsy) followed by contralateral foot drop (peroneal nerve palsy).
   Physical examination: Absence of tendon reflexes outside the distribution of weakness but **normal sensory examinations.**
   Laboratory findings:
   (i) Normal CSF protein (unlike GBS and CIDP).
   (ii) NCV: Conduction block suggests focal demyelination.

(iii) Elevated anti- GM_1 ganglioside antibodies in the serum: Nonspecific, but it is an important finding.

Most likely diagnosis: Multifocal motor neuropathy.

Treatment: Intravenous immunoglobulin or cytotoxic drugs, (Remember, plasmapheresis or corticosteroids is **not** effective).

87. A 35 year old man appears in a private doctor clinic with **H/O frequent ankle sprain. He denies any athletic** activities in his whole life. He has four brothers, one of them has similar problems.

Physical examination: Distal wasting of intrinsic muscles of the feet, anterior tibial and calves; **plus** high arches (pes cavus) of the feet, hammer toes, and loss of ankle reflexes.

Best diagnostic test: To examine his brother who has similar clinical problems.

Mode of transmission: Most of them are autosomal dominant associated with chromosome 17; sex-linked form is associated with **connexin-32 gene**.

Most likely diagnosis: Chercot-Marie-Tooth (CMT) disease.

CMT-type I: Abnormal peripheral myelination.

CMT-type-II: Axonal degeneration.

Treatment:

(a) Foot drop: Ankle brace.

(b) Genetic counseling and family education is important for reassurance and to avoid further diagnostic studies.

Prognosis: Most of them have normal daily occupational activities and life span.

88. **Most common clinical problem** in patients with amyloid neuropathies: **Painless injuries of the hands and feet** (osteomyelitis or infections) **due to loss of pain and thermal sensation;** other findings are postural hypotension, impotence, bladder and bowel incontinence are due to autonomic dysfunctions.

Clinical diagnosis: To identify the similar problem in other family members (autosomal dominant).

Specific diagnosis: Molecular genetic analysis.

Treatment: No definitive treatment but education to prevent pain and thermal injuries.

Pathogenesis: Deposition of amyloid (fibrillary protein) in peripheral nerve, sensory, and autonomic ganglia.

Important molecular findings: Substitution of methionine for valine at position 30 in the molecule results in transthyretin (prealbumin) gene protein.

89. Most common cause of peripheral neuropathy: **Diabetes.** Most frequent type is **diabetic polyneuropathy, other type is mononeuropathy.**

(A) **Signs and symptoms of diabetic polyneuropathy.**

(i) **Neurologic:** Initially asymptomatic, then symmetric distal sensory loss in both the feet, dysesthesias (unpleasant sensation when bedsheet touches the toes), burning, throbbing, or lightning pain in the feet and legs. Unlike other neuropathie, it reduces both small and large nerve fibre sensations.

(ii) **Others:** Sinus arrythmia, hypotension (postural), impotence, constipation or unpredictable diabetic loose stool, and fecal incontinence.

Treatment:

(a) Maintain the blood sugar as normal as possible is the most important therapy.

(b) Neuropathic pain: TCA, carbamazepine, or high dose of amitriptyline (do **not** use opiates).

(c) Prevention of painless injuries: Education, well-fitting shoes, frequent examination of the feet, avoid pain and thermal injuries.

(d) Diarrhea: Diphenoxylate.

(e) Impotence (most distressing problem): Intracavernous injection of yohimbine may be helpful.

(B) Mononeuropathy and multiple mononeuropathies.

Signs and symptoms:

(i) **Typical third cranial nerve palsy: Inability to adduct the eye or open the eye-lid and normal pupil.** (Remember, **pupil is always abnormal** in third nerve palsy due to intracranial mass or aneurysms).

(ii) **Diabetic lumbosacral plexopathy:** Hip pain with asymmetric weakness of proximal leg muscles plus weight loss; femoral neuropathy (quadriceps weakness and loss of knee reflex); typically involves hamstring and gluteal muscles.

(iii) **Diabetic truncal neuropathy:** Pain, hypesthesia, and numbness along the intercostal nerves.

Prognosis of all neuropathies: Patients recover within months.

90. **Uremic neuropathy** (creatinine clearance is <10% of normal):

Signs and symptoms: Footdrop and leg weakness are the most important findings, absence of ankle reflex is characteristic, sometimes parasthesia or burning sensation may be present.

Treatment:

Renal transplantation is better than dialysis to keep the peripheral nerve function.

91. **Outcome of critical care neuropathies:** Patients recover completly.
Etiology: Unknown; serious illness, or sepsis.
Signs and symptoms: Distal involvement with motor weakness.
Pathology: Axonal degeneration.
Treatment: None.
Difficulty: To wean the patients from ventilator.

92. **Most common cause of alcohol neuropathy:** Multifactorial **nutritional deficiencies (**thiamines multivitamins), sometimes it is due to alcohol.
Signs and symptoms: Initial symptoms are the **pain and paresthesia of soles of the feet,** followed by burning sensation. Examination reveals distal weakness and loss of reflexes first in the ankle.
Treament:
(i) Thiamine and multivitamins:
(ii) Avoid alcohol.

93. **HIV infections and neuropathies**.
(a) Most common neuropathic complication is **sensory neuropathy of AIDS.**
Signs and symptoms: Pain in the soles of the feet and difficulty in walking. **Typically the reflexes are exaggerated at the knees and lost at the ankle.**
Pathogenesis: Unknown; it is **not** due to HIV infection within the nerves.
Treatment: Symptomatic.
(b) Guillain-Barre syndrome (GBS) and chronic inflammatory peripheral neuropathy (CIDP): Both occurs in **early HIV infections (before the development of the AIDS),** usual CD4 counts between 250 to 500.
(c) CMV polyradiculopathy in AIDS patients: Pain in the back and legs with paraparesis and loss of reflexes.
CSF: Elevated polymorphs and protein.
Treatment: Ganciclovir and/or foscarnet.

94. A 50 year old female appears in the ER with H/O **paresthesia (pricking and tingling) of the first three fingers for last few days.** It is relieved by shaking or elevating the hands. She is working with the computer for the last few years.
Physical examination:
(i) Positive Tinel's sign: Paresthesias in the median nerve distribution while tapping the carpal tunnel or sustained flexion of the wrist.
(ii) Severe cases: Sensory loss and weakness in the median nerve distributed skin and muscles respectively.
Diagnostic study: NCV shows prolongation of nerve conduction across the carpal tunnel.

Most likely diagnosis: Carpal tunnel syndrome.

Treatment.

(a) Splinting of the wrist in slight dorsiflexion during sleep: It increase the cross- sectional area of the carpal tunnel.
(b) Injection of corticosteroids into the tunnel.
(c) Potassium-sparing diuretics may be helpful.
(d) **Severe cases:** Surgical release of the carpal ligament.

95. A 60 year old man noticed irregular facial features. He denies any pain behind the ears.

Most likely diagnosis: Facial paralysis (Idiopathic, unilateral).

Treatment:

(i) Oral corticosteroids with rapid tapering.
(ii) Protection of the cornea from becoming dry and injury.

Prognostic evaluation: Electrophysiologic study of the facial nerve after the first several days.

96. **Causes of facial nerve palsy**:

(i) **Most common is idiopathic.**
(ii) CNS: Multiple sclerosis, HIV infection.
(iii) Infection: Herpes zoster, meningitis.
(iv) Infiltrative: Carcinomatous meningitis.
(v) Infiltrative: Lyme disease and sarcoidosis.
(vi) Tumor: Primary tumors of the facial nerve.

97. **Important points in peripheral neuropathies associated with monoclonal gammopathies (due to monoclonal proteins IgM, IgG, and IgA):**

(a) **POEMS syndrome:** Polyneuropathy, **o**rganomegaly, **e**ndocrinopathy (hirsutism, testicular atrophy), **m**onoclonal IgM protein, and skin pigmentation. It is associated with **osteosclerotic myelomas.**
(b) Cryoglobulinemia, with or without monoclonal gammopathy, may cause neuropathy.
(c) The monoclonal proteins can cause **amyloid deposition in the nerve,** diagnosis is made by histologic findings.
(d) MAG (myelin-associated glycoprotein) is produced by the IgM monoclonal proteins with sugars on Schwann cells.

Treatment:

(i) Solitary plasmocytomas: Excision and radiation are curative.
(ii) Other neuropathies: Plasmapheresis.
(iii) Amyloid neuropathies: No treatment.

98. **Few important points in immune-mediated ataxic neuropathies**.
   (a) **First group is carcinomatous sensory neuropathy:** Most frequently associated with **occult or overt** (small cell) carcinoma of the lung, breast, and ovary. Presence of **anti-Hu antibody (**neither sensitive nor specific) with ataxic neuropathy indicates underlying cancer.
   (b) **Second group has features of** Sjogren's syndrome: Keratoconjunctivitis sicca, elevated antinuclear antibody titers. Patients may have Adie's pupil (large pupil and more reactive to accomodation than to light) or rarely joint disease.
   (c) **Third group is idiopathic sensory neuropathy:** No systemic disease, acute onset, may be misdiagnosed as GBS.
   (d) **Clinical presentation of all three groups: Gait ataxia, inability to localize arms or legs, absence of reflexes, normal motor strength, positive Romberg sign** (patients can stand on their feet together when eyes are open, but fall when eyes are closed).
   (e) **Diagnosis:** Electrodiagnostic study shows absence of sensory and preservation of motor functions.
   (f) **Treatment:**
      (i) Rehabilitation, physical therapy, and gait training.
      (ii) Rarely, cytotoxic or corticosteroid therapy is helpful.

99. **Most important associations in facioscapulohumeral dystrophy**:
   (a) Sensorineural hearing loss.
   (b) Coats syndrome: Progressive painless blindness and retinal telangiectasias.

100. **Signs and symptoms of facioscapulohumeral dystrophy (autosomal dominant)**: The name of the disease indicates that muscular dystrophy begins in the **face,** followed by **scapular muscles and that of humerous (upper arms).**
   Patients are unable to bury the eyelashes, appear with expressionless face, **winging of the scapulas when** arms are raised but absence of muscular hypertrophy.
   Serum CK level: Normal or mildly elevated.
   Treatment: Corticosteroids **cannot** alter the disease process.

101. **Abnormalities in myotonic dystrophy.**
   (a) **Frontal baldness.**
   (b) **Subcapsular cataracts.**
   (c) **Cardiac conduction defects and sudden death.**
   (d) Testicular atrophy and ovarian dysfunction.
   (e) End organ unresponsiveness to insulin.

(f) Extrathyroidal hypometabolism.
(g) Hypercatabolism of IgG.
(h) Mental changes.
(i) Reduced gastric motility and dilated colon.
(j) Rarely, retinal pigmentation and abnormal skull (small sella turcica, hyperostosis, large paranasal sinuses, and protruding mandible).

102. **Signs and symptoms of myotonic dystrophy:** It appears in childhood or **around 19 years of age. Myotonic symptoms appear before** or at the same time of weakness, subsequently **dystrophic process predominates and mytonia reduces.** It involves **distal part of the extremities,** levator palpebrae, facial, masticatory, cervical, pharyngeal, esophageal, and laryngeal muscles. It can also involves proximal muscles and **respiratory muscles results in hypercapnia, hypoxia, respiratory acidosis, and somnolence. Remember, usually** there is **no** external opthalmoplegia.
Preferred diagnostic mathod: Biopsy of the muscles.
Serum CK level: Normal or mildly elelvated.

103. **Most common cause of death in oculopharyngeal muscular dystrophy**: **Starvation or aspiration pneumonia.**

104. **Manifestations of oculopharyngeal muscular dystrophy (autosomal dominant)**: Patients appear, between age 50 to 70, with **progressive ptosis, dysphagia,** subsequently all external ocular and other voluntary muscles are affected.
Diagnosis is confirmed by: Muscle biopsy. Serum CK level: Normal or slighty elevated.

105. **Treatment and prevention of the muscular dystrophies**:
(A) Treatment: (Nonspecific therapy only).
  (i) Physical therapy to prevent contractures.
  (ii) Orthoses.
  (iii) Corrective orthopedic surgery.
  (iv) Cardiac conduction defects: Pacemaker.
  (v) Myotonia: Phenytoin or quinine.
(B) **Prevention:**
  (i) Antenatal diagnosis.
  (ii) Detection of carriers and genetic counseling.
  (iii) Future: Gene therapy.

106. Most common form of **HIV- associated myopathies:**

(a) **Polymyositis.** It appears **early** It is mediated by **T-cells.** Patients appear with **pseudothrombophlebitis and recurrent myoglobinuria** but pathogenesis is **unknown.**
(b) Other causes are: **Zidovudine** (used in HIV treatment) induced toxic mitochondrial myopathy coexistent with HIV-related myopathy; **HTLV-1** can be associated with chronic spastic paraparesis and polymyositis.

107. **Sporadic inclusion body myositis:** Patients are usually older than 50, male, appear with **slowly** progressing **weakness, atrophy, absence of reflexes,** in the proximal and distal muscles of the lower extremities (quadriceps) and **no** involvlement in facial, cervical, and pharyngeal muscles.
EMG: Myopathic changes plus abnormal electrical activities.
Serum CK level: Normal or mildly elevated.
Diagnosis is confirmed by: Muscle biopsy.
Treatment: No response to corticosteroids and other immunosuppressants.

108. **Similarities and differences between dermatomyositis and pure polymyositis**:
(A) **Similarities: Proximal muscles** weakness, mononuclear inflammatory exudate in muscle and myopathic changes.
EMG: Spontaneous electrical activities.
Treament: Corticosteroid.
(B) **Differences.**
(i) **The characteristic rash** is present in dermatomyositis, but absent in pure polymyositis.
(ii) Dermatomyositis always have **capillary injury and necrosis** which are absent in polymyositis.
(iii) **No** evidence of T-cell mediated cytotoxity in dermatomyositis, which is due to **humoral response against** vascular element.
(iv) Peripheral muscles atrophy and degenration are found in dermatomyositis.

109. **Difference** between scleroderma and other inflammatory myopathies:
(a) **Serum CK level: Normal or mildly elevated in** scleroderma.
(b) **EMG (resting): Normal** in scleroderma.
(c) **Inflammatory cells:** T cells and macrophages in scleroderma.

110. **Most common cause of eosinophilia- myalgia with L-tryptophan preparation**: It is due to **contaminant of** L-tryptophan [1,1- ethylidenebis (tryptophan)]. Patients appear with **eosinophilia** (>10^9 per liter), myalgia (severe), fascitis, sometimes pneumonitis, myocarditis, and encephalopathy.

111. **Most common cause of adult CPT (carnitinine palmitoyltransferase) deficiency:** Homozygous **Ser 113 Leu mutation in the CPT-II gene.**
Sings and symptoms: Muscle pain, fatigability, periodic myoglobinuria due to exertion, especially if associated with fasting and cold. Patients are asymptomatic between attacks.
Muscle lipid contents: Normal or slightly increased.

112. **Primary carnitine deficiency (PCD) syndrome:** Autosomal recessive. It is due to defective carnitine transport in **heart, muscle, kidney, intestinal epithelium, and fibroblasts.**
Signs and symptoms: Cardiomyopathy, weakness, and hypoketotic hypoglycemic encephalopathy.
Treatment: Carnitine.
(Myopathic form of PCD may respond to steroids).

113. A 35 year old short statured man appears with H/O **strokelike episodes**, focal or generalized seizures, dementia, episodic vomiting, and hearing loss.
ABG: Metabolic acidosis (due to elevated lactic acids in the serum).
MRI: Encephalomalacia outside the distribution of main cerebral arteries.
Most likely diagnosis: MELAS (mitochondrial encephalomyopathy, lactic, acidosis, strokelike episodes).

114. A 19 year old male patient was referred by a pediatrician to an internist with the **signs and symptoms of retinitis pigmentosa, progressive external opthalmoplegia (PEO), hearing loss, short stature, mental defect, and heart block**. The patient has a pacemaker and hearing aid.
Most likely diagnosis: Kearns-Sayre syndrome.
In this syndrome, **patients may also have** seizures, peripheral neuropathy, hypogonadism, hypoparathyroidism, diabetes, **renal Fanconi syndrome**, lactic acidosis, cystic changes or calcifications in the basal ganglia.

115. **Most common type of steroid-induced myopathy**: **Fluorinated drugs (e.g.,dexamethasone, triamcinolone) cause more myopathy** than nonfluorinated (e.g., prednisone) drug.

116. **Few important points in glucocorticoid- induced myopathy**:
(a) **Women are more** susceptible than men.
(b) Myopathy is **more common in divided daily doses** than single or alternate day doses.

(c) **Weakness** is more common in **proximal muscles** than distal, and **lower extremities are** more commonly involved than upper extremities. **Hip and ankle flexor** muscles are severely affected.
(d) **No** involvement in cranial nerves.
(e) Myopathy develops in almost all patients, if they are receiving steriods 60 mg daily divided doses for 3 months.
(f) Serum CK level is **normal.**
(g) **Treatment: Reduce the steroid doses to the minimum or discontinue** if possible.
(h) **Prognosis:** Regain normal muscles strength within 1 to 4 months after discontinuation of the steroid.

117. The periodic paralysis (PP): Two types are primary **(k is low, high, or normal)** and secondary (K is **low or high, never normal).**

(A) **Primary: Autosomal dominant,** serum k may be low or high but remains **normal during acute** attacks and **normal or low-normal between attacks.**

(i) **Primary hypokalemic (low k) periodic paralysis:** Patients **feel very weak in the morning** but improve as day progresses. **The symptom exaggerated by excitement, high sodium, and high carbohydrate in diet. The key features: Positive family history, and mildly low serum k during attack and normal k between attacks.** It begins in childhood and improves by 4th or 5th decade.

Treatment: Glucose plus insulin, oral Kcl.

(ii) Primary hyperkalemic periodic paralysis: It occurs in children (**not** important for the examination).

(B) **Secondary:** It is due to potassium wastage (urine, GI) or retention of serum k (renal and adrenal insufficiencies). Serum k is either **decreased or elevated during and between attacks.**

(i) Secondary hyperkalemic (high k) periodic paralysis: It is due to renal or adrenal insufficiency, acute attack of malaria, or spironolactone therapy.

Diagnosis: Very high serum k level (>7 mEq/L).

(ii) Secondary hypokalemic (low k) periodic paralysis: It is due to thyrotoxicities, barium intoxication, or wastage of k in the urine and GI tracts.

118. **Treatment of all periodic paralysis**:

(A) Primary:

(i) Acetazolamide: It can prevent attacks or decreases the frequency. (The complications of acetazolamide: renal stone, matabolic acidosis).
(ii) **Low k type- Oral kcl is the treatment of choice,** preventive therapies include acetazolamide, low-carbohydrate, and low-sodium diet.

(iii) **High k type:** Glucose plus insulin, inhalation of metaproterenol or albuterol in acute attacks. The preventive therapy include acetazolamide or thiazide diuretics, and high-carbohydrate diet.
(iv) Cold induced paramyotonic hyperkalemic PP: Tocainide.

(B) Secondary:
(i) Thyrotoxic low k type: Antithyroid drugs, kcl, low-carbohydrate, low-sodium diet (**no** acetazolamide).
(ii) Barium induced low k type: IV sodium sulfate.
(iii) Excessive wastage (urine and GI): Try to stop the wastage.
(iv) High k type due to renal insufficiency and adrenal insufficiency.

Treat the underlying causes plus treatment for hyperkalemia.

119. **Alcoholic myopathy.**
Alcohol causes acute necrotizing myopathy with myoglobinuria in chronic alcoholics. Initial hypokalemia (e.g., renal loss, vomiting, diarrhea, and sweating) is followed by high k due to the renal failure and myoglobinuria.

120. **Side effects of chloroquine**: Myopathy, peripheral neuropathy, macular and corneal degenerations.

121. **Side effects of emetine (ipecac alkaloid)**: Myopathy, cardiotoxicity.

122. **Most common causes of death in myoglobinuria**: **Renal or respiratory failure.**
Signs and symptoms of myoglobinuria: Patients complain of muscle pain, swelling, and weakness for few hours followed by **dark brown discoloration of the urine.** Remember, myoglobinuria can causes microscopic hematuria.
Urine immunoprecipitation assay: Positive for myoglobin. It is the **best diagnostic test.**
Patients with renal failure: **High k, high p, low ca.**
Treatment.
(a) Rest.
(b) Hydration and diuretics.
(c) $NaHCO_3$ to make the urine alkaline.
(d) Treatment for renal failure: Dialysis.

123. Causes of myoglobinuria:
(a) **Traumatic:** Rhabdomyolysis (acute, massive muscles breakdown).
(b) **Infectious:** Viral (e.g., influenza A, herpes, E-B virus, coxsackie); bacterial (sepsis), clostridial infection (gangrene).

(c) **Metabolic: Carbon monoxide** poisoning, severely low glucose and k, high Na and H_2O, other metabolic diseases.
(d) **Toxic:** Cocaine, barbiturates, other narcotics, amphetamine, lovastin, epsilon amino-caproic acid, and amiodarone.
(e) **Idiopathic.**

124. **Stiff-Man syndrome**: Patients appear with initial **intermittent spasms** of the axial and limb muscles followed by **continuous stiffness due to spasms of the agonist and antagonist muscles simultaneously.** Absence of cerebral or spinal cord disease.
EMG: Constant firing of normal motor units in the stiff muscles.
Treatment.
(i) **Diazepam or baclofen:** Increase GABA-mediated central inhibition.
(ii) **Clonidine:** Prevents norepinephrine release from nerve terminals.
Association: It is strongly associated with auto-immune diseases (insulin-dependent diabetes mellitus).

125. **Isaacs' syndrome (or generalized neuromyotonia)**: It is an **autoimmune disorder.** Patients appear with **stiffness, delayed relaxation of the affected muscles, and myokymia (**small undulating movements of the overlying skin).
EMG: High frequency recurring bursts of motor unit potential.
Treatment.
(i) Phenytoin or carbamazepine: Inhibit abnormal discharges.
(ii) Plasmapheresis may be effective.
Association: Thymoma, myasthenia gravis, exposure to penicillamine, and anti-acetylcholine receptor antibodies.

126. **Rippling muscles:** It is an autosomal dominant, benign condition. The patients appear with mild muscle pain and stiffness during exercise. Local percussion causes myoedema.
Serum CK level- Mildly elevated.

127. **Diagnosis and management of acquired syringomyelia (fluid filled cyst within spinal cord or medulla due to arachnoiditis, trauma, or tumor).**
(A) Diagnosis.
(i) MRI: It detects the size of the cavity, associated tumor, or arachnoiditis. It is the best diagnostic method.
(ii) CSF: Normal except protein which is elevated with tumor or arachnoiditis.
(iii) EMG: Denervation in the wasted muscles but normal sensory conduction in analgesic hand.

(B) Treatment: **Surgery: Decompression of the cyst** by syringoarachnoid, syringopleural, or syringoperitoneal shunt.

128. **Signs and symptoms of acquired syringomyelia:**
   (i) It depends upon the segment of the spinal cord affected.
   (ii) **Posttraumatic syringomyelia** patients appear with **weakness and impaired sensation** months or years after the trauma (results in paraplegia or quadriplegia).
   (iii) Arachnoiditis (due to subarachnoid hemorrhage, meningitis, trauma, surgery, or spinal anesthesia) usually involves **thoracic or lower cervical segments.**
   (iv) Syringomyleia is due to intramedullary spinal cord tumor: Signs and symptoms depends upon the extent and location of the tumor.

128. **Mental development and tuberous sclerosis:**
   (a) Majority of the patients have mild to severe mental deficiency.
   (b) **Remember, 33% of cases have normal or superior intelligence (Important).**

129. **Most common clinical presentation in tuberous sclerosis: Hypopigmented spots (100%) mostly over the trunk (easier to see with Wood's lamp),** next common is **adenoma sebaceum on the face,** then fibroma of the nail bed, mental deficiency, retinal hamartomams (50% of cases), renal tumors (66% of cases), cardiac rhabdomyomas (30% of cases), shagreen patches over the lower back, and seizures.

130. **Diagnosis and treatment of tuberous sclerosis:**
   (A) **Diagnosis:** Clinical (adenoma sebaceum, hypopigmented spots, ungual fibromas) and MRI is the procedure of choice.
   (B) **Treatment:**
      (i) Symptomatic: To control seizures.
      (ii) **Surgery:** It is done in hamartomas which are symptomatic and have gliomatous changes.

131. **Mode of inheritence and tuberous sclerosis**: **Autosomoal dominant,** location of gene on chromosome 9q and 16p.

132. **Most common intracranial tumor in neurofibromatosis 1**: **Gliomas of the optic nerve and chiasm.**
   Signs and symptoms of neurofibromatosis 1: **Cafe au liat spots (more than six spots each greater than 1.5 cm in diameter), axillary freckles (specific),**

peduncultated subcutaneous, or plexiform masses, hypertension (due to renal artery disease), and pheochromocytoma (5% of adult patients).

Diagnosis:

(i) Clinical diagnosis.

(ii) Intra or extraspinal tumor: MRI.

(iii) Intracranial and hamartomas: CT or MRI.

Treatment:

(a) Most patients are asymptomatic: No treatment is needed.

(b) Optic nerve gliomas: Radiation therapy.

(c) Symptomatic schwannomas (peripheral): Surgical removal.

(d) Symptomatic intraspinal or intracranial schwannomas: Surgical therapy.

Mode of inheritence: Autosomal dominant.

133. **Screening of family members of neurofibromatosis 2: Hearing test and BAER** (brain stem auditory evoked response) because **bilateral acoustic neuromas are the most common clinical presentation (Important)**. Other intracranial tumors are meningiomas and ependymomas. A few Cafe au lait spots are present (42% cases).

Mode of inheritance: Autosomal dominant, gene location on **chromosome 22q.**

134. **Most commonly involved organ in myasthenia gravis (MG)**: **Eyes (40% of cases);** others are generalized (40%), only extremities (10%), or only bulbar or bulbar plus eyes (10%).

135. Most common thymic abnormality in MG:

Thymic hyperplasia (66% of cases); other is thymoma (10 to 15%) which may results in myocarditis or giant cell myositis. MG is an autoimmune disease. MG (10%) is also associated **with other autoimmune diseases** (hyperthyroidism, SLE, polymyositis), ulcerative colitis, rheumatoid arthritis, sarcoidosis, pemphigus, pernicious anemia, Lambert-Eaton myasthenic syndrome, or Sjogren's syndrome.

136. Clinical presentations of MG (myasthenia gravis):

(a) Female >male, women appear in the third decade and men in the sixth or seventh decade.

(b) **Ocular muscles:** Bilateral, asymmetric, **characteristic ptosis and diplopia.**

(c) **The weakness of the muscles supplied by other cranial nerves:** Expressionless face, everted lips, drop jaw, nasal regurgitation of the fluids, chocking, slurred hypernasal speech, and snarl like smile.

(d) Patients may appear with general voluntary muscles weakness but **normal reflexes. (Important).**
(e) **Remember, symptoms are exaggerated** by exertion, high or low temperature, excitement, and infections.
(f) The weakness of the limb muscles: Difficulty in lifting objects, combing hairs, walking, running, and climbing stairs.
(g) **First 3 years are important:**
  (i) Most rapid progression and death occur.
  (ii) Most remissions occur during this period.

137. **Diagnosis and treatment for MG (myasthenia gravis):**
(A) Diagnosis:
  (i) History and physical examination.
  (ii) **Anticholinesterase test: Intravenous edrophonium** (actions last few minutes) improves the degree of ptosis, eye movements, and the force of the hand grip.
  Side effects of edrophonium: The cholinergic side effects are flushing, fasciculations, lacrimation, vomiting, diarrhea, and abdominal cramps. Patients with cardiac disease, it causes sinus bradycardia and A-V block. Treatment for toxicities: Atropine.
  Intramuscular neostigmine actions last for 2 hours.
  (iii) **Serologic tests:** Acetylcholine receptor (AChR) antibodies are positive in all patients with moderate to severe MG, 80% with mild generalized MG, 50% with ocular MG, and only 20% in patients with remission.
  (iv) **C3 localization: It is the easiest and most convenient way to confirm the diagnosis.**
  (v) EMG: Positive.
(B) Treatment for MG:
  (i) Anticholinesterases: **Pyridoxine bromide is most commonly** used because of its fewer muscarinic side effects, other drug is neostigmine bromide.
  (ii) **Treatment for cholinergic crisis** (abdominal pain, vomiting, lacrimation, flushing, and diarrhea): **Atropine.**
  (iii) **Treatment for myasthenic crisis:** Edrophonium.
  (iv) Patients who are **unresponsive (respiratory distress, profuse secretion) to the** increasing doses of anticholinesterases, it is sometimes **difficult to distinguish between** the cholinergic or myasthenic crisis: Stop the medications, ventilator therapy, and IV fluids.
  (**Remember, drug unresponsiveness usually disappears in few days).**
  (v) Prednisone (alternate day therapy).

(vi) **Thymectomy:** It is an absolute indication for thymoma. It is also used in severly ill patients unresponsive to other therapies.

(vii) Azathioprine: It is helpful in more than 50% of cases.

(**Side effects of the drug:** Leukopenia, pancytopenia, infections, and hepatocellular damage).

(viii) Intravenous immunoglobulin therapy is also helpful.

(ix) **Plasmapheresis is used only in fulminating or severely ill patients unresponsive to all other therapies.**

138. **Few important points in Lambert-Eaton myasthenic syndromes:**

(a) It is associated with cancer, particulary **small-cell cancer of the lung.**

(b) It is an **acquired autoimmune disorder,** produces autoantibodies which result in deficiency of calcium channel at motor nerve terminal. It is also associated with HLA-B8, DRw3 antigens, and other autoimmune diseases.

(c) Patients appear with weakness and **fatigability of proximal limb (mostly lower limbs)** and torso muscles **except** extraocular and bulbar muscles, absence or hypoactive reflexes, and autonomic presentations characterized by dry mouth, decreased sweating, postural hypotension, altered pupillary reflexes, or impotence.

(d) EMG: Smaller amplitudes when stimulation frequencies are less than 10 Hz.

(e) **Treatment: (**Anticholinesterases are slighty helpful).

(i) Guanidine hydrochloride: It is very toxic but reduces the symptoms.

(ii) **Noncancer patients:** Prednisone (alternate day) and azathioprine are the best treatment of choice.

(iii) Future theapy: 3, 4- diaminopyridine.

139. **Signs and symptoms of organophosphate insecticides intoxication**: (It inhibits cholinesterase irreversibly, results in accumulation of acetylcholine). Patients appear with seizures, alteration in mental status, coma, muscarinic side effects, weakness, cramps, and fasciculation.

Treatment:

(i) Gastric lavage (>100 L of water) followed by activated charcoal, oral cathartics.

(ii) Seizures: Anticonvulsants.

(iii) Respiartory failure: Ventilator management.

(iv) **Atropine is helpful,** and pralidoxime may be useful.

140. **Most common type of cerebrovascular stroke: Ischemic stroke (80 %),** other type is hemorrhagic stroke (20%).

141. **Few important values in CNS:**

(a) **Normal cerebral blood flow**: 60 ml/100 grams of brain per minute.

(b) Normal arterial O_2 tension and blood glucose levels: **CBF delivers** 350 mmol O_2 and 260 mmol glucose to 100 grams of brain each minute, but **the brain** 's consumption of O_2 is 156 mmol and glucose is 33 mmol.

(c) Normal cerebral blood volume (CBV) is 50 ml, mechanical hyperventilation ot a $Paco_2$ of **20 to 25 mm Hg reduces** CBV to 35 ml.

(d) **This is very important point**: **In normal patients CBF remain constant** when the MAP (mean arterial pressure) is between 50 (lowest level) and **150 (highest level) mm Hg.** In patients with chronic hypertension both the levels **are higher than normal.** When MAP is above 150, CBF increases and MAP is lower than 50, CBF decreases.

(e) **Focal cerebral ischemia** (most common cause is embolic or thromboembolic) **lasting 15 to 30 minutes** causes **irreversible damage** to specific neurones.

(f) **Generalized cerebral ischemia (**most common cause is cardiac asystole or ventricular fibrillation) lasting **more than 5 to 10 minutes** in a normothermic patient causes failure of recovery of consciousness.

(g) **Most commonly involved areas of brain due to anoxia:**

(i) Neocortex: 3, 5, 6 layers.

(ii) Hippocampus: CA1.

(iii) Cerebellum: Purkinje fibres.

(iv) Striatum: Small and medium sized neurones.

142. **Most common site of atherothrombosis of cerebral blood vessels:** Carotid artery bifurcation and origin of the internal carotid artery.

143. **Most common source of emboli** occluding middle cerebral artery (MCA) partly or completely: Emboli from the heart or extracranial carotid arteries.

144. **Signs and symptoms of MCA occlusion** (**ischemia**):

(A) **Superior branch: Weakness and sensory loss are maximum in the face and arm, rarely** inferior quadrantanopsia may present, **but vision is normal.** Hemianopsia is due to **visual inattention** than true blindness becuase MCA branches only supply the dorsal and parietal half of the optic radiation. **Impaired voluntary gaze** away from the side of the lesion may be present, but **normal** oculocephalic or oculovestibular reflex is noted.

(i) **Dominant hemisphere involvement: Expressive (Broca's) aphasia, abnormal naming, writing, and fluency but normal** comprehension.

(ii) **Nondominant hemisphere involvement:** Anosognosia (**not** aware of the deficit), unilateral neglect, and spatial disorientation.

(B) **Inferior branch:** Most important is the **sensory loss** particularly integreated sensations (**perception of shapes:** stereognosis).

(i) **Dominant hemisphere involvement:** Receptive (Wernicke's) aphasia with fluent speech characterized by jargon and paraphasias; **abnormal** naming, reading, writing, and comprehension.

(C) **Deep MCA syndrome (**Selective occlusion of the MCA main stem causing **ischemia in the territory of the lenticulostriate vessles** but **normal** superior and inferior branches): **Hemiparesis or hemiplegia** but **normal** sensory, language, and visual responses. The symptoms are due to infarction of the internal capsule due to occlusion of lenticulostriate vessels.

(D) **Proximal occlusions** of the MCA (may include both superior and inferior branches, perforating branches of **internal capsule, basal ganglia, and optic radiation):** Contralateral hemiplegia, hemianesthesia, dense homonymous hemianopsia.

(i) Dominant hemisphere involvement: Global aphasia.

(ii) Nondominant hemisphere involvement: Anosagnosia.

145. **Signs and symptoms of internal carotid artery (ICA) occlusion (ischemia):**

(a) It **mimics symptoms and signs of MCA occlusion** in severe ICA stenosis.

(b) **Transient monocular blindness (amaurosis fugax)** is due to obstruction in opthalmic artery blood flow.

(c) In severe bilateral internal carotid artery stenosis, there is hypoperfusion of cerebral hemisphere and **symptoms in border zones** between the major vascular areas.

(d) Patients may appear **with severe ipsilateral headache due to occlusion of ICA** than that of intracranial vessels.

(e) **Anterior circulation TIA** (transient ischemic attack) **is due to disease of the ICA than** that of intracranial vessels.

146. **Signs and symptoms of anterior cerebral artery (ACA) occlusion**:

(a) **ACA occlusion distal to anterior communicating artery: Contralateral hemiparesis and sensiory loss (worst in the lower extremities),** gait ataxia, and sometimes urinary incontinence is due to damage of parasagittal frontal lobe.

Language: Reduced spontaneous speech may be associated with depressed psychomotor acitivity.

Remember, acute syndrome is most likely either due to spinal cord disease or rarely occlusion of the superior sagittal sinus (which drains blood from the medial surfaces of both cerebral hemispheres).

147. **Signs and symptoms of posterior cerebral artery (PCA) occlusions:**

(a) **Occlusion distal to the penetrating branches: Complete contralateral loss of vision or quadrantanopsia** (superior or inferior is due to involvement of the lower or the upper calcarine arteries). **Central (or macular) vision may be spared** due to collateral supply from MCA.

Dyslexia (difficulty in reading) and **dyscalculia** (difficulty in calculations) may be present.

(b) **Proximal occlusion of the PCA: Hemisensory disturbances** may lead to intractable thalamic pain on the abnormal side. Bilateral occlusions cause **memory loss. Hemiballism** (wild, uncontrolled, and flailing limb movements) may develop with involvement of subthalamic nucleus.

148. **Signs and symptoms of basilar artery occlusion:**

(a) **Occlusion of the basilar apex:** Initially there **is reduction in arousal** followed by **bilateral blindness and amnesia** (due to occlusion of the flow into the PCA's), in addition to that **abnormal vertical gaze and pupillary reaction (due to tegmental damage).**

(b) **Occlusion of the basilar artery:** Contralateral hemiparesis and sensory loss, ipsilateral bulbar and /or cerebellar signs **with normal intelligence documented by the command through the movement of the eyes or eyelids.**

149. **Signs and symptoms of vertebral artery (VA) occlusion:**

(a) Occlusion of the **superior cerebellar artery** (supplies most of the cerebellar cortex): It is the **most common cause of cerebellar infarction** which is characterized by **ataxic gait, ipsilateral clumsiness, dysarthria, dizziness, headaches, and vomiting.** Subsequent **swelling of the brain** causes ipsilateral gaze paresis and/or mystagmus followed by **stupor, hydrocephalus** (due to obstruction of the fourth ventricle), and **herniation** (upward or downward) **of the cerebellum.**

(b) Occlusion of the **VA plus ipsilateral PICA (posterior inferior cerebellar artery): Lateral medullary syndrome: Ipsilateral Horner's syndrome, ataxia,** vertigo, nystagmus, and vomiting. There is **ipsilateral loss of facial pain,** and temperature sensations, and contralateral loss of pain and temperature sensations in the trunk and extremities.

(c) **Vertebrobasilar ischemia (VBI): Diplopia,** ataxia, facial weakness, vertigo, dizziness, and long tract signs.

(d) **Focal brain stem ischemia: Crossed syndromes: Ipsilateral cerebellar dysfunction (ataxia)** and **contralateral** dysfunction below the lesion involving pyramidal (hemiparesis), spinothalamic, and dorsal column pathways.

150. **Signs and symptoms of anterior choroidal artery**: Hemiparesis (face, arm, and leg), variable hemisensory loss, and sometimes hemianopsia (due to optic tract ischemia). It is difficult to differentiate from MCA ischemia.

151. **Investigation of choice in acutely ill patients with ischemic stroke**: **CT scan is better than MRI in acutely ill patients** because MRI requires longer time, needs to remove ferromagnetic materials, and difficulty in monitoring the patients in the scanner.

MRI is more sensitive than CT scan to detect the **changes in the tissue structures,** and it **provides more accurate and earlier measure of cerebral infarctions. MRI is the best when acute illness is over or CT scan is nondiagnostic.**

152. **Investigation of choice in primary cerebral hemorrhage: CT scan.** Remember, **hemorrhagic conversion of an ischemic infarct usually develops after 1 to 2 days** and maximum up to 4 weeks.

153. **Limitations of CT scan in cerebral infarctions:**
   (a) It **cannot** detect infarcts <5 mm in diameter.
   (b) It is difficult to **detect brain stem infarction** due to bony obstruction.
   (c) CT scan can detect only 5% of strokes within first 12 hours, 50% between 24 to 48 hours, and **90% by the end of one week.**
   (d) Do **not** use CT scan with contrast which is **mildly neurotoxic,** and also **the infarct becomes less visible** due to its hypodensity.

154. **Diagnosis of the stroke**:
   (a) **History: In stroke, neurologic deficit lasts more than 24 hours unlike TIA (transient ischemic attack) which lasts less than 24 hours.**

   Headache is common in hemorrhagic and embolic strokes but **absent in** atherothrombotic and ischemic stroke. H/O polycythemia or use of oral contraceptive is also important.
   (b) **Physical examination:** It includes BP, pulse, neurological, cardiovascular, renal, and opthalmoscopic examinations.
   (c) **Laboratory studies**: CBC plus platelets count, glucose, PT, PTT, lipid profile, renal functions, and serum electrolytes. **In elderly patients,** high ESR indicates gaint cell arteritis. **In young patients** antiphospholipid antibodies (immune- related diseases), parotein C and S, tests for collagen vascular diseases, platelet function, viscosity, and serum VDRL.
   (d) **CT scan is performed in acutely ill patients. MRI is the best after the acute stage or when CT scan is nondiagnostic.**

(e) **CVS:** Twelve leads ECG and rhythm strip should be done in all patients to rule out acute MI and arrythmias.

Remember, echocardiography is **not** indicated unless patients have history or physical examination suggest cardiac disease**. Stress testing can** be done in selected patients during convalescence to rule out ischemic cardiovascular disease.

(f) **Lumber puncture:** It is **not** recommended except in meningitis and neurosyphilis. If needed, it should be done **after the eye examination and CT or MRI to rule out increased ICP.**

(g) **Noninvasive CVS examination:**

(i) Duplex ultrasonography: It is the **best** method for **direct examination** of the common, internal, and external carotid arteries.

(ii) **Intracranial blood vessels** can be examined by CT, MRI, or MRA (magnetic resonance angiography). **Pulsed transcranial doppler** can detect direction and velocity of blood flow of the intracranial vessles orginating from circle of Willis.

(h) Cerebral angiography: It should **not** be done routinely. It is **only** indicated before the CVS surgery, and to look for an arterial dissection, cranial arteritis, and fibromuscular dysplasia.

155. **Most common cause of ischemic stroke in all age groups: Atherosclerosis of extracranial and intracranial arteries.** It causes stroke either by in **situ stenosis, occlusion, or embolization** of plaque material to distal branches of the cerebral vessels.

156. **Most common source of emboli in ischemic stroke**: **Cardiac (33% of all ischemic stroke);** noncardiac causes are vascultits, drug related, hematologic disorder, and different other conditions.

157. **Emboli of cardiac origin, few important points:**

(a) Most common cause of **mural thrombi is the myocardial infarction (anterior wall)** due to **dyskinetic myocardium,** other causes are atrial fibrillation and cardiomyopathy.

(b) **Valvular heart diseases** cause emboli: Important causes are **infective endocarditis,** rheumatic heart disease (mostly associated with atrial fibrillation), nonbacterial endocarditis (cancer of prostate, stomach, lung, pancreas, and ovary; Libman-Sacks endocarditis with SLE), mitral valve prolapse, and prosthetic valves.

(c) Remember, cardiac tumor most likely to embolize is **myxomas.** It may be associated with **hemolytic anemia** due to lysis of RBC's.

158. **Adult patients with HbSS (sickle cell disease) most common type of stroke: Hemorrhagic.**

159. **Most common form of multiple myeloma** causes increased viscosity and stroke: Multiple myeloma with predominance of **IgA.**

160. **Drugs causing stroke:**
   (a) **Over the counter:** Prolonged use of cold medications and nasal decongestants contain ephedrine, phenylpropanolamine, and phenoxazoline.
   (b) High-dose of estrogen contraceptives.
   (c) IV use of heroin, cocaine (infective endocarditis, mycotic aneurysms hepatitis B), pentazocine, and methylphenidate (Ritalin).

161. **Time to produce irreversible brain damage in focal vascular occlusion: Within 2 to 3 hours.**

162. **Most important risk factor for stroke: Hypertension.**

163. **Prevention of stroke.**
   (a) **To control the hypertension with antihypertensive therapy.**
   (b) To stop smoking and reduce alcohol intake.
   (c) To control diet and obesity.
   (d) To treat diabetes mellitus.
   (e) **Use of anticoagulants** for atrial fibrillation and selected MI.
   (f) **Use of antiplatelet agents (NSAID's) for atherosclerosis (carotid or vertebrobasilar).**
   (g) **Prophylactic surgery: Endarterectomy is the treatment of choice in carotid artery (70-99% stenosis) atherosclerosis (symptomatic patients).**
   Best treatment for 30-69% stenosis: Medical or surgical. It is under investigation.
   Best treatment for < 30% stenosis: Medical.
   (h) **Women:** Try to avoid estrogen containing oral contraceptives.

164. **Diagnostic evaluation of patients with acute focal neurologic dysfunction**:
   (a) **First stabilize the vital signs:**
      (i) Airway, oxygen, ventilation (prn).
      (ii) Maintain the normal vital signs plus BP.
      (iii) ECG with rhythm strip.
      (iv) Blood analysis: CBC with platelet count and differential, PT, PTT, ESR, SMA-6.

(b) Pertinent history is to be obtained.
(c) Medical examination: **Neurological,** CVS, hematological, and other systems. Neurological examination should include opthalmologic examination.
(d) Head CT Scan without contrast: To rule in hemorrhagic or ischemic stroke, focal diseases (e.g., tumor, abscess, and encephalitis).

165. **Management of patients with acute focal brain ischemia:**
(A) Initial general therapy:
(i) BP > 220/120 plus systemic organ dysfunction: IV nitroprusside or beta-blocker to reduce BP by 20-25%.
(ii) BP > 220/120 and normal organ functions: Oral ACE inhibitor or calcium channel blocker to reduce BP by 10 to 15%.
(iii) BP < 220/120: No antihypertensive treatment for 72 hours, then use antihypertensive but do **not** reduce BP below 160/90 for 1 week.
(iv) Maintain blood glucose between 75 to 200 mg/dL.
(v) Appropriate IV fluid therapy.
(vi) Appropriate therapy for fever (T >100° F).
(B) **Treatment of atherothrombotic stroke:**
(i) Complete/nonprogressing: ASA, ticlopidine.
(ii) Incomplete/ progressing: Heparin then ASA; thrombolysis then heparin/ASA.
(C) **Treatment for atherothrombotic TIA:** ASA, ticlopidine.
(D) **Treatment for cardioembolic stroke:**
(i) Nonhemorrhagic, small infarct: Heparin/warfarin at 48 hours.
(ii) Nonhemorrhagic, large infarct: Heparin/warfarin at 5-7 days.
(iii) Hemorrhagic infarct: Heparin/warfarin at 2-4 weeks.
(E) **Treatment for cardioembolic TIA:**
(i) Heparin.
(ii) Warfarin.

166. **Most dangerous form of venous stroke is due to**: **Superior sagittal sinus thrombosis.** Patients appear with **bilateral** weakness and sensory abnormalities in both legs. **Remember, bilateral involvement indicates venous origin** than arterial. Seizures occur more in venous occlusion than arterial.

Best diagnostic study for venous sinus thrombosis: Angiography; but MRI or CT scan can make the diagnosis.

Treatment: Heparin.

167. **Most common cause of diffuse brain ischemia:**

(a) **Prolong diffuse ischemia:** Cardiac asystole or other forms of cardiopulmonary failure.
(b) Brief diffuse ischemia: It causes syncope without any brain damage. Patients with prolonged ischemia appear with unconsciousness, coma, followed by eyes-open vegetative state.

Treatment: To restore the CVS functions.

168. **Most common cause of intracranial hemorrhage**: **Subarachnoid hemorrhage** (50%), rest (50%) is within the brain.

169. **Most common cause of subarachnoid hemorrhage (SAH): Rupture of saccular or 'berry' aneurysm (80% of all cases). Most commonly involved age** group is between **40 to 65, women are** more involved then men particularly **during pregnancy. Most common sites of saccular aneurysm is anterior at the bifurcation of the arteries.** It is mostly due to congenital **defects in the muscles and elastic tissues of the** arterial media which progressively deteriorates with hemodynamic stress.

170. **Risk factors of aneurysmal SAH.**
   (i) **Sudden rise in BP (**emotional excitement, athletic activities, and coitus) is detrimental.
   (ii) **Remember,** hypertension is **not** a risk factor.

171. **Familial saccular aneurysm is associated with:**
   (a) Polycystic kidney disease.
   (b) Ehlers-Danlos syndrome.
   (c) Other connective tissue diseases.

172. **Most common site of fusiform (or ectatic) aneurysms: Basilar artery.** Fusiform aneurysms **rarely rupture, difficult to treat ruptured aneurysms with surgical clipping** because of their shape and stiff walls.

173. **Most commonly involved cranial nerves in basilar artery aneurysms (fusiform): Cranial nerves V, VII, and VIII.** Patients appear with **facial pain, hemifacial spasm, and hearing loss with vertigo, respectively.** Patients symptom mimic tumors of the cerebellopontine angle, pituitary, or suprasellar mass.

174. **Most common cause of mycotic aneurysms:** It is due to **septic degeneration** of the distal cerebral arterial muscle and elastic tissues.

175. **Clinical presentation of aneurysmal SAH (subarachnoid hemorrhage)**:

(a) Patients appear with **focal headaches** or **sentinel headaches** with vomiting and meningeal irritations.

Remember, patients with sentinel headaches should have **CT scan done,** if negative **then spinal tap should be done.**

(b) Compression of the **third cranial nerve (oculomotor)** by the expanding aneurysms: Patients appear with ipsilateral ptosis, opthalmoparesis, **dilated pupil with loss of pupillary light reflex with or without orbital pain.**

(Remember, diabetes causes third cranial nerve paralysis, has all the above features **but normal pupil).** Patients may also have **amnesia along with third cranial nerve palsy.**

(c) **Giant aneurysms (>2.5 cm) of the internal carotid artery (ICA) lying within cavernous sinus:** Patients appear with **unilateral opthalmoplegia, and orbital pain which are** due to compression of the III, IV, VI, and the first division of V cranial nerves.

(d) Giant aneurysms of the **supraclinoid portion of ICA:** Patients appear with **unilateral vision loss or field defect** due to compression of the optic nerve or tracts.

(e) Rupture of the saccular aneurysms: Most common presentation is **unconsciousness which is preceeded by the 'most excruciating headaches'.**

(f) **Symptoms and signs of chemical meningitis:** Patients appear with fever, high BP, meningeal irritation, nuchal rigidity, with or without subhyaloid retinal hemorrhages.

176. **Diagnosis of aneurysmal SAH:**

(a) **Best diagnostic method is the head CT scan which detects blood in the basal cisterns (75% of cases)** within 48 hours of bleeding. (Remember, MRI is less sensitive).

(b) When CT scan fails to diagnose bleeding, **then lumbar puncture is diagnostic.** It shows xanthochromic CSF (onset 4 to 6 hours, duration for 6 weeks), **RBC counts are constant in all the tubes,** and slower blood clot formation.

(c) **Indications for cerebral angiography:**

(i) It is the most **definitive test** to detect the source of SAH.

(ii) **It should be done immediately** when diagnosis is **not** certain.

(iii) It is **recommended immediately** in **septic endocarditis and SAH to** rule in mycotic aneurysms.

(iv) It should be done in patients with **subacute bacterial endocarditis with systemic embolism.**

(d) General investigations:

(i) CBC plus platelets count, PT, PTT, SMA 6.
(ii) **ECG:** It may show tall T waves, short PR intervals, peaked or inverted T waves, and increased U waves.

177. **Treatment for aneurysms:**
(A) **Saccular aneuryms:**
(i) **Surgical clipping is the definitive therapy** to prevent rebleeding.
(ii) Medical therapies (to reduce the risk of rebleeding and cerebral vasospasms):
(a) Bed rest.
(b) Analgesics and mild sedation.
(c) Stool softeners to reduce straining (which increases the ICP).
(d) Nimodipine (calcium channel blocker) to keep the systolic BP 160 to 170 mm Hg and the diastolic BP 90 to 100 mm Hg.
(e) To overcome cerebral vasospasms by raising cerebral perfusion pressure: Increase plasma volume, phenylephrine, or dopamine. **Remember, it can be done only after surgical clipping.** Otherwise it may cause rebleeding.
(B) **Mycotic aneurysms:**
(i) Unruptured: Appropriate antibiotic is followed by angiography.
(ii) Single and surgically accessible aneurysms: **Surgical clipping should be done promptly**.

178. Incidence of aneurysmal rebleeding is highest: **First 2 weeks after onset of SAH.**

179. **Optimal time to do surgical clipping in ruptured aneurysms:** Controversial.
(i) Hunt grade of 1 to 3 (extend from asymptomatic or minimal headaches up to drowsiness, confusion, or focal deficits): **24 to 36 hours** of the onset of bleeding.
(ii) Most neurosurgeons prefer to operate within the **first 3 days** or **after days 10 to 14.** Avoid from 3rd to 10th days **due to vasospasms and poor outcome.**
(iii) Patients appear in the **hospital after 3 days,** or angiogram shows active vasospasms, or Hunt **grade 4 to 5 (stupor to deep coma):** Surgical clipping should be **delayed for 10 to 14 days.**
(iv) Rebleeding of aneurysms (highest during the first 2 weeks after SAH): **Surgical clipping should be done urgently** because mortility is up to 50%.
(v) **Repeating cerebral angiogram** is recommended prior to delayed (10 to 14 days) surgical clipping to rule out cerebral vasospasms.

180. **Sizes of saccular aneurysms and management (rupture is directly proportional to the size of aneurysm):**

(a) Less than 5 mm: Follow up carefully.
(b) Between 5 to 10 mm: Consider surgical clipping.
(c) Greater than 10 mm: Surgical clipping at earliest possible time.

Remember, unruptured aneurysms diagnosed incidentally can bleed at a **yearly rate of 1 to 3%.**

181. **Late medical and neurologic complications of aneurysmal SAH.**

(a) Medical:
  (i) Low serum Na is due to increase ADH secretion.
  (ii) Cardiac myonecrosis.
  (iii) Cardiac arrythmias.
(b) Neurologic:
  (i) **Rebleeding** from the same aneurysm (first 2 weeks).
  (ii) **Cerebral vasospasms (3 to 10 days after rupture).**
  (iii) **Communicating hydrocephalus is** due to blockage of CSF outflow.
  (iv) **Cerebral ischemia is** due to vasospasms.
  (v) Occasionally, seizures.

182. **AVM** (arteriovenous malformation). **Arteries are connected directly to veins** without intervening capillaries. AVM's can be present anywhere in the brain, usually have no brain tissues. It is due to **abnormality of the embryologic development.**

Other types of vascular malformations:

(i) Venous angiomas: Most common asymptomatic type (rarely causes seizures, headaches).
(ii) Cerebral varix: Single dilated vein and asymptomatic.
(iii) Cavernous angiomas: Large sinusoidal vessels receive blood supply from arteries and veins, mostly thrombosed, rarely bleed, symptoms are headaches and seizures, **best diagnosed by CT scan (not** angiogram).
(iv) Telangiectasias: Rare, composed or **dilated capillaries,** located deep inside the brain mostly asymptotic but may have serious bleeding.

183. **Signs and symptoms of AVM:**

(a) Most common presentation **is intracranial hemorrhage which apears first during 2nd to 4th decades of life.**
(b) Other presentations are **seizures** and neurologic deficit.
(c) Remember, **the decline in the incidence of rebleeding with time** (6% first year, 2% after 5 years, 1 to 2% thereafter) indicates **spontaneous thrombosis of arterial feeders.**

(d) Important point to remember, **small AVM's (< 2.5 cm) tend to bleed more often (unlike aneurysms) for unknown reasons.**

(e) Bleeding is **less severe** and **vasospasm is less often** than aneurysms.

(f) Focal neurologic deficit **without seizures** is due to vascular thrombosis and hypoperfusion of the brain tissues (**steal syndrome**).

(g) Headaches are found in AVM (10% cases), site of headaches may **not** coincide with the site of AVM or usually do **not** alternate between the sites of the head like migraine.

184. **Investigations and treatment for AVM:**

(A) Investigations.

(i) **Best diagnostic method is angiography.** It can demonstrate the feeding arteries which are usually unilateral, may be contralateral, or extracranial.

(ii) MR images are equal or more effective than CT scan.

(iii) CT scan with contrast can diagnose 85% of cases.

(B) **Treatment:**

(i) **Unruptured AVM with seizures or headaches over the age 55:** (Conservative management). Anticonvulsant for seizure, antihypertensive for high BP; avoid NSAID's and anticoagulant.

(ii) **Unruptured AVM** under age 55: Surgical resection is curative.

(iii) AVM deep inside the brain, or lies in language-vulnerable areas, or elderly patients (AVM must be < 3 cm in diameter): Focused gamma x-rays or proton beam radiation is effective and safe.

(iv) Arterial embolization is **not** very effective alone and it should be done with either surgery or radiation therapy.

185. Most common three causes of focal cerebral hemorrhage: **Hypertension is the most common cause,** other causes are **ruptured AVM's** and **amyloid** (or congophilic) angiopathy. It can occur in excessive use of anticoagulants (warfarin), fibrinolytic agents (tissue plasminogen activator), street drugs (cocaine, amphetamines), trauma, coagulation disorders (hemophillia, DIC), leukemia, and polycythemia.

186. Most common sites of focal cerebral hemorrhage: **Putaminal hemorrhage (35 to 50% of all hemorrhages),** others are cerebellar (10 to 30%), thalamic, pontine, and lobar cerebral hemorrhages.

187. Signs and symptoms of focal cerebral hemorrhages:

(a) **Putaminal hemorrhage**: Lethargy or coma, contralateral weakness including face, contralateral hemianopsia, and gaze paresis with eyes deviated toward the hemorrhage.
(b) **Cerebellar hemorrhage:**
  (i) **Occipital headache is the first symptom,** initially patients **remain conscious** because brain stem is spared. It is followed by ataxic gait, vomiting, and clumsiness.
  (ii) Progressively it causes brain stem compression: Contralateral hemiparesis, caloric-resistant ipsilateral gaze paresis, and **normal pupillary reflexes.**
  (iii) Finally herniation of the cerebellar tissue downward through the foramen magnum or upward across the tentorium or hydrocephalus.
(c) Thalamic hemorrhage (10 to 15%): Patients may lose consciousness early or remain awake with contralateral hemiparesis, sensory loss, and homonymous hemianopsia.
(d) Pontine hemorrhage (10 to 15%): Patients appear with **coma, small reactive pupils,** loss of oculovestibular response, bilateral extensor posturing, and quadriplegia. Remember, small hemorrhage may **not** produce coma.
(e) Lobar cerebral hemorrhage: It is found in amyloid angiopathy. Patients are mostly elderly, they appear with headache, nausea, and vomiting. Coma and seizure are usually absent because of small amount of subcortical bleed into the white matter.

188. **Investigations and treatment of focal cerebral hemorrhages**:
(A) Investigations.
  (i) Noncontrast CT scan: It is the best diagnostic method in acute condition.
  (ii) MRI: It can detect small hemorrhage; especially in the brainstem.
(B) Treatment:
  (i) Acute parenchymal bleeding:
    (a) Supportive.
    (b) To avoid herniation: **Hyperventilation is** to reduce cerebral edema and blood flow, plus mannitol is to reduce cerebral edema.
  (ii) Surgical evacuation of the hematoma:
    (a) **Cerebral bleed:** Surgical evacuation is not recommended for bleeding into cerebral hemisphere because it increases neurologic deficit and does **not improve** the mortality.
    (b) **Cerebellar bleed** (≤3 cm): Lateral ventricular shunt is better than surgical evacuation.
    (c) **Cerebellar bleed** (>3 cm): Lateral ventricular shunt plus surgical evacuation to relieve compression on the brain stem.

189. **Prevention of focal cerebral hemorrhage:**
   (a) To control the BP.
   (b) To control the anticoagulation therapy.
   (c) Avoid cocaine and amphetamines which cause bleeding.
   (d) **No** preventive therapy is available for amyloid angiopathy.

190. **Signs and symptoms of hypertensive encephalopathy:**
   (a) **Increased ICP:** Headaches, vomiting, blurring of vision.
   (b) **Focal neurologic signs, seizures, stupor, or coma.**
   (c) **Retinal findings:** Arteriolar narrowing, hemorrhages, or papilledema.

191. **Pathogenesis and management of hypertensive encephalopathy:**
   (a) Pathogenesis: **Focal or diffuse cerebral edema is due** to capillary leak of the plasma and cellular components of the blood. **The capillary leak** is due to high BP **which has exceeded the cerebral arterial autoregulation.**
   (b) Treatment: It is a medical emergency.
      (i) To control the BP: IV nitroprusside.
      (ii) Seizures and high $PaCO_2$ (both are vasodilators of CNS vessels): Controlled hyperventilation, diazepam is followed by phenytoin or carbamazepine.
      (iii) Eclampsia with hypertensive encephalopathy: Prompt delivery of the fetus plus anticonvulsants before delivery.

192. **Most common organisms of brain abscess**:
   (a) HIV patients: Toxoplasma.
   (b) Trauma patients: S.aureus.
   (c) Other patients: Anaerobe.

193. **Most common symptom of brain abscess**: **Headache of recent onset is the most common symptom.** Other symptoms and signs are lethargy, fever, focal signs (aphasia or hemiparesis), nuchal rigidity, vomiting, and seizures (when involves the cortical gray matter).
   Remember, patients may have **normal temperature, normal peripheral WBC counts,** and **absence of neck rigidity with normal ICP.**

194. **Diagnosis and treatment of brain abscess:**
   (A) **Diagnosis:**
      (i) **Best diagnostic studies: CT scan or MRI. MRI is better for posterior fossa abscess because bones are prominent in CT scan. MRI plus Gd (gadolinium)** is better for cerebritis, edema, and venous thrombosis.

MRI with or without Gd is better than CT scan of multiple abscesses.

(ii) Remember, CSF examination is **not** useful because **it may be normal unless** the abscesses are communicating or close to the ventricles, and lumbar tap **can enhance the process of herniation.** It should be deferred or cancelled until the CT or MRI was done.

(B) Treatment:

(i) **Antibiotics plus surgical aspiration or excision are the treatment of choice.**

(ii) **Antibiotics** (to cover **anaerobes, streptococci, or s.aureus** in trauma): Penicillin plus metronidazole and add vancomycin if S.aureus is suspected.

(iii) **Corticosteroids** may reduce the edema surrounding abscesses.

(iv) **Surgical aspiration is** performed stereotactically under CT guidance.

(v) **Surgical excision** by craniotomy.

(vi) **HIV patients with toxoplasma abscesses:** Sulfadiazine plus pyrimethamine or pyrimethamine plus clindamycin in patients are allergic to sulfar drugs.

195. A patients who is receiving 4 weeks antibiotics for brain abscess, **follow up CT scan or MRI shows same size of the brain abscess and the patient remains symptomatic.**

Diagnosis: Antibiotics failure.

Management: Surgical procedure should be performed plus change of antibiotics.

Few important points to remember:

(a) **Abscesses should shrink** with 4 weeks of appropriate antibiotics treatment.

(b) **Ring enhancement** may persist after clinical improvement and CSF normalization.

196. **CT scan findings in progression of brain abscess:**

(a) **Early cerebritis stage:** Low density lesions with partial ring enhancement.

(b) **Late cerebritis and early capsular stage:** Well-formed ring-enhancing lesions which are typically **thin walled and uniform.** Remember, thick, nonuniform, or nodular enhancing lesions indicate other diseases. Diffusion of contrast material into the lucent center is found in delayed contrast scan.

(c) **Late capsular stage:** Well-formed ring enhancing lesion **without** delayed diffusion of contrast material.

197. **Most common organism causing spinal epidural abscesses: S.aureus;** followed by streptococci, Gram-negative anaerobes, and TB (tuberculosis).

Most commonly affected populations: IV drug users.
Signs and symptoms: Fever, acute or subacute neck or **back pain, stiff neck, and headaches**.
Focal percussion tenderness is a very important finding. Undiagnosed patients develop **weakness and paralysis** distal to the spinal level of infections.
Diagnostic method:
(i) **Culture or Gram-stain of the pus obtained after exploration.** It is positive in 90% of cases.
(ii) Blood culture is positive (only 60 to 90% of cases).
(iii) CSF culture is positive (only 20% of cases).
(iv) **MRI plus Gd is the best diagnostic method,** if not available, then do CT with myelography.
(v) CSF: High protein, low glucose, and high lymphocytes count; **Gram stain is rarely positive.**

198. Treatment of spinal epidural abscesses:
(a) **Antibiotics:** Nafcillin or oxacillin plus gentamicin. Use vancomycin with or without rifampin (better penetration in abscess cavity) in confirmed S. aureus abscesses.
(b) Surgical decompression is **not** needed in early cases.

199. Most common organism causing septic cavernous sinus thrombosis: **S.aureus.**
Signs and symptoms: Headache, facial pain, fever, **chemosis and proptosis of the orbit,** third cranial nerve palsy, sensory loss in the distribution of the first and second branches of trigeminal nerve.
Best diagnostic method: MRI with or without Gd; (CT scan is **not** helpful, but CSF resembles meningitis).
Treatment:
(i) Prompt drainage of the infected paranasal sinuses.
(ii) Antibiotics: Nafcillin or oxacillin.
(iii) Heparin: Controversial therapy.

200. Most common source of infection in lateral sinus thrombosis: Acute or chronic infections in the **middle ear.**
Signs and symptoms of lateral sinus thrombosis: Ear pain, vertigo, fever, mastoid swelling, and sixth cranial nerve palsy.
CSF: Elevated pressure but normal composition.
Treatment:
(i) Antibiotics (to cover S. aureus and anerobes): Nafcillin or oxacillin with penicillin or metronidazole.

(ii) Surgical drainage of the mastoid.

201. Treatment of choice for septic sagittal sinus thrombosis: **Vancomycin plus third generation cephalosporin,** because most common organisms are **S.aureus, beta-hemolytic streptococci, pneumococci and Klebsiella.**
Signs and symptoms: (Middle and posterior third of sagittal sinus are **more rapidly progressive** and symptomatic than anterior third).
(i) **Increased ICP: Headaches, vomiting, stupor, and coma.**
(ii) **Cortical infarctions: Seizure, hemiparesis.**

202. **Most common source of neurologic complication of infective endocarditis: Valvular vegetations. Cerebral emboli (not** the systemic) **are most** commonly originated **from mitral valve endocarditis.**
Time of embolization depends upon the virulence of the organisms and acute or subacute disease.
(i) Acute endocarditis with staphylococci or enterococci: Embolization occurs early within 7 days.
(ii) Subacute endocarditis with streptococcus viridans: Embolization occurs during and after therapies.

203. **Warfarin causes intracerebral hemorrhages:** In **native valve endocarditis (not in** prosthetic valve).

204. **Most commonly involved artery in mycotic aneurysms: Middle cerebral artery in the distal portion** unlike congenital berry aneurysms.

205. **Most common source of infection causing subdural empyema: Infected paranasal sinuses are** due to retrograde thrombophlebitis; less frequently is due to chronic otitis media.
Signs and symptoms of subdural empyema: Most important is lateralized headaches, fever, vomiting, meningeal signs, focal neurologic signs (seizures, hemiparesis), and papilledema.
(To rule out meningitis, **papilledema and lateralizing deficits are** more common in empyemas).
Best diagnostic studies: MRI or CT scan shows extra-axial, crescent shaped mass with an enhancing rim over there cerebral cortex below the inner table of the skull or the interhemispheric fissures.
Treatment.
(i) Prompt surgical drainage.
(ii) IV antibiotics to cover organisms same as sinusitis or brain abscess.
(iii) Prophylactic anticonvulsants because seizures are common.

206. **Signs and symptoms of cranial epidural abscess:** Headaches, fever, focal neurologic signs because it is associated with subdural empyema (**not** with sinusitis or otitis).
Best diagnostic studies: MRI or CT with contrast shows peripherally enhancing lenticular-shaped lesion in the epidural space.
Treatment: Surgical drainage plus antibiotics.

207. **Most common organism in malignant otitis externa: Pseudomonas aeruginosa. (**It is a normal flora of the external ear).
Signs and symptoms: Ear pain, facial swelling, purulent meningitis, multiple cranial nerve palsies, and osteomyelitis of the base of the skull.
Treatment.
(i) Ticarcillin or ceftazidime plus aminoglycoside.
(ii) Surgical debridement and drainage.

208. **CDC (Centers for Disease Control and prevention) recommendations for patients with HIV and syphilis more than 1 year:** Lumbar tap and examination of the CSF irrespective of neurological symptoms.

209. **Treatment for neurosyphilis in HIV patients**: Same as in patients without HIV.
Duration: Penicillin for 2-3 weeks.
Normalization of CSF is the end point of therapy.
Proof of adequate therapy: **Normal CSF cell count and a falling protein at 6 months.**
Definitive diagnostic test for neurosyphilis: CSF inflammatory changes (high cell count and proteins, low glucose). Patients do **not** have neurosyphilis, **if CSF is normal.**
CSF-VDRL is usually positive in neurosyphilis but it can be **falsely negative** in rare cases (**very important point), so negative CSF-VDRL cannot** exclude neurosyphilis.

210. **Most definitive test for syphilis**: Serum FTA-ABS (**not** serum VDRL but rising VDRL titer indicates active infection). Remember, serum FTA-ABS will remain positive throughout life.

211. **CSF response to penicillin treatment in neurosyphilis:**
(a) **CSF cell counts progressively decrease and become zero at 6 months.**
(b) **CSF protein progressively decrease and become normal in day 7,** may increase a little bit in day 21, and finally become normal at 6 months.

(c) CSF glucose increases in day 7, may decrease in day 21, and finally increase at 6 months.
(d) CSF-VDRL should decrease (from 1: 2 to 1: 1) in day 7, should disappear at 6 months.
(e) Serum-VDRL may **not** decrease even at 6 months.

212. **Most common cause of progressive multifocal leukoencephalopathy: HIV-1 infection; other organisms are papovavirus, JC virus.**

Signs and symptoms of progressive multifocal leukoencephalopathy (PML).

Homonymous visual field defect, hemiparesis, hemisensory loss, aphasia, and apraxia. Patients have no fever, no malaise, and no loss of consciousness.

Diagnosis: MRI is better than CT scan.

CSF: Normal cell count, normal or mildly elevated proteins.

Definitive diagnosis: Brain biopsy.

Treatment.

(i) No definitive treatment is available.
(ii) Spontaneous remissions can occur.
(iii) Future therapy: Cytosine arabinoside.

213. An adult appears in ER with H/O **progressive dementia** and **myoclonus** but **absence of fever.** Lumbar CSF examination: Normal.

EEG: Diffusely slow background with superimposed complexes with or without myoclonus.

Most likely diagnosis: CJD (Creutzfeldt-Jakob disease).

Definitive diagnostic method: **Brain biopsy (**Remember MRI, CT scan, and laboratory tests are **not** helpful).

Treatment: None.

Prognosis: Fatal.

Prevention:

(i) A patient should **not** be isolated.
(ii) Fluids and secretion precaution by wearing gloves.
(iii) Accidental skin contact with contaminated fluids or materials should be followed by washing with sodium hydroxide or household chlorine bleach.
(iv) Appropriate disposal of needles.
(v) Autoclaving of surgical and pathological instruments.
(vi) Organs, or tissues should **not** be used for transplantation or replacement therapy.

Few important points in CJD:

(a) In advanced stage patients may develop cerebellar signs, pyramidal tract dysfunction, decorticate or decerebrate posture, stupor, and coma.

(b) Most cases are **sporadic** with unknown pathogenesis but two common mechanisms are genetic and infectious.
(c) Chromosomal location: **Chromosome 20** (mutation of Pr P gene on the short arm).
(d) Subtypes of CJD and presentations:
  (i) Optic type: Cortical blindness.
  (ii) Dyskinetic type: Extrapyramidal signs are prominent.
  (iii) Ataxic type: Cerebellar signs are prominent (It resembles kuru).
  (iv) Gerstmann-Straussler-Scheinker syndrome: Autosomal dominant, spinocerebellar ataxia, leucine is substitued for proline at PrP codon 102 which promotes brain amyloid accumulation.
  (v) Fatal familial insomnia: **Untreatable insomnia,** dysautonomia, motor deficit, atrophy of thalamic muclei, and specific PrP gene mutation.

214. **Most common presentation of acute disseminated encephalomyelitis (ADEM) in adults**: **Neurologic symptoms** (pyramidal tract and sensory dysfunctions, cranial nerve abnormalities, cerebellar signs, movement abnormalities, loss of muscle reflexes, in severe cases stupor and coma).
Best diagnostic study: MRI but **diagnosis of ADEM is made by exclusion (mostly CNS infections).**
Etiology- Viral illness, vaccinations or mycoplasma infection.
Treatment- Supportive, anticonvulsant for seizures.

215. **Acute necrotizing hemorrhagic encephalopathy (ANHE):** It is a very severe form of ADEM. Patients appear with or without URI symptoms, fever, severe headaches which is followed by seizures, lethargy, and coma.
CBC: Marked peripheral leukocytosis.
CSF: Pleocytosis (mostly polymorphs and sometimes bleeding).
Preferred diagnostic study: CT or MRI.
Therapy: Supportive.
Prognosis: Fatal.
Postmortem findings of the brain: Swollen plus petechial hemorrhages within the white matter.

216. **Most important presentation of Reye syndrome**: **Absence of jaundice, elevated serum ammonia and transaminases levels.** Patients appear with initial illness followed by vomiting, lethargy, seizures, transtentorial herniation, and hypoglycemia.
Diagnosis is made by: Clinical plus elevated ammonia and transaminases levels but normal bilirubin level. (**No** need for liver biopsy).
Treatment:

(i) In ICU, monitor and control ICP.
(ii) To correct hypoglycemia and electrolytes imbalance: Solutions with high glucose content.

Prevention: Avoid aspirin and viral illness.

Association: It is mostly associated with influenza A and B, herpes varicella zoster.

Defect: Mitochondrial fatty acid metabolisms (entry of fatty acid or beta-oxidation).

217. **Etiology of multiple sclerosis (MS): Unknown** but it is due to immune-mediated inflammatory demyelinations.

218. **The earliest event in the development of multiple sclerosis (MS):** Breakdown of the blood-brain barrier which is followed by perivenular mononuclear infiltrates, then breakdown of the myelin. In MS, there are **scattered areas of myelin loss** (1 mm. to several cm. in diameter) in the **brain, spinal cord, and optic nerves.**

219. **Signs and symptoms of multiple sclerosis**: **(Women** are affected more than men, most common age group is between **20 to 50).**

(a) **Younger patients:** Subacute or acute onset of **focal neurologic symptoms and signs** in optic nerves, posterior columns, pyramidal tracts, cerebellum, medical longitudinal fasciculus, or central vestibular system.
(b) **Older patients: Gradual onset of progressive myelopathy** which appears as progressive spastic leg weakness, axial instability, and bladder dysfunction.
(c) Most common **initial** presentation: **Sensory loss in one or more limbs.**
(d) **Eye findings:** Monocular loss of vision, oscileopsia, or double vision (diplopia).
(e) **Spasticity:** It includes hyperreflexia, increased muscle tone, limb spasms along with weakness and loss of dexterity.
Lower extremities are more involved than upper extremities manifested by clumsiness, cerebellar ataxia, or rarely spastic weakness.
(f) **Urinary symptoms:** Bladder malfunctions include urgency, hesitancy, incomplete emptying, or urge incontinence.
(g) **Neuropsychological manifestations:** Depression, cognitive difficulty, and emotional lability.
(h) Remember **transient reversible worsening of neurological functions** due to increased body temperature (even 0.5°c), fever, and strenuous physical exertions. Heat reduces the axonal conduction.

(i) Most important early findings are **exacerbations and remissions which progressively become fixed** with the advancement of the disease.

220. **Poor and favorable indicatiors in MS (multiple sclerosis):**

(a) **Poor indicators: Porgressive disease,** from the beginning, predominance of **motor and cerebellar signs, diagnostic MRI at** the initial presenatation.
(b) **Favorable indicators: High degree of remission** after the first attack, predominance of **sensory symptoms, and benign course in the first 5 years** after the onset of the diseases.
(c) Exaggeration of the symptoms: By infections of any kind and post partum period. Infections activate the immune system and the disease.
(d) Reduction of the symptoms: During pregnancy.
(e) **Remember,** progression of the MS is **not** affected by one or more pregnancies.

221. **Diagnostic studies in multiple sclerosis:** MS is diagnosed by **clinical presentations** supported by **the laboratory** tests.

(A) **The Schumacher clinical criteria to diagnose the MS:**
 (i) Neurological examination shows **objective abnormalities in CNS functions.**
 (ii) **Two or more areas of the brain are involved.**
 (iii) Predominant **white matter involvement.**
 (iv) Patients age is between **10 and 50.**
 (v) Clinical presentations **cannot be** explained by any other disease process.
 (vi) CNS involvement after two or more episodes, each lasts >24 hours, and a month or more interval; or CNS involvement after a slow or stepwise progression of clinical presentations over at least 6 months.

(B) Laboratory investigations:
 (i) CSF findings: **Elevated gamma globulin (**normal is <13% of the total CSF protein), **detection of OCB** (oligoclonal bands) in up to 80% of patients, **normal** CSF protein, **selectively increased IgG** levels, and **free kappa light chains** strongly suggest the diagnosis of MS.

 Remember, MBP (myelin basic protein is released due to myelin destruction) **elevation indicates only acute or active disease condition** and it is **normal** in quiescent period and in normal individuals.

 (ii) **MRI is better** than CT scan: It shows **multifocal, hyperintense images** in the periventricular white matter, corpus callosum, spinal cord, brain stem, cerebellum, and cerebellar peduncle. MRI findings are **nonspecific** particularly in patients older than 50 but it is the **best diagnostic study to rule out other diseases.**

(iii) Sensory evoked potential: Slower conduction velocity or conduction block is due to loss of myelin. Increased latency in VEP (visual evoked potential) is widely used but it is **not** useful to measure progression or response of the therapy.

222. **Possible diagnostic error or 'Red flag' in the diagnosis of multiple sclerosis:**
(a) Normal CSF examination.
(b) Absence of involvement of second, third cranial nerves, sensory, and urinary bladder.
(c) Absence of remission; steadily progressive disease.
(d) Syndrome could be explained by the localized disease.

223. **Treatment of multiple sclerosis:**
(A) Therapy for the diseases:
(i) Corticosteroid- IV methylprednisolone (MP) is followed by prednisone.
(ii) Immunomodulatory therapy:
(a) **Betaseron** [human recombinant interferon beta (1b) preparation]: It reduces the frequency of exacerbation and the progression of MRI lesions.
Side effects: Flulike symptoms, inflammation at the site of injection, rarely elevation of the AST, ALT.
(b) Avonex (interferon beta- 1a, human recombinant interferon): It also reduces the MRI disease process.
Side effects: Flulike symptoms.
(c) Partially effective immunosuppressive drugs (**only** used under controlled protocols): Methotrexate, cyclophosphamide, cyclosporine.
(B) Symptomatic therapy:
(i) To reduce spasticity: **GABA- agonist beclofen is the drug of choice,** diazepam may by used along with baclofen. Dantrolene is used in patients who do **not** respond to the baclofen and diazepam.
Side effect of dantrolene: Toxic hepatitis. It should be used cautiously in patients with myocardial diseases.
(ii) To reduce dystonic spasms: Carbamazepine or phenytoin.
(iii) To reduce intention tremor: Clonazepam. It is difficult to treat ataxia.
(iv) Fatigue: Amantadine or pemoline.
(v) Bladder problems.
(a) UTI: Antibiotics, prophylactic antibiotics, and urologic evaluations.
(b) Urinary retention (>100 ml) in non UTI: Oxybutynin or propantheline (both are anticholinergics).

(vi) Depression with anxiety and insomnia: **Amitriptyline.** Use **imipramine** if patients have associated bladder symptoms.
(vii) Memory loss or older patients: Desipramine or nontriptyline (tricyclic with reduced anticholinergic effects).
(viii) Emotional lability: Amitriptyline (low doses).
(ix) Trigeminal neuralgia or paresthesias: **Carbamazepine,** or alternative drugs are **amitriptyline,** phenytoin, and baclofen.
(x) Chronic low back or leg pain: NSAID's.
(xi) Cognitive dysfunction: Rehabilitation therapy.
(xii) Infections: Antibiotics.
(xiii) Heat sensitivity: Cool showers or air conditioning.

224. **The lifetime risk of a child whose mother has multiple sclerosis:** 3 to 5% (it is 30 to 50 folds higher than general populations).

225. **Pregnancy, postpartum, breast feeding, and education with multiple sclerosis:**
(a) In pregnancy: Symptoms are reduced.
(b) In postpartum: Symptoms are exaggerated.
(c) In breast feeding: It has almost **no relation** with postpartum symptoms exaggeration.
(d) Educations are the following:
(i) Women with mild to moderate diseases can have planned one or more babies.
(ii) Breast feeding is allowed, if feasible.
(iii) Women should **not** have babies only to reduce the symptoms of MS.
(iv) The physician should tell about the **unpredictable courses of the disease ranging** from neurologically intact for many years to severely ill patients.
(v) Patients should be seen by physician as needed, usually 6 to 12 months interval.
(vi) Patients should have faith on healthy diet and fitness activities.

226. **Signs and symptoms of acute transverse myelitis:** Patients appear with sudden or rapid onset of **back or radicular pain** which is followed by **ascending paresthesias** and **paralysis beginning in the feet, sensory loss below a particular dermatome** corresponding to the site of involvement, urinary or fecal incontenence. **All these symptoms are due to spinal cord dysfunction,** symptoms may progress **within minutes (**due to infarction) or **few days.**
Best diagnostic study: MRI to rule out other diseases.

Preceeding infections: Patients may have **URI (or flulike), measles, or mycoplasma** infection before the onset of neurological symptoms. Remember **transverse myelitis and progressive myelopathy are either the first or late manifestation of MS.**

Treatment:

(i) **Cord compression:** Surgical decompression, antibiotics, or corticosteroids.
(ii) Idiopathic transverse myelopathy, MS, or cord compression: Corticosteroids.
(iii) Neoplastic cord compression: Dexamethasone.
(iv) Idiopathic transverse myelitis: IV methylprednisolone.
(v) Ventilator management.
(vi) Urinary bladder catheterization.

227. **Most common cause of optic neuritis: Multiple sclerosis.** Other causes are tobacco- nutritional amblyopia, vasculitis, optic nerve compression, ischemic optic neuropathy, vitamin B_{12} deficiency, sarcoidosis, or Leber's disease.

228. **Signs and symptoms of optic neuritis:** Patients appear with acute or subacute, partial or complete loss of vision in one or both eyes; pain is present inside, around, or behind the eye.
   (a) **Retrobulbar neuritis:** Lesion is in the posterior two thirds of the optic nerve, so **normal opthalmological examination for initial 2 to 3 weeks, then disc becomes pale and atrophic.**
   (b) **Papillitis:** Lesion is in the anterior portion of the optic nerve, **papilledema and loss of vision are** noted by opthalmological examination. (Remember, papilledema is due to increased ICP and has normal vision).

229. **Patients with idiopathic optic neuritis, CSF oligoclonal bands, or MRI abnormalities indicate: Early conversion to MS.**

230. **Treatment of optic neuritis: Intravenous methylprednisolone for 3 days followed by prednisone with tapering doses within 8 days of the beginning of the disease.** It reduces the risk to conversion of MS by 50%.

231. **Devic's disease (neuromyelitis optica syndrome):** Patients appear with first loss of vision (optic neuritis) then paraplegia (partial or complete transverse myelopathy) or paraplegia is followed by loss of vision. It may be a part of MS or its variants. This syndrome may be due to acute disseminated encephalomyelitis, SLE, or sarcoidosis.

232. Patients appear with acute or subacute onset of **altered behavior,** headaches, apathy, mutism, and **difficulty in communication.**
CSF: Normal.
MRI: Extensive lesions in cerebral white matter.
Definitive diagnosis: Biopsy and histopathological findings of alternating bands containing demyelinated and partially demyelinated axons.
Most likely diagnosis: Concentric sclerosis.

233. Gene location in (ALD) adrenoleukodystrophy (x-linked): **Xq28.** (other recessive form is called neonatal ALD).
Adult patients appear with progressive dementia, adrenal insufficiency without CNS involvement or **asymptomatic male** with H/O affected family member.
Defect: Fatty acids accumulation in the tissues and body fluids are due to defective peroxisomal catabolism.
Diagnosis is confirmed by: Increased level of very long chain fatty acids in blood, tissue, or cultured fibroblasts.
Prenatal diagnosis: Biochemical and genetic screening of amniocytes.
Gene screening: DNA probe.
MRI: Symmetrical lesions in the posterior parietal and occipital white matters.
Adrenal functions: Decreased hormonal levels.
CSF: Same as in MS but higher proteins.
Treatment:
(i) Dietary restriction of long chain fatty acids.
(ii) Replacement of adrenal hormones.
(iii) **No specific treatment** but bone marrow transplantation may slow the disease progression.

234. **Enzyme deficiency in metachromatic leukodystrophy: Arylsulfatase A.** It is a lysosomal storage disease. **Adult patients appear with progressive mental deterioration to severe dementia,** pyramidal tract, cerebellar signs, absence of tendon reflexes, and elevated CSF protein.
Definitive diagnosis: Increased urinary excretion of sulfatide and **reduced enzyme activity in venous blood or cultured fibroblasts.**
Treatment: Bone marrow transplantation may slow or stop the progression of the disease.

235. Most common type and etiology of seizure in adults.
(a) **Type: Complex partial (39%),** next is generalized tonic-clonic type (25%).
(b) **Etiology**: **Idiopathic or cryptogenic (55%) means cerebral injury.**

236. **Uncinate fits are associated with: Brain tumors.** Uncinate fits are the type of complex partial seizures, preceeded by an olfactory aura because of their origin in or near the uncus of the medial temporal lobe.

237. **Most common source of complex partial seizures: Temporal lobe,** most commonly from **mesial temporal lobe structures (**hippocampus, amygdala, and parahippocampal gyrus**).**
   (A) **Presentation of complex partial seizures of temporal lobe origin: Motionless staring, impair consciousness followed by automatisms** (repetitive purposeless complex movements), **dystonic positioning of the upper extremities** contralateral to seizure discharge. **Gestural automatisms:** Fumbling, hand wringing, patting movements, picking at clothes or objects.
   Oroalimentary automatisms: Lip smacking, swallowing, sucking, and chewing movements.
   Clumpsy preservation of ongoing motor activities: Walking, eating, washing dishes, or drawing **seizures usually last for 45 to 90 seconds and are followed by confusion, disorientation for several minutes, and** postictal aphasia if involves the dominant temporal lobe. Patients do **not** remember the seizures episode that occurs after the aura.
   (B) Presentation of **complex partial seizures of frontal lobe origin:**
      (i) Begin and end aburptly.
      (ii) Postictal symptoms are absent or rarely present.
      (iii) Abnormal motor movements: Thrashing, pelvic thrusting, pedalling movements of lower extremities, flailing of arms and legs, or loud noise.
      (iv) Scalp EEG: Minimal or nonlocalizing changes.

238. **Treatment for temporal lobe epilepsy:**
   (a) Anticonvulsant drugs can suppress secondary generalized seizures, but >50% of patients continue to have parital seizures.
   (b) Drug-resistant cases: Temporal lobectomy is the treatment of choice.

239. **Few important points in post-traumatic epilepsy:**
   (a) It is directly proportional to severity of the head injury.
   (b) Majority of the patients with severe head injury develop seizures within 1 to 2 years.
   (c) Most common type is partial or secondarily generalized seizures.
   (d) Mild head injury does **not** cause seizure.

(e) Impact seizures (generalized convulsion at or immediately after injury) and early seizures (within first two weeks) are due to acute reaction of the brain to the trauma.

(f) **Remember, seizures begin after 10 to 14 days causes** increased risk of developing post-traumatic epilepsy.

(g) **Treatment:** Phenytoin is the drug of choice in early seizures. It **is used to prevent seizures** in severe head injury for 1 to 2 weeks, **after that phenytoin should be discontinued** in patients without seizures because phenytoin **cannot** prevent the development of later seizures (Important).

240. Treatment of EPC (epilepsia partialis continua- focal seizures which involve part or all of one side of the body): No treatment (anticonvulsants, corticosteroids, antiviral agents) is effective. **Some patients spontaneously improve.**

Causes of EPC in adults are following:

(i) Severe strokes.

(ii) Brain tumors (primary or metastatic).

(iii) Encephalitis.

(iv) Metabolic (hyperosmolar nonketotic hyperglycemia).

241. **Recurrent risk after first seizure:**

(a) Patients with idiopathic generalized seizures, normal EEG, and negative family history: Only 24 %.

(b) Patients with severe head injury and abnormal EEG (high-risk group): 65% in 2 years.

(c) Remember, person with first seizure does **not** have epilepsy.

242. Recurrent risk after second seizures: More than 80%, so it is a reliable indication of epilepsy.

243. Causes of death in epilepsy:

(a) Most common cause of death in idiopathic or cryptogenic epilepsy is **accident (most common is drowning).**

(b) Patients with symptomatic epilepsy: Mortality is due to **underlying disease condition.**

(c) Other causes of death: **Cardiac arrythmia, myocardial infarction, and pulmonary edema**.

244. Diagnosis of epilepsy:

(a) **A detailed history is the most important factor in the diagnosis.** It should be obtained from family members or other close observers.

(b) EEG: It is the most important diagnostic study for epilepsy.
Few important points about EEG:
(i) Up ot 50% of patients with epilepsy may have abnormal initial EEG.
(ii) Serial EEG's or sleep deprivation for 24 hours before the EEG increases the chances to make the diagnosis.
(iii) **Definitive diagnosis** can be made by documenting characteristic ictal discharge during a clinical attack.
(iv) Interictal abnormal EEG **cannot prove or refute** a diagnosis of epilepsy.
(v) Interictal abnormal EEG can be present in **2% of the normal populations.**
(vi) A small number of patients with epilepsy have **normal EEG's** despite utmost effort.
(vii) Simultaneous EEG, closed-circuit TV, and computer-assisted detection and analysis are very helpful in making accurate diagnosis of epilepsy and localizing epileptogenic foci for resective surgery.

(c) **MRI is more helpful than CT** scan in detecting epileptogenic cerebral lesions.
(d) Young adults with unexplained cause of seizure. should have blood and urine tests for substances abuse (cocaine and other drugs). Routine blood analysis for CBC, SMA-6, liver function tests are useful for baseline study.
(e) Lumbar tap is **not** helpful unless there is meningitis or encephalitis.

Remember, repeated seizures may increase the CSF protein and the cell counts up to 100 for 24 to 48 hours.

(f) ECG: It should be done in **young patients with first seizure** and family history of arrythmia, sudden death, or episodic unconsciousness. It is important in **any patients with arrythmias or valvular** disease of the heart.

245. **Definitive diagnostic method in psychogenic epilepsy**: Video/EEG study: **Normal.**

Patients appear with **atypical and nonstereotyped attacks,** precipitated by emotional or psychological factor, H/O psychiatric illness, **normal** EEG, and **unresponsive to anticonvulsant medications.**

246. **Medical management of seizure:**

(A) **First seizure:**
(i) Rule out any medical or neurologic illness.
(ii) Hospital admission is **not** needed but close follow up is needed.
(iii) EEG should be done but MRI or CT scan is **not** needed unless there is strong suspicion of intracerebral lesions.

(iv) Use of anticonvulsant medication is a matter of controversy. Recent evidence suggests that it may reduce the risk of relapse.

(v) Patients who have **two or more high risks** should be treated with anticonvulsant drugs. **High risk means** abnormal EEG, abnormal physical finding, H/O significant cerebral injury, positive family history of seizure, and abnormal MRI or CT scan.

(vi) Medications used are the following:

(a) Primary generalized seizure: Tonic-clonic, tonic, and myoclonic types: **Valproate is the drug of choice.** Absence type: **Ethosuximide is the drug of choice because valproate is more toxic.** Remember, do **not** use phenytoin, carbamazepine in **absence and myoclonic seizures** because they can exacerbate the seizure.

(b) Simple and complex partial: **Carbamazepine or phenytoin is the drug of choice** but phenytoin causes gingival hypertrophy, coarse facial features, and hirsutism. So, **carbamazepine is the drug of choice for younger and patients who are concerned about the facial cosmetic features.** Valproate, primidone, or phenobarbital can be used.

(c) Secondary generalized: Same as above.

247. **Side effects of antiepileptic drug:**

(a) **Most common side effects are dose related:** Monitor serum level of the drug.

(b) **Idiosyncratic reactions: It is the most serious and life-threatening side effect.** It includes rash, thrombocytopenia, agranulocytosis, aplastic anemia, hepatic failure, and **Stevens- Johnson syndrome.**

Remember, it is not dose related and no laboratory test can predict idiosyncratic reaction.

(c) Carbamazepine: **Benign leukopenia but no anemia and no increased risk of infection.**

(d) Remember, patients with epilepsy may have **normal asymptomatic elevation of SGOT, SGPT, and GTT.** No further intervention is needed.

248. **Management of treatment failure in epilepsy:**

(a) First use **only one anticonvulsant.**

(b) If failed, then change the anticonvulsant **to a new one.**

(c) If failed, then **use two medications** simultaneously.

(d) The following drugs can be used as an adjunctive therapy: Felbamate, gabapentin, and lamotrigine. (Felbamate causes aplastic anemia and hepatic failure).

249. **Most common cause of convulsion** in epileptic patients who are pregnant receiving antiepileptic medication: **Low antiepileptic drug level** because of physiologic increase of volume of distribution and clearance. **Seizure can be avoided by close monitoring of serum drug level, particularly after first trimester.** Remember, **epilepsy is not a contraindication of pregnancy** but physician should inform the patients regarding complications and appropriate management should be instituted.
Most of the patients (>90% have normal babies).

250. **Complications and management of epileptic patients during pregancy:**
   (A) Complications (Women have 1.5 to 3 times higher rates of complication irrespective of treatment).
      (i) Increased seizures (33% of cases), intrapartum bleeding, abruptio placentae, toxemia, premature delivery, and still birth.
      (ii) Major fetal malformations (e.g., cleft lip or plate, cardiac anomaly, spina bifida, and anencephaly):
         (a) Normal general population: 2%.
         (b) Patients is on one anticonvulsant drug: 5 to 6%.
         (c) Patients is on two anticonvulsant durgs: 10%.
         (d) Valproate and carbamazepine increase the risk of neural tube defects.
      (iii) Minor malformations (e.g., hypoplastic nails, hypertelorism, **low-set ears, andprominent lips**): It is due to genetic and drug related effects. **This is very important to remember that all anticonvulsants including phenytoin and valproate cause minor malformations.**
      (iv) Hemorrhagic complication of the newborn.
   (B) **Treatment.**
      (i) **To avoid bleeding in the newborn:** Mother should receive **oral vitamin K, 20 mg per day during the last month of pregnancy** plus baby should get routine 1 mg vitamin K intramuscular injection.
      (ii) To avoid neural tube defects: Mother should receive **folic acid before conception (very important point), 1 mg per day.**

251. **Surgical management of epilepsy:**
   (a) Ideal patients for resective surgery:
      (i) Seizures begin in an **identifiable localized area of cortex.**
      (ii) Surgical excision **can remove the epileptogenic region.**
      (iii) Surgery should **not** impair neurologic function.
   (b) Surgical therapy is the following:
      (i) **Focal cortical resection: Most common type of surgery used is in adults.**

(ii) Corpus callosotomy and hemispherectomy: These two procedures are used in selected patients who developed uncontrolled seizures **in childhood.**

(c) Surgery is done in **patients with failed medical treatment,** but many patients benefit from early surgical intervention.

252. **Treatment of status epilepticus:**

(i) Airway, oxygen, intubation, IV access, blood test, drug level.

(ii) Give **IV benzodiazepine (diazepam 10 mg, repeated once or lorazepam)** followed by **IV phenytoin (20 mg/kg** at a rate not exceeding 50 mg/minute).

(iii) If seizure continues, give **additional phenytoin 5 mg/kg. About 80% of patients respond with this management**.

(iv) If seizures continues, patients should be **admitted to the ICU** and **anesthetized with IV phenobarbital** 5 mg/kg, followed by 25 to 50 mg every 25 to 50 minutes prn to produce a burst- suppression pattern on continously recorded EEG.

(v) Ventilator management as needed.

(vi) Vasopressors for hypotension.

(vii) Patients with hypoglycemia: First give thiamine 100 mg, is followed by 50 ml of 50% glucose (IV push).

253. **Two types of status epilepticus:**

(a) Convulsive status epilepticus: It is a medical emergency. It may be either **idiopathic generalized onset** or bilateral spread from focal epilepsy. It is the first manifestation of epilepsy in 10% of patients and >50% of patients of status epilepticus do **not** have a H/O epilepsy.

Most of the death is due to underlying condition (not due to status epilepticus).

(b) Nonconvulsive status epilepticus: It is found in middle-aged or elderly **individual with no H/O seizures.** Patients appear with **sudden onset of fluctuating confusional state, clouding of consciousness,** bizarre behavior, delusion, paranoia, catatonia **but absence of stupor or coma.**

Etiology: Mostly unknown, it may be due to electrolyte imbalance, focal cerebral lesion (frontal lobe infarction), and drug toxicity (lithium).

Diagnosis: Abnormal discharge in EEG plus clinical presentation.

Treatment.

(i) IV diazepam or lorazepam causes dramatic improvement.

(ii) Long term seizure control: Valproate, phenytoin, or carbamazepine.

254. **Most common causes of loss of smell sensation**: Local obstructive disease, viral infection, or head injuries.

255. **Most common causes of loss of the taste sensation**: Drug ingestion (e.g., penicillamine, captopril, antirheumatic, and antiproliferative).

256. **Visual field defects due to damage of the visual pathways**: (Important).
    (a) **Optic nerve:** Unilateral blindness (amaurosis).
    (b) **Lateral optic chiasm:** Grossly incongruous, contralateral incomplete homonymous hemianopia.
    (c) **Central optic chiasm:** Bitemporal hemianopia.
    (d) **Optic tract:** Incongruous incomplete homonymous hemianopia.
    (e) **Temporal (Meyer's) loop of optic radiation**: Congruous partial or complete contralateral homonymous **superior** quadrantanopia.
    (f) **Parietal (superior) projection of optic radiation**: Congruous partial or complete contralateral homonymous **inferior** quadrantanopia.
    (g) **Complete parieto-occipital damage of optic radiation**: Complete contralateral congruous homonymous hemianopia with **macular sparing is** due to psychophysical shift of foveal point.
    (h) **Incomplelte (subtotal) damage of visual cortex**: Congruous homonymous **scotomas** encroaching **acutely or central vision.**

257. **Most common cause of acute or subacute monocular vision loss is due to following optic nerve disease**: Demyelinating disease (optic neuritis, papillitis, or retrobulbar neuritis), vascular obstruction (ischemic optic neuropathy), tumors invading the optic nerve, or space-occupying lesions.

258. **Anton's syndrome:** Cortical blindness with denial of visual defect. Patients **not only deny blindness but also confabulate the visual environment from memory.** Lesions are in the medial, temporal, parietal lobes, and calcarine cortex.

259. **Physiologic anisocoria (**or benign pupillary dilatation): Lifelong difference in the size of the two pupils with normal reflex reaction. **Disparity remains constant during dilatation and constriction.**

260. **Argyll-Robertson pupils:** Small (1 to 2 mm), irregular, unequal, fixed to light but constrict to accomodation. It is found in tertiary neurosyphilis, partial findings in **diabetes,** and some autonomic neuropathies.

261. Pupillary responses are due to lesions in the optic nerve, oculomotor, and pretectum:
   (a) **Optic nerve damage (B/L-bilateral):**
      (i) Baseline pupillary response: (B/L) dilatations.
      (ii) Light placed on affected side: (B/L) remains dilated.
      (iii) Light placed on normal side: (B/L) constrictions.
      (iv) Accomodation: (B/L) constrictions.
   (b) **Oculomotor nerve damage:**
      (i) Baseline pupillary response: Dilated affected side and other side is normal.
      (ii) Light placed on affected side: Dilated affected side and normal side is constricted.
      (iii) Light placed on normal side: Same as (ii).
      (iv) Accomodation: Same as (ii).
   (c) **Pretectum damage:**
      (i) Baseline pupillary response: (B/L) dilatations.
      (ii) Light placed on affected side: Same as (i).
      (iii) Light placed on normal side: Same as (i).
      (iv) Accomodation: (B/L) constrictions.

262. Drugs causing sensorineural hearing loss:
   (a) **Aminoglycoside antibiotics** (e.g., gentamicin, amikacin, kanamycin, tobramycin, streptomycin, and neomycin): Most commonly affect the **cochlea.**
   (b) Furosemide, ethacrynic acid.
   (c) Salicylates.
   (d) Antineoplastic agent: Cisplatin (severe ototoxicity).

263. **Evaluations of the hearing loss (step by step):**
   (A) **First, history** (drug, hereditary or family history, trauma, noise exposure, intrauterine factors) should be obtained.
   (B) **Second, examination of the ear:**
      (i) **Abnormal findings:** Cerumen, otitis media, drum perforation, trauma, cholesteatoma: Treat accordingly.
      (ii) Normal findings: Do pure tone audiometry.
   (C) **Third, pure tone audiometry.**
      (i) **Conductive hearing loss:** Do **impedance audiometry** to diagnose the following diseases– Eustachian tube malfunction, otosclerosis, serous otitis, and ossicular chain dysfunction.
      (ii) **Sensorineural hearing loss:** Do BAER study.
   (D) **Fourth, BAER study:**

(i) **Normal:** Do fistula test.
  (a) Abnormal fistula test: Diagnosis is perilymph fistula.
  (b) Normal fistula test: Diagnosis could be labyrinthitis, infarct of labyrinth, noise induced, **presbycusis** (progressive, bilateral hearing loss in advanced age), **Meniere's syndrome** (fluctuating hearing loss, tinnitus, recurrent vertigo, sensation of fullness or pressure in the ear; all these symptoms are due to endolymphatic hydrops or hypertension).

(ii) **Abnormal BAER study: Do MRI or CT scan** to diagnose the following diseases:
  (a) Brain stem infarct.
  (b) Multiple sclerosis.
  (c) Acoustic neuroma.
  (d) Other cerebellopontine angle tumor.

264. **Most sensitive diagnostic study to diagnose cerebellopontine-angle tumor: MRI.**

Patients appear with retrocochlear hearing loss (diagnosed by BAER study), sensation of disequilibrium, and rarely positional vertigo. C-P angle tumors are acoustic neuroma, meningioma, and epidermal cyst.

265. **Evaluation and method of diagnosis in patients with tinnitus:**

(A) **First,** history of taking any offending drugs (e.g., indomethacin, aminophylline, propranolol, levodopa, quinidine, salicylate, caffeine).

(B) **Second, examination of the ear:**
  (i) Audio sounds: (three types).
    (a) Continuous: Acoustic emissions, venous hum.
    (b) Synchronous with pulse: Aneurysm, venous, hum, vascular tumor, and malformation.
    (c) Synchronous with respiration: Patent eustachian tube.
  (ii) No audible sounds: Do neurologic examination.

(C) **Third,** neurological examination: (two types).
  (i) Brain stem signs: Multiple sclerosis, tumor, ishcemic infarction.
  (ii) Normal: Do audiogram.

(D) **Fourth,** audiogram: (three types).
  (i) Normal: Idiopathic tinnitus.
  (ii) Conductive hearing loss: Cerumen, otitis media, otosclerosis.
  (iii) Sensorineural hearing loss: Do BAER study.

(E) **Fifth, BAER study**:
  (i) Abnormal (neural): Acoustic neuroma, vascular compression, other C-P angle tumors.

(ii) Normal cochlear: Ototoxic drugs, noise, presbycusis, labyrinthitis, perilymph fistula, Meniere's syndrome.

266. **Evaluation and method of diagnosis in patients with vertigo:**
   (A) **First:** History of drugs intake, trauma, migraine, and hereditary factors.
   (B) **Second,** examination shows (three types):
      (i) Focal neurologic signs: Do MRI or CT scan to diagnose MS, tumor, infarction, degenerative disease.
      (ii) Normal: Do audiometry.
      (iii) Hearing loss: Do audiometry.
   (C) **Third:** Audiometry (two types):
      (i) Normal: Do ENG (electronystagmography) to diagnose benign positional vertigo, ototoxicity, physiologic, vertigo, and peripheral vestibulopathy.
      (ii) Sensorineural loss: Do BAER study.
   (D) **Fourth**: BAER study (two types):
      (i) Normal: Fistula, labyrinthitis, labyrinthine concussion, Meniere's disease.
      (ii) Abnormal: Acoustic neuroma, other C-P angle tumor.

267. **Most common cause of pathological vertigo**: BPV (benign positonal vertigo).
   Most common etilogy of BPV: **Unknown**, other causes are head injury, viral labyrinthitis, and vascular occlusion.

268. **Most common causes of physiologic vertigo**: Motion sickness, space sickness, and height sickness.

269. **Treatment of vertigo:**
   (A) **Specific therapies**.
      (i) Surgery: Acoustic neruoma.
      (ii) Anticoagulants: Vertebrobasilar insufficiency.
      (iii) Antibiotics: Bacterial or syphilitic labyrinthitis.
   (B) **Symptomatic therapy:**
      (i) Patients prefer to lie still with eyes closed in a quiet, dark room.
      (ii) Antivertiginous drugs with sedation: Phenargan or diazepam.
      (iii) To stop vomiting: Prochlorperazine.
      (iv) Antivertiginous drug with **less** sedation: Meclizine or transdermal scopolamine.
   (C) **Rehabilitative therapy**: Vestibular rehabilitation exercise is helpful.

270. **Treatment for tinnitus**:
 (a) Detailed inverview, examination, laboratory investigation, and then **reassurance.**
 (b) Patients with hearing loss: Hearing aid.
 (c) Cerumen of the external ear canal should be removed.
 (d) Tinnitus during sleep: To mask the tinnitus, FM clock radio tuned between stations and it should be off when patients go to sleep.
 (e) H/O drug intake: Stop the drug.
 (f) H/O alcohol, nicotine, or caffeine: Stop those items.

271. **The syndrome of classic migraine (four phases):**
 (a) **First, prodromal phase:** Alteration of mood approximately 24 hours or more before the headache, or red wine may precipitate the attack.
 (b) **Second, neurologic phase:** Patients noticed **bright flashing lights in the center of the visual field** and then radiate towards periphery, or may have unilateral paresthesias of the hand and perioral area, aphasia, hemiparesis, and hemisensory defects. **These may occur without headache in older** people.
 (c) **Third, characteristic neurologic symptoms: Unilateral throbbing frontotemporal headache opposite of the side of neurologic** symptoms, nausea, vomiting, **photophobia, phonophobia** (unable to tolerate noise), and diarrhea. Headaches may last **usually 4 to 6 hours or** longer, it consists of dull, aching, bilateral pain extends into the back of the neck and shoulder and it is relieved by vomiting or sleep.
 (d) **Fourth, postheadache phase:** Exhaustion, scalp tenderness, and recurrence of head pain on sudden head movement.

272. **Common migraine:** Same as classic migraine **without neurological symptoms. The attacks are precipitated by** vasodilators (nitroglycerine), reserpine (release serotonin), estrogens, and oral contraceptives.
Diagnosis: History of migraine.
Treatment: Sumatriptan or ergotamine.

273. **Diagnosis and treatment of classic migraine**:
 (A) Diagnosis:
  (i) **History of migraine;** physical findings are usually **absent** and **no** laboratory studies are diagnostic.
  (ii) Patients with neurologic findings: MRI or CT scan to rule out other diseases.
 (B) **Treatment:**
  (a) **Prevention: It is the best treatment.**

(i) Avoid food, medications, stress, fatigue, and excessive sleep. These may be the precipitating factors in different individuals.

(ii) **Pharmacologic prevention: Beta-adrenergic,** serotonin, calcium channel blockers, NSAID's, antidepressants, valproic acid.

(C) **Pharmacologic treatment:**

(i) Mild attacks: Analgesics and bed rest.

(ii) Moderate to severe attacks: Ergotamine or sumatriptan **(intravenously),** is therapeutic and diagnostic. Sublingual or rectal preparation of ergot is better than oral in effectiveness.

(iii) **Extremely severe headaches in the ER:** IV sumatriptan is the drug of choice.

(iv) **Prophylaxis** for headaches occur more than once a week- Ergotamine.

274. **The side effects of ergotism:** Muscle pain, mottled skin is due to vasoconstriction, peripheral gangrene, and multifocal encephalopathy.

275. A 50 year old woman appears in the ER in the spring or fall with H/O severe headaches (few times a day, mostly at night) which are characterized by sudden onset of **knife-like pain in the nostril or behind the eye including the forehead.** Patients also bang her head in the wall, threaten suicide during severe headache. Headaches last for 30 minutes to 2 hours and it **appears and disappears suddenly without any residual symptoms.**

Physical examination: Ipsilateral watery nostril and the eye. Horner syndrome may or may **not** be present.

Most likely diagnosis: Cluster headaches.

Diagnosis is made by the: History.

Treatment.

(i) **Acute attack: Oxygen inhalation** may reduce the headaches, analgesics may **not** help because by the time it absorbs the attack is over.

(ii) **Prophylactic: Oral ergotamine tartrate is helpful.** It should be **withdrawan every seventh day to avoid ergotism** and to see whether the cluster headaches are over.

276. **Chronic paroxysmal hemicrania (cluster variants)**: Patients appear with cluster headaches 10 to 20 times per day, each last 10 to 30 minutes, and exacerbated by exertion.

Treatment: Indomethacin is the drug of choice. If failed, then use tricyclic antidepressants.

277. **Chinese food headaches:** It is due to monosodium glutamate (MSG). Patients appear with postprandial headache, tight sensation around the face and head, rarely diarrhea and giddiness.
Treatment: Avoid chinese food which contains MSG.

278. **Causes of hangover headaches:** Alcohol withdrawal, dehydration, and toxic effect of various congeners present in different toxicants.

279. **Severe thunderclap headaches may be associated with: Subarachnoid hemorrhage** (SAH) but most of the time there is no pathological findings. Patients appear with severe, suddent onset of **exploding pain all over the head and it** resolved gradually over ther hours.
CSF: Lumbar tap to rule out SAH, if positive then **angiography** may be needed to look for **intracranial aneurysms.**

280. **Treatment of hypertensive headaches**: **Antihypertensive drug.** Patients appear with throbbing occipital headaches in the early morning.

281. **Tension-type headaches:** It is benign, found in majority of the individuals, usually bilateral, last minutes to days, but **absence of photophobia, phonophobia, and nausea.**
Treatment:
(i) First method is to treat the underlying causes.
(ii) **Asprin** is the better than acetaminophen because of its antiprostaglandin properties.
(iii) Massage may help.
(iv) Sharply localized painful areas: Injection of local anesthetic is helpful temporarily.
(v) Patients who are receiving chronic ingestion of analgesics: **Stop those medications** which may cause tension-type headaches.
(vi) Depressed patients: Amitriptyline (antidepressant).
(vii) Anxious patients: Diazepam relieves the symptoms, it is also diagnostic.
Remember, diazepam <30 mg per day for 2 to 3 weeks does not cause physical depedence.

282. **Treatment of post-traumatic headaches (dull, aching, generalized pain after head injury)**:
(a) Patients should return to work as soon as possible.
(b) Treatment is same as tension-type headaches.
(c) Reassurance and psychologic support.
(d) Mild analgesics or anxiolytic drug (diazepam).

283. **Post-traumatic syndrome:** Post-traumatic headaches **plus giddiness, unsteadyness, insomnia, fatigue, and unable to concentrate.**
Treatment: Same as pos-traumatic headaches.

284. **Treatment of trigeminal neuralgia:**
   - (a) **Carbamazepine:** It is mainly anticonvulsive, not analgesic, but it has sedative properties. It is also used in **glossopharyngeal neuralgia and lightning pains of tabes dorsalis.**
   - (b) Other medications may be effective: Baclofen, pimozide, and phenytoin; rarely effective drugs are valproate, lorazepam, and mexiletine.
   - (c) **Surgical procedures:**
     - (i) **Lesioning of the gasserian ganglion:** Radiofrequency or glycerol injections.
     - (ii) **Posterior fossa craniotomy**: To relieve compression of the trigeminal nerve by vascular structures.

285. **Signs and symptoms of trigeminal neuralgia or tic douloureux:** Sudden, paroxysmal (lightning- like) pain in the distribution of the one or more branches of the trigeminal nerve. It may be precipitated by touching the trigger zone around lips and buccal cavity.

286. **Most common cause of trigeminal neuralgia**:
   - (a) **Compression of the trigeminal nerve by normal but aging arteries or veins of the posterior fossa is the most common cause.**
   - (b) Sometimes it may be a **manifestation of** multiple sclerosis, gasserian ganglion tumor, or brain-stem infarct involving the descending root of the trigeminal nerve.
   - (c) Unknown.

287. **Most important part of the body to be examined in glossopharyngeal neuralgia**: **Tonsil to rule out tonsillar tumor and posterior pharynx.**
Signs and symptoms of glossopharyngeal neuralgia: Sudden, paroxysmal (lighting-like) pain in the distribution **of the glossopharyngeal and vagus nerves,** pain begins in the (triggering zone) tonsil or posterior pharynx, then **spread towards the angle of the jaw and the ear, rarely** patients may have bradycardia or cardiac arrest.
Treatment:
   - (a) **Carbamazepine is the drug of choice.**
   - (b) If failed, then use other drugs already mentioned.

288. **Diagnostic approach of patients with headaches in general:**
   (a) Patients with migraine or tension-type headache: History is most important and then physical examination.
   (b) Patients with recent onset of headache, worsening headache, post-traumatic or headaches begin after the age of 30: **MRI is the best diagnostic method,** next is CT scan.
   (c) Patients with headaches associated with fever or suspected subarachnoid hemorrhage: Lumbar tap is indicated.
   (d) Remember, EEG and brain scan are **not** useful.

289. **Treatment of different types of pain**:
   (a) **Postherpetic neuralgia:**
      (i) Topical application of lidocaine.
      (ii) Carbamazepine is helpful in mild pain.
      (iii) TCA or mexiletine, fluphenazine (neuroleptics) are useful in severe continuous pain.
      (iv) **Remember,** acyclovir and corticosteroids have **no** effects on postherpetic neuralgia but **both reduces pain in acute herpes.**
      (v) The pain may **disappear spontaneously** after one or two years.
   (b) **Fibromyalgia and myofascial pain:**
      (i) Mild analgesic medications, heat, and massage may help in some patients.
      (ii) Massage or injection of the trigger points **with local anesthetic** may help in others.
      (iii) Antidepressants are helpful for short term therapy in 20% of patients.
      (iv) Long term therapy includes psychological help to patients.
   (c) **Sympathetically maintained pain**:
      (i) Block sympathetic outflow to the affected site while stimulating and mobilizing the painful area.
      (ii) Phenoxybenzamine (sympatholytic drug) and short duration of corticosteroids may be helpful.
      (iii) **In unresponsive patients, drugs used for neuropathic pain** are the TCA (amitriptyline), carbamazepine, and mexiletine (oral local anesthetic). Patients should be referred to multidisciplinary pain center.
   (d) **Phantom limb pain**:
      (i) Cutaneous stimulation: By rubbing or electrical stimulation.
      (ii) Repeated anesthetic block of peripheral nerves proximal to the stump.

290. **Most common complication of osteoporosis: Vertebral compression fractures.** Patients appear with localized tenderness and muscle spasm at the level of the compressed nerve roots.

291. **Most common form of low back pain with radiculitis is associated with**: **Discogenic disease which includes prolapse, protrusion, or extrusion of intervertebral disc substances.** Patients may appear with acute pain which is preceeded by the chronic intermittent low back pain or H/O acute injury.
Most common site of disc herniation is between **L4-L5** or **L5-S1.**
   (a) **Symptoms and signs of L4 nerve root involvement:** Referred pain along the course of the femoral nerve during hip extension and knee flexion, absence or reduced of patellar reflex, or weak knee extention.
   (b) **Symptoms and signs of L5 nerve root involvement:** Classic sciatic pain (radiating along the posterior thigh, anteromedial leg and foot, weakness of the toe extensors).
   (c) **Symptoms and signs of first sacral radiculopathy:** Pain along the posterior thigh, calf, and heel; absence or reduced Achilles tendon reflex; weakness of the ankle and toe flexors.

292. **Investigations and treatment of back pain**:
   (A) **Investigations**:
      (i) Trauma: Plain x-ray. It also detects degenerative diseases.
      (ii) Suspected bony injury: X-ray or CT scan.
      (iii) Tissue injury: MRI.
      (iv) Planning for surgery: CT or MRI.
      (v) Metabolic: Ca, P, alkaline phosphatase.
      (vi) R/O neoplasms, infections, or inflammations: Anemia plus increased ESR.
      (vii) Osteomyelitis or neoplasms: Bone scan, vertebral biopsy.
      (viii) Nerve roots involvement: EMG.
   (B) **Treatment:**
      (i) Conservative therapy (bed rest, analgesics, anti-inflammatory medication, or moist heat).
      (ii) After bed rest, gradual walking, exercise, and back protection with lumbosacral support.
      (iii) **Most herniated disc respond to conservative management.** Unresponsive patients may require epidural steroids, nerve root or sleeve infiltration with steriods. Before surgery, psychological evaluation and exercise for back strengthening is helpful.
      (iv) **Surgery is indicated** in patients with progressive muscular weakness and neurologic deficit despite conservative management or cauda equina syndrome.

(v) **Prophylactic therapy after surgery or conservative management:** Postural education, avoid lower spine stress, daily exercise to strengthen the lumbar and abdominal muscles.
(vi) Spondylolisthesis or discogenic disease: Laminectomy, joint fusion may be needed.

293. **Signs and symptoms of parkinsonism**: **Tremor at rest, bradykinesia** (general slowing down of movement and daily activities), **rigidity** and **postural instability.** The **first two symptoms are the most typical** findings. It is more common in men above 55.

Two major subtypes of Parkinson's disease (PD):

(a) **Tremor subtype:** Earlier age of onset, normal mental status, and slower progression of the diseases than PIGD (postural instability and gait difficulty) subtype.
(b) **PIGD subtype:** Dementia, bradykinesia, and rapidly progressive disease.

Etiology: Unknown; genetic and environmental factor (meperidine analogue 1-methyl-4- phenyl 1,2,3,6- tetrahydropyridine- MRTP).

Pathogenesis: Neuronal loss (80% of dopaminergic neurons) with depigmentation of **substantia nigra** (SN) and dopamine depletion in the striatum must appear before clinical symptoms begin; presence of Lewy bodies (eosinophilic).

294. **Treatment of parkinsonism**:

(a) **Deprenyl:** It **increases the striatal concentration of dopamine** by blocking its metabolism by MAO (mono amino-oxidase) It **increases the energy and decreases the** bradykinetic symptoms, disease progression, and motor disability.
(b) **Trihexyphenidyl (anticholinergic drug)** should be added with deprenyl.
(c) Patients with depression: TCA (amitriptyline or nortriptyline) is helpful.
(d) **Amantadine may be used as an alternative** in elderly patients because anticholinergic and TCA cause urinary hesitancy, blurring of vision, and dry mouth.

Side effects of amantadine: Ankle edema, livedo reticularis, increase CHF, and mild anticholinergic effects.

(e) **The combinations of deprenyl trihexyphenidyl, and amantadine** may be used first, if the symtoms are **not** controlled adequately then use **levodopa plus carbidopa.**

Side effects of the levodopa: Psychiatric disorder, dyskinesis, and clinical fluctuation.

Contraindications of levodopa: Patients with melanoma; it should be used carefully in cardiac arrythmias, psychosis, dementia, or peptic ulcer disease.

(f) Bromocriptine pergolide (dopamine agonist) may be used **alone** without levodopa but **should be used together** as symptoms increases.

Side effects of bromocriptine pergolide: Same as levodopa plus erythromelalgia (painful erythema of the legs).

(g) Surgical management of PD (may be helpful).
  (i) Stereotaxic thalamotomy is rarely used to reduce the tremor.
  (ii) Pallidotomy and thalamic stimulation may reduce the symptoms.
  (iii) Experimental: Transplantation of fetal substantia nigra.

(h) Psychosocial support and education about the PD is important.

295. **Unresponsiveness to levodopa may occur (15% of patients) due to**:
  (a) **Wrong diagnosis: Patients may have postsynaptic parkinsonism** instead of PD.
  (b) **Drug interaction:** Between depamine receptor blocking agents and antiemetic drugs.
  (c) Pharmacokinetic causes: Inadequate doses, delayed emptying of the stomach, competitive absorption in small intestine and blood-brain barrier by the dietary amnio acids.

296. **Shy-Drager syndrome** (atypical parkinsonism) Patients appear with H/O orthostatic light headedness, sexual impotence, incontinence, and other autonomic symptoms **but no tremor.**

297. **Hallervorden- Spatz disease:** Autosomal recessive, patisents appear with dementia, bradykinesia, ataxia, choreoathetosis, retinitis pigmentosa, seizures, rigidity, and spasticity.
Pathology: Accumulation of iron in the globus pallidus (GP) and substantia nigra (SN). Cysteine (chelates iron) is also elevated in GP.

298. **Parkinsonism-plus disease or multliple system degeneration**:
  (a) Progressive supranuclear palsy: Parkinsonism plus supranuclear opthalmoparesis.
  (b) Alzheimer's disease with parkinsonism: Parkinsonism plus dementia.
  (c) Straitonigral degeneration: Parkinsonism plus laryngeal stridor.
  (d) Shy-Drager syndrome: Parkinsonism plus dysautonomia.

299. **Parkinsonism caused by drugs**:
  (a) Reserpine: Deplete presynaptic dopamine storage.
  (b) Antipsychotic and antiemetic drugs: Block the dopamine receptors.

300. **Most common type of tremor in the developed nations**: **Essential tremor.** It is an autosomal dominant. Patients do **not** have rigidity and hypokinetic features which are found in PD. Patients appear with **flexion-extension oscillation of the hands at the wrist or adduction-abduction movements of the fingers with outstretched hands.**

Treatment:

(a) Propranolol is the drug of choice.
(b) Other drugs which may be effective are primidone, lorazepam, alprazolam.
(c) Patients unresponsive to durgs: Local injection of botulinum may be effective or high frequency thalamic stimulation.
(d) **Surgery:** Thalamotomy is the last resort.

301. **Genetic marker of adult onset of primary dystonia**: Chromosome 9 (q32-q34 region), dopa responsive dystonia is linked to chromosome 14.

302. **Tardive dystonia (secondary dystonia)**: It is due to dopamine receptor blocking drugs (**tranquilizers** such as chlorpromazine, haloperidol, amoxapine, thioridazine), antiemetics (prochlorperazine, metoclopramide), and levodopa.
Treatment: Discontinue all the drugs or reduces the doses as needed.

303. **Treatment of dystonias**:

(a) **Supportive therapy:** Prosthesis, techniques of relaxation.
(b) **Trihexyphenidyl** (anticholinergic): It is the **most frequently used medication.**
(c) Dopamine-depleting and dopamine receptor blocking drugs **may be added in advanced cases.**
(d) Diazepam or lorazepam, baclofen, and carbamazepine may be helpful.
(e) Levodopa is effective in adolescent dystonia.
(f) Botulinum toxin injection into the contracted muscles causes paralysis.
(g) Surgical procedures are the following:
    (i) Cervical rhizotomy: Neck dystonia.
    (ii) Orbicularis myectomy: Blepharospasm.
    (iii) Thalamotomy: Hemidystonia or generalized dystonia.

304. **Most definitive diagnosis in Huntington's diseases (HD)**: Mutated Huntington gene consist of **unstable expanded CAG repeats.** The diagnosis is certain **when the repeat number exceeds 42.** It is done to confirm clinical diagnosis.

305. **Clinical presentation of Huntington's disease (HD)**:

(a) **Neurological presentation:** Gradual onset of clumsiness, and adventitious, randon, brief movement. **Initially distal chorea which becomes generalized.** Patietns have **difficulty in** maintaining **steady grip or tongue protrusion. Patients also have unsteady, irregular, dance like gait.**
(b) **Congnitive changes:** Impaired judgement and loss of recent memory.
(c) **Neuropsychological presentation:** Apathy, social withdrawal, agitation, depression, delusion, hallucination, or psychosis.

306. **Mode of inheritance and chromosome in HD**: Autosomal dominant, chromosome 4p 16.3.
Genetic counseling is important.

307. **Treatment of HD: (Symptomatic therapy).**
(a) **To control psychosis:** Use haloperidol, pimozide, thioridazine, and fluphenazine, if necessary.
Side effects: Tardive dyskinesia.
(b) To control chorea: Use reserpine.
Side effects: Depression, sedation, akathisia (inability to sit still), and parkinsonism.

308. **Consequence of group A streptococcus infection**: **Sydenham's chorea** which appears 6 months or after the infection unlike carditis and arthritis, both appear soon after infection.

309. **Neuroacnathocytosis (or Chorea-acanthocytosis):** Patients appear with chorea plus self mutilation (tongue and lip biting), lingual dystonia, motor and phonic tics.
Blood smear: Presence of acanthocytes.
CT or MRI: Caudate atrophy.
Mode of inheritance: Autosomal recessive.

310. **Gilles de la Tourette syndrome:** It is the **most common cause of tics. Genetic** is the most common cause of this syndrome. **The criteria of this syndrome:**
(a) Onset before the age 21.
(b) Both multiple motor and one or more phonic tics are usually present.
(c) Involuntary movement and noises **cannot** be explained by any medical condition.
(d) It occurs many times a day or everyday, often more than 1 year duration.
(e) The characteristics of the tics changes over time.
Treatment:

(a) Mild cases: Reassurance and behavioral theapy.
(b) Moderate to severe cases (social embarrassment of physical discomfort):
  (i) Dopamine receptor blocker: Fluphenazine, haloperidol, and pimozide. They reduces the frequency, severity of the tics, and also impulsive, aggressive behavior.
  Side effects of the drugs: Weight gain, sedation, depression, and tardive dyskinesia.
  (ii) Clonazepam, fluoxetine, clonidine, and clomipramine: They are useful in obsessive-compulsive disorder and other behavioral problems.

311. **Mode of inheritance and chromosome in adult-onset cerebellar ataxia:** Autosomal dominant; chromosome 6p, 12q, or 14q.

312. Signs and symptoms of adult onset cerebellar ataxia:
(a) Cerebellar ataxia, limb incoordination, dysarthria, and unable to walk, within 15 years from the onset of the disease between 20 to 50 years. These are the **most important findings.**
(b) Babinski signs and increased reflexes are usually present.
(c) Extrapyramidal findings may include chorea, athetosis, dystonia, and cogwheel rigidity.
(d) Retina: Pigmentary degeneration.
(e) Supranuclear oculomotor nerve disorder may be present: Ptosis, lid retraction, nystagmus, and upward gaze paresis.
Diagnosis: MRI shows **cerebellar atrophy plus** pons with dilatation of the fourth ventricle and pontine cisterns, but in **pure cerebellar atrophy only cerebellum is shrunken.**

313. **Amyotrophic lateral sclerosis.**
(a) **Chromosome: 21q** which is the location of the enzyme superoxide dismutase.
(b) **Incidence:** Mostly sporadic; males above 40.
(c) Pathology: Degenerative disorder of the CNS.
(d) Signs and Symptoms: **Progressive muscular weakness** of the limbs, trunk, respiratory muscles, throat, and tongue. Symptoms of both upper and lower motor neurones. **Normal** sensations (except vibration sense of the feet), **normal bladder, bowel, and sexual functions**.
(e) Most common cause of death: Lung infection and insufficiency.
(f) **Diagnosis:** No definitive test, **mostly clinical diagnosis.**
CSF: Normal or mildly elevated protein.
CT or MRI: Normal.
Serum creatine kinase: Normal or moderately increased.

EMG: Active and chronic denervation of the muscles involved, motor NCV is normal or reduced, and normal sensory conduction.

(g) **Conseling:**
- (i) Remember, physician should **not** make premature diagnosis.
- (ii) Physician should tell the patient and family **gradually, gently, and tactfully** regarding the disease.

(h) **Treatment:**
- (i) No medication is available.
- (ii) Physical therapy **cannot** delay the neuromuscular deterioration.
- (iii) Use cane or walker for impaired gait.
- (iv) Nasogastric tube feeding for dysphagia.
- (v) Mechanical ventilation for respiratory failure.
- (vi) Experimental medication may be used.

(i) **Prognosis**: Very poor.

314. **Narcolepsy and daytime hypersomnolence:**

(a) **Chromosomal location: 6** ; DQB1-0602 halotype is present.

(b) **Signs and symptoms:** It begins before the age of 25 and last a lifetime. Patients appear with **excessive daytime sleepiness without an increase in 24-hours sleep** is diagnostic plus catalepsy (Jelly-like bodily weakness plus laughter) with or without paralysis (brief period of feeling of paralysis and after sleep), presleep hallucinations-dream.

(c) Diagnosis: By history, age, and exclusion of other disease of hypersomnia.

(d) **Treatment:**
- (i) **Methylphenidate or dextroamphetamine (stimulants) is the best drug of choice to** counteract daytime drowsiness.
- (ii) TCA (imipramine or desipramine) is used to reduce catalepsy.

315. **Treatment of different sleep disorders**:

(a) **Insomina:**
- (i) Recent onset: Short acting benzodiazepines (triazolam for induction of sleep and flurazepan or quazepam for duration of sleep) are the drug of choice.
- (ii) Sustained, refractory, and chronic insomnia: Combined antidepressants and behavioral therapy; **avoid hypnotics.**

(b) **Parasomnias (motor or autonomic disorders which can delay or disrupt the normal sleep)**.
- (i) Bruxism (teeth grinding): Psychiatric consult to reduce stress and anxiety plus teeth shield.
- (ii) Somnoambulism: Lorazepam.
- (iii) REM behavior disorder: Clonazepam.

(iv) Restless leg syndrome: Carbamazepine, carbidopa, levodopa, oxycodone, or propoxyphene.
(v) Night terrors (rare in adults): R/O drug- alcohol, psychiatric disorder, or structural lesion.

316. **Alzheimer's disease and chromosomal link**: Chromosomes 14,19, and 21. Down syndrome may develop the disease in third or fourth decade of life.

317. **Risk factor of Alzheimer's disease:** Genotype for ApoE, particularly **homozygotes for $ApoE_4$ have higher risk** than with E_3 or E_2 homozygotes. E_3 heterozygotes have intermediate risk.

318. **Protective factor of** Alzheimer's disease: **High level of education** may be a protective factor.

319. **Signs and symptoms of Alzheimer's disease**: Gradual **impairment of memory and reasoning** usually begin after the age of 60. It can progress for decades or longer. Patients are unable to learn new events, failure to recognize familiar faces, unable to make correct decision regarding financial and nonfinancial matters, **but they can maitain their speech.** Some patients may **become suspicious** of family members, friends, or employer and show paranoid behavior particulary in the evening hours. Patients are **unable to visualize more than one object** in the visual field.

320. **Diagnostic method of Alzheimer's disease:**
Diagnosis: No reliable markers to make the diagnosis. **Patients must have the following features:**
(a) Documented dementia by bedside examination or neuropsychological test.
(b) Severe impairment of memory.
(c) Dementia should **not** be sudden or rapidly **progressive.**
Patients should **not** have the following features in early presentation:
(a) Motor abnormalities (gait disorder or hemiparesis): It is absent in Alzheimer's disease.
(b) Loss of somatic sensation: Absent.
(c) Visual field defect: Absent.
(d) Seizures: Absent.
Positron emission tomography: Diminished metabolic activity in the temporoparietal region.
CSF: Normal or mildly elevated protein.
CT or MRI: Normal or enlargement of sulci.
EEG: Normal in early stage or nonspecific slowing as disease progresses.

321. **Treatment of Alzheimer's disease**:
   (a) No drug is effective.
   (b) Tacrine is hepatotoxic and noneffective.
   (c) Early stage: Place cue cards around the house, it helps them to carry out their own care.
   (d) Appropriate motor skills (music playing, typing, card playing, dancing) give more pleasure.
   (e) Medicine is used for appropriate sleep.
   (f) Nursing home or facilities for dedicated service for long term care.

322. **Signs and symptoms of Pick's disease (degenerative loss of neurons in the frontal and anterior temporal regions)**:
   (a) Mostly women, over the age of 60, appear with impairment of judgements, socially inappropriate behaviors predominate over memory impairments. These symptoms are mostly due to involvement of frontal lobe.
   (b) Progressive aphasia without dementia: Most prominent or only symptom is the **language disorder.** It is called the left temporal form of Pick's disease.

   Diagnosis CT or MRI shows asymmetric lobar atrophy.

ENDOCRINOLOGY AND REPRODUCTIVE DISEASE

1. **Chromosomal location of the human gene for pro-pro ANP (atrial natriuretics peptide) which is derived from the heart: Chromosome 1.**

2. **Most common tumors affecting the hypothalamus**: **Pituitary adenomas**, and next most common is craniopharyngioma.

3. **Most common endocrine abnormality due to irradiation of the brain: Hyperprolactinemia,** but may also develop hypopituitarism.

4. **Most common hormonal defect of the pituitary in hypothalamic disease:** Loss of normal GH (growth hormone) secretion.

5. **Chromosomal defect in Prader- Willi syndrome**: Chromosome 15 deletion.

6. **Increased or decreased melatonin production is due to the following factors:**
   (a) **Increased:** Physical exercise, norepinephrine, psoralen, certain TCA, and manic states.
   (b) **Decreased:** Beta-blockers, alpha-2-agonists, and depressive phase.
   (c) Neither increased nor decreased: Diet and activity.

7. **Signs and symptoms of pineal tumors (e.g., pineoblastomas or pineocytomas, germinomas, embryonal carcinomas, and glial tumors)**:
   (a) It **decreases the production** of melatonin due to destruction of pineal tissues **except** pineocytomas which rarely may increase the melatonin level.
   (b) It may cause **hydrocephalus** due to obstruction of the aqueduct, may need a shunt to reduce ICP.
   (c) It may produce Parinaud's syndrome (paresis of upward conjugate gaze) due to pressure on the quadrigeminal plate.
   (d) Some germinomas and embryonal carcinomas cause delayed onset of puberty due to secretion of HCG (human chorionic gonadotropin).

8. **Treatment of pineal tumors**:
   (a) Surgical removal.
   (b) Radiation.
   (c) Chemotherapy.

   It depends upon the type, location, with or without metastases of the tumor.

9. **Best diagnostic study of pituitary tumors**: **MRI** because bone structures are **not** well defined and **less** radiation unlike CT scan.

10. **Most common cause of acquired hypopituitarism**: **Pituitary adenomas.** Few other important causes are:
    (a) **Neoplastic:** Metastatic tumors, craniopharyngiomas.
    (b) **Vascular:** Sheehan syndrome (postpartum necrosis), pituitary apoplexy, trauma, diabetic necrosis, vasculitis, and sickle cell disease.
    (c) **Infiltrative/ inflammatory:** Sarcoidosis, TB, syphilis, Histiocytosis X, and Hand-Schuller-Christian disease.
    (d) **Iatrogenic:** After surgery, radiation.
    (e) **Metabolic/ neurogenic:** Anorexia nervosa, amyloidosis, critical illness, and hemochromatosis.

11. **Sheehan's syndrome:** Pituitary infarction in the peripartum period due to excessive hemorrhage and hypovolemia.
    Pituitary apoplexy: It is due to bleeding into the tumor with associated infarction.

12. **Most common cause of radiation induced hypopituitarism**: The effects of radiation on **hypothalamic function,** but high-dose radiation can cause direct pituitary damage.
    Signs and symptoms: It can be delayed as much as several years. The first symptoms are usually **GH and gonadotropin deficiencies,** rarely ACTH or TSH deficiencies may develop initially.
    Management: Monitor high-risk patients at yearly intervals and try to avoid radiation induced injuries.

13. **Empty sella syndrome: (two types)**:
    (a) **Primary:** It is mostly found in **women,** may be associated **with benign intracranial hypertension, normal pituitary functions are usually present,** and 15% of patients have mild hyperprolactinemia.
    (b) Secondary or acquired: It may due to radiation, surgery, or pituitary infarction especially of the adenoma.
    Best diagnostic study: **MRI,** it shows **flattened rim of tissues** along the floor of sella.

14. **Mass effects of pituitary adenomas:**
    (a) Patients appear with **headaches** (retro-orbital or referred to the top of the skull), nausea, vomiting, and **altered level of consciousness which may be due to infarction of the adenoma.**

(b) **Pituitary apoplexy** (bleeding into the adenoma) may develop in severe cases. It needs **immediate surgical decompression.**

(c) **Eye: Bitemporal hemianopsia is the most common visual field defect** because adenoma causes pressure on the central region of optic chiasm which carries nasal fibres **which are responsible for temporal vision.** Large tumors may invade the optic nerve or cavernous sinus.

Treatment of visual fields defect:

(i) Recent onset of visual loss: Surgical removal of the tumor causes dramatic improvement.

(ii) Long standing visual loss: Surgery may **not** recover the visual losses.

(d) Hypopituitarism: **It is mostly due to compression of the hypothalamic-pituitary stalk** than from direct pressure or replacement of the normal pituitary. Patients appear with:

(i) **GH deficiency.**

(ii) **Hypogonadotropic hypogonadism.**

(iii) **Mildly elevated (<100 ng/ml) prolactin levels** occur in stalk compression, it is due to reduced inhibition by dopamine.

Best diagnostic imaging study: MRI. It may show **thin rim of normal pituitary tissue** due to compression by large adenomas.

[Remember, **diabetes insipidus (DI) due to vasopression deficiency** is **not** usually found in pituitary adenomas. DI is common in craniopharyngioma or other conditions causing hypothalamic dysfunction].

15. **Treatment of pituitary adenomas**:

(A) **Surgical therapy: Transsphenoidal approach to remove the pituitary tumors is the best surgical method.** Other method is transfrontal approach which is used only for extensive exploration.

Complications of transsphenoidal surgery: (<5% of cases) CSF leak, hemorrhage, hypopituitarism, optic nerve damage, and sinusitis.

Prognosis:

(i) Microadenomas (<1 cm in size): Hormonal hypersecretion is corrected up to 90% of patients.

(ii) Macroadenomas: Hormonal hypersecretion is corrected in <30% of patients.

Remember, surgery is the first treatment of choice except in prolactinoma.

(B) **Radiation therapy: It is most commonly used after incomplete transsphenoidal resection.** It may be used either with medical therapy or alone when patients refuse or cannot have surgery. There is **very slow response in** radiation therapy.

Complications of radiation: Mostly dose-related but may be due to idiosyncrasy.

(i) **Hypothalamic injury:** It is most common and causes partial or complete hypopituitarism.
(ii) Less common complications are: Brain necrosis, damage of optic nerve and blood vessels, **may develop sarcomas.**

(C) **Medical therapy.**
(i) **Prolactinomas:** Dopamine agonists, which includes ergot derivatives **bromocriptine, lisuride, pergolide,** and **D2 selective agonist (CV205-5O2) are the primary drug of choice.** There is a rapid reduction of prolactin levels and tumor size with therapies.
(ii) **Acromegaly: Dopamine agonists are useful but have less effect on GH responses and tumor sizes.** Somatostatin analogues (octreotide) is also useful, it reduces the secretion of GH and TSH.
(iii) TSH-producing tumors: Octreotide.
(iv) Gonadotropin-producing tumors: **GnRH antagonists** are more effective than agonists **in reducing the FSH** but have little effect on tumor growth.
(v) **Cushing's disease**: The primary target is to reduce the steriod biosynthesis. Ketoconazole, aminoglutethimide, metyrapone, and O, P, DDD (mitotane) are used.

16. **Location of the GH gene**: Chromosome 17.

17. **To measure GH (growth hormone) reserve, best laboratory test**: **Low IGF-1 level (**IGF means insulin like growth factor), **not GH levels.**

18. **GH deficiency is most frequenty assessed by**:
(i) **Insulin-induced hypoglycemia (<40 mg/dL):** It stimulates the CNS pathways, results in increase of GH (>10 microgram /L).
Contraindication: This test should **not** be done in patients with seizures and coronary artery diseases. Use L-Dopa or L-Arginine test.
(ii) L-Dopa or L-Arginine stimulation test: Normal response in GH >7 microgram/ L.

19. A 38 year old man appears in the clinic with H/O **progressively increasing shoe-size and width for last several months** and he is unable to wear his wedding ring as well. He went to a dentist who noticed malocclusion and increased spacing between the teeth. His wife also noticed sleep apnea and change of voice recently.
Physical examination: Enlargement of the lower jaw (prognathism), lips, nose, sinuses (frontal bossing), and tongue. **A moist, doughy, enveloping**

handshake is noted by the physician and it is characteristic of the disease. Patients also have arthralgias in both large and small joints.

Most likely diagnosis: Acromegaly.

Etiology: GH- producing tumor arises most commonly from pituitary, or rarely ectopic production of GRF from carcinoid or pancreatic islets.

Important associated clinical findings are:

(i) Premalignant polyps and colon cancer: Colonscopy is recommended.

(ii) **CVS:** Cardiac hypertrophy, CHF, or ischemia. **It is the most common cause of death in acromegaly** along with cerebrovascular disease.

Diagnosis:

(a) **Initial screening test:** Elevated serum **IGF-1 level.**

(b) **Most reliable diagnostic test is glucose tolerance test:** Increased glucose levels **fail to reduce GH levels below 2 ng/ml or may cause a paradoxical rise of GH levels.**

(c) MRI is to look for pituitary tumors, if absent then consider ectopic GRF secretion.

Treatment: The ultimate goal is to achieve normal GH and IGF-1 level, avoid hypofunction of the pituitary, and prevent the recurrence.

(a) **Transsphenoidal surgical approach is to remove the tumor: It is effective to reduce the GH levels <5 ng/ml in 60% of patients with microadenomas** and is only effective in <30% of patients with macroadenomas.

(b) **Medical treatment:**

   (i) Octreotide (somatostatin analogue): **It reduces GH and IGF-1 levels in** majority of the patients and decrease the tumor size in 50% of cases. It can be used as adjunctive therapy with surgery and/ or radiation.

   Side effects of octreotide: Diarrhea, cholelithiasis.

   (ii) Bromocriptine: It is less effective than octreotide, required high doses, some patients only respond to this than octreotide, or may be used together.

(c) **Radiation treatment: It is only used along with surgery and/ or medical therapy.** It is **not** used alone because of increased risk of hypopituitarism and may take up to 10 years to reduce the GH- levels.

20. **Location of prolactin gene**: **Chromosome 6.**

21. **Prolactin deficiency**: It is rare, found in combined hormone deficiencies.
Presentation: Absence of postpartum lactation.
Diagnosis: Low prolactin levels with or without TRH sitmulation.
Remember, prolactin deficiency have no effects on breast development or other tissues.

22. **Most common type of pituitary adenomas**: Prolactinomas (25 to 40% of all adenomas).

23. **Signs and Symptoms of hyperprolactinemia:**
   (a) Women (mostly premenopausal): **Galactorrhea, oligomenorrhea, amenorrhea, and infertility.** Estrogen deficiency can cause **dyspareunia, decreased libido, and osteopenia.** Few patients may have hirsutism due to elevated androgens.
   (b) Women (postmenopausal): Most patients appear with mass effects than hormonal effects.
   (c) **Men: Hypogonadism with reduced LH, FSH, and testosterone level.** Hypogonadism causes decreased libido, impotence, and rarely gynecomastia or galactorrhea.

24. Diagnosis and treatment of hyperprolactinemia:
   (A) **Diagnosis:**
      (i) Physiologic hyperprolactinemia (except in pregnancy or renal failure): Mild elevation of serum prolactin (<50 ng/ml) which may be normal in repeat testing.
      (ii) Rule out primary hypothyroidism: It causes mild hyperprolactinemia.
      (iii) Rule out **use of psychotropic durgs** which reduces dopamine production or by blocking its action: It causes serum elevation of prolactin (<100 ng/ml).
      (iv) **MRI or CT scan should be done in all patients with mild hyperprolactinemia** unless physiologic or drug induced causes are certain: **Imaging studies can differentiate between microprolactinomas and large mass lesions** which cause stalk compression.
      (v) Idiopathic hyperprolactinemia: It is either small microprolactinomas or altered hypothalamic regulatory function of prolactin secretion. **Remember, few microprolactinomas may develop large tumors.**
   (B) **Treatment:**
      (i) Microprolactinoma in asymptomatic patients: F/U prolactin levels and **no treatment is needed.**
      (ii) **Hyperprolactinoma causing hypogonadism, osteopenia, or infertility:**
         (a) **Bromocriptine (dopamine agonist) is the drug of choice**. It reduces the tumor size, normalize prolactin levels, correct amenorrhea and galactorrhea. If patients cannot tolerate bromocriptine use other dopamine agonist (e.g., pergolide).

(b) **Patients unresponsive to dopamine agonist: Transsphenoidal surgical removal of the tumor is the treatment of choice.**

(iii) Microprolactinomas: **No radiation therapy is recommended** because of slow, incomplete responses, and high incidence of hypopituitarism.

(iv) **Patients with infertility or pregnancy:**

(a) Bromocriptine can induce fertility. It should be stopped during pregnancy, although it does **not** causes any malformations.

(b) **Pregnant patients with visual field defects and headaches are** mostly due to macroadenomas and rarely microadenomas.

MRI should be done to confirm the tumor growth and bromocriptine should be started despite pregnancy.

Remember, to monitor the prolactin levels during pregnancy is **not** helpful because it is already elevated without tumor.

(c) **Patients with macroadenomas, wanted to become pregnant:** Transsphenoidal decompression before pregnancy and maintain the fertility.

(v) **Patients with macroadenomas:**

(vi) **With visual field defects: Bromocriptine is the drug of choice.**

(vii) **Rapid loss of visual acuity or recent tumor bleeding: Surgery is the treatment of choice.**

(viii) **Visual field defects unresponsive to bromocriptine:** Surgery is the next mode of therapy. Radiation therapy is used as an adjunct with bromocriptine and surgery.

25. **Most common cause of ACTH deficiency: Treatment with exogenous glucocorticoids which** causes suppression of the **HPA (hypothalamic-pituitary-adrenal axis).**

26. **Signs and symptoms of ACTH deficiency (secondary hypocortisolism)**: It is due to **decreased glucocorticoid but normal mineralocorticoid** activities. Patients appear with vomiting, fever, weakness, fatigue, and low BP.
Laboratory findings: Low cortisol, Na, and glucose, but high eosinophil counts. Absence of hyperpigmentation, hyperkalemia, volume depletion which are found in **primary adrenal hypofunction (hypocortisolism).**
Evaluations of ACTH reserve:

(i) Hypothalamic CRH (corticotropin-releasing hormone) stimulates the ACTH secretion.

(a) In hypothalamic dysfunction: Increased ACTH.

(b) In pituitary dysfunction: No change in ACTH.

This test can differentiate between hypothalamic and pituitary dysfunctions.

(ii) Insulin induced hypoglycemia causes neuroglycopenia which stimulates ACTH secretion.

(iii) Metyrapone test (alternative to insulin tolerance test): Metyrapone stimulates ACTH secretion by inhibiting cortisol production.

Treatment of ACTH deficiency:

(a) **Glucocorticoids replacement therapy.**

(b) **No need** to give mineralocorticoid.

(c) Patients should wear Medic Alert tag with warning signs of cortisol deficiency (vomiting, abdominal pain, fatigue, postural dizziness, and low grade fever): Stress dose of steroids should be given in symptomatic patients.

27. **Most common cause of Cushing's syndrome (excess of glucocorticoids): Cushing's disease (pituitary neoplasms) is 60 to 70% of all Cushing's syndrome.** Other causes are adrenal causes of cortisol excess, ectopic production of ACTH, and physiologic condition of overproduction of cortisol.

28. **Most common cause of Cushing's disease: Primary defect is at the level of pituitary (pituitary neoplasms)** and **rarely** due to hypothalamic disorders. Only 10 to 15% of pituitary tumors secrete ACTH. Unlike other pituitary tumors, **most of the ACTH- secreting tumors are locally invasive microadenomas** at the time of diagnosis because of the **clinical features of cortisol excess is present when the tumor is small.** The excess cortisol also inhibits the growth of the adenomas.

29. **Signs and symptoms of Cushing's disease (pituitary causes of increase ACTH)**:

 (a) The characteristic **centripetal distribution of fat, results in 'buffalo hump', 'moon facies',** fat deposition over the supraclavicular area, minimal fat deposition in the extremities; wide (>1 cm) and purple striae (due to steroid induced thinning of the dermis); osteopenia and hypokalemia (due to ACTH excess); hyperpigmentation (like Addison's disease but less severe), hirsutism and acne (due to excess adrenal androgens, **more severe** than in adrenal adenomas); high BP, glucose intolerance, and proximal muscle weakness (due to glucocorticoid excess).

 (b) Other symptoms are the following: Immune suppression, opportunistic infections, delayed wound healing, and increased incidence of suicide.

30. **Diagnosis of Cushing's syndrome**: It can be done in an outpatient setting in most cases.
   (A) **First step is to determine whether the cortisol excess is true or false:**
      (i) Remember, random cortisol levels are **not** useful because of diurnal variation of the hormone.
      (ii) **Overnight dexamethasone test:** It is most widely used initial screening test:
         (a) **Normal** dexamethasone suppression test: Patients do **not** have Cushing's syndrome.
         (b) **Abnormal** dexamethasone suppression test but patients do **not** have Cushing's syndrome: Patients who are depressed or up to 30% of all hospitalized patients.
         (c) **Abnormal** dexamethasone suppression test: Patients have Cushing's syndrome (pituitary, ectopic, or adrenal causes).
      (iii) Elevated 24-hours urine free cortisol (UFC): It is more sensitive and specific than overnight dexamethasone suppression test.
   (B) **The second step,** if the cortisol levels are high, is to perform **low-dose dexamethasone suppression test:**
      (i) Normal individuals (on the second day of the test): **It suppresses plasma cortisol to** <5 microgram/dl and reduces 17- hydroxysteroids to <2.5 mg/24 hours or (UFC) to < 20 microgram/24 hours.
      (ii) All forms of Cushing's syndrome: It does **not** suppress cortisol level.
   (C) **The third step,** if the cortisol levels are **not** suppressed, is to perfom **high dose dexamethasone test** to distinguish between **ACTH-dependent and ACTH-independent** or between **pituitary and ectopic causes of ACTH-dependent Cushing's syndrome.**
      (i) Adrenal cortisol excess (ACTH-independent): Plasma and urinary cortisol levels are **not** suppressed by dexamethasone suppression test even at high doses and plasma ACTH levels **are low** due to suppression of the hypothalamic- pituitary axis.
      (ii) ACTH-producing pituitary adenomas (ACTH-dependent): The 17-hydroxysteroids are suppressed to <50% of baseline and UFC is suppressed <90% of baseline in high-dose dexamethasone suppression test.
      (iii) The ectopic ACTH syndrome (ACTH- dependent): The plasma ACTH levels are very high (>200 pg/ml), low k levels (more common than other forms of Cushing's syndrome), and hyperpigmentations. The clinical features of Cushing's syndrome may be changed by the rapid rise of cortisol, results in fluid retention, weakness, glucose intolerance, and poor skin integrity. Remember, it is more common in patients with known malignancies (e.g., oat cell cancer, thymic, bronchial, or GI

carcinoids, medullary throid cancer, and islet cell tumors) and can exacerbate the symptoms of malignancies.

Remember, some subset of ectopic ACTH tumors particularly carcinoids may have **similar** results **like pituitary tumors** in dexamethasone suppression test. Carcinoids can be detected **by MRI or CT scan**.

(iv) To further distinguish between pituitary ACTH tumors and ectopic ACTH tumors: (Three methods).

(1) The metyrapone test which is the inhibition of 11 beta-hydroxylase which blocks cortisol synthesis → inhibits negative feedback → **increased ACTH production in pituitary tumors** → increased production of 11-deoxycortisol. The most ectopic ACTH tumors do **not** increased ACTH production with decreased cortisol levels, but the **subset of ectopic ACTH tumors** respond like pituitary tumors in dexamethasone suppression test, **have positive response (increase ACTH production)** like pituitary tumors.

(2) Inferior petrosal sinuses (central) and peripheral blood ACTH sampling simultaneoulsy: In pituitary tumors, there is a **gradient of 2:1** (central: peripheral) in ACTH levels but absence of gradient in ectopic ACTH tumors.

(3) MRI or CT scan: It should be done in suspected pituitary adenomas but as it is small in size (microadenomas), results are mostly normal.

31. **Treatment of Cushing's disease:**

(a) Transphenoidal surgery:

(i) Microadenomas: Surgery can cure up to 80% of the cases.

(ii) Macroadenomas: Surgical cure is less common.

(iii) Unsuccessful surgery: Reoperation can cause remission in up to 50% of the cases.

(b) Pituitary irradiation: It is the second line of treatment. It is done in patients with surgical failure or surgery cannot be perfomed.

(c) Bilateral removal of the adrenal glands after transsphenoidal surgery: It is done in patients with high cortisol levels. After surgery patients should get maintainance mineralocorticoids and glucocorticoids.

(d) Medical treatment with ketoconazole, metyrapone, aminoglutethimide, and mitotane: It is used to prepare the patients for surgery or to control the hypercortisolism during the interval when radiation treatment is becoming effective.

32. **Nelson's syndrome:** The development of pituitary adenomas after bilateral adrenalectomy. The patients have hyperpigmentation, very high ACTH level,

and other features of enlarging pituitary tumor. The patients should be followed up after bilateral adrenalectomy:

(i) ACTH levels.
(ii) MRI or CT scan.

Treatment of Nelson's syndrome.

(i) Transsphenoidal surgery.
(ii) Additonal radiotherapy may be helpful.

33. The functions of FSH and LH in males and females:
   (A) **In males:**
      (i) **FSH:**
         (a) **Locations of FSH receptors:** Sertoli cells and seminiferous tubules.
         (b) **Function:** Sperms maturation.
      (ii) **LH:**
         (a) **Locations of LH receptors:** Leydig cells of the testes.
         (b) **Function:** It stimulates androgen production.
   (B) **In females:**
      (i) **FSH:**
         (a) **Locations of FSH receptors:** Granulosa cells of the ovaries.
         (b) **Function:** It induces enzymes involved in estrogen biosynthesis.
      (ii) **LH:**
         (a) **Locations of LH receptors:** Thecal cells of the ovaries.
         (b) **Functions:** It stimulates the production of ovarian androgens and steroid precursors.

34. **Signs and symptoms of primary hypogonadotropic hypogonadism and treatment:**
   (a) In females (due to estrogen deficiency): Vaginal dryness, breast atrophy, and diminished libido. In addition to that hot flushes are common in **postmenopausal women**.
   (b) In males (due to testosterone deficiency without elevation of LH and FSH): Decreased libido and sexual function.

   Treatment:

   (a) Premenopausal women:
      (i) The combined estrogen and progestin preparation (for hormonal replacement and cyclical growth of the endometrium).
      (ii) Pusatile GnRH (for GnRH deficient individuals) or gonadotropins to induce ovulation and fertility.
   (b) Men:
      (i) Testosterone.

(ii) Pulsatile GnRH (for GnRH deficient individuals) or gonadotropins to induce spermatogenesis.

35. **Secondary hypogonadotropic hypogonadism**: The signs and symptoms are same as primary hypogonadotropic hypogonadism.
It has two types:
(a) Physiologic or reversible.
(b) Pathologic.

(a) **Physiologic**: It is found in stress, heavy exercise, weight loss, severe illness, or anorexia nervosa. It is **due to GnRH deficiency** and more common in women than men.
Treatment:
(i) To treat the underlying cause.
(ii) If it is **not** possible to correct the underlying cause use **hormonal replacement therapy to** protect from osteopenia and to cycle the endometrium.
(b) Pathological causes are the following:
(i) CNS radiation.
(ii) Hypothalamic lesions.
(iii) Pituitary tumors.
(iv) Hyperprolactinoma.
All of the above are due to GnRH deficiency.
(v) Rare causes are the following: Mutations in the LH-beta or FSH-beta genes, acquired isolated gonadotropin deficiency (autoimmune etiology).

36. **Few important points in FSH-and LH- producing pituitary tumors**:
(a) The majority of the tumors **produce low levels of intact glycoprotein** hormones or their uncombined alpha or beta subunits.
(b) **FSH is produced more** than LH and **alpha subunit is more than** beta subunit.
(c) Most of the patients are **asymptomatic.** The patients become symptomatic due to mass effect result in **visual loss, hypogonadism, and loss of libido.**
(d) Men with FSH-secreting tumors can paradoxically produce hypogonadism due to **Low** testosterone levels.
(e) Men with LH- secreting tumors (rare) have **increased** testosterone levels.
(f) Premenopausal women appear with menstrual irregularity or secondary hypogonadism.

(g) Postmenopausal women have **reduced gonadotropin levels** because mass effect of gonadotropin producing tumors cause stalk compression, result in **impairment of GnRH stimulation of gonadotropin.**

37. **Diagnosis and treatment of FSH- and LH- producing tumors**:
   (A) **Diagnosis:**
      (i) Tumors do **not** produce significantly elevated FSH and LH (gonadotropins), so hormonal levels may be normal with the diseases or low in many women particularly postmenopausal.
      (ii) GnRH stimulation tests are **not** helpful.
      (iii) **Paradoxically, TRH stimulates the** secretion of intact gonadotropins or in most patients with gonadotropin tumors.
      (iv) Men with proven tumors have **high-normal or elevated FSH levels, low levels of testosterone, and elevated levels of prolactin.**
      (v) **Postoperative diagnosis** is made by immunohistochemical analysis or gonadotropin gene expression.
      (vi) CT scan or MRI detects the tumor mass.
   (B) **Treatment:**
      (i) Transsphenoidal surgery is rarely curative but to reduce the size of the tumor mass which causes most of the symptoms.
      (ii) Postoperative radiation therapy is useful in patients with residual tumor.
      (iii) To monitor the tumor recurrence: Use visual field examination, CT or MRI, tumor markers (free alpha or beta subunit levels), TRH testing.
      (iv) Rapid recurrence of the tumor: Repeat surgery and /or radiation therapy is helpful.
      (v) Medical therapies are **not** very effective (e.g., bromocriptine, somatostatin analogues, GnRH agonists or antagonists).

38. **Central hypothyroidism:**
   (A) **Secondary (pituitary) hypothyroidism:** TSH deficiency.
   (B) Tertiary (hypothalamus) hypothyroidism: TRH deficiency.
   Laboratory diagnosis:
   (A) Secondary hypothyroidism: Low free T_4 (**not** total T_4**) without** elevated TSH.
   (B) Tertiary hypothyroidism: Low free T_4 **with** elevated TSH (but reduced bioactivity of TSH).
   (C) Sick-euthyroid syndrome: Low free thyroid hormone (T_4) with low TSH.
   (D) TBG deficiency: High T_3 resin uptake, with normal or low normal free T_4 and T_3.
   Treatment of central hypothyroidism: L-thyroxine (**not** the TSH).
   Follow up of the patients: To monitor serum levels of free T_4 and T_3.

39. **Signs and symptoms of TSH-secreting tumors**:
   (a) It resembles Grave's disease except autoimmunity (absence of opthalmopathy).
   (b) Diffuse goitre.
   (c) Mass effects of the tumor (visual field defects, headaches).

40. **Diagnosis and treatment of TSH- secreting tumors**.
   (A) **Diagnosis:**
      (i) In appropriately **elevated TSH levels along with elevated T_4 and T_3** (because bio-feedback mechanism is impaired), excess secretion (elevation) of free alpha subunit and/ or GH, elevated 24-hour uptake of radioiodine.
      (ii) CT or MRI is to detect the mass in the pituitary.
   (B) **Treatment:**
      (i) **Transsphenoidal surgery** is rarely curative because of the large size of the tumor.
      (ii) **Surgery is followed by radiotherapy** for remaining tumor mass.
      (iii) **Somatostatin analogues** (e.g., octreotide) decrease TSH and alpha-subunit levels but **no** effect on tumor growth.
      (iv) **Antithyroid drugs or radioiodine is** to treat hyperthyroidism.

41. **Null cell pituitary tumors:** It is nonfunctioning tumors. It produces low level of the free alpha subunit, FSH, and LH.
   Signs and symptoms: The tumor mass effect (visual field defects, headaches) and hypopituitarism.
   Treatment: Transsphenoidal surgery.
   Follow-up: CT or MRI, and visual field examination (absence of serum tumor markers).

42. **Normal values which are important**:
   (a) Normal plasma osmolality = 278 to 294 mOsm/kg of water.
   (b) Normal plasma vasopressin (AVP) = 0 to 5 pg/ml.
   (c) Normal urine osmolality = 70 to 1200 mOsm/kg.
   (d) Urine osmolality is highest (or maximum) 1200 mOsm/kg when plasma osmolality is highest normal 294 mOsm/kg and vasopressin level is highest normal 5 pg/ml.
   (e) Increase of plasma osmolality **above 294 mOsm/kg, increases the plasma vasopressin** above 5 pg/ml, but urine osmolality remains the **maximum 1200 mOsm/kg** because urine concentration capacity is limited by the renal inner medulla.

(f) Decrease of plasma osmolality below 282 mOsm/kg will not cause further decrease of vasopressin (O pg/ml) or increase in urine volume (maximum 20 L/day).
(g) Normal daily urine output is 1 to 2 L/day (maximum 20 L/day).
(h) Total daily intake and output of the fluid are the same 2100 to 3400 ml **(Intake includes** fluids from food 800-1000 ml, oxidation of food 300-400 ml, and water as a liquid 1000-2000 ml;.

Output includes urinary loss 1000-2000 ml, insensible loss 800-1000 ml, sweat 200 ml, and feces 100-200 ml).

43. Types of diabetes insipidus (DI): (Three).
   (a) **Hypothalamic DI**: **Low** vasopressin levels, large volume of diluted urine, **increased** serum osmolality results in thirst and polydipsia.
   (b) Nephrogenic DI: **High** vasopressin levels, kidneys do **not** respond to vasopressin, large volume of diluted urine, **increased** serum osmolality results in thirst and polydipsia.
   (c) Primary polydipsia: **Low** vasopressin levels, large volume of diluted urine, **decreased** serum osmolality due to ingestion of excessive water.

44. Signs and symptoms of hypothalamic DI:
   (a) **Acute onset** (e.g., head trauma with basal skull fracture, hypothalamic injury, or transcranial surgery):The patients are unconscious; hypernatremia, absence of thirst, and polyuria.
   (b) **Gradual onset** (e.g., idiopathic or diseases):Polyuria (patients complain when urine volume is > 4 L/day), polydipsia.
   (c) **Partial DI** (some ability to secrete vasopressin which is reduced in normal serum osmolality): The patients symptom and urine volume are moderately different from patients with complete DI.
   (d) **A variant of hypothalamic DI** (absence of osmostat and intact volume receptors):The patients have **essential hypernatremia but absence of thirst**. When the patients blood volume is **normal**, increase osmolality will **not** increase the vasopressin or thirst because of absence of osmotic receptors. When the patients blood volume is **low**, there is increase secretion of vasopressin. The patients are chronically dehydrated, rehydration produces typical DI symptoms.
   (e) Rarely, autosomal dominant type DI: It is due to substitution or deletion of vasopressin gene. Cell death may cause DI in early adult life.
   (f) Pregnancy with DI: It is due to rapid catabolism of vasopressin by placental enzyme cystine aminopeptidase.

(g) DI with myxedema or adrenal insufficiency: **The patients need less vasopressin** because both myxedema or adrenal insufficiency reduces the ability to excrete free water by the kidneys.

45. **Clinical presentation of nephrogenic DI**:The patients appear with large volume of diluted urine (polyuria), polydipsia, increased serum osmolality, and elevated levels of serum vasopression.The gene for V_2 receptors are located at **Xq 28 region of X-chromosome**. Nephrogenic DI may be due to certain **drugs** (e.g., demeclocycline, fluoride, lithium) or **diseases** (sarcoidosis, sickle cell disease, multiple melanoma, pyelonephritis, or analgesic nephropathy).

46. **Clinical presentation of primary polydipsia**:
Most patients appear with gradual or acute onset due to trauma. The patients may drink > 20 L/day and even sleep throughout the night. The symptoms exacerbate during stress. The patients may have strong family history of excessive thirst, psychiatric disorder. Laboratory studies are all normal including serum sodium which may be low normal.

47. Water deprivation tests followed by vasopressin, the responses in different DI:
    (a) **Normal individuals**: Increase in urine osmolality with dehydration and no change with vasopressin.
    (b) **Nephrogenic DI**: No increase in urine osmolality with dehydratioon and vasopressin.
    (c) **Complete central DI**: No increase in urine osmolality with dehydration but increase osmolality with vasopressin.
    (d) **Partial central DI:** Partial increase in urine osmolality with dehydration and further increase with vasopressin.
    (e) **Primary polydipsia**: Partial increase in urine osmolality with dehydration but no change with vasopressin.

48. **Etiologic diagnosis of DI**: NMR (nuclear magenetic resonance) is the best diagnostic study, it shows **loss of the hyperintense signal of the posterior pituitary**. Remember, DI is symptomatic only when 80 to 90 % of the vasopressin producing cells (paraventricular and supraoptic nuclei) are destroyed.

49. Treatment of DI (diabetes insipidus):
    (a) Adequate water replacement to avoid metabolic complications.
    (b) Desmopressin (vasopressin agonist): It is avilable as intranasal spray, preferably given at night **to have undisturbed good night sleep. It has longer half life than vasopressin.**

(c) Orally administered medications are the following:
   (i) Chlorpropamide: It enhances the effect of vasopressin at the renal tuble. It is mostly useful in partial hypothalamic DI.
   (ii) Carbamazepine: It releases vasopressin.
   (iii) Clofibrate: It stimulates the release of endogenous vasopressin.
   (iv) Thiazide diuretics: It decreases urinary volume by increasing proximal tubular reabsorption and sodium depletion.
   (v) Ibuprofen: It is not used as a primary drug. It blocks the normal inhibitory action of PGE on vasopressin action on the kidney.

(d) **Patients who are chronically hypernatremic**: Remember, very rapid reduction of osmolality (**no more than 1 mEq every 2 hours**) in the ECF (extra cellular fluid) results in shift of water into the brain, cause cerebral edema and herniation. In this patient, **desmopressin and water regulation** should be done.

(e) Pregnancy with DI: Use desmopressin.

(f) Postsurgery or posttrauma patients with DI: Long term therapy is unpredictable.

50. **Triphasic response of the pituitary stalk to trauma or postsurgical patients**:
   (a) The first phase (first 6 days diuretic phase): DI is due to an axon shock and reduced vasopressin release. There is increased urine output, high to normal serum sodium values.
   (b) The second phase (7 to 10 days, antidiuretic phase): It is due to increased vasopressin release from posterior pituitary, urine volume is reduced, and low plasma sodium levels. Hyponatremia is treated with fluid restriction.
   (c) The third phage (after day 10, diurectic phage): The return of DI, increased urine output, serum sodium levels are upper limit of normal.

51. **Follow-up of DI:** DI should **not** be considered idiopathic until after 4 years of follow-up.
   CT or NMR should be done annually to detect the recurrence of the tumor or infiltrative process.

52. **Sites of production of thyroid hormone:**
   (a) T_4: It is produced only in the thyroid gland.
   (b) T_3: The 80% is derived from peripheral conversion of T_4 to T_3, and only 20% is produced by the thyroid gland.

53. **Values of thyroid hormone in normal, hypothyroid, hyperhyroid, and NTI conditions**:

(A) **Normal**: T4 (4.5-12.5 microgram/dl), free T4(0.9-2 ng/dl), T3(80-220 ng/dl), TSH (0.3-6 micro u/ml).
(B) **Hypothyroid:** Low T4 (<4.5), low free T4 (< 0.9), low T3 (<80), high TSH (>6), **low reverse** T3 **(<20 ng/dl)**.
(C) **Hyperthyroid**: High T4(>12.5), high free T4(>2), high T3(>220), low TSH (<0.3).
(D) NTI (nonthyroidal illness syndrome): **Elevated reverse T_3 > 40 ng/dl** (normal 20-40 ng/dl), **unlike** hypothyroid, but some patients have low T4, free T4, T3 and high TSH **like** hypothyroid. **Reverse T_3 can differentiate between between NTI and hypothyroidism**.

54. **Sick patients (NTI) and thyroid functions:** These are important points to remember:
   (a) A TSH level **above 20** micro U/ml in a NTI patient: Diagnosis is hypothyroidism Treatment: L-thyroxine.
   (b) A TSH level **below 0.03** micro U/ml in a NTI patient: Diagnosis is hypothyroidism **Treatment:** Propylthiouracil (PTU) and methimazole (MMI).

55. **Most common cause of thyrotoxicosis**: **Graves' disease** (60 to 90% of all cases). It is most likely an autoimmune disorder.

56. **Signs and symptoms of Graves' disease (Basedow's or Parry's disease)**:
   (A) **Feature of thyrotoxicosis**:
      (i) **Metabolic**: Weight loss with increased appetite (rarely weight gain), heat intolerance.
      (ii) **Thyroid**: Diffuse enlargement is most likely, or nodule(s).
      (iii) CVS: Palpitations, sinus tachycardia, increased difference between systolic and diastolic BP, atrial fibrillation.
      (iv) CNS: Fine tremor of hands, nervousness, emotional lability.
      (v) Skin: Warm moist smooth skin, excessive sweating, hair loss, fine hair, onycholysis.
      (vi) GI: Diarrhea.
      (vii) Muscles: Hyperreflexia, proximal muscle weakness, muscle atrophy.
   (B) Features specific for Graves' disease:
      (i) **Eye**: It usually affects both eyes or sometimes one eye only.
         (a) Proptosis: It is due to swollen retroorbital connective tissues.
         (b) Diplopia: It is due to swollen, fibrotic ocular muscles cause lid retraction and restrict eye movement particularly upward gaze.
         (c) Periorbital edema and chemosis: It is due to impaired orbital venous drainage.

(d) Visual field defects, papilledema: It is due to pressure on the optic nerve.
(e) Photophobia and easy tearing.
Best diagnostic study for eye disease: CT scan.
(ii) Dermopathy.
(iii) Acropachy.

57. **Diagnosis and treatment of Graves' disease**:
(A)Diagnosis:
(i) Clinical manifestation is characteristic in severe cases.
(ii) Laboratory findings: Markedly elevated T_3 levels, elevated T_4 levels, elevated free T_4 level, low TSH levels. The term T_3 toxicosis is used when T_4 is normal with elevated T_3 levels.
(iii) In typical Graves' disease: Do not perform radioactive iodine test or TSI levels.
(iv) To differentiate between NTI and hyperthyroidism: Elevated TSI confirms the diagnosis of hyperthyroidism and rule out NTI.
(v) Radioactive iodine scan:
(a) Cold thyroid nodule (decreased uptake) surrounded by high uptake tissues suggest **Graves' disease** with cold nodule. It needs biopsy.
(b) Hot nodule surrounded by decreased uptake (cold areas) suggests **toxic adenoma**.
(c) Very low uptake with pain on palpation indicates **thyroiditis**.
(d) No palpable thyroid tissues and no thyroid uptake indicates **ectopic thyroid**.
(vi) Euthyroid opthalmopathy or euthyroid Graves' disease: Patients with bilateral or unilateral opthalmopathy with minimal or no signs of thyrotoxicosis, T_4 and T_3 levels are upper normal and TSH levels are low normal or decreased.
(B)**Treatment of Graves' disease**:
(i) Antithyroid drug or radioactive iodine is the treatment of choice.
(ii) Surgery.
Follow-up: Life long follow-up is recommended. Up to 20% of patients may remit spontaneously and up to 50% become hypothyroid due to autoimmune destruction of the thyroid glands after 20 to 30 years without treatment.
(C)**Treatment of thyrotoxicosis**:
(i) **Propylthiouracil (PTU) and methimazole (MMI) are the best initial treatment of choice.** MMI is more potent than PTU and longer intrathyroidal residence time. MMI is used in moderate thyrotoxicosis,

but it depends upon the institution. PTU and MMI are thionamide derivatives.

Follow-up: Thyroid hormone values are **checked after 4 weeks** from the onset of treatment. Once thyroid hormone becomes normal, the dose is decreased. **Most relapses occur within 3 to 6 months after** discontinuation of the medication.

(ii) The patients can be initially treated with **MMI until euthyroid**, then combination of **MMI plus thyroxine (T_4) for 12 to 24 months** until all signs of Graves' disease disappered, then discontinue MMI and **only use T_4 for another 12 months.**

(iii) Radioactive iodine (RAI): It is used most frequently in the USA. It is the drug of choice in single or multinodulor toxic goitre, elderly patients, moderate thyrotoxicosis, allergic to PTU or MMI. RAI plus glucocorticoids are used for Graves' opthalmopathy.

Contraindication:

(a) Large retrosternal goitre: RAI can induce acute thyroiditis and airway obstruction.

(b) In pregnancy: Fetal thyroid can accumulate iodine.

Complications: The patients should be aware of these complications.

(a) Painful thyroiditis and worsening thyrotoxicosis.
Treatment: Aspirin with or without glucocorticoids.

(b) Hypothyroidism: It develops mostly with one year of treatment.

(iv) **Surgery (subtotal thyroidectomy)**:

(a) **Preoperative preparations**: The patients must be euthyroid before surgery. This is achieved with **PTU on MMI therapy for 6 weeks** before surgery, and to reduce the thyroid gland vascularity **use potassium iodide for 10 days prior** to surgery.

(b) **Indications**: Large obstructing glands, malignant or equivocal findings in needle aspiration, pregnancy, young uncooperative patients, or patients cannot or refuse medical therapies.

(c) Postoperative complications: Hypoparathyroidism, hemorrhage, recurrent laryngeal nerve paralysis, hypothyroidism, recurrent hyperthyroidism, transient low calcium, wound infection, and keloid formation.

(v) Alternative and supportive therapies:

(a) Iopanoic acid or sodium iopodate (oral cholecystographic agents). It is used in few patients who have toxic reactions to PTU or MMI, poor RAI uptake is due to excess iodine exposure or pregnancy, or **not** fit to have surgery.

(b) Propranolol (beta-blocker): It is used for tachycardia, tremor, anxiety, and heat intolerance **Contraindications**: Asthma or CHF.

(c) Multivitamin supplements for severe thyrotoxicosis and inadequate nutrition.

(D)**Treatment of opthalmopathy and dermopathy**:

(i) Mild opthalmopathy (only supportive care):

(a) Elevation of the head at night.

(b) Wearing of tinted glasses to protect the eyes from foreign body and sunlight.

(c) Methylcellulose eye drops (1%).

(d) Diuretics to reduce periorbital swelling.

(ii) Severe opthalmopathy (managed with opthalmologist and endocrinologist):

(a) Prednisone alone is most commonly used.

(b) Prednisone plus cyclosporine.

(c) External x-ray therapies to retroorbital areas (less popular treatment).

(d) Surgical decompression (transantral approach): To relieve the pressure on the optic nerve.

(e) After the acute process is over, the corrective surgeries (e.g., retroorbital muscle surgery, eyelid surgery) may be undertaken.

58. **Most common complications of antithyroid drugs (PTU and MMI): Allergy (skin rashes). Major serious complications are agranulocytosis. Routine monitoring of CBC is not recommended**, but a baseline CBC should be done before the onset of therapy.
Recommendation: Discontinue the medications if patients develop fever and infections (especially oropharyngeal), start antibiotics for infections.

59. **Jodbasedow effect**: The thyrotoxicosis can be precipitated by excess iodine intake in a toxic nodular goitre and also reported in Graves's disease. In the USA, it is due to exposure to iodinated **radiographic contrast material** or **iodinated drug (amiodarone** is antiarrythmic). It is typically found in iodine-deficient areas when iodine supplementation is given.
Treatment:
(i) MMI.
(ii) **Potassium perchlorate**: It inhibits iodine uptake and thyroid hormone formation.

60. **Thyroid storm**:
It is found in patients with severe thyrotoxicosis who develop infection, sepsis, or underwent surgical procedure.

Signs and symptoms: High fever (41°C, 105°F), severe tachycardia, restlessness, tremor, may develop low BP, CHF, acute abdomen, psychosis, delirium, and even coma.

Diagnosis:

(a) No acute increase in thyroid hormone in the serum, so **no laboratory test is helpful**.

(b) It is a clinical diagnosis.

Etiology:

(a) Increase tissue availability of thyroid hormone.

(b) Decrease plasma binding protein.

(c) Increase cytokines (e.g., TNF-alpha and IL-6).

Management:

(a) Inhibition of thyroid hormone formation and secretion:
 (i) PTU.
 (ii) Sodium iodide or KI.

(b) Sympathetic blockade:
 (i) Propranolol except in asthma and CHF.

(c) Glucocorticoid therapy:
 (i) Hydrocortisone.

(d) Supportive therapy:
 (i) Antibiotics for infection.
 (ii) Oxygen for hypoxia.
 (iii) Digitalis for CHF.
 (iv) Acetaminophen, and cooling blankets for fever (do **not** use salicylates).
 (v) IV fluids containing glucose, electrolytes, and multivitamins.

61. **Most common cause of thyrotoxicosis during pregnancy**: **Graves' disease;** next is toxic multinodular goitre, rarely increase hCG production by hydatiform moles or choriocarcinoma. Hyperemesis gravidarum leads to elevated T_4 but normal T_3 values.

Treatment:

(a) PTU or MMI is the drug of choice (do **not** give RAI).

(b) Subtotal thyroidectomy in the second trimester is the best time, if PTU or MMI fails.

(c) Do **not** give propanolol because it causes low birth weight in newborn, postnatal bradycardia, hypoglycemia, and poor response to hypoxia.

(d) **Nursing mother with thyrotoxicosis**:
PTU can be given because it does **not** impair mewborn's thyroid function (do **not** use MMI because it has a higher concentration in breast milk).

(e) Mild neonatal thyrotoxicosis: It is self-limiting, no treatment is needed.

(f) Severe neonatal thyrotoxicosis:

PTU should be given with or without propranolol.

62. **Most common cardiac disease is associated with Graves' disease**: **MVP (mitral valve prolapse)**. The patients with preexisting cardiac disease particularly elderly with multinodular goitre, can develop atrial fibrillation, ventricular tachycardia, CHF. The patients without cardiac disease can develop angina pectoris and high output cardiac failure.

63. **Treatment of cardiac diseases with thyrotoxicosis:**
    (a) PTU is the drug of choice.
    (b) Digitalis is used to reduce the ventricular tachycardia.
    (c) Propranolol or atenolol (beta-blocker) is used to reduce the heart rate.
    (d) Aspirin or warfarin sodium (anticoagulant) is used for atrial fibrillation.
    (e) Use diltiazem (calcium channel blocker) when propranolol is contraindicated (asthma, CHF).
    (f) If sinus rhythm has **not** returned after a euthyroid period of 4 months: Then cardioversion may be necessary.
    (g) Patients with angina pectoris: Patients should receive antithyroid drugs before coronary angioplasty or bypass surgery because of the danger of thyroid storm.

64. **Most common type and cause of hypothyroidism:**
    (a) **Primary hypothyroidism (disease of the thyroid gland) is the most common type(90-95% of cases)**, the rest is secondary hypothyroidism (pituitary hypofunction) or tertiary hypothyroidism (hypothalamic hypofunction).
    (b) **Most common cause of hypothyroidism is autoimmune disease** (goitrous or thyroprivic Hashimoto's disease). In the USA, next common causes are iatrogenic destruction of thyroid tissue by RAI, surgery, or external beam radiation. Iodine deficiency and goitrogens are the most common cause in rest of the world.

65. **Wolff-Chaikoff effect**:
    Iodine excess can also cause goitrous hypothyroidism due to iodine induced inhibition of thyroid hormone formation.

66. **Signs and symptoms of hypothyroidism:**
    (a) Skin: Dry, rough, hyperkeratotic, and nonpitting edema due to mucopolysaccharide deposits.
    (b) Muscle: Delayed tendon reflexes (especially Achilles tendon), weakness, stiffness, cramps, and increased muscle volume.

(c) **General**: Less active, sleepy, loss of hair, weight gain, and feeling cold.
(d) CNS: Forgetfulness, dementia, cerebellar ataxia.
(e) CVS: High BP, bradycardia, pericardial effusion, and high cholesterol levels.
(f) GI: Constipation.
(g) Respiratory: Sleep apnea, decreased ventilatory drive, pleural effusion.

67. **Diagnosis of hypothyroidism**:
(a) Primary hypothyroidism: Low free T_4, high TSH is diagnostic (T_3 is **not** helpful because it is normal in mild hypothyroidism and very low in NTI syndrome).
(b) Secondary hypothyroidism: Low free T_4, Normal or low TSH.
(c) Thyroid hormone resistence causing hypothyroidism: High free T4 and high TSH.
(d) Tertiary hypothyroidism: Low free T_4, normal or low TSH.
(e) To differentiate between secondary (pituitary) and tertiary (thalamic) hypothyroidism: Absence of TSH response in TRH stimulation test in secondary but presence of TSH response indicates tertiary hypothyroidism. In pituitary hypothyroidism, patients may have associated low FSH, LH, sex hormones, and ACTH levels.
(f) **Failing gland syndrome or subclinical hypothyroidism (minimal or no signs of hypothyroidism because normal T_3 maintains the normal metabolic status)**: T_4 and free T_4 lie just below the lower normal range, T_3 is normal, and TSH is very mildly elevated. Remember, TSH levels always lag behind the changes of T_4 and T_3 levels.
(g) Elevated cholesterol, CPK, LDH, and AST (aspartate transaminase) levels in hypothyroidism.

68. **Treatment of patients with low ACTH and low TSH in pituitary** hypothyroidism: Remember, **cortisol replacement therapy should be started first**, before the thyroid hormone replacement therapy.

69. **Treatment of hypothyroidism**:
(a) **Levothyroxine (T4) is the drug of choice.** It should be given probably rest of the patient's life and periodic evaluation is indicated.
(b) **During pregnancy** particularly in third trimester, **levothyroxine doses should be increased by 30 to 50 %.** After delivery, doses should be reduced to normal.
(c) Higher replacement doses of levothyroxine are needed in the following conditions:

Malabsorptions, antacids with aluminium preparation, rifampin, ferrous sulfate, and cholestyramine.

(d) Use of T3 is recommended in the following special situation:

(i) Short-term therapy of patients with thyroid cancer after thyroid operation.

(ii) Before the administration of RAI.

(iii) Myxedema coma.

(iv) Rare condition such as 5′ deiodinase deficiency. (Half life of T3 is 1 day and T4 is 7 days).

70. **Responses of treatment and follow up of hypothyroidism**:

(A) **Responses of treatment are the following**:

(i) **Clinical improvement begins 2 to 3 weeks** after the onset of therapy.

(ii) **T_4 and T_3 levels become normal within 2 to 3 weeks** after the onset of therapy.

(iii) **TSH levels become normal after 3 to 4 weeks or longer** because of increased number of thyrotrophs in the pituitary after prolonged hypothyroidism.

(iv) Complete clinical recovery like euthyroid takes **several months.**

(B) **Follow-up of patients on thyroid drug (T4)**:

(i) Free T4, T3, and TSH determination every 6 to 12 months.

(ii) **Diagnosis of over treatment**: TSH levels is below normal.

(iii) **Diagnosis of under treatment**: TSH levels is above normal.

(iv) Effects of chronic over treatment:

(a) Thinning of the bone.

(b) Cardiac hypertrophy.

(c) Arrythmias.

71. **Management of patients with hypothyroidism and angina pectoris**:

(The coronary artery disease is more common in hypothyroiodism. The treatment with thyroid hormone increases the angina because of increased cardiac demand and oxygen consumption.).

(a) **Levothyroxine (T_4) should be given because** it reduces BP, cholesterol, and produce euthyroid state. Adequate replacement therapy is difficult because of progressive angina.

(b) **Add propranolol** which may be helpful in angina but causes bradycardia.

(c) Patients with mild to moderate hypothyrodism **with angina pectoris**: Percutaneous coronary transluminal angioplasty or coronary bypass surgery can be performed without complication.

72. **Treatment of myxedema coma**: (Coma precipitates in severe myxedema due to infection, cold exposure, sedatives, or analgesies).
   (a) Avoid all the above mentioned precipitating conditions.
   (b) Admit to the ICU.
   (c) Vigorous thyroid hormone replacement therapy: Intravenous T_4 is followed by oral T_4 therapy or IV T3 is followed by oral T_4 therapy. **The use of T_3 may be beneficial because T_4 is converted to T_4 which may be affected in very ill patients**.
   (d) Glucocorticoid: IV hydrocortisone should be started, before that assesment of adrenal function should be evaluated because it can disturb the pituitary-adrenal feedback.
   (e) Intubation and mechanical ventilation: Patients are usually obtunded and **have high Pco_2 retention which indicates immediate thyroid hormone therapy, even when the level of T_4 and TSH are not avialable.**
   (f) Antibiotics for infections.
   (g) IV fluids, glucose, and electrolytes but avoid overhydration.

73. **Most common cause of severe thyroid pain or tenderness**: Quervain's thyroiditis (subacute nonsuppurative thyroiditis, granulomatous thyroiditis, or giant cell thyroiditis). It is associated with **HLA-B35**, presence of **thyroid antibody titers** (antimicrosomal, anti-TSH receptor, antithyroglobulin) in subacute phase (up to 20 % of patients) but disappear with improvement of the disease. It is preceded by viral infection (mumps, measles, influenza, coxsackie, adenovirus, echovirus, enterovirus).

74. **Signs and symptoms, diagnosis, and treatment of subacute painful granulomatous thyroiditis (or Quervain's thyroiditis)**:
   (a) The symptoms begin 1 to 3 weeks after viral infection. The patients appear with severe pain over the thyroid area, radiates to the ear, fever, muscle aches, anorexia, and painful swallowing. **Physical examination**: Very tender, may be enlarged thyroid gland but **no** cervical lymphadenopathy.
   (b) **Diagnosis**:
      (i) Elevated ESR > 100 mm/hour.
      (ii) Decreased RAI uptake (< 2% at 24 hours).
      (iii) Early stage: High T_4 levels.
      (iv) Late stage: Low T_4 levels and high TSH levels (like hypothyroidism, but rarely. develops permanent hypothyroidism).
      (v) Acute phase: Elevated thyroglobulin.
   (c) **Treatment:**
      (i) Mild cases: No treatment or aspirin for pain.
      (ii) Severe cases: Prednisone.

(iii) Thyrotoxic patients: Propranolol.

75. **Hashimoto's thyroiditis (chronic lymphocytic thyroidits) and histocompatibility antigen: HLA-B8.**
   (a) Goitrous variant: HLA-DR5.
   (b) Atrophic variant: HLA-DR3.
   It is the **most common type of thyroid autoimmune disease,** mostly affects women between third and fifth decades of life.

76. **Signs and symptoms, diagnosis, and treatment of Hashimoto's thyroiditis (chronic lymphocytic thyroiditis)**:
   (a) **Signs and symptoms: Euthyroid goitre is the most common clinical manifestation** (up to 75% of cases), the rest are atrophic variety. Hypothyroidism is found in 20% and hyperthyroidism is noted in < 5% cases. It is associated with other autoimmune diseases (adrenal, pituitary, parathyroid, beta-cells of pancreas, and gonads). It may occur with pernicious anemia, SLE, ITP, or Sjogren's syndrome.
   Physical examination: Firm, rubbery, painless, symmetrically enlarged, irregular surface thyroid gland which may cause tracheal obstruction.
   (b) **Diagnosis**:
      (i) Positive antiperoxidase antibodies (90% of cases).
      (ii) Positive anithyroglobulin antibodies (50% of cases).
      (iii) T_4 and TSH levels can be normal.
      (iv) In hypothroid form: Low T_4 and free T_4 levels, and high TSH levels.
      (v) Do **not** perform RAI.
      (vi) Fine-needle aspiration and biopsy is **not** routinely needed but may be helpful to differentiate from cancer or benign thyroid adenoma.
   (c) **Treatment:**
      (i) Thyroxine (T_4) replacement therapy in hypothyroid and potential hypothyroid states. It cannot reduces the size or obstruction caused by the gland.
      (ii) Surgery is needed to reduce the size and obstruction.
      (iii) Transient hyperthyroidism: Propranolol.
      (iv) Nontransient hyperthyroidism: Antithyroid drugs (PTU or MMI).

77. **Difference between Hashimoto's thyroditis and Graves' disease (both are autoimmune diseases)**:
   (i) TSI is specific for Graves' disease.
   (ii) TSH receptor blocking antibodies are present in Hashimoto's thyroditis.
   (iii) **Heavy lymphocytic infiltration** destroys the normal follicular structure is predominant in **Hashimoto's disease** than Graves' disease.

78. **Hashimoto's thyroiditis and thyroid cancer**: The incidence of cancer in **not** increased except **lymphomas**.

79. **Signs and symptoms, diagnosis, and treatment of subacute painless (lymphocytic) thyroiditis with transient hyperthyroidism**:
   (a) **Signs and symptoms**: The patients appear with sudden onset of **acute thyrotoxicosis** (weight loss, tachycardia, nervousness, and heat intolerance) and painless firm nodular goitre. Some patients appear with **hypothyroidism** after brief unnoticed period of hyperthyroidism. Postpartum thyroiditis occurs 3 to 6 months after delivery, initially hyperthyroid state (2 to 4 months) is followed by hypothyroid (which lasts for 1 to 3 months), then spontaneous recovery in most cases. **Absence** of signs of Graves' disease (eye signs and pretibial myxedemas).
   (b) **Diagnosis:**
      (i) Hyperthyroidism: Elevated T_4 and T_3 levels, low TSH levels.
      (ii) Positive antiperoxidase antibody (low titers).
      (iii) ESR is normal or mildly elevated (markedly elevated in subacute painful thyroditis).
      (iv) RAI uptake is suppressed.
      (v) Biopsy is **not** needed to make the diagnosis, it shows abundant lymphocytes infiltrate.
      (vi) TSI is normal (elevated in Graves' disease).
   (c) **Treatment**:
      (i) Propranolol: It is used in thyrotoxic state.
      (ii) Thyroid hormones: It is used in hypothyroid state.

80. **Most common thyroid disease in USA**: **Nontoxic goiter** (or simple goiter). It is a replication of benign epithelial cells **stimulated mostly by TSH** ; or IGF-1 and EGF.
   (a) **Signs and symptoms of nontoxic goiter**: The patients are **asymptomatic** or **symptoms of mechanical pressure** exerted by the enlarged thyroid gland (particularly substernal goiters) on the trachea, esophagus, recurrent laryngeal nerve, and large cervical veins.
      (i) Pressure on the recurrent laryngeal nerve: It causes hoarseness, rule out cancer.
      (ii) Pressure on the trachea: Respiratory distress begins when trachea is narrowed to 20 to 30 % of its normal size.
      (iii) **Pemberton's sign:** Livid suffusion of the face and discomfort due to obstruction of venous return of the external jugular veins.

(iv) Sudden onset of pain in a painless goiter: It indicates bleeding into the thyroid nodule.

(b) **Diagnosis of nontoxic goiter**:

(i) Elevated **TSH level is the best diagnostic test**; with normal or low-normal T_4 and mid-normal T_3.

(ii) **CT scan or MRI is the best diagnostic** method to evaluate the substernal extension of the thyroid gland.

(iii) Endemic goiter: Low T_4, normal T_3, and elevated TSH. **The amount of iodine intake can be detected by measuring the iodine excretion in the urine** which is reduced with reduced intake.

(c) **Treatment of nontoxic goiter**:

(i) Thyroxine (T_4) therapy for hypothyroid state.

(ii) Iodine supplementation is the best treatment of choice in endemic goiter.

(iii) Endemic goiter with obstructive symptoms or goiter size is **not** reduced with thyroxine: Partial thyroidectomy is followed by thyroxine therapy.

(iv) Iodine supplementation can cause Jodbasedow effect (thyrotoxicosis). RAI therapy has modest success in large goiter.

(v) Multinodular goiter (especially in older person): Do **not** give thyroxine if the TSH levels are suppressed or low-normal. Thyroxine is given if the TSH levels are elevated or high-normal. If the thyroxine therapy for 6 to 12 months could **not** decrease the nodular size, thyroxine should be stopped results in temporary hypothyroidism which begins 1 month after the discontinuation and lasts for 1 month.

81. **Procedure performed to distinguish between benign and malignant thyroid nodules**: **Fine needle aspiration.**

82. **Most common cause of single thyroid nodule**: Thyroid adenoma (85 % are benign, 15 % are malignant).

83. **Signs and symptoms, diagnosis and treatment of thyroid adenoma:**

(a) **Signs and symptoms**: Euthyroid adenomas Physical examination: Palpable nodule, lymph nodes should be examined.

(b) **Diagnosis and management**:

(i) **Fine-needle aspiration is the best diagnostic study** to distinguish between benign and malignant: (three findings).

(a) Malignant lesion: Surgery.

(b) Benign lesion: Thyroid hormone (T_4) and reaspirate 1-2 years.

(c) Hypercellular follicular neoplasm: RAI scan shows cold nodule (85 % of cases) which needs surgery and hot nodule (15% of cases) needs observation. 20 % of cold nodules are malignant and < 1 % of hot nodules are malignant. Recent report has suggested that mutant TSH **receptors** always stimulate thyroid hormone formation even when it is **not** occupied by TSH. If these patients are euthyroid, they should be followed. About 25 % of them become hyperthyroid, they should be treated with PTU or MMI followed by surgery, if surgery is contraindicated nodules should be ablated with RAI.

(ii) Large nodule with other nodules and H/O ionizing radiation: Surgery.

(iii) Thyroid function test should be done.

84. **Genetic factors and thyroid cancer**:
   (a) Mutation of the **ras kinase gene**: It occurs in papillary cancer.
   (b) Mutation of the p53 repressor gene: It occurs in anaplastic cancer.
   (c) Activation of the kinase genes (ret and trk): It occurs in thyroid cancer.

85. **Radiation and thyroid cancer**:
   (a) Radiation (up to 1500 rad) to the head and neck particularly during childhood: It has 30-fold increase in thyroid cancer.
   (b) **Remember**, radioactive iodine therapy (5000 rad or more) in Graves' disease do **not** increase the risk of thyroid cancer.

86. **Most common type of thyroid cancer**: **Papillary cancer (70 %, least aggressive type)**, next is follicular cancer (15 %), others are medullary cancer, lymphomas, and anaplastic cancer.

87. **Signs and symptoms, diagnosis, and treatment of thyroid cancer**:
   (a) **Signs and symptoms**: Rapid, painless, nodular growth, particularly in a male over 60 is characteristic.
   Physical examination: A single hard nodule which is fixed to the surrounding tissues plus firm, poorly mobile lateral lymph nodes is characteristic.
   (b) **Diagnosis**:
      (i) **Fine-needle aspiration of thyroid nodule and cytological examination are the best diagnostic method.**
      (ii) Thyroid ultrasonography can detect (fluid) cystic or solid lesion. **Remember, incidence of cancer is same in both cystic and solid lesions.**
      (iii) Thyroid scan is done to detect cold nodule when experienced cytopathologist is **not** available.
      (iv) Most patients have normal T_4, T_3, TSH.
      (v) Elevated T_4 and T_3 level **indicate follicular cancer**.
      (vi) Elevated calcitonin and calcitonin-related peptides in medullary cancer.

(c) **Treatment:**

(i) **Thyroid surgery is the best treatment of choice. It should be done by an experienced thyroid surgeon**: Near-total throidectomy or lobectomy is controversial.

Advantages of near-total thyroidectomy:

(a) The patient can be followed by measuring **thyroglobulin levels which are elevated in a recurrence of thyroid cancer after surgery**.

(b) Small amount of thyroid tissues can be ablated with RAI, normal thyroid tissues accumulate RAI more avidly than cancer tissues, so it is **difficult to treat cancer tissues with RAI in presence of large amount of normal tissues (in lobectomy)**.

(ii) **RAI (Radioactive iodine) ablation after near-total thyroidectomy is done in patients with papillary or follicular cancer**.

(iii) **Medullary cancer** should be treated with **surgery plus external radiation and chemotherapy**. It does **not** respond to RAI.

88. **Most common cause of Cushing's syndrome: Cushing's disease** (pituitary tumor) up to 80% of cases.

89. **Most common cause of ectopic ACTH secretion: Small cell carcinoma of the lung** (50% of all cases); next is endocrine tumors of foregut origin (islet cell tumor, thymic carcinoid, medullary carcinoma of thyroid, bronchial carcinoid), pheochromocytoma, and ovarian tumors.

90. **Signs and symptoms, diagnosis of Cushing's syndrome (glucocorticoid excess):**

(A) **Signs and symptoms**: The patients appear with **weight gain (most common presentation), 'Moon facies', high BP, violaceous striae,** hirsutism, plethora, proximal muscle weakness (unable to rise from squatting position unassisted), and glucose intolerance. **The characteristic truncal weight gain and buffalo hump** (doricervical fat deposition) are present.

(B) **Diagnosis:**

(i) The characteristic clinical features plus elevated urine free cortisol is diagnostic. Normal physiologic activation (stress, depression) causes elevation of urine free cortisol up to 250 microgram per day.

(ii) The 'Weak' clinical features plus urine free cortisol above 250 microgram/day.

(iii) The Cushing's syndrome with cancer (particularly small cell cancer of the lung): The patients appear with cachexia (instead of weight gain) due to malignancy, plus very high levels of urine free cortisol.

(iv) The 'strong' clinical features but normal urine free cortisol levels: It may due to iatrogenic or surreptitiouos exogenous glucocorticoid administration. The history should be suggestive.

91. **Causes of Cushing's syndrome**:
 (A) ACTH-dependent causes.
  (i) **Cushing's disease (ACTH-secreting pituitary tumor) is the most common cause**.
  (ii) Ectopic ACTH-secretion.
 (B) ACTH-independent cause.
  (i) **Adrenal adenomas are the most common** among the ACTH-independent causes.
  (ii) Adrenal carcinoma.
  (iii) Micronodular adrenal disease.
  (iv) Factitious or surreptitious glucocorticoid administration.

92. **How to distinguish between adrenal tumor and adrenal cancer?.**

Adrenal tumor	Adrenal cancer
1) Unilateral.	1) Bilateral.
2) < 4 cm in diameter.	2) > 6 cm in diameter.
3) Produce only one hormone (cortisol).	3) Produce more than one hormones (glucocorticoid plus mineralocorticoid or glucocorticoid plus androgen).
4) No metastases.	4) May have metases.
5) CT or MRI: Unilateral lesion with no metastases.	5) CT or MRI: Bilateral lesions with or without metastases.

93. **Treatment of different adrenal tumors**:
 (a) Small unilateral lesion with no metastases: Unilateral flank excision or laparascopic procedure to remove the tumor.
 (b) Large lesion with no metastases: Transabdominal operation to remove the tumor plus liver biopsy and careful examination of other organs.
 (c) Micronodular adrenal dysplasia: Bilateral adrenalectomy.
 (d) Lesion with metastases: Surgical excision plus chemotherapy OP'DDD (ortho, para'-DDD).
 Side effects of chemotherapy: Reduced attention span, somnolence, ataxia, and diarrhea.

94. **Difference between ACTH-dependent and ACTH-independent causes of Cushing's syndrome**: Measurement of ACTH levels after CRH administration:
    (a) ACTH-dependent diseases: > 10 pg/ml.
    (b) ACTH-independent diseases: < 10 pg/ml.

95. **Signs and symptoms, diagnosis of mineralocorticoid excess**:
    (a) **Signs and symptoms**: The patients have signs of arterial hypertension and dependent edema.
    (b) **Diagnosis**:
        (1) Serum electrolyltes: High Na, low k.
        (2) ABG: Metabolic alkalosis.
        (3) Resting plasma renin activity:
            (a) High renin levels: Renin-angiotensin dependent mineralocorticoid excess.
            (b) Low renin levels: Renin-angiotensin independent mineralocorticoid excess.

96. **Two important causes of renin-angiotensin-independent mineralocorticoid excess**: (aldosterone mediated).
    (a) Aldosterone secreting adenoma.
    (b) Aldosterone secreting bilateral hyperplasia. Other causes are adrenal cancer, licorice (chewing tobacco) intoxication, CAH (congenital adrenal hyperplasia), and 11 beta-hydroxysteroid dehydrogenase deficiency.
    How to differentiate between aldosterone mediated and other mineralocorticoid mediated condition:
        (1) Elevated or normal aldosterone levels in the urine and plasma indicate aldosterone mediated disease.
        (2) Low aldosterone levels indicate other mineralocorticoid mediated disease.

97. **How to differentiate between aldosterone mediated adrenal adenomas versus hyperplasias**: **The most definitive diagnostic test is to measure the cortisol-aldosterone ratios in adrenal venous blood sampled** at the same time from both adrenal glands after the administration of ACTH:
    (a) High levels of aldosterone from one adrenal gland and none from the other: It indicates adenoma.
    (b) Equal aldosterone levels in both adrenal glands: It indicates hyperplasias.

98. **Treatment of adrenal adenomas and hyperplasias**:
    (a) Unilateral adenomas: Surgical excision.

(b) Bilateral hyperplasias: It is best treated with **spironolactone** which inhibits the mineralocorticoid excess. Use **antihypertensive drugs** if BP is **not** controlled with spironolactone.

99. **How to distinguish the different non-aldosterone mediated renin-angiotensin-independent mineralocorticoid excess ?**:
   (a) Adrenal cancer: CT or MRI is the best diagnostic method.
   (b) CAH: Symmetrically moderately enlarged adrenal glands detected by CT or MRI.
      (i) 11-hydroxylase deficiency: High BP and elevated serum 11-deoxycortisol levels.
      (ii) 17-hydroxylase deficiency: High BP, delayed puberty, genital ambiguity, and elevated plasma progesterone levels.
   (c) 11 beta-hydroxysteroid dehydrogenase (HSD) deficiency: This enzyme converts active cortisol to inactive cortisone. Enzyme deficiency results in elevated cortisol levels and high BP.
   Treatment: Dexamethasone or predinisone to suppress the cortisol levels.
   (d) Licorice (chewing tobacco) has active ingredients **glycyrrhizic acid** which is a competitive inhibitor of 11-beta HSD: Licorice intoxication results in high BP and elevated cortisol level as mentioned in item (c).

100. **Treatment of all cases of non-aldosterone-mediated renin-angiotensin-** independent mineralocorticoid excess, **except cancer**: All of them should respond to adrenal suppression with dexamethasone **except cancer**. The successful adrenal suppression should be followed by **long term hydrocortisone therapy**.

101. **Causes of renin-angiotensin-dependent mineralocorticoid excess**:
   (a) Vomiting.
   (b) Diuretics.
   (c) Bartter's syndrome.
   (d) Renin-secreting tumors.
   (e) Renal ischemia.
   (f) Edematous condition: CHF, nephrotic syndrome, cirrhosis.

102. **Signs and symptoms, diagnosis of glucocorticoid deficiency**:
   (A) **Signs and symptoms:**
      (a) Chronic syndrome: It is characterized by anorexia, malaise, postural hypotension, weight loss, and hyperpigmentation.
         (1) **Laboratory findings:** Normocytic normochromic anemia, relative lymphocytosis with eosinophilia.

(2) SMA-6: Low Na, high BUN (prerenal azotemia).

(b) **Acute syndrome:** It is characterized by agitation, confusion, fever, abdominal pain, low BP, shock; untreated patients quickly lead to coma and death.
Laboratory findings: Same as in chronic syndrome.

(B) **Diagnosis**:

(a) ACTH challenge test (IV administration of 250 microgram ACTH) and measurement of serum cortisol after 45 to 60 mintues: Cortisol level < 20 indicates adrenal hypofunction (normal value is 20 or more). Baseline ACTH plasma level should be drawn before ACTH administration.

(b) Low ACTH plasma levels: It means ACTH-dependent causes of glucocorticoid deficiency.

(c) High ACTH plasma levels: It means ACTH-independent causes of glucocorticoid deficiency.

103. **Causes of glucocorticoid deficiency**:

(a) ACTH-independent causes:
- (1) TB (tuberculosis).
- (2) Autoimmune (idiopathic).
- (3) Rare causes are the following: Fungal infection, metastases, adrenal hemorrhage, HIV infection, ketoconazole, OP′DDD, and sarcoidosis.

(b) ACTH-dependent causes:
- (1) Hypothalamic-pituitary-adrenal suppression:
  - (a) Exogenous: Glucocorticoid, ACTH.
  - (b) Endogenous: Cure of Cushing's syndrome.
- (2) Hypothalamic-pituitary lesion:
  - (a) Tumors: Primary pituitary tumor and metastatic tumor.
  - (b) Infection: TB, actinomycosis.
  - (c) Craniopharyngioma.
- (3) Head injury.
- (4) Isolated ACTH deficiency.
- (5) Sarcoidosis.

104. **Most common cause of ACTH- dependent glucocorticoid deficiency**: Hypothalamic-pituitary-adrenal suppression by exogenous administration of **glucocorticoids either iatrogenic or factitious**. It depends upon the **dose** (20 mg or less/day hydrocortisone, 5 mg/day or less prednisone, 0.5 mg/day dexamethasone are less likely to cause suppression), **duration** (< 3 weeks less likely to cause suppression), and **single dose first thing in the morning** is

also less likely to cause adrenal suppression. The clinical manifestations may be **'chronic' or 'acute' syndrome**.

Recommendation to avoid adrenal suppression: To give lower doses, less than 3 weeks, and single dose in the morning are the ideal method to give steroid therapy.

Other causes of glucocorticoid deficiency are due to hypothalamic-pituitary disease: It is **rare** but is important to diagnose early **by CT or MRI** to avoid blindness.

105. **Treatment of chronic ACTH-dependent glucocorticoid insufficiency**: To replace the missing hormone, glucocorticoid should be replaced with **hydrocortisone.**

Monitor the efficacy of treatment with **hydrocortisone**:

(1) **Under replacement therapy**: Weight loss, anorexia, low Na.

(2) **Over replacement therapy**: Weight gain, plethora, supraclavicular fat deposition.

Doses of cortisol during stress (fever, trauma such as laceration, fracture, vomiting, surgical procedures, and dental extraction): The doses should be **doubled** for **the duration of the stress** and **reduced to normal replacement doses after the stress is over.**

106. **Most common cause of primary adrenal insufficiency**:

(1) Autoimmune process in USA and other western world.

(2) TB in rest of the world.

107. **Autoimmune destruction or primary adrenal insufficiency**: Two types are I and II.

Type I.	Type II.
1) Children (12 years). 2) Autosomal recessive. 3) NO HLA association. 4) Dominant features are: Adrenal insufficiency, hypoparathyroidism, mucocutaneous candidiasis.	1) Adults (24 years). 2) Autosomal dominant. 3) Associated with DR 3/DR 4. 4) Dominant features are: Adrenal insufficiency, insulin dependent diabetes mellitus, autoimmune thyroid disease.

108. **All the clinically important fungi cause adrenal suppression except: Monilia.**

109. **Most common fungal cause of adrenal suppression**: **Histoplasmosis**; next is South American blastomycosis followed by North American blastomycosis, coccidioidomycosis, and cryptococcosis.

110. A patient appers with **H/O back pain for few days followed by signs and symptoms of adrenal suppression**. The patient is receiving anticoagulants for pulmonary emboli, cardiac emboli, or other thrombotic phenomenon.
Most likely diagnosis: Adrenal hemorrhages. Diagnosis: CT scan.

111. **AIDS patients with adrenal suppression, most common associated infections**:
CMV, Mycobacterium avum –intracellulare.

112. **Treatment of ACTH-independent glucocorticoid deficiency: Hydrocortisone** which is also used in ACTH-dependent glucocorticoid deficiency.
   (a) Fludrocortisone acetate (Florinef), it is a mineralocorticoid and equipotent of aldosterone.
   Monitor the drug effects: Serum k levels which may be low.

113. **Signs and symptoms of mineralocorticoid deficiency**: Hyponatremia, hyperkalemia, mild metabolic acidosis which leads to profound muscle weakness and cardiac arrythmias. The patients may appear with **combined mineralocorticoid and glucocorticoid deficiencies.** ACTH-stimulation test is **normal in isolated mineralocorticoid deficiency** and **abnormal in glucocorticoid deficiency,** so this test is helpful to distinguish these two conditions.

114. **Most common cause of selective aldosterone (mineralocorticoid) deficiency**: **Renin deficiency (hyporeninemic hypoaldosteronism)**. It is common in elderly patients, appear with mild, nonoliguric renal failure, may be associated with insulin-dependent diabetes mellitus and diabetic nephropathy. Other causes of renin-angiotensin-dependent hypoaldosteronism include **autonomic neuropathy with prolonged bed rest**, rarely due to use of indomethacin (PGE inhibitor).

115. **Renin-angiotensin-independent causes of isolated hypoaldosteronism**:
   (a) Inhibition of aldosterone synthesis: Heparin, cyclosporine, calcium channel blocker.
   (b) After removal of an aldosterone-secreting adenoma.
   (c) Pseudohypoaldosteronism (aldosterone resistance).

(d) All causes of ACTH-**independent** adrenal insufficiency (TB, autoimmune, other rare causes are fungal infection, metastases, adrenal hemorrhage, HIV infection, ketoconazole, OP′DDD, and sarcoidosis): Hypoaldosteronism is found **if the treatment is limited to glucocorticoid only**.

(e) 18- hydroxylase deficiency. This enzyme converts corticosterone to aldosterone.

116. **Treatment of isolated hypoaldosteronism**: (Isolated aldosterone deficiency does **not** produce symptoms **unless there is salt deprivation**. In adults, **more than 4 grams/day** is adequate to keep the paitents asymptomatic).

(1) Adequate salt intake: More than 4 grams/day.

(2) Fludrocortisone is used when patients **cannot** maintain adequate oral salt intake for any reason. It is given as **single oral dose in the morning**.

117. **Signs and symptoms, diagnosis, and treatment of 21-hydroxylase deficiency in CAH**: It is an autosomal recessive disorder.

(A) **Signs and symptoms**: Although it is congenital but patients may appear at the onset of puberty with **hirsutism, cystic acne, and oligomenorrhea**. The clinical presentation is **identical** as idiopathic hirsutism-polycystic ovarian disease.

How to differentiate the two conditions, just mentioned above:

(i) ACTH-stimulation test:

(a) Normal individual: 17-hydroxyprogesterone levels are < 350 ng/dl.

(b) 21-hydroxylase deficiency: 17-hydroxyprogesterone level are > 1500 ng/dl.

(B) **Diagnosis**:

(i) Elevated 17-hydroxyprogesterone levels in the plasma.

(ii) ACTH-stimulation test.

(C) **Treatment**: Glucocorticocoid replacement therapy with cortisol (Cortef) single morning dose.

Diagnosis of overtreatment: ACTH-stimulation test 3 to 6 months after the onset of therapy would detect overtreatment or adrenal suppression.

118. **von Hippel-Lindau syndrome (VHLS)**: Autosomal dominant, chromosomal location 3p25-p26, clinical manifestations include pheochromocytoma, retinal angioma (fundus examination is important), ranal cysts and cancer, pancreatic cysts, cerebellar hemangioblastoma, and epididymal cystadenoma.

119. **Signs and symptoms, diagnosis, and treatment of pheochromocytoma**: **Most of the tumor is solitary, unilateral, intra-abdominal, and adrenal medullary origin**.

(A) **Signs and symptoms**: Paroxysmal hypertension, episodic palpitations, headaches, and diaphoresis. Family H/O pheochromocytoma, VHLS, MEN (retinal angiomas, mucosal neuromas, enlarged thyroid gland), carbohydrate intolerance, labile, refractory high BP, orthostatic hypotension, and sometimes cholesterol gallstones.

(B) **Diagnosis:**

(1) **Routine test:** Hyperglycemia (50 % of cases).

(2) **Urine tests**:

(a) **Elevated urinary metanephrine (catecholamine metabolites) is the most sensitive and specific test for pheochromocytoma.**

(b) Elevated VMA (catecholamine metabolites).

(3) **Blood tests:**

(a) Elevated plasma catecholamines (norepinephrine plus epinephrine): **More than 2000 pg/ml strongly suggest pheochromocytoma** (normal values are < 1000 pg/ml, between 1000 to 2000 pg/ml may be due to pheochromocytoma, physical or mental stress).

(b) The clonidine suppression test: It is done when plasma catecholamine levels are **between 1000 to 2000 pg/ml** or equivocal:

Absence of pheochromocytoma: Plasma norepinephrine levels should fall to < 500 pg/ml after clonidine.

Presence of pheochromocytoma: Plasma norepinephrine levels should **not** fall after clonidine i.e., positive test.

(4) **Anatomic localization**:

(a) CT scan: It is done most frequently but it is **nonspecific.**

(b) MRI: It may be better for extra-adrenal tumors but it is **nonspecific**.

(5) **Functional test:** MIBG (metaiodobenzylguanidine) scan: It is highly specific (98%) for chromaffin tissue (pheochromocytoma) but less sensitive than CT or MRI.

(C) Treatment of pheochromocytoma:

(i) **Preoperative preparation and management**:

(a) **Alpha-blocker (phenoxybenzamine)**: It is used to control the BP (to keep < 160/90 mm Hg), prevent paroxysmal hypertension, and avoid tachyarrythmias.

Side effects of phenoxybenzamine: Orthostatic hypotension, tachycardia, diplopia, nasal congestion, dry mouth, and ejaculatory dysfunction.

(b) **If BP or tachyarrythmias is not controlled with phenoxybenzamine**: Use propranolol (beta-blocker) or metoprolol as an alternative, they are useful for **predominant epinephrine-secreting tumors**.

(c) **If combined alpha and beta blockers are not fully effective**: Use tyrosine hydroxylase inhibitor (alpha-methyl-paratyrosine).

Side effects of the drug: Sedation, extrapyramidal reaction, diarrhea, fatigue, and anxiety.

(d) **Severe hypertensive crisis: IV nitroprusside is the drug of choice**, phentolamine, or sublingual nifedipine (calcium channel blocker) may be used.

(e) **Avoid the following drugs**: Opiates, naloxone, histamine, glucagon, indirect sympathomimetic amines (tyramine, phenylpropanolamine), TCA, **cocaine**, guanethidine, metoclopramide, or sulpiride. **All of them can enhance high BP**.

(ii) **Operative and perioperative management**:

(a) **Surgical resection of the tumor and entire adrenal gland**: It provides cure in majority of the cases because 90% of pheochromocytomas are benign. Up to 25% cases may have lesser degree of hypertension.

How to diagnose residual tumor after surgery: Elevated urinary catecholamine 1 to 2 weels after surgery is suggestive of residual tumor.

(b) Intraoperative glucose (to avoid hypoglycemia) and saline solution to expand the intravascular volume.

(c) Intraoperative IV nitroprusside, phentolamine, or nicardia may be needed to control the BP.

(d) Postoperative management: **For hypoglycemia**: Glucose infusion.

For hypotension: Volume replacement is the most important, norepinephrine prn.

For hypertension: Rule out residual tumor, renal damage hypertension, or essential hypertension. The management should be appropriate.

120. **Diagnosis and treatment of malignant pheochromocytoma**: Remember, only 5 to 10% are malignant, extraadrenal tumors are most likely to metastasize than primary adrenal tumors, most common sites of metastases are retroperitoneum, bone, liver, and lymph nodes.

(A) **Diagnosis:**

(1) Biopsy of the tumor: It shows adjacent tissue invasion or metastatic spread.

(2) Elevated plasma DOPA indicates malignancy.

(3) Elevated HVA in the urine (DOPA and dopamine are metabolized to HVA) indicates malignancy.

(B) **Treatment:**

(1) **Phenoxybenzamine and propranolol** are the mainstay of the treatment of catecholamine excess.

(2) If **not** controlled, then use alpha-methylparatyrosine.

(3) Chemotherapy: It is **not** very effective but combination of vincristine, cyclophosphamide, and dacarbazine may be helpful in many patients.

(4) **Radiotherapy**: **Irradiation to skeletal metastases is helpful**, but the tumor itself is **not** radiosensitive.

(5) **Experimental**: High dose radiation with MIBG.

121. **Adrenal myelolipoma:** It is a benign, incidental mass due to accumulation of bone marrow elements in an otherwise normal functioning adrenals.
Diagnosis: Fatty mass is detected by CT or MRI.
Treatment: No treatment is needed.

122. **Different types of diabetes**:

(a) Type I or insulin-dependent (IDDM): Chromosome 6.

(b) Type II or non-insulin-dependent (NIDDM).

(i) Obese (80%).

(ii) Non-obese (15%).

(iii) MODY (maturity onset diabetes of the young).

(c) Secondary diabetes:

(i) Drugs: Glucocorticoids, thiazide, propranolol, phenytoin, pentamidine, and oral contraceptive.

(ii) Pancreatic disease: Chronic pancreatitis, pancreatic cancer, hemochromatosis, and cystic fibrosis.

(iii) Endocrine disease: Cushing's syndrome, acromegaly, pheochromocytoma, glucagonoma, and polycystic ovary syndrome.

(iv) Defective insulin receptor or antibodies against insulin receptor.

(v) Genetic: Turner's syndrome, ataxia-telangiectasia, myotonic dystrophy, and Huntington's disease.

(vi) Malnutrition: It is mostly found in developing countries.

123. **Risk factors of diabetes**:

(a) Gestationoal diabetes-Up to 40% can develop type II diabetes within 10 years. Rarely, pregnancy can precipitate type I diabetes.

(b) Impaired glucose tolerance: Up to 25% can develop type II diabetes.

124. **Diagnosis of diabetes mellitus**:

(a) **Random plasma glucose 200 mg/dL or more is diagnostic.**

(b) The patients with suspected diabetes but not confirmed by random glucose testing (< 200 mg/dL). Overnight fasting plasma glucose levels should be done:

(1) If **glucose levels equal or exceeds 140 mg/dL** on two separate occasions **are diagnostic.**

(2) If fasting glucose levels **are between 115 to 140 mg/dL**: This is a suspicious result but **not** diagnostic. **Next step is to do OGTT (oral glucose tolerance test). OGTT level at 2 hour > 200 mg/dL is diagnostic.**

(c) Impaired glucose tolerance (IGT):

(1) Fasting glucose levels is < 140 mg/dL.

(2) 2-hour OGTT level is between 140 to 200 mg/dL.

(3) An intervening glucose is 200 mg/dL or more.

IGT patients should be tested **annually** using **fasting glucose measurement** because they have **high risk of premature cradiovascular disease** like diabetes and **about 25%** of IGT patients **will become diabetic.**

(d) Testing a normal pregnant woman for diabetes:

(1) **Screening test of 50 grams OGTT between 24 to 28 weeks of gestation**: If fasting glucose is 105 mg/dL or 1-hour OGTT level is > 150 mg/dL, then an extended test of 100 grams **OGTT should be done. The diagnosis of gestational diabetes is made if two values equal or exceed the upper limit of normal (Normal values are the following**: Fasting 105 mg/dL, 1 hour 190 mg/dL, 2 hour 165 mg/dL, 3 hour 145 mg/dL).

125. **The characteristic of IDDM and NIDDM**:

	IDDM	NIDDM
1) Chromosome	6	Unknown
2) Age of onset	<40	≥40
3) Obesity	Absent	Present
4) Wasting	May be present	Absent
5) Plasma insulin	Low to absent	Normal to high
6) Plasma glucagon	High, suppressible	High, resistant
7) Insulin treatment	Responsive	Resistant to responsive
8) Sulfonylurea treatment	Unresponsive	Responsive
9) Complication	Ketoacidosis	Hyperosmolar coma
10) HLA molecules (class II)	DR3, DR4; DQ (Caucasians)	No

11) Islet cell antibodies (ICA)	Present in 80% of new onset diabetes	No

126. **Leprechaunism syndrome**: It is due to mutation in insulin receptors results in severe growth retardation and insulin resistance.

127. **Abdomial fat cells and insulin resistance**: It is **more resistant to insulin and have higher lipolytic rate** than fat derived from peripheral deposits **Detection of intra-abdominal visceral fat**: CT or MRI.

128. **Most important marker of endogenous insulin secretion: C-peptide.** It is the most important marker because it is **not** metabolized by the liver unlike insulin.

129. **Hormones producing opposite action of insulin (counter regulatory hormones)**: Glucagon (produced by alpha cells of pancreas), GH, cortisol, and catecholamines.

130. **Type I diabetes and viral epidemics (Important)**: Type I diabetes is associated with viral epidemics. Viral infection provoked insulin-resistance in a patient with marginal beta cell function. **Mumps, coxsackievirus, and congenital rubella epidemics cause type I diabetes**.

131. Insulin receptor function: Insulin receptor has **both alpha and beta chains**. Its function depends upon the intrinsic protein tyrosine **kinase activity (phosphorylation) on beta subunit**. **Insulin binds with alpha subunit** which is present on the extracellular surface.

132. **Incidence of diabetes in identical twins**:
    (1) Type I diabetes: 30 to 50 %.
    (2) Type II diabetes: Almost 100 %.
    (3) Nonidentical twins: Incidence is much lower than identical twins.

133. **Advantage of human insulin over animal insulin (beef, pork, and beef/pork combination): Human insulin is less antigenic, rapid onset of action, and shorter duration of action.** Human insulin is most commonly used.

134. **Insulin preparations and their action**:

Insulin	Onset of action	Duration of action

1) Regular (short acting)	30 minutes	5-8 hours
2) NPH or Lente (intermediate acting)	1-2 hours	16-24 hours
3) Human (ultralente)	4-6 hours	24-28 hours

135. **Goal of treatment of diabetes:**

(a) **Short term:**

(1) To keep metabolic control as normal as possible.

(2) Improve sense of well-being.

(b) **Long term:** Reduce the risk of complications (atherosclerosis, retinopathy, neuropathy, and nephropathy).

136. **'Honey moon period'** in type I diabetes: Partial recovery of the beta-cell function of the pancreas, secretion of endogenous insulin improves, and **need for reduction of insulin doses.** Remember, glycemic control is important to preserve the beta-cell function.

137. **Insulin injection therapy in type I diabetes**:

(a) **During the first few years of diabetic life (some** degree of beta cell function persists): **(Two daily injections,** injection should be given **same region** but **different loctaions at the same time each day** i.e, in the **abdomen in the morning to slow and optimize insulin delivery** and in the buttock or leg in the night **to slow absorption. Daytime leg or buttock movements enhances insulin absorption**).

(1) Mixture of rapid-acting plus intermediate-acting insulin **before breakfast**.

(2) Same combinations **before dinner**.

Initial adjustment should be made with the doses of intermediate acting insulin to optimize the predinner and fasting glucose values. After that, doses of **rapid-acting insulin should be adjusted according to prelunch and bedtime glucose values**.

1) Increased GL level in A.M.	Increase P.M. dose of NPH
2) Decreased GL level in A.M. (fasting)	Decrease P.M dose of NPH
3) Increased GL level in noon	Increase this A.M. dose of regular insulin
4) Decreased GL level in noon (pre-lunch)	Decrease this A.M. dose of regular insulin
5) Increased GL level in evening	Increase this A.M. dose of NPH
6) Decreased GL level in evening (pre-dinner)	Decrease this A.M. dose of NPH

7) Increased GL level at night	Increase this P.M. dose of regular insulin
8) Decreased GL level at night (bed time)	Decrease this P.M. dose of regular insulin

(b) **Several years after the onset of type I diabetes (twice daily injection is not enough because residual insulin secretion stops which is measured by decreased c-peptide). Most important is to control fasting glucose levels.** Fasting hyperglycemia is mostly due to glucose overproduction by the liver, inadequate overnight doses of insulin, and sleep associated GH release.

Three injections schedule: (Combinations).

First approach:

(1) Before breakfast: Mixture of intermediate and short-acting insulin.
(2) Before dinner: Short-acting insulin.
(3) At bed time: Intermediate acting insulin.

Second alternative approaches are the following:

(1) Ultralente: Before breakfast and dinner.
(2) Regular insulin: Before breakfast, lunch, and dinner.

Third alternative approach:

(1) Regular insulin: Before breakfast, lunch, and dinner.
(2) Intermediate acting insulin: At bed time.

138. **Dawn phenomenon and Somogyi phenomenon**:

(a) **Dawn phenomenon**: Early morning hyperglycemia, usually without preceeding hypoglycemia.

Etiology:

(1) Nocturnal rise of GH.
(2) Increased clearance of insulin.

Treatment: Increased insulin doses (evening dose of NPH).

(b) **Somogyi phenomenon**: (Rare in adults) Early morning rebound hyperglycemia which is preceeded by hypoglycemia.

Etiology:

(1) Release of counter regulatory hormones.
(2) Overdose of insulin (last evening dose of NPH).

Treatment: Decreased insulin doses (evening dose of NPH).

How to distinguish these two phenomenon?

(1) Decreased 3 A.M. blood glucose levels: Somogyi phenomenon.
(2) Normal 3 A.M. blood glucose levels: Dawn phenomenon.

139. **Hypoglycemia in type I diabetes:**

(a) **Causes of hypoglycemia:**

(1) Missing meals.
(2) Excessive exercise.

(b) Signs and symptoms of hypoglycemia:
(1) **Daytime:** Autonomic symptoms such as sweating, tremor, nervousness, and hunger.
(2) **During sleep:** Asymptomatic or night sweats, unpleasant dreams, and early-morning headaches.

(c) **Mechanism of protection from hypoglycemia:**
(1) Cessation of insulin release.
(2) Release of counter regulatory hormones. It increases hepatic glucose production and decreases glucose utilization in nonhepatic tissues.
Remember, **glucagon is the most important** primary counter regulatory hormone, epinephrine, and norepinephrine are the major back up when glucagon is **not** available. Cortisol and GH do **not** function in acute hypoglycemia but they do in prolonged fasting or sustained hypoglycemia.

(d) Treatment:
(1) Ingestion of carbohydrate immediately (sugar, candy, and sugar containing beverage).
(2) Unarousable patients: IV glucose, glucagon.

140. **Diet and exercise plan of diabetes:**

(A) **Diet plan:**
(1) Reduce weight, if necessary.
(2) Carbohydrate intake (45-60 %): It depends upon the severity of hyperglycemia and triglyceride level.
(3) Increased monosaturated fat (olive, peanut, and canola oils).
(4) Decreased saturated fat (animal fat) to < 10 % of calories.
(5) Decreased cholesterol intake to < 300 mg/day.
(6) Restriction of salt in patients prone to high BP.

(B) **Exercise plan:**
(1) **Type:** Aerobic is the best exercise. Avoid straining and heavy lifting.
(2) **Frequency:** 3 to 4 days/week.
(3) **Duration:** 20 to 30 minutes before and followed by stretching and flexibility exercise for 5 to 10 minutes.

141. **Management of type II diabetes**:

(a) **Diet and exercise:** It is the most important and the only therapy may be required to control the blood sugar. It is very helpful particularly obese and sedentary patients. Diet and exercise plan were discussed in the last item.

(b) **Weight loss for obese patients**: Approximately 5 kg weight loss from the baseline weight is very helpful to reduce the blood sugar levels. The weight loss should be achieved with adequate nutrition. The restriction of 500 kcal/day and 3500 kcal/week, results in 1 lb. weight loss/week. The obese patients who are failed to loss weight, very low calorie diet (600 to 800 kcal/day) should be prescribed with supervision.

(c) The daily calorie intake for sedentary patients: **As low as 25 to 30 kcal/kg body weight/day**.

(d) **Carbohydrate intake (few important points):**

(i) **Mild hyperglycemia**: Diet high in carbohydrate (50-60 %) can improve insulin action and glycemic control.

(ii) **Severe fasting hyperglycemia or with triglyceride elevation:** Moderate carbohydrate (45-50 %) intake is recommended.

(iii) Total amount of carbohydrate is more important than source of carbohydrate. **Remember, complex carbohydrate (starch) and simple sugar would increase the blood sugar levels similarly in diabetic patients.**

(iv) **The optimum source of carbohydrate are the following**: Food containing **water soluble fibers** (e.g., oats, legumes, fruit, pectin, gums) have better control of blood sugar levels.

Mechanism of action of fibres:

(a) It increases the gastric emptying time.
(b) It reduces the meal absorption.

(v) Modest amount of sucrose and complex carbohydrate should be added to the glucose.

142. **Effect of exercise in diabetes**:

(A) Improves insulin action.
(B) Enhances weight loss appropriately.
(C) Lower the cardiovascular disease.
(D) Fall in VLDL-triglyceride levels.
(E) Rise in HDL-cholesterol levels.
(F) Increase fibrinolytic activity.

143. **Pharmacologic therapy of Type II diabetes:**

(A) **Oral glucose-lowering agents:**

Indications:

(1) Mild diabetes, elderly patients.
(2) Pronounced obesity.
(3) Unresponsive to diet and exercise.

Contraindications:

(1) Allergy.
(2) Severe insulin deficiency.
(3) Pregnancy.

Oral glucose-lowering agents are following: Sulfonylurea drugs: Mechanism of action: Enchance insulin secretion by binding to k channel on the beta cell surface.

(i) **Tolbutamide** (sulfonylureas):
Advantages: Shortest duration of action, metabolized by the liver, and used in elderly patients with impaired renal function.
Disadvantages: Less effective due to poor compliance because doses 2 to 3 times/day.

(ii) **Chlorpropamide (sulfonylurea)**:
Advantages: Longest acting, once per day dosing.
Disadvantages: **Hyponatremia** is **due** to increased ADH particularly in elderly patients, **hypoglycemia** in patients who has renal impairment and skip meals because it is partially metabolized by the liver and excreted by the kidney.

(iii) The patients who are unresponsive to sulfonylurea drugs (tolbutamide, chlorpropamide, tolazamide, glipizide, or glyburide):
Use insulin or **add metformin (biguanide)**. **It is rarely helpful to switch from one oral drug to another**.

(iv) **Metformin**: **Mechanism of action**: Reduces hepatic gluconeogenesis, decrease intestinal glucose absorption results in reduce serum glucose as well as insulin indirectly. It is excreted by the kidney.
Advantages: Enhance weight loss (helpful in obese patients), reduce atherosclerosis (because hyperinsulinemia is atherosclerotic), absence of hypoglycemia.
Disadvantages: Anorexia, nausea, rarely causes lactic acidosis (cannot be used in renal insufficiency), short half life (given 2 to 3 times/day).

(B) **Insulin therapy in type II diabetes**:
Indications:
(1) Unresponsive to oral glucose-lowering drugs.
(2) **It is the first line of drug** in young, nonobese, severely hyperglycemic, or pregnant patients.
(3) Temporarily used during stress (surgery, infection, and injury).
(4) **Newly diagnosed patients or mild diabetes** who still has some endogenous insulin secreting capacity.
(5) **In practice, most insulin treated patients are obese, who have severe hyperglycemia and failed oral therapy due to high insulin deficient and resistant.**

Contraindications:

(1) Poorly compliant patient.
(2) Patients with high risk of hypoglycemia.
(3) Obese patients with insulin resistance. Patients need very high dose of insulin.

Goal of therapy:
To reduce the morning hyperglycemia.

Type of insulin:
Intermediate acting, preferably splitting doses, particularly before dinner or at bedtime to control morning glucose. **Remember, combination of insulin and oral drugs are not more effective than insulin alone, to lower the blood sugar levels.**

144. **Self-monitoring of blood glucose (SMBG) recommendation**:
(A) **Type I diabetes**:
(1) To monitor before each meal and at bedtime.
(2) Periodic monitoring 90 to 120 minutes after meals to check postprandial hyperglycemia.
(3) Occasional monitoring in the middle of the night (e.g., 3 A.M.) to avoid nocturnal hypoglycemia.

(B) **Type II diabetes on insulin**:
Daily SMBG, before breakfast, before dinner, and at bedtime.

(C) **Type II diabetes on oral agents**:
SMBG every 2 or 3 days, before breakfast or dinner.

(D) **Type II diabetes on diet:**
Patients should learn SMBG, monitor periodically to avoid metabolic decompensation and learn their glucose fluctuation with food.

145. **Glycohemoglobin (HbA_{1C}) and few important points**:
(a) It is the '**gold standard**' by which glycemic control is measured **except** in acute cases.
(b) It represents glycemic control during the **preceeding 6 to 12 weeks**.
(c) It is formed when glucose reacts nonenzymatically with hemoglobin A molecules particularly HbA_{1C}.
(d) **Falsely low HbA_{1C} levels are found:**
(i) Pregnancy.
(ii) Hemolytic anemia.
(iii) Sickle cell disease or trait.
(iv) Hemoglobin C or D disease.
(e) **Falsely high HbA1c levels are found:**
(i) Thalassemia.
(ii) Myeloproliferative disease.

(iii) Large dose of aspirin.

(f) It **cannot** help to determine the specific changes in therapy.

(g) The discrepancies between SMBG and HbA_{1C}, **the problem lies with SMBG** than HbA_{1C}.

146. **Therapeutic targets for nonpregnant diabetic patients**:
   (a) BP < 130/85 (normal < 140/90).
   (b) Premeal glucose (mg/dL) 80-120 (normal < 115).
   (c) Bedtime glucose (mg/dL) 100-140 (normal < 115).
   (d) HbA_{1C}(%) < 7 (normal < 6).
   (e) Fasting triglyceride (mg/dL) < 150 (normal < 150).
   (f) LDL-cholesterol (mg/dL) < 130 (normal < 130).
   (g) HDL-cholesterol (mg/dL) > 35 (normal > 35).

147. Indications of pancreas/islet transplantation:
   (a) Type I diabetes patients on immunosuppression for renal allografts.
   (b) Chronic pancreatitis patients who have undergone total pancreatectomy followed by intraportal injection of their own islets.

148. Formula to calculate osmolality:
   Osmolality (mOsm/L)=2[Na+K(mEq/L)]+{Plasma glucose (mg/dL)}/18.
   (i) Value > 320 mOsm/L = Hyperosmolality.
   (ii) Value > 350 mOsm/L = Severe hyperosmolality.

149. **Etiology, signs and symptons, diagnosis, complications of diabetic ketoacidosis (DKA):**
   (A) **Etiology:** It is more common in **type I diabetes.**
      (i) Diabetes with infection.
      (ii) Missed insulin injection.
      (iii) Inappropriate reduction in insulin dosage.
   (B) **Signs and symptoms of DKA:**
      Patients appear with severe dehydration (due to osmotic diuresis), hyperglycemia, abdominal pain (periumbilical and constant in nature), anorexia, nausea, and vomiting.
      Physical examination:
      Signs of dehydration and metabnolic acidosis which includes dry skin and mucous membrane, tachycardia, postural hypotension, depressed mental status, **Kussmaul respiration (deep and rapid breathing)**, decreased jugular venous pressure, and sweet-sickly smell of patient's breath (ketosis).
   (C) **Diagnosis of DKA:**

(i) Hyperglycemia (250 to > 1000 mg/dL).
(ii) Low pH (mild cases, 7.20 to 7.35; severe cases, 6.8 to 6.9).
(iii) Low serum $NaHCO_3$.
(iv) Increased anion gap [Na-(cl + HCO_3)].
(v) Presence of qualitative assesment ketone bodies in the serum (rapid diagnosis).
(vi) Quantitative elevation of beta-hydroxybutyrate and acetoacetate are **not** readily available.
(vii) Elevated serum Na, BUN (prerenal azotemia), amylase level.
(viii) Normal, elevate, or reduced serum k, phosphate, and magnesium level.

(D) **Complications**: Mortality is between 5-10 %. **Death is due to underlying serious illness in elderly, cerebral edema for children**.

150. **Etiology, signs and symptoms, diagnosis, complications of nonketotic hyperosmolar syndrome (NKHS)**:

(A) **Etiology**: It is more common in elderly with mild or undiagnosed type II diabetes.
(i) The patients cannot drink enough to cope with osmotic diuresis due to hyperglycemia.
(ii) Impaired renal function that decreases glucose loss in the kidney, results in hyperglycemia.
(iii) The patients may be receiving thiazide diuretics (diuretic effects and decrease insulin secretion), or unable to recognize the thirst or have access to fluids.

(B) **Signs and symptoms**:
The patients apperar with severe dehydration, hyperglycemia, may be altered level of consciousness (depends upon the duration and severity of hyperosmolarity), sometimes reversible neurologic abnormalities (grand mal or focal seizure, extensor planter response, hemisensory or motor deficit, aphasia, delirium, and enhancement of pre-existing organic mental syndrome).
Physical examination: Severe dehydration (dry mouth and mucous membrane), less frequent GI symptoms unlike DKA.

(C) **Diagnosis**:
(i) Hyperglycemia (> 600 mg/dL).
(ii) Elevated serum osmolarity (> 320 mOsm/L).
(iii) Elevated hemoglobin, BUN, LFT's, and triglyceride.
(iv) **Pseudohyponatremia is due to elevated triglyceride**, or Na may be normal or elevated due to severe dehydration.

(D) **Complications**: Mortality is between 10-20 %, it depends upon the age, elevated BUN and sodium levels. Other complications are thromboemoblic events, rhabdomyolysis, and aspiration. It rarely causes cerebral edema and acute renal failure unlike DKA.

151. **Management of DKA and nonketotic hyperosmolar syndrome (NKHS): The goal is to correct the metabolic disturbance and replace fluid and electrolytes.**

(i) **Initial stages of therapy is to restore vascular volume** (water deficit 5 to 12 liters) and correct hyponatremia (sodium deficit 5 to 10 mEq/kg). The deficit is more in NKHS than DKA. The water loss is more than sodium. **First give isotonic normal saline (0.9% Nacl solution)**. The fluid therapy varies, give **1 liter of normal saline in first 30 to 60 minutes followed by another liter for next 1 hour**. The saline or half-normal saline should be given at the rate of **0.5 liter per hour** which should be adjusted **over the next 6 hours and thereafter** according to the patients response, CVS status, and oliguria.

(ii) **All patients of DKA except elderly**: **Alternate normal saline and hypotonic solutions** (only hypotonic solution can cause cerebral edema due to intracellular shift of water, particularly in young patients).
All patients of NKHS and elderly DKA patients: Use **hypotonic solutions** because sodium requirement is less (normal saline can cause hypernatremia).

(iii) **The glucose should be added to the solution when blood glucose falls to 250 to 300 mg/dL** to avoid hypoglycemia and cerebral edema.

(iv) Insulin therapy (insulin resistance is present in both DKA and NKHS, but do not give large doses which can produce low k, phosphate, and delayed low glucose): IV bolus 0.1 U/kg regular insulin is followed by 0.1 U/kg/hour. **This is very important to remember that glucose should fall about 100 mg/dL/hour (rapid fall may cause cerebral edema**).

(v) **Potassium replacement therapy:** (Initial k deficit is about **5 mEq/kg but** serum k may be **normal, low, or high** especially with metabolic acidosis or renal failure. **Insulin causes low serum k by shifting k into the intracellular space. Fluid therapy causes low serum k by dilution and enhances k excretion through kidney by improving renal perfusion)**.

(a) **Low serum k:** Give k 30-40 mEq per hour.

(b) Normal serum k with adequate urine output: Give k 20 mEq/hour.

(c) Normal serum k with **inadequate urine output**: Do not give k.

(d) ECG should be done to know intracellular K level (peaked T wave means **high**, flat or inverted T wave means **low**). Remember, intracellular K deficit in renal tubular cells cause further loss of k by the kidney.

(vi) Sodium bicarbonate therapy for metabolic acidosis in DKA: It is **not** necessary to give $NaHCO_3$ amount (44 mEq every 1 to 2 hours) is given when there is severe acidosis (pH < 7.0 to 7.1) and it should be **stopped when pH is 7.1**.

(vii) Prophylactic use of phosphate in DKA is not very helpful. Hypocalcemic tetany may complicate phosphate therapy unless magnesium is given. In NKHS, severe phosphate loss is due to longer prodromal period: **Treatment**: Give k phosphate with magnesium.

(viii) Remember, high WBC count (leukocytosis) may be present in DKA and NKHS: Do not give prophylactic antibiotics.

(ix) The close monitoring is very important:
  (a) Strict I and O (intake and output).
  (b) Urine catheterization in unconscious or oliguric patients.
  (c) Gastric decompression in unconscious patients to avoid aspiration.
  (d) Monitor CVP (central venous pressure) in severe hypovolemia or renal insufficiency.
  (e) Laboratory measurement (every 1 to 2 hours) of pH, glucose, and electrolytes.

(x) To treat the underlying medical illness is extremely important.

152. **Signs and symptoms, diagnosis, and treatment of alcoholic ketoacidosis:** H/O large amount of alcohol consumption and abstain from food or drink for long period of time.

(A) **Signs and symptoms:** The patients are anorectic and have nausea, vomiting. **Physical examination**: Dehydration and malnutrition.

(B) **Diagnosis**: H/O alcohol use plus characteristic severe ketoacidosis (low pH, large ketone bodies in the blood). Hyperglycemia may or may not be present.

(C) Treatment:
  (i) Fluid and glucose administration intravenously.
  (ii) Rarely, need insulin for hyperglycemia except in diabetic patients.

153. **Most frequent complication of type I diabetes**: **Severe hypoglycemia**. Hypoglycemia also occurs with oral glucose-lowering drugs particularly long acting sulfonylureas or in elderly patients with impaired renal function.

154. **Normal protective response to hypoglycemia which is converted to normoglycemia**:

(i) Secretion of the counter regular hormones.

(ii) Dissipation of insulin.
(iii) Subjective awareness of hypoglycemia, results in ingestion of carbohydrates.

Rememeber, brain cannot synthesize or store more than a few minutes supply of glucose. Brain needs constant infusion of glucose.

155. **Difference between DKA and NKHS:**

DKA	NKHS
(i) Found in type I diabetes.	(i) Found in type II diabetes.
(ii) Presence of severe acidosis and ketosis.	(ii) Absence of severe acidosis and ketosis (except in some type II diabetic patients with low endogenous insulin).
(iii) Increased anion gap.	(iii)Normal anion gap.
(iv)GI symptoms are more frequent.	(iv)GI symptoms are less frequent.
(v) Acute renal failure is common.	(v)Acute renal failure is uncommon.
(vi) Cerebral edema is common.	(vi)Cerebral edema is uncommon.
(vii) Alternate use of normal saline and hypotonic solutions	(vii) Hypotonic solutions are commonly used

156. **Similarities between DKA and NKHS:**

DKA	NKHS
(i) Hyperglycemia.	(i) Same
(ii) Increased osmolarity.	(ii) Same
(iii) Dehydration.	(iii) Same
(iv) Low serum Na due to increased osmolarity.	(iv) Low serum Na due to increased triglyceride.
(v) Fluids, electrolytes, and insulin are the treatment of choice	(v) Same.

157. **Most common cause of blindness between the age 30 to 65:**

Diabetes type I, the blindness is due to retinopathy. First sign of diabetic retinopathy is **microaneurysms**. Most common contributing factors for blindness are **due to retinal detachments and hemorrhages**.

158. **Phases of diabetic retinopathy**:
(A) **The earliest nonproliferative phase has the following findings:** Microaneurysms, retinal blot hemorrhages, hard exudates, cotton wool spot or soft exudates (infarctions of the nerve fiber layer). **Visual acuity is usually normal.**
(B) **Proliferative phase:** Proliferation of new blood vessels and fibrous tissue from retinal vessels to vitreous, results in retinal detachments and hemorrhages which leads to severe visual loss or blindness.
(C) Some patients develop severe visual loss without proliferative changes: It is a **macular edema which** is due to deposits of hard exudates surrounding the macular area. It is more common in type II diabetes.

159. **Treatment of diabetic retinopathy**:
(i) Adequate control of hyperglycemia.
(ii) To control high BP adequately.
(iii) Surgery: Retinal photocoagulation is the treatment of choice in progressive retinopathy, with new vessels formation, and macular edema. Vitrectomy may be required for more advanced proliferative retinopathy.

160. **Opthalmologic follow-up of diabetic patients**:
(i) Type I diabetes: Within 5 years of the onset of disease.
(ii) Type II diabetes: From the onset of the disease. Retinopathy affects **up to 20% of patients in type II diabetes at the time of detection of the diabetes because it was undiagnosed. In type I diabetes, retinopathy is absent at the time of diagnosis of diabetes**. Up to 25% at 5 years, 70% at 10 years, and > 95% after 15 years develop retinopathy in type I diabetes.

161. **Most common cause of ESRD (end stage renal disease) in USA**: **Diabetes mellitus**. ESRD is more common in type I (up to 35%) than type II diabetes (up to 20%).

162. **Presentation of diabetic nephropathy: Four stages of presentation**:
(i) **Gross proteinuria (> 0.3 gram of albumin/day)** begins approximately **15 years after** the diagnosis of diabetes with **normal renal function**, with or without high BP.
(ii) Decreased GFR (about 3 years after), increased serum creatinine, **massive proteinuria** and **nephrotic syndrome (clinical nephropathy)**.

(iii) **Progressive decline** in GFR(40 to 50% decline) and **rise of serum creatinine**.

(iv) After that, **ESRD develops within 10 years**.

In type II diabetes, presentation varies such as moderate proteinuria may persist for long time without significant deterioration of renal function.

163. **How to monitor the progression of renal failure ?**: To plot the **reciprocal of serum creatinine** as a function of time.

164. **Renal diseases associated with diabetes**:
   (a) **Asymptomatic bacteriuria and pyelonephritis** are common. It is due to glycosuria, autonomic bladder dysfunction, and decreased perfusion.
   (b) Papillary necrosis.
   (c) Renal artery stenosis.
   (d) Other associated complications are due to decreased renal function:
      (i) Hyperkalemia in patients receiving ACE inhibitors.
      (ii) Hyporeninemic hypoaldosteronism, particularly in elderly patients.

165. **The marker of essential hypertension in some type I diabetes with nephropathy**:
   Increased erythrocyte sodium-lithium countertransport.

166. **Treatment of (diabetic) nephropathy**:
   (a) **Early stage** (no microalbuminuria):
      (i) Optimize glycemic control.
      (ii) Treat hypertension, if present.
      (iii) Routine screening for UTI and bladder dysfunction.
   (b) **Stage with microalbuminuria**:
      (i) Strict glycemic control.
      (ii) Ace inhibitors: It reduces the proteinuria that are independent of BP lowering effects.
   (c) **Stage with clinical nephropathy**:
      (i) **Most important to control the hypertension and intraglomerular pressure**: Use ACE inhibitors with or without **calcium channel blocker**.
      (ii) **Aggressive glycemic control has little value in this stage (please remember this point)**.
      (iii) Dietary protein restriction (0.8 gram/kg body weight/day) has **limited benefit** once GFR becomes abnormal.
   (d) **Stage with ESRD**: The treatment is the same as nondiabetic patients but instituted early:

(i) Renal transplantation is the treatment of choice in younger patient. It is better than dialysis.
(ii) Dialysis (CAPD or hemodialysis) is used for older type II patients.

167. **Most common cause of morbidity and mortality after renal transplantation in diabetic patients: Cardiovascular disease.**

168. **The different types of diabetic neuropathy:**
(A) **Distal sensorimotor neuropathy is the most common type. It is due to axonal loss.** Patients appear with **symmetric numbness, tingling in the extremities particulary lower extremities**, worsen **at night** and as the time progresses. The signs may be complicated by **ulceration and cellulitis.**
Physical examination: Distal symmetrical loss of sensation, variable loss of reflexes (e.g., ankle), and **muscle wasting of the intrinsic muscles of the hands and feet**.
The clinical picture is not distinguishable from other causes of distal neuropathy such as alcohol, uremia, heavy metals, and amyloidosis.
(B) **Acute sensory neuropathy**: It is a less common, self-limiting variety, characterized by **severe pain (worsening at night) and hyperesthesia**.
(C) **Proximal motor neuropathy or femoral neuropathy or diabetic amyotrophy**: It is more common in **male, elderly, type II diabetic patients,** characterized by weakness and wasting of the **major proximal muscle groups of the pelvis, may be with sensory deficit along the femoral nerve**.
(D) Mononeuropathies: It is characterized by the asymmetric involvement of the cranial nerves (oculomotor, trochlear, and abducens nerves) and peripheral (median, radial, and lateral popliteal nerves). Etiology is unknown or vascular compromise. Nerve entrapment may cause peripheral lesions.
(E) **Autonomic neuropathy:** It has a **poor prognosis** and is due to **disturbed regulation of the local blood flow**.
(i) **CVS**: Orthostatic hypotension (most disabling effect), myocardial ischemia or infarction, prolonged QT interval.
(ii) **GI**: Constipation (most common), diarrhea (most distressing), fecal incontinence (loss of sphincter control), and bloating.
(iii) **Bladder dysfunction**: It is due to **neuropathy** results in infrequent urination, dribbling, overflow incontinence, incomplete emptying and residual urine (> 150 ml may result in UTI).
(iv) Heat stroke and hyperthermia.

(v) Impaired sexual function such as male impotence, retrograde ejaculation.

Please remember that symmetric neuropathies are similar in type I and II, but focal neuropathies are common in type II older patients.

169. **Treatment of diabetic neuropathy**:

(i) **Most important is the pain control:** Analgesics, TCA (may be effective), IV lidocaine or analogue oral mexiletine (severe pain), rarely opiates are used.

(ii) Orthostatic hypotension: Stocking supports, 9 alpha-fluorohydrocortisone, pindolol, and clonidine.

(iii) Gastroparesis: Metoclopramide, cisapride, or erythromycin are used to stimulate gastric emptying.

(iv) **Diarrhea**: Avoid high fiber diet; use broad spectrum antibiotics, clonidine, diphenoxylate or Imodium.

(v) Bladder emptying: It is stimulated by **bethanechol**.

(vi) Male impotence: Vacuum erection aids, intracorporeal papaverine or phentolamine injection, and penile prosthetic implants.

170. **Presentation, prevention, and treatment of diabetic foot**:

(A) **Presentation**: It is characterized by **planter ulcers that heals slowly, loss of normal** sensation of the foot, results in **gangrene** in severe cases. It is due to neuropathy and vascular insufficiency.

(B) **Prevention**:

(i) Education.

(ii) Inspect feet daily (use mirror for planter surface).

(iii) Never walk barefooted.

(iv) Do **not** applyl hot water or heating pads to feet.

(v) Wear properly fitting soft shoes.

(vi) Break in new shoes slowly.

(vii) Use second pair of shoes at night.

(viii) Keep feet clean, dry between toes.

(ix) Lubricate dry skin using a nongreasy lotion or cream to avoid cracking.

(x) Cut toe nails.

(xi) Visit foot care specialist routinely.

(xii) Do **not** smoke.

(C) **Treatment for ulcers**:

Antibiotics, dead tissue debridement, appropriate dressing, cast immobilization (to distribute body weight away from an ulcerated areas), and amputation, if necessary.

171. **The medications are used to control hypertension in diabetic patients**: The following medications are indicated if BP is not lowered below 130/85 mm Hg.
   (i) **ACE inhibitors**: It is especially used if patients have associated renal disease.
   (ii) Alternative medications are calcium channel blockers, alpha-adrenergic blockers, and vasodilators.
   (iii) **Avoid** thiazide diuretics and beta-blockers: They can complicate lipid and glycemic control.
   (iv) Use diuretics if there is volume component of high BP.

172. The major cause of death in diabetes are due to the following: Atherosclerosis involves the arteries of the **heart, lower extremities, and brain.**

173. **The syndrome X (Reaven hypothesis), effects of insulin resistance results in hyperinsulinemia**:
   (i) Glucose intolerance.
   (ii) Increased VLDL and lowered HDL.
   (iii) Increased high BP.
   Hyperinsulinemia directly or indirectly (all three effects mentioned above) causes **increased coronary artery disease**. This observation suggests **evenly distributed and smaller doses of insulin are biologically more effective** than unevenly distributed large doses.

174. **The comprehensive management plan of diabetes**:
   (A) **Improve sense of well-being**:
      (i) Glycemic control.
      (ii) Regular exercise.
   (B) **Reduce macrovascular risk**:
      (i) Lipid control (reduce LDL-cholesterol levels < 130 mg/dL, or < 100 mg/dL in patients with vascular disease).
      (ii) Glycemic control.
      (iii) Weight control.
      (iv) BP control.
      (v) Avoid smoking (active and passive).
      (vi) Appropriate exercise.
   (C) Minimize microvascular/neuropathic complications:
      (i) Glycemic control.
      (ii) BP control.
      (iii) Urine test for albuminuria.
      (iv) Foot care.

(v) **Regular eye examination by an opthalmologist.**

175. **Signs and symptoms of hypoglycemia**:
   (A) First adrenergic symptoms are due to secretion of adrenal hormones and epinephrine: **Sweating, palpitations**, weakness, anxiety, tremor, and hunger.
   (B) **Second neuroglycopenic symptoms of CNS (glucose < 45 mg/dL in serum)**: Headache, dizziness, altered mental status, visual and motor disturbances, unconsciousness, and convulsion.

176. **Most serious form of reactive hypoglycemia (Important): Alimentary hypoglycemia.** The patients had H/O gastrectomy, gastrojejunostomy, pyloroplastomy, or vagotomy. They appear with symptoms of **hypoglycemia 30 to 120 minutes after a meal**, may result in **seizure or coma.**
   Pathogenesis:
   (i) Rapid absorption of glucose results in brisk and inappropriate elevation of insulin.
   (ii) Gut-derived **incretins** stimulates insulin secretion.

177. **Idiopathic reactive hypoglycemia has two syndromes**:
   (A) Idiopathic postprandial syndrome or pseudohypoglycemia: **It is more common,** characterized by either adrenergic symptoms or mild neuroglycopenia **2 to 5 hours after meals** while serum glucose levels are normal.
   (B) True idiopathic reactive hypoglycemia: It is rare, characterized by adrenergic symptoms of hypoglycemia after meals but do **not** cause neuroglycopenic symptoms.
   Mechanism: Unknown.
   Treatment: Ingestion of carbohydrate relieves the symptoms.

178. **Hypoglycemia**:

Reactive	Fasting
(i) Hypoglycemia after meals	(i) Hypoglycemia after fasting
(ii) More common	(ii) Less common
(iii) Less serious	(iii) More serious
(iv) Hypoglycemia never occurs after fasting	(iv) Hypoglycemia may occur within 6 hours after meals
(v) Does not need thorough search for a specific etiology	(v) Needs thorough search for a specific etiology

179. **Fasting hypoglycemia**:
   (A) Rates of glucose production and utilization during fasting:
      (a) Glucose production: 2 mg/kg/minute.
      (b) Glucose utilization: 12 mg/kg/minute.
   (B) Pathogenesis:
      (a) **Decreased rate of glucose production by the liver is due to:**
         (i) Decreased gluconeogenesis due to hormonal defects.
         (ii) Defect in enzymes causing gluconeogenesis.
         (iii) Liver disease.
         (iv) Decreased gluconeogenic substrate.
         (v) Drugs.
      (b) A combination of decreased production and increased utilization of glucose.
         Increase utilization is due to:
         (i) Insulin (endogenous or exogenous).
         (ii) Insulin-like factors.
         (iii) Certain metabolically active tumors.
         (iv) Unavailability of fat for energy production.

180. **Drug induced hypoglycemia:**
   (a) **Insulin and sulfonylureas are the most common cause** of hypoglycemia in patients receiving those drugs.
   (b) Other drugs are propranolol, pentamidine, quinine, and alcohol ingestion.

181. **Signs and symptoms and diagnosis of insulinoma:**
   (A) **Signs and symptoms**: The patients appear with diplopia, palpitation, confusion or bizarre behavior. The symptoms may occur **five or more hours after a meal or after an overnight fast**. Some patients may **have refractory seizure disorder without other symptoms (Important)**.
   (B) **Biochemical diagnosis: Whipple's traid, it consists of**:
      (i) The symptoms of hypoglycemia which is relieved by the elevation of blood glucose levels.
      (ii) Inappropriately elevated plasma insulin and C-peptide levels.
      (iii) Absence of sulfonylurea in the plasma.
      How to make diagnosis when a patient has H/O hypoglycemia but neither symptoms nor blood glucose levels suggest hypoglycemia: Next step is to supervise fasting and to **document hypoglycemia and hyperinsulinemia at the same time** (**Remember**, high insulin levels have **no values** when serum glucose levels are normal or elevated).

(i) Gold standard is to evaluate as an **inpatient fast for 72 hours or when symptoms begin** (most of the patients develop symptoms when glucose level is <46 mg/dL).
(ii) Extended overnight fasts may be useful initial test as an outpatient.

(C) **Localization of the insulinoma**:
(i) CT scan is the best procedure of choice.
(ii) Preoperative and intraoperative sonogram.

182. **Treatment of insulinoma:**
(i) Removal of the tumor mass in the pancreas.
(ii) If the tumors cannot be identified even during surgery, **then distal pancreatectomy may be successful** because tumors are evenly distributed in the pancreas.
(iii) Malignant insulinoma (it metastasizes to regional lymph nodes and liver but **rarely** cause distant metastases): If tumors cannot be identified or the patients refuse surgery:
(a) **Diazoxide** (inhibits insulin release) **is the best treatment of choice.**
(b) Phenytoin, propranolol, and verapamil are useful in some patients.
(c) Somatostain, octreotide may be helpful in some patients.
(d) Chemotherapeutic drugs (streptozotocin plus flurouracil or chlorzotocin) may have some benefits.

183. Important points in differential diagnosis of hypoglycemia:
(a) Sulfonylurea causes hypoglycemia: **Sulfonylurea must be present in the blood**. It is **absent** in exogenous insulin and insulinoma causing hypoglycemia. **Sulfonylurea drugs have similar findings like insulinoma**: Low glucose, inappropriately high insulin, elevated c-peptide and proinsulin, absence of insulin antibodies.
(b) **Exogenous insulin**: It has the almost same features of insulinoma **except low or normal c-peptide and proinsulin**, may have insulin antibodies. **Absence of sulfonylurea in the blood**.
(c) **Insulinomas:** Already discussed. Absence of sulfonylurea and insulin antibodies; elevated c-peptide, proinsulin, and insulin; low plasma glucose.

184. **Most common extrapancreatic tumors causing hypoglycemia**: **Sarcomas and fibromas of mesenchymal or epithelial origin**. Renal, adrenal, and GI cancers, and hepatomas may cause hypoglycemia.
The mesenchymal tumors are found in retroperitoneal areas or thorax.
Laboratory findings: Low glucose and characteristic low insulin levels. Some patients may have high levels IGF-II mRNA (insulin-like growth

factor). IGF-II cause hypoglycemia through receptors of IGF-I and insulin, and also reduces GH levels.

185. **Most common islet cell tumor: Insulinoma**; second most common is **gastrinoma associated with Zollinger-Ellison syndrome**. This syndrome produces recurrent gastric ulcers **due to hypersecretion of gastric acids**.

186. **Most common islet cell tumors in MEN I**: **Gastrinomas and insulinomas**. The pancreatic tumors in MEN I are **mostly multiple and malignant**.

187. **A patient with islet cell tumors with hypercalcemia due to hyperparathyroidism, most likely diagnosis: MEN I.**

188. **Verner-Morrison syndrome**: Watery diarrhea, hypokalemia, achlorhydria (WDHA), and pancreatic cholera.

189. **Clinical features, diagnosis, and treatment of VIPoma**:
   - (A) **Clinical features:** The patients appear with **watery diarrhea** (**> 3L/day in 80% of patients**), **volume depletion, hypokalemic metabolic acidosis** (loss of k and HCO_3 in the stool) results in severe weakness, flaccid paralysis, and hypokalemic nephropathy. **Diabetes or glucose intolerance** is due to glucagon-like effect of VIP or hypokalemia causing inhibition of insulin secretion. **Hypercalcemia** (50% of cases) **is due to parathyroid hormone related peptide** (**not** due to parathyroid adenomas). (**Low k, pH, HCO_3, fluid volume; gastric hypochlorhydria or achlorhydria; elevated glucose and calcium**).
   - (B) **Diagnosis:**
     - (i) Elevated levels of VIP in the plasma.
     - (ii) To localize the tumor: CT scan or intraoperative ultrasonography.
   - (C) **Treatment:**
     - (i) Surgical removal of the primary tumor is the treatment of choice.
     - (ii) If the tumor cannot be localized, then **blind distal pancreatectomy should be done.**
     - (iii) The patients with metastases: Surgical removal of the primary tumor or local effects is controversial.
     - (iv) Medical treatment includes the following:
       - (a) Fluids and electrolytes.
       - (b) Octreotide: It reduces the tumor output of VIP and reduces intestinal chloride secretion in response to VIP.
       - (c) Glucocorticoids: It reduces diarrhea without affecting levels of VIP.
       - (d) Transient response to diarrhea with clonidine and indomethacin.

(e) Chemotherapy in inoperable tumors: Combinations of streptozotocin and fluorouracil or streptoxotocin and doxorubicin can lower VIP levels and the symptoms.
(f) Hepatic embolization can be used to reduce VIP production by hepatic metastases.

190. **Clinical features, diagnosis, treatment, and follow-up of glucagonoma**: The glucagon is produced by the A cells located in the periphery of the islets.

(A) **Clinical features:** The patients appear with characteristic **necrolytic, erythematous** rash (>80% of cases) **over the face, extremities, and intertriginous areas**. The rash is initially erythematous, scaly followed by bullous then crusty, and heals as hyperpigmented, indurated lesions or superimposed infections. The patients may have thin hair, **dystrophic nails, stomatitis, glossitis, and angular stomatitis**. The rash is due to increased glucagon, associated deficiency of amino acids or may be zinc. The patients may appear with mild **asymptomatic diabetes mellitus** (abnormal glucose tolerance test without ketosis), weight loss, anemia, thromboembolism, and psychological depression.

(B) **Diagnosis**:
(a) Severely elevated glucagon levels are > 1000 pg/ml (normal 50 to 150 pg/ml).
(b) To localize the tumor and metastases: CT scan should be done.

A patient appears with rash, thomboembolic disease, and new-onset diabetes: Rule out glucagonoma.

(C) **Treatment:**
(i) Surgical removal of the tumor mass is important.
(ii) Octreotide: It reduces the glucagon levels and symptoms particularly rash.
(iii) Zinc supplementation and amino acid infusions may reduce the rash.
(iv) Arterial embolization to reduce hormonal production.
(v) Chemotherapy: Combinations of streptozotocin, fluorouracil, doxorubicin, and dacarbazine also reduces hormone production and causes partial remission.

(D) **Follow-up**:
(i) Tumors may increase despite all these therapies for a period of 2 to 10 years.
(ii) Enhance gastrin hormone production.

191. **Clinical features, diagnosis, and treatment of somatostatinoma**: The somatostatins are produced by D cells of the islet.

(A) **Clinical features:** The patients appear with **mild diabetes mellitus, diarrhea, steatorrhea, cholelithiasis, jaundice, weight loss, anemia, and hypochlorhydria**. The somatostatin inhibits insulin release, gallbladder motility, pancreatic enzyme, and bicarbonate secretions.
(B) **Diagnosis**: It is difficult because it is **rare**, symptoms are **nonspecific** and **mild**. Hepatic metastases are found (66% of cases) at the time of diagnosis. Elevated levels of somatostatin **except in duodenal somatostatinomas which may be associated with neurofibromatosis**.
(C) **Treatment:** Same as other islet cell tumor **except** octreotide which is **not** effective.

192. **Islet cell tumors producing other hormones**:
(i) ACTH secretion: It causes Cushing's syndrome.
(ii) GH secretion: It causes acromegaly.
(iii) Parathyroid hormone related peptide: It causes hypercalcemia.
(iv) Pancreatic polypeptide (PP) hormone: Most of the patients are asymptomatic.

193. **The testis-determining gene (SRY) is located on the**: Short arm of human Y chromosome.

194. **Male differentiation of the genital tract**:
(i) **Testosterone**: It is produced by the Leydig cells, maintain the Wolffian ducts (**male ducts**) results in **formation of male internal genital organs**. It is converted intracellularly by 5 alpha-reductase to **dehydrosterone which forms the external genital** organ. **Please remember this**:
Testosterone: It forms male **internal** genital organs.
Dehydrotestosterone: It forms male **external** genital organs.
Male anatomic development: Completed by 90 days.
Penile development: Only between 20 weeks and term.
(ii) **AMH (anti-Mullerian hormone)**: It is produced by sertoli cells and **inhibits the formation of Mullerian ducts (female ducts)**. It started to regress at 8 weeks and the process is completed around 10 to 12 weeks. AMH is located on chromosome 19 but acts through receptor located on chromosome 12.

195. **Female differentiation of the genital tract**: It is formed by the **degeneration of the Wolffian ducts** (male ducts) around 10 weeks and proliferation of the mullerian ducts (female ducts) to form fallopian tubes, uterus, and upper vagina.

196. **Turner syndrome and GH**: The treatment of Turner syndrome with GH has improved the final height. The patients have short stature, normal genitalia, dysgenetic ovaries, primary amenorrhea, infertility, web neck, but normal mental development.

197. **The karyotype of mixed gonadal dysgenesis**: 46, XY or mosaic 45, X/46, XY. It is characterized by testis on one side and a fibrous streak on the other with ambiguous genitalia. It is better to raise as female and to remove the testis and gonadal streaks because of high incidence of malignancy.

198. **The most common karyotype of true hermaphroditism**: **46, XX (68% of cases)**, others are 46, XY and mosaic. It is rare, characterized by the **presence of ambiguous genitalia** (rarely completely masculine or feminine), **ovotestis** with normal ovarian tissues and dysgenetic testicular tubules, uterus (90% of cases). The patients may have **breast development, ovulation, and menstruation**. Normal childbirth is possible when testicular tissues are removed by surgery.

199. **Pure gonadal dysgenesis (testicular regression syndrome)**: It is characterized by **normal female phenotype** (**normal uterus and fallopian tubes but streak** gonads), attains **normal height** (unlike Turner syndrome), has **46, XX** or 46, XY karyotype. Some testicular tissues were functional up to 10 weeks then regressed, so it is called fetal testicular regression syndrome.

200. **Femal pseudohermaphroditism:** It is characterized by ambiguous external genitalia, two normal ovaries, 46, XX karyotype. It is the **most frequent type of intersex**. The patient also has normal uterus, tubes, and upper vagina. The reconstruction of the lower vagina and proper medical treatment leads to normal childbirth.

201. **Congenital adrenal hyperplasias**:
   (a) Classic type or 21-hydroxylase deficiency: The patients appear with ambiguous genitalia at birth with or without salt-loss, gene located on the short arm of **chromosome 6.**
   Prenatal diagnosis: Molecular genetic (DNA) approach of CVS or amniotic fluid cells, measurement of 17-OHP or AD in amniotic fluid. (AD is androstenedione, 17-OHP is 17-hydroxyprogesterone).
   Prenatal treatment: Oral dexamethasone is given to the mother before 9th week of gestation to term for affected female but is discontinued for male or unaffected female.

Postnatal diagnosis: Elevated 17-OHP (17-hydroxyprogesterone) levels in the serum or ACTH stimulation test.

Postnatal treatment: Life long hormonal therapy:

(i) Infancy and childhood: Hydrocortisone.

(ii) Adolescence and adulthood: Dexamethasone or prednisone (glucocorticoids), plus 9-alpha-fluorohydrocortisone (mineralocorticoid) and added salt to the diet for salt-wasting group of patients.

(iii) Surgical genital repair for ambiguous genitalia.

(b) 11-beta-hydroxylase deficiency: Hypertension with or without hypokalemic alkalosis, gene located in the long arm of chromosome 8.

Prenatal diagnosis and treatment: Same as in 21-hydroxylase deficiency.

Postnatal diagnosis: Elevated serum 11-deoxycortisol (compound S) and deoxycorticosterone.

Postnatal treatment:

(i) Glucocorticoids.

(ii) Surgical genital repair for ambiguous genitalia.

202. A 20 year old patient appears with normal breast development, amenorrhea, absent or scanty pubic and axillary hairs.

Physical examination: Vagina ends blindly, with or without palpable gonads in the labia majora.

Laboratory tests:

(i) Elevated testosterone, LH, and estrogen levels in the serum.

(ii) Abdominal sonogram: Absence of uterus, tubes, and ovaries but presence of testes.

(iii) Chromosome: 46, XY.

Most likely diagnosis: **Male pseudohermaphroditism due to androgen insensitivity (abnormalities of testosterone receptors).**

203. **Reifenstein syndrome or partial androgen insensitivity**: The patients have male phenotype with gynecomastia and infertility at puberty and chromosome is 46, XY.

204. **Male pseudohermaphroditism is due to 5 alpha-reductase deficiency: This enzyme converts testosterone to dehydrotestosterone (DHT).**

(A) **Signs and symptoms**: **Severe penoscrotal hypospadius**, may be blind vaginal pouch, female habitus, no breast development and internal genital male organs (testosterone maintains the Wolffian ducts such as normal vasa deferentia, seminal vesicles, and epididymides). DHT- mediated virulization of the urogenital sinus and external genitalia is **impaired** and prostate is small or absent. **At puberty testosterone causes masculinization, growth of the phallus, rugation, and hyperpigmentation of the scrotum**. Chromosomal study shows 46, XY.

(B) **Diagnosis**: Elevated or normal plasma testosterone and decreased DHT levels.

(C) **Treatment**:

(i) Repair of the genitalia in infancy.

(ii) In adults: **High dose of testosterone esters**.

205. Maximum number of germ cells (6 to 7 millions) are present in ovaries: **Around 4 to 5 months of intrauterine life**. It started to form around 6 to 7 weeks of intrauterine life, peak around 4 to 5 months then rapidly reduced until birth, then progressively reduced until the age of 50 and above.

206. **First sign of puberty in girls**: **Breast budding (median age of onset 9.8 years). Menstruation begins after 2 years from the** onset of breast budding.

(i) Breast development: It is due to ovarian **estrogen.**

(ii) Axillary hairs: It is due to ovarian **androgen.**

(iii) Pubic hairs: It is due to ovarian **androgen and estrogen.**

207. **Precocious puberty**: Pubertal changes before the age of 8 years.

(i) Isosexual: Development is the characteristic of the **same sex**.

(ii) Heterosexual: Development is the characteristic of the **opposite sex**.

208. **Delayed puberty**:

(i) Absence of any secondary sex character by the **age of 13 years**.

(ii) Absence of menarche by **the age of 16**, or **5 or more years have passed since the breast budding**.

209. **Most common cause of primary amenorrhea:**
Imperforate hymen.
Treatment: Surgical resection. Most common cause of secondary amenorrhea is pregnancy.

210. **The single most common chromosomal disorder in human**: **Turner syndrome (45, X)**. More than 95% of such fetuses are aborted.

211. **Most common chromosomal anomaly in all aborted fetus**: Turner syndrome.

212. **Most common trisomy in all aborted trisomy fetuses**: Trisomy 16 (100% mortality).

213. A less than 30 year old intellectual woman appears with H/O abrupt cessation of menstruation along with psychosexual problems or socioenvironmental trauma. The patient does **not** have any anatomical abnormalities of the hypothalamic-pituitary-ovarian axis and **no** other endocrine abnormalities.
Laboratory test: Low to normal levels of gonadotropins and relatively low estrogens.
Most likely diagnosis: Hypothalamic chronic anovulation (HCA).
Treatment:
(i) Psychological counseling.
(ii) Change in life style particularly those engaged in strenuous exercise programs.
(iii) Clomiphene citrate can induce ovulation and can be used in woman who wants to become pregnant.
(iv) Human menopausal gonadotropin and human chorionic gonadotropin (hMG-hCG) or GnRH may be effective in women unresponsive to clomiphene.
(v) Exogenous steroids may be used to avoid osteoporosis. (Amenorrhea may occur with discontinuation of steroids).
(vi) A combination of oral conjugated estrogens, ethinyl estradiol or micronized estradiol or transdermal estradiol daily, with oral medroxyprogesterone acetate added for the first 12 to 14 days of each month.
(vii) Oral contraceptive agents can be used as an alternative in sexually active women.
(viii) Contraception is advised for sexually active women with HCA, because the functional defect is mild and may resolve any time.
(ix) Ingestion of calcium is needed.

214. **Most common cause of heterosexual pubertal development**:
Polycystic ovary (PCO) syndrome. PCO causes anovulation due to inappropriate feedback signals to the hypothalamic-pituitary unit. PCO begins at or near puberty with hirsutism, irregular menstruation, normal breast development, typical female habitus with masculinization. (**In contrast**, patients with congenital adrenal hyperplasia show very little if any female development at puberty).
Laboratory findings of PCO: Mild elevation of basal LH and moderate elevation of all androgens.

Treatment of PCO: It is a benign disorder, no ideal therapy is available, therapy should be directed to hirsutism, induction of ovulation if pregnancy is desired, and prevention of estrogen-induced endometrial hyperplasia and cancer.

(i) Anovulatory, non hirsute women, not desiring pregnancy: Intermittent progestin (medroxy progesterone acetate for 10 to 14 days each month) or oral contraceptives to reduce the risk of endometrial cancer. Remember, intermittent progestin does not inhibit ovulation, so contraception is needed.

(ii) Anovulatory, hirsute women, not desiring pregnancy: Oral contraceptive agents are the first drug of choice.

(iii) Patients desiring pregnancy: Clomiphene citrate is the first drug of choice to induce ovulation. Other drugs to induce ovulation are hMG-hCG, purified FSH, pulsatile GnRH.

(iv) **Surgical therapy is indicated** when medical therapy fails, ovarian tumor or fertility is **not** an issue. Surgical therapy includes wedge resection by laparotomy or laser/cautery destruction of follicles by laparoscopy.

215. Most common cause of **hirsutism** in women: **Increased androgen production without any serious underlying problem**. The patients appear with hair growth **over the lower abdomen, on the breast, and over the upper lip**. Presence of hair over the upper back, upper chest, and upper abdomen indicates **severe hyperandrogenism**. Presence of only facial hair or unusual pattern of hirsutism is due to **local variation in skin 5 alpha-reductase activity.**

Diagnosis of hirsutism:

(i) Patients with normal menstruation and no signs of Cushing's syndrome: Hormonal evaluation is **not** needed (Important).

(ii) Patients with **irregular** menstruation: Measure serum testosterone, 17-OHP, prolactin, LH, and FSH.

(a) Testosterone levels <170 ng/dL: No androgen secreting tumors.

(b) Testosterone levels >170 ng/dL: Rule out PCO (polycystic ovarian syndrome) and 21-hydroxylase deficiency.

(c) Serum 17-hydroxyprogesterone levels measured between 7 and 9 A.M. during the first week of menstruation:

-Value <200 ng/dL **excludes** 21-hydroxylase deficiency.

-Mildly elevated values (<1000 ng/dL) are found in **both homozygous and heterozygous 21-hydroxylase deficiency.** (Remember, heterzygous disorder is **not** associated with hirsutism) and PCO.

-To differentiate between these two conditions: Measure 17-hydroxyprogesterone levels 30 to 60 minutes after the ACTH, **levels are**

>1500 ng/dL in homozygous 21-hydroxylase deficiency and **not** in PCO.

(d) Elevated prolactin levels in prolactinoma.
(e) Elevated LH in PCO.
(f) Remember, measurement of DHEAS (dehydroepiandrosterone sulfate) is **not** helpful.

Treatment of hirsutism: It is a cosmetic **problem** but may have serious psychosocial **effects**. The risk and the bebefits should be considered in each cases.

(i) Mechanical hair removal: **Electrolysis** is safe in mild to moderate hirsutism, **bleaching and mechanical hair removal** are safe in mild cases.
(ii) Drug treatment (no drug is approved by FDA for hirsutism).
  (a) **Antiandrogens (spironolactone, cyproterone acetate, flutamide)** block the androgen receptors and the **drug of choice for hirsutism.**
  Side effect of the drugs:
  -Flutamide and cyproterone: They cause drug induced hepatitis.
  -Spironolactone: It causes increased frequency of menses which is controlled by using oral contraceptives together. It is **contraindicated** in renal insufficiency.
  (b) Finasteride (5 alpha-reductase inhibitors): It blocks the formation of DHT (dehydrotestosterone). **It is used in benign prostatic hyperplasia**. It is **contraindicated** during pregnancy because it causes **ambiguous genitalia in a male offspring.**
  (c) Oral contraceptives: It is **not** effective alone. It is used with spironolactone or hirsutism in PCO.

216. **Most common organism in mastitis**:
S.aureus. Mastitis is a complication of lactation, usually after the first pregnancy.
Treatment:
(i) Continuation of the breast feeding.
(ii) Antistaphylococcal antibiotics.
If the patients do **not** respond to the above management: Rule out breast abscess.
Treatment:
(i) Incision and drainage under general anesthesia
(ii) Appropriate antibiotics.

217. A 40 year old woman appears in the private clinic with H/O breast pain and lump particularly before menstruation.

Physical examination: Irregular thickening particularly in the upper outer quadrant.
Most likely diagnosis: **Fibrocystic changes of the breast**. It is an exaggerated physiological response to a changing hormonal environment.

218. **Drugs causing hirsutism (androgen-independent)**:
(i) Minoxidil.
(ii) Cyclosporine.
(iii) Diazoxide.
(iv) Glucocorticoids.
(v) Phenytoin.
Treatment: Avoid the drugs.

219. **Nipple discharge**:
(A) **Postmenopausal women**: Always rule out carcinoma of the breast.
(B) **Serous or bloody discharge**: Most common cause is **benign intraductal papilloma**, but carcinoma occurs 10 to 15% cases. This type of discharge must be investigated.
(C) **Galactorrhea**: It is a spontaneous milky discharge. Prolactin levels may be elevated (>20 ng/ml is abnormal).
(i) Physiological causes of elevated prolactin: Breast stimulation, exercise, eating, sleep, coitus, stress, and pregnancy.
(ii) Prolactinomas, or prolactin secreting pituitary adenoma (microadenoma < 1 cm, and macroadenoma > 1 cm): MRI or CT scan is the best diagnostic imaging study.

220. **Evaluation of patients with breast mass or lump**:
(A) The careful examination of the breast in sitting or standing position plus examination of the axilla and supraclavicular area. After that breasts should be examined in supine position. (Approximately 80% of American women discover their own lesions, while taking a shower). It is difficult to discover lesion in very large breast by routine examination in obese person, **so mammography is indicated**.
Remember, **once a lesion is discovered** the diagnosis has to be made except in the teenager for whom **elective excisional biopsy of fibroadenoma is recommended.**
(B) The following different ways the diagnosis can be made:
(i) **Cyst aspiration**: If the fluid is clear or cloudy, no residual mass is left after aspiration, then **reassurance** and **routine follow-up after 1 month** and monthly self examination of the breast is recommended.

If the fluid is bloody, residual mass is left after aspiration, or residual mass in first follow-up examination, then **open biopsy is mandatory** which is also done for any solid mass **except** in teenager.
Remember, cytologic examination of cyst fluid or nipple discharge is not helpful. Microscopic examination of the unilateral bloody or serosanguinous discharge may be helpful.

(ii) Fine-needle aspiration (FNA): It is better to **perform mammogram before the FNA**. FNA is helpful for **dominant mass**. **It is reliable only if positive**.

(iii) **Mammography**: It is **very useful screening test** in the asymptomatic patients or to confirm the physical examination finding. False-negative results may be up to 10 to 25%.
Remember, presence of dominant mass but negative mammography in a patient, appropriate referral and an open biopsy is indicated (Important for the Board examination).

(iv) **Breast biopsy**: It should be done in **an operating room by the trained medical team**, under local anesthesia.

221. **Management of benign breast conditions**:

(i) **Reassurance** is indicated for patients with mild symptom or mild fibrocystic changes.

(ii) Sometimes, a well-fitting brassiere, mild analgesic, and salt restriction are helpful.

(iii) The patients with greater discomfort: Most important is reasonable and rational explanation. The topical use of progestational agents, tamoxifen, primrose oil, various vitamins, and bromocriptine may be helpful.

(iv) When conservative measures fail, then use **danazol** in symptomatic patients.

(v) Galactorrhea with pituitary microadenoma: Use bromocriptine for indefinite period of time.

(vi) Galactorrhea with pituitary macroadenoma: Use bromocriptine followed by surgery.

(vii) Excessive galactorrhea without pituitary adenoma and normal serum prolactin levels: Bromocriptine may be helpful. Asymptomatic patients do **not** need any treatment. The patients **do need** further **endocrine work up** and **refer to reproductive endocrinologist for fertility, if desired**.

222. **Incidence of breast cancer in a daughter or sister of breast cancer patients:**

Two-to three fold greater risk than in women without an affected first-degree relative.

The relative risk is 1.4 = One first-degree relative is affected.
The relative risk is 4 to 6 = Two first-degree relatives are affected.

223. **Genes and their relation with breast and ovarian cancer:**
   (i) Mutation of BRCA 1 gene on chromosome 17: Female breast and ovarian cancers.
   (ii) Mutation of BRCA 2 gene on chromosome 13: Female and male breast cancers but **not** ovarian cancer.

   Mutation in either BRCA 1 or BRCA 2 is found in 1% of all women, the risk of breast cancer exceeds 50% before age 50 and 80% by age 65.

224. **Risk factors of breast cancer, besides family history and genetic mutation**:
   (A) **Increased risk of breast cancer**:
      (i) Diet:: Fatty food.
      (ii) Moderate amount of alcohol consumption.
      (iii) Therapeutic radiation of mastitis or repeated chest fluroscopy for TB.
      (iv) Postmenopausal estrogen replacement.
      (v) Early menarche, late menopause, and late or no pregnancy.
      (vi) Long term use of contraceptive pills.
      (vii) Male with klinefelter's syndrome.
      (viii) Breast biopsy shows atypical hyperplasia.
   (B) **Decreased risk of breast cancer**:
      (i) Early menopause, late menarche, and early or more numerous pregnancies.
   (C) **No increased risk of subsequent breast cancer**:
      (i) Breast biopsy shows benign disease.

225. **Clinical presentation and diagnosis of breast cancer**:
   (A) **Clinical presentation**: The patients appear with painless lump with or without bloody discharge (bloody discharges are found in intraductal papillomas).

   Physical examination: Hard, irregular mass, skin dimpling, or niple retraction with or without involvement of the axillary, supraclavicular, or infraclavicular lymph node.
   (B) **Diagnosis**:
      (i) Mammogram should be done first.
      (ii) Fine-needle aspiration cytology is done as an outpatient. Remember, a negative mammogram or needle aspiration does **not** always rule out cancer. If there is a concern, then do:
      (iii) Excisional biopsy under local anesthesia as an outpatient.

The first step is to do item number (ii) or (iii). **The second step** is to discuss the treatment options if the cancer is diagnosed.

226. **Screening methods of breast cancer**: **Three ways** to detect the breast cancer early which improves the chances of successful treatment.
   - (A) **Self-examination**: It is simple, no cost, free of risk, can detect early cancer, but it does **not** reduce the mortality.
   - (B) **Examination by a physician**: **The American Cancer Society recommends that every women over the age of 40 have a routine breast examination annualy**.
   - (C) **Breast imaging techniques**:
     - (i) Sonography can distinguish cystic from solid lesions.
     - (ii) Guidelines for mammography in asymptomatic women:
       - (a) Mammography every 1 to 2 years for women aged 50 or older.
       - (b) Mammography annually for women at any age with a personal history of breast cancer.
       - (c) **Mammography annually for women aged 40 and over who have family history of breast cancer or increased risk.**

227. **Sites of metastasis of breast cancer**: Lymph nodes, skin, lung, pleura, liver, brain, pericardium, eye, bone, ovary, and adrenal. **Breast cancer is the most common source of metastases to the eye in women.**

228. **Most common type of breast cancer**: **Infiltrating ductal cancer** derived from mammary epithelium.

229. **Methods of spread of breast cancer**:
   - (i) Directly to the blood stream.
   - (ii) Through draining lymphatics.

230. **The complications of metastatic breast cancer**:
   - (A) Hypercalcemia is due to bone metastases. **Treatment of hypercalcemia**:
     - (i) Saline and furosemide: Enhances calcium excretion.
     - (ii) Pamidronate and gallium nitrate: Inhibit bone resorption.
   - (B) Leptomeningeal metastases:
     Diagnosis: The demonstration of breast cancer cells in CSF.
     Treatment: Intrathecal or intraventricular chemotherapy.
   - (C) Epidural metastases:
     Diagnosis: MRI.
     Treatment: Radiation therapy.

231. **Most common cause of male infertility**: **Hypogonadism** (90% of cases) results in impaired spermatogenesis (abnormal sperm count or semen quality) and up to 90% of these men have **isolated deficiency of sperm production with normal androgen production** (i.e., idiopathic oligospermia or azoospermia).

232. A 55 year old adult male underwent routine physical examination which revealed bilateral breast masses **up to 3 cm in diameter**:
Most likely diagnosis: **Normal physiologic gynecomastia**. It is found in 40% of healthy adult men, increasing in prevalence with advancing age.

233. **Drug – induced gynecomastia**:
(A) Exogenous estrogen:
(i) Diethylstillbestrol is used in metastatic prostate cancer.
(ii) Accidental ingestion, use, contact, or occupational exposure.
(B) Drugs altering androgen production or action:
(i) Spironolactone.
(ii) Ketoconazole.
(iii) Cimetidine.
(iv) Cytotoxic drugs.
(C) Drugs interacting with estrogen receptors:
(i) Digitalis.
(ii) Marijuana.
(D) CNS active drugs:
(i) Sedatives.
(ii) Amphetamines.
(iii) Antidepressants.
(iv) Tranquilizers.
(v) Antihypertensive drugs.

234. **Systemic disorders causing gynecomastia**:
(i) Hepatic cirrhosis.
(ii) Thyrotoxicosis.
(iii) Renal failure.

235. **Tumors causing gynecomastia**:
(A) Estrogen-secreting tumors:
(i) Adrenal carcinoma.
(ii) Leydig cell or Sertoli cell tumor of testis.
(B) Gonadotropin-secreting tumor:
(i) Lung cancer.

(ii) Testicular cancer.
(iii) Liver cancer.

236. A 18 year old male appears for routine physical examination which revealed bilateral firm testicular sizes < 2 cm in length (normal testicular size is 3.5 cm and above) and bilateral gynecomastia.
Most likely diagnosis: **Klinefelter's syndrome (47, XXY)**.
Other clinical features are: **Azoospermia** (>95% of cases), **majority of them have normal intelligence.**
Laboratory findings: Low serum testosterone, elevated estradiol, FSH, and SHBG (sex-hormone binding globulin).
Treatment:
(i) Testosterone replacement therapy.
(ii) Mammoplasty for gynecomastia.
(iii) No treatment for infertility which is irreversible.

237. **Disease associated with klinefelter's syndrome**:
(i) Chronic obstructive pulmonary disease.
(ii) Malignancy (breast cancer, lymphoma, germ cell cancer).
(iii) Autoimmune disease (SLE, Hashimoto's throiditis).

238. **Testicular atrophy in adolescents or adults**: **Mumps**. It can be prevented by giving vaccine. Mumps, other infectious agents, thermal trauma, radiation, cytotoxic drugs, and environmental toxins often-cause **severe germ cell damage results in decreased spermatogenesis but normal** Leydig cell function results in normal androgen function.
(i) Irradiation only 15 rad: Temporary suppression of spermatogenesis.
(ii) Irradiation > 600 rad: It causes permanent infertility.
(iii) Irradiation > 800 rad and cytotoxic agents: Androgen deficiency.
(iv) **Sulfasalazine**: It causes oligospermia, reduced sperm motility, and infertility.
(v) MOPP therapy (chemotherapy) for Hodgkin disease: Permanent infertility is due to severe seminiferous tubular damage. (MOPP therapy includes nitrogen mustard, vincristine or Oncovin, procarbazine, and prednisone).

239. **Treatment of hypogonadism**:
(A) Androgen therapy:
(i) **In adults, testosterone enanthate or cypionate is the drug of choice**. It stimulates libido, increase potency, increase male hair growth, enhances energy level, and increases hemoglobin concentration.

(ii) **Recently, a transdermal patch containing testosterone applied to the scrotum** in hypogonadal men.

(B) Gonadotropin and LHRH therapy:

(i) **Use of hCG** (have LH-like biologic activity) **and hMG** (have both FSH and LH activities). Both of them are more expensive than testosterone. Testosterone stimulates and maintains androgenization in patients with hypogonadotropic hypogonadism when fertility is **not** required. For fertility or spermatogenesis, **both hCG and hMG** may be required to use as long as 2 to 3 years. Initial treatment should begin with hCG, if the sperm counts are not adequate then add hMG along with hCG therapy.

(ii) Therapy of Kallmann's syndrome (hypogonadotropic hypogonadism, micropenis, anosmia or hyposmia, aspermia, color blindness, nerve deafness, short fourth metacarpals, and craniofacial asymmetry): **Pulsatile administration of LHRH stimulates** endogenous gonadotropin secretion and spermatogenesis to induce fertility.

240. **Contraindication of androgen therapy in men**:

(i) Prostatic cancer.

(ii) Male breast cancer.

Both are androgen-sensitive cancer.

241. **Few important points of testicular tumors:**

(i) Most common testicular tumors arise from **germ cells (seminomas and nonseminomas) (95% of cases) and most of them are malignant**. The peak age of testicular cancer is 20 to 35.

(ii) The remaining 5% are **non-germ cells tumors** (derived from Leydig or Sertoli cells) and most of them are **benign (90% of cases)**, remaining 10% are malignant which metastasize by lymphatics.

(iii) **The risk of cancer is high** in an undescended testis and also in contralateral descended testis.

(iv) Seminomas are **sensitive to the radiation therapy unlike nonseminomas**.

(v) Seminomas usually **metastasize via regional lymph nodes** to retroperitoneal, mediastinal, and supraclavicular lymph nodes but **nonseminomas metastasize by both lymphatic and hematogenous routes** (particularly to liver and lungs).

(vi) Most patients with germ cell tumors appear with **painless testicular mass** but bleeding into the tumor causes pain. It is diagnosed by ultrasonography or MRI. The patients with non-germ cell tumors appear with gynecomastia, isosexual, or heterosexual precocious pseudopuberty.

(vii) A testicular mass in a **patient over 50 indicates lymphoma** than germ cell tumor.

(viii) **The treatment of advanced seminomas**: **Orchiectomy and radiation** to the periaortic and iliac lymph nodes or **combination chemotherapy** results in cure up to 80 to 95% of cases.

The treatment of advanced nonseminomas: Orchiectomy plus chemotherapy (add cisplatin to multiple-drug chemotherapeutic regimen) plus removal of retroperitoneal lymph nodes (advanced cases) results in response rate of > 90% and long term remission in 50 to 90% of patients.

The treatment of non-germ cell tumors: **Orchiectomy**.

242. **The function of zinc in prostate**: Zinc may protect the prostate against infection. Zinc concentration in prostate is highest than any other tissues of the body.

243. **The most important marker of prostate cancer**: **PSA (prostate-specific antigen)**. Other marker is **acid phosphatase**. Both are secreted by the prostate. PSA is useful in **screening, staging, and monitoring response to treatment. An elevated serum prostatic acid phosphatase is diagnostic for metastatic prostate cancer**.

244. **Most common cause of prostatitis**: **Unknown (95% of cases)**, only 5% cases are due to bacterial infection. **Most common bacterial infection is due to Escherichia coli**. Most common source of bacterial prostatic infection is previous baceterial urethral infection. It is due to **direct ascent of** bacteria from the urethra to prostate.

245. **Diagnosis of bacterial prostatitis**:

(i) The best diagnostic method is to perform **quantitative simultaneous bacterial cultures of** urethral urine, bladder urine, and EPS (expressed prostatic secretion). **Four different specimens are collected and cultured separately**:

(a) VB1 (the first voided 10 ml of urethral urine).
(b) VB2 (the midstream urine of bladder).
(c) EPS.
(d) VB3 (the first voided 10 ml immediately after prostatic massage).

The diagnosis of bacterial prostatitis is confirmed **when EPS and VB3 bacterial counts significantly exceeds** those of VB1 and VB2 by at least one logarithm.

(ii) **Initial diagnostic method** to examine the EPS under high-powered field (hPF) and should compare with the spun sediment of first 10 ml of urethral urine are midstream bladder urine. **The presence of > 20 WBC/hPF and oval fat bodies (lipid laden macrophages)** indicate prostatitis.

246. **Clinical presentation, diagnosis, and treatment, and follow-up of acute bacterial prostatitis**:

(A) **Clinical presentation**: The patients between age 20 to 40 appear with **fever, chill, pain in the suprapubic, lumbar and perineal regions**, and urinary irritative and obstructive symptoms.
Physical examination: Suprapubic tenderness is due to urinary retention, rectal examination shows hot, enlarged, and tender prostate (presence of fluctuant prostate indicates abscess). **Please remember, vigorous rectal examination of the prostate results in septicemia or secondary epididymitis, so it should be examined very gently and carefully.**

(B) **Diagnosis**:
(i) Urinalysis and urine culture show increased WBC and bacterial counts respectively.
(ii) Pelvic ultrasonography or CT scan to diagnose prostate abscess.
(iii) IVP or abdominal sonogram is helpful in recurrent bacterial prostatitis to rule in upper urinary tract abnormalities.

(C) **Treatment**:
Initially the patients should be admitted to the hospital for the following therapy:
(i) Intravenous gentamicin (gram negative coverage) plus ampicillin (to cover enterococci) **should be started initially.**
(ii) IV antiboitics are followed by oral **trimethoprim, trimethoprim-sulfamethoxazole, and quinolone derivatives which are the drug of choice. It should be continued for 4 to 6 weeks**.
(iii) For urinary retention: Urinary catheter or temporary suprapubic cystostomy is useful.

(D) **Follow-up**: To examine the EPS and VB3, 6 to 12 weeks after the onset of therapy to confirm that the infection has resolved.

247. **Granulomatous acute bacterial prostatitis**: It is due to previous bacterial infection, prior transurethral resection, or TB (tuberculosis).
Signs and symptoms: Irritative and obstructive urinary symptoms. The palpable induration mimics prostatic cancer.
Diagnosis: The biopsy can confirm the granulomatous lesion and can differentiate from the cancer.
Treatment:
(i) The symptoms may resolve spontaneously.
(ii) Use of antibiotic is controversial.

248. **Clinical presentation, diagnosis, and treatment of chronic bacterial prostatitis**:

(A) **Clinical presentation**: The symptoms are **similar but milder** than acute bacterial prostatitis. The patients appear with **urinary frequency, dysuria, vague lower abdominal, lumbar, and perineal pain** but fever and urethral discharge are **uncommon.**

(B) **Diagnosis**:

(i) **Initial EPS study**: More than 10 WBC/hPH and > 1 or 2 lipid-laden macrophages/hPF are abnormal.
Please remember that 5 to 10% of men without prostatic symptoms have > 10 WBC/hPF and have normal EPS with prostatitis while receiving antibiotic therapy.

(ii) **In first office visit**, quantitative culture of VB2 (bladder urine) and nonquantitative culture of EPS: Presence of **Gram-negative organism in either of this culture** indicates the **possibility** of chronic bacterial prostatitis. The next step should be in item number (iii).

(iii) **In second office visit**, conventional bacterial localization cultures should be done **to confirm the chronic bacterial prostatitis.**

(C) **Treatment**:
It is very difficult to treat. Antibiotic alone can cure only 30 to 50% of cases, but **suppressive antibiotic therapy results in complete symptomatic relief** and **reduces the risk of serious illness.**

(i) **Initial antibiotic therapy:** Trimethoprim-sulfamethoxazole, ciprofloxacin (or norfloxacin), or carbenicillin is the **drug of choice**. It is given for 4 to 12 weeks.

(ii) **Suppressive antibiotic therapy**: Trimethoprim, trimethoprim-sulfamethoxazole, or nitrofurantoin is effective.

(iii) **Experimental therapy**: Direct injection of thiamphenicol or aminoglycosides into the prostate is helpful in patients who are unresponsive to antibiotic therapy.

249. **Chronic abacterial prostatitis and prostatodynia:**

(A) **Signs and symptoms**: It is similar to chronic bacterial prostatitis.

(B) **Diagnosis**:

(i) Chronic abacterial prostatitis: EPS are **abnormal** but all cultures are normal (rarely positive).

(ii) **Prostatodynia**: EPS and all cultures are normal.

(C) **Treatment**:

(i) **Majority of them are treated only with stress management** because of psychological basis. **It is the therapy of choice.**

(ii) **Only some patients** in both the conditions may respond to antibiotics.

250. **Clinical presentation, diagnosis, and treatment of benign prostatic hyperplasia (BPH)**:

(A) **Clinical presentation**: It is either obstructive or irritative.

(i) **Obstructive symptoms** (due to narrowing of bladder neck and prostatic urethra): **Hesitancy** to initiate voiding, straining to void, **decreased force and caliber** of the urinary stream, and **incomplete urinary bladder emptying.**

(ii) Irritative symptoms (due to reduced bladder compliance, incomplete bladder emptying, or UTI secondary to obstruction): Urinary frequency, nocturia, dysuria, urgency, amd urge incontinence. **Please remember irritative symptoms could be due to UTI, bladder cancer, and neurogenic bladder**.

Physical examination: Enlarged (no more than 2 to 3 times of normal), rubbery/fleshy prostate by DRE (digital rectal examination). DRE gives a rough estimate of prostatic size but it is not reliable to rule out prostatic obstruction.

(B) **Diagnosis of BPH**:

(i) Transrectal ultrasonography to know the degree of enlargement of the prostate.

(ii) Abdominal ultrasonography to detect the hydronephrosis (or obstructive uropathy), prostatic size, and postvoid residual urine volumes are helpful.

(iii) Most important physiologic test to document urinary obstruction is **to measure the urinary flow rate. Please remember, decreased flow rate only is not an indication for prostatectomy**.

(iv) Cystourethroscopy is **misleading** in prostatic obstruction.

(v) Retrograde urethrogram may be helpful in patients with BPH and urethral stricture.

(C) **Treatment of BPH**:

(i) **Partial prostatectomy is the treatment of choice. Transurethral resection of prostate (TURP)** is safe and effective. Transabdominal approach when adenoma is large (>70 grams).

Indications of prostatectomy:

(a) Troublesome voiding symptoms.
(b) Recurrent UTI.
(c) Obstructive uropathy due to enlarged prostate.
(d) Gross hematuria due to enlarged prostate.
(e) Urge incontinence.
(f) Urinary retention.

Risk factors of prostatectomy:

(a) More than 80 years.
(b) Prostatic size > 45 grams.
(c) Preoperative urinary retention.
(d) Surgical time > 90 minutes.

(ii) Transurethral laser ablation and transurethral hyperthermia are new treatments of BPH.

Advantages of these procedures: Less morbidity than TURP.

Disadvantages of these procedures: Prostatic tissues are not obtained to rule in cancer and may be less effective than TURP.

(iii) **Alternative therapy of BPH**:

(a) Transurethral incision of the bladder neck: It is done as an outpatient, under local anesthesia, less blood loss, but **less** effective for larger prostate.
(b) Alpha-adrenergic blockers (terazosin, doxazosin): Both **decreases** smooth muscle tone of prostatic capsule and bladder neck, effective in 70% of cases.
(c) 5 Alpha-reductase inhibitors (it inhibits the conversion of testosterone to DHT which is a most active prostatic androgen): It is effective in 30% of cases, decrease prostatic size by 30% after 3 to 6 months of therapy, but prostate **quickly regrows to its original size after cessation of therapy**.

(iv) For patients who are **poor surgical candidates** and unresponsive to medical therapies:

(a) Clean, intermittent catheterization.
(b) Long term use of indwelling catheter.
(c) Intraurethral placement of metal alloy prostatic stent.

251. **Most common cancer in men in the USA: Prostatic cancer**. It is the second most common cause of cancer death in men.

252. **Risk of prostate cancer in men with a first-degree relative with prostate cancer:**

Two fold increase. It is transmitted as an **autosomal dominant** like breast and nonpolyposis colon cancers.

Etiology of prostate cancer: **Unknown,** environmental factors are important, positive family history. **Remember, BPH do not cause prostate cancer**.

253. **Absence of prostate cancer:**

(i) Men castrated before puberty.
(ii) Men with estrogen therapy.

254. **Most common type of prostate cancer**: **Adenocarcinomas (95% of cases)**, other types are squamous cell cancer, transitional cell cancer, and sarcomas.

255. **Most common sites of metastases of prostate cancer**: **Pelvic lymph nodes, pelvic bones, and lumbar spine**. In some patients the disease progress very rapidly and in others it progress very slowly.

256. **Clinical presentation, diagnosis, and treatment of prostate cancer**:

(A) **Clinical presentation**: Initially the patients are asymptomatic, followed by urinary obstruction (due to urethral invasion), uremia (due to ureteral obstruction), skeletal pain and pathologic fractures (due to metastases). **Physical examination:** DRE appears harder, indurated prostate with obscured boundaries, urinary retention, signs of uremia, lymphadenopathy, and CHF.

(B) **Diagnosis of prostate cancer:**

(i) The best screening method is a **combination of DRE and serum PSA determination.**

(a) If the DRE is **normal**, the chances of having prostate cancer are about **2%, 15%, and 35% for a serum PSA of <4, 4 to 10, or >10 ng/ml respectively**.

(b) If the DRE is abnormal, the chances of having prostate cancer are about **10%, 35%, and 67% for a serum PSA of < 4, 4 to 10, or >10, respectively**.

(c) Transrectal ultrasonography (TRUS) is **not** accurate for initial screening study, only 30% of the abnormal lesions detected on TRUS are malignant.

(d) The patients with **abnormal DRE and/or PSA**, the TRUS is much more accurate than digitally guided blind biopsy.

(ii) **Whitmore staging of prostatic cancer**:

(a) T1 = Microscopic disease in a clinically benign gland.

(b) T2 a-b = Nodule involves less than one posterior lobe.

(c) T2 c = Nodule involves one entire lobe or both posterior lobes.

(d) T3 = Extension beyond the peripheral capsule of the prostate.

(e) T4 = Invaded adjacent structures (bladder neck, pelvic walls, levator muscles, and external sphincter).

(iii) **Staging evaluation:** It is done by DRF, TRUS, and MRI of the prostate.

(a) Serum prostatic acid phosphatase: Elevated levels are 70% sensitive and 100% specific for metastatic disease.

(b) **Serum PSA levels**: It replaces the prostatic acid phosphatase in prostate cancer. The higher the level of PSA, the greater the likelihood of advanced disease. **PSA is also important to evaluate the response to therapy** such as, after radical prostatectomy measurable level of PSA indicates **residual or recurrent disease results in treatment failure**.

(c) **The radionuclide bone scan is the best method to detect bony metastases**.

(d) **To detect the staging of pelvic lymph nodes, best procedure is to perform pelvic lymphadenectomy** either before radical surgery or at the time of surgery with frozen-section biopsy (CT scan or lymphangiography is **not** reliable).

(C) **Treatment of prostate cancer:**

(i) **Watchful waiting**: It is the best treatment of choice for men with a life expectancy of < 10 years who have moderate or well-differentiated tumors. It is **not** appropriate for younger patients.

(ii) **Surgery:** Radical prostatectomy (removal of entire prostate plus both seminal vesicles) is the best treatment of choice.

Complication of radical prostatectomy:

(a) Urinary incontinence.

(b) Sexual dysfunction.

(iii) **Radiation:** It is indicated in the following condition:

(a) Localized disease in a patients who either refuses radical surgery or is not a candidate for surgery.

(b) Stage T3 disease: It is **not** cured surgically. Radiation therapy is done either by external beam or implantation of radioactive seeds inside the prostate.

(iv) **Hormonal therapy**:

(a) **LHRH** (luteinizing hormone releasing hormone) **agonists** (that inhibits testosterone) **alone** or the **addition of antiandrogen** are the best **hormonal therapy for advanced prostatic cancer**. The timing of hormonal therapy has **little effect** on the course of the disease, so it is preferably delayed until the patients become symptomatic.

(b) DES (diethylstilbestrol) is **not** used for complications of gynecomastia and CVS disease.

Relapse after LHRH/antiandrogen therapy indicates continued growth of hormone-insensitive cells.

(v) **Chemotherapy**: It is **not** effective in prostate cancer.

257. **Multiple endocrine neoplasia type 1 (MEN-1) (3P stands for parathyroid, pancreas, and anterior pituitary involvement): It is an autosomal dominant disorder.**

(A) **Parathyroid disorder**: **Hyperparathyroidism** is the most common abnormality. The patients age between 20 to 40 appear with **hypercalcemia** or **remain asymptomatic** or develop Zollinger-Ellison syndrome (peptic ulcer with gastrin producing tumors).
Treatment: Parathyroidectomy (removal of either three glands or four glands with a portion of one gland should be implanted in the forearm for future accessibility).

(B) **Pancreatic islet disease**: The pancreas is involved with microadenomas, macroadenomas, and hyperplastic lesions.

(a) The Zollinger-Ellison syndrome (peptic ulcer disease associated with gastrin producing tumors) is the most common disease.

Diagnosis: CT scan or intraoperative ultrasonography can diagnose macroadenomas.

Treatment:

(i) **Medical**: H_2-receptor antagonists and H+, K+ ATPase inhibitors can control the secretion of stomach acid.

(ii) **Metastatic lesion**: It is a slow growing tumor, metastases to the liver. Chemotherapy is only partially effective.

(iii) **Surgery**: It has limited use because of very high recurrence rate after surgery.

(a) **Insulinomas:** It is the second most common disease, tumors are small, multiple, and less malignant than the gastrinomas.

Diagnosis: The dominant insulin production can be diagnosed by selective portal venous sampling.

Treatment: Removal of the tumor or subtotal pancreatectomy.

(C) **Pituitary disease:** The patients may appear with symptoms of hypersecretion syndrome, sellar mass, or hypopituitarism. **Prolactinomas are the most common tumors**. The patients may appear with **acromegaly** either due to pituitary tumor or growth hormone-releasing hormone by pancreatic islet tumors. **The adrenocortical hyperfunction** due to pituitary adenomas or from production of ACTH or corticotropin-releasing hormone by a foregut carcinoid.

258. **Multiple endocrine neoplasia types 2a and 2b**:

(A) **MEN type 2a:** Autosomal dominant, chromosome 10, the patients appear with medullary cancer of the thyroid (MCT), pheochromocytoma, and less commonly, hyperparathyroidism. Most common cause of death is MCT which can be prevented by complete thyroidectomy. Point mutation in the

RET proto-oncogene, **so, carrier can be detected by direct** genetic testing (**RET lesion) which has replaced calcitonin testing.**

(B) **MEN type 2b**: Chromosome 10, the patients appear with MCT, pheochromocytoma, and rarely hyperparathyroidism. **Presence of mucosal neuromas of the tongue, lips, eyelids, and GI tract, and a marfanoid features which are absent in type 2a**. The patients have point mutation that changes methionine-918 to a threonine. The carrier can be detected by the same method as described in type 2a.

259. **McCune-Albright syndrome:** It is a triad of polyostotic fibrous dysplasia, Café-au-lait spots, and endocrinopathy (usually precocious puberty which is more common in girls and is gonadotropin-independent). The point mutation is at **arginine-201 in the Gs alpha subunit**.

260. **Autoimmune polyglandular syndromes: (Type 1 is found in children, type 2 is found in adults):**

(A) **Most frequent clinical manifestation of type 2**: **Insulin-dependent diabetes mellitus** and **thyroid disease** (autoimmune hypothyroidism or Grave's disease). **Addison's disease is the next common disorder. Pernicious anemia, alopecia, vitiligo, celiac disease, myasthenia gravis**, and less commonly hypophysitis and primary hopogonadism are found.

(B) **Treatment of type 2:**

(i) Treatment of each condition should be done.

(ii) Thyroid hormone therapy can precipitate symptoms of adrenal insufficiency.

(C) **Inheritance of type 2**: HLA association.

(D) **Organ specific antibodies in type 2:** They appear before the clinical manifestation and predict subsequent disease.

261. **Carcinoid syndrome:** It is a slow growing malignant neoplasm of **enterochromaffin cells**. These tumors typically contain **5-hydroxytryptamine (serotonin), and tachykinins (substance P). The metastatic tumors** associated with carcinoid syndrome usually arise **primarily from tumors of the ileum**. Carcinoid tumors **usually metastases to the liver, bones,** lungs, pancreas, ovaries, adrenal, and spleen.

(A) **Clinical manifestations**:

(i) **Cutaneous flushing is the most common clinical features**. The erythematous flush involves the head and neck. It may be associated with tachycardia but the **BP is low or normal.** Telangiectasias are found over the face (malar areas) and neck.

(ii) **GI symptoms:** Explosive diarrhea and abdomial cramps are common symptoms.
(iii) **Cardiac symptoms**: Endocardial thickening, tricuspid incompetence, and PS (pulmonic stenosis).
(iv) **Pulmonary symptoms**: Bronchoconstriction is found during flushing attack.
(v) **Other symptoms:** Intestinal obstruction, GI bleed, hepatomegaly (due to metastases), and necrosis of the hepatic tumors.

(B) **Mechanism of the flush:**
(i) **Tachykinins** (particularly neuropeptide K) cause carcinoid flush. It is a vasodilator.
(ii) Flushing may be stimulated by **catecholamines** during exercise and emotional stimuli.
(iii) Flushing may be stimulated by **pentagastrin** during eating.
(iv) Flushing may be stimulated by **histamine** in gastric carcinoids that secrete histamine.
(v) **Please remember that serotonin does not cause flushing**.

(C) **Diagnosis of carcinoid syndrome**: Overproduction of 5-hydroxyindoles plus increased excretion of urinary 5-HIAA (hydroxyindoleacetic acid) (> **25 mg of 5-HIAA is diagnostic**; normal is < 9 mg, between 9 to 25 may be found in acute intestinal obstruction, nontropical sprue, or carcinoid syndrome). Remember, bananas and walnuts cause elevated 5-HIAA in urine because they contain serotonin.

(D) **Treatment of carcinoid syndrome**:
(i) Octreotide (somatostatin anologue): It improves the flushing and endocrine manifestation. It also reduces excretion of 5-HIAA in urine and tachykinin levels in the blood.
Side effect of octreotide: Hypoglycemia is due to inhibition of glucagon and GH secretion.
(ii) H_1 and H_2 histamine receptor blockers are helpful in histamine-secreting gastric carcinoids.
(iii) **Complete surgical cure** is possible in a few patients with early diagnosis of carcinoid syndrome due to tumors in ovary, testis, or bronchus.
(iv) Surgical debulking of tumor in the liver is helpful in some patients.
(v) Embolization of hepatic artery can reduce inoperable hepatic metastases.
(vi) Chemotherapy is only helpful when given intra-arterially along with embolization of hepatic artery.
(vii) If patients are not responsive to above measure, then **interferon-alpha may be used as an adjunctive therapy**.

(E) **Causes of death in carcinoid syndrome**:

(i) Cardiac failure.

(ii) Hepatic failure.

DERMATOLOGY

1. **Atopic Dermatitis:** Scaly, dry, lichenified lesions over the antecubital and popliteal fossa, face, neck, and upper extremities; face with diffuse erythema, perioral pallor, and redundant creases below the eyelids.
   Etiology: Unknown but elevated IgE reagenic antibodies.
   Treatment: Topical steroids (best therapy), emollients (best therapy for dryness), systemic antihistamines. Oral antibiotics cover staphylococcal infection, if present.
   Associated Lesions: Anterior subcapsular cataract and keratoconjunctivitis.

2. **Stasis dermatitis:** It is due to peripheral venous insufficiency. The patients appear with inflammatory, edematous, red, hyperpigmented petechial scaling or weeping reaction around the medial malleolus and distal third of the lower leg.
   Treatment: Supportive hose (to prevent venous stasis edema), topical steroids (to treat eczema), wet compresses (for oozing and crusting), weight loss (for obese), antibiotics (for superimposed infection).

3. A patient appears with recurrent coin-shaped patches mostly on the external surface of the arms and legs.
   Physical Examination: Vesicles and papular patches plus scaling and thickening, rarely central clearing (like fungus infection).
   Most likely diagonsis: Nummular eczematous dermatitis.
   Treatment:
   (i) The combination of topical steroids, 3% crude coal tar and ultraviolet light to control the eczema.
   (ii) Avoid wool, soap, and frequent bathing. There are irritants.

4. A **nervous patient appears with H/O constant scratching and lesions** over the neck, lower legs, and groin.
   Physical Examination: Chronic, pruritic, lichenified eczematous eruption over the nape of the neck, lower legs, and groin areas.
   Most likely diagnosis: Lichen simplex chronicus.
   Treatment: Steroid injection into the lesion is more helpful than topical steroids, oral antihistamines, and to stop rubbing and scratching.

5. **Seborrheic dermatitis**: **It is more common in patients with neurologic disorders (e.g. Parkinson's disease or stroke)**. The patients appear with **erythematous, eczematous patches with yellow, greasy scales** especially in the middle of the face, nasolabial folds, and eyebrows.

Treatment: Antiseborrheic shampoos (containing tar, sulfur, selenium sulfide, zinc pyrithion, or salicylic acid) **are the best treatment**, in addition to that some patients need **topical steroid lotion or gel in hairy areas** and **hydrocortisone cream to apply in face**.

6. **Hand eczema:** It is common in housewives, cooks, food handlers, and medical personnal. It is due to irritants (soap and water), atopy, and frequent hand washing. It involves the **dorsum of the hands unlike** dyshidrotic eczema (pompholyx) which involves the **palm and sole**.
   Treatment: Topical steroids, emolients, and avoid soap, detergents, and water.

7. **Exfoliative dermatitis (erythroderma)**: The patients appear with **total body erythema, edema, scaling, and fissuring** due to increased blood flow through the skin and vasodilatation.
   Etiology: Idiopathic, cutaneous (psoriasis, atopic or contact dermatitis, seborrheic dermatitis, pityriasis rubra pilaris), systemic (mycosis fungoides, leukemias, lymphomas), or drugs (antibiotics, antiepileptic drugs, barbiturates, gold).
   Treatment: Oral steroids (in severe cases), topical steroids with plastic sauna suit (in less severe cases).

8. **Fungal infection of the skin:** It is due to dermatophytes (Trichophyton, Microsporum, Epidermophyton), candida, and tinea versicolor.
   (a) Dermatophytosis: Annular inflammed patches with elevated scaling and central clearing. It is found in diabetic and immunosuppressed patients.
   (b) **Candidiasis:** It appears in the groin, perineum, gluteal folds, digital webs, axillae, and inframammary areas. It is found in diabetic, obese patients using antibiotics.
   (c) **Tinea versicolor:** It appears as scaling, red to brown or white oval patches over the neck, trunk and upper arms. It appears hypopigmented in summer months.

9. **Diagnosis of all fungal infection:** KOH preparation and fungal culture.
   Treatment:
   (i) Localized dermatophytic or candidal glabrous skin infection – Use **econazole, miconazole, clotrimazole, and ciclopirox creams, ointments, or lotions.**
   (ii) Tinea versicolor: It can respond to the above mentioned drugs but **selenium sulfide antidandruff shampoo (locally) is effective**.
   (iii) Severe widespread fungal infection or patients resistant to local antifungal drugs – **Griseofulvin is the drug of choice** (not effective in Candida),

micronized form (Ultra fine) is very effective.

(iv) Candida infection – **Ketoconazole** (orally) is useful. It is hepatotoxic, so LFT's should be done. It is effective against dermatophyte but should **not** be used initially.

10. **Rubella (German measles):** It is preceeded by prodrome of **fever and constitutional** symptoms. The patients appear with **erythematous, maculopapular rashes begin on the face then spread to the trunk and extremities, finally fading with desquamation on third day**.

11. **Verruca vulgaris and molluscum contagiosum**: Both viruses cause **unique papular lesions confined to the skin**. Wart papilloma virus form different forms of warts. Molluscum contagiosum (DNA poxvirus) form papules with central umbilication.

    Treatment:

    (i) **For warts:** Liquid nitrogen cryotherapy, combination of salicyclic and lactic acids, podophyllin and cantharidin.

    (ii) **For molluscum contagiosum lesions:** Curettage of the central core, liquid nitrogen freezing, or cantharidin application.

12. **A postoperative surgical patient appears** with sudden onset of fever, rashes (erythematous, macular, diffuse eruption that blanches with pressure followed by desquamation), vomiting, hypotension, renal insufficiency, and strawberry tongue.

    Most likely diagnosis: Toxic shock syndrome due to Staphylococcus aureus.

    Treatment: Antistaphylococcal antibiotics.

13. Most common forms of drug reaction:

    Hives and morbilliform rashes: The erythematous macules and papules often confluent which can begin **within a week from the onset of the therapy**.

    Diagnosis: It is made by history of itching, rashes, and fever (rarely). It can be differentiated from viral exanthem by the absence of viral prodromal symptoms and less mucous membrane rashes.

    Drugs causing rashes: Trimethoprim-sulfamethoxazole, penicillin, ampicillin, and gentamicin.

    Treatment: Stop the drugs, antihistamines, occasionally systemic steroids, and topical steroids.

    Mechanism of drug reaction:

    (i) Unknown in most of the cases.

    (ii) Only 10% of cases are immunologically mediated. Type I is IgE mediated, type II is cytotoxic antibody reaction, type III is circulating immune complexes, and type IV is delayed hypersensitivity.

(iii) Nonimmunologically mediated drug reaction includes toxic overdose, idiosyncratic responses, drug interaction, and pharmacologic side effects.

14. **Psoriasis: Erythematous papules and plaques surmounted by silvery, thick scales that mimic mica. Lesions are distributed symmetrically over the elbows, knees, trunk, scalp, palms, soles, and nails**. Nails may have pitting and red-brown discoloration (onycholysis).
Koebner phenomenon (intense trauma to the skin causes new skin lesions) is helpful diagnotic feature.
Pathogenesis: Unknown, may be multifactorial, associated with **HLA antigens BW17, B13, and BW37**.
Treatment: No curative drug is available for psoriasis.
(i) Topical steroids (intermediate and strong potency) or **add** topical tars and anthralin preparation or ultraviolet light (UVB with tar or UVA with oral psoralens).
(ii) Calcipotriene ointment (Dovonex) is a new effective treatment. This vitamin D ointment inhibits the hyperproliferative reaction.
(iii) **The patients with severe disease unresponsive to topical therapies**:
Antimetabolites: Methotrexate, azathioprine, and hydroxyurea.
Retinoid: Etretinate is useful in pustular and erythrodermic form of psoriasis.
Contraindication of antimetabolites and retinoid: Pregnancy and women of childbearing age.
Side effects: Bone marrow suppression; elevated triglycerides and LFT's.

15. **Pityriasis rosea (Christmas tree pattern of rashes):** The patients first appear with **'herald patch', (single lesion mimic ringworm lesion)** anywhere especially neck or lower trunk area and is followed by **generalized rashes** (oval or round, tannish pink or salmon colored, scaling papules and plaques) **over the trunk, upper extremities**, neck, and legs.
Treatment: Self-limited disease but topical corticosteroids, antihistamines, and ultraviolet light (UVB) are helpful.

16. **Lichen planus:** Pruritic, inflammatory, papulosquamous lesions usually over the ankle, wrist, mouth, and genitalia. Presence of **Wickham's striae** (white reticulated lines or fine white dots) surmounting the shiny, flat tops (mimic the appearance of lichen). Remember, Koebner phenomenon occurs in lichen planus. It can also involve the mucous membrane.
Etiology: Unknown.

Two conditions mimic lichen planus:

(i) **Drugs:** Thiazides, phenothiazine, quinidine, antimalarials, and gold.

(ii) Graft-verus-host disease: It causes dermal sclerosis, ulceration, reticulated pigmentation, and cicatricial alopecia.

Most common complication of recurrent herpes simplex infection: Erythema multiforme. It is a hypersensitivity reaction of skin and mucous membrane which develops 1 to 2 weeks after herpetic recurrence. It is due to herpesvirus containing immune complex reaction to herpes antigen.

17. **Erythema multiforme (target or bull's-eye lesion):** It is an immunologic reaction in the skin and mucous membrane results in **erythematous plaques, blisters, and target or bull's-eye lesions**. Involvement of **eye and mucous membrane of the mouth** are known as **Steven-Johnson syndrome**.
Etiology: Unknown (50% of cases), drugs (penicillins, phenytoin, barbiturates, sulfonamides), or infections (herpes simplex, streptococcus, Mycoplasma pneumoniae).
Treatment:
(i) To treat the underlying infections.
(ii) To stop the medications.
(iii) Use of systemic steroid is controversial.
(iv) The patients with severe oral lesions need IV fluids and topical anesthetics such as viscous Xylocaine.

18. **Bullous pemphigoid:** It is an autoimmune disorder. Elderly persons appear with **tense, large blisters on normal or erythematous skin** usually in the axillae, groin and flexure areas. Itching may be severe or absent.
Treatment: Prednisone and rarely immunosuppressive agents.

19. **Herpes gestationis** (It is a misnomer because it has **no** relation with herpes): It is a rare autoimmune disorder that occurs mostly during **the second and third trimester of pregnancy** and **subsides within a few weeks after delivery**. It appears as pruritic, vesicular lesions (first appear on the abdomen then spread all over the body) on the normal or erythematous skin.
Associated complications: Fetal mortality (up to 30% of cases), premature live births, sometimes transient vesicobullous lesions of the healthy newborn.
Treatment: Oral prednisone is used in throughout pregnancy with intermittent tapering, sometimes topical steroids and diphenylhydramine are used for pruritus and extensive bullae.

20. **Pemphigus vulgaris (or a variant pemphigus vegetans):** Both are acquired autoimmune diseases involving skin and mucous membrane (oral) results in

rupture bullae, bleeding, weeping, and crusted lesions.
Complications of untreated Pemphigus vulgaris: Extensive denudation, fluid and electrolytes imbalance, sepsis, and death.
Treatment: High doses of systemic steroids (prednisone) for long period of time, methotrexate, or intramuscular injection of gold.

21. **Pemphigus erythematosus:** It appears with superficial blisters, erosions, crusting, and oozing over the scalp and face. It mimics seborrheic dermatitis or butterfly rash like SLE. It does **not** involve the mucous membrane.
Treatment: Low doses of systemic steroids are helpful.

22. **Familial benign pemphigus or Hailey-Hailey disease:** It is differentiated from other form of pemphigus by its **dominance inheritance, absence of mouth lesions, intracellular antibodies,** and benign course. It appears with groups of **blisters** in neck, axillae, and groin. Warm weather and superimposed bacterial infections cause exacerbations and remissions.
Treatment:
(i) Antibiotics (systemic and topical) for bacterial infections.
(ii) Topical antifungal drug for superimposed candida infections.

23. **Acne:** It is the most common pustular disease of the skin affecting pilosebaceous units of the face and upper trunk.
Pathogenesis: Androgens stimulate sebum production, proliferation of anaerobic bacteria (Propionibacterium acnes), and obstruction of sebum flow.
Treatment:
(i) **Topical application of benzoyl peroxide and vitamin A** allow the sebum to flow freely onto the surface of the skin.
(ii) **Topical and oral antibiotics (tetracycline or erythromycin)** are used for inflammatory papules and pustules.
(iii) **Oral 13-cis retinoic acid (Accutane)** decreases sebum production and sebaceous gland size. It is **only** used in severe acne.
(iv) Spironolactone (antiandrogenic property) is used in difficult cases.
Factors enhances acne:
(i) **Drugs:** Androgens, phenytoin, systemic corticosteroids, high-progestin birth control pills, iodide-and bromide-containing agents.
(ii) Oil based cosmetics.
(iii) Tumors secreting excessive androgen: Adrenal tumors, ovarian tumors, and polycystic ovarian disease.

24. **Rosacea:** It is an inflammatory disorder of blood vessels and pilosebaceous units of the face. Middle-aged individuals appear with **papules, pustules,**

erythemas, and telangiectasias over the middle of the face. History of **flushing and blushing** of the face while using alcohol, hot-spicy foods, and caffeine. Long standing rosacea in the nose leads to rhinophyma.
Rhinophyma: Large, red, bubous nose is due to hyperplasia of the Sebaceous glands, connective tissues and blood vessels of the nose.
Ocular complications of Rosacea: Blepharitis, keratitis, conjuctivitis, and chalazion.
Treatment:
(i) Tetracycline and/or metronidazole must be continued for life at low doses orally because it reccurs when therapy stops.
(ii) Do not use high-potency topical corticosteroids for long period of time on the face because it may induce or aggravate the pre-existing rosacea.

25. A group of people developed generalized pruritic follicles all over the body **except head and neck regions**. Few days ago they went for swimming in a swimming pool.
Most likely diagnosis: Hot tub folliculitis or swimming pool folliculitis. It is due to contaminated water with **Pseudomonas aeruginosa infection**.
Treatment:
(i) Most cases resolved within 10 days **without any treatment**.
(ii) If no improvement, use appropriate antibiotics.

26. Most common organism in folliculitis: **S.aureus**.
The important clinical finding is a **thin hair within the pustule**.
Furuncle: It is a single deeper pustule.
Carbuncle: It is a multiple deeper pustule with multiple openings.
Treatment:
(i) Dicloxacillin or erthromycin.
(ii) Mild folliculitis: Use topical antiseptic cleansers (povidone-iodine or chlorhexidine).
(iii) Abscesses: Incision and drainage plus antibiotics.

27. A patient appears with **indurated, boggy, inflammatory plaques** studded with pustules over the face.
Most likely diagnosis: Tinea barbae. It is called kerion if it occurs in the scalp.
Organism causing the infections: Dermatophytes (especially T.verrucosum).
Treatment:
(i) Griseofulvin is **the drug of choice**.
(ii) Short course of oral corticosteroids is helpful.

28. **Most common organisms**:
    (a) **Cellulitis:** Group A streptococci and S. aureus.
    (b) **Erysipelas:** Group A streptococci. Erysipelas has well-defined painful border and 'orange-peel' epidermal surface. Cellulitis does **not** have well-defined border.
    Treatment: Systemic antibiotics, dicloxacillin or cephalosporins are used in both the conditions.
    (c) **Necrotizing fascitis:** Mixture of aerobic and anaerobic Gram-negative organisms. It is a special form of deep fascial structures cellulitis, mostly found in diabetes and immunosuppressed patients.
    Treatment: Surgical debridement and broad-spectrum antibiotics.

29. **Urticaria:** It appears as **wheals**, erythematous,and edematous swelling of the dermis due to increased permeability of capillaries and small venules.
    Pathogenesis: Increased vascular permeability is due to release of **histamine** and **other chemical substances** from cutaneous mast cells by **type I IgE hypersensitivity reaction** and by non-immunologic mechanisms.
    Acute urticaria: The duration is less than 6 weeks. It is due to drugs (aspirin, opiates) and other identifiable causes.
    Chronic urticaria: The duration is greater than 6 to 8 weeks. The causes are difficult to identify.
    Angioedema: Hives covering large areas and causes deep tissues (tongue, throat, airways) swelling result in respiratory difficulty due to obstruction of the airways.
    Treatment:
    (i) Try to identify and avoid the etiologic agents.
    (ii) Antihistamines or oral steroids for Urticaria.
    (iii) Acute angioedema or laryngeal edema is treated with epinephrine, diphenhydramine, and intubation if needed.

30. **The characteristic of skin rash in Lyme disease**: Erythema chronicum migrans. It is an annular skin lesion caused by spirochete (Borrelia burgdorferi).
    Treatment of Lyme Disease: Doxycycline, cefuroxime, clarithromycin, or azithromycin.

31. **Keratoacanthomas:** Ii is a self-limited epitheliomas appears over the sun-exposed areas as flesh colored papules. It is difficult to differentiate from squamous cell cancer.
    Treatment:
    (i) Usually spontaneously subside within 6 to 8 weeks but **leaves a scar**.

(ii) Surgical excision is recommended to avoid scar formation.

32. **Epidermal cancers (Basal cell and Squamous cell cancers)**: Both the cancers are found in **sun-exposed areas** (face, neck, arm, and hands) and more common in **immunosuppressed individuals**.
    (a) **Basal cell cancer:** It causes extensive local destruction but **rarely** metastasize. Nodular type is the most common type, other types are superficial, pigmented, and sclerosing (or scarring) basal cell cancers.
    Treatment: It depends on the location, size, type, and primary or recurrent.
    (1) Curettage and electrodesiccation.
    (2) Scalpel excision.
    (3) Radiation therapy.
    (4) Cryotherapy.
    (b) **Squamous cell carcinoma:** It is **less** common, more aggressive, locally invasive, and commonly metastasize.
    (c) **Bowen's disease:** It is squamous cell cancer in situ (e.g. penis).
    (d) Squamous cell cancer is ulcerated, crusted, and easily friable lesion.
    (e) **Actinic keratosis:** It is a precancereous lesion, may convert into squamous cell cancer. It appears as red, ill-marginated macules, and papules with yellow-brown adherent scales in sun-exposed skin.
    (f) Diagnosis of squamous cell cancer: Biopsy confirms the diagnosis.
    Treatment:
    (i) Excision is the treatment of choice.
    (ii) Actinic keratosis is treated with liquid nitrogen freezing or if numerous use topical 5 fluorouracil (1 or 5% cream or solution) over 2 to 4 weeks.

33. A 50 year old man appears with the complain of changing size, shape, and color of the existing nevi. The patient also complains of pruritus.
    Immediate investigation of choice: Biopsy.
    Most likely diagnosis: Malignant melanoma.
    Prognosis: The depth of malignant melanomas **less than 0.76 mm have 100% cure rate** and greater than 1.6 mm depth have 20 to 30% of survival for 5 years.
    Treatment:
    (i) Surgical excision and biopsy of small lesion.
    (ii) In large lesion: First incisional biopsy, then complete surgical excision.
    Few important points in malignant melanomas:
    (i) Suspicious pigmented lesions should have **full-thickness tissue biopsies** for diagnostic and prognostic evaluation. In suspected pigmented lesions shave-biopsy, shave-excision and electrocautarization are contraindicated.
    (ii) Malignant melanomas occur in families with dysplastic nevus syndrome.

34. **Kasabach-Merritt syndrome (K-M syndrome):** Platelet consumption by large cavernous hemangiomas.
Cavernous hemangiomas usually do **not** resolved spontaneously like capillary hemangiomas (90% resolve by 90 years of age).
Treatment of hemangiomas:
(i) Capillary hemangiomas – Resolves spontaneously.
(ii) Cavernous hemangiomas or large hemangiomas which ulcerate, bleed, and impinge on vital structures or K-M syndrome – **Oral prednisone**, if no response use **alpha-interferon.**

35. A 49 years old male, homosexual and drug abuser came for routine office visit.
Physical examination: A small painless red nodule over the lower extremity.
Most likely diagnosis: Kaposi's sarcoma.
Prognosis: Extremely poor.
Few important points in Kaposi's sarcoma:
(i) It is more common in **men** than women, average age is seventh decade, associated with lymphedema, average survival is 10 years.
(ii) It appears in fourth decade in AIDS patients, average survival less than 2 years.

36. **Pyogenic granuloma (no infectious process is involved and no cancer)**: It is bright red, **raspberry-like** growth, friable, bleeds easily, and rapid growth within weeks. It represents capillary hemangiomatous proliferation and follow injury or surgery.
Treatment: Excision, curettage, and electrocautarization or cryotherapy.

37. A patient appears with multiple, red, painful, tender, deep nodules (1 to 5 cm in sizes) in pretibial regions of both feet. The patient has no other medical problem.
Most likely diagnosis: Erythema nodosum.
The factors causing erythema nodosum: Unknown, sarcoidosis, inflammatory bowel disease, streptococcal infection, TB, Yersinia enterocolitis, deep fungus infections, oral contraceptives, and pregnancy.
Treatment:
(i) To treat the underlying causes if any.
(ii) Symptomatic therapy with aspirin, non-steroidal anti-inflammatory drugs, potassium iodide, or short courses of systemic steroids (prednisone).

38. A 50 years old patient appears with **tender, red nodules on the lower legs and thighs**. The patient denies any abdominal symptoms. The lesions are **subcutaneous fat necrosis**.
Serum amylase and lipase values: Elevated.
Next investigation of choice: Biopsies.
Most likely diagnosis: Pancreatic cancer or pancreatitis.

39. **Dermatomyositis rashes:** Heliotrope (violaceous edema of eyelids), Gottron's papule (flat-topped papules over the knuckles), reticulated patches of hyper and hypopigmentation, erythema, and telangiectasia noted on the V of the neck, face, knees, and elbows.

40. **Rashes of lupus erythematosus**:
    (i) Butterfly rashes on the face is found in SLE.
    (ii) Psoriasiform skin rashes on the face and trunk in subacute lupus.
    (iii) Periungual telangiectasias are found in SLE and other connective tissue disorders.
    (iv) Discopid lupus (lupus localized to the skin): It appears as red plaques with white scales. Subsequently plaques atrophy, hypopigmentation in the centre, and hyperpigmentation on the rim of the lesions.

41. **Complication of X-radiation skin changes (atrophy, irregular pigmentation, telangiectasias, and finally ulceration)**: **Cancer formation** in the radiated skin areas.

42. A 45 years old immunosuppressed patient appears with **painless lesions begin as hemorrhagic bullous patches** in the axillary and anogenital regions. Bulluos patches subsequently become necrotic and ulcerated, **central gray to black eschar surrounded by erythema**.
Culture of the skin lesion: Pseudomonas is present.
Most likely diagnosis: Ecthyma gangrenosum.

43. **Behcet's syndrome:** Multiple genital and oral, small painful ulcers with iridocyclitis. It may cause neurologic and GI involvements, arthiritis, and erythema nodosum.

44. **LEOPARD syndrome (dominantly inherited condition)**:
    (a) L = Lentigines (hyperpigmented macules) on the head, trunk, palms, soles, and extremities.
    (b) E = ECG abnormalities.
    (c) O = Ocular hypertelorism.

(d) P = Pulmonary stenosis.
(e) A = Abnormal genitalia.
(f) R = Retarded growth.
(g) D = Deafness.

45. A middle aged construction worker appears with lentigines over the face, arms, and dorsum of the hands. Those areas were exposed to the sun.
Most likely diagnosis: Actinic lentigines which is a benign lesion.

46. **Melasma (chloasma) of women:** Symmetrical hyperpigmentation over the malar eminence, forehead, and upper lip.
Etiology: Pregnancy, birth control pills, or ultraviolet radiation.
Treatment:
(i) Use of hydroquinone (bleaching agent) is controversial.
(ii) Sunscreens may be useful.
(iii) May resolve spontaneously after delivery in pregnant patients.

47. **Albright's disease (polyostotic fibrous dysplasia):** The patients also have three or four large hyperpigmented macules usually distributed **unilaterally** on the buttocks or cervical area.

48. **Xeroderma pigmentosa**: Inability to maintain the integrity of DNA results in multiple freckles over the face, lips, conjunctiva, and extremities. Variable sizes hyperpigmented patches interspersed with hypopigmented areas.
Complications and sequel: Basal and squamous cell cancers, malignant melanomas leads to early death. Other complications are keratoses and keratoacanthomas.

49. **Neurofibromatosis (von Recklinghausen's disease):** Multiple neurofibromas all over the body. Café-au-lait spots, six or more, each 1.5 cm in diameter are diagnostic for this autosomal dominant disease. Isolated Café-au-lait spots are prsent in 10% of normal populations.

50. **Few important points in vitiligo**:
(i) Most patients of vitiligo are healthy.
(ii) It is associated with autoimmune disorders (thyroiditis, hyperthyroidism, diabetes mellitus, pernicious anemia, and Addison's disease).
(iii) Spontaneous partial repigmentation occurs in one third of cases in sun-exposed areas.
(iv) Use of PUVA helps in some repigmentation.
(v) 36% of cases are familial.

51. **Tuberous Sclerosis:**
   (i) Autosomal dominant.
   (ii) Hypopigmented macules (oval or mountain ash-leaf configuration) are present over the trunk or buttocks.
   (iii) Periungual fibromas.
   (iv) Adenoma sebaceum.
   (v) CT scan of the brain to diagnose tumorous dysplasia.
   (vi) Mental retardation and unexplained seizures in newborn.

52. **Piebaldism:**
   (i) Autosomal dominant.
   (ii) A white forelock is typical presentation or hypomelanosis of the anterior surface of the chest, forehead, central scalp, and extremeties.

53. **Treatment of fungal nail infections:**
   (i) Oral griseofulvin is used for dermatophyte infection until the nails appear clear.
   (ii) Ketoconazole is used for Candida infections or in patients unresponsive to griseofulvin.
   (iii) Oral therapy needs 4 to 6 months for fingernails and 12 to 16 months for toenails.
   (iv) Topical antifungal powders are helpful for long-term prophylaxis in elderly patients with toenails fungal infections. Toenails funguses are difficult to eradicate in elderly patients because nails grow very slowly.

54. **Most common organism in paronychia (or painful red swelling of the nail fold)**: **C.albicans**. It is due to wet hands.
   Treatment:
   (i) Avoid water.
   (ii) Use of antifungal solutions locally 2 to 3 times per day for 1 or 2 months.

55. (a) **Yellow nail syndrome:** It is found in COPD, pleural effusion, and bronchiectasis.
   (b) **Splinter hemorrhages of the nail:** It is more commonly found in trauma than bacterial endocarditis.
   (c) **Hypertrophic osteoarthropathy (clubbing plus bone pain and proliferative periosteitis):** It is found in bronchogenic squamous cell cancer.
   (d) **Clubbing of the fingers:** It is found in lung abscess, bronchiectasis, and lung cancer.

56. **Alopecia areata:** Round or oval patches of hair loss usually on the scalp, beard, eyebrows, or eyelashes.
Alopecia totalis: Total hair loss in the scalp.
Alopecia universalis: Total body hair loss.
Treatment:
(i) Topical, intralesional, and systemic steroids may be helpful.
(ii) Recent mode of therapy includes **topical** minoxidil, photochemotherapy with PUVA, induction of allergy or irritant contact dermatitis with 1% anthralin and topical dinitrochlorobenzene.

57. **Tinea capitis:** It appears as one or more patches of hair loss with mild scaling, erythema, and broken hairs.
Etiologic agents: Trichophyton tonsurans.
Treatment: Griseofulvin is the drug of choice.

58. **Androgenic alopecia (or male pattern of baldness):** It involves the frontal, vertex, and upper occipital region. There is **no actual loss of hair** but conversion of normal hairs by fine, unpigmented, poorly seen vellus hairs. It is absent in male with **low** testosterone levels (Klinefelter's syndrome).
Treatment: Hair transplantation or scalp reduction is helpful.

59. **Trichotillomania (or traumatic, self-induced):** It is due to compulsive twisting and rubbing results in breaking and epilation of the hair shafts.
Treatment:
(i) Mild cases: Self-limited.
(ii) Severe cases: Psychiatrist should evaluate for emotional problems.

60. **Traction alopecia:** It is due to excessive traction or traumatic hair styling techniques result in **hair-thinning** at the margins of the scalp.
Treatment: Avoid excessive traction or trauma to the hairs.

61. **Diffuse or generalized alopecia:**
(a) **Stress alopecia or telogen effluvium:** This diffuse hair loss is due to severe emotional and physiologic stress (major surgery, high fever, systemic illness, crash diet), drugs convert growing hairs to resting hairs and finally shed (beta-blocker, coumarin, heparin, allopurinol, thiouracil, probenecid, lithium, amphetamines). **Excessive shedding means more than 5 hairs are lost when 12 hairs are grasped.**
Treatment: To treat the underlying stress and avoid the underlying conditions. Hairs regrow within 4 to 6 months.

(b) Hypothryoidism, seborrheic dermatitis may cause diffuse hair loss.
(c) **Toxic alopecia (or disrupted hair growth due to toxic agents):** Anticancer drugs (doxorubicin and others) and radiation therapy cause damage of the cells of hair bulb. Hypervitaminosis A and retinoids interfere with keratinization.

62. **Ultraviolet light from the sun and effects**:
(a) UVC = shorter than 290 nm, **absorbed by the ozone layer**, does not reach the earth.
(b) UVB = 290 to 320 nm, it causes **cancer, burning, tanning, and aging**.
(c) UVA = 320 to 400 nm, it needs 1000 times more energy than UVB to cause hyperpigmentation (melanogenic) and erythrogenic effects. UVA causes chemical inflammatory reactions through window glass.

Few important points regarding ultraviolet lights:
(i) UV lights do penetrate shades and clouds, so they are **not** protective.
(ii) Avoid sun exposure between 11 A.M and 2 P.M when 50% of UV lights are received.
(iii) Aspirin, indomethacin, or PGE synthesis inhibitors can reduce the burns (PGE are elevated in sun burnt skin).

63. **Dermatologic effects of exposure of the UV sunlights**:
(a) **Chronic exposure:** Keratoses, keratoacanthomas, basal cell cancer, squamous cell cancer, and may be melanomas.
(b) 3 to 4 days exposure: Cellular, molecular changes, and new melanin formations.
(c) ½ to 1 day exposure: Inflammation and edema formations.

64. **Exogenous factors (chemical agents taken orally or applied locally on the skin) causing two kinds of photosensitivity reactions when exposed to the sun**:
(a) **Phototoxic reaction:** Nonimmunologic, free radicals **cause redness, swelling, pain, and rarely blister formation**. Most phototoxic agents absorb UVB light. It is due to drugs (sulfonamides,phenothiazines), plant derivatives (furocoumarine or psoralens),dyes; plants, fruits, and vegetables (causing phytophotodermatitis).
(b) **Photoallergic reaction:** Acquired, type IV delayed hypersensitivity immunologically altered response to light. **Eczematous** and sometimes urticarial skin lesions after 24 hours exposure to the sun is due to UVA light. It is due to perfumes, chemicals (fragrances, sunscreens, blankophores, salicylanilides, laundry soaps, and bleaches).

Treatment of photosensitivity reactions:

(i) Avoid the photosensitizing agent.
(ii) Avoid the sun exposure and use sunscreens.
(iii) Topical or oral steroids.

65. A 45 year old male patient appears with history of **eczematous patches, red to violaceous papules or plaques, and urticarial lesions over the back of the hands, face, the nape and V of the neck**. It occurs in late spring and early summer after he typically spends few hours exposed to the sun and the patient gets better in the winter months.
Most likely diagnosis – Polymorphous light eruption (PMLE).

66. **Risk of skin cancer in patients with transplantation**: Seven times greater than normal. Cutaneous neoplasms both benign and malignant (basal cell and squamous cell cancers) are higher than normal. **Biopsy of skin lesions should be done as soon as possible**.

67. Skin infections in immunocompromised patients:
(a) **Primary skin infections:** Most common bacterial organisms are group A streptococci and S.aureus (cause cellulitis), less common organisms are Pseudomonas and anaerobe. Primary infection with viruses (herpes, papillomavirus) and dermatophytes (fungus) are common.
(b) Disseminated infection metastatic to the skin by hematogenous route: Most common organisms are Pseudomonas, other Gram-negative bacilli, Histoplasma, Coccidiodis, Candida, Aspergillus, and Mucoraceae. The skin infections may appear as vesicles, bullae, necrosis, gangrene, or pustules.
(c) Skin disease characteristic of HIV infections: Kaposi's sarcoma, oral hairy leukoplakia, bacillary angiomatosis (red, raised, nodular lesions with a scaling base), eosinophilic folliculitis (extremely pruritic follicular papules on the head, neck, and extremities).

67. **Most common occupational disease in USA:** Skin disease. Occupational contact dermatitis is the most common (95% of cases) cause. It is due to external contact with chemical, physical, and biologic agents.

68. **Clinical manifestations, diagnosis, and treatment of occupational contact dermatitis**:
(a) **Clinical manifestation:** Most common sites of involvement are the hands in addition to other parts of the body.
(i) **Acute irritant dermatitis:** Acute onset of erythema, papules, vesicles, edema, or large bullae in severe cases may be followed by hyper or hypopigmentation.

(ii) **Allergic contact dermatitis:** There is a latent period of 7 to 10 days between the contact with allergens and the development of dermatitis. Acute or Chronic eczematous reaction with erythema, papules, vesicles, scaling, and pruritus.

(iii) **Cumulative insult dermatitis:** It develops after a long period of contact (rings, earrings, watchbands) results in dry, fissure and eczematous reaction.

(b) **Diagnosis:**

(i) Occupational history is the most important to make the diagnosis.

(ii) Personal or family history of dermatitis.

(iii) Complete physical examination.

(iv) Allergic contact dermatitis is confirmed by diagnostic patch testing.

(v) No confirmatory test for irritant contact dermatitis.

(c) **Treatment:**

(i) Avoid the irritants or allergens.

(ii) Symptomatic treatment with antihistamines and topical steroids.

(iii) Acute contact dermatitis: Cold wet dressing with Burrow's solution.

(iv) Severe dermatitis: Use systemic steroids.

(v) Dry and chronic eczema: Topical steroids and emollients.

(vi) Antihistamines are used for pruritus and mild sedation.

(vii) A temporary or permanent change of job and vocational training may be needed.

(viii) Some states require reporting of occupational diseases.

(d) **Prognosis:** Poor, if not treated early and adequately.

70. **Chloracne:** It is the first and most constant finding in **chronic dioxin poisoning**. It appears as small straw-colored cysts and comedones behind the ears and malar areas.

71. **Cutaneous T cell lymphomas (mycosis fungoides):** It is found in people working in heavy industry or have industrial chemical exposure.

EYE DISEASES

1. Legal visual acuity for driver's license in most states: At least 20/40.

2. Different types of cataract and causes:
   (i) Posterior subcapsular cataract: Systemic corticosteroids.
   (ii) Sun flower cataract (orange copper deposits in the anterior capsule): Wilson's disease.
   (iii) Christmas tree cataract (red, green, and blue opacities in the lenticular cortex): Myotonic dystrophy.
   (iv) Nuclear sclerotic: Senile cataract. It is often **familial** but the cause is **unknown**.

3. Most common cause of acquired cataract: **Unknown**, other causes are trauma, metabolic (diabetes, hypoglycemia, galactosemia), hypocalcemia, or radiation.

4. **Treatment of cataract.**
   (i) **Removal of the cataract**. Most cataracts are removed for visual reasons (a driver needs surgery if vision is **below 20/40**, an old person may not need surgery even with **20/200**).
   (ii) Cataract should be removed in mature, hypermature cataracts, and immature swollen cataract causing angle-closure glaucoma.
   Please remember, removal of a lens in advanced glaucoma or macular degeneration does **not** improve the vision.

5. **Complications of cataract surgery**: It is **rare** and the complications are hemorrhage, infection, corneal decompensation, retinal detachment, and cystoid macular edema with reduced vision.

6. **Clinical manifestation, diagnosis, and treatment of glaucoma**: (Open-angle is a failure of absorption of aqueous humor by trabecular meshwork, angle-closure is a shallow anterior chamber between cornea and iris).
   (A) **Open-angle glaucoma**: (Normal maximum intraocular pressure is 21 mm Hg).
      (i) **Most common type**: Chronic open-angle glaucoma.
      (ii) **Signs and symptoms**: Mostly asymptomatic until the disease is advanced. Initial symptom is **only the peripheral vision loss** and **absence of pain**.
      (iii) **Diagnosis**: Elevated intraocular pressure (> 21 mm Hg), optic disc edema, and visual field defect. Gonioscopy can distingusih between open-angle and angle-closure glaucoma.

(iv) **Treatment**.

(a) Medical: Topical use of parasympathomimetics (pilocarpine, carbochol), beta-blockers (timolo), and sympathomimetics (epinephrine, dipivefrin); **if the above medications fail**, use topical indirect parasympathomimetics (echothiophate), systemic carbonic anhydrase inhibitors (acetazolamide, methazolamide).

(b) **Surgical**: It is indicated when medical therapy fails. Laser trabeculoplasty or surgical fistula between anterior chamber and subconjunctival space is helpful.

(B) Angle-closure glaucoma.

(i) **Signs and symptoms**: Red, painful eye with decreased vision, pupil is about 6mm and fixed, dull corneal light reflex, diaphoresis, nausea, and sometimes vomiting. **Please remember, fixed mid-dilated pupil with decreased vision in absence of pain and redness, always rule in glaucoma**.

(ii) **Diagnosis.**

(a) Slit-lamp examination with tonometry (elevated intraocular pressure, may be above 50 mm Hg).

(b) Gonioscopy may be needed to distinguish from open-angle glaucoma.

(iii) **Caution**.

(a) Pupil dilating agents can precipitate the attack of angle-closer glaucoma.

(b) Short action pupillary dilator (tropicamide) may be used and the patient should be observed carefully.

(c) **Nonopthalmologist should not routinely dilates adults pupil in out patient.**

(iv) **Treatment: It is an emergency**.

(a) **Initial treatment**: Parenteral acetazolamide, mannitol, oral glycerol, isosorbide (in diabetes), plus topical pilocarpine, and beta-adrenergic agonist.

(b) **Surgery**: It is indicated when acute attack is broken with medications. **Laser iridotomy of the affected and nonaffected eye (prophylactic)** because it is mostly bilateral.

(C) Secondary glaucomas.

(i) **Causes:** Trauma (blood), diabetes, vascular discrders (new vessels are formed and causedobstruction of the angle), JRA (chronic inflammation), or lens-induced glaucoma.

(ii) **Treatment**.

(a) Same as primary open-angle glaucoma **except** removal of the lens in lens-induced glaucoma.

(b) Ischemia causes neovascularization: Photocoagulation of ischemic tissues.

(c) Tissue proliferation closes surgical fistula: **Put a plastic valve connecting** anterior chamber with subconjunctival sac to avoid this complication or use **antimetabolites** to inhibit the tissue growth.

(d) Destruction of the ciliary body by thermal, laser, or ultrasound to control intraocular pressure but **rarely** preserves useful vision.

(D) **Treatment of absolute glaucoma of any cause**.

(i) Enucleation (removal of the eye) is the definitive treatment of blind, and painful eye.

(ii) Topical medications or retrobulbar injection of alcohol may relieve the pain and allow the eye to be retained.

7. **Vision and papilledema**.

(i) Acute papilledema: **Normal** visual acuity.

(ii) Chronic papilledema: Optic atrophy and permanent loss of vision.

Treatment: Surgical fenestration of the optic nerve sheath in eyes may halt progression of visual loss.

8. **True and pseudopapilledema**:

True	Pseudo.
(i) Accumulation of axoplasms in the optic disc	(i) Accumulation of hyaline materials in the prelaminar optic nerve.
(ii) Increased ICP	(ii) Normal ICP
(iii) Diagnosis: By opthalmoscopy.	(iii) Diagnosis: If opthalmoscopy cannot diagnosis, then CT or ultrasonography should be done
(iv) Presence of physiologic cup except in advanced cases	(iv) Frequent absence of physiologic cup.

9. **Papilledema** and **optic neuritis** (anterior optic neuritis is papillitis and posterior optic neuritis is **retrobulbar optic neuritis**).

Papilledema	Optic neuritis.
(i) Disc is swollen, elevated, and may be hemorrhagic.	(i) Papillitis: Same as in papilledema. Retrobulbar neuritis: Normal disc by opthalmoscopy.
(ii) Acute-No visual loss. Chrome-Loss of vision	(ii) Loss of vision in both anterior and posterior neuritis.

(iii) Usually bilateral	(iii) Usually unilateral
(iv) Treatment: Surgical fenestration of the optic nerve sheath may halt the progression of visual loss.	(iv) Treatment: Controversial. Corticosteroids cannot alter visual outcome but decrease the demyelination.

10. **Anterior ischemic optic neuropathy**: Elderly patients appear with acute onset of loss of vision and swollen disc due to infarction. It may involve superior or inferior half of the optic disc and corresponding loss of vision.
    Etiology.
    (i) Idiopathic is the most common cause.
    (ii) Initial manifestation of giant cell arteritis in elderly persons.
    Nonarteritic type usually occurs **in discs with small cups and may involve the second eye** in two fifths of cases.
    Treatment.
    (i) To treat the underlying giant cell arteritis.
    (ii) Surgical incision of the optic nerve sheath is **not** effective in nonarteritic type.

11. Most common intrinsic tumors of the optic nerve causes disc swelling and loss of vision: Glioma and meningioma.

12. A 45 year old man came for routine physical examination. Opthalmoscopic examination shows **temporal pallor of the optic disc**. The patient is asymptomatic.(Important).
    Most likely diagnosis: Normal eye.
    Recommendation: No further intervention is necessary.

13. **Optic atrophy**: It is due to death of the axons in the retina and optic nerve. Three types of optic atrophy.
    (A) **Primary**: Progressive pallor without loss of disc substance. It is due to retrograde or anterograde degeneration from compression, vascular injury, or toxic metabolites.
    (B) **Secondary**: It is due to swelling of the optic disc which has an irregular border with milky gray appearance from vascular and glial changes.
    (C) **Glaucomatous**: Increased cupping and loss of disc substance.
    Diagnosis of optic atrophy: It is difficult because some normal disc may **appear pale**. In patient with nuclear sclerotic cataract, disc pallor may be missed due to cataract. **Please remember that the diagnosis of optic atrophy should not be made unless it is associated with loss of vision or visual acuity**.

14. **Pseudooptic atrophy**: It is found in retinitis pigmentosa. It is called pseudooptic atrophy because **axons are preserved** and **ganglion cells are intact**. Dystrophy of rods and cones, vascular, and gliotic changes produce **pseudoatrophic (waxy pallor) finding.**

15. A 20 year old man appears with history of acute or subacute visual loss, recently he lost bilateral central vision.
    Opthalmoscopic examination: Optic atrophy.
    Most likely diagnosis: **Leber's hereditary optic neuroretinopathy.**
    Treatment: No effective treatment, some patients spontaneously improve.
    Mode of transmission: Through abnormal maternal mitochondrial DNA.
    Diagnosis: Study of mitochondrial DNA from peripheral leukocytes. Please remember, men cannot transmit the disease and all women in the pedigress are either carrier or affected.

16. An adult male has survived retinoblastoma in the childhood, he may develop: **Osteogenic sarcoms** or other cancers.

17. **Most common primary intraocular tumor of the adulthood**:
    Malignant melanomas of the choroid. It is most commonly found in **middle-aged whites**. Most common site of metastases is in the **liver**. Skin melanomas metastasize to the eye and orbit.
    Treatment of malignant melanomas of the choroid.
    (i) Enucleation is the traditional therapy.
    (ii) Other treatments are photocoagulation, local resection, and radiation therapy.
    Please remember, many benign conditions mimic malignant melanomas, the diagnosis should be certain before enucleation.

18. **Most common ocular malignancy of adulthood**:
    Metastatic cancers. Most common primary site of cancer origin is the breast followed by lungs, kidneys, GI tract, prostate, and testis. Metastatic cancers is more common than malignant melanomas of the choroid.
    Treatment of metastatic cancer of the eye:
    (i) Removal of the eye is rarely needed particularly when the eye is blind and painful.
    (ii) **Palliative radiation or chemotherapy** is the treatment of choice.

19. **Graves' orbitopathy (few important points):**

(i) The clinical manifestation includes exophthalmos, lid retraction, increased IOP (intraocular pressure), diplopia, decreased eye movement, reduced vision from optic neuropathy, or exposure keratitis.
(ii) The patients may be **hyper, hypo, or euthyroid** when orbitopathy first manifest.
(iii) It can develop in patients **previously treated** with hyperthyroidism.
(iv) **Opthalmic Graves' disease**: Graves' orbitopathy with **normal thyroid functions**.
(v) Diagnosis: Coronal CT or MR1 shows characteristically enlarged ocular muscles.
(vi) **Treatment**.
  (a) Systemic steroids reduce exophthalmos and temporarily reduce optic nerve pressure.
  (b) Surgical decompression is the definitive therapy.
  (c) Orbital irradiation is also helpful.
  (d) Surgery of the extraocular muscles and lids improves diplopia and lid retraction. It is done after the orbitopathy has stabilized.

20. **Most common cause of unilateral or bilateral exophthalmos: Graves' orbitopathy**.

21. **Central retinal artery occlusion (CRAO)**.
  (A) **Signs and symptoms**: Sudden loss of vision in one eye, opthalmoscopy reveals arteriolar narrowing and vascular stasis.
  (B) **Causes of CRAO**: **Emboli** (atheromatouos, myxomatous, and material from diseased or artificial heart valves), disease of small vessels, carotid occlusion, giant cell arteritis, polyarteritis nodosa, or sickle cell trait after trauma or stress.
  (C) **Management of CRAO**: It is an emergency because prompt action may dislodge the embolus, restore the circulation of the retina, and preserve the vision.
    (i) **Management by nonopthalmologist**.
      (a) Firm, intermittent pressure on the globe with heel of the hand, alnernating raising and lowering **intraocular pressure (IOP)**.
      (b) Mixture of 95% oxygen and 5% carbon dioxide are administered by mask for several minutes at a time.
    (ii) **Management by opthalmologist.**
      (a) Retrobulbar injection of local anesthetic to dilate the arteries plus item number(b).
      (b) Anterior chamber paracentesis to reduce the pressure in the vascular bed of the eye.

22. **Branch retinal artery occlusion (BRAO):**
    (A) **Signs and symptoms:** Partial loss of vision and wedge-shaped pale areas in the retina by opthalmoscopy.
    (B) **Etiology of BRAO**.
        (i) **Older individuals**: Source of emboli is ipsilateral carotid artery.
        (ii) **Young individuals**: Migraine, increased IOP, coagulation defects, and oral contraceptives may cause vascular occlusion.

23. **Central retinal vein occlusion (CRVO).**
    (A) **Signs and symptoms**: Loss of vision with dilated tortuous veins, retinal hemorrhages, and disc swelling in one eye are characteristic findings. It is **not** an emergency.
    (B) **Treatment.**
        (i) No accepted immediate therapy.
        (ii) Panretinal photocoagulation may reduce the risk of neovascular glaucoma.

24. **Branch retinal vein occlusion (BRVO)**.
    (A) Signs and symptoms: Blurred vision, hemorrhage, cotton-wool spots in the fundus, and macular edema.
    (B) Treatment: Photocoagulation is helpful in macular edema.

25. A patient appears with ocular pain, opthalmoscopic examination shows exudative retinal detachment and diagnosis of **scleritis** (inflammation of the deep scleral tissues) has been made. The patient may have the following systemic disorders:
    SLE, dermatomyositis, rheumatoid arthritis, polyarteritis nodosa, systemic selerosis, relapsing polychondritis, and Wegener's granulomatosis. The most common cause of episcleritis (inflammation of the superficial scleral tissues) is **idiopathic** but it may be associated with the above mentioned systemic disorders.
    Treatment of scleritis.
    (i) Systemic steroids and other antirheumatic drugs are useful in some patients.
    (ii) Local steroid injection may cause perforation.

26. **Treatment of keratoconjunctivitis sicca (corneal inflammation is due to dry eyes)**:
    (i) Artificial tears perferably without preservatives.
    (ii) Temporary or permanent occlusion of the lacrimal punctata to decrease tear outflow.

(iii) Contact lenses, moisture chambers, or goggles over the eyes to decrease evaporation.

27. **Sjogren's syndrome**: Keratoconjunctivitis sicca, dry mouth (xerostomia), plus a connective tissue disorder.

28. **Most common vascular retinopathy**: **Diabetic retinopathy**. It is classified into **background** or **proliferative**. Background retinopathy is subdivided into **simple background** and **preproliferative form**.
    (A) **Simple background:** Microaneurysms, dot/blot hemorrhages, and hard exudates.
    (B) **Preproliferative**: Cotton-wool spots, numerous intraretinal hemorrhages, beading of veins, and intraretinal microvascular abnormalities.
    (C) **Proliferative**: Neovascularization, fibrovascular proliferation, and subsequently vitreous hemorrhages.
    Treatment.
    (i) Good diabetic control.
    (ii) Ablation of ischemic retina by photocoagulation.
    (iii) Removal of the vitreous and its contents in advanced proliferative retinopathy.

29. **Most common type of retinopathy in type 2 diabetes over age 50**: **Background retinopathy**. It is the most common cause of **new onset of blindness when associated with macular edema.**

30. **Most common retinal changes in hypertension: Arteriolar narrowing** (normal ratio of the diameter of arteriolar and venous blood vessels is 2:3 or 3:4), othre findings are **microaneurysms, hemorrhages, edema, lipid deposits**, exudates, and cotton-wool spots.
    Consequence of hypertensive vascular changes.
    (i) Retinal vascular occlusions.
    (ii) Ischemic optic neuropathy.
    (iii) Acclerates atherosclerosis but atherosclerosis does not require hypertension.

31. **Retinal changes in atherosclerosis: Atheromas (yellow-white plaques)** of the retinal arteriole are the only absolute findings. It is larger and found in **central central artery and its first branches** (please remember, **calcific or lipid emboli** are smaller and found in the peripheral retina).

32. **Different types and causes of retinal emboli**:

(i) **Talc emboli (small white flecks)** in heroin abusers.
(ii) **Septic emboli (white-centered hemorrhages, Roth spots)** in subacute bacterial endocarditis.
(iii) **Cardiac myxoma** is a rare but important cause of retinal emboli.
(iv) Platelet-fibrin emboli can cause transiet monocular blindness.
(v) Calcific or lipid emboli.

33. **SLE and retinal findings**: It is **nonspecific**, most frequent findings are hemorrhages and cotton-wool spots. Cotton-wool spots are **not** exudates but represent axoplasmic stasis due to ischemic vasculitis.

34. **Causes of hyperviscosity retinopathy (vascular occlusions, dilated and tortous veins, retinal hemorrhages):**
(i) Leukemia.
(ii) Sickle-cell anemia.
(iii) Polycythemia.
(iv) Multiple myeloma.
(v) Waldenstrom's macroglobulinemia.

35. **Reiter's syndrome**: It is a traid of initial onset of **nonbacterial urethritis** followed by **polyarthritis** and ocular inflammations (mostly conjunctivitis followed by anterior uveitis and keratitis).

36. **HLA-B 27 positive**.
(i) Reiter's syndrome.
(ii) Ankylosing spondylitis.
Both causes **uveitis**, other causes are **Behcet's syndrome** (hypopyon uveitis, a layer of white cells in the lower portion of anterior chamber), **lymphoreticular cancers** (CNS lymphomas, reticulum cell and histiocytic sarcomas), and **Vogt-Koyanagi-Harada syndrome** (uveomeningitis).

37. **Treatment of uveitis.**
(i) Initial therapy with topical predinisolone or dexamethasone.
(ii) Topical use of mydriatic-cycloplegics in anterior uveitis is helpful.
(iii) Periocular corticosteroids or oral predinisone in severe uveitis or posterior uveitis.
(iv) Immunosuppressive therapy is needed sometimes.

38. **Ocular infections and treatment.**
(A) **Herpetic keratitis:** Characteristic dendritic ulcer.

Treatment: Topical antiviral therapy. No treatment is required for dendritic keratitis due to herpes zoster opthalmicus.

(B) **Gonococcal conjunctivitis**: Sexually promiscuous adults appear with copious discharge and swollen eyelids.

Treatment: Parenteral ceftriaxone and saline lavage of eye secretion.

(C) **Chlamydia conjunctivitis** (or inclusion blennorrhea): It causes subacute conjunctivitis with urethritis in developed countries. It causes trachoma and blindness in developing countries.

Treatment.

(i) Systemic tetracycline or erythromycin.

(ii) Topical antibiotic is not adequate.

(D) **Corneal ulcers:** It is due to bacterial or fungal infection, trauma, after surgery, contact lens wear, preexisting corneal disease.

Treatment.

(i) Refer to an opthalmologist as soon as possible.

(ii) Topical antibiotics and other measures.

(E) **Bacterial endopthalmitis**: It is most commonly found after perforation (accident or surgery).

Diagnosis: Cultures and smears from anterior chamber or vitreous cavity by aspiration.

Treatment.

(i) Antibiotics (intravitreal, systemic, topical, and periocular) according to Gram stain.

(ii) Surgical vitrectomy may be needed.

(F) **Candida endopthalmitis**: Most common organism in metastatic (endogenous) endopthalmitis is **Candida albicans**. It may due to prolonged use of intravenous catheters or parenteral drug abuse results in multiple white fluffy choreoretinitis.

Treatment.

(i) Antifungal drugs (systemic or intravitreal).

(ii) Spontaneous improvements may occur.

39. **Medications and side effects**

(i) Carbonic anhydrase inhibitor (used to reduce intraocular pressure). **Paresthesias is the most common**, other are urolithiasis, systemic acidosis results in anorexia, depression, and weight loss.
Treatment: Sodium bicarbonate.

(ii) Corticosteroids.

(a) Systemic administration for prolonged periods: Posterior subcapsular cataracts.

(b) Topic steroids: Increase IOP in genetically predisposed person and enhance herpetic keratitis.

(iii) **Ethambutol**: Optic neuropathies are very common when dose exceeds 15 mg/kg.

(iv) **Thioridazine**: Degeneration of retinal pigments.

(v) **Amiodarone**: Disc swelling and visual loss like anterior ischemic optic neuropathy, pigmentation in corneal epithelium.

(vi) Quinine: Acute blindness, dizziness, hearing loss, and tinnitus.

(vii) Chloroquine: Bull's eye pattern of parafoveal loss of pigmentation and visual loss.

GENETICS

1. **Fragile X syndrome:** Macroorchidism, mental retardation, and sometimes autistic features. Most common site is Xq 27. A molecular test is available to detect the female carrier.

2. **Turner syndrome (45, X)**: Delayed puberty, infertility, aortic coarctation, biscuspid aortic valve (most common cardiac lesion), short and/or webbed neck, and short fourth metacarpals. Hormonal therapy is needed for pubertal development.

3. **Klinefelter syndrome (47, XXY)**: **It is the most common cause of male infertility**. Other features are microorchidism, gynecomastia, mental retardation, immature behavior, and tall stature with long limbs. Incidence is 1 in 500 males.

4. **47, XXX females**: Normal appearance, low IQ, delayed language development, usually normal sexual development but the **behavioral, social, and emotional problems are the key findings**.

5. **47, XYY males:** Temper outburst, impulsive behavior, tall stature, may have lower IQ and more criminal behavior than general males.

6. **Kallman syndrome** (microdeletion Xp 22): Anosmia (inability to smell), hypogonadotropic hypogonadism, ichthyosis, short stature, and mental retardation.

7. **Down syndrome (95% have trisomy 21, 5% have translocation mostly 14/21)**: Mental retardation, brushfield spots, nystagmus or strabismus may be present, fissured tongue, upward and outward slanting of the palpebral fissures, congenital heart defects (most common is endocardial cushion defect), increased susceptibility to infection and immunoglobulin imbalance, increased **incidence of hypothyroidism due to antithyroid antibodies**.

8. **Down syndrome and presports investigation**: Lateral x-ray of the neck to rule out atlantoaxial joint subluxation/dislocation that may cause spinal cord compression and paralysis.

9. **Velocardiofacial (VCF or Sprintzen) and DiGeorge's syndrome:** Both are due to **deletion of chromosome 22(q 11)**. The patients appear with mental

retardation, hypernasal speech without clefting (due to velopharyngeal incompetence), with or without phobias and psychosis.

10. **Pradder-Willi syndrome (deletion of the chromosome 15 q)**: Hypogonadism (in males), truncal obesity, almond-shaped eyes, narrow bifrontal diameter, stubbornness and obsessive-compulsive behavior. The chromosomal deletion is same as in Angelman syndrome.

11. **Angelman syndrome (deletion of the chromosome 15 q): Happy appearance, ataxia, microcephaly**, flat occiput, wide spaced teeth, and prominent nose. Deletion occurs **in the maternally transmitted chromosome**.

12. Retinoblastoma and chromosome: Autosomal dominant and 5% of cases have constitutional deletion of **chromosome 13**, band q14.

13. **Specific cancers and chromosome:**
    (i) Synovial sarcoma: **Chromosomes X and 18**, translocation between the proximal short **arm (p) of the X chromosome** and proximal **long arm (q) of chromosome 18**.
    (ii) **Clear cell sarcoma: Chromosome 12 and 22**, breakpoint near the centromere of chromosome 12 q, the materials distal to breaksite is translocated to chromosome 22.
    (iii) **Chronic myleogenous leukemia**: **Chromosome q and 22**, breakpoint and exhange of chromosomal material results in new fusion gene (BCR on chromosome 22 and ABL oncogene on 9).
    (iv) Metastatic malignant melanoma: Abnormalities in chromosmes 1, 3, 4, 6, 8, 9, 14, and 21; (ring chromosome and missing short arms).

14. **Current recommedation of folic acid in prevention of neural tube defects (NTD)**:
    (i) **All women** of reproductive age should receive at **least 0.4 mg of folic acid/day**.
    (ii) **Women who are at increased risk** for recurrence of NTD's should receive **4.0 mg of folic acid/day** while planning pregnancy and for the first three months of pregnancy.
    (iii) **Folic acid supplementation of 0.8 mg/day** for women of reproductive age may also decrease the incidence of other congenital malformations due to maltifactorial inheritance.

15. **Incidence of pyloric stenosis in first child**, when either of the parents had pyloric stenosis.

(i) Mother had pyloric stenosis: Incidence is 18%.
(ii) Father had pyloric stenonsis: Incidence is 5%.

16. **Sotos syndrome: Increased mandibular growth, long narrow chin, mild mental retardations**, and sometimes abnormal glucose tolerance test. **Mostly sporadic** cases or may be autosomal dominant. This syndrome may be associated with hepatocellular cancer, intestinal polyposis, mixed parotid tumor, osteochondroma, cavernous hemangioma, hariy pigmented nevi, and Wilms' tumor.

17. **Stickler syndrome: Most common is myopia and retinal detachment**, others are mitral valve prolapse, progressive degenerative arthropathy (may require total hip replacement), both conductive and sensorineural hearing losses (need hearing aid).

18. **Beckwith-Wiedemann syndrome** (BWS or overgrowth syndrome): **The gene is located at chromosome 11 p 15.5**. Height ($\geq 95^{th}$ percentile), weight (between 75th and 95th percentile), creases on the ear lobes, pits on the posterior rim of the helix, cardiovascular defects (33% of cases), and normal pubertal development. It may be associated with hepatoblastoma, adrenal cancer, and Wilms' tumor.

19. **Noonan syndrome** (46, xy or male Turner syndrome): Normal chromosome, mental retardation, pulmonic stenosis, malignant hyperthermia may occur, hematologic abnormalities (thrombocytopenia, von Willebrand disease, or Factor XI deficiency). **In young adult**, face is triangular and sharp facial features **but in older adult,** skin is wrinkled and transparent, higher anterior hairline.

20. **William syndrome**: It is due to **deletion of one elastin allele located within chromosome subunit 7 q 11.23**. Mental retardation, supravalvular aortic stenosis, hypercalciuria results in hyperparathyroidism, ectopic calcium deposits. It may be associated with GI problems (obesity, diabetes mellitus, peptic ulcer, diverticulitis, chronic constipation, and cholelithiasis), GU problems (infections, bladder diverticulum, ureteral reflux, renal insufficiency, and nephrolithiasis), and musculoskeletal problems (lordosis and restricted joint movements).

21. **Bardet-Biedl syndrome (autosomal recessive)**: **Severe retinal dystrophy results in blindness**, constricted visual fields, abnormal color vision, mental retardation, **genital hypoplasia** (small testis and penis in males, infertility) is

due to primary germinal hypoplasia and also hypogonadotrophic hypogonadism, **structural and functional changes in the kidneys with hypertension**.

22. **Saethre-chotzen syndrome (autosomal dominant)**: Craniosynostosis, mostly normal intelligence, and deviated nasal septum.

23. **Werner syndrome (chromosome 8p)**: **First sign is gray hair which appears approximately 20 years of** age, followed by loss of hair, atrophic skin (in the face and extremities), cataract, high pitched or hoarse voice, skin ulcers, **finally diabetes at a mean age of 34**, hypertension (50% of cases), vascular calcification, **testicular atrophy, reduced fertility**. Two most common cause of death are cancers (sarcomas and meningiomas) and vascular accidents.

24. **Autosomal recessive**: Affected individual (homozygous) should receive one mutant gene from each parents (heterozygous). Here, only homozygous state has the disease and heterozygous is the carrier. When both parents are heterozygous then offspring can have four different conditions:
    (i) The offspring can receive normal allele from both parents and become normal.
    (ii) The offspring can receive a normal allele from the father and a mutant allele from the mother and become unaffected but heterozygous.
    (iii) The offspring can receive a normal allele from the mother and a mutant allele from the father and become unaffected but heterozygous.
    (iv) The offspring can receive the mutant alleles from both parents and become affected or disease (homozygous).
    So, the chances are 1 in 4 is homozygous, 1 in 2 is heterozygous for mutant gene, and thus 2 in 3 heterozygous.
    The offspring of the diseased (homozygous) person are all carrier (heterozygous) when the spouse is not affected. The offspring could be affected (homozygous) when the spouse is also carrier (heterozygous) which is rare.
    Only one generation of the family will have the disease, that means one individual or his/her sibling (brother or sister) has the disease. Affected person's parents, offspring, cousin, nephew, niece, uncle, or aunt will not have the disease. In description of family tree, when anybody other than the individual's own sibling is affected, it is not autosomal recessive. Diseased (25%), carrier (50%), normal (25%); **males and females are equally affected. It is the most common type**.
    Calculation of carrier and disease in autosomal recessive disorders or cystic fibrosis: Let us assume the person A has autosomal recessive

disease, his sibling is B married to an unrelated spouse C, wants to know the chances that his children will get the disease. The B has 2/3 chances of being heterozygous.

p = Frequency of normal allele.

q2 = Frequency of CF phenotype.

$p + q = 1$

$(p + q)^2 = 1$

$q^2 = 1$ in 2000 (let us assume the frequency of CF gene in the general population).

$$q = \sqrt{\frac{1}{2000}} = \frac{1}{45}$$

$$p = 1 - q = 1 - \frac{1}{45} = \frac{44}{45}$$

The proportion of carriers (frequency of heterozygote) is 2 pq.

$$= 2 \times \frac{44}{45} \times \frac{1}{45} = \frac{1}{22} = 5\% \text{ (approximately)}$$

So, C has 1/22 chances of being heterozygous (carrier).

Both B and C will be heterozygous =2/3 X 1/22 = 1/33 (3%).

The probability of first child will be affected = 1/4 X 1/33 = 1/132 =< 1% (1/4 = autosomal recessive)

The person A has a sister D married to an unrelated spouse. They want to know about the risk of her first child being affected: The same as above i.e., <1%. The risk of birth defect in a newborn of unrelated parents, is 2-3%. The risk of birth defect, in a newborn of related (first cousin) parents, is 4-6% (double).

25. **Autosomal dominant:** Each individual who inherits the gene will have the disease. Affected individual will inherit the gene from his/her affected one parent except in fresh mutation which is rare. Other parent is normal. The affected individual (e.g., he) is heterozygous. He will probably marry a girl who is **not** affected. His children will inherit normal allele from his wife and either the normal or mutant (abnormal) allele from him, so his children will each have 1: 1 chance of having the mutant gene and the disease. (Rarely, if both parents carry the gene, i.e., heterozygous, then their children can inherit either normal or mutant allele from each parent and become homozygous. So, the chances of children become normal 1 in 4, heterozygous 2 in 4, or homozygous 1 in 4 ; so 3 out of 4 being affected.).

    Generation after generation is affected. That means mother or father or uncle or aunt or brother or sister or nephew or niece or cousin is affected. More than one generation is affected. Diseased (50%), normal (50%), no carrier. Male and female are equally affected. It is the second most common type.

26. **X-linked recessive**: Each son of a carrier female has a 50% (1/2) chance of having the disease and each daughter had 50% (1/2) chance of being carrier. All daughters of affected male are carriers of the mutant gene but all sons are normal. Carrier daughter may have affected sons. In each pregnancy the female carrier has a 25% chance of having affected son, 25% chance of carrier daughter, and 50% chance of normal children (son and daughter).
    Only male is affected and female is the carrier. More than one generation is affected. Person's brother, male cousin, nephew, or grandfather has the disease, but sister, niece, female cousin, uncle, aunt, father, mother are not affected. If female is affected, exclude X-linked recessive.
    Diseased (25%), carrier (25%), normal (50%). In each pregnancy of a carrier, 50% of male children are affected and 50% of female children are carrier.
    Example: X-linked recessive (e.g., hemophiliac A).
    (i) A consultand's female whose mother is a carrier and father is normal, but maternal grandfather had the disease and grandmother was normal. The risk that she is a carrier is ½ (50%) and the risk of having an affected son is ½ (carrier) x ¼ (X-linked recessive transmission risk) = 1/8.
    (ii) A consultand's female whose sister become a carrier from her mother and rest of the conditions are same as above. The risk of her become the carrier and her son being affected are the same as above.
    (iii) A consultand's female whose mother is not a carrier and father is normal, but maternal uncle had the disease and grandmother was the carrier but grandfather was normal. The risk that she is a carrier is 1/33 (3%) and risk of having an affected son is 1/33 X ¼ = 1/32 =< 1%.
    (iv) A consultand's male whose brother has the disease, one sister is the carrier, and other sister is not a carrier. The chances that he is a carrier zero because male cannot be the carrier and the chance of having an affected son is zero if the mother is not a carrier.
    (v) A consultand's female who is a carrier, the chances of having an affected child already been discussed.

27. **X-linked dominant:** Generation after generation, more than one generation is affected. Person's father or mother, brother and/or sister, nephew and/or niece, uncle and/or aunt has the disease. All daughters of the affected father will be affected, but none of his sons. If mother is affected, both the sons and daughters will be affected, and it will then be difficult to differentiate this from autosomal dominant.
    Diseased (50%), normal (50%), no carrier; equal incidence in male and female, but males are seriously affected.

28. **How to detect mode of transmission when family pedigree is given.**
    (a) See if more than one generation has been affected: Exclude autosomal recessive.
    (b) See if a female has the disease: Exclude X-linked recessive.
    (c) See if mother and father are not affected: Diagnosis is autosomal recessive or X-linked recessive.
    (d) See if mother or father is affected: Diagnosis is autosomal dominant or X-linked dominant.
    (e) See if the father and all his daughters are affected but non of his sons are affected: It is X-linked dominant.
    (f) See if the father and half of his daughters and half of his sons are affected: It is an autosomal dominant.
    (g) See if the mother and half of her daughter and half of her sons are affected: Either autosomal dominant or X-linked dominant. In X-linked dominant sons are affected more seriously.

29. **Important points in genetic counseling.**
    (A) **First step in genetic counseling: To confirm the diagnosis**. The diagnosis is confirmed by the following.
        (i) To review the medical records.
        (ii) To obtain medical history.
        (iii) Physical examination.
        (iv) Conventional laboratory test: Bone X-ray, alpha-1 antitrypsin serum levels.
        (v) Molecular genetic analysis: Specific DNA markers.
    (B) **Second** important part of genetic counseling is **putting the risk in perspective**. The perception of risk may have more importance in family decision making than actual numerical value of the risk. Physical handicap may be a severe burden and mental handicap is unacceptable.
    (C) **Third** is presymptomatic diagnosis of inherited disorders (e.g., breast cancer, Huntington's disease, and alpha-1 antitrypsin deficiency).
    (D) **Fourth** is the description of the disorder in booklets, pamphlets, and other informative literature.

30. **Gene therapy:** The alteration of pathopsysiologic state by introducing nucleic acids into a cell. These nucleic acids may be genes, portion of genes, oligonucleotides, or RNA.
    Different strategies of gene therapy in cancer patients:
    (i) Inhibitory genes construct for over expressed or dysregulated dominant oncogenes.
    (ii) A wild-type tumor suppressor gene for recessive oncogene mutations.

(iii) Toxin genes selectively delivered to cancer cells to destroy and eradicate them.
(iv) Immunomodulatory genes to enhance the immunogenicity of tumors.

31. **Different diseases and mode of transmission.**
   (A) **Autosomal recessive.**
      (i) Alpha-1 antitrypsin deficiency.
      (ii) Cystic fibrosis.
      (iii) Albinism.
      (iv) Wilson's disease.
      (v) Hemochromatosis.
      (vi) Homocystinuria.
      (vii) Sickle-cell anemia.
      (viii) Tay-Sachs disease.
      (ix) Cystinuria.
      (x) 21-Hydroxylase deficiency.
      (xi) Phenylketonuria.
      (xii) Galactosemia.
      (xiii) Glycogen storage disease.
   (B) **Autosomal dominant**.
      (i) Familial hypercholesterolemia.
      (ii) von Willebrand's disease.
      (iii) Marfan syndrome.
      (iv) Acute intermittent porphyria.
      (v) Huntington's disease.
      (vi) Polycystic kidney disease.
      (vii) Hypertrophic obstructive cardiomyopathy.
      (viii) Hereditary spherocytosis.
      (ix) Osteogenesis imperfecta tarda.
   (C) **X-linked**.
      (i) Fragile X syndrome.
      (ii) G6PD deficiency.
      (iii) Hemophilia A, B.
      (iv) Duchenne muscular dystrophy.

32. **Different diseases and chromosomes**.

Diseases	**Chromosomes**.
(i) Familial polyposis of the colon	5 q
(ii) Cyctic fibrosis	7 q
(iii) NF2 (bilateral acoustic neuroma)	22 q
(iv) Alzheimer disease I	21 pter-q 21

(v) Myotonic dystrophy	19 q
(vi) Wilson disease	13 q
(vii) Huntington's disease	4 q
(viii) Alagille syndrome	20 p
(ix) Neurofibromatosis	17 q
(x) Adult type polycystic kidney disease	16 p
(xi) Charcot-Marie-Tooth neuropathy 1	1 q
(xii) Kidd blood group	18 q
(xiii) Xeroderma pigmentosa	15
(xiv) Variegate porphyria	14 q
(xv) von Hippel-Lindau syndrome	3 p
(xvi) Pradder-willi syndrome	15
(xvii) Werner syndrome	8 p
(xviii) Velo-cardio-facial syndrome (VCF)	22 q
(xix) Beckwith-Wiedemann syndrome (BWS)	11 p

STATISTICS

1. **Null hypothesis**: When we compare two groups in a study and notice some differences between them, the null hypothesis may suggest that the observed differences are due just to random variation in the data. If you accept null hypothesis, you think that observed differences are due to such random variations, but if you reject the null hypothesis, you think that observed differences are not due to random variations. **Null hypothesis may be true or false**.
   Type I (alpha) error means null hypothesis is true, but rejected.
   Type II (beta) error means null hypothesis is false, but accepted.
   No error means either null hypothesis is true and accepted or is false and rejected.

2. **The P value:** P value < 0.01 means the result is statistically significant because the probability of random variation alone is very small.

3. **Incidence of the exposed and non exposed group**:
   (Disease is cancer, exposure in smoking).

	Disease present	**Disease absent**
Exposure present	A (80)	B (20)
Exposure absent	C (30)	D (70)

   Incidence rate of exposed group = A/A+B = 80/80+20 = 80%
   Incidence rate of non exposed group = C/C+D = 30/30+70 = 30%
   Incidence rate = Only new disease cases over a period of time is divided by population at risk, so incidence means new cases.
   Prevalence rate = Total number of cases at a given time is divided by total populations, so prevalence means all cases.

4. **Sensitivity and specificity**: (test of VDRL for syphilis).

	Disease present	**Disease absent.**
Positive screening	A (90)	B (20)
Negative screening	C (10)	D (80)

   Sensitivity = A/A+C = 90/100 = 90%
   Specificity = D/B+D = 80/100 = 80%
   Positive predictive value = A/A+B = 90/110 = 81%
   Negative predictive value = D/C+D = 80/90 = 88%
   Sensitivity = Persons with the disease and positive screening test divided by number of persons tested with disease (100), i.e., sensitivity of test means it gives a positive finding when the person has the disease.

Specificity = Persons without the disease and negative screening test is divided by number of persons tested without diseases (100), i.e., specificity of a test means it gives a negative result when the person does **not** have disease.
Positive predictive value = Persons with the disease and positive screening test divided by the total number of positive screening test.
Negative predictive value = Persons without the disease and negative screening tests divided by the total number of negative screening test.
In syphilis, RPR and VDRL have high sensitivity, so the test can give high false positive and few false negative results, but FTA-ABS has high specificity which gives correct diagnosis.
A = True positive, D = True negative.
B = False positive, C = False negative.

5. **Case control studies.**

	Liver failure	**Normal liver.**
Alcoholic	A (70)	B (20)
Non-alcoholic	C (30)	D (80)

Cases = A/A+C = 70/100 = 70%
Controls = B/B+D = 20/100 = 20%
Incidence of exposed group = A/A+B = 70/90 = 77%
Incidence of non-exposed group = C/C+D = 30/110 = 27%

6. **Relative risk** = Incidence rate among exposed group is divided by incidence rate among non-exposed group = 77%/27% = 2.9% (calculated from liver failure and alcohol abuse).
Attributal risk = Incidence rate among exposed group minus incidence rate among non-exposed group = 77%-27% = 50% (calculated from liver failure and alcohol abuse).
Absolute risk = Same as incidence.
= A/A+B = 70/90 = 77% (calculated from liver failure and alcohol abuse from item 5 in case control study).

7. **Mean** = Sum of the numbers associated with the observations is divided by the number of observations.
Median = Middle number.
Mode = Most frequently occuring number.

8. **Probalility of a disease condition.**

Probability = Total number of times disease occurs is divided by total number of times disease can occur (e.g., total number of AIDS patients = 60, total number of pneumocystis pneumonia = 20, so probability = 20/60 = 33%).

9. **Chi-square test**: This test is most commonly used for differences between proportions, i.e., comparing effects of two different drugs used in two different groups.

PHARMACOLOGIC PRINCIPLES

1. Volume of distribution of drug (Vd): It means total amount of drug is present in the body in relation to its serum concentration.

   Formula:

$$Vd = \frac{\text{Dose (mg)}}{\text{Plasma level (Cp)}}$$

   Example: (Drug X) Plasma level (Cp) = 10 microgram/ml.

   Volume of distribution (Vd) = 100 L =100,000 ml.

$$\text{Dose} = Vd \times Cp$$
$$= 100{,}000 \text{ X } 10 \text{ microgram}$$
$$= 1000 \text{ mg}$$

   (i) So, the dose of the drug X can be calculated if the volume of distribution and plasma levels are given.

   (ii) The plasma level can be calculated when the Vd and dose are given.

$$Cp = \frac{\text{Dose (mg)}}{Vd} = \frac{1000 \text{ mg}}{100 \text{ L}}$$
$$= \frac{1000{,}000 \text{ microgram}}{100{,}000 \text{ ml}}$$
$$= 10 \text{ microgram / ml}$$

   (iii) The loading dose of the drug should be calculated from this formula.

   (iv) When the volume of distribution of the drug is reduced from 100 L to 50 L and the dose given (1000 mg) then the plasma level will be.

$$Cp = \frac{1000 \text{ mg}}{50 \text{ L}} = \frac{1000{,}000 \text{ microgram}}{50{,}000 \text{ ml}}$$
$$= 20 \text{ microgram / ml}$$

   The higher drug level may induce toxicity.

2. **Half-life of drug (T ½).**

$$T\tfrac{1}{2} = \frac{0.693 \times Vd}{\text{Cl (clearance)}}$$

   (0.693 = extra cellular fluid volume). It is a time when drug serum level drops by half (50%). In order to calculate the half-life, Vd and Cl values should be provided.

   Example

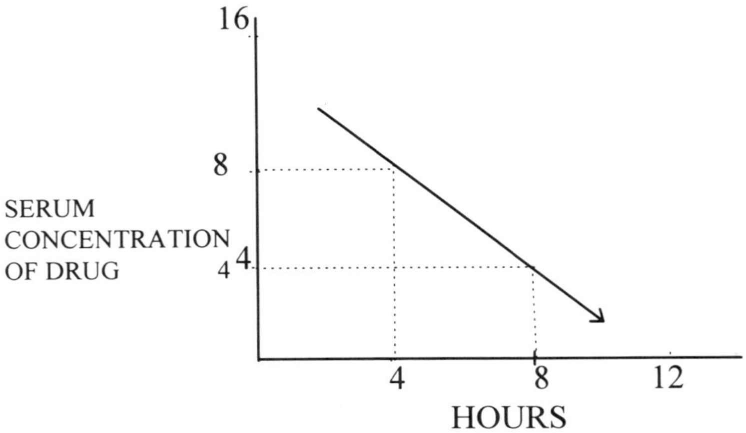

Serum concentration of drug is 8 at 4 hours and is 4 at 8 hours, the drug level is reduced to half in 4 hours, serum half-life is 4 hours.

3. **Clearance (Cl)**: It is the amount of drug removed per unit of time from the body.

$$Cl = \frac{0.693 \times Vd}{T\frac{1}{2}}$$

In order to calculate the clearance, Vd and T ½ values should be provided.

4. **Steady state concentration of drug.**

$$\text{Steady state (Css)} = \frac{\text{Rate of infusion (Rinf)}}{\text{Cl (clearance)}}$$

It is **4 to 5 times** of half life. Approximately 94% steady state is achieved in 4 half life and **97% steady state is achieved in 5 half life**. The 5 times of the half time is the correct answer.
Example: Drug X has half life is **30 minutes**, so steady state will be achieved in **120 to 150 minutes**. In 'steady state', tissues are in equilibrum i.e., amount of drug infused is equal to amount of drug eliminated. When serum half life is not given then Css can be calculated from the values of Rinf and Cl.

5. **Calculation of Css (steady state) when medication is given by mouth (PO):**
Example: A 70 kg weight asthmatic receiving theophylline 480 mg Q.12.H, the calculation of serum steady state maximum (Css, max) and steady state minimum (Css, min). The physician wants to maintain the plasma concentration 15 mg/L

$$\text{Css, max} = \frac{\text{F.dose / Vd}}{1\text{-}\exp(\text{-kT})} = \frac{480 \text{ mg / 35 L}}{0.65} = 21 \text{ mg / L}$$

[F.dose = 480 mg, Vd = 0.5 l/kg = 0.5 X 70 = 35 L, 1 = oral availability, exp(-KT) = 0.35, the fraction of the last dose (corrected for bioavailability) that remains in the body at the end of a dosing interval].
Css, min = (Css, max) X [exp(-KT)]
= 21 X (0.35) = 7.4 mg/L

6. **First-order (or linear) kinetics and zero-order (or nonlinear or dose-dependent) kinetics:**

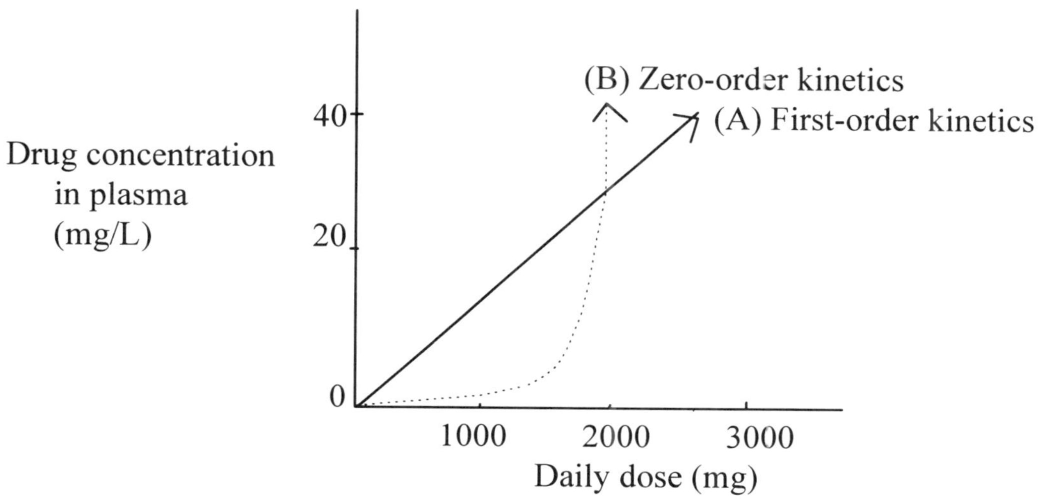

(A) **First-order kinetics**: The amount of drug eliminated is directly proportional to the concentration of drug in the plasma. Most of the drugs follow the first-order kinetics. These drugs do not cause rapid toxicities.
(B) **Zero-order kinetics:** The elimination of the drug does not increase with the increase in doses, results in rapid rise of drug plasma levels (e.g., phenytoin, salicylates, and ethanol) results in toxicity.

7. **First-pass effect**: When a drug crosses the intestinal wall or passes through the liver, it can be bound further or metabolized. This process is called first-pass effect (or elimination). If the GI absorption is complete, this effect equals the liver extraction rate.

8. **Distribution and elimination phases of a drug.**

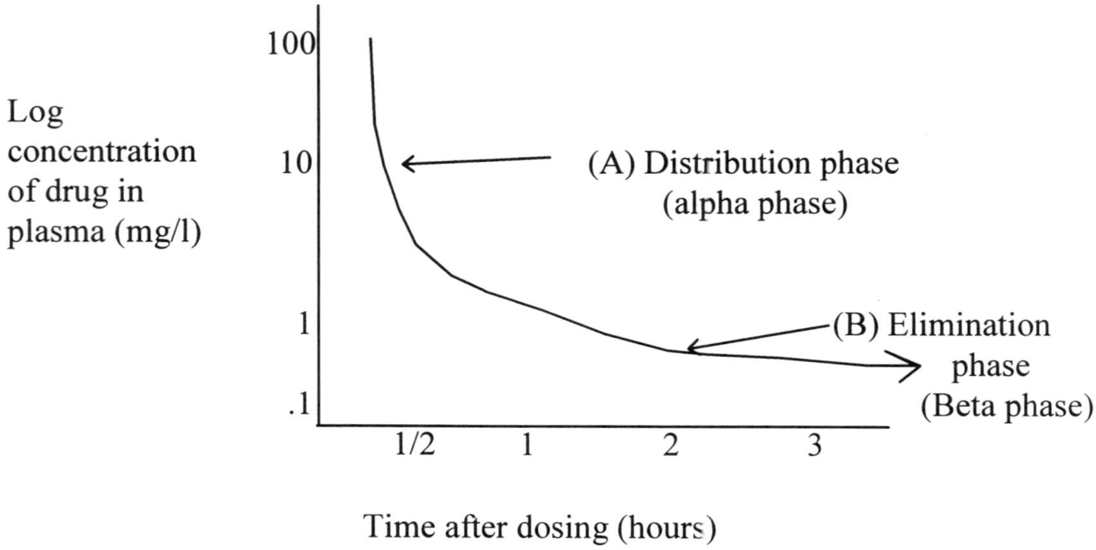

(A) **Distribution phase:** Initial portion when cencentration of the drug decreases rapidly.
(B) **Elimination phase:** The later portion when concentration of the drug decreases slowly.

9. **Pharmacokinetic changes in the elderly:**
   (i) Most typical is the **increase in the total body fat** but **decrease in lean body mass, total body water, plasma**, proteins, and albumin.
   (ii) Vd (volume of distribution) is reduced in water-soluble drugs and Vd is increased in lipid-soluble drugs.
   (iii) Both cardiac output and blood flows to the kidneys (reduced GFR as much as 50%) and liver (less affected except drugs with high hepatic clearance, e.g., lidocaine).

10. **Pharmacodynamic changes and recommedations in the elderly:**
   (i) Elderly patients may have increased target-organ sensitivity, **so the lowest effective dose should be used** (e.g., anticoagulants may cause increased bleeding and antianxiety, sedative-hypnotic drugs may cause increased CNS depression with the doses well tolerated by young adults).
   (ii) Increased drug interactions and adverse drug responses for both prescription and over the counter medications.
   (iii) The drugs which are eliminated by the **kidneys may be reduced by 50%**.
   (iv) The drugs which are eliminated by the **liver** may **not** need the adjustment except drugs with high hepatic clearance.

11. **Few important points in drug interactions:**

(i) The risk of drug interaction in critically ill patients usually increased when receiving **more than 10 medications** especially AIDS patients.
(ii) The 6-mercaptopurine (**antileukemic drug**) inhibits the metabolism of allopurinol (used to control hyperuricemia), results in allopurinol toxicities (Important).
(iii) **Amiodarone (half life is 1 to 2 months) inhibits the metabolism** of calcium-channel blocker, flecainide, **warfarin**, quinidine, and phenytoin **for several months after being discontinued**.
(iv) **Cimetidine** can inhibit the metabolism of warfarin, **diazepam, propranolol, theophylline,** quinidine, imipramine, and lidocaine.
(v) **Phenytoin** metabolism is inhibited by **valproic acid, INH**, clofibrate, dicoumarol, chloramphenicol, and phenylbutazone.
(vi) Probenecid inhibits penicillin transport, decreases its clearance, and increases the effectiveness of penicillin.
(vii) The **renal excretion of methotrexate is inhibited** by salicylates, probenecid, and phenylbutazone.
(viii) The blood pressure lowering effect of guanidinium-type of antihypertensives **are blocked** by TCA, phenothiazines, and ephedrine.
(ix) **Cigarette smoke and the following drugs** (e.g., ethanol, phenobarbital, phenytoin, rifampin, griseofulvin, and glutethimide) **can increase the hepatic metabolism through P-450 system of the following drugs** (e.g., **theophylline, beta-blockers, warfarin, corticosteroids**, cyclosporine, and cyclophosphamide) result in reduced effectiveness.
(x) Colestipol and cholestyramine can bind with digoxin and warfarin in the GI tract like iron-binds with tetracycline.

12. **Few important items in toxic or immunologic response to drugs:**
(i) **Penicillin** allergy is due to penicilloic acid, or penicilloyl-polylysine (**Important**).
(ii) Most severe form of drug allergy is anaphylaxis, which is due to an **IgE-mediated hypersensitivity (Important).**
(iii) Immunologic reaction of the drug occurs when it binds with protein to form drug-protein complex (compounds with low molecular weight < 1000 are **not** antigenic).
(iv) **Cisplatin** causes **direct toxicity** to the kidney and VIII cranial nerve.
(v) **Acetaminophen undergoes oxidative metabolism** to **form toxic reactive metabolites** which is detoxified by glutathione. **N-acetylcysteine forms complex with reactive metabolites** and reduces hepatic toxicity in acetaminophen overdose.

PAIN

1. **Characteristic of pain:**
   (i) **Acute pain**: It is due to hyperactivity of the autonomic nervous system results in **tachycardia, diaphoresis, and hypertension**.
   (ii) **Subacute pain**: It develops over several days, and episodic pain appears for a set period of time on a recurring basis.
   (iii) **Chronic pain**: It is the persistence of pain for 3 months or longer.

2. **Etiologic characteristics of pain:**
   (i) Chronic pain with structural diseases (e.g., metastatic cancer, rehumatoid arthritis, sickle cell disease): To treat the underlying disease and the pain.
   (ii) Psychophysiologic disorders causing pain (e.g., herniated disc, torn ligament): The best management is through a **structured rehabilitation program designed to modify pain behavior but not** through medical management. Use of analgesics are **not** very effective.
   (iii) **Pain without structural or physiologic basis (e.g., psychiatric illness)**: To treat the underlying psychiatric disorder is important. The patients do **not** respond to pain treatment.

3. **Few important points in assessment of pain:**
   (i) All patients with pain should be evaluated adequately.
   (ii) History, physical, and neurological examination should be done.
   (iii) Appropriate diagnostic procedures should be done and therapy should be instituted.
   (iv) Provide continuity of care to reduce patient's anxiety, to ensure patient's compliance, and to asses patient's response to therapy.
   (v) Patients with pain can have psychiatric syndromes (e.g., anxiety, depression).
   (vi) Alternative method of pain control (such as temporary use of local anesthetic via epidural catheter in vertebral body collapse) should be started initially rather than using as a last resort.
   (vii) Painful diagnostic procedures should **not** be done in advanced cancer patients or terminally ill patients.
   (viii) Discuss advance directives for managing pain of dying patients.

4. **Side effects of opioid medications and management**: Opioid (agonist are morphine, codeine, meperidine, oxycodone, propoxyphene hydrochloride; mixed agonist/antagonist are pentazocine, butorphanol).
   (i) Respiratory depression: Treated with naloxone.
   (ii) Nausea, vomiting: Use antiemetics.

(iii) Constipation: Appropriate diet, cathartics, stool softeners.
(iv) Seizures: It is mostly due to **nonmeperidine** which is a metabolite of meperidine. Multifocal myoclonus occurs more commonly in patients with renal insufficiency receiving meperidine.
Treatment: Stop the meperidine, use alternative drugs such as fentanyl or methadone which are **not** mostly excreted by the kidneys.

5. **Management of pain:**
(A) **Mild to moderate pain:** Use nonopioid analgesics (e.g., aspirin, acetaminophen, and NSAID's). The patients should receive the maximum dose of one drug before switch to another drug. If the pain is **not** controlled then switch to opioid analgesics.
(B) **Moderate to severe pain.**
(i) Use opioid agonist or antagonist plus nonopioid.
(ii) Opioids plus adjuvants (e.g., hydroxyzine and dextroamphetamine).
(C) **Management of tolerant patients**.
(i) Use combination of nonopioid and opioid drugs.
(ii) Use combination of drug therapy, anesthetic, and neurosurgical procedures.
(iii) Use alternate opioid analgesic starting with ¼ to ½ of the analgesic dose and titrate to analgesia.
(iv) Use epidural local anesthetic alone or in combination with opioids.
(D) To prevent and treat physical dependence (withdrawal signs after abrupt withdrawn of the drugs) and psychological dependence (craving a drug for other than pain relief, involvement to get it and use it).
(E) Best route of administration is oral, any other routes can be used.
(F) Do **not** use placebos to asses the pain.
(G) Alternate methods of pain control.
(i) Physical therapy.
(ii) Cognitive behavioral therapy.
(iii) Anesthetic and neurosurgical therapy.

6. **Management of cancer pain:**
(A) **First-step**: Non-opioid with or without adjuvant for pain.
(B) **Second-step**: Weak opioid with or without non-opioid with or without adjuvant for pain persisting or increasing.
(C) **Third-step:** Strong opioid with or without non-opioid with or without adjuvant.
(D) If the pain is unresponsive to above therapies.
(i) Localized pain: Neurolytic blocks is used in tumor infiltration in the chest wall or other local infiltrations.

(ii) Pain is unilateral and below the waist: Cordotomy may be considered.
(iii) Diffuse pain: Nitrous oxide inhalation may be used.
(iv) **Chronic pain**: Behavioral approaches include relaxation techniques, breathing exercises, and cognitive control of pain, used as an adjuvants.

(E) The physician is responsible for providing continuing care, constantly reassessing both the diagnosis and treatment to achieve maximum relief of pain and suffering for both the patient and the family.

7. **A nonmalignant patient is on chronic opioid therapy, the physician should assess the following in each visit:**
(i) Opioid-related side effects.
(ii) Degree of analgesia or comfort.
(iii) Functional status (physical and psychosocial).
(iv) Watch for aberrant drug-related behaviors.

PREVENTIVE HEALTH CARE

1. Common **misconception** in preventive health care:
   (i) Disease with a strong heritability component **cannot** be altered. **It is not true** because genetic traits for disease often result from the influence of multiple genes and need environmental factors for expression.
   (ii) Prevention is less useful in older persons. **It is not true** because elderly persons have a greater absolute risk of disease and preventive measures are helpful.

2. Most common cause of death in USA of all age groups: **Heart disease (35.7%), next is cancer (22.4%)**.
   (i) Between age 25-44 = Accidents.
   (ii) Between age 45-64 = Cancer.
   (iii) Between age 65-74 = Heart disease.
   (iv) Between age 75 + = heart disease.

3. US PS TF (United States Preventive Services Task Force) recommendations:
   (a) **Lung cancer screening**: Routine CXR is **not recommended** because early detection does not usually alter patient's prognosis.
   (b) **Prostate cancer screening**: Determination of PSA and rectal examination are **not recommeded** for prostate cancer screening.
   (c) **Colon cancer screening.**
      (i) Fecal occult blood/sigmoidoscopy (age 50 and above): Annual fecal occult blood and/or periodic flexible sigmoidoscopy.
      (ii) Fecal occult blood/sigmoidoscopy (high risk group): Person age 50 or older who have first-degree relatives with colorectal cancer; a personal history of breast, ovary, or endometrial cancer; or a previous diagnosis of inflammatory bowel ldisease, adenomatous polyps, or colorectal cancer.
      (iii) Colonoscopy (high risk, age 19-39): Persons with a family history of familial polyposis coli or cancer family syndrome.
      (iv) Fecal occult blood/colonoscopy (high risk, age 40 and above): Person with a family history of familial polyposis coli or cancer family syndrome.
   (d) **Breast cancer screening**: Mammography (high risk age 35-49, and 50 and above): Women aged 35 and older with a family history of premenopausally diagnosed breast cancer in a first-degree relative; otherwise every 1 to 2 years beginnig at age 50.

(e) **Cervical cancer screening (age 19-64, high risk 65 and over)**: Pap smear every 1 to 3 years. At 65 and over only women have **not** had previous documented screening in which smears have been consistently negative.
(f) **Osteoporosis screening (high risk 40-64)**: Determination of bone mineral content in premenopausal women at increased risk for osteoporosis (e.g., bilateral removal of the ovary before menopause, slender build) and for whom estrogen replacement therapy would otherwise not be recommended.
(g) **HIV infection screening (high risk 19-64)**: Persons with STD; homosexual and bisexual men; past or present IV drug abusers; history of prostitution and multiple sexual partners; women whose past or present sexual partners were HIV infected, bisexual, or IV drug users; persons with long-term residence or birth in an area with high prevalence of HIV infection; or persons with history of transfusion between 1978 and 1985.
(h) **Heart disease screening (age 19 and above):** Men > 40 with two or more cardiac risk factors (high BP, high blood cholesterol, cigarette smoking, family history of coronary artery disease, and diabetes mellitus), or sedentary or high-risk men planning to begin a vigorous exercise program, or men who would endanger public safety (e.g., airline pilots).
(i) **TB screening (high risk 19 and older)**: PPD testing should be done in household members of persons with TB or **others at risk for close contact with the disease** (e.g., staff of TB clinics, shelters for the homeless, substance abuse treatment facilities, nursing homes, correctional institutions, and dialysis units); residents of homeless shelters, nursing home, or correctional facilities; recent immigrants or refugees from countries in which TB is common, migrant workers; or **persons with HIV infection**.
(j) **Thyroid function tests (women 65 and over) and glaucoma testing by an eye doctor (65 and over, both men and women)**.
(k) **Hearing test (high risk 19-64)**: Persons exposed regularly to excessive noise.
(l) **Nonfasting total cholesterol (age 19 and over).**
(m) **Fasting glucose (high risk 19 and over)**: The severely obese, persons with family history of diabetes, or women with history of gestational diabetes.
(n) **Rubella antibodies (high risk 19-39)**: Women lack evidence of immunity.
(o) **VDRL (high risk 19-64)**: Prostitutes, persons who engage in sex with multiple partners, or contact of persons with active syphilis.
(p) **Gonorrhea culture (high risk 19-64)**: Prostitutes, persons with multiple sexual partners, or sexual contacts with a persons who has culture-proven GC, or persons with history of repeated GC.
(q) **Chlamydial testing (high risk 19-64)**: Persons attend clinics for STD, other high-risk health care facilities, or have risk factors for chlamydial

infection (e.g., multiple sexual contacts or a sexual partner with multiple sexual contacts, age less than 20).

4. **Goals for Americans to achieve the following dietary recommendations:**
   (A) **Fat**.
      (i) Total (% of calories) = < 30 (< 25).
      (ii) Saturated (% of calories) = < 10 (< 7).
      (iii) Cholesterol (mg/day) = < 300 (< 200).
   (B) **Carbohydrates** (% of calories) = ≥50 (≥55).
   (C) Vegetables and fruits (1/2 cup servings/day = 5(7) or more.
   (D) Whole grain products/legumes (servings/day) = 6 or more.
   (E) Fiber (grams/day) = 20-30.
   (F) Red meat (3-0z servings/week) = < 3.
   (G) Alcohol (as ethanol, 0z/day) = < 1.
   (H) Salt (grams/day) = < 6.
   (Fat has 9 Kcal/gram, carbohydrate and protein have 4 Kcal/gram); hence, **reduce fat intake is the best way to reduce energy intake** and **to reduce the risk of obesity and diabetes. Reducing total fat intake may reduce the risk of cancers (e.g., colon, prostate, and breast); Reducing saturated fat specifically lowers risk of coronary artery disease. Recent study suggests too much reduction of fat is not needed.**

5. **Alcohol and dietary supplements recommendations**:
   (a) Less than 1 0z/day (equivalent to two cans of beer, two small glasses of wine, or two average cocktails). Some studies suggest that moderate alcohol intake reduces the risk of coronary artery disease, this does **not mean that nondrinkers should start drinking because 1 0z of alcohol has 200 Kcal.**
   (b) Routine use of nutritional supplements is of **little or no benefit**, and **unprescribed daily use of supplements in amount exceeding the recommended allowances should be avoided**.

6. **Exercise and its benefit:**
   (a) **Moderate and vigorous exercise has health benefits**. Moderate exercise means brisk walking at 3 to 4 miles per hour, vigorous exercise means jogging, singles tennis, and moving heavy furniture.
   (b) Only 40% of American adults are physically active on a regular basis (20 minutes or more at least 3 times/week), 30% of adults are completely sedentary during their leisure time.
   (c) **The most direct benefits of physical activity are CVS and musculoskeletal adaptations**.

(d) **The regular physical activites are helpful** in CHD (coronary heart disease), bone density, glucose metabolism, and mental health.
(e) **Mental health:** Exercise reduces anxiety and depression.
(f) **Cancer**: Exercise lowers the mortality from cancers of **colon** (by reducing intestinal transit time) and **breast. Excercise alters endocrine functions**.
(g) **Osteoporosis**: Bone density is reduced by bed rest and increase by weight-bearing activity. **Postmenopausal women who walk approximately 1 mile/day have higher bone mineral density and slower rate of bone loss than sedentary women**. The combination of physical activity, calcium supplementation, and estrogen replacement therapy may or may not be helpful for women.
(h) **Diabetes**: Exercise may **also prevent non-insulin dependent diabetes mellitus (NIDDM)** by increasing the muscle glucose uptake and also increases insulin sensitivity.
(i) **Weight control**: Most effective methods to maintain ideal body weight are the **diet and regular** physical activity.
(j) **CHD (coronary heart disease):** Physical activity prevents CHD by the following mechanisms:
    (i) **Reduces the following:** Systolic BP, diastolic BP, triglycerides, weight gain, platelet adhesion, thrombosis, myocardial oxygen demand, and ventricular arrythmias.
    (ii) **Increased the following:** HDL cholesterol, glucose uptake, insulin sensitivity, fibrinolysis, and myocardial oxygen supply.

7. **Most common negative effect of physical activity: Musculoskeletal overuse injuries of the lower extremities. Three factors are strongly associated with this injury:**
   (i) Previous injury is the strongest predictor of future injury.
   (ii) Exercise intensity.
   (iii) Increased duration of activity or mileage.
   Physician's advice to patients to avoid this injury:
   (i) Tell the patients about the risk factors causing injuries.
   (ii) Advice moderate physical activity.
   (iii) Gradual increase in duration of activity or mileage.
   Other negative effects of exercise.
   (i) Exacerbation of asthma.
   (ii) Exacerbation of diabetes.
   (iii) Rarely, the risk of cardiac arrest is **transiently elevated** for both those who are **not regularly active and regularly active**. However, **the overall risk of cardiac arrest is reduced in active group**.
   Physician's advice to patients to avoid those illnesses:

(i) Reduce the physical activity from vigorous to moderate.

8. Most common cause of sudden death during jogging: **Underlying coronary heart disease**.

9. **Medical examinations before participation in exercise:**
   (i) **Men over age 40 and women over age 50** should undergo medical examination before participating in **vigorous exercise program**.
   (ii) Persons with **multiple risk factors for** CVS disease should undergo medical examination.
   (iii) **Persons with sympotmatic CVS disease** should undergo physician-supervised, symptom-limited exercise with BP and EKG monitoring.
   (iv) **No medical examination** is needed for persons free of disease and wanted to participate in moderate-intensity physical activity (e.g., walking).

10. **The exercise recommendation of CDC (Centers for Disease Control) and Prevention and the American College of Sports Medicine**: "Every American adults should accumulate 30 minutes or more of moderate intensity physical activity on most, preferably all, days of the week".

11. **Tobacco smoke may produce illness by**.
    (i) Systemic absorption of toxins.
    (ii) Local lung injury by oxidant gases.

12. **Tobacco withdrawal symptoms**: The long term users may **develop physical dependence and associated with increased number of nicotine cholinergic receptors in the brain**. The patients develop the **following symptoms**: Anxiety, irritability, restlessness, difficulty in concentration, craving for tobacco, hunger, disturbed sleep, and sometimes depression.

13. **The highest number of mortality in cancer due to smoking in both men and women: Lung cancer**; other sites of cancers are esophagus, oral cavity, larynx, pancreas, bladder, kidneys, stomach, crevix, and blood (leukemia).

14. **Tobacco related illnesses are the following**.
    (A) **CVS: Coronary heart disease results in sudden death**, cerebrovascular disease, peripheral vascular disease (e.g., aortic aneurysm), atherosclerosis, and acute ischemic episodes.
    Mechanism of damage by smoking:

(i) **Increase of the following:** BP, heart rate, endothelial injury, LDL, oxidized LDL, coagulability, arrythmia, polycythemia, and blood viscocity.
(ii) **Decrease of the following**: HDL, relatively low oxygen is due to elevated carbon monoxide.

(B) **Pulmonary disease**: **More than 80% of COPD in USA is due to cigarette smoking**, other diseases are the following: respiratory infections (mostly viral, also bacterial), chronic bronchitis, emphysema, airway obstruction, **and cancer.**
Mechanisms of pulmonary injury from smoking.
(i) Direct injury of oxidant gases.
(ii) Decreased antiprotease activity.
(iii) Increased elastase activity (a protein that breaks down elastin and other **connective tissues**).

(C) **GI symptoms:** Esophageal reflux, duodenal and gastric ulcers, and cancers (e.g., esophagus, stomach).
Mechanisms of ulcer formation:
(i) Increase acid secretion.
(ii) Decrease of the following: Pancreatic bicarbonate secretion, pyloric sphincter tone, and gastric mucosal barrier (due to decreased PGE synthesis and gastric mucosal blood flow).

(D) **Osteoporosis**: Cigarette smoking **reduces the peak bone mass** attained in early adulthood and **increases the rate of bone loss in late adulthood.**

(E) Increased risk of cataract, olfactory dysfunction, facial wrinkling, and fire-related injuries.

15. **Interaction between cigarette smoking and drugs:**
(i) **Propranolol**: Reduced antianginal and antihypertensive effects.
(ii) **Nifedipine (and other calcium channel blocker)**: Reduced antianginal effect.
(iii) **Oral contraceptives**: Enhanced thrombosis, stroke, and myocardial infarction.
(iv) **Cimetidine and other H_2 blockers**: **Lower rate of ulcer healing and higher rate of ulcer recurrence**.
(v) Diazepam, chlordiazepoxide, and chorpromazine: Reduced sedation.
(vi) Propoxyphene: Reduced analgesia.

16. **Higher doses of following drugs are needed in smokers due to enhanced metabolism of drugs by smoking: Theophylline, propranolol, heparin, flecainide, imipramine**, desmethyldiazepam, oxazepam, estradiol, estrone, phenylbutazone, pentazocine, phenacetin, antipyrine, and caffeine.

17. **Treatment of nicotine addiction:**
    (a) **National Cancer Institute developed a office smoking cessation program (4 A's):**
        (i) **Ask** about smoking at every opportunity.
        (ii) **Advice** all smokers to stop.
        (iii) **Assist** the patient in stopping and maintaining abstinence.
        (iv) **Arrange** follow-up to reinforce non-smoking.
    (b) Nicotine replacement medications (e.g., nicotine gum and transdermal nicotine patch): All smokers should be instructed to quit smoking completely before the onset of nicotine replacement therapy.
        Side effects of nicotine gum: **Hiccups, upset stomach**, jaw fatigue, sore mouth and sore throat.
    (c) Physician advice to quit smoking, minimal intervention programs, and more intensive treatment (e.g., smoking cessation clinic) help in reducing the incidence of smoking.
    (d) Remember, 70% of smokers would like to quit and 70% or more relapse even after the best treatment. Advice them to try again and again.

18. **Few important points in injury:**
    (i) **Injuries** are the leading cause of death for all American aged 1 to 44.
    (ii) **Unintentional injury** is the most common, next is suicide then homicide.
    (iii) **Firearm deaths exceed** motor vehicle deaths for **men from age 25 to 84**, the peak among **young men is mainly homicide** and the peak among **older men is mainly suicide**.
    (iv) **Motor vehicle deaths exceed** firearm deaths among the young (< 25 years) and very elderly (> 84 years). Both groups are vulnerable to pedestrian and vehicle occupant deaths.
    (v) **Alcohol consumption is a major risk factor** for all types of injury, both intentional (homicide and suicide) and unintentional (motor vehicle accidents).
    (vi) **Falls** accounted for 1/3 of all injury-related admission.
    (vii) **Violence against girls and women by intimates, and relatives are more common** than by strangers. **Women usually report violence by strangers** than nonstrangers.

19. **Physicians participation to reduce the injury and violence:**
    (i) Counsel patients about injury risk and prevention (e.g., gun control, airbags, seatbelts, child car seats, helmets, smoke detectors, window guards, avoid alcohol, and avoid excessive hot water).

(ii) Identify and refer abused patients to appropriate authorities (social and legal services).
(iii) Emphasize rehabilitation and community follow-up: Patients should return to productive lives by appropriate physical and occupational therapy.
(iv) Improve the injury database for research and prevention.
(v) Focus on agent and environmental factors: Host is the victim; agents are the motor vehicles, guns, and bullets; environmental factors are the social (laws, customs, regulations) and physical (energy absorbing, protective barriers and surfaces).

20. **Immunizations for adults**:
(A) **General considerations**.
(i) All adults should have a **primary series of tetanus and diptheria toxoids** with boosters **combined toxoids (Td) every 10 years**. Recent report suggests that a single Td booster at age 50 may be sufficient who have received a primary series.
(ii) Rubella vaccine should be given to susceptible female of child bearing age.
(iii) Persons born after 1957 should have immunity against measles and mumps.
(iv) **Pneumococcal vaccine and annual vaccination against influenza** should be given in all adults aged 65 and older.
(v) Health care workers exposed to blood or blood products should receive **hepatitis B vaccine**.
(vi) Persons caring for patients at high risk of complication from influenza should **receive annual influenza vaccine**.
(vii) Health care workers if come in contact with persons transmitting measles, mumps, or rubella should be immune to those diseases.
(B) **Pregnancy**.
(i) Live vaccines **are contraindicated** (e.g., oral polio, yellow fever, and MMR).
(ii) Women who receive MMR **should wait 3 months before becoming pregnant**.
(iii) **Td** should be given in pregnant women who are inadequately vaccinated to prevent neonatal tetanus in their infants.
All vaccinations should be given after the first trimester. All pregnant women should be **screened for hepatitis B surface antigen**, offspring of carrier mother should receive both hepatitis B vaccine and hepatitis B immunoglobulin and offspring of noncarrier mother should receive **only** hepatitis B vaccine.
(C) **Immunocompromised patients**.

(i) Live vaccines are contraindicated **except** in HIV patients (**asymptomatic patients should receive MMR** and **MMR should be considered for symptomatic patients as well**).
(ii) **Enhanced potency inactivated polio vaccine (eIPV)** should be given to HIV infected patients instead of oral polio.
(iii) Patients with leukemia on remission who did **not** receive any chemotherapy for at least 3 months **may receive live-virus vaccines (polio, MMR)**.
(iv) **Pneumococcal vaccine and annual influenza vaccine** should be given to HIV infected patients.
(v) Inactivated vaccines and toxoids can be given in immunocompromised patients but the efficacy may be diminished.
(vi) **Live vaccines are not usually contraindicated** in short-course therapy (< 2 weeks) with corticosteroids, alternate day regimens with low or moderate doses of short-acting corticosteroids, tendon injections, or topical applications of steroids.

21. **Indications of Td (tetanus and diptheria) vaccination following a wound:**
(i) Persons with **unknown immunization status** or those who received **less than 3 doses of** tetanus toxoid should **receive a dose of Td regardless of the severity of the wound**.
(ii) Persons who have received **3 or more doses but last dose was given more than 10 years ago**, should receive Td even **with clean, minor wounds**.
(iii) Persons who have received 3 or more doses but last dose was given **more than 5 years ago**, should **not** receive Td with clean, minor wounds but should **receive Td in all other wounds**.
(iv) **TIG (tetanus immunoglobulin)** should be given at the same time but in different sites to persons who have **not received 3 doses of toxoid** and have wounds which are **unclean and major**.

22. **Complications of Td vaccination**.
(i) Local inflammation and low-grade fever are the most common findings.
(ii) Rarely develops Guillain-Barre syndrome (GBS).

23. **Indications of MMR (measles, mumps, and rubella) in adults.**
(A) **To protect from measles.**
(i) Persons embarking on foreign travel should have received two doses or should have serologic evidence of immunity.
(ii) High risk adults such as students in colleges, direct patients contact, or international travelers.

(iii) Patients with **anaphylactic reaction to eggs should be vaccinated carefully** under established protocols.

Side effects of measles vaccine: Rash, encephalopathy, encephalitis, or **thrombocytopenia (in MMR)**.

(B) **To protect from rubella:** It should be given in all adults particularly women in child bearing age without prior history of vaccination and immunity.

Side effects of rubella vaccine.

(i) **Arthralgias** (mostly small peripheral joints in 40% of cases), **arthritis** (up to 20%). Joint symptoms begin **1 to 3 weeks after vaccination** and **persist for 1 day to 3 weeks**.

(ii) Rarely develops transient peripheral neuritis and pain in the arms and legs.

(iii) Rubella vaccine **can be given in persons who are allergic to eggs without problems**.

(C) **To protect from mumps**: It should be given to all persons, particularly susceptible male without prior history of vaccination and immunity.

Side effect of mumps vaccine.

(i) Fever, allergic reactions, and **parotitis**. Thrombocytopenic purpura develops in MMR vaccine.

(ii) Patients with anaphylactic **reaction to eggs** should be vaccinated carefully under established protocols.

24. **Hepatitis B vaccine**: **It is the only vaccine which can prevent cancer (hepatitis B- related liver cancer)** and prevent acute/chronic complications of hepatitis B infection.

Side effects of hepatitis B vaccine: Soreness at the injection site; **GBS is** found **in plasma derived vaccine** and absent in recombinant vaccine. **There is no risk of getting HIV infection from either vaccine**.

25. **Influenza vaccine**.

(a) **Indications for annual influenza vaccination**.

(i) Persons aged 65 and older.

(ii) Chronic cardiopulmonary disorders.

(iii) Residents of nursing home or other chronic care facility.

(iv) Chronic diseases such as diabetes, renal insufficiency, hemoglobinopathies, and immunosuppression.

(v) Children on long term aspirin therapy.

(vi) Transmission of influenza to high risk patients can be reduced by vaccinating health care workers and house hold contacts exposed to high risk patients.

Side effects in influenza vaccine.

(i) **Soreness at the site of injection** is the most common, others are fever, malaise, myalgia, and rarely severe allergic reaction.

(ii) Do **not** produce GBS.

(iii) Persons with anaphylactic reaction to eggs should **not** be vaccinated without careful evaluation.

26. **Pneumococcal vaccine:**

    (a) **Indications**: CVS disease, and pulmonary disease, cirrhosis, diabetes, **spleenic dysfunction or asplenia**, alcoholism, CSF leak, Hodgkin disease, lymphoma, multiple myeloma, **nephrotic syndrome, chronic renal failure**, HIV infection, immunosuppression, and all adults, 65 and above.

    (b) **Effectiveness:** It is effective against **Streptococcus pneumoniae** responsible for 88% of the bacteremic disease in USA.

    (c) **Booster dose:** It is given **6 years after** the initial vaccination in patients with highest risk (e.g., asplenia, renal failure, or nephrotic syndrome).

    (d) **Side effects**: Local reactions, fever, and malaise.

    (e) **Important point:** Approximately 2/3 of patients admitted with pneumococcal disease had been hospitalized for other reasons within last 5 years.

27. **Polio vaccine:**

    (a) **Indication in adults.**

    (i) Traveling to areas where wild polio virus is endemic or epidemic: Partially vaccinated adults should receive 3 doses of either eIPV or OPV and completely vaccinated adults should receive booster dose of eIPV or OPV.

    (ii) Health care workers exposed to wild viruses should be immuned to polio. EIPV is vaccine of choice for **both recipient** and **immunocompromised patient with** whom the health care worker has contact from exposure to OPV.

    (b) **Contraindication**: OPV should never be given **to immunocompromised patients** or to **a child living in a household with immunocompromised persons.**

28. **Meningococcal vaccine**: It is **not** routinely given in USA.

    (a) **Indications.**

    (i) Asplenia (functional or anatomic).

    (ii) Terminal complement component deficiences.

    (iii) Travelers who will stay in areas with hyperendemic or epidemic disease.

29. **Rabies vaccine.**
    (a) **Indications.**
        (i) High-risk persons including animal handlers.
        (ii) Selected laboratory and field workers.
        (iii) Travelers traveling for more than 1 month in high risk areas for rabies.
    (b) **Duration**: It should be given on day 0,7,28.

30. **Vaccines recommended for international travelers**:
    (a) **Yellow fever vaccine**: This disease occurs in South America and Africa. The vaccine should **not** be given in immunocompromised persons, persons with anaphylactic reaction to eggs, and pregnancy.
    (b) **Typhoid vaccine:** The vaccine is recommended for travelers to areas with contaminated food and water. Food and water precautions are very important. The vaccine is also recommended for family or other intimate contacts of typhoid carrier and laboratory workers handling Salmonella typhi.
    (c) **Cholera vaccine:** It is recommended for travelers visiting in some countries.
    (d) **Japanese encephalitis vaccine**: It is recommended for travelers to Asia who will spend a month or more in endemic areas. Travelers are advised to take precaution **from mosquito bites**.
    (e) Other vaccines used selectively are the following: Smallpox vaccine, oral adenovirus vaccines types 4 and 7 (for use in the military), anthrax vaccine, plague vaccine, BCG vaccine, and trivalent botulism antitoxin (ABE).

31. **Genetic factors in alcoholism:**
    (i) Alcoholism in the biologic father is a much **greater predictor for alcoholism in the son even he was raised in adoption**. It is difficult to stop drinking for those male offsprings of alcoholic father.
    (ii) In other types of familial or non-familial alcoholism (no genetic factors) the alcoholic individuals **may be able to stop drinking without difficulty**.

32. **Ethanol:**
    (A) **Absorption.**
        (i) Intestine: 75% are absorbed.
        (ii) Stomach: 25% are absorbed.
    (B) **Metabolism.**
        (i) Ethanol is oxidized to **acetaldehyde** by alcohol dehydrogenase in the liver.

(ii) **Alcohol-flush reaction**: It is characterized by vasodilatation with **facial flushing, hot sensations, tachycardia, and hypotension**. All these findings are **due to elevated acetaldehyde level**.

(iii) In peripheral tissues, **acetate** is formed from acetaldehyde by acetyl coenzyme A and finally to CO_2 and H_2O.

(C) **Excretion**: Up to 98% are excreted by the **liver**, the rest by the kidneys. It follows **zero-order kinetics and** is independent of concentration **results in rapid rise in plasma levels and toxicity.**

33. **Clinical manifestation, evaluation, and management of acute alcohol intoxication:**

(A) **Clinical manifestation.**

(a) Blood ethanol levels (50-100 mg/dL).
- (i) Sporadic drinkers: Euphoria, incoordination.
- (ii) Chronic drinkers: Minimal or no effect.

(b) Blood ethanol levels (100-200 mg/dL).
- (i) Sporadic drinkers: Slurred speech, ataxia, drowsiness.
- (ii) Chronic drinkers: Incoordination.

(c) Blood ethanol levels (200-300 mg/dL).
- (i) Sporadic drinkers: Lethargy, stupor, vomiting, incoherent speech.
- (ii) Chronic drinkers: Mild emotional and motor changes.

(d) Blood ethanol levels (300-400 mg/dL).
- (i) Sporadic drinkers: Coma.
- (ii) Chronic drinkers: Drowsiness.

(e) Blood ethanol levels (>500 mg/dL).
- (i) Sporadic drinkers: Respiratory depression and death.
- (ii) Chronic drinkers: Lethargy, stupor, and coma.

(f) **Alcoholic blackouts:** Loss of memory of new events for several hours, normal long term memory and consciousness.

(B) **Evaluation and management.**

(a) History of quantity of alcohol intake, rate of drinking, use of other drugs, other medical or psychiatric disorders, and previous alcohol abuse or alcoholism.

(b) **Stuporous patients**: Airway must be evaluated immediately. The patient should be intubated for severe hypoventilation, accumulating secretions, or coma.

(c) Routine head CT scan is **not** needed unless history of head trauma or focal neurologic signs.

(d) Gastric lavage (after intubation) is helpful if patient is obtunded due to recent, massive alcohol consumption.

(e) **Hemodialysis** is indicated if blood alcohol level exceeds 600 mg/dL.
(f) The patient with acceptable mental status and no other disorders can be kept calm under observation until sobriety returns.
(g) Routine blood tests to rule out anemia, **low k, Mg, phosphate, and glucose. Elevated serum ammonia level indicates hepatic encephalopathy**.
(h) If the laboratory results are **not** quickly available then **IV glucose** (12.5 to 25 grams) and **infusion of 5% dextrose in 0.5 normal saline** for alcoholic ketoacidosis.

34. **Clinical manifestation and management of alcohol withdrawal syndrome:**
(A) **Clinical manifestation**.
(i) 8 hours: Tremor, anxiety, irritability, nause, and vomiting.
(ii) 24 hours: Hyperexcitability, disordered perception, insomnia, and convulsion.
(iii) 2-5 days: Delirium tremens.
(B) **Management**.
(i) Thiamine (100 mg) IV to prevent or treat Wernicke's encephalopathy followed by daily multivitamins.
(ii) **Tremor and disordered perceptions:** Use benzodiazepine.
(iii) **Convulsion**: It is brief and self-limited, no specific anticonvulsant is needed but **sedating dose benzodiazepines are helpful in recurrent seizures** unlike phenytoin.
(iv) **Complete evaluation for a convulsive disorder is indicated** in focal seizures, more than six seizures, seizures persist beyond 6 hours, prolonged postictal state, and suspicion of other CNS disorders.
(v) **Delirium tremens**.
(a) Hospital admission and emergency management.
(b) Volume depletion with delirium tremens: Fluid therapy (4 to 10 liters in first day).
(c) To control the behavior and reduce symptoms without endangering the patient: IV diazepam (5 to 10 mg or more every 5 to 15 minutes until the patient is calm, then maintenance therapy).

35. **Rehabilitation in alcoholics.**
(i) The most successful treatment deserves active participation of family members, friends, and peers.
(ii) Local support groups such as Alcoholics Anonymous and Al-Anon are very helpful.
(iii) 50 to 70% success rate in socially stable middle-class alcoholics is **not** due to special kind rehabilitation program.

(iv) The prognosis is better if alcoholics enter the treatment program before the onset of medical problems.
(v) Most alcoholics do **not** admit the problems of drinking and most primary care physicians do **not** recognize the problems.
(vi) Alcoholic problems are recognized by the medical problems and socioeconomic status.

36. **Drug abuse and treatment**:
  (A) **Sedatives (e.g., barbiturates, diazepam, lorazepam, and alprazolam)**.
    (i) **Uses**: For seizure, insomnia, and anxiety. Benzodiazepines (e.g., diazepam, alprazolam) are the most effective drugs for anxiety.
    (ii) **Abstinence syndrome**: Irritability, diaphoresis, sleep disturbances, and peculiar sensations.
    Treatment.
    (a) **Acute withdrawal symptoms**: Hospital admission, close monitoring for cardiac arrythmias or seizures, a test dose of 20 to 40 mg diazepam may stop slurred speech which indicates higher level of dependence and daily dose should be adjusted accordingly.
    (b) Gradual detoxification by using diazepam over 1 to 3 weeks, some centers prefer phenobarbital.
    (c) After detoxification patients should be in a treatment program to prevent recurrence.
  (B) Stimulants (e.g., cocanie, dextroamphetamine, methylphenidate, and phenmetrazine).
    (i) **Mechanism of action of cocaine**: It blocks reuptake of dopamine at central synapses results in enhanced dopaminergic synaptic activity.
    (ii) **Toxicity.**
      (a) **Acute cocaine toxicity**: High BP, tachycardia, hyperthermia, arrythmias, followed by seizures, brain stem depression, stroke, vasculitis, cardiorespiratory collapse, and coma.
      (b) **Acute amphetamine toxicity:** Paranoid behavior, tactile hallucinations (**bugs crawling under the skin**), visual or auditory hallucinations, and compulsive behavior.
      (c) **Chronic intranasal cocaine use:** Ulceration or perforation of nasal septum.
      (d) **Chronic stimulant use:** Schizophrenic disorders.
      (e) Intense craving for cocaine is the most important withdrawal symptoms and it is due to dopamine depletion in CNS.
    (iii) **Treatment**.
      (a) **Anxiety and irritability**: Use benzodiazepines.

(b) **Acute psychotic reactions:** Use **haloperidol** if amphetamine is involved but it is self limited if cocaine is involved.

(c) Supporting environment and stop cocaine supply.

(C) **Opioids (agonists: morphine, methadone**, heroin, fentanyl, codeine, propoxyphene, oxycodan, meperidine, hydromorphone; **antagonists**: naloxone, naltrexone; **partial agonist-antagonists**: pentazocine, buprenorphine, nalbuphine, butorphanol).

(i) **Metabolism**: Heroin is hydrolyzed to morphine which is the active metabolite at opiate receptors.

(ii) **Toxicity.**

(a) **Acute opioid overdose: Pulmonary edema, cyanosis, respiratory distress,** reduced consciousness, increased ICP, cerebral edema, seizures, **fever, leukocytosis, pinpoint pupil** (sometimes dilated nonreactive pupil due to hypoxia or multiple drug use).

(b) **Adverse effects of opioid use are due to unsterile practice and adulteration in street drugs**: Skin abscesses, cellulitis, thrombophlebitis, embolisms (peripheral and pulmonary) and **S.aureus endocarditis**.

(c) **Complications of heroin use**: Hepatitis, pulmonary (pneumonia, abscess, TB, and infarct), disseminated extrapulmonary TB, angiothrombotic pulmonary hypertension, mycotic aneursysms, phlebitis, necrotizing angitis, neurologic problems (**meningitis, brain, subdural, or epidural abscesses, transverse myelitis,** polyneuroathy, and tetanus), **rhabdomyolysis, and myoglobinuria**.

(iii) **Treatment**.

(a) **Acute overdose: Naloxone** intravenously should be given. It increases pupil size, respiratory rate, and alertness. Remember, absence of response to repeated dose of naloxone excludes opioid overdose.

Side effects of naloxone.

It can **precipitate withdrawal symptoms** in opioid-dependent persons.

Management: Titrate the doses with the clinical symptoms.

The rapid metabolism of naloxone results in recurrence of overdose is due to long acting drugs (e.g., methadone, LAAM).

Management: Same as above.

(b) Opioid withdrawal symptoms (**heroin withdrawal** occurs 6 to 10 hours after last injection, patients appear with craving, restlessness, sweating, **rhinorrhea, yawning** followed by **dilated pupils, abdominal cramps,** vomiting, diarrhea, tremor, piloerection, bone and muscle pain. The symptoms mimic severe 'flu', peaks at 36 to

48 hours, and subsides over 5 to 10 days ; **long acting opioids such as methadone and LAAM** produce an abstinence syndrome that develops more slowly, less intensity, and long lasting):**Methadone is the drug of choice**, alternative drug is **clonidine.**

(D) **Cannabis (Marijuana and Hashish)**.

(i) **Active metabolites: Δ-9-Tetrahydrocannabinol** cause most of the pharmacologic effects.

(ii) **Adverse effects:** Acute panic, paranoid reaction, **distortion of body image,** inflammation of bronchi and sinuses. **Schizophrenic patients should avoid** cannabis because of increased sensitivity of adverse reaction. The chronic users are **failing in school or employment**.

(iii) **Treatment**.

Acute symptoms: Benzodiazepines are used in severe cases, **supportive and reassurance**.

Chronic heavy users: No medication is needed; hospitalization or entering into a therapeutic community, **remove the cannabis and then psychotherapy**.

(E) Hallucinogens [**LSD**, **PCP**, DMT (dimethyltryptamine), mescaline, psilocybin, MDMA (5-methoxy-3-4- methylene dioxyamphetamine, ectasy).

(i) **Adverse reactions:** The **acute reaction such as panic or psychosis ('bad trip')** are the most common complications of psychedelic use. LSD causes more **suicide or self-injury**, PCP causes **suicide mostly by drowning**.

'Flash backs' symptoms: The brief reappearance of **hallucinations or distortions days or weeks after** the last hallucinogenic dose. It is common in heavy users and usually **disappears without treatment**.

LSD producing symptoms (within 20 minutes after oral ingestion): **Dilated pupils, fever**, tachycardia, high BP, piloerection, and increased alertness. Psychoactive effects (hallucinations, mood swing) within 1 to 2 hours.

(ii) **Treatment**.

Acute panic reaction: Observation, reassurance, and supportive environment.

In severely agitated patients: IM lorazepam or haloperidol is needed. Prolonged psychosis needs hospitalization and treatment with neuroleptics.

PCP overdose: Support of vital signs, **gastric lavage with activated charcoal** to prevent absorption, acidification of the urine with **IV ammonium chloride.** In mild cases use cranberry juice with ascorbic acid.

(F) **The symptoms of anticholinergic drugs** (ingestion of alkaloids atropine, hyoscyamine, and scopolamine in natural plant form e.g., herbal tea and medications): Dilated pupils, dry mouth, flushing, fever, and tachycardia. **Treatment**: Symptomatic treatment includes fluids, antipyretics, and protect from self-injury. **In sever cases use cholinesterase inhibitors and lorazepam**. Remember, phenothiazine is **contraindicated** for their anticholinergic effects.

(G) **Inhalants** (gasoline, toluene, kerosene, amyl nitrite, carbon tetrachloride, and nitrouos oxide) **producing symptoms:** Cardiac arrythmias (it is the most common cause of death during exercise or upper airway obstruction), bone marrow supression, cerebral degeneration, damage to liver, kidneys, and peripheral nerves are found in prolonged exposure or daily doses. **Amyl nitrite liquid**: It is smooth muscle dilators used by male homosexuals for orgasm. It causes palpitations, headache, and postural hypotension, and loss of consciousness. It is found **in room deodorizers**. **Treatment: Acute** episodes are brief and **no treatment** is needed. **Chronic** users or associated psychiatric disorders should be referred to **psychiatrist** and measures to **prevent relapse**.

37. **Treatment of drug dependence**.

(A) **Acknowledgement of the problems**: The patients do **not** admit or seek for treatment. The concerned persons (family members, friends, or relatives) **must confront to patients in a firm but supportive way.**

(B) **Detoxification**: **Outpatient management is equally effective** like inpatient management if the drug taking is interrupted and it is cheaper. The continued therapy is usually lasting for months or years.

(C) **Pharmacotherapy.**

(i) The drugs used are already discussed previously.

(ii) Pharmacotherapy is to treat specific psychiatric disorder.

(iii) Do **not** use antianxiety drugs or sedatives because the patients who have abused one drug probably have abused prescribed psychoactive drugs.

(iv) **Naltrexone (opiate antagonist) reduces relapse rate in alcoholics** (Important).

(v) **Methadone** is used for opioid-dependent patients.

(vi) The patients **must be thoroughly detoxified before using naltrexone otherwise it precipitate withdrawal symptoms (important)**.

(vii) Comprehensive rehabilitation program including psychotherapy is important.

(D) **Psychotherapy**: It is **similar** in all classes of drugs and should **begin as early as possible** but **little values** when patients are still intoxicated or confused. It is compatible with medications used e.g., **methadone,**

naltrexone, disulfiram, or nicotine patch. Psychotherapy involves counseling regarding job-finding, family therapy, group therapy, individual therapy, behavioral therapy, self-help program such as Narcotic Anonymous and legal problems.

38. **The diseases caused by environmental and occupational factors: To obtain appropriate history is the most important**.
   (i) **Mesothelioma and laryngeal cancer**: Asbestos.
   (ii) **Lung cancer:** Asbestos, radon, or beryllium.
   (iii) **Lymphoma:** Benzene.
   (iv) **Renal failure:** Cadmium.
   (v) **Dementia**: Alcohol.
   (vi) **Abdominal pain**: Lead.
   (vii) **Hepatic angiosarcoma**: Vinyl chloride.
   (viii) **Urinary bladder cancer**: Aniline dye workers.
   (ix) **Kidney cancer**: Coke oven workers.
   (x) **Lymphoid and myeloid leukemia**: Radiologist (ionizing radiation) and rubber or chemical industry (benzene).
   (xi) **Bone cancer**: Radium chemist and processor.
   (xii) **Nasal cavity cancer:** Woodworkers, furniture makers (hardwood dust and fromaldehyde).
   (xiii) **Scrotal cancer:** Automatic lathe operators, metal workers, petroleum refiners, and coke oven workers.
   (xiv) **Trachea, bronchi, or lung cancer:** Asbestos, radon, coke oven, mustard gas, arsenic, and nickel.
   (xv) **Raynand's phenomenon:** Vibration, vinyl chloride.
   (xvi) **Asthma** (extrinsic): Bakers (flour), woodworkers (wood dust), platinum, isocyanates.
   (xvii) **Pneumoconiosis**: Coal workers (coal dust).
   (xviii) **Ornithosis**: Poultry workers, veterinarians, zoo staff, and pet shop workers.
   (xix) **Parkinson's disease (secondary)**: Manganese processing, welders, battery makers.
   (xx) **Male infertility**: Pesticide (diabromochloropropane).
   (xxi) **Byssinosis**: Cotton industry workers.
   (xxii) **Toxic hepatitis**: TNT, carbon tetrachloride, phosphorus, and ethylene dibromide.

39. **Few important points in radiation injury:**
   (i) Ionizing radiation produces biologic effects by **damaging the DNA**.

(ii) The **maximum permissible radiation dose (50 mSv) in any given year, radiation workers** in USA receive < 1 mSv yearly.

(iii) **Us residents** receive most (55%) of ionizing radiation from **radon** which is a natural source.

(iv) **The clinical manifestations are the following:**

(a) **Acute radiation syndrome (or whole boby radiation injury > 1 Sv**.

< 1 Sv: Safe.

1-2 Sv: Nausea, vomiting, leukopenia; **excellent prognosis; no treatment** is needed.

2-6 Sv: Hemorrhage, leukopenia, epilation; guarded prognosis; **need transfusion of WBC and platetes, and antibiotics**.

6-10 Sv: Same as above but more severe injury; need transfusion, **bone marrow transplantation** and antibiotics.

10-20 Sv: **Diarrhea, electrolytes imbalance, fever**; poor prognosis, and need fluids and salts, and possible bone marrow transplantation.

> 50 Sv: **Ataxia, coma, convulsion**; very poor prognosis; only palliative therapy.

(b) **Skin**: Erythema, desquamation, necrosis, and ulceration.

(c) **Lens**: Cataract.

(d) **Testis**: Permanent sterility.

(e) **Ovary**: Permanent sterility.

(f) **Lung**: Pneumonia.

(g) **Bone marrow suppression**: Leukopenia, thrombocytopenia.

(h) **Intestine**: Dysentry-like syndrome.

(v) Genetic: **At least 1.0 Sv** is needed to double the rate of heritable **mutations** in human germ cells.

(vi) Growth of tumors: Both **benign and malignant** growths occur by irradiation.

(vii) Effects of prenatal irradiation: Embroyonic death, fetal malformations, carcinogenic effect, mental retardation, and dose dependent decreased IQ test.

40. **Few important points in nonionizing radiation:**

(i) UVR (ultraviolet radiation) is subdivided into UVA, UVB, UVC .

(ii) **UVC** (ultraviolet band C) **is germicidal.**

(iii) Major source of UVR is sunlight, **UVR only damages the skin and eyes.**

(iv) **UVR is absorbed in DNA** results in formation of **pyrimidine dimers** which **causes mutational changes.**

(v) The **decrease in ozone layers causes increase in nonmelanotic skin cancers.**

(vi) **Infrared radiation** (ovens, furnaces, welding, lamps) causes **burn of the skin and cataract.**

(vii) **Please remember that microwave radiation** (electromagnetic waves but different frequencies than infrared radiatioon) **can interfere with cardiac pacemakers and other medical devices.**

(viii) **Persons wearing pacemaker should avoid EMF's** (electromagnetic fields > 0.5 mT such as exist around transformer, accelerators, NMR systems, and electrical devices).

41. **Few important points in electrical injury:**

(i) AC (alternating current) is the more common and more dangerous than DC (direct current).

(ii) Low-voltage injury is < 1000 volts and high-tension electrical injury is > 1000 volts.

(iii) Electrical injury is caused by four mechanisms: direct contact, conduction, arc, and secondary ignition.

(iv) **In low-voltage injury skin and subcutaneous tissues at the site of contact** are most commonly involved, **rarely** muscle and bone beneath the cutaneous burn are involved.

(v) **In high-voltage injury skin, subcutaneous tissues, and tissues conducting the electricities through the body are damaged**.

(vi) Clinical manifestations of high-voltage electrical injuries.

(a) **Heart: Cardiopulmonary arrest is common** particularly in lightning injuries, **temporary arrythmias, permanent conduction delays, and infarct patterns** may be present.

(b) **Burn wound:** It is typically **charred, excavated, visible deeper anatomic structures**, subsequently **edema** formation, **increased tissue pressure beneath the muscle fascia, and signs of vessels and nerves compression. Loss of pain, sensation, and decreased pulses indicates compartment syndrome**.

Diagnostic method of compartment syndrome: Doppler ultrasonography of distal pulses and direct measurement of compartment pressure (> 30 to 40 torr indicates tissue damage).

(c) **Acute renal failure: It is due to direct effect of myoglobin and indirect effect of hypovolemia**. Necrotic tissues release **myoglobin** which is **directly toxic to renal tubular cells results in reddish brown urine without red blood cells** and **hypovolemia enhances the toxicity of myoglobin.**

(d) **Nervous system: Both CNS and peripheral nervous** systems may be affected. **Motor involvement** are more common than sensory abnormalities. A **syndrome of polyneuritis** affecting nerves away from

the sites of surface injury may occur after several days or weeks. Immediate onset of spinal cord symptoms **are temporary and reversible**.
Delayed onset of spinal cord symptoms are often **permanent or partially reversible** appears as **transverse myelitis, ascending paralysis, hemiplegia, or related syndromes**.

(e) **Internal organs**: Dysfunction of the liver, pancreas, and gut usually indicates patient's underlying condition.

(f) **Bony fractures: Long bone fractures** are due to fall and **vertebral column fractures** are **due to spasm of the paraspinous muscles**.

(vii) **Treatment.**

(a) Cardiopulmonary resuscitation for cardiac arrest, patients should be monitored for 48 hours and treat for **arrythmias accordingly followed by thorough cardiologic investigation** once the acute injury has healed.

(b) **Fluid management: Ringer's lactate** solution to maintain urinary output 50 to 75 ml/hour; in gross myoglobinuria urinary output should be increased 100 to 150 ml/hour by **increasing fluid infusion, mannitol** is used when urine output is low despite adequate fluid therapy.

(c) **Wound management**.

(i) Second and third degree cutaneoous wounds should be debrided, cleansed, and application of topical antibacterial burn creams preferably sulfamylon (mafenide acetate).

(ii) Do **not** use prophylactic antibiotics.

(iii) **Tetanus prophylaxis** should be up to date.

(iv) **Surgical decompression** is done if the compartment pressure > 30 to 40 mm Hg.

(v) **Escharotomy** is done for circumferential third-degree burn of the extremities.

(vi) Fasciotomy is done for compartment syndrome.

(vii) In first 24 hours **technetium-99 m pyrophosphate scintigraphy is the most common diagnostic technique** to determine the nonviable tissues which exhibit no uptake. **Nonviable tissues should be removed to avoid infection**.

(viii) Viability of the deep tissues are determined by **serial surgical explorations**.

(ix) Amputation is the last choice. It is indicated in severe hyperkalemia, severe myoglobinuria, or infection.

42. **Post-traumatic stress syndrome:** It is a late complication develop in a few months or several years after the electrical injuries, **especially if a body part has been lost**.
    Signs and symptoms: Cataract, contractures, cholelithiasis, or psychiatric symptoms.
    Treatment: Removal of the cataract; extensive rehabilitation and reconstructive surgery for contractures; removal of the symptomatic gallstones; or psychotherapy and medications for psychiatric disorders.

43. **Lead poisoning**: (Workers exposed to lead such as miners, welders, auto and paint manufacturing, demolition workers).
    (A) **Signs and symptoms**.
    - (i) **GI tract**: Crampy, diffuse abdominal pain, nausea, vomiting, anorexia, constipation, or rarely diarrhea.
    - (ii) **Blood:** Basophilic stippling, usually microcytic hypochromic anemia or normocytic normochromic anemia.
    - (iii) **Nervous system:** Wrist drop, foot drop, memory lapses, incoordination, sleep distrubances, in severe cases ataxia, cranial nerve palsies, syncope-like attacks, psychosis, seizures, blindness, or coma.
    - (iv) **Tetraethyl lead paisoning:** Euphoria, nervousness, insomnia, convulsion, hallucinations, and frank psychosis.
    - (v) **Kidneys:** Interstitial nephritis, dysuria.
    - (vi) **Joints:** Polyarthritis.

    (B) **Diagnosis**: Elevated whole-blood lead levels (> 40 microgram/dl), whole-blood erythrocyte protoporphyrin or zinc protoporphyrin (> 50 microgram/dl) plus anemia and basophilic stippling.
    (C) **Treatment:** EDTA, BAL, or penicillamine plus removal from the exposure.

44. **Mercury poisoning:**
    (A) **Signs and symptoms.**
    - (i) **Metallic mercury (dental offices, industries)**: Cough, **chest pain, hemoptysis, chills, fever**, diffuse pulmononary infiltrates; **abdominal pain, diarrhea, dermatitis, metallic taste; insomnia, nervousness, depression, mental deficiency, loss of sexual drive may appear early**; polyneuropathy, amblyopia, acrodynia, joint pains, swollen gum with blue line around the teeth **and nephrotic syndrome**.
      Diagnosis: Increased excretion of mercury in urine by giving chelating agent; blood and urine levels are **not** reliable.
      Treatment: Chelating agents plus removal from the source.

(ii) **Inorganic mercury (ingestion from industrial contamination):** Abdomial pain, diarrhea, **proteinuria, nephrotic syndrome, rhabdomyolysis, acrodynia, and elevated** muscle enzymes.
(iii) Organomercurials (industrial contamination of water): CNS (paresthesias, ataxia, hearing loss, blindness, dysarthria, spasticity, paralysis, and coma) plus milder symptoms listed in metallic mercury poisoning.

45. **Arsenic poisoning (industries, herbicides, insecticides, rodenticides, veterinary medicine).**
(A) **Signs and symptoms.**
(i) **Arsenic gas poisoning** (serious clinical manifestations **between 1 to 6 hours** after exposure): Fever, headache, vomiting, explosive diarrhea, epigastric pain, hemolytic anemia, encephalopathy, renal failure (ATN), myocardial damage, bone marrow suppression, and CVS collapse followed by chronic renal failure those who survived.
(ii) **Arsenic ingestion.**
(a) **First week after ingestion: Garlic odor in the breath (also found in selenium, phosphorus, tellurium, dimethyl sulfoxide poisoning)**, diarrhea, cramping abdominal pain, **dysphagia, cyanosis, hematuria,** muscle cramps, peresthesia, **epistaxis**, excessive thirst, **conjunctivitis**, periorbital swelling, jaundice, hepatomegaly, **rhabdomyolysis**, cardiomyopathy, pericarditis, pulmonary edema, respiratory muscle paralysis, renal failure with ATN, and seizure.
(b) **After the first week**: Symmetric polyneuropathy is the most common presentation, burning sensation in a stocking-glove distribution, motor weakness, and absent reflexes.
(c) **Subacute poisoning: Aldrich-Mees lines (transverse white bands)** on the nails and garlic odor.
(d) **Chronic poisoning:** Hyperpigmentation and hyperkeratoses on the palms and soles; alopecia and rain-drop depigmentation; **skin cancers in USA is mostly due to medicinal use of Fowler's solution (inorganic arsenic).**
(e) Workers exposed to arsenic (miners, vineyard workers, smelter worker): Higher incidence of squamous cell cancer of the lung and bronchogenic cancer.
(B) **Diagnosis of arsenic poisoning:** Measurement of arsenic in blood, urine, hair, or nails but the interpretation is difficult.

(C) **Treatment: BAL (dimercaprol) is the drug of choice within 24 hours of exposure. Exchange transfusion or dialysis may be helpful in acute illness**. DMSA or penicillamine may be useful.

46. **Zinc toxicity: Renal failure with ATN**, low BP, anemia, abdominal pain, elevated serum amylase levels with or without pancreatitis.

47. **Aluminium toxicity: Speech disturbance is a characteristic feature,** memory loss, seizure, abnormal EEG, myoclonic twitches, and dysarthria. It may be due to repeated dialysis.
Diagnosis by DFO mobilization test: Deferoxamine (DFO) forms complexes with aluminium and enhances excretion.
Treatment: Deferoxamine. Reverse osmosis and deionization treatment may reduce dialysis induced dementia. **DFO can temporarily enhance encephalopathy**.

48. **Cobalt toxicity: Cardiomyopathy, cor pulmonale, pulmonary interstitial fibrosis, goiter** resulting from blockage of iodine uptake, peripheral neuropathy, **sensorineural deafness, optic atrophy**, renal tubular damage, **and hyperlipidemia**.

49. **Copper toxicity**: Hemolytic anemia, jaundice, necrosis of liver and pancreas, abdominal pain, fever, chills, and severe leukocytosis.

50. **Iron toxicity:** Hemosiderosis, rarely hemochromatosis, and proximal myopathy.
Treatment: Deferoxamine.

51. **Cadmium toxicity.**
(A) **Signs and symptoms.**
(i) **Acute toxicity:** The characteristic clinical features **appear 4 to 10 hours after exposure**, manifest with **dyspnea, substernal discomfort**, cough, vomiting, in severe cases wheezing, **hemoptysis, pulmonary edema, low BP, and renal failure**.
(ii) **Chronic toxicity:** Over 10 years of aerosol exposure causes **emphysema without bronchitis** and proteinuria. **The most common long term toxicity in both oral and aerosol exposure is benign proteinuria**.

52. **Nickel toxicity**.
(A) **Signs and symptoms**.

(i) Substernal pain, drowsiness, vomiting **followed by a latent period of 1 to 5 days** then appearance of fever, chills, dyspnea, and blood-tinged sputum. In severe cases cyanosis, convulsion, respiratory failure, and death may occur.
Treatment: Diethyldithiocarbonate is the drug of choice, or BAL.
(ii) High incidence of nasal, laryngeal, and lung cancers.
(iii) Nickel contact dermatitis.

53. **Thallium toxicity.**
(A) **Signs and symptoms.**
(i) **Acute toxicity: Hematemesis, vomiting, diarrhea with or without blood,** muscle pain, fever, excessive thirst, hyperhidrosis, delirium, seizures, respiratory failure, and coma.
(ii) **Patients survive after 1 week:** Alopecia (**total in the head**, sparing inner 1/3 of eyebrows, facial, and axillary); peripheral neuropathy, ascending neuropathy **mimicking** Guillain-Barre syndrome; abdominal pain and vomiting mimicking acute appendicitis; **multiple cranial nerves involvement (palsy) sparing VIII cranial nerve**; blindness is due to optic neuritis, postural hypotension, impotence, amenorrhea, and **blue discoloration of the gums**.
(B) **Diagnosis: Determination of thallium in 24 hours urine is diagnostic;** blood and urine levels could be misleading.
Key features: Unexplained abdominal pain, neurologic presentation, and alopecia.
Treatment: Hemodialysis can remove 50% of the total body thallium, **prussian blue or activated charcoal** enhance absorption and excretion in the stool, **repeated dialysis** are needed because the half-life of thallium is one month.

54. **Selenium deficiency and toxicity:**
(A) **Deficiency:** Cardiomyopathy (Keshan disease).
(B) **Toxicity.**
(i) **Acute:** Vomiting, diarrhea, pallor, depression, **garlic odor in breath**, nervousness, sometimes sore throat, dyspnea, and cough.
(ii) **Chronic: Bronze color of the skin, brittle nails and hairs**; abdominal pain vomiting, and diarrhea; garlic odor in breath, **diffuse dermatitis,** and **dental caries**.

55. **Barium toxicity: Profound hypokalemia** is due to intracellular displacement of k in systemic absorption of barium. **Low k causes** cardiac arrythmias, flaccid paralysis, renal failure, and respiratory paralysis. Chronic aersol

exposure **cause bilateral bengin pneumoconiosis (pulmonary nodules up to 0.5 cm in diameter** without fibrosis) **in an asymptomatic persons**.
Treatment.
(i) Potassium for hypokalemia.
(ii) Avoid occupational aerosol expoure.

56. **Manganese toxicity**: **Compulsive behavior** (singing, dancing, running, fighting), cerebellar signs (ataxia, rigidity, and Parkinson-like facies), **hypersomnia**, memory loss, impotence, speech dfficulty, and **sometimes psychosis**.
Treatment: No effective therapy.

57. **Antimony toxicity: Adams-stokes syndrome**, cardiac arrythmias, **metal fume fever**, acute renal tubular insufficiency, electrolytes abnormalities, hematemesis, and circulatory collapse.
Treatment: Gastric lavage, activated charcoal, and **dimercaprol** or less toxic dimercaptosuccinic acid or dimercaptopropanesulfonic acid.

58. **Boron toxicity**.
(i) **Ingestion of boron: Seizures,** vomiting, anemia, **alopecia**, skin eruption (erythema, desquamation, and exfoliation).
(ii) **Exposure to liquid boron**: Cortical blindness, **deafness, seizures,** dementia, acidosis, and cardiac arrest.

59. Tin toxicity (foods from tin cans, used in agricultural products).
(i) **Ingestion**: **Ataxic dysmetria, nystagmus,** seizures, loss of hearing and vision, **increased intracranial pressure**, paresis, and polyneuropathy.
(ii) **Aersol:** Benign asymptomatic mild pneumoconiosis (bilateral pulmonary nodules) with normal pulmonary function.

GERIATRIC MEDICINE

1. **Chromosomal involvement in Alzheimer's disease**: **Chromosome 14 and 21 are dominant, chromosome 19 implicate the blood protein apolipoprotein E (apo E)**. The apo E is also associated with **atherosclerosis** results in **stroke and heart attack**.

2. **Beneficial effects of exercise in geriatric age groups (> 65 years):**
   (i) Improves cardiac performance.
   (ii) Reduces the risk of hypertensive disease.
   (iii) Improves skeletal muscles strength.
   (iv) Reduces age related bone loss and fractures.

3. **Declining of physiologic functions in elderly persons:**
   (i) **Decrease** in renal clearance, vital capacity, bronchiolar ciliary movement, immune function, and sexual activities.
   (ii) **Increase** in heart attacks, infections, arterial wall stiffness, vascular disease, diabetes, and impotence. **Remember beta-blocker reduces penile erection**.
   (iii) The brain imaging of < 70 years old Alzheimer's disease (AD) patients have clear distinction from nondemented patients of same age group in the numbers of plaques and tangles. In advanced age it is difficult to distinguish the brain imaging findings between AD and normal persons.

4. **Few important points in neurologic problems associated with aging:**
   (i) **Alzheimer's diseases and related dementias** are found in 50% of patients above 80 years of age.
   (ii) **Delirium** is a common problem in hospitalized patients admitted for acute problems.
   Definitive diagnostic features are acute onset, decreased arousal, inattention, fluctauting course, and disorganized thinking. **Neuroleptics and narcotics pain relievers** can impair the cognition in the elderly.
   (iii) The treatment for delirium are the following: **The most important is the staff understanding and patience, bedroom lights should be left on at night**, **restraints** should be minimized but patients should **not** fall from the bed, **neuroleptics** should be kept at low doses, caregivers should be **gentle**, presence of loving concerned family members are helpful, patients **should be kept out of bed** as much as possible during waking hours.
   (iv) Most common **nonspecific symptom** is **recent loss of memory over 70 years of age,** other symptoms are **depression or hopelessness, insomnia-fatigue**. There is **no treatment** for organic memory loss, but that due to

anxiety or inattention may be helped by **counseling** or **referrel to concerned lay or religious support system**. Remember, benzodiazepines or other tranquilizers are **not** helpful or **may be harmful**. Low dose **antidepressant medications** are useful.

(v) Musculoskeletal wear and tear can be reduced by **exercise even walking with briskly swinging**.

(vi) Dizziness, giddiness, orthostatic dysequilibrium are common but true vertigo **is uncommon**. Vertigo occurs in extreme head **extension results in vertebral artery compression**. Avoid excessive head extension to reduce vertigo. Anxiety plays an important role in all of the above symptoms except vertigo.

(vii) Ringing tinnitus indicates gradual high-tone hearing loss but **no effective** treatment is available. **Progressive** nerve deafness should be **referred to otologist or neurologist**.

(viii) Most serious visual problems (cataracts, glaucoma, or macular degeneration) should be **referred to opthalmologist**.

(ix) **Please remember that extensor planter responses are not normal findings** but reduction of deep-tendon reflexes and disappearance of Achilles tendon jerks are normal.

(x) Patients with peripheral neuropathy should be evaluated for **metabolic disorders** or **nerve root compression**. Most of the causes remains unknown and treatment is symptomatic.

5. **Drugs which cause neurotoxic effect in elderly, mostly are dose related:**
   (i) Cimetidine, H_2 blockers, histamine: Confusion.
   (ii) Aspirin: **Tinnitus,** confusion.
   (iii) Nonsteroidal anti-inflammatory drugs: **Aseptic meningitis**, confusion.
   (iv) Carbamazepine, phenytoin: Confusion, **ataxia**.
   (v) Levodopa, bromocriptine: Confusion, **postural hypotension, dyskinesias**.
   (vi) Digitalis: Confusion, **hallucinations**.
   (vii) Benzodiazepines: **Depression, amnesia, falls, drowsiness**.
   (viii) Corticosteroids: **Delirium**.
   (ix) Anticholinergics (atropine, metoclopramide, TCA, tranquilizers): Hallucination, urinary retention, glaucoma, constipation, hypothermia.
   (x) Antihypertensives: Postural hypotension, giddiness, falls.

6. **Impairment of cognitive functions in elderly indicate: Brain disease.**

7. **Clinical features and diagnosis of dementia:**
   (A) **Clinical features.**
      (i) Impairment of short-term and long-term memories.

(ii) Impairment of judgement in interpersonal, social, and work-related problems.
(iii) Impairment of abstract thinking.
(iv) Aphasia (language problems), apraxia (motor skill problems despite physical capacity), agnosia (failure to recognize familiar object despite intact sensory function).
(v) Personality change (e.g., alteration or accentuation of premorbid traits).

(B) **Diagnosis:** Mini-Mental State Examination (MMSE, 19 items/30 points), a score of **25 or more is normal** and **score of 20 or less indicates dementia** even with low educational levels.

8. **A patient complains of memory loss; mental status test is normal or nearly normal suggest**: **Mental illness** (**not** organic congnitive loss).

9. **An elderly person complaining of memory loss that is not apparent to others, Most likely cause**: **Depression** (**not** cognitive impairment).

10. **Excess disability and management:**
    (A) **Excess disability:** Physical disability causes depression, anxiety, psychosis **plus associated dementia**, the compounded problems are known as excess disability.
    (B) **Management:** Treat the depression, agitation, delusion, anxiety; psychosocial intervention and psychotropic medications.

11. **Causes of sleep disorder in elderly**: Arthritis, urologic, cardiac, and mental disorders are the common causes. **Remember, mere aging is not the cause.**

12. **Most common cause of impotence in elderly**: **Psychogenic,** other causes are depression, social situation (opportunity for sexual relation), drug, alcohol, metabolic (hypothyroid), medical, or surgical conditions.

13. **Few important points of depression in elderly**:
    (i) Most of them are **not** depressed.
    (ii) Depressed patients **stay in bed and unable to carry out the task.**
    (iii) Elderly men have **highest rate of suicide**.
    (iv) Depression is diagnosed by measuring the geriatric depression scale (15 questions, each has one point), **scores greater than 5 indicates probable depression**.
    (v) Treatment of depression includes pharmacologic, behavioral, and pharmacological interventions.

(vi) Depressed persons have higher mortality than nondepressed persons in nurisng home.

14. **Pseudodementia: It is really a depression appears as dementia**. Pseudodementia is clinical state in which **mental disorders** (**not** the dementing diseases) **impair cognitive functions in elderly**.

15. **Difference between depression (pseudodementia) and dementia:**

Depression.	Dementia.
(i) Rapid onset and brief duration of cognitive impairment.	(i) Gradual onset and longer duration of cognitive impairment.
(ii) Past and family history of depression usually present.	(ii) Past and family history of depression usually absent.
(iii) Depressed mood is more prominent than cognitive impairment.	(iii) Cognitive impairment is more prominent than depressed mood.
(iv) Patients complain more of cognitive impairment.	(iv) Patients complain more of depression.
(v) Cognitive symptoms is more influenced by fluctuation of mood.	(v) Cognitive impairment is less influenced by fluctuation of mood.
(vi) Antidepressants are effective.	(vi) Antidepressants are not effective.

16. **Fear (or dread) of death in elderly:**
    (i) Fear of death is **not** the same as thinking of death.
    (ii) Fear of death is more common in midlife crisis.
    (iii) **Fear of death in elderly** is **more commonly associated with terminal illness or personal loss**.
    (iv) **Death anxiety** in elderly is either the effect of **depression** or the **initial awareness of dying (not due to awareness of aging)**.
    (v) Fear of death is a sign of distress.
    (vi) Depression should be treated with antidepressants.

17. **Psychiatric consultation in major medical and surgical illnesses**: It **reduces the hospital stay** and **helps in returning home quickly** than entering in a nursing home facility.

18. **Pharmacologic therapies for older persons**:

(i) **SSRI's** (selective serotonin uptake inhibitors) such as fluoxetine, paroxetine, and sertraline **are the drug of choice for depression.** SSRI's do **not** have sedative, hypotensive, anticholinergic, and cardiac (arrythmias) side effects **unlike** tertiary amines (imipramine, doxepin, amitryptyline) and secondary amines (desipramine, nortriptyline, amoxapine). **SSRI's can produce nausea, insomnia, anxiety, drowsiness, and headaches**.

(ii) **ECT** (electroconvulsive therapy) is a **safe and effective treatment** for depression.

(iii) MAO (monoamine oxidiase) inhibitors are **not** used for their potential toxic effects.

(iv) **Oxazepam and lorazepam are used for sleep disorders in elderly**.

(v) **Preferred antipsychotic drugs** for elderly patients are **low-dose/high-potency** (e.g., haloperidol, trifluoperazine) neuroleptics or **intermediate range** (e.g., trilafon). **The side effects** of haloperidol, trifluoperazine are **extrapyramidal activities and parkinsonism.** The side effects of high-dose/low-potency neuroleptics (e.g., thioridazine, chlorpromazine) are sedation, postural hypotension, and anticholinergic reactions.

(vi) Most psychoactive drugs (e.g., long acting benzodiazepines) are lipid soluble and metabolized in the liver **except** lithium which is water soluble and excreted by the kidneys.

19. **Pharmacokinetic changes in the elderly:**

(i) **Renal:** The most consistent age-related change is **renal**. GFR declines approximately 50% between the third and ninth decades of life. **Please remember serum creatinine does not reflect age-related decline in GFR because** of age-related declining of muscle mass which is a source of creatinine.

(ii) The doses of the drugs with **narrow therapeutic index** (ratio of doses producing the desired effect and toxic effect) such as **digoxin and aminoglycosides** should be adjusted according to actual renal function.

(iii) **Liver**: **Reduction of hepatic blood flow and probably phase I metabolism** (hepatic oxidative process and may be cytochrome P-450 causes oxidation) but **no** change in phase II metabolism (hepatic conjugation) in elderly.

(iv) **Fat and lean body mass: Increase in fat** and **decrease in lean body mass.** The volume of distribution of **fat-soluble drugs are higher, delayed steady-state, and delayed unexpected toxicity.** The volume of distribution of water-soluble drugs are **lower, earlier steady-state, and earlier toxicity**.

(v) **Serum albumin:** It is normal in healthy elderly but **decreases during illness**. Drugs highly bound to albumin (e.g., phenytoin) **may develop**

toxicity in **normal serum therapeutic levels (bound plus free drugs) because of disproportionate increase of free drugs.**

20. An elderly patient appear with H/O **constipation, fever, agitation, altered mental status, urinary retention,** or H/O paradoxical diarrhea following constipation.
Most likely diagnosis: Fecal impaction. The clinical presentation may lead to misdiagnosis and wrong treatment.
Treatment: Suppositories, enemas, or manual disimpaction.
Prevention of constipation: Strict attention to bowel habits, adequate (**not** excessive) dietary fibers, proper hydration, and laxative prn.

21. **Medications which cause constipation**: TCA, anticholinergics, calcium channel antagonists, opioid, some antihypertensive drugs, aluminium-containing antacids, and bile-acid resins.

22. **Most common cause of urinary incontinence in elderly:**
(A) **Overactivity of urinary bladder detrusor muscles (also called detrusor hyperreflexia or instability) is the most common cause**. It is due to lack of inhibition from higher cerebrocortical centers to brain stem detrusor reflex. **Remember, most patients do not have neurological disease**.
Treatment: Bladder training (prolonging the interval between voidings by using behavioral technique), physically disabled or cognitively impaired should **be toileted on time and use adult diapers. Oxybutinin** (antispasmodic drug) relaxes bladder wall and promote urine storage. **Remember, urodynamic studies are not needed** in all patients prior to therapy but **it is important to rule out 'over flow incontinence' prior to therapy**.
(B) Other causes of urinary incontinence is **'true stress incontinence'** (i.e., without detrusor contraction). It is found in postmenopausal women (**loss of** pelvic musculature support of bladder neck) typically occurs after a cough, sneeze, or rising from a sitting position.
Treatment: Pelvic musculature exercises, alpha-adrenergic drug (e.g., phenylpropanolamine) to increase urethral tone, and exogenous steroids (controversial).

23. **Urinary incontinence and indwelling bladder catheter**: **Chronic indwelling catheter should not be used in urinary incontinence because UTI is almost 100%**. Suprapubic catheter and incidence of bacteriuria for short term but **no effect on long term. Chronic use of antibiotic produces reistant organisms**. Intermittent catheterization is used for urinary retention, failure of intermittent

catheterization results in **use of indwelling catheter**. Antibiotics should be reserved for symptomatic illness (fever, lower abdominal pain, bacteriuria).

24. **Most common cause of urinary retention in elderly men: Benign prostatic enlargement**. In women **it is rare** and due to immobility, bedridden state, fecal impaction, or anticholinergic drugs (TCA, diisopyramide, first-generation antihistamine) and **drug used to treat urinary incontinence**.
Remember, diuretics can cause urinary retention due to large volume of urine incapacitate compromised bladder. Diabetes mellitus, diabetes cystopathy, or cystocele may cause urinary retention.

25. **Difference between urinary retention (inability to void) and increased residual urine (post void residual volume >50 ml)**: The former condition **needs immediate attention and therapy,** the later condition is **asymptomatic and dose not require therapy.**

26. An elderly women is unable to bear weight after fall and has severe pain on weight bearing joint. Hip fracture should be ruled out until proven otherwise.
Most likely diagnosis: Hip fracture.
First investigation of choice: X-ray of the hip (frondal and lateral view), if it is negative then **bone scan or MRI** should be done as soon as possible.
Treatment: Surgery should be performed as soon as possible after the patient is stabilized because morbidity and mortality are very high if surgery is delayed beyond 24 to 48 hours.
Assesment of patient: To find the reason for the fall is very important.
Causes of fracture: Bone loss and the tendency to fall.

27. **Few important points in falls and fractures in elderly:**
    (i) Hip fractures are more common in women than men.
    (ii) **First** manifestation of bone loss is found in **trabecular bone of the vertebrae and extreme ends of long** bones.
    (iii) Osteoporosis **is a proportional loss of both mineralized and nonmineralized defect** which **is due to vitamin D deficiency in elderly**. In elderly osteomalacia is associated with osteoporosis and mimic clinical appearance of osteoporosis.
    (iv) **Treatment for osteomalacia is exposure to sunlight** (only 15 minutes exposure twice a week is sufficient for light-skinned persons, more time is needed for elderly and dark-skinned persons) and **vitamin D 800 IU/day or higher doses for vitamin D deficient** patients.
    (v) Treatment **for osteoporosis**. There is **no effective** treatment for elderly. **Estrogen and calcitonin** may prevent the bone loss but **cannot** replace the

bone already been lost. **Etidronate (biophosphonates) inhibits bone resorption but impairs mineralization when given for long term**. **The cyclical use of etidronate plus calcium** may reduce the fracture risk. **Calcium (inhibits bone resorption) plus vitamin D** (enhance intestinal calcium absorption) **reduce the fracture risk in elderly** patient.

(vi) **Prevention of osteoporosis**:

(a) Most important is to identify and address preventable causes of bone loss (e.g., vitamin D deficiency, primary hyperparathyroidism, phosphate depletion, **use of heparin or corticosteroids,** alcohol, cigarette, and inadequate calcium intake). Daily recommended calcium intake is **1500 mg elemental calcium for both men and women to correct negative calcium balance**.

(vii) Prevention of fall is the most important in elderly patients.

28. **Electrolyte imbalance in elderly patients:**

(i) **Hyponatremia is very common**. It is due to increased APV (arginine vasopressin), decreased excretion of water, decreased GFR. It may be due to **CHF, central neurologic impairments, syndrome of inappropriate antidiuretic hormone secretion (SIADH).** Inappropriate ADH secretion is **due to increased physiologic release of AVP as well as** exposure to other pharmacolgical drugs which cause an increase ADH secretion. Hyponatremia could be due to enteral feeding and hypotonic feeding.

29. **Management of pressure sores**:

(A) **Prevention**: It is the most important and main goal is to avoid the pressure.

(i) Lift (**not** slide) bedridden patients.
(ii) Keep the skin dry.
(iii) Early identification of vulnerable patients.
(iv) Correct nutritional deficiencies.

(B) **Treatment**:

(i) Do **not** use topical antibiotics in ulcers, it causes antibacterial resistance.
(ii) Systemic antibiotics are used in cellulitis or systemic infections.
(iii) Uncomplicated blisters should be managed without debridement or dressing.
(iv) Superficial ulcer craters should be kept clean and covered with a dressing if needed.
(v) Ulcers with subcutaneoous necrotic tissues should be debrided.
(vi) Ulcers involving muscles, bones should be debrided surgically and skin grafting may be required.

30. **Few important points in medical decision making for cognitively impaired elderly:**
   (i) Patients have the **right to refuse** unwanted medical treatment plus life-sustaining treatment. This can be done through an **advance directive** (written or oral) or **an authorized surrogate** decision maker or DNR (do **not** resuscitate) order.
   (ii) Remember, tube feeding is **an active** treatment.
   (iii) Withdrawal of **tube feeding and water** will **not** cause painful death. **Dehydration** causes early development of **hyperosmolarity,** release of **endorphins (analgesic)**, and rapid development of coma.
   (iv) Tube feeding, gastrostomy, or jejunostomy feeding **can cause aspiration**.
   (v) Physicians should know the rules of individual states regarding patients right.
   (vi) **Physician who object withdrawal of** life sustaining treatment should transfer **the patient in an another facility** which will respect and obey patient's decision.
   (vii) Physicians are **not** required to provide futile treatment, CPR in terminal cancer patients are **not** futile.
   (viii) Physicians should provide the following palliative care:
      (a) **To relieve pain** and **not** to kill the patient by administering lethal drugs.
      (b) Subjective or objective evidence indicates that terminally ill patient is experiencing pain.
      (c) Physician's therapeutic response is proportional to patient's level of pain.

RENAL DISEASE

1. Few important points in renal function and size:
   (i) Urine specific gravity < 1.008 indicates hypo-osmolality and > 1.020 indicates hyperosmolality.
   (ii) Glucosuria occurs once serum glucose levels exceed 160 to 200 mg/dL.
   (iii) Normal urinary protein excretion rates are < 40 mg/24 hours, but **up to 150 mg/24 hours are considered normal** by most nephrologist in nondiabetic patients.
   (iv) Protein excretion > 150 mg/24 hours indicates renal or extrarenal causes.
   (v) Protein excretion rates **> 3.5 grams/ 24 hours /1.73 sq. meter of body surface** are known as nephrotic range proteinuria.
   (vi) Nondiabetic patients with isolated proteinuria **40 to 150 mg/ 24 hours** but completely asymptomatic should have **annual** follow up evaluation.
   (vii) **Microscopic hematuria** is **> 2 to 3 RBC's per high-power field** in 12-ml spun urine.
   (viii) Pyuria means > 3 WBC's per high-power field and a positive leukoesterase dipstick, **both are abnormal**.
   (ix) Normal kidney size is between 11.5 to 12.5 cm (L > R).

2. **GFR (glomerular filtration rate) and Ccr (endogenous creatinine clearance)**:
   GFR can be estimated by measuring **Ccr from 24-hour urine.**

$$Ccr = \frac{Ucr \times V}{Pcr}$$

   Ucr = Urinary concentration of creatinine.
   V = Urine volume in 24 hours.
   Pcr = Plasma concentration of creatinine.
   Serum creatinine is a much better index than BUN of renal function. Serum BUN values depend upon the protein intake, liver function, and urea excretion rates from the kidney. In prerenal failure, there is increased tubular reabsorption of urea results in **disproportionate rise in BUN with respect to creatinine.**

3. Fractional excretion of electrolytes (Na or k) or FE_{Na}/FEk calculation: It is calculated from spot urine (not 24-hour urine).

$$FE_{Na} = \frac{U_{Na}/P_{Na}}{Ucr/Pcr} \times 100$$

   U_{Na} = Urinary Na, P_{Na} = Plasma Na, Ucr = Urinary creatinine, Pcr = Plasma creatinine.

(i) **Prerenal cause** = FE_{Na} < 1, urine sodium < 20 mEq/liter, urine osmolality > 500 mOsm/kg H_2O.
(ii) **Parenchymal or renal cause** = FE_{Na} > 1, urine sodium > 40 mEq/liter, urine osmolality < 350 mOsm/kg H_2O.

$$FE_K = \frac{Uk / Pk}{Ucr / Pcr} \times 100$$

(iii) **FE $_k$ rises with decrease in renal function (GFR).**
(iv) **FE $_k$ is low with extrarenal losses and decrease in dietary** intake.
(v) **Uk of 40 mEq/liter suggests renal losses of k,** associated with primary aldosterone secretion, Bartter's syndrome, renal artery stenosis, and **diuretics**.

4. **Indications for renal ultrasonography:** Hydronephrosis, renal cysts, calculi, and guide needles.

5. **Indications and contraindications of renal biopsy:**
   (A) **Indications:**
      (i) Hematuria if persistent for > 6 months.
      (ii) Nephrotic syndrome.
      (iii) Acute renal failure from unknown cause (**not** due to ATN).
      (iv) Transplanted kidney to manage posttransplant therapy.
      (v) SLE (systemic lupus erythematosus).
      (vi) Diabetes mellitus (only atypical coondition).
      (vii) Wegener's granulomatosis (unknown etiology).
      (viii) Goodpasture's syndrome (unknown etiology).
   (B) **Contraindications**:
      (i) Bleeding abnormalities (PT > 3 seconds from control, prolonged bleeding time).
      (ii) Platelets count < 60,000.
      (iii) Single kidney.
      (iv) Diastolic BP < 90 mm Hg before biopsy.
      (v) Patients are **not** cooperative.

6. **Please remember the following:**
   Angiotenisin I = **Decapeptide**, synthesized in the **kidneys**.
   Angiotenisin II = **Octapeptide**, synthesized in the **lungs, CNS,** and vessels.
   Angiotenism III = **Heptapeptide**, synthesized in the circulation by angiotensinase.

7. **Responses of the body in volume depletion:**

(i) **Tachycardia,** increased peripheral resistence, decreased venous capacitance.
(ii) **Increased** catecholamines, **ADH** (when volume is reduced > 8 to 10%), **angiotensin II,** and **endothelin I (prostaglandin H_2, throboxane A_2)**. ADH causes water retention and hypoperfusion; catecholamines cause hypoperfusion and sodium retention.

8. **Formations and functions of angiotensins**:
(A) **Formations:**

Renin substrate
↓renin
Angiotensin I (decapeptide)
↓pulmonary converting enzyme
Angiotensin II (octapeptide)
↓circulating angiotensinase
Angiotensin III (heptapeptide)

(B) **Functions of angiotensin II:**
(i) More potent vasoconstrictor than norepinephrine.
(ii) It stimulates aldosterone secretion and sodium retention.
(iii) Angiotensin II is formed in CNS, it stimulates thirst.
(iv) It is also synthesized locally in the vessels, functions of those are unknown.

(C) **Functions of angiotensin III:**
(i) Less potent vasoconstrictor than angiotensin II.
(ii) It stimulates thirst.
(iii) It is not a potent stimulator of aldosterone secretion.

9. **Clinical manifestation, diagnosis, and treatment of volume depletion**:
(A) **Clinical manifestation:** It depends upon the rate, volume, and type of fluid loss.
(i) **Mild volume loss:** Weakness, postural giddiness, and tachycardia.
(ii) **Severe volume loss:** Tachycardia, peripheral vasoconstriction, and hypotension.

Please remember that **lack** of physical findings does **not** exclude the presence of mild to moderate volume loss. **History is very important**.

(B) **Diagnosis**:
(i) **Initial assesment:** Pluse, BP, clinical estimate of venous pressure, and skin temperature. These findings are **not** conclusive in moderate degree of fluid loss. **The fluid challenge is helpful to evalute critically ill patients** in whom **the volume deficit results in reduced cardiac output**. Give 500 ml of normal saline over 1 to 3 hours.

(ii) Patients with **normal** cardiac reserve: Monitor pulse, BP, and urine output after the fluid challenge.

(iii) Patients with **impaired** cardiac reserve: Monitor **pulmonary capillary wedge pressure** through Swan-Ganz catheter or cardiac output. It can detect **fluid overload** due to fluid challenge. **In volume loss** there are pulmonary vasoconstrition of both venous and arterial circuits. **During volume expansion** (fluid challenge), the pulmonary capillary wedge pressure **rises initially** (which should **not** be misinterpreted as an adequate volume replacement) and **subsequently falls**.

(iv) CVP is **not** reliable to measure pulmonary vascular volume.

(v) **Severe** degree of volume loss **also reduces GFR and FE_{Na} but increases prerenal azotemia.**

(C) **Treatment**:

(i) Goal is to increase ECV (extra cellular fluid volume):

(a) **Solution containing sodium is the best fluid to expand ECV** (infusion of 1 liter of normal saline solution increases the blood volume approximately 300 ml or 6%).

(b) Patients with hypertonic volume-contraction (e.g., diabetes insipidius, excessive sweating) should be treated **with D_5W** (infusion of 1 liter of D_5W increases the blood volume approximately 75 to 100 ml or 2%).

(c) **Colloid-containing solutions** (e.g., iso-oncotic albumin and plasma) are used in **patients with burn,** in which cutaneous protein losses are significant.

(d) **Blood**: In **most** hemorrhagic conditions, combination of **PRBC** (packed RBC) with **either normal saline or colloid solutions** is used. In massive hemorrhagic shock, whole blood therapy is used.

10. **Difference between septic shock and hypovolemic shock**: (Pulmonary capillary wedge pressure is **reduced** in both conditions).

Septic shock	Hypovolemic shock
(i) Warm extremities, low BP, and oliguria.	(i) Cool often cyanotic extremities, low BP, and oliguria.
(ii) Reduced systemic vascular resistance (SVR).	(ii) Increased SVR.
(iii) Treatment: Antibiotics plus appropriate fluids	(iii) Treatment: Isotonic saline solutions.

11. **Calculation of serum osmolality**:

Osmolality = $2[Na^+] + [Glucose]/18 + [BUN]/2.8$

$$= 2 \times 140 + \frac{90}{18} + \frac{28}{2.8} \quad (\text{Na} = 140,\ \text{glucose} = 90,\ \text{BUN} = 28)$$

$$= 280 + 5 + 10 = 295$$

12. **Diuretics which cause hearing loss**: **Loop diuretics** (e.g., furosemide, bumetanide, and ethacrynic acid), they also cause **hypokalemic alkalosis**.
Mechanism of diuresis: Inhibit the absorption of Na^+, Cl^-, K^+ in ascending limb of Henle.
They are the most potent diuretics, so named as **'high-ceiling' diuretics.**
Other types of diuretics:
(A) Proximal tubule diuretics (e.g., acetazolamide, metolazone).
Acetazolamide (carbonic anhydrase inhibitor): It blocks proximal reabsorption of sodium bicarbonate.
Metolazone (thiazide class of diuretics): It blocks NaCl absorption in early distal and proximal tubules.
Side effects:
Acetazolamide: Hyperchloremic acidosis, low k.
Metolazone: Hypokalemic alkolosis.
(B) **Early distal diuretics** (e.g., thiazide, metolazone): Inhibit NaCl absorption in early distal tubles.
Side effects: Hypokalemic alkalosis, hyperglycemia, hyperuricemia.
(C) Late distal diuretics (e.g., aldosterone antagonist is spironolactone, nonadlosterone antagonists are triamterene, amiloride): Inhibit NaCl absorption in late distal diuretics.
Side effects: Hypokalemic acidosis.

13. **Electrolyte disorders in different clinical and laboratory conditions (Important):**
(i) **Low** serum Na, **high serum lipid,** normal serum glucose, normal serum osmolality: Hyperlipemia (laboratory artifact). The test should be repeated because of pseudohyponatremia.
(ii) **Low** serum Na, **high serum protein,** normal serum glucose, normal serum osmolality: Hyperproteinemia (laboratory artifact). The test should be repeated because of pseudohyponatremia.
(iii) **Low serum Na, high serum glucose, increased** serum osmolality: Hyperglycemia. In true hyperglycemia avoid excessive glucose administration. In pseudohyperglycemia the specimen should **not** be contaminated with glucose.
(iv) **Low** serum Na, **normal** serum glucose, **increased** serum osmolality, after diuretic therapy: Mannitol therapy. The treatment is to discontinue or

judicious use of mannitol. Both item (iv) and (v) are due to increased nonsodium ECF solutes.

(v) **Normal** serum Na, **increased serum osmolality**: Increased nonsodium ECF and ICF solutes (e.g., ethanol, methanol, ethylene glycol, isopropyl alcohol). **'Osmolar gap'** means normal serum Na and increased serum osmolality which is helpful **in diagnosis of ethanol intoxication** or in azotemia.

(vi) **Lower serum Na,** tubular loss of Na in the urine, **volume expansion without edema,** increased GFR, **reduced** tubular absorption of creatinine and uric acid, normal thyroid and adrenal functions: **These are the major characteristic of syndrome of inappropriate ADH secretion (SIADH).**

14. **Different types of ADH responses:**
    (i) **Appropriate ADH secretion**: Increased ADH secretion when serum osmolality is **elevated** (e.g., dehydration, volume loss) to maintain the normal physiologic fluid volume. **ADH secretion curve is nonlinear but rapid rise of ADH secretion in > 7 to 10 % of volume loss (Important).**
    (ii) **Inappropriate ADH secretion (SIADH)**: Increased endogenous ADH or ADH like substance release when serum osmolality is **normal or low** (e.g., cancer, different drugs, CNS infection, trauma, tumors, pulmonary infections, and ventilators with positive pressure). **ADH secretion curve is linear with normal osmolality (285 to 315) (Important). Four different patterns of plasma ADH secretion in SIADH patients**:
        (a) **Normal relation** between ADH secretion and serum osmolality: ADH is secreted when serum osmolality is **normal (285 to 315)**.
        (b) **Erratic ADH release (37% of SIADH)**: Increased ADH secretion even with very low serum **osmolality (50 to < 200 approximately)**.
        (c) **Reset osmostat (33% of SIADH)**: Increased ADH secretion (abnormally low threshold) when serum osmolality is mildly low **(between 240 to 280 approximately)**.
        (d) ADH leak pattern (14% of SIADH): Increased ADH secretion when serum osmolality ranges from below normal to normal (**240 to 285 approximately**).

15. **Beer potomania**: Decreased solute delivery to the collecting duct is called beer potomania. Beer has **low concentration of salts and other solutes but high carbohydrate content. Normal individual** with normal diet without beer produces approximately 1000 mOsm of solutes for urinary excretion, 50 mOsm of solutes need 1 liter of free water, (1000/50 = 20 liters) **a normal person can consume 20 liter of water without developing hyponatremia.**

16. **Clinical manifestations, diagnosis, and treatment of hyponatremia:**

(A) **Clinical manifestations**:

(i) Acute hyponatremia: Lethargy, somnolence, seizure, coma, and death. CNS symptomps and signs are due to cerebral edema from rapid fall of serum Na. It is a medical emergency.

(ii) **Chronic hyponatremia**: CNS manifestations are **less common** even serum Na as low as 100 mEq/liter because of loss of brain solutes (particularly k) reduces brain cell swelling.

(B) **Diagnosis**: History (intake of drugs, beer, excessive water, infections, weight loss, cancer) and physical examination are very important.

(i) **Appropriately increased ADH secretion**:

Low = Plasma Na, **urine Na** (< 10 to 15 mEq/liter), **FE_{Na} (< 1%)**, serum osmolality, and **blood volume.**

High = **Plasma uric acid,** urine osmolality, BUN, and plasma creatinine.

Normal =None.

(ii) **Inappropriately increased ADH secretion**:

Low = Plasma Na, **plasma uric acid,** serum osmolality.

High = **Urine Na** (> 30 mEq/liter), **FE_{Na} (> 1%)**, urine osmolality.

Normal = BUN, plasma creatinine; blood volume is either **normal or increased.**

(iii) **Edema plus hyponatremia:** It is due to **reduced** arterial blood volume and **increased** ECF volume.

(iv) The results of fluid restriction (600 to 800 ml daily):

(a) **In SIADH:** Weight loss (2 to 3-kg over 2 to 3 days), correction of hyponatremia, cessation of urinary loss of Na.

(b) **Renal salt-wasting disease, Addison's disease**: Weight loss **fails to correct** hyponatremia and urinary loss of Na.

(C) **Treatment**:

(i) **Acute correction of hyponatremia (serum Na < 120 mEq/liter) with CNS manifestations is a medical emergency**: Goal is to increase the serum Na up to levels of **120 to 125 mEq/liter over 6 hours period** by **administering hypertonic 3 to 5% saline.** The following formula is used:

The required mEq of sodium =[125- measured serum Na^+] X 0.6 X body weight in kg.

=(125-115) X 0.6 X 60.

= 10 X 0.6 X 60 = 360 mEq of sodium.

(measured Na =115, total body water volume = 60% or 0.6 of body weight, body weight = 60 kg).

Physicians who are unable to remember the formula: Administer **250 ml of either 3 or 5% saline over 4 to 6 hours**. This will increase serum Na by 10 to 15 mEq/liter and control clinical manifestations.

(ii) **Chronic correction of hyponatremia**:

(a) **Asymptomatic non-volume depleted hyponatremia**:
First approach is to restrict electrolyte free water intake < 1 liter/day plus high dietary salt intake.
Alternative second approach is to **use normal saline plus must use loop diuretic** (diuretics enhances urinary loss of salts results in decrease in ECF volume). This approach is **faster** than the first approach. **Please remember** isotonic saline infusion without loop diuretic **may reduce the serum Na** in patients with SIADH. **Loop diuretic must be used with infusion of normal saline.**
Alternative third approach is to use lithium carbonate or demeclocycline (both block effects of ADH in collecting ducts and enhance excretion of free water) when first two approaches fail.

17. **Complication of too-rapid correction of hyponatremia:**

(A) **Osmotic demyelination syndrome**: It is due to selective loss of myelin (sparing neurons and axial cylinders) any part of the brain specifically the pons.
Signs and symptoms: It appears several days after too-rapid correction of hyponatremia. Patients appear with **fluctuating level of consciousness, behavioral disturbances, ataxia, speech difficulty, and pseudo-bulbar palsy**.
Prognosis: In nonfatal cases, the recovery may take weeks and residual defect may persist.
How to avoid this complications ?:
Two-step method should be followed.
(i) First step is the acute correction of symptomatic hyponatremia.
(ii) Second step is the chronic correction of asymptomatic or residual hyponatremia.

18. **Clinical manifestations, diagnosis, and treatment of hypernatremia:**

(A) **Clinical manifestations**: It is produced by **brain shrinkage** because high Na (high osmolality) in ECF draws water out of the brain cells into the ECF. The symptoms of hypertonicity produced either **by high Na or high glucose levels. The clinical manifestations are somnolence, confusion** when ECF osmolality exceeds **320 to 330** mOsm/kg of H_2O. It depends upon the degree and rate of development of hypertonicity. The patients have decreased ICF and **increased or normal ECF volumes**.

(B) **Diagnosis**: Elevated serum Na and serum osmolality.

(C) **Treatment**:

(i) **Acute hypernatremia: Intravenous infusion of normal saline has two advantages**: It **avoids rapid fall of serun Na levels** and provides **fluid resuscitation** in impending CVS collapse. (**Total body water is 60% of body weight, 2/3 of that is intracellular, and 1/3 is extracellular which** includes plasma and interstitial fluids).

19. **Complication of rapid correction of hypertonicity or hypernatremia to normal serum osmolality (Important)**:

(A) **CNS damage is due to brain swelling**: Accumulation of **idiogenic osmoles by brain cells** is a compensatory mechanism for **maintaining brain volume** in hypertonicity. Normal serum osmolalilty is **relatively hypotonic** to brain cells that have accumulated idiogenic solutes.
Signs and symptoms: Increased ICP, seizures,herniation, coma.
How to prevent this complication ?: Serum Na levels should **not drop more than 1 mEq/liter every 2 hours for the first 2 days of treatment**.

20. **Essential hypernatremia:** Mildly elevated serum sodium levels in conscious patients. It may be due to **insensitivity of thirst centers** and osmoreceptors to osmotic stimuli but thirst and antidiuresis occurs when fluid volume is reduced. It may be found in histiocytosis involving CNS.

21. **Hypernatremia is due to inadequate thirst**: It is found in **comatose** patients, primary hyperaldosteronism, or Cushing's syndrome.

22. **Osmotic diuresis**: It is caused by diabetic ketoacidosis (DKA), nonketotic hyperosmolar coma, and mannitol.

(i) DKA patients receiving normal saline infusion: Usually do **not** cause hypernatremia because patients are young and have **increased** urine concentrating capacity.

(ii) Nonketotic hyperosmolar coma should be treated with **half-normal saline** because patients are **older** and have **decreased** urine concentrating capacity. Do **not** use normal saline.

23. **Chronic European licorice ingestion**: It cause a syndrome that mimics **primary hyperaldosteronism because glycyrrhizic acid** (present in licorice) have properties similar to aldosterone. **It causes hypokalemia**.

24. **Liddle's syndrome**: It is a rare tubular defect characterized by hypokalemia, hypertension, metabolic alkalosis, and normal aldosterone secretion.

Treatment: Traimterence (remember aldosterone antagonist spironolactone is **not** effective).

25. **Most serious side effect of hypokalemia (< 3.5 mEq/liter): Neuromuscular system disorder.**
Serum k levels (2 to 2.5 mEq/liter) = Musculer weakness.
Serum k levels (< 2 mEq/liter) = Areflexic paralysis and respiratory insufficiency.
Loss of large amount of k from skeletal muscles may result in **rhabdomyolysis and myoglobinuria**. These are common in athletes and military recruits due to excessive exercise, sweating, and ECF volume contraction. **Remember loss of k 1 mEq/liter means loss of 300 mEq of total body k.**
Treatment of hypokalemia: Potassium salts plus treat the underlying disorder. EKG should **not** be used as a guide for k replacement therapy. Oral Kcl causes GI **irritation** and enteric coated Kcl causes **SI ulceration**.

26. **Hyperkalemic-periodic paralysis:** Autosomal dominant, patients appear with myotonia and acute muscle paralysis.
Treatment:
(i) Acute paralysis: Intravenous calcium gluconate or glucose and insulin.
(ii) Chronic hyperkalemia: Diuretics (acetazolamide) reduces the attack.

27. **Psedohyperkalemia**: It is found in **thrombocytosis, leukocytosis** because blood clotting enhance k release from these cells (e.g., myeloproliferative disorders).
Diagnosis: Elevated serum k and normal plasma k.

28. **Clinical manifestations, diagnosis, and treatment of hyperkalemia:**
(A) **Clinical manifestations**: The most important EKG findings are **alternation in cardiac excitibility**. The management depends upon the EKG findings.
(B) **Diagnostic study of EKG**:
 (i) K levels (> 6.5 to 7 mEq/liter) = Peaked T waves.
 (ii) K levels (> 7 to 8 mEq/liter) = Prolonged PR interval, followed by loss of P wave and wide QRS complex.
 (iii) K levels (> 8 to 10 mEq/liter) = Sine wave pattern and cardiac standstill.
(C) **Treatment**:
 (i) **Glucose (25 grams) plus insulin (10 units)** infusion. **Insulin promotes k entry into cells and glucose prevents hypoglycemia.** (Do **not** use 50% glucose which may increase k if given rapidly. Use 10% glucose over 30 minutes).

(ii) **Sodium bicarbonate** (40 to 150 mEq IV over ½ to 1 hour interval) **promotes k entry into cells**. (It can cause hypernatremia, increased ECF volume in renal compromised patients).

(iii) **Beta-2 agonists (e.g., albuterol)** is used in mild hyperkalemia in chronic disorders (e.g., chronic renal failure, hyperkalemic periodic paralysis). **It promotes shift of k from ECF to ICF**.

(iv) Severe hyperkalemic cardiotoxicity (absent P wave and wide QRS complex): Use of **calcium gluconate** (10 to 30 ml of 10% solution over 10 to 20 minutes) inhibits effect of k on cardiac muscles. (It can **unmask** digitalis toxicity and **precipitates with $NaHCO_3$ solution**).

(v) **Enhance k removal from GI tract by sodium polystyrene sulfonate or kayexalate**: Each 1 mEq of Na is exchanges for 1 mEq of k. Kayexalate is either used with sorbitol (osmotic diarrhea) or as enema.

(vi) Acute hemodialysis or peritoneal dialysis. It is used in acute renal failure, CHF, burns, and rhabdomyolysis.

29. **Acid-base disorders**:

DISORDERS	pH	Pco_2	Bicarbonate
Respiratory acidosis	↓ 7.20	↑60	↑35
Respiratory alkalosis	↑7.55	↓18	↓10
Metabolic alkalosis	↑7.55	→35	↑35
Metabolic acidosis	↓7.20	↓20	↓10
Compensated respiratory acidosis	→ 7.35	↑60	↑35
Compensated respiratory alkalosis	→7.35	↓18	↓10
Acidosis (respiratory + metabolic)	↓ 7.00	↑60	↓10
Alkalosis (respiratory + metabolic)	↑7.65	↓18	↑35

-↓CO_2 is always associated with ↓HCO_3 and vice versa.
-Compensated means pH is normal, but CO_2 and HCO_3 are abnormal .
- ↓ = Low, ↑ = high, → = Normal.

How to remember easily ?:

(i) First look at pH (low, high, or normal).

(ii) **Low pH (acidosis):** Metabolic (↓HCO_3); respiratory (↑CO_2); combined (↓ HCO_3, ↑ CO_2).

(iii) **High pH (alkalosis):** Metabolic (↑HCO_3); respiratory (↓CO_2); combined (↑HCO_3, ↓CO_2).

(iv) **Normal pH (compensated):** Respiratory acidosis (↑CO_2, ↑ HCO_3); respiratory alkalosis (↓CO_2, ↓ HCO_3).

30. **Anion gap**:
   (A) Serum anion gap = $Na^+ - (cl^- + HCO_3^-)$
      (i) **Normal** value of serum anion gap is **10 to 12** mEq/liter (e.g., RTA, diarrhea, dilutional acidosis, carbonic anhydrase inhibitors, primary hyperparathyoridism, small bowel drainage, ureterosigmoidostomy).
      (ii) **Increased anion gap (> 12 mEq/liter)**: Endogenous cause (uremic acidosis in renal failure, lactic acidosis, ketoacidosis, beta-hydroxybutyric acidosis), exogenous causes (methanol, ethylene glycol, salicylates, paraldehyde).
      (iii) **Decreased anion gap (< 10 mEq/liter): Multiple myeloma of IgG variety, rarely lithium toxicity**, hypercalcemia, hypermagnesemia; hyperviscosity syndrome shows decreased anion gap is due **to laboratory artifact**.
   (B) Urinary anion gap = $(Na^+ + K^+) - Cl^-$
      (i) Positive urinary anion gap is found in **RTA** (urinary **Na^+ plus k^+ together is more** than Cl^-)
      (ii) Negative urinary anion gap: Urinary Cl is more than **Na^+** and **k^+** together (e.g., **hypercholremic metabolic acidosis due to GI loss**, normal renal response is to excrete more cl).

31. **Hypoglycemia in alcoholic ketoacidosis is due to: Decreased NAD** (nicotine adenine dinucleotide) dependent gluconeogenesis, decreased glucose results in increased insulin secretion is followed by increased free fatty acids and finally **increased ketogenesis** inside the mitochondria.

32. **Most important clinical finding in metabolic acidosis**: **Hyperventilation** and in severe cases **Kussmaul's** respiration. It is difficult to detect hyperventilation in patients with chronic metabolic acidosis. Lactic acidosis causes decreased cardiac output results in poor tissue perfusion and more metabolic acidosis.

33. **Calculation of bicarbonate deficit in metabolic acidosis**: (24 mEq/L – measured plasma HCO3) X 0.6 X Body weight. **Bicarbonate is given when pH falls below 7.1**. It is better to **raise plasma bicarbonate level up to 16 mEq/L over 12 to 24 hour period,** rather than to correct complete bicarbonate deficit.

34. **Clinical manifestations, diagnosis, and treatment of metabolic alkalosis** (e.g., ECF volume loss, low k, hypercapnia, excess mineralocorticoid).

(A) **Clinical manifestations**: No specific signs and symptoms are present. **Cardiac arrythmias and hypoventilations** (with reduced renal function) are found. Associated hypokalemia causes **muscular weakness and hyporeflexia**.
(Tetany and muscular irritability are **rare** in metabolic alkalosis but **common in respiratory alkalosis**).

(B) **Diagnosis:**
- (i) Measuring serum electrolytes and ABG: **Elevated serum bicarbonate and pH; low k and cl** in the serum.
- (ii) Metabolic alkalosis with volume loss: Urinary **chloride < 10 mEq/liter**.
- (iii) Volume loss patients with Bartter's syndrome or receiving diuretics: **Urinary chloride > 20 mEq/liter plus postural hypotension and hypokalemic metabolic alkalosis**.

(C) **Treatment**:
- (i) **Chloride-responsive patients** (e.g., after diuretic therapy, after hypercapnea, gastric fluid loss): **Intravenous administration of 0.9% Nacl** to correct tachycardia and hypotension. **Potassium salts** should be given to k deficient patients.
  Patients with severe metabolic alkalosis and hypoventilation ($Paco_2$ > 60 mm Hg): **Dilute hydrochloric acid or other acidifying salts** (e.g., lysine or arginine hydrochloride) may be needed. Acidifying agents should **not** be used in significant liver disease.
- (ii) **Chloride-resistant alkalosis** (urine chloride > 20 mEq/liter, normal or increased ECF volume; Bartter's syndrome, Liddle's syndrome, mineralocorticoid excess, hypercalcemia, selective dietary k depletion): Metabolic alkalosis is best treated by **treating the underlying disease.**

35. **Metabolic acidosis, metabolic alkalosis, and combined disorders:**

Disease condition	HCO_3^-	Cl^-	Anion gap
(i) Metabolic alkalosis	High	Low	Normal
(ii) Hyperchloremic acidosis	Low	High	Normal
(iii) Anion gap acidosis	Low	Normal	High
(iv) Anion gap acidosis plus hyperchloremic acidosis	Low	High	High
(v) Metabolic alkalosis plus anion gap acidosis (DKA is complicated by vomiting)	Normal, low, or high	Low	High

(vi) Metabolic alkalosis plus hyperchloremic acidosis	Normal	Normal	Normal
(vii) Metabolic acidosis plus hyperchoremic acidosis (vomiting plus interstitial nephritis)	Low	High	Normal

36. **Clinical manifestations, diagnosis, and treatment of respiratory acidosis:**
   (A) **Clinical manifestations:** It depends upon the severity of CO_2 retention and rate of rise of CO_2. Patients appear with somnolence, confusion, CO_2 narcosis, asterixis, and dilated, totuous fundic vessels or papilledema.
   (B) **Diagnosis**: Elevated Pco_2 and decreased pH in ABG.
   (C) **Treatment**:
      (i) To treat the **underlying disorder and ventilator support**.
      (ii) **Naloxone** should be given to all comatose patients in the ER for an **unknown** cause of respiratory depression.
      (iii) Drug abuse should be ruled out.
      (iv) **Patients with chronic hypercapnia**:
         (a) Treat the underlying cause such as pneumonia.
         (b) **Minimum oxygen should be given very cautiously** to avoid tissue hypoxia. Hypoxia is the stimulus for respiration. Excessive use of oxygen may suppress respiration.
         (c) **Never use alkali** in respiratory acidosis.

37. **Clinical manifestations, diagnosis, and treatment of respiratory alkalosis:**
   (A) **Clinical manifestations**:
      (i) Chronic hyperventilation patients: Asymptomatic.
      (ii) **Acute hyperventilation syndrome**: It is characterized by light-headedness, circumoral numbness, tingling of the extremities, paresthesias, and neuromuscular excitability due to low ionized calcium and magnesium.
   (B) **Diagnosis:** Low PCO_2, high pH in ABG.
   (C) **Treatment:**
      (i) Acute respiratory alkalosis: To correct the underlying disorder.
      (ii) Patients with severe anxiety provokes hyperventilation syndrome: **Air rebreathing with a paper bag** is very helpful, if fails use **sedation**.
      (iii) **Patients in high altitude**: Pretreatment with acetazolamide (500 mg daily) produces mild metabolic acidosis which can prevent respiratory alkalosis.

38. **Fractional excretion of sodium (FE_{Na}):**

$$FE_{Na} = \frac{\text{Urine Na / serum Na}}{\text{Urine creatinine / serum creatinine}}$$

39. **Difference between prerenal and acute tubular injury which cause acute renal failure:**

	Prerenal	Acute tubular injury
(i) FE_{Na}	< 1	> 1
(ii) Urinary osmolality (mOsm/kg H_2O)	> 500	< 350
(iii) Urinary sodium (mEq/L)	< 20	> 40
(iv) Urinary/plasma creatinine ratio	> 40	< 20
(v) BUN/creatinine ratio	> 10 to 1	10 to 1

40. Diseases associated with **FE_{Na} < 1% despite intrinsic renal damage**:
   (A) **Vascular inflammation**: Renal transplantation rejection, acute glomerulonephritis, and acute vasculitis.
   (B) **Severe intrarenal vasoconstriction:** CHF, severe burns, sepsis, liver disease, acute bilateral ureteral obstruction, norepinephrine/dopamine infusion, NSAID's, and iodinated radiocontrast materials.

41. **Clinical manifestations, diagnosis, and treatment of acute renal failure:**
Clinical manifestations: Most common presentations are **weight gain and edema** due to Na and H_2O retention, rarely kidney pain (**except** with urolithiasis, acute pyelonephritis, or tumors). It is also associated with **increased k, metabolic acidosis** (impaired renal excretion of k and H ions) followed by **hypocalcemia, hyperphosphatemia, hyperuricemia, anemia** (hypercalcemia may occur in myoglobinuric ARF), finally **vomiting, irritability, hyperreflexia, asterixis, seizures, coma, and coagulation disorders** (GI bleeding and ecchymoses) **are called uremic syndrome due to accumulation of unexcreted waste products**. Flank pain or urethral pain is usually present in postrenal obstruction. Rapid weight loss and postural hypotension are found in hypovolemic prerenal failure.
   (A) **Diganosis of acute renal failure**:
      (i) **Urinalysis**:
         (a) **Prerenal**: Presence of hyaline casts but **no** RBC or WBC; FE_{Na} < 1, urine osmolality > 500, urinary Na < 20.
         (b) **Renal:** Presence of granular casts, proteinuria, RBC's and WBC's; FE_{Na} > 1, urinery osmolality < 350, urinary Na > 40.

(c) **Postrenal:** Presence of WBC's (infection), RBC's or proteinuria/hematuria (venous occlusion).

(ii) **Serum**: High (K, urea, p); low (pH, Ca, hematocrit).

(iii) BUN/creatinine ratio: Prerenal (> 10 to 1), renal (10 to 1).

(iv) Urinary and plasma creatinine ratio: Prerenal (> 40), renal (< 20).

(B) **Treatment of acute renal failure**:

(i) **Correction of reversible causes**:

(a) **Avoid nephrotoxic drugs** (e.g., NSAID's reduces renal blood flow) and **nephrotoxic radiocontrast agents**.

(b) Monitor plasma drug levels and adjust the doses accordingly.

(c) Prerenal hypovolemic, hypotensive patients: Maintain BP by discontinuing antihypertensive, isotonic saline to increase ECF volume, blood for anemia or bleeding.

(d) Elderly patients with longstanding high BP, presently recorded BP 100/70: IV isotonic saline (500 to 1000 ml) to increase the plasma volume.

(e) Patients with edema or ascites: Do **not** give saline. Edema or ascites means **positive sodium** balance and **intrarenal vasoconstriction**. Infusion of saline causes worsening of edema and ascites.

(f) **Patients with obstructed uropathy**: Urologic consultation plus maintenance of zero fluid balance.

(g) Patients with low FE_{Na} (< 1%) and **no** edema: Fluid challenge with 500 ml of saline plus 40 to 80 mg IV lasix may reverse **an oliguric phase to a nonoliguric phase**.

(h) **Patients with edema plus oliguria:** A trial of 2 to 10 mg lasix (furosemide) may **reverse an oliguric phase to a nonoliguric phase**, if urine flow **exceeds 20 to 30 ml/hour, lasix is used to achieve fluid balance**. Low dose **dopamine** (1 to 3 microgram/Kg/minute) may increase the urine output by renal vasodilatation. **Discontinue lasix and dopamine** if no improvement in urine output.

(ii) **General support**:

(a) **Avoid** indwelling urinary catheter in uncomplicated patients. Intermittent catheterization (sterile technique) is used in oliguric, obtunded patients.

(b) **Maintenance of fluid balance is the most important: Daily weight measurement is the best method of maintaining accurate fluid balance** (fluid intake/output is **less** accurate and **more** cumbersome). Patients should receive **fluid (500 ml** of water, tea) **plus total amount of last 24-hour urine output**. Patients with fever may receive more fluid but **no** weight gain is accepted. Severely catabolic patients may lose about 0.5 kg/day.

(c) **No** extra Na, k, and cl are allowed **besides food**.

(d) Patients with weight gain: Restrict the Na.

(e) Patients with normal Na: No restriction of H_2O.

(f) Patients with low Na: Restriction of H_2O.

(g) Dietary protein: **Restriction to 0.8 gram per Kg/body weight/day** and **energy** intake (carbohydrates plus fats) should **provide 35 kcal/kg/day**. Patients who are NPO should receive IV amino acids and glucose.

(h) Measurement of serial BP (supine plus upright), serum electrolytes, BUN, creatinine, and hematocrit are important.

(i) Hyperkalemia (> 6 mEq/L) should be treated with **sodium polystyrene sulfonate exchange resin with sorbitol**. EKG changes of widened QRS complex on A-V dissociation should be **treated urgently with IV calcium gluconate or calcium chloride**. Administration of glucose plus insulin, hypertonic $NaHCO_3$ (patients with acidosis) can reduce the serum K levels **within 30 to 60 minutes**.

(j) **Hemodialysis**: **It is indicated in hyperkalemia unresponsive** to above mentioned therapy, **severe metabolic acidosis**, **pulmonary edema, azotemia** (SUN > 100 mg/dL), **bleeding, pericarditis, uremic enteropathy, encephalopathy, and seizures**.

(k) **Peritoneal dialysis (PD):** It is the method of choice in patients with severe cardiac failure but do **not require rapid removal** of k or other waste products. PD **avoids rapid** shifts in blood volume and does **not** require anticoagulants.

(iii) **Recovery of renal function:**

(a) **Prerenal ARF:** It is **reversible** if the underlying disorder is corrected.

(b) **Postrenal or obstructive ARF:** Renal function is **stabilized or improved** if the obstruction is relieved.

(c) **Intrinsic or renal ARF**: It has variable outcome. Glomerulonephritis and vasculitis have complete recovery after immunosuppressive therapy. Tubular damage due to ischemia or toxin is **reversible. Nearly normal recovery of renal function in nonoliguric** than oliguric renal failure. **Maximum improvement in renal function occurs in the second week**, mild defects may **persist for months or years** after acute tubular damage.

42. **Prevention of acute renal failure (ARF):**

(i) **Avoid** NSAID's and nephrotoxic antibiotics in ARF patients.
(ii) **Intravenous saline** should be given in patients receiving **cisplatin** and other nephrotoxic medications.
(iii) **Use of allopurinol** reduces the uric acid production in leukemia or massive tumors.
(iv) **Intravenous saline** should be given before giving iodinated radiocontrast material and before surgery.

43. **Most common causes of chronic renal failure (CRF) in USA: First is diabetes, second is hypertension.**

44. **Clinical manifestations of chronic renal failure (CRF):**
(i) Patients are **not** aware of advancing renal failure until the GFR decreased to < 15 ml/minute.
(ii) **Azotemia** indicates retention of nitrogenous waste products due to renal insufficiency.
(iii) **Uremia indicates final stages of progressive renal insufficiency** and clinical manifestations of complex, multiorgan system involvements.
(iv) **The uremic syndrome includes the following**:
(a) Metabolic acidosis: **Increased anion gap (20 to 24 mEq/L), low serum bicarbonate** (**not** below 12 to 15 mEq/L), another form is type IV RTA (most characteristically found in diabetes with CRF, high k level is due to hyporeninemic hypoaldosteronism).
(b) Hyperkalemia but total body k depletion.
(c) **Salt-losing nephropathy** (patients need dietary salt supplementation), **sodium retention** results in increased ECF volume causing high BP, cardiomegaly, pulmonary edema, and peripheral edema.
(d) Low calcium, high phosphate, secondary hyperparathyroidism, and vitamin D deficiency. Patients tolerate low calcium very well, tetany can be precipitated by infusion of $NaHCO_3$ but **muscle cramping and twitching in CRF** are **not** due to hypocalcemia.
(e) Accumulation of magnesium and aluminium are **due to excessive intake**.
(f) **CVS: Accelerated atherosclerosis** (**elevated triglycerides** are due to inadequate removal and normal or mildly elevated plasma cholesterol), **hypertension (most importantly due to Na retention and volume expansion,** and alteration of renin-angiotensin axis), **pericarditis (associated with uremia or dialysis; uremic pericarditis is due to unknown etiology but associated with uremia**, patients appear with pain in the left side of the chest, tamponade, pericardial friction rub, or **diastolic collapse in severe cases that needs emergent surgical**

drainage. Uremic pericarditis responds to peritoneal dialysis. Pericarditis due to dialysis should be treated with hemodialysis), and myocardial dysfunction.

(g) **Hematologic abnormalities: Anemia** (due to erythropoietin and iron deficiencies), **hemorrhagic disorders** (prolonged bleeding time is due to platelet dysfunction or peripheral destruction of platelets, **treated with hemodialysis which removes uremic toxin guanidinosuccinic acid**), **enhanced staphylococcal or Gram-negative infections** (due to deranged or deficient humoral or cellular immunity, leukocyte dysfunction, decreased inflammatory reaction, or increased exposure to bacteria or virus. Aggressive vaccination **particularly hepatitis B vaccine should be given. Staphylococcal infection is due to cutaneous contamination through the arteriovenous hemodialysis access**). Anemia producing symptoms and signs of **pallor, tachycardia, systolic ejection murmur, and wide pulse pressure.**

(h) **GI disorders:** Anorexia, nausea, vomiting, alteration of taste, and **GI bleeding. The later is due to scattered petechiae, ulceration, peptic ulcer disease, angiodysplasia**, or platelet dysfunction.

(i) **Renal osteodystrophy** includes osteomalacia, osteosclerosis, osteoporosis, and osteitis fibrosa (secondary hyperparathyroidism). Patients appear with bone pain and spontaneous fracture.

(j) **Neurologic disorders: Peripheral neuropathy** (sensory loss in a **stocking-glove distribution,** diminished deep tendon reflexes, muscular weakness, **restless leg syndrome**, painful paresthesias of extremities, and twitching; **lower extremities are more involved** than upper extremities) and **CNS** (insomnia, fatigue, asterixis, and psychological problems).

(k) **Endocrine disorders:** Fasting blood glucose is either normal or slightly elevated but abnormal glucose tolerance (insulin resistance, insulin degradation, hypoglycemia; **amenorrhea and infertility** in women, **impotence and oligospermia** in men, **hypothermia** is due to reduced metabolic rate.

(l) **Myopathy:** Muscular wasting and weakness develop slowly (**proximal** muscles are mostly affected) in end-stage renal disease (ESRD).

(m) Pruritus: Generalized pruritus, uremic frost, and soft tissue calcifications.

Treatment: Frequent dialysis, dietary restriction of protein, correction of secondary hyperparathyroidism, and parathyroidectomy.

(n) Hyperuricemia: It occurs when GFR has decreased to 20% of normal. **Pseudogout (due to crystalline deposits** other than uric acid and deposition of amyloid and beta-2 microglobulin), arthritis, and rarely clinical gout are present.

45. **Diagnostic approach in uremia patients:**
   (i) A **detailed history** (such as hematuria, nocturia, dysuria, polydipsia, polyuria, exposure to toxins, infections, and family history of renal disease) has to be obtained and can **lead to the diagnosis**.
   (ii) **The physical examination should include (BP, edema,** nailbed findings, **retina, CVS, renal auscultation for bruits and palpation for size**, rectal examination for prostatic evaluation, gynecologic examination for pelvic masses, and musculoskeletal examination) and it is very important.
   (iii) Laboratory tests: CBC, urinalysis; **in CRF, hematocrit is low, phosphate is high, and benign urinary sediment is present**. These are all **nonspecific** findings to distinguish from AFR.
   (iv) **Renal sonogram** to determine the size (**small size indicates chronicity and irreversibility, normal size usually means acute** process) and to rule out hydronephrosis or cystic masses.
   (v) It is important to differentiate between prerenal, renal, and postrenal causes of azotemia. Lower urinary tract obstruction (**most common cause is enlarged prostate in men**) is diagnosed **by measuring postvoid residual urine** which is increased. Upper urinary tract obstruction (**most common cause is renal stone, bladder cancer**) is diagnosed by sonogram (dilated pelvis, ureter, and calices **above** the obstruction) and normal postvoid residual urine.
   (vi) Patients with **renal parenchymal disease** (hypertensive, analgesic, or hypercalcemic nephropathy; hemolytic-uremic syndrome; lupus and interstitial nephritis; multiple myeloma, pyelonephritis, progressive glomerulonephritis): **Renal biopsy is the definitive diagnostic method. Contraindications to renal biopsy**:
      (a) If the biopsy findings will **not** influence in the management.
      (b) Bleeding disorders (uncorrectable).
      (c) Severe hypertension (uncontrolled).
      (d) Infection, abscess (perinephric).
      (e) Hydronephrosis.
      (f) Extreme obesity.

46. **Management of patients with chronic renal failure (CRF):** Three categories are the following: treatment of aggravation factors, treatment of specific complications of uremia, and long-term care.
   (A) **Treatment of aggravating factors**:

(i) **Volume depletion:** It is one of the most common cause of **worsening kidney function**. Look for physical signs, measure urinary electrolytes, and rise of serum creatinine.
Etiology: Absolute (aggressive use of diuretics, dehydration, GI fluid losses), effective (nephrotic syndrome, ascites, low cardiac output, low renal perfusion).
Treatment: Adequate hydration and avoid or treat the underlying cause.

(ii) **Avoid the nephrotoxic drugs** (e.g., aminoglycosides, excessive diuretics, prostaglandin synthesis inhibitors) **or adjust the doses.**

(iii) **Appropriate intervention for obstruction:** Tubular (uric acid crystals, Bence Jones protein) or posttubular (ureteral stone, prostatic hypertrophy, necrotic papillae).

(iv) **Hypertensive crisis:** It causes worsening of kidney function. **Rapid and adequate control of BP** is very important.

(v) **Toxins:** Vasodilators, nephrotoxic antibiotics, and radiocontrast materials **may cause rapid rise of creatinine. These toxins should be avoided**. CRF patients with **diabetes or multiple myeloma causes** worsening of renal **function due to volume depletion.**
Treatment: Adequate hydration reverses the renal function.

(vi) **Infection:** UTI; and sepsis with hypotension causes worsening of renal function.
Treatment: Appropriate antibiotics and maintenance of normal BP (in case of hypotension).

(vii) **Hypercalcemia and hyperphosphatemia** cause worsening of renal function and soft tissue calcification. It is found in **multiple myeloma.**
Treatment: Vitamin D supplementation, calcium-carbonate as a phosphate binder, and restriction of dietary phosphate.

(B) **Treatment of complications of uremia**:

(i) **Hyperkalemia:** Serum k level up to 6 mEq/L does **not** need therapy. **Modest elevation of k** (> 6 mEq/L) **require dietary restriction as a first step** plus to correct the underlying cause or factor (volume depletion, acidosis, high intake of k, fever, medications such as spironolactone, Kcl, NSAID's, beta-blocker, triamterene, amiloride, and trimethoprim), **severe hyperkalemia** with EKG changes should be treated with calcium gluconate, glucose plus insulin, $NaHCO_3$, and kayexelate.

(ii) **Sodium imbalance:**

(a) Patients with volume depletion: Administer adequate volume **but avoid** hypertension, pulmonary edema, and peripheral edema.

(b) Orthostatic hypotension: Liberalized salt intake.

(c) Metabolic acidosis: Give $NaHCO_3$.

(d) **Patients with volume expansion:** Give diuretics (**furosemide alone** or in **combination with thiazide**), uncontrolled patients need **peritoneal dialysis or hemodialysis**.

(e) **Hyponatremia or hypernatremia:** The treatment protocol (**water restriction or administration of free water**) **is the same** as in any other patients.

(f) **Severe hyponatremia with CNS symptoms**: Administration of **hypertonic saline solution** but the resultant volume expansion may be treated with **urgent dialysis**.

(iii) **CVS: Hypertriglyceridemia** and **high BP** are the most important risk factors **for atherosclerosis and high CVS mortality. Please remember that successful patients with renal transplantation have increased CVS death.**

(a) **Treatment for hypertriglyceridemia:** Same dietary principles for CRF and non-CRF patients; clofibrate or cholesterol synthesis inhibitors if used, doses should be adjusted.

(b) **Treatment for hypertension:** The most important is to **decrease the intravascular volume** by dietary restriction of salt and water, judicious use of diuretics (furosemide, thiazide) or dialysis in severe cases.

Antihypertensive medications (clonidine, calcium channel blockers, beta-blockers, ACE inhibitors, or minoxidil) may be needed. **Uncontrolled malignant** hypertension may respond **to bilateral nephrectomy**.

(c) **Treatment of uremic pericarditis: The best initial therapy is daily dialysis for approximately one week.** Unresponsive patients need **drainage and intrapericardial injection of nonabsorbable steroids**. Failure of medical management necessciates **partial pericardiectomy**.

(iv) **Treatment for anemia:** Goal is to increase the hematocrit between 30 to 33% (higher level may cause high BP, headaches, sometimes seizures). **Oral iron supplementation (ferrous salt)** or in some **unresponsive patients use intravenous iron dextran is recommended. Folic acid supplementation is also recommended. Recombinant human erythropoietin is effective in anemia with ESRD.**

(v) **Treatment for infections:** Use of nonnephrotoxic or less nephrotoxic antibiotic is recommended.

(vi) **Treatment for renal osteodystrophy** (due to hyperparathyroidism, decreased vitamin D metabolites, and chronic metabolic **acidosis**): **Use calcium carbonate** (to bind phosphate) **and calcitriol** to control secondary hyperparathyroidism. **Monitor PTH levels which are elevated long before** the radiographic changes. **Use $NaHCO_3$ to correct metabolic acidosis**.

(vii) **Treatment for neuropathy**: **No specific** treatment is available but symptomatic improvement is noted after dialysis or renal transplantation.

(viii) **Treatment for myopathy: Active vitamin D analogues, nutritional supplements, and erythropoietin** are useful. Some patients may improve after parathyroidectomy for secondary hyperparathyroidism.

(ix) **Treatment for high uric acid:** Asymptomatic patients do **not** need any treatment. **Allopurinol is the drug of choice** (up to 100 mg per day) becausse CRF do **not** respond to uricosuric medications. Patients with gout need chronic therapy with **cholchicine (0.6 mg/day)**.

(x) **Treatment for pruritus:** The goal is to treat secondary hyperparathyroidsm. To **lower serum phosphate use dialysis and restrict phosphate intake** or **rarely** parathyroidectomy for intractable pruritus. **Topical emulsified oils or oral antihistamines** is useful in some patients.

(C) Treatment for long term care:

(i) **Diet: Restriction of protein intake** (**0.6 gram/kg body weight/day**), of which **at least 60% contains protein rich in essential amino acids** (e.g., lean meat, eggs, and milk). Approximately **30 Kcal/day is adequate**, but it is reduced for obese and increased for under weighed patient.

Remember severe protein restriction is **not** recommended. **Adequate nutritional support plus dialysis prn reduce morbidity and mortality**.

Water-soluble B vitamins plus vitamin C, and folic acid are recommended (**no** need to give vitamin A or E). **Vitamin D** is used only for renal osteodystrophy. Severe dietary restriction of sodium is **not** needed unless high BP or edema is present.

If the urine output is > 1 liter/day, **no need to restrict dietary k**.

Patients on chronic hemodialysis should have appropriate diet therapy.

47. **Follow-up of patients with CRF**:

(i) All patients should be seen at least every 3 months.

(ii) History, physical examination, and monitor CBC, SUN, **creatinine, and electrolytes**.

(iii) **Serum creatinine is an indirect index of GFR**, alternatively 24-hour urine to measure creatinine and urea clearance is an approximation of GFR and indication of dietary protein intake.

(iv) **Serum creatinine of 10 mg/dL** (or reciprocal of serum creatinine 0.1 or less) is an indication of dialysis.

48. Most common cause of death in dialysis patients: **Myocardial infarction and cerebral vascular accidents (50% of deaths)**. Chronic dialysis may cause a **syndrome of acclerated atherosclerosis,** other causes are **hypertension, anemia, hypertriglyceridemia** due to heparin in dialysis, **acetate** in the dialysate is toxic to myocardium, and **hyperparathyroidism** may **induce vascular calcification**.

49. **New clinical problems with long term dialysis (both PD and hemodialysis):**
    (i) Dialysis dementia or aluminium intoxication (aluminium from dialysate plus phosphate binders): It is characterized by intermittent speech problems, stuttering, personality alteration, myoclonus, seizures, auditory and visual hallucinations, followed by mute, coma, and death.
    (ii) Myocardial infarction.
    (iii) CVA (cerebral vascular accidents).
    (iv) **Acquired cystic kidney disease** (at least 4 cysts in each native kidney, small size kidneys, and absence of family history will differentiate from polycystic kidney disease). Acquired cysts may turn into malignancy. Death rate in cancer are the same in both dialysis and nondialysis patients.
    (v) **Amyloidosis** (deposition of beta-$_2$ microglobulin in the bone and joints) causes **carpal tunnel syndrome** and **severe problem of erosive spondyloarthropathy**.

50. **Other complications of PD and hemodialysis:**
    (A) **Complications common to both types:** Infection, hepatitis, heart disease, and osteodystrophy.
    (B) **Complications of PD:** Hyperglycemia, peritonitis, diminished peritoneal ultrafiltration, abdominal hernias, and protein malnutrition.
    (C) **Complications of hemodialysis:** Hypotension, hypoxia, nausea, headaches, vomiting, trace metal intoxication, and air embolism.

51. **Indications for kidney transplantation:**
    (i) Diabetes mellitus with renal failure (Kimmelstiel-Wilson disease) **is the most common cause**.
    (ii) Hypertensive renal disease with renal failure is the **seconod** common cause.
    (iii) Glomerulonephritis with end-stage renal disease.

52. **Chromosomal location of the major histocompatibility complex (MHC): Chromosome 6.**

53. **Type of glomerulonephritis which has high incidence of graft loss due to recurrent disease (up to 30%)**: Focal glomerulosclerosis (FGS).

54. **Contraindications of kidney transplantation:**
    (i) **Absolute contraindications**: Malignancy, severe atherosclerosis, severe pulmonary disease, active liver disease (hepatitis B and C may cause eventual liver failure in some patients after transplantation).
    (ii) **Relative contraindication:** Infection with HIV virus (patients may progress from carrier state to clinical AIDS due to immunosuppressive therapy).

55. **Most common cause of immediate nonfunction of the allograft of kidney: Acute tubular necrosis like syndrome** that is **reversible ischemic** damage to the allograft. Other causes in **primary nonfunction** are obstruction, vascular thrombosis, and hematoma which cause ureteral compression.

56. **Management of patients after allograft of the kidney:**
    (i) **Immediate nonfunctioning kidney:** First find out the cause and correct the underlying problem. **Most patients have reversible** renal problems which does **not** need surgical intervention. Renal sonogram can rule out obstruction.
    (ii) Immediate functioning kidney.
    (iii) Careful observation of rejection in both functioning and nonfunctioning kidneys.

    Treatment for both functioning and nonfunctioning kidneys:
    (i) Primary immunosuppressive therapy: OKT3 (monoclonal antibody) or ALG (antilymphocyte globulin) is used **until the allograft functions** well. After that, **cyclosporine, azathioprine,** and prednisone are added, and OKT3 or ALG is discontinued.
    (ii) Some groups begin **tripple-drug therapy** (cyclosporine plus azathioprine plus prednisone) **immediately before the kidney transplantation.**
    (iii) Some groups use **cyclosporine plus prednisone** or **cyclosporine alone**.
    (iv) **Experimental drugs FK-506, rapamycin, and RS-61443** are promising.

57. **Toxicity of cyclosporine:**
    (i) Nephrotoxicity: Acute reversible and chronic kidney damage.
    (ii) Other toxicities are **tremor, hyperglycemia,** palmer and planter **paresthesia, hyperkalemia,** hepatotoxicity, **hypertrichosis,** and gingival hypertrophy.

58. **Complications of OKT3:**
    (i) Many patients do **not** respond after the initial course of therapy.
    (ii) Development of murine antibodies which limit its effectiveness.

59. **Most common opportunistic infection after the kidney transplantation**: **Cytomegalovirus infections**. Some believe it is due to OKT3 therapy. **Signs and symptoms of CMV infections**: It may range from **asymptomatic** to severe illness **leads to coma and death**. Most of the patients appear with **fever, malaise, and lenkopenia**, symptoms last **for 1 to 2 weeks and them resolve without sequelae**. Opportunistic infections usually occur **a month or more after operation**.

60. **Most serious long term complications after kidney transplantation**: Vascular disease, infections, cancer, and chronic liver disease.

61. **Glomerular disease with reduced serum complement levels**: SLE, subacute bacterial endocarditis, post streptococcal glomerulonephritis, idiopathic membranoproliferative glomerulonephritis, and cryoglobulinemia.

62. **Glomerular diseases with normal serum complement levels: IgA nephropathy, MCNS** (minimal change nephrotic syndrome), **FSG** (focal segmental glomerulosclerosis), **membranous nephropathy, polyarteritis nodosa,** anti-GBM dissease, pauci-immune rapidly progressive glomerulonephritis, **Wegener's granulomatosis,** and **Henoch-Schonlein purpura**.

63. **Most common type of idiopathic nephrotic syndrome** (proteinuria > 3 to 3.5 grams/day, hypoalbuminemia, edema, hperlipidemia includes elevated levels of total and LDL cholesterol with low or normal HDL cholesterol): **Membranous nephropathy (25-30% cases). Other causes of nephrotic syndrome are** MCNS, FSG, other proliferative and sclerosing glomerulonephritis, and rarely membranoproliferative glomerulonephritis. Renal biopsy is the best guide for treatment and prognosis of nephrotic syndrome.

64. **Most common type of nephrotic syndrome associated with thrombotic events, especially renal vein thrombosis: Membranous nephropathy**.

65. A patient who is diagnosed to have membranous nephropathy suddenly **develops flank pain, chest pain with respiratory difficulty**, and deterioration of renal function (**Important**).
    Most likely diagnosis: Renal vein thrombosis and pulmonary embolism.

66. **Clinical presentation and EM (electron microscopic) findings of membranous nephropathy**:
    (A) It is typically present with **onset of proteinuria and edema with or without microhematuria and high BP**. Initially GFR and renal function are **normal. Serum complement levels are normal**. Renal vein thrombosis and pulmonary embolism are very common.
    (B) **EM findings:** Subepithelial electron-dense deposits all along the glomerular capillary loops.

67. **Membranous nephropathy may be associated with the following diseases**: **SLE, drugs** (gold salts, trimethadione or tridione), **infections** (hepatitis B and C, lues), and **tumor** (solid tumors and lymphomas).

68. **Treatment of membranous nephropathy:**
    (i) Remember spontaneous remission rate is 20 to 30%.
    (ii) **Recent studies** show **cyclophosphamide plus steroids can reverse progressive renal failure and achieve remission of heavy proteinuria**.

69. **MCNS (minimal change nephrotic syndrome)** or 'nil disease' or lipoid nephrosis:
    (A) **Clinical presentations:** Typically present with **periorbital** and **peripheral edema due to proteinuria with or without** high BP, microscopic hematuria, and azotemia are due to hypoalbuminemia and intravascular volume loss.
    (B) **Laboratory findings:** Complement levels and serologic tests **are normal.**
    (C) **EM (electron microscopic) study**: No immune deposits, normal GBM, but **fusion of the visceral epithelial foot process. Similar** histologic pattern may be seen in adverse effect of drugs (NSAID's, lithium), leukemias, and Hodgkin disease.
    (D) **Treatment:**
        (i) Remissions and relapses are commonly found.
        (ii) **Prednisone** (60 mg per day or 120 mg alternate day) for **2 months**, if the response is slow continue treatment for **4 months** before the **diagnosis of steroid-resistant have been made**. **Tapering** of the steroid dose should begin 1 to several weeks **after complete remission** and should continue gradually over 1 to 2 months.
        (iii) Treatment of first relapse: Same as initial treatment.
        (iv) Patients who relapses third time or steroid-dependent (cannot tolerate lower prednisone dose beyond a certain level without recurrence of proteniuria): **Use cyclophosphamide or chlorambucil**, (alternative

therapy is to use low-dose cyclosporine but it is nephrotoxic and has high rate of relapse).

70. **FSG (Focal segmental glomerulosclerosis)**:
    - (A) **Etiology:** Idiopathic or other causes (e.g., **heroin abuse, HIV disease, obesity, sickle cell disease, urinary reflux,** and **lesions associated with single or remnant kidneys**).
    - (B) **Clinical presentations: Asymptomatic proteinuria, edema,** or **nephrotic syndrome (66% of cases)** with non selective proteinuria (< 1 to 30 gram/day), microscopic hematuria (50% of cases), and high BP (30 to 50% of cases).
    - (C) **Laboratory findings: Decreased GFR** (up to 30% of patients), **normal** complement levels, and serologic tests.
    - (D) **EM findings: IgM and C3 are commonly found in areas of glomerulosclerosis**.
    - (E) **Treatment:**
        - (i) Immunosuppressive therapy (6 to 12 months) **with steroids and cytotoxic drug**.
        - (ii) Patients unresponsive to above therapy: **Use low-dose cyclosporine**.
    - (F) **Prognosis**:
        - (i) **Most patients develop ESRD** in 5 to 20 years from the onset of presentation.
        - (ii) Few patients develop spontaneous remission or proteinuria.

71. **MPGN (membranoproliferative or mesangiocapillary glomerulonephritis): It is not common.**
    - (A) Clinical manifestation: **Most patients appear with nephrotic syndrome**, others may appear with asymptomatic microhematuria and proteinuria or acute nephritic picture with urinary sediments. Poor prognosis include high BP, low GFR, and nephrotic syndrome.
    - (B) **Laboratory findings**: Low serum complement levels are found **intermittently in type I MPGN** and **C3 levels are always low** in type II MPGN.
    - (C) **Histologic findings:** Proliferation of glomerular mesangial cells along the capillary wall and split the GBM. Type II MPGN is dense deposit with autoantibody (IgG, C3).
    - (D) **Treatment: No effective therapy in adults** but corticosteroids, other immunosuppressive drugs; anticoagulants, and antiplatelet agents to reduce glomerular damage from coagulation; and NSAID's have been used.

72. **Most common form of idiopathic glomerulonephritis**: **IgA nephropathy**. It is more common in **male** than female, **peak incidence in the second and third decades of life**.

73. **IgA nephropathy**:
   (A) **Clinical presentations:** Most common presentation is **asymptomatic microscopic hematuria and/or proteinuria**. Hypertension is present (20 to 50% of cases). Some patients may have **normal GFR over decades** and others may develop **high BP, nephrotic syndrome, and renal failure**. **Please remember clinical presentations have no corelation with elevated serum IgA levels.**
   (B) **Laboratory diagnosis:** Elevated serum IgA levels (33 to 50% of cases).
   (C) **Treatment: No effective therapy is available** but **glucocorticoids and cytotoxic drugs** are recommended for patients with **crescentic IgA nephropathy**. Physicians should treat patients at highest risk **for progression to renal failure**.
   (D) **Factors causing poor outcome in IgA nephropathy: Absence of gross hematuria**; presence of hypertension, persistent and severe proteinuria, elevated serum creatinine, male with older age of onset, features of severe proliferation and sclerosis, and/or tubulo interstial damage and crescent formation.
   (E) **Complications after renal transplantation:**
      (i) Morphologic recurrence in the allograft is significant.
      (ii) Recurrence does **not** cause graft loss.

74. **Henoch-Schonlein purpura**: It is **less** common in adults. It is small-vessels vasculitis.
   (A) **Signs and symptoms:**
      Skin: Macular rash on the ankles which extends to the legs and thighs, purpuric lesions.
      GI: Cramps, diarrhea, in severe cases melena and bloody diarrhea.
      Arthralgias: Knees, wrists, and ankles.
      Renal: Features of acute proliferative glomerulonephritis.
   (B) Histologic findings: Similar as IgA nephropathy.
   (C) **Treatment: No proven therapy like IgA nephropathy**. Rash, arthralgias, and abdominal symptoms **usually resolves spontaneously**. Some patients with abdominal symptoms may be treated with **short course of steroids**. Patients with severe glomerular disease should be treated with **glucocorticoids and cytotoxic drugs** like IgA nephropathy.
   (D) **Prognosis:**
      (i) Most patients recover completely.

(ii) Patients with severe glomerular disease have an unfavorable long-term outcome.

75. **Post-streptococcal glomerulonephritis (PSSGN)**: Severe disease can occur in adults, most commonly occurs in **winter months following episodes of pharyngitis** or **streptococcal infections at any site**. Subclinical cases are more common than clinical cases.
   (A) **Clinical presentations: Hematuria and proteinuria** after latency period of **10 days to several weeks** after throat infection or even longer after skin infection. **Hypertension is present in most cases**.
   (B) **Laboratory findings:** Throat or skin culture may **not** be positive, but **positive ASLO (anti-streptolysin O), AHT (antihyaluronidase), antistreptokinase, and anti-DNase titers. Normal C4 levels** but **decreased** C3 **and total hemolytic component levels during the episode of acute glomerulonephritis**.
   (C) Histologic findings: Glomerular hypercellularity, coarse granular deposition **of IgG, IgM, complement (especially C3) along the capillary wall.**
   (D) **Nephritogenic strains of group A beta-hemolytic streptococci: M types** 1,2,4,12,18,25,49,55,57, and 60.
   (E) **Treatment:**
      (i) PSGN is a **self-limited disease;** hematuria and proteinuria may resolve slowly over months.
      (ii) **Symptomatic therapy to control hypertension and fluid retention**: Antihypertensive and diuretics are used.

76. **Most common organism in glomerulonephritis due to bacterial endocarditis**: **Staphylococcus aureus especially in drug addicted population**. Approximately 40 to 80% of patients with **S.aureus endocarditis develop proliferative glomerulonephritis.** (Previously most common organism was Streptococcus viridans). Glomerulonephritis is more common in **acute** than subacute endocarditis.
   Signs and symptoms: Hematuria, RBC caste, proteinuria (< 1 gram to nephrotic range), and progressive renal failure.
   Laboratory findings: Reduced C3 and total serum complement levels.
   Treatment: Appropriate antibiotics.

77. **Types of glomerulonephritis in visceral abscesses, pneumonias, and infections:**
   (i) Proliferative glomerulonephritis: Deep visceral abscesses, osteomyelitis, pneumonias.
   Treatment: To treat the underlying cause.

(ii) Immune complex form of glomerulonephritis: Pneumonias (bacterial, mycoplasma), infected cerebral ventriculoatrial shunts for hydrocephalus. Treatment: To treat the underlying cause.

78. Different types of RPGN (rapidly progressive glomerulonephritis): RPGN causes **renal failure within weeks to months and crescent formations** (extensive extracapillary proliferation).
    (A) **Primary type**:
    Type I: **Anti-GBM** (glomerular basement menbrane) antibody disease (plus pulmonary disease is called **Goodpasture's syndrome**).
    Type II: **Immune complex deposition** (e.g., SLE, post-streptococcal).
    Type III: **Pauci-immune** (antineutrophil cytoplasmic antibody postive).
    (B) **Secondary type**: SLE, IgA nephropathy-H-S purpura, membranoproliferative glomerulonephritis, post-streptococcal glomerulonephritis, polyarteritis nodosa, and hypersensitivity angitis.

79. **Anti-GBM disease:** It is more common in **young adults men.**
    (A) **Signs and symptoms: Pulmonary hemorrhage, hemoptysis** (anti-GBM antibodies damages the pulmonary capillaries), renal function deteriorates from **normal to renal failure within days to weeks**.
    (B) Diagnosis: **Positive anti-GBM antibodies,** immunoflurescent (IF) study **shows linear deposition of immunoglobulin along the GBM**, crescent formation with proliferative glomerulonephritis.
    (C) **Treatment**: **No** proven effective therapy.
        (i) **Pulmonary bleeding:** High dose oral or intravenous corticosteroids can stop pulmonary bleeding **but** are **not** effective in renal lesions.
        (ii) **To reduce** production of anti-GBM antibodies: Cyclophosphamide and corticosteroids are effective.
        (iii) **To remove** circulating anti-GBM antibodies: **Plasmapheresis** is effective.
        (iv) **To prevent irreversible renal damage**: Rapid intensive therapy should be done.

80. Type III RPGN (rapidly progressive glomerulonephritis):
    (A) **Signs and symptoms**: Progressive renal failure and nephritic presentations.
    (B) **Diagnosis:** Positive antineutrophil cytoplasmic antibody.
    (C) **Treatment:** Oral cyclophosphamide plus corticosteroids. They are also used in Wegener's granulomatosis and polyarteritis nodosa. **Steroids plus cytotoxic agents** are **useful in both oliguric and patients on dialysis**.

81. **Important marker for different renal disease associated with pulmonary disease**:
    (i) Uremic lung: High BUN and creatinine.
    (ii) SLE: Positive anti-DNA antibodies, low complement.
    (iii) Goodpasture's syndrome: Positive anti-GBM antibodies.
    (iv) Wegener's granulomatosis, polyarteritis: Positive anti-neutrophil cytoplasmic antibodies.
    (v) Pneumonia with immune complex glomerulonephritis: Low complement, circulating immune complexes.
    (vi) Nephrotic syndrome, pulmonary embolism, renal vein thrombosis: Positive lung scan.

82. The routine urinalysis in an **asymptomatic patients reveals proteinuria and microscopic hematuria**. The subsequent laboratory investigations **reveal < 1 gram/day proteinuria, glomerular microhematuria**, and **normal** GFR (measured by creatinine clearance). **The next step of initial management should be: Close observation only,** monitor proteinuria and GFR. **Biopsy is indicated with progressively increasing proteinuria or decreasing GFR**.

83. **Lupus nephritis and treatment:**
    (A) **Lupus nephritis (WHO classification)**:
        (i) Class I = **Normal** glomeruli and no renal findings.
        (ii) Class II = **Mesangial disease**, mild to moderate proteinuria (never nephrotic), and may have active serology.
        (iii) Class III = **Focal** proliferative glomerulonephritis, active proteinuria (25% nephrotic), active serology, and with or without high BP.
        (iv) Class IV = Diffuse proliferative glomerulonephritis, **heavy** proteinuria (frequently nephrotic), **very active serology, often reduced GFR, and high BP**.
        (v) Class V = Membranous glomerulonephritis, significant proteinuria (often nephrotic) **but** less active lupus serology.
    (B) **Treatment of severe lupus nephritis**:
        (i) Recent studies at the NIH shows **intravenous cyclophosphamide (cytoxan) can prevent long term renal failure**. It is the **most** effective drug.
        (ii) **Intravenous pulse methylprednisolone is most effective** in patients with recent decline in GFR, with greater serologic activity, plus diffuse proliferative lesions.

84. Most common cause of glomerular damage in developed countries: **Diabetes mellitus.** Remember, **both insulin dependent (30 to 40%) and non-insulin**

dependent can have progressive renal involvement. Diabetes is the most common cause of new patients included in ESRD programs.

Histologic findings in diabetic nephropathy: Thickening of the GBM, mesangial sclerosis, nodular intercapillary glomerulosclerosis (**Kimmelsteil-Wilson nodules**).

Treatment in diabetic nephropathy:

(i) **Prevention by controlling high blood sugar and high BP.**

(ii) **Use ACE inhibitors** to reduce intracapillary glomerular pressure.

(iii) Renal transplantation in ESRD.

85. **Amyloidosis with renal disease**: About 80% of amyloidosis patients have renal involvement, it is a multisystem involvement disease.
   (A) **Signs and symptoms**: Albuminuria, decreased renal functions, and 25% develops nephrotic syndrome.
   (B) **Preferred diagnostic study of amyloidosis:** Organ biopsy **other than kidney** e.g., gingival biopsy, rectal biopsy, or fat pad biopsy.

86. **Light chain deposition disease (LCDD) of the kidney**: LCDD is a systemic disease caused by overproduction and extracellular deposition of monoclonal extracellular light chain. **LCDD is more common in male with lymphoplasmacytic B cell disease like multiple myeloma.**
   (A) **Signs and symptoms:** Albuminuria, nephrotic syndrome (50% of cases), high BP, and renal insufficiency. Some patients have **classic Bence Jones cast nephropathy plus acute renal failure**.
   (B) **Treatment:** Chemotherapy used for multiple myeloma.

87. **HIV nephropathy** (Important).
   (A) **Precipitating factors for acute renal failure**: Drugs (NSAID's, pentamidine, trimethoprim-sulfamethoxazole, aminoglycosides), **pyrexia and dehydration superimposed on sepsis-hypotension-respiratory failure**.
   (B) **Signs and symptoms:** HIV nephropathy is a unique pattern of glomerular disease **characterized by heavy proteinuria and rapid progression to renal failure**. It is found in both **asymptomatic carriers** of **HIV and AIDS patients**.
   (C) **Histologic findings:** Minimal change pattern, mesangial hyperplasia, glomerulopathies associated with **immune complex deposition and/or IgA deposition, most important is HIV nephropathy**.
   (D) **Differential diagnosis from heroin nephropathy**: Heroin nephropathy is **FSGS** and has **less fulminant** course of renal failure than HIV nephropathy.
   (E) Treatment of acute renal failure: Dialysis helps in regaining renal function.

88. **Thrombotic microangiopathies (microthrombosis of glomerular capillaries and small arterioles):**
   (A) **These includes the following conditions:** Hemolytic-uremic syndrome, thrombotic thrombocytopenic purpura, antiphospholilpid syndrome, and **use of drugs (e.g., mitomycin, cyclosporine).**
   (B) **Signs and symptoms: Gross or microscopic hematuria, proteinuria (< 2 grams/day)** but may reach nephrotic levels, renal insufficiency, oliguric or nonoliguric acute renal failure.
   (C) **Treatment:**
      (i) To correct hypovolemia, control high BP.
      (ii) Dialysis for severe renal failure.
      (iii) Antiphospholipid syndrome with thrombotic angiopathy: Use anticoagulants (heparin and then warfarin).

89. **Glomerulonephritis due to mixed cryoglobulinemia:**
   (A) **This is important to remember, hepatitis C-associated renal disease could be misdiagnosed as mixed cryoglobulinemia glomerulonephritis.**
   (B) **Signs and symptoms:** Proteinuria, high BP, hematuria, renal insufficiency, nephrotic syndrome (20% of cases), or acute nephritic picture (up to 33% of cases).
   (C) **Characteristic laboratory findings:** Lows serum complements (C1q-C4).

90. **Clinical and laboratory manifestation, diagnosis, treatment, and prognosis of tubulointerstitial disease of the kidney:**
   (A) **Clinical and laboratory manifestations**:
      (i) **Tubular dysfunction is much more** than glomerular dysfunction (low GFR).
      (ii) **Tubular abnormalities:**
         (a) **Polyuria and nocturia** are due to reduced urinary concentrating capacity.
         (b) **Renal tubular acidosis** (hyperchloremic metabolic acidosis).
         (c) Serum: High k, low Na.
         (d) **Partial or complete Fanconi's syndrome**: Increased urinary excretion of glucose, uric acid, amino acid, phosphate, and bicarbonate.
      (iii) **Renal endocrine deficiencies**:
         (a) Hyporeninemic hypoaldosteronism (high k, metabolic acidosis).
         (b) Erythropoietin deficiency (anemia).
         (c) Calcitriol deficiency (renal osteodystrophy).
      (iv) **Urinalysis:**

(a) Modest proteinuria (< 3.5 grams/day) which consists largely of low-molecular-weight tubular proteins (e.g., lysozyme, beta-$_2$-microglobulin).

(B) **Diagnosis**:

(i) **Renal biopsy is the most definitive method** but this is **not** always needed.

(ii) **History, physical examination, and laboratory tests** are helpful to make the diagnosis.

(C) **Treatment:** General supportive therapy, correct the electrolyte disorders, and management of acute and chronic renal failures.

(D) **Prognosis**: It depends upon the specific cause of tubulointerstitial disorder.

91. **Most important cause of toxic nephropathy**: **Drugs,** other causes are **direct or indirect** injury of the kidneys from exogenous chemical and physical factors (**environmental agents**) and excessive levels of **calcium and uric acid** in the body. **Indirect injury** could be due to **immunologic reactions, drug induced hypotension, or hemolysis**. Toxic nephropathy **may results in tubulointerstitial disease but they are not the same**.

92. **Toxic injury of the kidneys are due to the following factors**:

(i) **Kidneys are exposed to more blood-borne materials** than any other organs **except lungs.**

(ii) **High metabolic rate** of renal tubules for active transport.

(iii) **Large glomerular capillary area for trapping immune complexes**.

(iv) Precipitation of **less soluble forms such as uric acid** from urate.

(v) Some substances (**e.g., aminoglycosides**) **concentrated in the renal cortex** and other (**e.g., phenacetin**) **concentrated in the renal medulla,** results in renal toxicites.

93. **Most common cause of acute interstitial nephritis (AISN)**: **Drugs** (e.g., **NSAID's, penicillin, allopurinol, sulfonamides, antituberculous drugs**), other causes of AISN are **idiopathic, SLE, acute glomerulonephritis with** anti-tubular basement membrane antibodies and/or secondary interstitial nephritis, **renal transplantation rejection**, renal **infections** (bacterial, TB, fungal), **systemic infections** (mycoplasma, CMV, toxoplasma, syphilis, streptococci, infectious mononucleosis, and Legionnaire's disease).

94. A male patient is receiving **amoxicillin** for fever and sore throat, both the symptoms improve after 3 days of antibiotic therapy. Subsequently patient develops **gross hematuria,** proteinuria (less than nephrotic range), azotemia, **fever, pyuria plus eosinophiluria (characteristic)**.

Laboratory values: Presence of eosinophil in the urine, renal loss of sodium, **hypercholremic metabolic acidosis with high k (distal RTA)**, and **elevated serum IgE levels**.
Most likely diagnosis: Amoxicillin induced acute interstitial nephritis.
Treatment: Discontinuation of amoxicillin, use another appropriate medicine for underlying problem, **some patients may need interval dialysis**. A short course of **high-dose of prednisone** may enhance **the recovery** but can exaggerate the underlying infection.

95. **Few important points in nephropathy (AISN) caused by penicillins** (amoxicillin, ampicillin, methicillin, nafcillin, oxacillin, penicillin G, mezlocillin, and carbenicillin):
    (i) AISN has **no relation with drug doses.**
    (ii) Symptoms and signs usually **begins 2 weeks** (may range from 2 days to several weeks) **after drug therapy**.
    (iii) AISN should **not** be confused with the recurrence of the underlying disease.
    (iv) Recovery may require several weeks.

96. **Most important and frequent cause of drug induced AISN**: **NSAID's. The diagnosis is made** from history of taking NSAID's, clinical manifestations, and improvement with discontinuation of the drug. Rarely biopsy (renal) is need to confirm or exclude the diagnosis.

97. **Clinical manifestations of any drug induced acute interstitial nephritis**: Hematuria, proteinuria, fever, eosinophilia, pyuria, eosinophiluria, and azotemia.

98. **Few important points regarding drug related acute interstitial nephritis (AISN):**
    (i) Both sulfonamide diuretics (**furosemide, thiazide, acetazolamide**) and sulfonamide antibiotics can cause **AISN**. Few patients develop **skin rash** along with other presentations. A **short course of corticosteroids** may hasten the recovery.
    (ii) Antituberculous drugs (rifampin, INH, ethambutol, PAS) cause AISN, **rifampin is the most common among anti TB drugs. Transient hypercalcemia of unknown cause** has been reported along with AISN during antituberculous therapy. **Remember corticosteroid is not useful**.
    (iii) **Allopurinol** causing AISN appears with **exfoliative maculopapular skin rash**, fever, **eosinophilia, decreased renal function,** and **acute hepatic injury (elevated AST > 1000 units/L)** followed by **mortality (20% of**

cases) from severe systemic reactions, sepsis, GI bleeding, hepatic or renal failure.

Treatment of allopurinol AISN: Discontinue the medication, supportive therapy, dialysis, and corticosteroids may be helpflul.

Prevention: Do **not** use allopurinol for asymptomatic hyperuricemia.

(iv) Cephalosporins, ciprofloxacin, erythromycin, vancomycin, tetracyclines, polymyxin B can cause AISN.

(v) **Most frequent or clinically important drugs causing AISN are the following**: NSAID's, penicillins group of drugs, sulfonamides, allopurinol, and rifampin.

(vi) **Group A beta- hemolytic streptococci is the most common** organism causing AISN. **Acute bacterial pyelonephritis is the most common infection causing AISN**. Patients appear with **fever, chills, flank pain, and bacteriuria**. AISN is also caused by fungus and mycobacterium. **All these infections can cause renal scarring** but **rarely** cause ARF.

(vii) AISN associated immune disorder such as SLE is **diagnosed by renal biopsy unlike drug induced AISN is diagnosed by characteristic history, clinical presentations, and laboratory findings**.

99. **Proteinuria and drug induced AISN (Important)**: All the drugs produce mild proteinuria **except NSAID's. NSAID's particularly fenoprofen cause heavy proteinuria often in the nephrotic range (> 3.5 grams/day)**.

100. **Chronic interstitial nephritis (CISN)**:

(A) **Histopathologic findings: Interstitial fibrosis, atrophy, loss of renal tubules,** interstitial infiltrates of inflammatory cells. The glomeruli may be **normal** but contracted.

(B) **Few important etiologic factors:**

(i) **Urinary tract obstruction is probably the most important factor, second is nephrotoxin** such as **drugs** (analgesics e.g., acetaminophen, phenacetin, aspirin, and nitrosoureas), **hypercalcemia, oxalate, uric acid, low k; neoplasms** (leukemia, lymphoma, multiple myeloma); **immune disorders** (SLE, chronic rejection of renal transplantation, chronic glomerulonephritis with interstitial nephritis); **cystic disease** (medullary cystic disease, polycystic disease); **diabetes, sickle cell disease, vascular disease, and idiopathic**.

(C) **Clinical presentations**: It is mostly due to **renal tubular functional defects** such as **polyuria, nocturia, RTA, partial or complete Fanconi's syndrome (increased renal excretion** of glucose, sodium, phosphate, bicarbonate, uric acids, amino acids), and **hyperkalemia with hyponatremia. Please remember, there is no eosinophilia or**

eosinophiluria but sterile pyuria may be present (**AISN have eosinophilia, eosinophiluria, and pyuria**).

(D) **Diagnosis:** History, physical examination (flank tenderness), laboratory findings are diagnostic. Renal sonogram is helpful to rule **out obstructed uropathy**.

101. **Few important points in analgesic nephropathy (AN):**

(i) Most important drugs causing AN are **phenacetin, acetaminophen**, used **in combination with aspirin**. (Phenacetin is converted to acetaminophen soon after ingestion).

(ii) In USA, 2 to 10% of all ESRD are due to AN.

(iii) AN more frequently occurs in **middle aged women**.

(iv) **Patients appear with anemia, UTI with pyuria**, hematuria, flank pain (ureteral colic), renal insufficiency, proteinuria (< 2 grams/day), increased atherosclerosis (especially coronary artery disease), renal artery stenosis, and hypertension.

(v) Anemia is due to renal insufficiency, hemolysis, GI blood loss from peptic ulcer disease or gastritis.

(vi) Kidneys are **normal size and shape in early stages** and reduced size, thin cortex plus irregular surfaces in late stages.

(vii) **Radiologic demonstration of papillary necrosis** (which is more common in diabetes, sickle cell disease, UTI, and urinary tract obstruction) **may suggest AN** if the above mentioned diseases are absent.

(viii) **Please remember** AN patients have increased risk of **developing transitional cell cancer of the urinary tract particularly of the pelvis**.

(ix) **Prevention**: Avoid those drugs; education, encouragement, and often psychological counseling.

(x) **Treatment:** To treat the underlying conditions (high BP, UTI, dehydration, and obstruction).

102. **The effects of NSAID's on kidneys:**

(i) **Most common renal side effect is sodium retention as well as retention of fluids.** These do **not** cause any problems in patients with **normal** renal and cardiac functions but **cause worsening of preexisting CHF and hypertension**.

(ii) **Acute renal failure is due to hypoperfusion of the kidneys** by NSAID's (**indomethacin** and **triamterene** are more likely to cause problems). Patients appear with **oliguria, low FE_{Na}** mimc prerenal azotemia. **Renal biopsy shows ATN. The treatment is to discontinue the drugs and rarely temporary dialysis**.

(iii) **AISN (acute interstitial nephritis) with acute renal failure** are found in some patients with NSAID's, **particularly fenoprofen. Please remember, NSAID's causing AISN results in heavy proteinuria (often in the nephrotic range > 3.5 grams/day)** and **absence of eosinophilia, eosinophiluria, and skin rashes unlike other drugs causing AISN** which **have mild proteinuria and presence of eosinophilia, eosinophiluria**.

(iv) **Hyperkalemia and metabolic acidosis** are found in patients with renal insufficiency and sodium depletion.

103. **Antibiotics which cause renal damage**:

(i) **Aminoglycosides:** Most important manifestation **is acute renal failure** due to direct toxic effect **on glomeruler filtration and tubular toxicity**, elevated serum creatinine levels, **reduced serum k and magnesium due to renal wasting**. Most nephrotoxic aminoglycoside drug is neomycin and least toxic is streptomycin. **Calculation of aminoglycosides doses in older patients:** Older patients have **low GFR but normal creatinine levels**. The doses **should be adjusted** despite **normal creatinine levels to avoid ARF (Important).**

Treatment of ARF due to aminoglycosides:

(a) Discontinue the drug.
(b) Give alternative appropriate nonnephrotoxic antibiotic.
(c) Supportive measures, monitor serum creatinine levels.
(d) When **no** alternative antibiotic can be found, monitor aminoglycoside levels, and administer with low doses.

(ii) Cephalosporins alone are **rarely** nephrotoxic but combination with aminoglycoside is nephrotoxic, monitoring of renal of function is needed.

(iii) **Tetracycline is nephrotoxic,** it inhibits protein synthesis and shunts amino acids into urea results in **elevation of BUN but normal** creatinine. Doxycycline and minocycline are **less** nephrotoxic. **Outdated tetracyclines can cause Fanconi's syndrome. Demeclocycline** can cause ARF particularly when given to hyponatremic patients with hepatic cirrhosis.

(iv) **Amphotericin B** is nephrotoxic, it causes **distal RTA, renal k wasting, nephrogenic diabetes insipidus,** progressive renal insufficiency, and acute renal failure in volume depleted patients (diuretics, vomiting, diarrhea). **When BUN > 50 mg/dL, temporary discontinuation or alternate day therapy is recommended**.

104. **Nephrotoxicity and iodinated radiographic contrast materials**:

(i) **Risk factors: Diabetes with renal insufficiency has the highest risk,** older age, dehydration, prior history of contrast induced renal failure, and probably multiple myeloma.

(ii) **Pathogenesis:** ARF is due to **ischemia,** renal arterial **vasoconstriction** due to hypertonicity, **tubular obstruction** by protein precipitation, and **direct tubular toxicity**.

(iii) **Diagnosis**: History of contrast study and elevation of serum creatinine within 24 hours of study, peak within 7 days.

(iv) **Treatment:**

(a) **Mild to moderate** renal insufficiency: Only conservative management, resolves within few days.

(b) **Severe** renal insufficiency: Temporary dialysis may be required.

(v) **Prevention:**

(a) **To correct the dehydration.**

(b) **Minimize the amount** of contrast or do ultrasonography**.**

(c) **Hypertonic mannitol immediately after exposure** to contrast material in high risk patients may reduce the incidence of ARF**.**

105. **Antineoplastic drugs which cause nephropathy**:

(i) **Cisplatin: Hypomagnesemia** (renal Mg wasting is found in 50% of patients, may persist for several weeks following therapy), **hypokalemia** (renal k wasting), **low-molecular weight proteinuria. ARF can be avoided** by adequate hydration, slow infusion of cisplatin, and saline diuresis prior and during administration of cisplatin.

(ii) Administration of **recombinant interleukin-2** in advanced cancer patients may develop **acute renal insufficiency** due to prerenal azotemia.

(iii) Renal injury from radiation does **not** occur **with < 1000 to 2000 cGy. Excessive radiation** may cause mild proteinuria, benign to malignant hypertension, and urinary concentration defects.

(iv) Methotrexate with **high doses** causes direct tubular damage. Toxicity may be reduced by **intravenous hydration and alkali administration**.

(v) **Mitomycin C**: Initially mild proteinuria, azotemia, followed by **thrombocytopenia, microangiopathic hemolytic anemia, and ARF** (**mimic hemolytic uremic syndrome**) (**Important**).

(vi) Nitrosoureas [**streptozocin**, carmustine (BCNU), lomustine (CCNU), methyl CCNU]: **Streptozocin** causes proteinuria, azotemia, proximal RTA, glycosuria, aminoaciduria, and phosphaturia. Other nitrosoureas develop **CISN and glomerulosclerosis**.

106. Patients with acute lymphoblastic leukemia or poorly differentiated lymphomas have received chemotherapy or radiotherapy. Patients subsequently developed **acute obstructive renal failure**.
Laboratory findings: Ratio of urinary uric acid/creatinine concentration > 1:1.

Most likely cause of renal failure: Uric acid precipitation in the renal tubules and tumor lysis syndrome.

Treatment:

(i) **Prevention** of ARF due to massive tumor cell killing: **Intravenous hydration to** maintain the urine output 3 liters or more per 24 hours **plus high dose of allopurinol before the onset** of cytotoxic treatment.

(ii) Urinary alkaliniztion usefulness is **not certain**. It increase the solubility of uric acid but precipitation of **phosphate salts in renal tubules**.

(iii) **Hemodialysis** is useful to remove uric acid and other cellular products.

107. **Few important renal side effects of certain drugs:**

(i) **Methylsergide** (used for migraine headaches): Retroperitoneal fibrosis and ureteral obstruction.

(ii) **Heroin abuse: Focal sclerosing glomerulopathy is** followed by nephrotic syndrome.

(iii) **Nifedipine:** Prerenal azotemia due to hypotension.

(iv) **Captopril:** Allergic interstitial nephritis (skin rash, eosinophilia, and eosinophiluria).

(v) **Acyclovir:** ARF due to precipitation of the drug in renal tubules.

(vi) **Cyclosporin A (for several months):** Occlusion of renal arterioles, reduced GFR, and CISN.

(vii) **D-Penicillamine**: Proteinuria, nephrotic syndrome, **rarely** pulmonary bleeding with glomerulonephritis.

(viii) **Methoxyflurane** (fluorinated anesthetic agent, but **enflurane is rarely toxic**): Dose-related postoperative diabetes insipidus and acute renal failure (ARF).

108. **Few important points in obstructive uropathy:**

(i) **Upper** urinary tract obstruction means lesions are located **above the ureterovesical junction** and **lower** urinary tract obstruction means lesions are **below the ureterovesical junction**.

(ii) **Upper** obstruction can be **subdivided** into **intrinsic** (intraluminal or intramural) and **extrinsic**.

(iii) **In middle aged women, cervical cancer** is a common cause of **extrinsic ureteral or ureterovesical junction obstruction. In elderly men (over 60), most common cause is benign prostatic hyperplasia and prostatic carcinoma. Urolithiasis** is predominant in young adults (ages 25 to 45, men > women). **Hydronephrosis** is found in adults (3.6%).

109. **Clinical manifestations of urinary tract obstruction:**

(i) **Acute complete obstruction:** Patients appear with acute renal failure and anuria in bilateral complete obstruction.
(ii) **Chronic partial obstruction (e.g., chronic hydronephrosis)**: Patients may be completely asymptomatic, or asmptomatic with elevated levels of BUN and creatinine, or symptomatic with intermittent pain, or symptoms of **polyuria and /or nocturia** with or without elevation of BUN and creatinine.
(iii) **Lower urinary tract obstruction:** Distended, palpable, and occasionally tender bladder particularly in prostatic hypertrophy.
(iv) **Upper urinary tract obstruction:** Flank tenderness is noted in acute obstruction. Kidney is palpable in long standing obstruction.
(v) **Classic 'renal colic':** Steadily increasing severe **flank pain** (stones lodged in the **upper third** of ureter), or **radiating to the testes, groin, or labia (stones lodged in the lower tow-thirds of ureter). It is associated** with **vomiting and sweating**.
(vi) **Vesicoureteral reflux:** Pain radiates into the flank during micturition.
(vii) Partial or incomplete obstruction of urinary tract: **Normal urine output or polyuria, sometimes severe polyuria may cause hypernatremia (diabetes insipidus like syndrome). Please remember, symptoms of oliguria or anuria alternating with polyuria or acute anuria suggests obstructive uropathy**.
(viii) Gross hematuria is present in obstruction **particularly due to stones**.
(ix) **Hypertension** is commonly present in **obstructive renal disease** due to fluid retention, increasede ECF volume, decreased medullary vasopressor substances, and **increased renin secretion.** In **chronic** bilateral obstruction, hypertension is due to decreased sodium excretion, increased ECF volume, but **decreased renin levels**.
(x) **UTI is more common in lower urinary tract obstruction** (than upper) due to **increased bacterial adherence** to the bladder and **decreased bacterial washout. Please remember, urinary tract obstruction should be ruled out in recurrent UTI, unresponsive UTI to antibiotics,** and **presence of proteus or peseudomonas in urine culture of noninstrumented patients**.
(xi) **Lower urinary tract obstruction**: Reduced force and caliber of urine stream, hesitancy, urgency, intermittency, incontinence, and postvoid dribbling.
(xii) **Rarely** develops polycythemia due to increased erythropoietin.

110. **Diagnosis of urinary tract obstruction**:
(i) **Laboratory findings:** Eleveated SUN and creatinine, high k, hyperchloremic metabolic acidosis.

(ii) Ultrasonography is the **initial procedure of choice in suspected obstruction.**
False-negative results can occur in dehydration and early obstruction**K**.
(iii) **UB (kidney, ureter, bladder):** It can detect **calculi**, **dilated bladder, and morphologic difference in two kidneys**.
(iv) Do **not** use IVP (intravenous pyelogram) in compromised kidney function (creatinine > 3 to 4 mg/dL) because of nephrotoxicity and delayed excretion of contrast materials. **IVP is used to investigate acute renal colic**.
(v) **Retrograde pyelography** is used. **IVP is contraindicated** to visualize the ureter and collecting system. **It can detect the site and cause of obstruction**.
(vi) Isotopic renography (intravenous radionuclide injection followed by imaging with gammascintillation camera) is used for **upper urinary tract obstruction**.
(vii) CT scan and MRI are useful to find the **cause of obstruction**.
(viii) **Whitaker test (pressure flow studies)** is helpful when upper urinary tract obstruction **cannot** be diagnosed by above mentioned studies. It is a measurement of **pressure difference between renal pelvis and bladder**.
(ix) **The following investigations are useful for lower urinary tract obstruction**:
   (a) **VCUG** (voiding cystourethrogram) is used to diagnose **vesicoureteral reflux** causing urinary tract dilatation.
   (b) Cystoscopy to inspect the bladder.
   (c) **Retrograde urethrography is to evaluate anterior urethra** (**cannot** evaluate posterior urethra.
   (d) **Excretory or retrograde cystogram is the best diagnostic study to evaluate posterior urethra**.
   (e) **Urodynamic studies:** Debimetry (urinary flow rate), cystometrography, electromyography, and urethral pressure profile.

111. **Treatment of urinary tract obstruction:**
(i) **Acute complete obstruction distal to the bladder** (lower): **Placement of urethral catheter** usually relieves the symptoms, some patients **need suprapubic cystostomy**.
(ii) **Acute complete obstruction in the upper urinary tract: Percutaneous nephrostomy** tubes or **passage of retrograde ureteral catheter**.
(iii) **Acute complete obstruction with sepsis: Appropriate antibiotic and prompt relief of obstruction,** sometimes **dialysis** before surgery or instrumentation in ARF.
(iv) Management of calculi (it is **the most common cause of ureteral obstruction**): Pain is controlled by intramuscular **narcotic analegesic,**

stones < 5 mm in diameter do not need surgery or instrumentation because majority of these stones pass spontaneously; stones between 5 to 7 mm, only 50% pass ; and stones > 7 mm usually are **not** passed spontaneously. **High fluid therapy** to increase the urine volume **at least 2 liters/day** may help to mobilize the stone. **Surgery** is indicated when a **stone completely blocks the ureter** and does **not** move. **Endourologic method is successful to remove the obstruction up to 98% of cases. Extracorporeal shock wave or ultrasound lithotripsy** is effective (up to 90% of cases) for ureteral calculi of 7 to 15 mm that lie above the pelvic brim. **All patients should be followed** up for **recurrence of stone and should receive preventive therapy**. Calculi located **distal to the pelvic brim should be removed from below. Appropriate antibiotic** should be used for infection.

(v) Patients with chronic partial obstruction: Surgery could be **delayed for weeks or months except** in repeated UTI, progressive renal damage, urinary retention, dysuria, flank pain, and voiding dysfunction.

(vi) **Management of lower urinary tract obstruction:**

(a) **Bladder neck and urethral obstruction** with reflux, marked urinary retention, bleeding, or renal parenchymal damage: **Surgery is indicated**.

(b) **Benign prostatic hypertrophy without** infection, **normal** urinary tract, and **mild** symptoms: **Nonsurgical** management and **follow up** can be done until the patient and physician agree that surgery in needed.

(c) **Urethral strictures in men** (**not** common in women)**: Dilation** of urethra or **direct visual internal urethrotomy.**

(d) **Obstruction of neuropathic bladder** (**atonic** bladder due to **lower** motor neuron disease e.g., **diabetes**): **Void at regular intervals** to achieve satisfactory emptying, sometimes respond to **bethanecol chloride** (cholinergic agent), (alpha-adrenergic blocker relaxes urethral sphincter but is **not** used for side effects). **Please remember, the best treatment for patients with significant residual urine and UTI is intermittent (4 to 5 times/day), clean, regular self-catheterization. Long-term indwelling catheterization should be avoided for infections and other complications**.

(e) Obstruction of neuropathic bladder (**hypertonic** bladder due to **upper** motor neuron disease): To improve **bladder storage function,** may use **anticholinergic agents**. Occasionally long-term, clean, intermittent self-catheterization may be needed **but it should be avoided for infections and other complications**.

(vii) **Management of post obstructive diuresis** (natriuresis and diuresis after relief of obstruction results in loss of Na, k, Mg, and other solutes):

(a) **It is self-limited, replacement of fluid and electrolytes are not usually required except in excessive loss of sodium and water which are inappropriate for the volume status (low volume)** or **due to intrinsic tubular defect of sodium and water absorption**. Please do **not** give excessive fluid that enhances postoperative diuresis and natriuresis.

112. **Renal cortical thickness and prognosis in obstructive uropathy (chronic hydronephrosis):** Thin cortex has **poor** prognosis. Renal function **recovery** depends upon the severity, duration, infection, pre-existing renal disease, and underlying causes of obstruction.

113. **Proximal RTA (renal tubular acidosis):** Proximal (type II) RTA is a **hyperchloremic, hypokalemic metabolic acidosis.**
   (A) Pathophysiology: Normally 85 to 90% of filtered bicarbonate is absorbed by proximal tubule, and 10 to 15% by distal tubule. In **proximal RTA**, 15% or more bicarbonate is excreted by the kidney. Initial plasma bicarbonate is normal, urine pH is alkaline; subsequently plasma bicarbonate **falls between 15 to 18 mm**, distal tubules are capable of reabsorbing all the filtered bicarbonate, urine pH becomes **acidic**.
   (B) **Clinical presentations: Acidemia** (causing growth failure, anorexia, malnutrition, volume depletion), **low k** (polyuria, nocturia, polydipsia, muscular weakness), and defective mineral, parathyroid, vitamin D metabolism (osteomalacia).
   (C) **Diagnosis:**
   Plasma: High cl, low k, low pH. (Proximal RTA is **not** an isolated diagnosis, usually associated with Fanconi's syndrome).
   (D) **Treatment: To treat the underlying cause** (e.g., multiple myeloma, offending drugs, toxins like heavy metals). If the underlying cause **cannot** be treated, **give large quantities** of **sodium and potassium bicarbonate**. **Thiazide diuretics** cause volume contraction and **stimulate proximal tubular bicarbonate reabsorption.**

114. **The Fanconi's syndrome (generalized proximal tubular dysfunctions):** This syndrome is characterized by **glucosuria, generalized aminoaciduria,** and **uricosuria. Recently,** it is associated **with depletion of mitochondrial DNA, particularly in a mitochondrial myopathy with generalized tubulopathy.**
   (A) **Etiology: Multiple myeloma** is the most common cause in **older** adults; **dysproteinemias, heavy metal toxicities** (chronic cadmium, acute lead)

are most common acquired form in adults, cystine crystals may deposit in cornea and conjunctiva, or hereditary fructose intolerance.

(B) Clinical presentations: Polyuria, muscle weakness, osteomalacia, conjunctival and corneal irritations.

(C) **Diagnosis**: Documentation of global tubular dysfunction, serum and urine electrophoresis should be done, and try to find the underlying cause.

(D) **Treatment:**

(i) Supplementation of sodium and potassium (up to 10 to 15 mEq/kg/day), phosphate, magnesium, and vitamin D.

(ii) To treat the underlying cause.

(iii) Removal of heavy metals by environmental changes or chelation.

(iv) Cysteamine is effective in cystinosis.

(v) Fructose restriction in hereditary fructose intolerance.

(vi) D-penicillamine is effective in Wilson's disease.

115. **Bartter's syndrome (functional disorder of the ascending limb of the loop of Henle** results in **hypokalemia, metabolic alkalosis**, and **hyperreninemic hyperaldosteronism** but **absence** of edema and high BP):

(A) **Pathophysiology**: Reduced ECF volume causes hyperreninemic hyperaldosteronism results in **sodium retention** and **k excretion.**

(B) **Clinical presentations:** Hypokalemia, muscle weakness, polyuria, nocturia, metabolic alkalosis results in hypocalcemia with Trousseau and chvostek signs, (**remember, absence of edema and high BP**).

(C) **Differential diagnosis: Excessive use of diuretic or laxative** can mimic clinical and laboratory findings of Bartter's syndrome. **Other causes of** hyperreninemic hyperaldosteronism are **associated with high BP unlike** Bartter's syndrome.

(D) **Diagnosis:** Urinary chloride > 20ml/L, **negative screening test** for diuretics in the urine and laxatives in the stool (phenolphthalein test).

(E) **Treatment:**

(i) Supplementation of k and magnesium.

(ii) Propranolol, spironolactone, captopril, prostaglandin inhibitors (e.g.,aspirin or indomethacin).

116. Classic distal RTA (renal tubular acidosis or type I): It is characterized by hypokalemic, hyperchloremic metabolic acidosis associated with selective defect in distal acidification.

(A) **Pathophysiology**: Normally 10 to 15% of filtered bicarbonate is absorbed by distal tubule. In distal RTA, bicarbonate reabsorption is reduced results in metabolic acidosis, low k and cl. **Distal nephron is not capable of**

lowering the luminal pH below 5.5 after challenge by metabolic acidosis.

(B) **Clinical presentations:** Nephrocalcinosis and nephrolithiasis are **either cause or result of distal RTA**. The symptoms of hypokalemia (muscle weakness) and metabolic acidosis are present. Bone disease occurs **less** than proximal RTA.

(C) **Etiology and mode of genetic transmission**: Autoimmune diseases, drugs, toxins, and tubulointerstitial disease; autosomal dominant.

(D) **Diagnosis:** Plasma (high cl, low k and pH), urine pH > 5.5 and reduced urinary acid excretion. **Urinary anion gap** (urinary sodium plus k minus cl, proportionate to the negative value of urinary ammonium NH_4+) is **positive or zero** in distal RTA (**unlike** in diarrhea, **negative or large** urinary anion gap, **high urinary ammonium results in high urine pH**).

(E) **Treatment:** Alkali therapy (1 to 3 mEq/kg/day), it also reduces urine k wasting **unlike** proximal RTA.

117. **Generalized distal (type IV) RTA**: **Aldosterone deficiency or antagonism** causes **hyperkalemic,** hyperchloremic metabolic acidosis due to subnormal net acid excretion and **often by salt wasting**.
Diagnosis: Plasma (**high k, low pH,** low Na, **high cl**), **reduced** GFR, urinary pH < 5.5, urinary anion gap is **positive or zero (like proximal RTA, distal RTA, and glomerular insufficiency).**

(A) **Treatment:**

(i) **9-alpha-flurocortisone** is used for mineralocorticoid deficiency.

(ii) **High dose of synthetic mineralocorticoid** is needed in hyporeninemia due to mineralcorticoid resistance.

(iii) Loop diuretic (furosemide or ethacrynic acid) is used when high BP precludes administration of mineralocorticoid.

(iv) Along with diuretic include **restriction of dietary potassium (<50 mEq/dl), therapy with sodium bicarbonate** (1 to 3 mEq/kg/day), and rarely **short course of cation-exchange resin**.

118. **Clinical presentations of diabetes with kidney involvement:**

(i) Patients are often **asymptomatic until** the GFR is **reduced 10 to 30% of normal values. During this interval, arterial hypertension is common** and protein excretion rates can reach to the levels of nephrotic syndrome results in **edema, hypoalbuminemia,** and **hypercholesterolemia**.

(ii) **Uremic symptoms** appear when the GFR is already reduced to **10 to 30% of normal values. The nausea and vomiting of uremia is difficult to distinguish** from the same symptoms of diabetic autonomic gastroparesis. **Diabetic peripheral neuropathy may mimic uremic neuropathy,** but

painful hypesthetic neuropathy are mostly due to long standing diabetes than uremia.

(iii) **Orthostatic hypotension** is a complication in treating patients of **hypertension with diabetic autonomic neuropathy**.

(iv) Patients with **IDDM plus renal disease almost always have diabetic retinopathy**. Patients with **NIDDM plus renal disease develop diabetic retinopathy up to 60 to 70% of cases.**

(v) Cardiovascular complications are **more severe in NIDDM than** IDDM.

(vi) **Both IDDM and NIDDM patients with renal disease have high incidence of myocardial infarction, stroke, and peripheral vascular disease results in amputation** than in patients **without** renal involvement.

119. **Treatment of diabetic nephropathy:**

(A) **Prevention**:

(i) **To control the blood sugar** adequately.

(ii) **Antihypertensive** can prevent or stop progression of diabetic nephropathy.

(iii) **Use of converting enzyme inhibitors** at the stage of microalbuminuria **with or without significant high BP**, can **delay or probably prevent significant proteinuria. It is also effective in advanced degree of nephropathy** for both IDDM and NIDDM patients. Try to achieve BP $<$ 130/90 mm Hg. **The complications** of using converting enzyme particularly in NIDDM are **hyperkalemia and elevated serum creatinine due to renal artery stenosis**.

(iv) **Restriction of dietary protein** is also indicated.

(v) Intensified glycemic control and lipid-lowering agents may be justified in advanced stage.

(B) Treatment for advanced stages of diabetic nephropathy: **The decision to perform dialysis or renal transplantation** depends upon the symptoms rather than the laboratory values. Diabetic nephropathy plus cardiomyopathy patients **may need early therapy** because of poor tolerance of high BP and excessive ECF volume. **Patients with diabetes do not tolerate** these procedures well unlike nondiabetic patients.

120. **Few important points in UTI and pyelonephritis**:

(i) UTI includes both **asymptomatic** microbial colonization in the urine and **symptomatic** infection with **microbial invasion and inflammation** of the urinary tract.

(ii) **Bacteria is the most** common organism but yeast, fungi, and viruses can cause UTI.

(iii) **Escherichia coli is the most common organism** (80 to 90% of cases); staphylococcus saprophyticus is most common (10 to 20% of cases) in young women among gram-positive organism.

(iv) Suprapubic aspiration of the urine is the **best diagnostic study**.

(v) Bacterial colony forming unit (CFU) ≥ **100, 000 /ml is** significant and suggestive of an infection.

(vi) Bacterial CFU low counts **1000 to 10,000 /ml may be clinically significant** when voided specimens are collected from **males,** under conditions of **suppressive antibiotic therapy, brisk diuresis**, and for slow growing organism **such as staphylococci**.

(vii) **Pyuria/dysuria (urethral) syndrome** is characterized by **low bacterial CFU counts with pyuria and dysuria**. This syndrome indicates **early phase of UTI**, found in **females** (33 to 55% of cases), and clinically indistinguishable from urethritis (e.g., Chlamydia trachomatis, Neisseria gonorrhoeae, or herpes simplex).

(viii) **Asymptomatic bacteriuria** is most commonly found in **asymptomatic females** with **large numbers of bacteria in urine**.

(ix) **Asymptomatic infection** means **asymptomatic bacteriuria plus pyuria. Pyuria** means **10 or more leukocytes per high power field** in the centrifuged specimen, or **5 or more when uncentrifuged**.

(x) **Acute pyelonephritis** means pyogenic, focal infection of the renal parenchyma with local and systemic symptoms.

(xi) **Chronic pyelonephritis** means cortical scarring, tubulointerstitial damage, and deformity of the calyx. **Active** chronic pyelonephritis means **persistent infection** and **inactive** type means focal sterile scars of a past infection. (Remember, **hypertension can cause cortical scars** like pyelonephritis and **analgesic nephropathy can cause papillary necrosis**).

(xii) **Organisms commonly produce infections**: E. coli, Pseudomonas species, Staphylococcus species, enterococci, other gram-negative and gram-positive bacteria, and yeast.

(xiii) **Organisms are considered contaminant**: Lactobacillus, alpha-hemolytic streptococci, and anaerobes.

(xiv) **Candida albicans and cryptococcus neoformans infections** are found **in immunosuppressed patients, diabetes, and in patients receiving corticosteroids**.

(xv) **UTIs are the most common cause of gram-negative infection** in hospitalized patients. **Approximately 50% of all hospital acquired infections begin in the urinary tract** in association with the urologic catheter and urologic procedures.

(xvi) UTI occurs most commonly by an ascending route.

121. Relationship of instrumentation and UTI:
   (i) **More than 90% will develop infection within 3 to 4 days after indwelling catheter placement**.
   (ii) After single catheterization, approximately **1 to 2% healthy individual will develop persistent bacteriuria**, the risk is higher in the debilitated patient, prostatic obstruction, and at the time of delivery.

122. **Clinical manifestations and laboratory findings of UTI:**
   (A) Clinical manifestations:
      (i) **Lower urinary tract (urethritis or cystitis):** Frequency, urgency, burning sensation during urination, suprapubic pain or discomfort, low-grade fever, and cloudy or blood tinged urine.
      (ii) **Upper urinary tract (acute pyelonephritis):** Acute onset of fever, shaking chills, flank pain, leukocytosis, and with or without urinary symptoms. **Atypical presentations** may be **backache without flank tenderness**, pain in the upper or lower abdomen with GI disturbances, or **only general fatigue**.
   (B) **Laboratory findings**:
      (i) **Lower urinary tract involvements:**
         (a) Positive urine culture is the best diagnostic method.
         (b) Leukocyte esterase test is positive.
         (c) Nitrite test may be positive.
         (d) Gram stain of uncentrifuged urine: leukocytes (≥ 5/hpf), Gram-negative rods or Gram-positive cocci (≥ 1/hpf).
      (ii) **Upper urinary tract involvements**:
         (a) Same findings as mentioned above plus.
         (b) Leukocytosis.
         (c) Blood culture is positive only 20% of cases.
         (d) Minimal effect on serum creatinine.
         (e) Decreased ability to concentrate urine.

123. **Urologic and radiologic studies of UTI**:
   (i) **Ultrasonography** with bladder voiding studies and **radionuclide studies** are more commonly used. Invasive studies (e.g., IVP, VCUG, and cystoscopy) are less commonly needed.
   (ii) Urologic studies are less useful in females, even with recurrent infections.
   (iii) CT scan is helpful to detect renal abscesses.
   (iv) **Cystoscopy is done to detect** bladder tumors, interstitial cystitis, and anatomic abnormalities. **It should not be done to see the response of therapy.**

124. **Management of UTI**:

(A) **Asymptomatic bacteriuria**:

(i) It should **not** be treated in otherwise healthy or elderly females **without** structural or neurologic abnormalities.

(ii) **Urease producing bacterias** (Proteus, Providencia, S. saprophyticus, Morganella, and corynebacterium D2 are virulent) **should be treated adequately** because they can produce **urinary calculi**.

(iii) Antibiotics should **not** be used for patients **with indwelling catheter** because of **superinfections with more resistant microorganisms**.

(iv) **Antibiotics should be used for high risk patients** (e.g., diabetes, before urologic procedures, renal transplantation, anatomic or neurologic abnormalities, or polycystic kidneys).

(v) Antibiotic treatment in asymptomatic bacteriuria in early pregnancy can prevent acute pyelonephritis in third trimester.

(B) **Acute symptomatic UTI:**

(i) **Pretreatment urine cultures** are desirable, but **not** mandatory; **in young women** with acute dysuria and pyruria **most common diagnosis is uncomplicated bacterial cystitis**: Treated with short-course **of antibiotics**.

Response to treatment is determined by **disappearance of bacteria by 24 to 48 hours (microscopic examination) but pyuria may persist up to a week (Important). Failure** of treatment is determined by presence of bacteria after 48 hours, pyuria > 1 week, and persistence of symptoms: **Antibiotic should be changed immediately.**

(ii) **Pretreatment urine cultures should be obtained** in young men, the elderly; suspected pyelonephritis or complicated infection; symptomatic catheter related or instrument associated; relapsing infections; pregnant women with bacteriuria.

(iii) Oral antibiotic (most commonly used for uncomplicated cases) are **trimethoprim, trimethoprim – sulfamethoxazole,** nitrofurantoin, **amoxicillin – clavulanate, ciprofloxacin,** norfloxacin; or carbenicillin indanyl (for pseudomonas infection).

(iv) Acute **uncomplicated** symptomatic infections (urethritis or bacterial cystitis): **Oral antibiotic therapy for 3 days is recommended** because it is equally effective as 7 to 10 days.

(v) Acute **complicated** symptomatic infections: Antibiotic therapy **for 7 to 14 days or even longer**.

(vi) **Symptomatic Chalmydia trachomatis urethritis**: Oral doxycycline or tetracycline for 7 day.

(vii) **Acute uncomplicated pyelonephritis: Single drug therapy for 7 to 14 days** is recommended. **Parenteral antibiotic** (trimethoprim-sulfamethoxazole, ampicillin-sulbactam, a cephalosporin, or an aminoglycoside) **is used for severely ill patients** or patients **with vomiting but switch to oral antibiotic as soon as possible**.

(viii) Patients with **active chronic pyelonephritis** (e.g., obstruction, foreign body, or abscess): Antibiotic is **not** effective alone. To relieve the obstruction, **removal of foreign body, or drainage of abscess plus antibiotic therapy is effective**.

(ix) Hematogenous pyelonephritis needs specific treatment for invading organism.

(x) Negative urine culture after 1 week of completion of therapy indicates cure.

(C) **Treatment of recurrent infections**:

(i) In diabetes, patients with transplantation, and elderly men: **Antibiotic for 4 to 6 weeks** should be given.

(ii) **Frequent recurrent infections**: **Repeated short-courses for each symptomatic episode** or long-term prophylaxis with **trimethoprim, trimethoprim – sulfamethoxazole, or nitrofurantion as a single bed time dose**. Prophylaxis for 6 months or longer is very effective **but resistant strains infrequently emerge as a complication**. Urinary antiseptic drugs (methenamine and its salts) are used as prophylaxis when **no other drug is effective**.

(iii) **Postcoital use of prophylactic antibiotic is very effective, voiding after sexual intercourse** is effective, **double voiding** is recommended in vesicoureteral reflux patients, and high-volume of fluid intake may be effective.

(D) **Treatment of complicated infections**:

(i) To relieve the obstruction, remove the foreign body plus appropriate antibiotic therapy.

(ii) Discontinue the ineffective antibiotic STAT.

(iii) Sometimes it is **best to leave the infection untreated** but to treat the acute episodes.

(iv) **Suppressive therapy is not recommended** unless it markedly reduces the bacterial numbers in the urine.

125. **Few important points in thromboembolic occulsion of the renal arteries**:

(i) **Most common source of renal thromboemboli (90% of cases) is left atrial thrombi** in patients with atrial fibrillation. Embolization is the most common cause and mostly involves one renal artery.

(ii) In patients age 60 and over, **localized (in situ) thrombosis** of renal artery is a **complication of progressive thrombosis**.

(iii) In patients **under** the age of 60, most common cause of renal thrombosis is **blunt trauma which damages the intima** (mostly in middle third of renal artery) **results in thrombosis**.

(iv) Renal thrombosis could be due to **inflammatory changes** in large arteries (systemic vasculitis, syphilis, thromboangitis obliterans, and Takayasu's arteritis) or **structural changes** (e.g., renal artery aneurysms, fibromuscular dysplasia).

(v) Clinical manifestations depend on the **extent, time, course,** and **pre-existing status of renal circulation**. Acute thrombosis and infarction appear with **sudden onset of flank pain** (**mimic renal colic**), **fever, nausea, vomiting; leukocytosis and elevated AST, LDH, and alkaline phosphatase** (due to infarction); hypertension (due to increased renin levels), microscopic hematuria, elevated BUN and creatinine.

(vi) **The definitive diagnostic study for renal artery occlusion is renal arteriography**. CT scan, MRI with angiography, and duplex doppler studies are also helpful.

(vii) **Management**:

(a) **Acute arterial thrombosis** requires surgical revascularization, adequate hydration, anticoagulation, controlling high BP, and dialysis if needed; alternative method of **thrombolytic therapy are being used more often**.

(b) **Traumatic** renal artery occlusion **requires surgery within 12 hours** after injury.

(c) **Nontraumatic unilateral** occlusion is managed more conservatively.

(d) In **chronic ischemic renal disease, surgical revascularization is** helpful.

(e) Hypertension is treated with **ACE** (angiotensin-converting enzyme) **inhibitors** or, if unresponsive, use balloon angioplasty.

126. **Most common cause of renal artery stenosis**:

(i) **In middle-aged and elderly patients**: **Atherosclerosis** is the most common cause (60 to 70% of cases.).

(ii) **In younger women: Fibromuscular dysplasis** is the most common cause.

127. **Clinical presentations, diagnosis, and treatment of renal artery stenosis**:

(A) **Clinical presentations**: **The development of hypertension in** a **previously normotensive** patient **over age 55 or under 30,** or **accelerated hypertension in a controlled hypertensive patient indicates renal artery stenosis (Important)**. Patients may appear with persistent **hypokalemia, metabolic alkalosis,** recurrent pulmonary edema, **unexplained decreasing renal function with or without high BP**, signs and symptoms of

peripheral vascular disease, unequal kidney size, and presence of epigastric bruit on physical examination.

(B) **Diagnosis of renal artery stenosis:**

(i) **The captopril renal scintigram (scan)** is the best **noninvasive function test to screen** for renal artery stenosis.

(ii) **Three-dimensional phase-contrast MRI** has sensitivity and specificity > 90%.

(iii) **Renal arteriography** may be required to **confirm the diagnosis and define the vascular anatomy** before any surgical or nonsurgical intervention.

(iv) **The ratio of renin** from the stenotic side versus the normal side renal **vein is > 1.5 in unilateral renal artery stenosis.** (Remember, peripheral vein renin levels have **no** value).

(C) **Treatment of renal artery stenosis**:

(i) **Percutaneous transluminal angioplasty is the initial treatment of choice** in both fibromuscular dysplasia and atherosclerotic renal artery stenosis. It is effective approximately 50% of cases in each of both conditions. It is ideal for **elderly patients who are at high risk for surgical intervention**.

(ii) Surgical revascularization should be done when angioplasty fails.

(iii) Medical conservative management **should be the last choice**. It should be reserved for patients with **definite contraindication to surgery or angioplasty**.

128. **Few important points in atheroembolic disease of the renal arteries**:

(i) **Embolization of cholesterol crystals** into renal arteries are **most common in elderly** persons **with widespread atherosclerosis**.

(ii) **Atheroemboli could be a complication** after surgery or manipulation of abdominal aorta or renal artery; and postangiography or postangioplasty.

(iii) Clinical presentations include **high BP** and **renal insufficiency**; or **evidence of cholesterol embolization** in the muscles, skin (livedo reticularis), or retina. It can cause CVA, ischemic bowel disease, acute pancreatitis, and gangrene of the extremities. Urinalysis shows proteinuria, and eosinophiluria.

(iv) Treatment includes **dialysis, adequate hydration, antihypertensive** for high BP, but should avoid hypotension.

129. **Renal vein thrombosis**:

(A) **Etiology: Nephrotic syndrome,** renal cell cancer with invasion of renal vein, extrinsic compression (tumor, lymph nodes, retroperitoneal fibrosis, aortic aneurysm), pregnancy or estrogen therapy.

(B) **Clinical presentations**:
  (i) **Acute renal vein thrombosis**: Flank pain, hematuria, enlarged kidney size, vomiting, leukocytosis, and decreased renal function.
  (ii) **Adult nephrotic patients with chronic renal vein thrombosis**: Increased proteinuria, glycosuria, aminoaciduria, phosphaturia, and decreased urinary acidification.

(C) **Diagnosis**: It is confirmed by **selective renal venography** (invasive study), **MRI with angiography** is helpful noninvasive study.

(D) **Treatment:**
  (i) Acute and chronic renal vein thrombosis: Anticoagulation with **heparin** for 7 to 10 days is followed by **oral warfarin (Coumadin)** for at least one year.
  (ii) Patients with recurrence or continued risk factors: Anticoagulation is continued indefinitely.
  (iii) Acute renal vein thrombosis with ARF: Fibrinolytic therapy may be needed.

130. **Few important points in Alport's syndrome**:
  (i) It is a **chronic progressive hereditary nephritis with hematuria and sensorineural hearing loss** (Important). **More severe in males** than females.
  (ii) **X-linked dominant** inheritance, mutations of **COL 4A5**, gene located in **Xq 22** which codes for the alpha-5 chain of type IV collagen.
  (iii) **Etiology: Absence of a 28-KD peptide (Goodpasture antigen) component** of the NC1 (noncollagenous) domain of the alpha-3 chain of type IV collagen of GBM (glomerular basement membrane).
  (iv) **Clinical presentations: Hematuria** (microscopic or gross), **sensorineural** hearing loss, **proteinuria** (70% mild, 30 to 40% nephrotic range), eye disorders (spherophakia, anterior and posterior lenticonus); **severe and progressive renal disease, high BP, and chronic renal failure in males**; mild and nonprogressive disease in females.
  (v) **Diagnosis: The documentations of** progressive renal disease, hematuria, with or without proteinuria, azotemia, or high BP, and **sensorineural hearing loss in one family member younger than 50 other than the proband**.
  (vi) **Treatment:**
    (a) No specific treatment is available.
    (b) To control the hypertension.
    (c) Renal failure: Peritoneal dialysis, hemodialysis or transplantation.
  (v) **Posttransplantation effects**:
    (a) **Goodpasture's syndrome** due to antibody against the GBM.

(b) **Improvement of hearing deficit**.
(c) **No** improvement in recurrence of renal lesions.
(vi) **Differential diagnosis**:
(a) Berger's disease: IgA nephropathy, mesangial deposits of IgA and variable amount of C3, IgM, or IgG.
(b) Benign familial hematuria: Thin GBM, nonprogressive disease.

131. **Nail-patella syndrome** (or osteo-onychodysplasia) (Important): **Mode of genetic transmission**: Autosomal dominant.
Clinical presentations: **Absent or atrophic fingernails, hypoplasia or absent of the patella,** subluxation of the radial bone heads, thickening of the scapula, accessory conical iliac horns, mild proteinuria (40% of cases), rarely hematuria, nephrotic syndrome and renal failure (27% of cases).
Treatment: **No specific therapy** is available. **Renal transplantation** has been done without evidence of recurrence of the disease in the transplanted organ.

132. **The radiographic (x-ray) appearance of kidney stones (Important)**:
(i) Radiologically **not** visible: Uric acid stones.
(ii) Radiologically **poorly** visible: Cystine stones (Uric acid and cystine stones require CT scan, ultrasonography, or IVP for detection).
(iii) **Radiologically visible**: Calcium phosphate, calcium oxalate, struvite (magnesium ammonium phosphate), when it complexes with calcium carbonate or phosphate.

133. **Clinical manifestations, diagnosis, treatment, and prevention of renal stones:**
(A) **Clinical manifestations**: **Renal colic** (sudden onset of acute pain beginning in the flank curving anteriorly towards the groin), **hematuria**, nausea, vomiting; urinary **frequency and dysuria** as the stone reaches the **ureterovesical** junction. **The pain disappears** when stone moves into the bladder or inside the ureter. Stones can cause **painless obstructive uropathy** which may **remain undiagnosed for long period of time**.
(B) **Diagnosis:**
(i) Plain X-ray (KUB) can diagnosis most of the stones **except** uric acid stones and sometimes cystine stones.
(ii) **Intravenous urography is the first step in evaluating patients with renal colic** but should be careful in patients with decreased renal function. **It is most useful to detect the degree and extent of urinary tract obstruction**.

(iii) Ultrasonography is the **safest**, can **detect hydronephrosis or hydroureter**. It **cannot detect the site** of obstruction and may **not** detect small stone.
(iv) Retrograde pyelography needs cystoscopy, it is useful in patients **when intravenous urography is contraindicated** (renal insufficiency or contrast dye allergy).
(v) CT scan is useful to detect uric acid stones and sometimes cystine stones.

(C) **Treatment of renal colic**:
(i) **IV fluid hydration, analgesic, and** radiologic assesment.
(ii) **Patients with significant obstruction: Observation** for movement of the stone during IV fluid hydration.
(iii) **Urologic intervention is indicated** if the evidence suggest that the stone will **not** pass within 2 to 3 days.
(iv) **Stones lodged in the proximal ureter or ureteropelvic junction:** The best methods to push stone into renal pelvis and disrupt it by ESWL (extracorporeal shockwave lithotripsy). If the stone **cannot** be pushed back, **it is bypassed with a stent to** provide urinary drainage and is **followed by ESWL disruption therapy. Percutaneous nephrolithotomy** is done in case of failure of ESWL.
(v) Stones (< 5 mm in diameter) in an asymptomatic patient: No intervention is needed.
(vi) Stones (> 5 mm and < 2 cm in diameter): **ESWL is the best method** of therapy.
(vii) Stones (> 2 cm), or stones (> 1 cm in the lower pole): **Percutaneous nephrostolithotomy is the best method of therapy** because lithotripsy alone, leaves residual stones (35 to 50% of cases).
(viii) Cystine stones: **Percutaneous nephrostolithotomy is required** because lithotripsy disrupts these stones poorly.
(ix) **Struvite and uric acid stones:** ESWL and percutaneous nephrostolithotomy are effective.

(D) **Prevention of recurrent renal stones:**
(i) **First step** is to make **correct diagnosis** of the cause of renal stones.
(ii) **Diagnosis requires** several urine and blood tests which should be done approximately **2 weeks after** the patients resume **normal activity and diet**.
(iii) Repeated sampling of **24-hour urine specimens** from patients on their **normal** diets and **test** diets are needed. (Test diet includes **400 mg calcium diet used** for 1 week before calcium challenge test). **Urine specimens** should be examined for pH, volume, creatinine, Ca, p, Mg, uric acid, k, Na, citrate, oxalate, and urinary urea nitrogen. **The addition**

of ammonia, chloride, and sulfate helps in calculation of relative supersaturation. The addition of **exogenous calcium oxalate or phosphate** is helpful to determine the formation of products for different crystal nucleation events.

(iv) Blood samples should be tested for Na, k, cl, HCO_3, p, PTH, and vitamin D_3 levels.

(v) Recent studies indicate that **recurrence** is common in patients with **first stone plus detectable metabolic abnormalities**.

134. **Treatment which is recommend for different types of renal stones**:

(i) **All stones:** High fluid intake to maintain urinary volumes between 2 to 3 liters.

(ii) Calcium oxalate, calcium phosphate stones, idiopathic hypercalciuria: Thiazide diuretics and related drugs; oral phosphate; controlled protein, Na and Ca diets; Na cellulose phosphate.

(iii) **Hyperoxaluria**:

(a) Primary: Pyridoxine.

(b) Dietary: Reduced oxalate diet.

(c) Enteric: Ca supplement, cholestyramine, and low-fat diet.

(iv) **Hypocitraturia**:

(a) RTA: Potassium citrate.

(b) Ileostomy or small bowel malabsorption: Potassium citrate.

(v) **Uric acid stones**: Postassium citrate, allopurinol.

(vi) **Hyperuricosuria:** Allopurinol, potassium citrate.

(vii) **Struvite stones:** Extracorporeal shockwave lithotripsy or percutaneous nephrostolithotomy, acetohydroxamic acid.

(viii) **Cystinuria, cystine stones:** Tiopronin, penicillamine.

135. **Most common type of cystic disease of the kidney: Simple renal cysts.** Other cystic disease **in adults** are **ADPKD** (autosomal dominant polycytic kidney disease), **medullary sponge kidney**, and medullary cystic disease (early adolescence). (Autosomal recessive polycystic kidney disease and medullary cystic disease are more **common in children, so those are not important for the examination**).

136. **Simple renal cysts**: It is most common, benign, increase in frequency with age. Most patients are **asymptomatic,** but sometimes appear with flank pain or hematuria. **Diagnosis is made by ultrasonography**. Cysts with pain or hypertension can be punctured with US guidance, drained, and sclerosed with instillation of alcohol within the cyst.

137. ADPKD (autosomal dominant polycystic kidney disease): It is the **most common hereditary cystic disease of the kidneys.** Most common type is **ADPKD 1**.

(i) **Chromosomes:** ADPKD 1 is on chromosome 16, ADPKD 2 gene is on chromosome 4.

(ii) Mode of inheritance: Autosomal dominant.

(iii) **Clinical manifestations:** Flank and back pains, hematuria (gross and microscopic), infection, hypertension, renal stones (36% of cases, urate or calcium), normal to very large size kidneys.

Extrarenal manifestations of ADPKD: Colonic diverticulosis (80% of patients with ESRD), **hepatic cysts** (50% of cases), **cardiac valve (mitral valve prolapse) defects** (26% of case), pancreatic cysts (10% of cases), intracranial aneurysms (5 to 10% of cases), and arachnoid cysts (5% of cases).

(iv) **Diagnosis: Ultrasonography** (may miss 2 to 6% of patients with cysts), **CT scan** (may miss rare patients with small cysts); and **the definitive diagnosis is made by gene linkage analysis.**

(v) **Treatment of ADPKD:**

(a) **Education** of patients and family members regarding the inheritance and manifestations of the disease.

(b) **Hematuria** is managed with **bed rest, hydration, and analgesics**.

(c) **Avoid** urinary tract instrumentation and Foley catheter to minimize infections.

(d) Infections should be treated with **antibiotics. Urine and blood cultures** should be obtained before antibiotic therapy.

(e) Unresponsiveness to antibiotic means cysts infection, **give trimethoprim – sulfamethoxazole, fluroquinolones, or chloramphenicol, these antibiotics can penetrate cysts fluid**.

(f) Infected hepatic cysts: Drainage of cysts and antibiotics are needed.

(g) Antihypertensive for high BP.

(h) **Percutaneous or surgical decompression of the cysts: It can reduce the pain** but **cannot** improve or preserve renal function.

(i) **Patients with renal failure:** Renal replacement therapy.

(j) **Patients with new clinical symptoms or develop complications** (malignancy, stones, intracystic or retroperitoneal bleeding): **CT scan is the best method of choice**.

(vi) **Differential diagnosis between multiple simple cysts and ADPKD:** Multiple simple cysts are usually **unilateral** (ADPKD is bilateral), **cortical cysts** (both cortical and medullary in ADPKD), **cysts size usually < 2 cm** (early ADPKD is < 2 cm), **normal kidney size** (ADPKD is normal or enlarged), **absence** of extra renal manifestations, genetic linkage, and family history.

138. **Medullary sponge kidney:** It is a **common disorder** of **unknown cause** with tubular dilatations within the medullary collecting ducts.
   (i) **Clinical manifestations:** Recurrent hematuria, renal stones, or UTI. **Presence of renal colic indicates obstruction**.
   (ii) **Diagnosis:** Excretory urography reveals normal size kidneys with medullary ductal ectasia ('bouquet of flowers' or 'paintbrush' appearance). Plain abdominal film can detect **calculi or calcification in the cystic lesions**. **Associated hypercalcuria and hyperparathyrodism may be present. Remember, serum electrolyte levels are normal. Renal function remains normal in absence of obstruction**.
   (iii) **Treatment:** Antibiotic for infections and therapy for calculi.

139. **VHL (von Hippel-lindau) disease**: It is an autosomal dominant disorder, characterized by **multiple tumors of the CNS, pheochromocytomas, and bilateral renal cell cancers.**

140. **Relationship of VHL gene and renal cell cancer**: Loss of VHL gene patients are associated with the deletion of short arm of chromosome 3.

141. **Clinical manifestations, diagnosis, and treatment of renal cell carcinomas**: It is typically diagnosed **during sixth and seventh decades** (male > female).
   (A) **Clinical manifestations: Hematuria is the most common symptom,** others are **pain and abdominal mass**. Systemic manifestations include **weight loss, anemia,** fever, **polycythemia, hypercalcemia, and nonmetastatic hepatic dysfunction.** Systemic manifestations may be the **only** presentation in renal cell cancer and **surgical removal of the primary tumor can relieve systemic manifestations.**
   Hormones producing systemic manifestations: Cytokines, interleukin-6, transforming growth factor alpha and beta, erythropoietin like substance, and parathyroid hormone-like substance.
   (B) **Diagnosis**:
      (i) Intravenous pyelography will detect **renal mass** but **cannot** differentiate cystic from solid.
      (ii) Ultrasonography (US) can differentiate cystic mass from solid mass:
         (a) **Complex cyst, solid mass,** or criteria for sonographic simple cyst are **not** met: **Next investigation of choice is contrast enhanced CT scan which is the best investigation of choice in renal cell cancer (Important). CT scan or MRI can** detect important useful

informations such as local and regional spread of the cancer, renal vein involvement, local lymph nodes involvement, and perirenal extension of the tumor.

(iii) Renal arteriography is **not** indicated unless planning for nephron-sparing surgery.

(C) **Treatment of renal cell cancer.**

(i) **Localized renal cell cancer: Redical nephrectomy** (removal of the kidney, Gerota's fascia, ipsilateral adrenal gland, and often regional **hilar** nodes) **is the treatment of choice. Extended** regional lymph nodes resection, or radiation therapy either before or after surgery is **not recommended**. Removal of the ipsilateral adrenal gland **is recommended only** if cancer involves **upper or mid pole of the kidney**.

(ii) Nephrom-sparing surgery is indicated in which radical nephrectomy will result in an anephric patient requiring dialysis such as **bilateral renal cell cancers** and renal cell cancer in a **solitary functioning kidney**.

(iii) Patients with solitary metastasis (at the time of diagnosis or after removal of the kidney): **Most common site of metastasis is the lung, resection** of the metastasis should be done.

(iv) Patients with stage IV disease (tumor in the adjacent or distant organs):

(a) Asymptomatic patients: No nephrectomy.

(b) Symptomatic patients: Nephrectomy is recommended.

(v) Postnephrectomy **adjuvant therapy** (or additional systemic therapy): **No** definitive role of this therapy but **stage IV patients may be treated with immunotherapy and chemotherapy**.

Immunotherapy: Interferon, recombinant human interleukin-2 (rh IL-2) can induce tumor regression (up to 13 to 14% of cases).

Toxicity of rh IL-2: The vascular leak syndrome characterized by generalized increase in vascular permeability, hypotension, and fluid retention. The treatment is to **lower the doses** of rh IL-2.

Chemotherapy: Most drugs are **not** effective but **limited success** with **vinblastine** and **floxuridine** which can **induce tumor regression** (up to 16% of cases). The hormones **tamoxifen** and **medroxyprogesterone acetate** can induce tumor regression < 10% and 1 to 2% cases respectively.

142. **Kidney cancer and lung cancer**:

(i) **Most common site of metastasis in kidney cancer is the lung (50% of cases); other sites are bone (49%)**, skin, liver, and brain.

(ii) A variety of cancer can metastases to the kidney, **most common primary site is the lung (cancer)**. Metastases to the kidney are **most commonly multiple**.

143. **A patient develops solitary renal mass, he has prior history of malignant disease without evidence of metastases:**
Most likely diagnosis: Primary renal cell cancer. The appropriate investigations and mangement should be done immediately.

144. **Most common malignant urothelial tumor: Bladder cancer.**

145. **Clinical manifestations, diagnosis, and treatment of bladder cancer:**
(A) **Clinical manifestations: Hematuria** (mostly gross, sometimes microscopic), **dysuria, frequency of urination, urgency,** and **large tumor can cause obstruction** of ureter or bladder outlet. (**Remember,** a patient appears with dysuria, urgency, frequency, **no** hematuria, and **no** infection, **bladder cancer should be ruled out**). **Pelvic pain appears** when it involves adjacent nerves and bone.
(B) **Diagnosis:**
(i) **IVP** should be done to locate the filling defect in the bladder and upper part of the urinary tracts.
(ii) **Cystoscopy** should be done **to locate** the tumor, **depth of invasion,** and to **obtain biopsy**.
(iii) Urinary cytology is helpful as **an initial** assesment and **follow up** of patients with muscular layer involvement and beyond.
(iv) To evaluate the metastases: CXR, abdominal and pelvic CT, and bone scan should be done.
(C) **Treatment:**
(i) Bladder cancer confined to the transitional cell layer: **Only transurethral excision**.
(ii) Bladder cancer most commonly recurs **in another site** within the bladder: Frequent cystoscopy and excision of recurrent cancers.
(iii) **Higher-grade cancers confined to the transitional cell layer and high-grade flat tumors (CIS):** Use intravesical **chemotherapy or immunotherapy with BCG** (bacille Calmette-Guerin) can **prevent or deter** the development of **invasive cancers**.
(iv) Bladder cancers invading the deeper layers of the bladder: **Radical cystectomy** (total removal of the bladder) **plus urinary diversion** (formation of ileal loop, continent reservoir, or orthotopic neobladder). Alternative therapy is **partial cystectomy or chemotherapy with radiation therapy**.

(v) Bladder cancers invading deeper layers plus high chances of **future recurrence or distant spread**: Cystectomy is followed by chemotherapy.

(vi) Patients with metastatic bladder cancer: **Polyagent chemotherapy** may prolong the life.

146. **Recurrence of bladder, ureter, and renal pelvic cancers:**

(i) **Bladder cancer commonly recurs in another site of bladder (rarely** recurs into renal pelvis or ureter).

(ii) **Cancer of ureter and renal pelvis most commonly recurs in the bladder** (25% of cases).

Recent studies have suggested that these multifocal or polychronotropic tumors **are clonal in origin,** possibility of **common malignant cell abnormality and /or reimplantation of tumor cells are the causes of tumor recurrence**.

147. **Clinical presentations, diagnosis, and treatment of transitional cell cancers of ureter, renal pelvis, and calices:**

(A) **Clinical presentations:** Hematuria (gross or microscopic), **ureteral obstruction,** and **pain** due to renal colic.

(B) **Diagnosis:**

(i) IVP shows **filling defect** in the calix, infundibulum, renal pelvis, or ureter.

(ii) Cystoscopsy with retrograde pyelography plus cytology or ureteroscopy may be needed to confirm the lesions.

(C) **Treatment:**

(i) **Low-grade, superficial lesions** confined to the transitional cell layer: Less radical therapy (segmental resection) is required.

(ii) **High-grade, deeper lesions** into the wall of the ureter or renal pelvis with greater potential of metastases: Definitive radical therapy (nephroureterectomy plus removal off a cuff of bladder), additional chemotherapy may or may not be helpful.

(iii) **Invasive lesions** in the renal pelvis, calices, and ureter plus metastatic spread: **Multi drug** chemotherapy may be helpful.

CARDIOVASCULAR DISEASES

1. **Raynaud's phenomenon**: It is a syndrome characterized by **attacks of pallor and cyanosis** of the digits in response **to cold or emotion** followed by **redness** after the attack.
   (i) **Primary disorder** is called **Raynaud's disease**
   (ii) **Secondary disorder** (means secondary to another cause or disease) is called **Raynaud's phenomenon.**
   (iii) **Pathophysiology:** First **intense vasconstriciton** or spasm of the digital arteries causes **pallor,** followed by **less severe** vasoconstriction results in partial filling up of capillaries and veins with deoxygenated blood **causes cyanosis**, followed by rewarming with reactive hyperemia **which causes redness**.

2. **CREST syndrome**: It includes calcinosis, Raynaud's phenomenon, abnormal esophageal motility, sclerodactyly, and telangiectasia.

3. **The relationship of angina pectoris, Raynaud's phenomenon, and migraine**:
   (i) 24% patients with angina pectoris develop Raynaud's phenomenon.
   (ii) 26% patients with angina pectoris develop migraine.

4. **Clinical manifestations, diagnosis, and treatment of Raynaud's phenomenon**:
   (A) **Clinical manifestations**:
      (i) **Typical attacks: Pallor and cyanosis** of the digits in response to cold or emotion. The attack may be **terminated spontaneously or by rewarming**, then the color of the hands **become red**. It usually affects all digits (mostly upper extremities) **symmetrically**.
      (ii) **Atypical attacks: Asymmetric** involvement **(one to two) of the digit, a portion of the** digit (most commonly distal part) may be affected.
      (iii) **Severe progressive cases:** Trophic changes occurs few years after the onset. The skin may **be thin, atrophic, and tight** (sclerodactyly) followed by **painful ulcer** formations which results in **small, pitted scars. The nails grow slowly, become brittle and deformed. The hairs disappear** from the dorsal aspect of the digits.
   (B) **Diagnosis**:
      (i) **Typical cases**: History of attack, precipitated by cold, and relieved by warming.
      (ii) **Atypical cases:** Provocation of an attack by immersing the hands in cold water temp 10 to 15°c or whole body exposure to cold is more effective. **Remember, a negative result cannot exclude the diagnosis**.

(C) **Treatment:**

(i) All patients benefit from **reassurance and protective measures against exposure to cold.** Protective clothing should cover not only to **cover hands and feet** but **also the face and trunk**; when exposure to cold is unavoidable then **use hand and foot wormers**; **prompt rewarming** (warm environment, warm water, warm air-blower) **can terminate the attack; avoid vibrating-tools** if those are the underlying cause (**remember**, avoid exposure to vibration- tool is **not** always effective).

(ii) **Rare or mild attacks:** Protective measures as mentioned above, cessation of smoking, and **no** drug therapy.

(iii) **Frequent or severe attacks without** trophic changes: Protective measures and calcium antagonists (nifedipine, diltiazem).

(iv) Frequent attacks with trophic changes but **no** open ulcers: Protective measuers **plus calcium antagonist** (nifedipine, diltiazem) **or oral reserpin** (interfere with sympathetic nerve activity) **plus sodium liothyronine or triiodothyronine** (iatrogenic hyperthyroidism causing vasodilatation of the digits).

(v) Frequent attacks with active, painful ulcers: **Intravenous PGE_1 (vasodilator), intra-arterial reserpine** followed by calcium antagonists (nifedipine, diltiazem); or reserpine plus liothyronine; or **misoprostol (vasodilator).** (Remember, surgical procedues such as preganglionic sympathectomy is not effective or stripping of palmar and digital arteries is under investigation).

5. **Drugs or chemicals can cause Raynaud's phenomenon**:

(i) Beta-adrenergic receptor blockers (propranolol).

(ii) Anticancer drugs (bleomycin, cisplatin, vinblastin).

(iii) Other are ergotamine, ergotism, methysergide, polyvinyl chloride. (**Remember**, beta-blockers block the beta-adrenergic vasodilating effects in the digits and also enhance vasoconstricting effects of norepinephrine).

6. **Raynaud's phenomenon and acrocyanosis**:

Raynaud's phenomenon	Acrocyanosis
(i) Episodic in nature.	(i) Sustained.
(ii) Pallor then cyanosis then redness.	(ii) Cyanosis is typical finding.
(iii) Only the digits are involved.	(iii) Involves whole hands, feet, and sometime proximal limbs.
(iv) Skin of the palm is dry.	(iv) Skin of the palm is wet, clammy, and sweaty.
(v) Trophic chanes and ulceration occur in digits	(v) No trophic changes and ulceration.

7. **Few important points in acrocyanosis**:
   (i) **Rare** disorder, more common in **women** than men, occur in **middle-aged and young adults,** it is due to arteriolar constriction.
   (ii) **Higher incidence in psychiatric patients**.
   (iii) Patients appear with **blue-colored hands** (less commonly involved feet) **which are exaggerated by exposure to cold** but **improved to purplish or red color by exposure to heat**. Patients also complain of **coldness** and occasional numbness.
   (iv) **Differentiation from Raynaud's phenomenon** is aleady discussed in item number 6.
   (v) **Differentiation from arterial obstruction** which appear with **absence** of pulses (acrocyanosis has **normal** pulses and arteriography shows **absence** of obstruction) and **obstruction** in arteriography.
   (vi) Acrocyanosis has **normal** arterial oxygen saturation **unlike** generalized cyanosis.
   (vii) Acrocyanosis does **not** need any drug therapy.

8. **Sneddon's syndrome** ; Generalized livedo reticularis and ischemic cerebrovascular manifestations, **elevated anticardiolipin antibodies** (25 to 33% cases).

9. **Livedo reticularis**: It is a **lacy, reticular, bluish discoloration** of the skin of the extremities. Most common **before age 20 to 30,** unknown etiology, probably **due to arteriolar constriction is** followed by stasis and dilatation of capillaries and veins.
   Treatment:
   (i) No treatment is needed in most cases.
   (ii) Protection from cold and avoid smoking are helpful.
   (iii) Severe cases may need **nifedipine and reserpine therapy**.
   (iv) Aspirin may be helpful in some patients of Sneddon's syndrome.

10. **Frostbite (polonged exposure to temperature below 0°c)**:
   (A) **Clinical manifestations:** Initial **prickling** sensation is followed by **numbness**, skin appear **white and cold** followed by **swelling, redness, increased temperature**. After 24 to 48 hours **blisters** (serous yellow or hemorrhagic) appear, may be followed by **necrosis** and **gangrene**.
   (B) **Treatment:**
      (i) **Avoid exercise or massage** which enhances the edema and pain.
      (ii) **Rewarming** should be done immediately (if frostbite involves deep tissues, rewarming should be done with 40 to 44°c water).

(iii) The limb should be left **exposed**, vesicles should **not** be touched.
(iv) Sympathectomy is helpful.
(v) Antibiotic for superimposed infection.

11. **Chilblain (Pernio)**: It is characterized by **erythema, itching, and ulceration** of the skin due to exposure to cold. It is **more common in women** than men **before the age 20.**
    (A) **Clinical manifestations**:
        (i) Acute forms: **Bluish-red discoloration, edema** of the lower extremities are associated with **burning, warmth, and itching** sensations lasted for 7 to 10 days followed by clear up with or without residual skin pigmentations. Severe cases may develop blebs, hemorrhage, and infections.
        (ii) Chronic forms (due to repeated exposure to cold): Ulcerative, erythematous, hemorrhagic lesions with bleb formations.It heals in the summer with permanent pigmented spots.
    (B) **Diagnosis:**
        (i) Acute forms: Characteristic distribution of rash produced by exposure to cold.
        (ii) Chronic form should be distinguished from erythema induratum of Bazin caused by Mycobacterium tuberculosis: **Erythema induratum** affects the **upper part** of the leg (chilblain affects the lower part), **lesions are nodular, deeper, infiltrative**, and associated with fever, arthralgias, and does **not** improve in the summer (**chilblain improves in the summer**).
    (C) **Treatment:**
        (i) **Mild cases:** Protect the skin from the cold, local anti-inflammatory ointments, avoid scratching and smoking.
        (ii) **Severe cases:** Reserpine or nifedipine may be effective.

12. **Most common cause of arterial obstructive disease of the extremities**: **Arteriosclerosis obliterans.** Most commonly affected vessel is the **superficial femoral artery, next most common sites are** distal aorta, its bifurcation into two iliac arteries, and popliteal artery.

13. **Clinical manifestations, diagnosis, differential diagnosis, and treatment of arteriosclerosis obliterans**:
    (A) **Clinical manifestations:** Intermittent claudication (pain during exercise and disappears during rest) followed by **pain at rest** and **trophic changes of bilateral extermities**. **Most commonly involved part is the calf muscles because of femoral arterial involvement**, the muscles of the

lower back, the buttocks, the thighs, and the feet may also be involved. **Pain at rest** indicates severe disease (**75% or more** reduction in cross-sectional area of the vessels), **pain during exercise** means less severe disease (**60% or more** reduction in cross-sectional area of the vessels). Physical examination reveal **reduced or absent arterial pulses** distal to the obstruction, **audible bruits** over the arteries involved, **changes of skin** (ischemic changes include cold, pallor,or cyanosis; trophic changes include dry,scaly,shiny skin), toe nails become brittle, loss of hair, finally ulcer and gangrene formations.

Leriche's syndrome: It is an isolated **aortoiliac disease** characterized by **claudication** of the lower back, buttocks, thigh or calf muscles, **atrophic limbs, pale skin of the feet and legs,** with or without impotence. **Physical examination** of this syndrome reveal **absent or weak** femoral pulses, **audible bruits** over the lower abdomen and femoral arteries.

(B) **Diagnosis of arteriosclerosis obliterans:**

(i) **Palpation of** the arterial pulses and auscultation of bruits can determine the **presence and site of arterial obstruction**.

(ii) **Leg elevation test**: Leg is elevated 45 angle in supine position, pallor of the planter surface indicates arterial insufficiency.

(iii) **Doppler velocimetry** to determine the pressure of dorsalis pedis or posterior tibial arteries: **Pressures < 30 mm Hg indicate severe ischemia and possibility of gangrene**.

(iv) **Aortography confirms** arterial obstruction.

(C) **Differential diagnosis**:

(i) **Arterial embolism:** Sudden onset and unilateral involvement.

(ii) McArdle's syndrome (muscle phosphorylase deficiency), venous disease, severe anemia can cause **intermittent claudication**: Patients have **normal** pulses.

(iii) Ergotamine or methysergide toxicity can cause severe vasospasm: History of drug ingestion; angiography shows **generalized vasospasm** and **absence** of segmental obstruction.

(D) **Treatment of arteriosclerosis obliterans**:

(i) Patients with arteriosclerosis obliterans **without evidence of ischemia: Medical** treatment only, limited physical activity, regular exercise program, avoid smoking, treat diabetes, and hyperlipidemia. The **affected extremity** should be kept clean, dry, soft, and **avoid trauma and cold**.

(Remember, vasodilator therapy is **not** effective and **may be harmful**). **Pentoxifyline** (increases RBC membrane deformability and therapy reduces blood viscosity) **is effective**. Patients are able to walk more and do more exercise with this medication.

(ii) **Patients with ischemia unable to do regular activity**:

(a) Surgical therapy includes **endarterectomy of the stenotic artery or a bypass surgery. Axillofemoral or femorofemoral grafts** are useful in **aortoiliac disease**.

(b) **Nonsurgical revascularization procedures** such as **balloon angioplasty, laser angioplasty,** and **rotational atherectomy** are useful alternatives. **Intravascular stent is used for iliac artery disease**. Long-term anticoagulants are used with revascularization procedures.

(iii) **Patients with ischemia but surgery is not possible** for anatomical problems: Bed rest, affected extremity should be kept **20 to 30° below the horizontal level, avoid** direct application of heat but extremity should be **kept warm by placing it** under a cradle (< 38°c temperature). The ulcers should be **debrided and kept clean with warm saline soaks. Antibiotic** is used for infection. Intraarterial administration of PGE_1 is **experimental. Finally amputation is performed to arrest advancing gangrene**.

(iv) **Preganglionic lumbar sympathectomy** is performed as an **acute intervention** to treat ischemic manifestations. **Before surgery local anesthetic should be injected** to demonstrate that temporary blocking of sympathetic nerves will improve limb circulations, **this is important in diabetes where peripheral neuropathy have already produced spontaneous sympathectomy**.

(v) Infusion of low-dose thrombolytic agents are used in acute and chronic thrombotic lesions, followed by revascularization surgery. Thrombolytic agents **can cause bleeding**.

14. **Most common cardiac complication in Marfan's syndrome**: **Aortic aneurysm and aortic dissection**. (Aortic dilatation may occur any time between 5 years and **sixth decade** of life). It commonly extends to innominate artery or may involve whole aorta (annuloaortic ectasia). Mitral valve or tricuspid valve regurgitation is also found in some patients.
Diagnosis: Echocardiography or MRI.
Treatment:
(i) **Beta-blocker** can inhibit the pace of aortic dilatation.
(ii) **Prophylactic operations** (replacement of ascending aortic aneurysm with **a composite tube graft** with is attached to prosthetic valve) is performed when **aortic root enlarges to 6 cm on echocardiography**.
(iii) Operation during **acute dissection is hazardous**.

15. **Most common cause of death in Marfan's syndrome**: **Complications** (rupture, dissection) **of aneurysms in the ascending aorta**.

16. **Buerger's disease (or thromboangitis obliterans)** (It is **less** common in USA, so **less** important for examination): It is an **inflammatory and proliferative** disease of the **medium and small arteries** and **veins of the limbs**. It is more common in **men** than women, between age **20 to 40**, almost all of the patients are **smokers**, associated with **HLA-A9 and HLA-B5 antigens**.

    (A) **Clinical manifestations:** Raynaud's phenomenon with digital **ulcerations, pain at rest due to ischemia with cold extremities** or typical intermittent claudication pain (mostly in the **arch of the feet** and sometimes pain in forearm or hand). **Migratory superficial thrombophlebitis** also occur, it subsides within several weeks.

    Physical examination shows diminished arterial pulsations, cold, pale, cyanotic, ulcerated, gangrenous, and edematous extremities.

    (B) **Diagnosis**:

    (i) **History of** young male, smoker; disease involves **both lower and upper** extremities, ischemia of the extremities from arterial occlusion plus migratory superficial thrombophlebitis.

    (ii) **Arteriography shows** segmental multiple occlusions of medium and small-sized arteries plus visualization of collateral vessels.

    (iii) **Preferred diagnostic study: Biopsy** which shows inflammatory and proliferative lesions.

    (C) **Treatment:** Stop smoking, protection from cold, local care of the ulceration or gangrene or finally amputation if needed. Sympathetomy may be useful temporarily. Vasodilator therapy may be used in Raynaud's phenomenon with ulceration.

    Remember, if the patient stops smoking, new lesions either do not develop or develop rarely.

17. **Most common source of embolism of the artery**: **Heart.** Emboli arises from thrombi in **left atrium with atrial fibrillation**, mitral valve disease **mostly stenosis, mural thrombi from myocardial infarction or cardiomyopathy, septic emboli from bacterial endocarditis due to vegetation in mitral or aortic valve**.

18. **Clinical manifestation, diagnosis, and treatment of sudden arterial occlusion:**

    (A) **Clinical manifestation: Sudden onset of severe pain plus ischemia** in 50% of cases, or **gradual onset of mild pain, numbness, paresthesias** in other 50% of cases. Muscular weakness or paralysis may be present. A saddle thrombus occluding **aortic bifurcation** can cause **shock-like state, abdominal pain, nausea, and vomiting.**

Physical examination shows **diminished or absent pulses distal to occlusion**; cold, pallor, or cyanosis of the extremity: superficial artery occlusion **causes localized tenderness.**

(B) **Diagnosis**:

(i) **It is easy to diagnose** in patients with sudden onset of severe pain plus ischemia.

(ii) It should be differentiated from **acute thrombophlebitis which appears with distended veins, edema, and feeble pulses**.

(C) **Treatment:**

(i) **Urgent surgical embolectomy** is recommended for large artery occlusion like aortic artery bifurcation.

(ii) Thrombolytic therapy (streptokinase or urokinase) **is used for smaller vessels occlusion or in patients with unstable general condition**. It is more effective with earlier onset of therapy and **used before surgery for bleeding**.

(iii) Anticoagulants are used after thrombolytic therapy.

(iv) Patients are **not** fit for surgical or thrombolytic therapy: The patients should be treated with **rest**, **dependent position of the limb under a cradle** whose temperature is between 30 to 35°, **anticoagulation with heparin STAT** (to prevent extension of thrombus or additional emboli), **lumbar sympathectomy** in vasospasm to improve blood flow.

(v) Sudden deterioration of patients treated conservatively: **Immediate surgical embolectomy preferably within few hours**, otherwise gangrene may supervene and finally amputation may be necessary.

19. **Arteriovenous fistula**:

(A) **Etiology:** Most common is **iatrogenic** created to perform renal dialysis; **trauma** from penetrating wound or surgical procedures.

(B) **Clinical manifestations:** Patients may be completely **asymptomatic** or pain near the fistula, edema, asymmetry of the limbs, varicosities; in some cases cardiac decompensation with palpitations, dyspnea on exertion, and orthopnea.

Physical examination shows positive Branham's sign: Temporary compression of the artery proximal to the fistula increases systemic vascular resistance and decreases heart rate.

(C) **Diagnosis**:

(i) Large superficial fistula can be diagnosed easily.

(ii) **Definitive diagnosis by arteriography**.

(iii) Venous blood oxygen saturation is higher in the affected limb than the nonaffected side.

(D) **Treatment**:

(i) **Surgical procedure of choice is to close the** fistula and re-establish the continuity of the involved artery and vein.

(ii) If the above procedure is **not** possible, then ligation of artery or vein, or both may be needed, but results in arterial or venous insufficiency.

(iii) **Anomalous artery fistula** is treated with ligation of the artery and obstruct the vein with sclerosing agent.

(iv) **Multiple fistula** are **not** possible to treat surgically, so managed conservatively such as local care, elastic bandage, and analgesics.

(v) Inoperable fistula with cardiac decompensation: Amputation may be needed.

20. **Most common site of glomus tumor (glomangioma): Nail beds**; other sites are upper and lower extremities. Glomus tumor consists of benign hypertrophied arteriovenous anastomosis.

(A) **Clinical manifestations:** Severe burning pain near the tumor or pain may precede the appearance of the tumor. Limbs become atrophic from lack of use due to fear of pain.
Physical examination shows reddish, purplish, or bluish well defined mass; or deformed nail and the phalanx when it is located under the nail bed; or sometimes tumor may not be visible or palpable.

(B) **Diagnosis**: Large tumor can be diagnosed by physical examination, small tumor needs US or MRI.

(C) **Treatment:** Surgical excision causes cure of this tumor.

21. **Most frequent and serious complication of deep-vein thrombosis**: **Pulmonary embolism (80 to 90% of cases)** arise from deep-vein thrombosis of the lower extremities. Deep-vein thrombosis usually begins in the calf **but serious pulmonary embolisms occur when it extends above the knee**.

22. **Thrombophlebitis and deep-vein thrombosis**: Thrombophlebitis is a venous thrombosis with inflammation of venous wall.

(A) **Thrombophlebitis**: It is most common in patients with **varicose veins**, and also common after pregnancy. Migratory superficial thrombophlebitis occurs with thromboangitis obliterans.

(i) **Clinical manifestations**: Superficial veins are red,hot, and tender. Septic thrombophlebitis appear with fever, chills, and leukocytosis. Remember, it does **not cause embolic complication** unlike deep-vein thrombosis.

(ii) **Diagnosis:** It is diagnosed from clinical manifestations. Ileofemoral thrombophlebitis appears with acute swelling with signs of inflammation of the involved lower extremity.

(iii) **Treatment:** Local therapy plus sometimes antiinflammatory drug (indomethacin). **No** anticoagulation is needed.

(B) **Deep-vein thrombosis**: It is more common in women over age of 40, history of major surgery, paralyzed limb, after thrombotic stroke, and acute myocardial infarction; malignangy, pregnancy,and use of oral contraceptives.

(i) **Pathogenesis**: Venous stasis, venous wall injury, hepercoagulable state. **Recurrent thrombophlebitis could be due to deficiency of anticlotting factors (antithrombin III, protein C, protein S, and heparin cofactor II)**.

(ii) **Clinical manifestations: Asymptomatic** (50% of cases) or symptomatic patients appear with **pulmonary embolism** (frequent and serious complication), **pain** in the region of thrombosed veins at rest or with exercise, **tenderness** on palpation, **positive Homan's sign** (pain on voluntary dosiflexion of the foot), **edema (pitting)** of the malleolar area, and difference in maximal circumferance (> 1.4 cm in men and > 1.2 cm in women) is suggestive.

Subclavian vein thrombosis: Swelling of the involved upper extremity plus collateral veins.

Superior vena cava thrombosis: Distended veins in the neck and upper part of the chest.

Axillary vein thrombosis: History of using crutches or sleeping on a sitting position with arms behind the back rest. Swelling of upper extremity plus collateral veins in axilla.

Ileofemoral veinous thrombosis: The characteristic presentations of rapidly advance swelling of the ipsilateral limb plus collateral distended veins.

(iii) **Diagnosis:**

(a) **X-ray venography is the most accurate** test and it is considered the '**Gold standard**'.

(b) **Duplex ultrasonography** (US plus doppler evaluation) is the **best noninvasive substitute for venography** particularly for thrombosis above the knee.

(c) US is used for above the knee thrombosis.

(d) **Impedance plethysmography:** It has high sensitivity and specificity. It is used as an alternative to duplex US.

(e) **Radionuclide venography:** It is used when X-ray or contrast is **not** advisable but **less** sensitive and specific than X-ray venography.

(iv) **Prophylactic therapy**:

(a) **Most commonly used medicine is low-dose heparin**. It is used in **surgical patients** (heparin 5000 IU subcutaneously **2 hours before surgery** and then every **8 to 12 hours until the patient is ambulatory) such as pelvic surgery, hip fracture, extensive orthopedic surgery, or hip replacement (not** effective in urologic procedures). Heparin reduces deep-vein thrombosis and pulmonary embolism.

High-dose heparin is more effective than low-dose when a-PTT (activated partial thromboplastin time) **is maintained in upper limit of therapeutic range.**

(b) **Low-dose heparin plus dihydroergotamine mesylate is more effective** in preventing **deep-vein thrombosis in surgical patients than low-dose heparin alone**. Ergotamine causes vasoconstriction and prevent coagulation.

(v) **Treatment of deep-vein thrombosis**:

(a) **Full anticoagulation is the best treatment. Initial drug of choice is heparin** (binds and activates anithrombin III, an inhibitor of activated factor X). It is given **preferably IV (intravenously)** or alternatively subcutaneously to **maintain a PTT two times of normal control** (monitor a-PTT initially 4 to 6 hours then once a day). **Oral warfarin** is started after 24 hours of heparin therapy (**monitor PT after 48 hours from the onset of warfarin** therapy to keep **international normalized ratio** in the PT test **between 2 and 3). Warfarin decreases the level of Factors II, VII, IX, and X**. Anticoagulation therapy for 3 months can prevent the recurrence of deep-vein thrombosis.

(b) IV administration of **streptokinase or urokinase** (dissolving the thrombus by **activation plasminogen to plasmin**) is more effective than conventional anticoagulants. **Human recombinant** tissue-type plasminogen activator can dissolve **pulmonary emboli and venous thrombi**.

Please remember, thrombolytic therapy is the best method of treatment in iliofemoral or subclavian-axillary vein thrombosis. Heparin is the best method of treatment in more distal deep-vein thrombosis for its high effectiveness and less bleeding complications.

(c) Patients in whom anticoagulation therapy **is contraindicated**:

(i) **Low-risk of pulmonary embolism in deep-vein thrombosis below the knee**: Local application of heat and elevation of the extremity are adequate.

(ii) **High-risk of pulmonary embolism in deep-vein thrombosis above the knee**: Local heat, elevation of the limb plus **implanting IVC** (inferior vena cava) filter or ligation if IVC. These procedures can be used when **anticoagulation therapy cannot be continued** for complication or **recurrent thrombophlebitis unresponsive to** anticoagulation or **septic thrombophlebitis unresponsive to antibiotics**.

(d) Activity in deep-vein thrombosis:

(i) Bed rest should be continued until the local signs of inflammation subside.

(ii) After 1 to 2 weeks, patient is allowed to walk wearing elastic stocking.

(iii) Resumption of full activity is allowed after 1 to 2 weeks if there is no discomfort.

23. **Management of bleeding due to heparin therapy: Protamine** (1 mg per 100 IU of heparin), in severe bleeding use blood or fresh frozen plasma.

24. **Management of bleeding due to warfarin therapy**: **Vitamin K_1** (0.25 to 1.0 mg IM) to reduce the PT to therapeutic range, in severe bleeding use blood or fresh frozen plasma.

25. **Varicose veins**:

(A) **Clinical manifestation:** Most patients have **asymptomatic dilated tortuous veins,** in some cases itching, postural edema, **postphlebitic syndrome (induration, fibrosis, and sustained edema)**, and finally **brownish discoloration and ulceration** of the skin.
Remember, patients have no signs of ischemia and have normal peripheral pulses.

(B) **Diagnosis:** Clinical presentation is adequate but **Trendelenburg test** can detect defective venous valves.

(C) **Treatment:**

(i) **Uncomplicated varicose veins**: Frequent periods of rest, elevation of the limbs, external pressure with elastic stockings or bandages. Do **not** obstruct the veins with garments (girdles).

(ii) **Complicated or advanced varicose veins: Ligation and stripping of the saphenous** veins, or **injection of sclerosing agent is** to **prevent postphlebitic syndrome**.

(iii) Stasis ulcers should be treated locally with warm, wet dressing prn.

(iv) Fibrosis should be treated with excision of the entire area and skin graft.

(v) Infection is treated with local and systemic antibiotics.
(vi) Postphlebitic syndrome is usually progressive and resistant to treatment.

26. **Most common organisms which cause lymphangitis: Hemolytic streptococcus or S. aureus**.

27. **Lymphangitis:**
  (A) **Clinical manifestations:** Local area of red streak along the lymphatics, swollen-tender lymph nodes, or surrounding area of cellulitis or systemic manifestations.
  (B) **Diagnosis:** Physical findings, leukocytosis with elevated neutrophils, and **confirmed by culture of the organism** from portal of entry or subcutaneous tissues.
  (C) **Treatment:** Appropriate antibiotics, surgically draining the focus of infection, elevation of an affected limb, local warm and wet dressing, and elastic support hose for several weeks to prevent lymphedema.

28. **Most common causes of lymphedema:**
  (i) Primary type: **Congenital** (**not** familial, present at birth). **Lymphedema praecox is congenital type but appears at puberty**.
  (ii) **Secondary type**: **Trauma is the most common,** other causes are **surgical removal of lymph nodes, radiation induced fibrosis** in cancer patients, **lymphoma or metastatic carcinoma involving lymph nodes**. (Filarial infection is common in tropical countries).

29. **Lymphedema**:
  (A) **Clinical manifestations:** Very slow enlargement of the limb which is **soft and pitting, initially edema subsides at night** followed by thickened skin and persistent edema.
  (B) **Complications:** Lymphangitis, cellulitis, or lymphangiosarcoma (in long standing cases).
  (C) **Diagnosis:**
    (i) Radioisotope lymphogram is confirmatory, it shows **reduced uptake in lymphedema** (increased uptake in venous obstruction).
    (ii) Lymphangiography can differentiate primary type (absence or hypoplasia of lymphatics) from secondary type (hyperplasia of lymphatics).
  (D) **Treatment:**
    (i) **Elevation of the limb, using elastic stocking,** and **diuretics** may be helpful.

(ii) If not controlled by the treatments above, **use benzopyrones.** (These drugs break down protein by activating macrophages, reduce viscosity, and enhance lymph flow).

(iii) **Surgery is done in advanced cases**. Surgery includes removal of subcutaneous.
tissues, induce new lymph vessels formation, and microsurgery to anastomose lymph vessels with veins.

30. **Types of cardiac tumors**:
   (A) **Primary**:
      (i) **Benign: Most common is myxoma**; others are rhabdomyoma, fibroma, and lipoma.
      (ii) **Malignant:** Sarcomas, lymphoma, and mesothelioma.
   (B) **Secondary: It is more common than primary**. All secondary tumors are malignant. **Most common secondary tumor is direct extension from lung cancer or breast cancer into the pericardium**.
      (i) **Direct extension:** Lung cancer, breast cancer, esophageal cancer, and mediastinal tumors.
      (ii) **Metastatic spread:** Melanoma, leukemia, and **lymphoma. These tumors can spread into the myocardium through blood or lymphatic spread**.
      (iii) **Venous extension:** Renal cell cancer, adrenal cancer, and liver cancer. **These tumors particularly renal tumors typically spread through IVC and involves right atrial cavity**.

31. **Most common intracavitary cardiac tumor**: **Myxoma**. It is located inside **the left atrium attached to the interatrial septum**. It is more common in **women** and may be associated with pigmented skin lesions and noncardiac tumors.

32. A women appears with history of fever, malaise, arthralgias, and cardiac signs and symptoms mimic rheumatic mitral stenosis. She denies any past history of rheumatic fever. Echocardiography reveals cardiac tumor.
    Most likely diagnosis: Left atrial myxoma. (It can also cause embolization. It may not be clinically symptomatic when small. It causes **mitral valve obstruction** during diastole. Myxomas can be multiple or recurrent).
    Treatment: Surgical removal of the tumor.
    Follow up: Close surveillance is indicated for recurrence.

33. **Rare intracavity (cardiac) tumors**:
    (i) **Renal cell cancer** spreads through IVC into the right atrial cavity.

(ii) **Angiosarcomas** occur more commonly in men than women, causes right sided congestive failure.
(iii) **Papillary fibroelastomas** arise from cardiac valves produce symptoms of systemic or coronary embolism.

34. **Most common intrapericardial tumors**: **Direct and contiguous spread of lung cancer or breast cancer**. Patients appear with pericardial effusion, tamponade, and may involve the myocardium as well.
Treatment:
(i) **Pericardiocentesis, balloon pericardiotomy, or surgical drainage and limited pericardiectomy (pericardial window)** are life saving short-and intermediate-term palliative procedures.
(ii) **Subxiphoid pericardiectomy** is a brief palliative procedure useful in very debilitated patients.

35. Intramyocardial tumors: Rare tumors, patients may be clinically silent, produce arrythmias, or obstructive features.
(i) Primary may be clinically silent, produce arrythmias, or obstructive features.
(ii) Primary malignant tumor: Sarcomas (angiosarcomas, fibrosarcomas, rhabdomyosarcomas) can also involve pericardium and endocardium.
Treatment: No good therapy for these primary tumors.
(iii) Secondary malignant tumors are melanoma, leukemia, and lymphoma.

36. Most common cardiac trauma:
(i) Nonpenetrating injury: Automobile accident.
(ii) Penetrating injury: Bullet and stab wounds. **Most common cause of death** in cardiac trauma is **hemopericardium, cardiac tamponade, or massive bleeding**.

37. **Few important points in nonpenetrating and penetrating cardiac injury (Important):**
(A) **Nonpenetrating injury**:
(i) **Most common clinical manifestation is myocardial contusion** due to impact of chest wall against the steering wheel.
(ii) **Diagnosis is made** by **new EKG changes,** or **arrythmias**, abnormalities in left ventricular wall motion by echocardiography, radionuclide ventriculography, or positive radionuclide scan.
(iii) Traumatic rupture of descending aorta just distal to the ligamentum arteriosum **occurs** because **aortic arch moves anteriorly** and

descending aorta is fixed. Surgical repair should be done STAT but **rarely** patients may survive long time without operative repair.

(B) **Penetrating injury**:

(i) **Most common clinical manifestations are hemopericardium, tamponade, or severe hemorrhage**.

(ii) Associated cardiac injuries include intracardiac shunts, valvular regurgitation, and rarely coronary artery injuries.

(iii) **Immediate thoracotomy should be** done **for tamponade and hemorrhages**.

(iv) Associated cardiac injuries can wait for definitive diagnosis and future repair.

38. **Cancer therapy and cardiotoxicity:**

(i) **Chronic radiation therapy**: Pericardial inflammation and effusion, **chronic constrictive pericarditis**, myocardial fibrosis, and accelerated coronary artery atherosclerosis.

(ii) **Doxorubicin (Adriamycin)**: Dose-related systolic and diastolic dysfunction, CHF with or without ventricular arrythmias (**Important**).
Preclinical diagnosis of cardiotoxicity: Radionuclide ventriculorgraphy shows fall in left ventricular ejection fraction, echocardiography, or right ventricular endomyocardial biopsy shows myofibrillar dropout and sarcotubular dilatation.
Treatment: Discontinue doxorubicin and treat CHF with digitalis, diuretics, and vasodilators.

(iii) **Cyclophosphamide**: Fatal hemorrhagic myocardial necrosis.

(iv) **5-fluorouracil:** Myocardial ischemia and infarction.

(v) **Taxol:** Asymptomatic arrythmias and abnormalities in the conducting system.

39. **Cardiac manifestations and systemic diseases**:

(i) Ankylosing spondylitis, psoriatic arthritis, Reiter's syndrome: Aortic regurgitation.

(ii) Rheumatoid arthritis: Pericarditis is most common plus pericardial effusion.

(iii) SLE: Pericardititis, myocarditis (inflammation and scarring), Libman-Sacks endocarditis (clinical myocarditis plus MI and AI).

(iv) Progressive systemic sclerosis: Focal myocardial necrosis, fibrosis, and dilated cardiomyopathies.

(v) **Carcinoid syndrome: Right side** of the heart is more commonly involved than left, thickening and scarring of **tricuspid and pulmonary valves** results in **stenosis and regurgitation, finally right heart failure**.

Treatment: Somatostatin analogue and in some patients valve replacement are helpful.

(vi) **Myotonic dystrophy**: A-V conduction defect with syncope and sudden death.

(vii) **Duchenne's muscular dystrophy**: Selective myocardial necrosis of posterobasal portion of left ventricle and adjacent papillary muscles.

(viii) **Friedreich's ataxia**: Symmetric or asymmetric left ventricular hypertrophy mimic hypertrophic cardiomyopathy.

(ix) **Cardiac amyloidosis**: It is the most common cause of death in amyloidosis. It produces **diastolic** (restrictive cardiomyopathy) dysfunction, **systolic** dysfunction, **arrythmias, conduction** disturbances, and **orthostatic hypotension**.

(x) **Hemochromatosis (iron overload) should be ruled out in cardiomyopathy with diabetes or hepatic cirrhosis**: Restrictive cardiomyopathy (reduced ventricular filling) and reduced systolic functions.

(xi) Myocardial sarcoidosis: Arrythmias and A-V conduction defects.

(xii) Diabetes mellitus: Restrictive cardiomyopathy with reduced ventricular filling.

(xiii) Pheochromocytomas: Focal myocardial contraction band necrosis, fibrosis, and rarely CHF.
Treatment: Initially use alpha-adrenergic blocker then beta blocker.

(xiv) **Hypothyroidism**: Pericardial effusion mostly without tamponade, high BP, and low heart rate.

(xv) **Hyperthyroidism**: Increased cardiac output, reduced systemic vascular resistance, atrial fibrillation, and rarely CHF.

40. **Most common cause of aortic aneurysms: Atherosclerosis** ; other causes are trauma, infection, and cystic medial necrosis. (**True** aneurysm is a widening of the vessel. **Pseudo or false aneurysm** is a localized rupture of the artery with sealing over the clot or adjacent structures). **Marfan's syndrome is characterized by cystic medial necrosis**.

41. **Most common site of aortic aneurysms: Abdominal aorta**. Abdominal aortic aneurysms are **most commonly present below the renal artery**, most common cause is **arteriosclerosis**, and **more common in men** than women.

42. **Clinical manifestations, diagnosis, and treatment of aortic aneurysms**:
(A) **Clinical manifestations**:
(i) **Abdominal aortic aneurysms**: Initially **lower back pain, rupture** causes hypotension and shock, and embolization can cause symptoms ranging from digital infarctions to anuria.

(ii) **Thoracic aortic aneurysms: Most common symptom is the pain. Pain is gradual, boring, and deep in gradually enlarging aneurysm. Increasing intensity of pain is an ominous sign of rupture (Important).**

(a) **Aneurysms of ascending aorta**: It causes aortic valve regurgitation, murmur of AI, and acute pulmonary edema.

(b) **Aneurysms of transverse aortic arch**: It is **less** common, symptoms include **dyspnea, stridor, hoarseness, cough, chest pain, and hemoptysis. These are due to associated important vital structures** such as SVC, PA, bronchi, trachea, lung, and left recurrent laryngeal nerve.

(c) **Aneurysms of descending thoracic aorta: Most common site** is between the origin of left subclavian artery and diaphragm. **Most common cause is arteriosclerosis**, other causes are **smoking and hypertension**.
Remember, pain in the interscapular region, hoarseness, hemoptysis, and it can rupture like abdominal aortic aneurysms.

(B) **Diagnosis of aortic aneurysms**:

(i) Abdominal aneurysms should be examined first by palpation.
(ii) **Ultrasonography (US) is the best, noninvasive diagnostic** study and it can detect aneurysm **as small as 2 to 3 mm in size.**
(iii) CT scan with contrast is equally effective like US.
(iv) Aortography may **not** detect the accurate size of aneurysm because of clots.
(v) Sometimes lumbar spine x-ray can detect the margins of abdominal aneurysms.

(C) **Treatment**: Surgical management of aneurysms with possible rupture or acute expansion.

43. **The risk of rupture** and **sizes of aneurysms**:

(i) The risk of rupture is **directly proportional to the size of** aneurysms (95% of patients die with aneurysms > 10 cm in size).
(ii) The risk of rupture is **low** in aneurysms 5 cm or less in size.

44. **Most common cause of dissecting aneurysms of the aorta: Hypertension; other causes are coarctation** of the aorta, **valvular aortic stenosis particularly bicuspid aortic valve**, trauma, relapsing polychondritis, **Marfan's syndrome, and Ehlers Danlos syndrome**.

45. **Types of dissecting aneurysms of the aorta**:

(i) Type I: Dissecting hematoma extends from ascending aorta (within few cm. of aortic valve), aortic arch, and descending aorta.
(ii) Type II: Dissecting hematoma restricted to the ascending aorta.
(iii) Type III: Dissecting hematoma restricted to the descending aorta.
(iv) **Acute**: Dissection occurs **within 2 weeks** from the onset of therapy.
(v) Chronic: Dissection occurs **more than 2 weeks** from the onset of therapy.

46. **Clinical presentations, diagnosis, and treatment of dissecting aneurysm of the aorta**:

(A) **Clinical manifestations**: Most common symptom is **pain in the anterior chest, sometimes severe** in nature or **increases with each heart beat. Pain occurs in the neck, jaw, or teeth if the aortic arch is involved. Aortic regurgitation causes diastolic AI murmur and CHF**. Other less common physical findings include **loss of peripheral pulses, syncope,stroke, paraplegia** (loss of blood supply to spinal cord), **vocal cord paralysis and hoarseness** (due to pressure on recurrent laryngeal nerve), **SVC syndrome** (due to pressure on SVC), **dyspnea** (due to pressure on trachea and bronchus), hemorrhagic pleural effusion, myocardial infarction, **persistent fever, or Horner's syndrome** (due to compression of the superior cervical ganglia).

(B) **Diagnosis**:
(i) **Aortic angiography** is the definitive procedure of choice.
(ii) **Transesophageal echocardiography should be considered first among noninvasive procedures** (CT scan or MRI) if it is available.
(iii) CT scan is an alternative when transesophageal echocardiography or MRI is not available.
(iv) **MRI is little more accurate** than transesophageal echocardiography but its use is **not practical** because patient may be intubated or is receiving IV antihypertensive drug.

(C) **Treatment**:
(i) **To control the hypertension (keep systolic BP between 100 to 120 mm Hg): IV sodium nitroprusside drip**. Add **propranolol** (intermittent IV boluses) to keep the heart rate **around 60 beats per minute**.
(ii) To place an intra-arterial line, central-venous line, or Swan-Ganz catheter.
(iii) **Aortography** should be done as soon as the patient's vital signs and clinical conditions become stable.
(iv) Echocardiography or CT scan is helpful while waiting for aortography.

(v) **Operative management**: It is indicated for types I and II (both involves ascending aorta) because these types are **unstable and prone to rupture.**

(a) If involves aortic root and aortic valves: To replace aortic root and aortic valve with a composite conduit.

(b) **If only ascending aorta is involved** but aortic root and aortic valves are intact: To replace the aneurysmal portion **with a synthetic tubular graft**. The same method is used for discending aortic dissection.

(vi) Type III (involves descending thoracic aortia): Long term medical therapy is used. Surgery is indicated in impending rupture, increasing in size, uncontrolled pain, or bleeding into the pleural space.

(vii) Follow up of patients **are the same** in both surgically and medically treated patients:To control the BP < 130 mm Hg with antihypertensive drug and heart rate < 72/minute with propranolol.

47. **Most common causes of death** in dissecting aortic aneurysms: The effects of **propagation of dissecting hematoma** (not due to initial intimal tear). Rupture into the **pericardial or pleural space** is fatal complication. Aortic regurgitation causes CHF.

48. **Few important causes of pericarditis**:

(i) Most common viruses are **coxsackie B, AIDS, and Echo**.

(ii) Most common bacterial organism is **Staphylococcus. Mycobacterium tuberculosis** is common in immigrants and high-risk populations.

(iii) Fungal infection is common in AIDS patients.**Histoplasma capsulatum** should be considered in patients reside in **Ohio Valley** and **coccidioidomycosis** should be considered in patients reside in **San Joaquin Valley of California (Important).**

(iv) **Chylopericardium** could be due to idiopathic, **post surgical, and other trauma to the thoracic duct (Important).**

(v) Blunt or sharp trauma is an important cause of pericarditis.

(vi) Pericardial effusion fluid due to myxedema may contain cholesterol crystals.

(vii) Radiation therapy causes pericarditis after several years of therapy.

(viii) Patients on chronic dialysis develop pericarditis, cardiac tamponade, but rarely develop constrictive pericarditis.

(ix) **SLE and its therapeutic drug procainamide** cause pericarditis.

(x) Myocardial infarction causes **acute, dry fibrinous** pericarditis due to inflammation or reaction to myocardial injury. **Dressler's syndrome** is the development of pericarditis (mostly with effusion) after weeks or months in **myocardial infarction** patients **due to autoimmune reaction**.

49. **Clinical manifestations, diagnosis, and treatment of acute (fibrinous) viral or idiopathic pericarditis**:
    (A) **Clinical manifestations**: Initial malaise and **fever** followed by **characteristic sharp or crushing precordial** (sometimes shift to the left side like pleurisy) **pain which is relieved by sitting up and increased by deep inspiration. Referred pain to the ridge of right trapezius is characteristic** but less common finding.
    Physical examination shows **characteristic pericardial friction rub (over the precordium)** which does **not** disappear with effusion.
    (B) **Diagnosis**:
    (i) **EKG: ST-segment elevation** (in lead I, II, aVF, V4, V5, V6) and depression (aVR, V1) are more common than PR-segment depression. **It is the diagostic test**.
    (ii) Echocardiogram: To detect pericardial effusion.
    (iii) Elevated ESR and leukocytosis.
    (iv) The following tests should **not** be done routinely: Viral titers, gallium scan, and determination of cardiac enzymes.
    (C) **Treatment**:
    (i) **NSAID's (e.g., indomethacin or ibuprofen) are the drug of choice**.
    (ii) Sometimes even **aspirin** is helpful.
    (iii) Resistant cases require **prednisone**.

50. **Pericardial effusion:**
    (A) **Lax percardial effusion**: Asymptomatic pericardial effusion is due to low intrapericardial pressure (< 3 or 4 mm Hg). CXR shows enlarged heart size. Diagnosis: Echocardiography confirms the diagnosis. (Remember, normal intrapericardial pressure is **subatmospheric** and almost equal to pleural pressure).
    (B) Pericardial effusion complicating acute pericarditis: Routine echocardiogram shows pericardial effusion in many patients with acute pericarditis and it can **differentiate pericardial effusion from myocarditis** (enlarged cardiac chambers). **Remember, echocardiogram is not needed** if the heart **size remains normal** in CXR, **no** evidence of tamponade, or myocarditis; clinical manifestations resolve **within 2 to 3 days after the onset of therapy**.

51. **Pericardiocentesis**:

(A) **Indications: Cardiac tamponade unresponsive to medical therapy**, suspected **purulent effusion**, and **rare** cause of bacteriologic or tissue diagnosis. It is less traumatic and less expensive than surgical drainage.
(B) **Indications of surgical drainage: Pericardial biopsy is needed to establish the diagnosis** and when lax pericardial effusion becomes **large and chronic** (idiopathic chronic effusive pericarditis).
(C) **No need for pericardiocentesis**: When venous pressure is **normal, absence** of hypotension, and etiology of effusion is known.

52. **Cardiac tamponade**:
   (A) **Clinical manifestations**: It should be suspected in patients with pericardial disease **develop heart failure or heart disease**. In severe cases patients appear with unconsciousness, severe hypotensive shock, and olilguria. **Conscious patients** complain of **sensation of fullness of the chest** and may be dyspnea with or without precordial pain.
   (B) **Diagnosis**:
      (i) Venous pressure: **Elevated jugular venous pressure** and **prominent x descent** (sharp inward movement of internal jugular pulse synchronous with the carotid pulse) are present.
      (ii) **Pulsus paradoxus** (pulse decreases or disappears during inspiration) **is present**.
      (iii) Friction rub may be present.
      (iv) Echocardiogram confirms the pericardial effusion and may show compression of the right atrium and ventricle.
      (v) EKG is not very helpful except small QRS complex in large effusion.
   (C) **Treatment**:
      (i) **Prompt removal of pericardial fluid is mandatory** unless the tamponade is mild and response to medical therapy. Pericardiocentesis is **safe** in experienced hands. **A small amount of fluid is removed in acute cases** because of steep pressure-volume curve of the pericardium.
      (ii) **Subxiphoid surgical drainage is indicated** in recurrent tamponade, to obtain biopsy, and in **less** experienced hands.

53. **Most common causes of constrictive pericarditis in USA**: **Idiopathic**, post-traumatic, secondary to neoplasms or radiation, or connective tissue diseases.

54. **Constrictive pericarditis**:
   (A) **Clinical manifestations**:
      (i) Elevated filling pressure of the **right side of the heart** results in peripheral edema, enlarged liver (congestion and dysfunction), and ascites.

(ii) Elevated filling pressure of the **left side of the heart** results in dyspnea and pulmonary edema.

(iii) **Pericardial knock (loul third heart sound) is audible and nonpalpable** apical beat.

(iv) Patients with severe hepatic congestion appear with **mild jaundice, palmer erythema, and spider angiomas**.

(B) **Diagnosis**:

(i) **Systemic venous congestion is present** and it is **not** explained by heart failure or other causes.

(ii) **Elevated venous pressure in the neck** is due to cardiac or pericardial causes (venous pressure is normal in liver disease).

(iii) **Echocardiogram** shows **normal** systolic function, normal cardiac valves, **small ventricles fill rapidly in early diastole only** (**no** filling in remainder of the diastole), and **abnormal motion of the interventricular septum**.

(iv) **EKG**: Inverted T-wave; wide, notched P wave; atrial fibrillation in long standing cases.

(v) **MRI is more accurate than CT-scan** to detect **thickened pericardium**.

(vi) To differentiate from restrictive cardiomyopathy: Endomyocardial biopsy or rarely exploratory throracotomy may be needed.

(C) **Treatment**:

(i) **Pericardiectomy is the treatment of choice**.

(ii) **Diuretic** is used to prepare the patient.
(Full clinical improvement may take 3 months after surgery).

55. **Most common cause of sudden death in athletes: Hypertrophic cardiomyopathy** (Important). It includes marked **left ventricular hypertrophy, asymmetric septal hypertrophy, supranormal contractility, and decreased left ventricular systolic cavitary dimension**.
Remember, left atrium is enlarged in hypertrophic, dilated, and restrictive cardiomyopathies.

56. **Hypertrophic cardiomyopathy**:

(A) **Genetic transmission**: Autosomal dominant; myosin heavy chain on chromosome 14.

(B) **Few important findings**:

(i) Ejection fraction is > 60% (normal ≥55%).

(ii) Left ventricular diastolic dimension is decreased (normal < 55 mm).

(iii) LV wall thickness is markedly increased.

(iv) Left atrium is enlarged.

(C) **Clinical manifestations:** Most patients are between ages 20 and 40, appear with **dyspnea on exertion, palpitation, syncope, or chest pain. Syncope occurs during or shortly after heavy exercise. It is the most common cause of sudden death in athletes**. Physical examination shows palpable, audible presystolic sound (S_4), and harsh murmur best heard at the left lower sternal border.

(D) **Diagnosis**:

(i) **EKG**: Left ventricular hypertrophy (LVH), increased Q waves (misdiagnosed as infarction). Left atrial abnormality is found in P waves, short PR interval with slurred QRS upstroke (misdiagnosed as preexcitation).

(ii) **Echocardiography shows LVH, asymmetric septal hypertrophy, and confirms the diagnosis**.

(iii) **Enhanced alpha wave** in the jugular venous pulse is due to abnormal septum causing decreased right ventricular compliance.

(E) **Treatment**:

(i) Asymptomatic patients with nonsustained ventricular tachycardia, to prevent suddeen death: **Amiodarone is used but it may increase the mortality in severely symptomatic patients. (Beta-adrenergic blocker and calcium channel blockers could reduce hypertrophy and sudden death but have no clear benefit in asymptomatic patients).**

(ii) **Mild to moderate symptomatic patients with exertional dyspnea and chest pain: Beta-adrenergic blocker and calcium channel blocker are useful. Verapamil improves left ventricular diastolic filling. Disopyramide** is useful for its negative inotropic effect. Amiodarone improves the clinical condition. (**Please remember do not use digoxin**).

(iii) **Severely symptomatic patients with high filling pressures which cause fluid retention: Diuretic therapy; combined medical therapy**, if fails to maintain adequate functional capacity use dual-chamber pacing. **Ventricular septal myotomy - myectomy is performed in patients with gradients > 50 mm Hg and refractory symptomos**. Mitral valve replacement may be useful in patients with a typical distribution of hypertrophy. (**Please remember do not use amiodarone**).

57. **Exercise, sudden death, and hypertrophic cardiomyopathy**:

(i) **Competitive sports are contraindicated due to sudden death**.

(ii) Sudden death is common in < 35 years with positive family history and syncope.

(iii) **Majority (66%) of sudden death occurs during rest or mild activity**.
(iv) **Majority of the patients with sudden death are asymptomatic or mildly symptomatic**.

58. **Apical hypertrophic cardiomyopathy**: It is characterized by **systolic apical obliteration in angiography** (spade-like cavity), **large negative T waves in precordial EKG, absence of** intraventricular gradient, and **mild** symptoms. Some patients, particularly elderly women appear with **severe symmetrical cardiomegaly** which is disproportionate to the degree of high BP.

59. **Dilated cardiomyopathy**: **It is the most common among all cardiomyopathies**.
   (A) **Few important causes: Infection** (viral is most common), **noninfection** (collagen vascular disease), **toxic** (alcohol, doxorubicin, cyclophosphamide, and interferon-alpha), **metabolic** (deficiencies of carnitine, thiamine, selenium; **diabetes**, and thyroid disease), and idiopathic.
   (B) **Few important findings:**
      (i) Ejection fraction is $< 30\%$ (normal $\geq 55\%$).
      (ii) Left ventricular diastolic dimension is ≥ 60 mm (normal < 55 mm).
      (iii) Decreased LV wall thickness.
      (iv) Increased LA size.
   (C) **Clinical manifestations:**
      (i) Exertional intolerance is the first symptom.
      (ii) **Left-sided pulmonary congestive symptoms** (exertional dyspnea, paroxysmal nocturnal dyspnea, and orthopnea) **occur before right-sided systemic congestive symptoms** (peripheral edema, enlarged liver, ascites, and discomfort on bending) except in young adults when right is more prominent than left.
      (iii) Ventricular tachyarrythmia, atrial fibrillation, and conduction block in chagas disease.
   (D) **Diagnosis**:
      (i) **Echocardiography is the initial investigation of choice**. It shows **dilated LV and often RV dilatation and poor contractility. Focal wall motion abnormalities** are common in **chagas disease, sarcoidosis**, or any other cardiomyopathies. Disproportionate LVH indicates prior hypertension.
      (ii) Thallium is **not** effective.
      (iii) Coronary arteriography is important to exclude coronary artery disease or atherosclerosis.
      (iv) Cardiac catheterization may be helpful to determine cardiac output, filling pressures, valvular defects, and to guide future therapy.

(v) The **only definitive indications** for endomyocardial biopsy are **transplantation rejection**, **anthracycline cardiotoxicity**; other indications are giant-cell myocarditis, hemochromatosis, amyloidosis, sarcoidosis, and hypereosinophilic syndrome.
(vi) EKG shows LV dilatation with poor R wave progression, higher voltage in V6 than in V5, and may be atrial fibrillation and LBBB (left bundle branch block).

(E) **Treatment**:
(i) Medical therapy with ACE inhibitors, diuretics, digoxin, and vasodilators are useful.
(ii) Beta-blocker may be useful in some patients.
(iii) Cardiac transplantation for patients unresponsive to medical therapy.
(iv) **Avoid vigorous exercise for next 3 to 6 months** in patients with history of alcohol, new-onset cardiomyopathy, and peripartum cardiomyopathy.
(v) **Avoid excessive bed rest and to remain mobile.**

60. **Restrictive cardiomyopathy**: It is the **least** common variety of cardiomyopathy.

(A) **Few important causes**: **Infiltrative** (**amyloidosis is most common**, sarcoidosis), storage (**hemochromatosis is most common**), **fibrotic** (radiation), **metabolic** (carnitine deficiency), **endocardial** (radiation, doxorubicin, carcinoid syndrome, Loffler's endocarditis or hypereosinophilic syndrome), and **idiopathic**.

(B) **Few important findings**:
(i) Ejection fraction is between 25 to 50% (normal $\geq$ 55%).
(ii) LV diastolic dimension is < 60 mm (normal < 55 mm).
(iii) LV wall thickness is normal or increased.
(iv) LA size is enlarged or massive.

(C) **Clinical presentations**:
(i) Exertional intolerance is the first symptom.
(ii) Frequent mitral and tricuspid regurgitations.
(iii) Right-sided systemic venous congestion (peripheral edema, enlarged liver, ascites, and discomfort on bending) often exceeds left sided pulmonary congestion (exertional dyspnea, paroxysmal nocturnal dyspena, and othopnea).
(iv) Atrial fibrillation; conduction block in amyloidosis and sarcoidosis; ventricular tachyarrythmias in sarcoidosis.

(D) **Diagnosis of restrictive cardiomyopathy:**
(i) Amyloidosis: Evidence of systemic disease plus **decreased voltage** in EKG, **increased wall thickness** in echocardiography, positive

monoclonal protein in either serum or urine; **biopsy of subcutaneous fat or rectum confirms the diagnosis**. Endomyocardial biopsy can perforate the heart.

(ii) **Sarcoidosis usually involves the lung**. Echocardiography may show global or regional ventricular dysfunction without severe dilatation. Endomyocardial biopsy **can miss** the focal lesion.

(iii) **Hemochromatosis:** Clinical pictures, serum iron proteins; **diagnosis can be confirmed by endomyocardial biopsy tissue stained for iron**.

(iv) Radiation induced fibrosis has H/o radiation for long period of time (up to 15 years), **(adriamycin) doxorubicin** may enhance the process of radiation injury.

(v) Loffler's endocarditis: **Persistent high eosinophil counts > 1500/cubic millimeter**.

(vi) **Carcinoid syndrome: Tricuspid valve and RV endocardium** are affected by the release of **5-hydroxyindoleacetic acid by** carcinoid tumors.

(E) **Treatment of restrictive cardiomyopathy**:

(i) Amyloidosis: **Treatment of CHF, use colchicine or combination of melphalan and prednisone** (digoxin is **not** useful, cardiac transplantation is not done for high incidence of recurrence).

(ii) **Sarcoidosis: Steroid** therapy decreases dysrhythmias and improves ventricular functions in some patients.

(iii) **Hemochromatosis: Phlebotomy and iron chelation therapy** can improve cardiac function before the irreversible cellular injury. (**Remember, death from hemochromatosis** is due to cirrhosis and liver cancer than from cardiac disease),.

(iv) **Endocardial restrictive disease**: **Diuretic** can reduce congestive symptoms but cannot resolve it. **Extensive surgical resection was performed for refractory cases** with high perioperative morbidity and mortality.

(v) **Loffer's endocarditis**: Immunosuppressive therapy is useful.

(vi) **Alcoholic cardiomyopathy**: Abstinence from alcohol plus symptomatic therapy.

(vii) **Idiopathic restrictive cardiac disease**: **Diuretic** is helpful but not curative (calcium channel blockers are **not** useful), **cardiac transplantation should be performed on time.**

61. **Few important points in dilated cardiomyopathy**:

(i) **Chagas' disease** (infection with Trypanosoma cruzi): It slowly causes myocarditis, right bundle branch block, and apical aneurysms. The organisms are not detected in tissues. It causes **autoimmune reaction**. **Destruction** of **parasympathetic ganglia** causes cardiac dysfunction. **Treatment**: No specific therapy; **pacemaker implantation** reduces death from heart block; **cardiomyoplasty is also useful**.

(ii) **HIV**: It causes **lymphocytic myocarditis** up to 50% of cases. Cardiomyopathy is due to HIV associated CMV and their related cytokine secretion.

(iii) **Toxoplasmosis**: It causes **myocarditis** with apical chest pain, arrythmias, followed by pericarditis and cardiac failure. Endomyocardial biopsy shows **focal lymphocytic infiltration** (cysts are found **very rarely**), diagnosis from rising antibody titers Treatment: Pyrimethamine and sulfadiazine.

(iv) Adriamycin (doxorubicin): It causes characteristic **vacuolar degeneration and myofibrillar loss** in endomyocardial biopsy. Cardiotoxicity is due to release of **free radicals, histamines, and catecholamines**.

(v) **Peripartum cardiomyopathy:** It shows **lymphocytic myocarditis** (30 to 50% of cases) due to **immune cross-reactivity** between uterine and cardiac myosite proteins.

62. **Most common causes of aortic stenosis in adults**:
    (i) **Rheumatic aortic stenosis**.
    (ii) **Degenerative aortic stenosis** is due to calcium deposits in the sinuses and annulus except margins of the leaflets.

63. **Most common cardiac defect** of aortic stenosis in adults: **Bicuspid aortic valve** but fibrosis and calcification produce difficulty in identifying bicuspid or **tricuspid (normal) valves**.

64. **Clinical presentations, diagnosis, and treatment of aortic stenosis (AS):**
    (A) **Clinical presentations: Chest pain, syncope, and cardiac failure are the characteristic symptoms. Most common** associated finding **is coronary artery disease in patients over age 40. All the symptoms are due to myocardial ischemia results in arrythmias which leads to syncope and sudden death. Please remember**, patients with AS have higher incidence of **GI bleeding from angiodysplasia, infective endocarditis, and aortic valve calcification is associated with hemolytic anemia (RBC destruction).**

    Physical examination reveals **diamond-shaped crescendo-decrescendo systolic murmur best** heart over the aortic area and along the left sternal border, **harsh murmur may be transmitted to carotid arteries, palpable thrill** over the aortic valve area, ejection click, atrial (S_4) gallop, and decreased peripheral pulses.

(B) **Diagnosis of AS**:

(i) **Echocardiography confirms** the diagnosis, estimates the size of the aortic office, and **doppler study** detects systolic pressure gradient across the valve.

(ii) **EKG** shows LVH with increasse in QRS amplitude and ST-T changes of strain pattern.

(iii) CXR shows **normal** heart size initially, subsequently enlarged LV, pulmonary edema due to cardiac failure.

(iv) **Cardiac catheterization is primarily indicated to rule out associated coronary artery disease**. It also detects pressure gradient between LV and aorta, and also mitral regurgitation.

(C) **Treatment of AS**:

(i) **Medical therapy**:

(a) **Prophylactic antibiotic** for dental, GI, and GU procedures in asymptomatic patients with stenotic or prosthetic valve to reduce the incidence of infective endocarditis.

(b) **AS with SVT**: Digoxin plus antiarrythmic drug to slow the ventricular response.

(c) **AS with chest pain**: Catheterization to rule out coronary artery disease, **nitrates** should be used very carefully because fall of arterial pressure can further reduce coronary blood flow.

(d) **Asymptomatic patients with significant AS** should be followed very closely because of high risk of cardiac events within 2 years.

(ii) **Surgical therapy**:

(a) **Only AS: Valvuloplasy, aortic-valve replacement**. Mechanical valve requires long-term anticoagulation therapy. Porcine valve lasts 10 years, it can be used in adults, older patients, and in whom anticoagulation is contraindicated (not used in adolescent and children).

(b) **As with coronary artery disease**: Aortic valve replacement with coronary artery bypass should be done.

(c) **Severely ill or elderly patients: Valvuloplasty** is an option but the rate of restenosis is high.

65. **Antibiotic prophylaxis in aortic stenosis and prosthetic valves (Important):**

(i) **Dental, oral, upper respiratory tract procedures**:

(a) **Amoxicillin** (3 grams 1 hour before and 1.5 grams 6 hours later).

(b) **Penicillin-allergy: Erythromycin or clindamycin** (Erythromycin ethylsuccinate 800 mg or E-mycin stearate 1 gram orally 2 hours before and ½ dose 6 hours later; clindamycin 300 mg orally 1 hour before and 150 mg 6 hours later).

(ii) **GI and GU procedures and instrumentationos**:
   (a) **Ampicillin plus gentamicin** (ampicillin 2 grams IV plus gentamicin 1.5 mg/kg IV 30 minute before procedure, and ampicillin 1.5 grams 6 hours later).
   (b) **Pencillin-allergy: Vancomycin and gentamicin** (vancomycin 1 gram IV over 1 hour plus gentamicin 1.5 mg/kg IV 1 hour before procedure and may be repeated 8 hours later).

66. **Aortic regurgitation (AR):**
(A) **Etiology:**
   (i) **Acute:** Endocarditis, aortic dissection, ruptured sinus of Valsalva, and prosthetic valve.
   (ii) **Chronic**: Rheumatic fever, hypertension, atherosclerosis, connective tissue disorders, cystic medial necrosis (Marfan's syndrome), and aortic ectasia.
(B) **Clinical manifestations**: Patients may **remain asymptomatic** for long period of time, **symptomatic** patients appear **with angina, cardiac failure, or sudden death when pulse pressure > 140/40 mm Hg and LV enlargement are present**. LV failure causes **dyspnea, paroxysmal nocturnal dyspnea, and orthopnea**. **Chest pain** is commonly associated with underlying coronary artery disease, and syncope is caused by arrythmias. Severe chest pain in acute aortic incompetence is probably due to **dissection**.
Physical examination reveals high-pitched, blowing, decrescendo diastolic murmur heard best along the left sternal border, **in severe AR diastolic murmurs or Austin Flint murmur is heard at the apex; bounding peripheral pulses** and clinical manifestations of wide pulse pressure includes bounding carotid pulse, pulsatile retinal arterioles, and head bobbing.
(C) **Diagnosis of AR:**
   (i) **Echocardiography is the best diagnostic method** to detect the abnormality of aortic valve, ascending aorta, annulus, end-diastolic dimension of LV > 55 mm is surgically irreversible dilatation, **so aortic valve replacement should be done before that.**
   (ii) EKG show LVH with increased QRS voltage amplitude and ST-T wave changes of strain pattern.
   (iii) **CXR: Enlarged heart size**, prominent ascending aorta, LV failure with pulmonary congestion.
   (iv) **Exercise testing**:It is clinically used in combination with radionuclide angiography. **Exercise ejection reduced by 5% or more** is an indication for surgery even in asymptomatic patients.

(v) **Cardiac catheterization**: To detect associated coronary artery disease and mitral regurgitation.

(D) **Treatment of AR**:

(i) **Medical therapy**:

(a) Antibiotic prophylaxis is indicated to prevent endocarditis.

(b) Heart failure with AR: Hydralazine and ACE – inhibitors are useful but benefits are rarely maintained. Digitalis, diuretics, and afterload-reducing agents have short-term benefits.

(ii) **Surgical therapy**:

(a) Aortic valve replacement should be done.

(b) **Aortic dissection**: Ascending aorta should be replaced.

67. **Mitral stenosis (MS)**:

(A) **Etiology: Most common cause is rheumatic fever** which causes fibrosis and scarring; other causes are **calcification** in elderly persons, rarely **left atrial myxoma or thrombus formations.**

(B) **Clinical manifestations**: Most common in **women** than men between ages 25 and 30. **Most common symptom is dyspnea due to pulmonary venous hypertension initially precipitated with exercise or fever, finally dyspnea may occur even at rest. Dyspnea can be** precipitated by paroxysmal atrial fibrillation which also causes **systemic** embolization. Hemoptysis may occur due to rupture of small vessels in the bronchi. **Physical examination reveals diastolic rumbling murmur**, opening snap, and accentuated first sound at the apex; **distended neck veins are due to RV failure with TR (tricuspid regurgitation).**

(C) **Diagnosis of MS:**

(i) Echocardiography is the best noninvasive diagnostic study for MS. **It shows characteristic square wave motion** of the E-to-F slope of the valve during diastole and **concordant movement of anterior and posterior mitral valve leaflets are the most important finding**.

(ii) **EKG shows** LA enlargement, RV hypertrophy, **characteristic notched and prolonged P wave** are most prominent in leads II, III, and aVF.

(iii) CXR shows **double contour along the right heart border** due to enlarged left atrium, and **Kerley's B lines** (transverse linear densities at the lung bases above the diaphragm) is due **to fibrosis and lymphatic engorgement.**

(iv) Cardiac catheterization can measure **the diastolic pressure gradient across the mitral valve. Coronary arteriography should be done in patients older than age 40.**

(D) **Treatment of MS**:

(i) **Medical therapy**:

(a) Patients should receive rheumatic fever prophylaxis until age 30.
(b) **To control ventricular response in atrial fibrillation**: Use digoxin, beta-blockers, and calcium channel blockers.
(c) **MS with atrial fibrillation**: All patients should receive anticoagulation therapy.
(d) **MS with atrial fibrillation plus pulmonary edema: Cardioversion** should be done. Patients should be **anticoagulated 2 weeks before to elective cardioversion** and **antiarrythmic drug should be started 2 days before the cardioversion, and if patients is on digoxin that should be stopped 1 day before the cardioversion**. If cardioversion is successful, patients should receive **long-term anticoagulation and antiarrythmic drug**.
(e) Patients with thromboembolism originates from left atrium: **Anticoagulation is indicated.**
(f) **Patients with acute embolisms to the abdomen or extremities: Surgical embolectomy** may be useful.
(g) **Valvuloplasty through catheter** is used in selective patients of MS such as elderly patients with high surgical risk and in young women desire to become pregnant at later date.

(ii) **Surgical therapy:**
(a) **Mitral commissurotomy is the procedure of choice** with pliable mitral valve without calcification and mitral regurgitation. This should be done in young women who wants to become pregnant.
(b) **If symptoms recur after commissurotomy: Mitral valve replacement should be performed.** Porcine valve does not need anticoagulation. **Prosthetic valve is preferred** in patients with calcified valve or had previous commissurotomy.
(c) **Patients with prosthetic valve**: Anticoagulation and antibiotic prophylaxis are needed.
(d) **Patients with atrial fibrillation**: Drug used to slow the ventricular response is needed.

68. **Mitral regurgitation (MR)**:
(A) **Etiology:**
(i) **Mitral valve prolapse is the most common cause of mitral regurgitation**. MR can be produced by coronary artery disease, annular calcification, and connective tissue disorders.
(ii) **Acute mitral regurgitation** could be due to **ruptured mitral valve** chordae from endocarditis, **trauma, acute MI is due to rupture of papillary muscles**, perforation of valve leaflet or chordae **from infective endocarditis.**

(B) **Clinical presentations:**

(i) Patients remain **asymptomatic with normal exercise tolerance** despite LVH. **Fatigue** due to reduced forward cardiac output is more common than dyspnea.

Atrial fibrillation develops from left atrial enlargement.

Ischemic cardiomyopathy syndrome occurs in patients with coronary artery disease plus MR appear with symptoms of impaired LV functions such **as fatigue, dyspnea, and orthopnea**. Acute syndrome of MR appears with **pulmonary edema**.

Physical examination reveals characteristic holosystolic murmur best heard over the mitral area radiates into the axilla.

In acute MR which is due to rupture of mitral valve, the murmur is **loud and harsh plus palpable thrill at the apex.**

(C) **Diagnosis of MR:**

(i) Echocardiography with doppler study can detect the intensity of MR and **LV end-systolic dimension < 50 mm can determine the optimal time for mitral valve replacement**.

(ii) Exercise testing and radionuclide angiography can detect **early onset MR.**

(iii) **Cardiac catheterization with left ventriculography confirms the diagnosis of MR**. It also detects coronary artery disease and aortic valve defect.

(iv) EKG shows LVH with increased QRS voltage and ST-T wave changes in lateral precordial leads. LA enlargement produces negative P wave in lead V_1.

(v) CXR shows LV enlargement initially, then LA enlargement (prominence along the right sternal border).

(D) **Treatment of MR:**

(i) **Medical therapy:**

(a) **Early MR without symptoms**: The same antibiotic prophylaxis as mentioned in mitral stenosis (MS) should be given.

(b) **MR with atrial fibrillation**: Use digoxin to slow ventricular response.

(c) **To maintain the forward stroke volume**: Use **nitrates** (afterload reducing drug) **and antihypertensive drugs**.

(d) **MR with cardiac failure**: Surgery is indicated.

(ii) **Surgical therapy:**

(a) Valvular reconstruction.

(b) Mitral valve replacement (prosthetic valve with anticoagulation or porcine valve).

Indications for surgery:

(i) It should be done before the patients become extremely symptomatic.
(ii) Echocardiographic systolic dimension < 50 mm is a predictor of MV replacement.

69. **Mitral valve prolapse (MVP): The synonyms are Barlow's syndrome and click murmur syndrome**. It is most common in women. MVP is due to myxomatous degeneration of the mitral valve.

(A) **Etiology:**
(i) MVP is found in 5% of adult population.
(ii) Connective tissue disease such as **Marfan's** syndrome and osteogenesis imperfecta.
(iii) Rarely with coronary artery disease.

(B) **Clinical manifestations**: Palpitations, fatigue, chest pain, orthostatic changes, and psychological problems. MVP causes slightly higher incidence of infective endocarditis than general population. Remember, sudden death usually does **not** occur in MVP.
Physical examination reveals thin habitus, narrow AP diameter of the chest, early to midsystolic click and a mid- or late systolic (crescendo and decrescendo) murmur.

(C) **Diagnosis of MVP**:
(i) **Echocardiography is the best diagnostic study. It shows inverted question mark or hammock type of configuration of MV. Color doppler** study detects the **amount** of regurgitation.
(ii) EKG shows **slightly inverted T wave** in the inferior and lateral precordial leads plus occasional ST segment depression. **Holter monitoring shows runs of premature beats arise from atrium and ventricle.**
(iii) CXR shows **elongated shaped heart.**
(iv) Exercise testing **can precipitate or aggravate the cardiac irritability and also documents patients fatigue and musculoskeletal symptoms**.
(v) Cardiac catheterization in **not** needed **unless** coronary artery disease has to be ruled out.

(D) **Treatment of MVP:**
(i) **Reassurance and conservative follow-up are the best treatment of choice in majority** of the patients.
(ii) **Palpitation and ventricular ectopy: Use beta-blockers** but fatigue can be aggravated with this drug.
(iii) Patients with prolong QT interval or syncope: **Use antiarrythmic drug**.
(iv) **Prophylactic antibiotic** should be given only to those patients with **audible click and murmur**. **Please remember, patients with MVP**

demonstrated by echocardiography without click and murmur **do not need antibiotic prophylaxis.**

(v) **Surgical management:**

(a) Mitral valve reconstruction or annuloplastomy is the surgical treatment of choice.

(b) MV replacement is an alternative surgical method.
Indications for surgery in MVP: Progressive mitral valve regurgitation with enlarged cardiac chambers or with ruptured chordae.

70. **Tricuspid stenosis (TS):**

(A) **Etiology: Most common cause is rheumatic fever** which also involves the mitral and aortic valves; rare causes are endocardial fibroelastosis, right atrial myxoma.

(B) **Clinical manifestations:** Dyspnea, fatigue, neck veins pulsation, and peripheral edema. **Physical examination reveals diastolic murmur increases with inspiration heard best along the left lower sternal border**. TS offers a protective mechanism for pulmonary vessels of mitral stenosis, so symptoms of MS is reduced with associated TS (Important).

(C) **Diagnosis:**

(i) Echocardiography with doppler study **confirms the diagnosis** and estimates the gradient across the tricuspid valve.

(ii) EKG shows tall, tented P wave in leads II, III, and aVF; **absence of RV hypertrophy.**

(D) **Treatment:**

(i) Antibiotic prophylaxis should be given as described in mitral stenosis.

(ii) Surgical repair or replacement of the tricuspid valve. It is done in association with the left sided valvular surgery.

71. **Tricuspid insufficiency (TI)**:

(A) **Etiology: TI is most commonly due to RV dilatation and hypertrophy**; it could be due to myocardial infarction, trauma, infective endocarditis, or prolapse.

(B) **Clinical manifestations**: Hepatic congestion and periperal edema. Physical examination reveals **holosystolic murmur increases with inspiration heard best along the left sternal border**; atrial fibrillation is common.

(C) **Diagnosis:**

(1) Echocardiography plus doppler study confirms the diagnosis and detects the degree of TR (tricuspid regurgitation).

(2) EKG shows sometimes atrial fibrillation without other features.

(3) CXR shows prominent RA and RV.

(D) **Treatment:**
   (1) To treat the underlying conditions leading to RV failure.
   (2) Annuloplasty is the surgical treatment of choice when valve leaflets are normal.
   (3) Rarely valve replacement is needed.

72. **Pulmonary regurgitation (PR)**:
   (A) **Etiology**: It is most commonly **due to severe pulmonary hypertension** which is produced by pulmonary embolism, mitral stenosis, and chronic lung disease.
   (B) **Clinical manifestations**: Graham steell murmur (high-pitched diastolic flow) along the left sternal border.
   (C) **Diagnosis:**
      (1) Echocardiography with doppler study confirms the diagnosis.
      (2) CXR shows prominent pulmonary artery.
      (3) EKG is mostly normal.
   (D) **Treatment:**
      (1) To treat pulmonary hypertension with drugs.
      (2) Rarely, surgery is performed along with mitral valve surgery.

73. **Pulmonic stenosis (PS)**: (**Not important for examination**): It is **rare**, caused by hypertrophic cardiomyopathy obstructing pulmonary outflow tract.

74. **Most common cause of death in USA**: **Heart disease** (25% of all deaths), most common cause is **acute myocardial infarction which can cause sudden death**.

75. **Most common cause of acute myocardial infarction (MI)**: **Thrombotic occlusion superimposed on severe coronary atherosclerosis**; other causes are coronary emboli, coronary vasospasm, coronary vasculitis, coronary ostial occlusion, trauma, augmented myocardial oxygen requirements exceeding oxygen delivery, infiltrative and degenerative coronary vascular diseases.

76. **Risk factors for acute myocardial infarction: Hypercholesterolemia, hypertriglyceridemia, hypertension**, diabetes mellitus, elevated LDL cholesterol, decreased HDL cholesterol, elevated plasma homocysteine, elevated lipoprotein levels, **truncal obesity, smoking, and genetic predisposition (strong family history) to atherosclerosis**.

77. **Most common cause of death in acute MI**: **Ventricular fibrillation** (> 85% of all deaths). Ventricular premature complexes can trigger ventricular fibrillation. Most common cause of late cardiac death is sudden arrythmias.

78. **Effect of myocardial infarction on organs other than heart**:
    (1) **Lungs**: Increased pulmonary venous pressure causes diminshed pulmonary compliance, dyspnea, pulmonary edema, and hypoxemia.
    (2) **Brain**: Cerebral hypoperfusion causes restlessness, confusion, combativeness, or rarely psychosis.
    (3) **Pancreas**: Decreased blood flow results in decreased insulin secretion.
    (4) **Fluid retention and hyponatremia** are due to increased vasopressin, angiotensin, and aldosterone.
    (5) **Blood**: Elevated ESR, leukocytosis, elevated plasma fibrinogen, circulating PAI-1, alpha-2 globulin, and viscosity.

79. **Clinical manifestations, diagnosis, and treatment of acute myocardial infarction:(Important).**
    (A) **Clinical manifestations:**
        (1) **The prodromal symptoms of 'Typical' Q-wave** infarction is manifested by **fatigue, malaise, or chest discomfort in the days before the acute onset.**
        (2) **Acute infarction occurs often early in the morning** (**not** associated with severe exertion) due to **increased catecholamine induced platelet aggregation and reduced plasma concentrations of PAI-1 after awakening.**
        (3) **The pain is severe, intense, unremitting for 30 to 60 minutes, crushing or squeezing in nature, retrosternal, and may radiate along the ulnar side of left arm, neck, jaw, or teeth.** Sometimes pain is noted **only in the epigastric region (commonly misdiagnosed as indigestion). Diaphoresis, restlessness, confusion, hiccup** (diaphragmatic irritation), palpitation, nausea, and vomiting are present.
        (4) Decreased LV function results in dyspnea, tachypnea, orthopnea, and pulmonary edema.
        (5) Decreased RV function results in edema, enlarged congested liver, and systemic venous hypertension.
        (6) **Myocardial infarction is clinically silent in approximately 1% of cases with positive EKG findings**.

        Physical examination reveals the following:
        (1) **General appearance**: Diaphoresis, pallor, and restlessness.
        (2) **Vital signs:**
            (a) **Temperature:** Fever occurs within 24 to 48 hours.

(b) **Heart rate**: Tachycardia, ventricular ectopic beat, ventricular tachycardia, atrial flutter or fibrillation; bradyarrythmias are due to impaired sinus node function or A-V nodal block.

(c) **BP**: Initial elevation of blood pressure is due to arterial vasoconstriction.

(3) **Fundoscopic eye examination:** Atherosclerosis (copper wiring of arterioles), diabetes with microaneurysms, hypertensive retinopathy with **hemorrhages which is a relative contraindication of fibrinolytic therapy**.

(4) **Abnormal pulses:**

(a) Jugular venous distension in RV failure.

(b) Pulsus alternans in LV failure.

(5) **Chest examination:**

(a) Pleural effusion in biventricular failure.

(b) Rales are present in LV failure.

(6) **Heart examination:**

(a) **LV failure**: Soft S_1, palpable S_4, dyskinesis, lateral displacement of apical impulse.

(b) **Left bundle branch block**: Paradoxical splitting of S_2 is present.

(c) **Papillary muscle dysfunction or rupture**: Mitral regurgitation is present.

(d) Pericardial friction rub may be present.

(7) **Extremities:** Peripheral edema, cyanosis, or pallor is due to RV failure.

(8) **Abdomen**: Positive hepatojugular reflex.

(9) **Neurological examination**: CVA (cerebrovascular accident) is due to embolization of ventricular mural thrombi. Please remember, **myocardial infarction is greater and worser with depression and infarction also precipitate depression without** beta-blockers and CNS active drugs.

(B) **Diagnosis of acute MI:**

(1) **Invasive monitoring**:

(a) Patients with MI **but hemodynamically stable without complications** (tachycardia, refractory arrythmias, pericarditis, cardiac rupture, compromised pulmonary, CNS, renal, and hepatic systems): Do **not** need invasive monitoring.

(b) Patients with **pulmonary venous hypertension and congestion**: Balloon flotation right heart catheter hemodynamic monitoring should be done but many patients may be managed conservatively.

(c) Patients with **peripheral hypoperfusion even after fluid administration** and those with CHF (refractory or progressive), hemodynamic instability, arrythmias, or persistent pain: Balloon flotation right heart catheter hemodynamic monitoring should be done.

(d) Monitoring catheter **should be removed within 72 hours** to avoid infection.

(e) In some patients **continuous monitoring** are **not** needed for subsequent management; **cardiac output, systemic, and pulmonary venous pressure, peripheral vascular resistance** are sufficient to manage the patients.

(f) In other patients continuous monitoring **are needed to see the effects of** vasodilators, diuretics, positive inotropic drugs, and therapeutic alteration of vascular volume for 2 to 3 days.

(2) **Patients are categorized with hemodynamic subsets:**

(a) **Systemic arterial BP** (normal, increased, or decreased) with systemic vascular resistance (increased or decreased).

(b) **Cardiac output** (normal, increased, or decreased).

(c) **Pulmonary venous hypertension (present or absent) or increased pulmonary arterial wedge pressure**.

(d) **Patients with elevated left ventricular filling pressure may have relative hypovolemia**. CVP is **not** reliable to asses the vascular volume.

(e) Systemic hypotension (arterial) may cause relative or absolute hypovolemia or to RV infarction (elevated systemic venous pressure).

(f) **RV failure with or without** tricuspid regurgitation leads to increased CVP without increased PV or PA occlusive pressure.

(g) **PV hypertension** with normal systemic BP **indicates LV failure**. LV failure is called mild with normal cardiac output and **severe** with decreased cardiac output.

(h) Severe systemic hypotension and PV hypertension indicate **cardiogenic shock with decreased cardiac output**. These patients should be managed with **immediate thrombolytic therapy, angioplasty, or surgery.**

(3) **Laboratory findings in acute MI:**

(a) **Sequential ECG findings are the important diagnostic study: Typical ST elevation persists** for hours, followed by **T waves inversion within the first few days and subsequent development of Q waves.**

Initial ST **depression** or T-wave inversion is difficult to differentiate from ischemia without infarction. ST-segment **depression** followed **by T-wave inversion** without formation of Q waves can be due to **non-Q-wave infarction or subendocardial ischemia without**

infarction. Q-wave infarction cannot be differentiated from non-Q-wave infarction initially if ST-elevation and Q-waves are absent. ECG abnormalities may be nonspecific in some patients with MI. Presence of abnormalities in large number of ECG leads indicates **extensive injury or associated pericarditis. Remember, LV myocardium is mostly involved by anterior and anterolateral infarcts than** inferior or true posterior infarcts.

(b) **CBC and platelet counts are normal initially, increase within 2 hours, and peaks within 2 to 4 days with predominance of polymorphonuclear leukocytes.** (Remember these counts may decrease after heparin). Elevation of ESR occurs within 48 hours.

(c) Fingertip pulse oximetry is important to know the oxygenation status but arterial blood gas should be done if necessary.

(d) CXR to assess cardiomegaly, pulmonary edema, pleural effusion, and Kerley B lines.

(e) **The definitive diagnosis of MI is done by measuring MB-CK (MB isoenzyme of CK). MB-CK is elevated above normal within 4 hours, peak (2-to 10-folds) in 16 to 24 hours, and return to baseline within 3 to 4 days. The extent of infarction can be estimated by the magnitude and persistence of elevation of MB-CK. Please remember these points, patients may have normal MB-CK with acute MI: Early onset of infarction** (so patients should not be discharged home early from ER when there is H/O MI), or **if MI occurs with modest degree more than 24 hours before admission because rate of clearance of MB-CK exceeds the rate of release from myocardium**. Determination of myosin light chains, **troponin I, or the LDH_1: LDH_2** isoenzyme ratio, which remains **elevated for several days after infarction because of slow clearance of LDH and these findings are nonspecific but may be helpful when MB-CK values are not elevated in suspected MI.**

(f) **Recently it has shown that earlier diagnosis** (within 2 to 3 hours of MI) can be made by **determining post-translational conversion of individual isoenzyme of CK to isoform**.

(g) Imaging studies: Most commonly used is **echocardiography and color doppler study. Abnormal wall motion is an important criteria in patients with first episode of MI**. It also detects the MR to TR, ventricular functions, ruptured septum, and calculates cardiac output.

99 m Tc-pyrophosphate and radiolabeled antimyosin antibodies can detect infarction **usually 24 hours after** the onset of infarction.

Perfusion scintigraphy with thallium 201 or 99m Tc- sestamibi (isonitrite) is sometimes useful when diagnosis is difficult. **Positron emission tomography** with tracers can detect the **quantitative** assessment of the **distribution and extent of myocardial impairment of perfusion and oxidative metabolism, and also differentiate reversible from irreversible injury**.

(C) **Treatment of acute MI**:

(1) **Prehospital phase:**

(a) **It is very important because 65% of deaths occurs within first hour. Majority of these patients can be saved by defibrillation instituted by policeman, fireman, or trained personnel**.

(b) **Use morphine** for analgesia.

(c) Prophylaxis and treatment of ventricular arrythmias: **Use lidocaine**.

(d) Support of systemic BP, cardiac output, and respiration.

(e) **Atropine** is used when heart rate is low with respect to BP.

(f) Coronary thrombolysis under medical supervision is becoming important.

(2) **Treatment in CCH:**

(a) Continuous ECG monitoring, liquid diet for 24 hours, stool softeners to avoid constipation, prophylaxis with oral sucralfate, H_2 antagonist (e.g.,famotidine, ranitidine, or cimetidine) for stress ulcers.

(b) Patients with **uncomplicated** infarctions should be confined to **bed for only 24 hours**. Physical activity should be **restricted to bed-chair regimen for 2 to 3 days in CCU stay, then gradual resumption of ambulatory activity in the late hospital phase.**

(c) Use of anxiolytic, sedative, or hypnotic **drug at night** may be useful.

(d) Patients on ventilator should be managed appropriately.

(e) **Oxygen** should be given to avoid hypoxemia.

(f) **Patients with severe or refratory pain**: IV morphine, pentazocine, or meperidine. (**Morphine toxicity** is treated with naloxone, **morphine-induced hypotension without pulmonary edema** can be treated with elevating the legs, supine position, fluids, and use of atropine for low heart rate).

(g) **Patients with continuous chest pain due to ischemia**: IV nitroglycerin is used carefully. It causes beneficial effect by reducing afterload, preload, and decreasing LVEDP results **in improves myocardial perfusion. (Remember, higher doses cause low BP, decreased myocardial perfusion, and decreased systemic venous tone).**

(h) **Oral calcium channel blocker** (e.g., nifedipine, diltiazem) may be useful.Nifedipine reduces ventricular after load and diltiazem reduces cardiac contractility and heart rate.

(i) **Oral or IV conventional or ultra-short-acting beta-blockers such as esmolol** may reduce ischemia and pain by **reducing heart rate and hence myocardial oxygen demands.**

(j) Use of nitrous oxide (20 to 50%) plus oxygen for analgesia is **not widely used in USA unlike Europe.**

(k) **To limit the infarct size**: Use **beta-blockers** (to reduce heart rate), **arterial vasodilators** such as nifedipine, nitrates, or ACE inhibitors (to reduce ventricular after load), **diuretics** such as furosemide and ethacrynic acid (to reduce LV pre load). **Beta-blockers are used in most patients** except in bronchoconstriction, heart failure, and bradycardia.

(l) **Coronary thrombolysis: First-generation drugs** are streptokinase,urokinase, and APSAC (acetylated plasminogen streptokinase activator complex) induces **activation of free plasminogen and clot-associated plasminogen indiscriminately, so increases the risk of bleeding** due to lack of clot selectivity. **Second-generation drugs are** t-PA and single-chain urokinase plasminogen activator. **These are the drug of choice for acute MI**. They induce clot lysis without producing systemic clot lysis, so **less chance of bleeding** than first generation drugs. **Recanalization is more rapid (with 1½ hour) and more frequent (80% to 90%) in the second-generation drugs than first-generation. Use of t-PA plus IV heparin have more benefits and less cardiovascular complications** than use of streptokinase with or without heparin. **Please remember that thrombolytic agents causing cerebrovascular accidents are the same with conservative management without thrombolytic drugs. Most common bleeding by plasminogen activators are limited to sites of vascular access.**

Contraindications of using plasminogen activators: Bleeding disorders, active internal hemorrhage, aortic dissection, hemorrhagic retinopathy, recent surgery, traumatic CPR, hypertensive crisis, or intracranial neoplasm. **Relative** contraindications are pregnancy, peptic ulcer disease, remote CVA, and hepatic failure.

Indications of thrombolytic agents: Patients (≤ 75 years of age) with suspected Q-wave infarction within 6 hours after the onset of symptoms. **It may be helpful** even if patients **appear after 6 hours**.

Its usefulness is not clear in non-Q-wave infarction, very advanced age, and unstable angina.

(m) **Adjunctive and conjunctive therapies: IV heparin is the drug of choice plus oral aspirin. Hirudin** (direct-acting antithrombins) is an experimental but promising drug.

Calcium antagonists are anti-injury drugs in the setting of reperfusion injury, as antiplatelet agents, and as coronary vasodilators.

Nitrates may reduce excess coronary reactivity and ischemia.

Lidocaine is used in reperfusion injury causing ventricular fibrillation. Acclerate idioventricular arrythmias may not require drug therapy.

Most important is conjunctive anticoagulation with antithrombin (heparin or hirudin) and conjunctive use of antiplatelet agents (aspirin or anibodies), antagonists to platelet glycoprotein II b/ III a receptor, prostacyclin and PEE_2 analogues,thromboxane receptor antagonists, synthetase inhibitors and serotonin antagonists (**all are experimental drugs**).

The TIMI group studies in NEJM showed that **outcome after invasive therapy (angiography and angioplasty)** versus conservative management after treatment with IV t-PA in acute MI was **not** superior than conservative management.

(n) **Mechanical revascularization (angioplasty or bypass surgery):**

(1) Mechanical revascularization is used as **primary therapy only for patients with contraindications to thrombolytic agents**, those patients with **cardiogenic shock refractory to coronary thrombolysis, and those with infarction resulting from occlusion of previously placed coronary bypass grafts amenable to angioplasty.**

The value of **rescue angioplasty** (angioplasty for occlusion which is refractory to fibrinolysis) has **not** yet established because of **irreversible injury by the time failure of thrombolysis was recognized**.

(o) **Prophylaxis and treatment of arrythmias:**

(1) Ventricular fibrillation should be treated STAT with **defibrillation therapy.**

(2) If ventricular fibrillation **cannot** be distinguished from true asystole: Fibrillation should be assumed and **defibrillation therapy** should be done STAT.

(3) **Electrical countershock (defibrillation therapy) should be done before endotracheal intubation** and other emergency procedures.

(4) **True asytole is present: Immediate external, transvenous, or transthoracic cardiac pacing should be done.**

(5) Ventricular fibrillation in acute MI**: Lidocaine is the drug of choice to prevent recurrence**. Prophylactic lidocaine is not needed when defibrillation and lidocaine are available for STAT use.

Side effects of prophylactic lidocaine: Seizures, CNS depression, cardiac-depression, proarrythmic, and asystole.

(6) Young patient with first heart attack within few hours of attack have a risk of fibrillation: Lidocaine can be used.

(7) After successful defibrillation therapy: **Lidocaine should be used by** continuous infusion particularly when associated with ventricular premature complexes or ventricular tachycardia.

(8) Recurrent ventricular fibrillation refractory to lidocaine: IV bretylium or amiodarone (still experimental in USA) can be used.

(9) High-grade ventricular ectopy or ventricular tachycardia: **Lidocaine should be used initially**. If persist more than few hours, **procainamide and quinidine are the drug of choice.**

(10) Torsades de pointes should be treated with override or IV magnesium sulfate.

(11) **Accelerated idioventricular rhythm:** It should **not** be treated unless hemodynamic decompensation occurs, then use **sequential or atrial overdrive pacing or atropine.**

(12) **To reduce** the incidence of primary lethal arrythmias and mortality in patients treated **with or without** thrombolytic drugs: Use IV magnesium sulfate.

(13) **Atrial fibrillation or atrial flutter (supraventricular arrythmias) without Wolff-Parkinson-White syndrome**: This condition should be treated with **calcium channel blockers (verapamil), digoxin, or short-acting beta-blockers (esmolol) to control ventricular rate**. **Procainamide or quinidine** is used to maintain sinus rhythm. **Rapid atrial pacing to stop atrial flutter** or electrical cardioversion to stop either atrial fibrillation or flutter in patients with progressive deterioration.

Patients with compromised hemodynamics or threatened myocardial viability plus SVT (supraventricular tachycardia) should be treated **initially** by stimulating vagal tone with **carotid sinus compression or the Valsalva maneuver, verapamil, IV**

adenosine, or electrical cardioversion. Use of adenosine is controversial.

(14) **Bradyarrythmias**: Bradycardia is common in inferior MI and it should be treated with **atropine**, if unresponsive then use **temporary transvenous pacing**.

First-degreee AV block or wandering atrial pacemaker does **not** usually require specific treatment. **Higher-degree of AV block or AV block plus hypotension unresponsive to atropine is treated with sequential pacing** to maintain the hemodynamics.

Long-term pacing is indicated when heart block persists throughout the hospital phase, impaired sinus node function, Mobitz II second-or third-degree block occurs intermittently or associated with newly acquired bundle branch block. **Temporary pacing** is used to maintain the hemodynamics and **prophylactic long-term pacing is used for high-risk patients.**

(p) **Treatment to maintain the hemodynamics:**

(1) **Hypertensive patients with increased cardiac output and normal pulmonary artery wedge pressure: Use esmolol** (beta-blocker) to reduce myocardial oxygen requirement.

(2) Hypotension with relative or absolute hypovolemia indicated by lack of adequate elevation (> 18 mm Hg) of LV filling pressure: **Use IV fluids, monitor pulmonary artery wedge pressure to avoid pulmlonary edema**.

(3) Hypotension with RV infarction (eleveated RV diastolic, RA, and central venous pressures): **Use IV fluids, dobutamine, dopamine, or beta-adrenergic agonists. Systemic arterial vasodilators** decrease RV outflow if LV failure is ameliorated and can be used when systemic arterial diastolic pressure is normal.

(4) **Severe hypotension** is due to pulmonary embolisms, ruptured ventricular septum, hemopericardium, or ruptured LV papillary muscles: Immediate surgical intervention after stability with pharmacologic and circulatory support. Surgery can delayed for 1 to 2 weeks if stability can be maintained without such measures and the patient can be monitored closely.

(5) Hypotension with severely elevated pulmonary artery wedge pressure is due to impaired LV function and cardiogenic shock: **Coronary thrombolysis, angioplasty, or surgery should be done because cardiotonic drugs** are **not** effective without the above mentioned therapy. **Intra-aortic balloon**

counterpulsation or circulatory support with a LV assist device is useful as temporary therapy before cardiac transplantation.

(6) Pulmonary venous hypertension with normal systemic BP indicates relative or absolute increase in vascular volume and LV failure: Use IV nitroprusside, nitroglycerin, or (IV or oral) ACE inhibitors. **If pulmonary edema is present with normal systemic BP and cardiac output**, then fluid is removed by phlebotomy with reinfusion of blood cell elements, slow continuous ultrafiltration, or rarely peritoneal dialysis. **If pulmonary congestion persists with low systemic BP and cardiac output, then use loop diuretics** (removes fluids plus pulmonary venodilation).

Do **not** use hemodialysis because it can alter filling pressures and cardiac performance.

Patients with CHF plus reduced cardiac output and hypotension, use of cardiotonic drugs (e.g., digoxin, dopamine, dobutamine, amrinone, or milrinone) are not effective alone and also produce risk of imbalance between myocardial oxygen demand and supply.

(7) **Hypotension with or without pulmonary venous hypertension due to LV failure usually associated increased peripheral vascular resistance**. In rare cases, pulmonary vascular resistance is **decreased**, then use dopamine or epinephrine. **Antibiotic** should be used in sepsis causing decreased pulmonary vascular resistance. Patients with severe ventricular failure, use intra-aortic balloon counterpulsation or LV assist devices followed be diagnostic catheterization and surgery.

(q) **Patients care in the step-down unit for acute MI**:

(1) **Uncomplicated MI** patients usually stay in the CCU **not** more than 72 hours, then transfer to **step-down unit**: Telemetry for **continuous ECG monitoring, daily physical examination**, and **laboratory monitoring** to detect early recognition of complication and to institute appropriate therapy.

(2) Patients with **fever** should be treated with **aspirin** (**not** with **NSAID's or corticosteroids** which causes impairment of infarct healing**). Patients can develop post MI** pericarditis (friction rub), deep venous **thrombosis** (fever plus positive Homan's sign), pulmonary **embolisms, infections, ventricular thrombi or aneurysms.**

(3) Patients should be assessed for LV function, exercise tolerance, and the severity of spontaneous or inducible ischemia.
(4) Gradual and judicious progressive ambulation then discharge with rehabilitation therapy.
(5) Patients received thrombolytic therapy, **heparin can be stopped** after 5 to 7 days and **daily aspirin** can be given to prevent thrombosis.
(6) Patient with ventricular mural thrombus or extensive hypokineseis, CHF, or ventricular aneurysm predispose to mural thrombus: **Anticoagulation with warfarin** should be given for 6 months.
(7) Patients **with non-Q-wave infarction without CHF**: **Use calcium channel blockers** (verapamil) to prevent recurrence.
(8) Patients with **Q-wave infarction** without failure or other contraindications: **Use beta-blockers** (to reduce the sympathomimetic activity and reinfarction; enhance survival).
(9) Patients with **complications** (**telemetry** which detects ischemic ST-deviation, heart block, arrythmia, new bundle branch block, tachycardia with minimal exertion; physical examination reveals CHF; echocardiography or radionuclide ventriculography reveals recurrent coronary occlusion): **Next step is to perform coronary arteriography and mechanical revascularization if indicated.**
(10) Patients **without** complications and particularly **those received thrombolytic drugs for submaximal period (7 to 10 days),** or limited-symptoms: **Next step is to perform exercise testing before discharge to determine whether coronary arteriography should be done.**
Indications of coronary arteriography after exercise testing: Exercise-induced ischemia (ST-depression ≥1 mm), **hypotension** with modest workloads, **reversible thallium perfusion defects, ventricular arrythmias**, wall motion defects with or without angina pectoris is an **indication of coronary arteriography**.
(11) Patients with **baseline** ECG findings are difficult to interpret: **Next step is to perform thallium scintigraphy or exercise echocardiography** for proper diagnosis.
(12) Patients who are **unable to exercise** for noncardiac reason: Use **dipyridamole thallium scintigraphy or dobutamine stress echocardiography**.
(13) Ambulatory continuous ECG monitoring to detect ventricular ectopy is associated with postinfarction LV dysfunction.

(D) **Management during convalescence**:

(1) **To prevent recurrent infarction**: Continued use of **beta-blockers** after **Q-wave** infarction, **calcium channel blockers** after **non-Q-wave** infarction with preserved LV function, and **aspirin** (to prevent thrombosis) is used for both Q-wave and non-Q-wave infarctions.
(2) **To prevent late complications of infarction** (cerebral or peripheral embolus from ventricular mural thrombus): Continued use of **anticoagulation therapy for 3 to 6 months.**
(3) **To prevent sudden cardiac death: Use beta-blocker** (if there is no contraindication).
(4) Do **not** use antiarrythmic drugs indiscriminately to suppress asymptomatic ventricular ectopy because it enhances mortality.
(5) Stop **smoking; treat** hypertension, diabetes, and hyperlipidemia (reduce LDL cholesterol to 100 mg/dL) appropriately.
(6) **Promptly detect** the signs and symptoms of ischemia including angina pectoris and **evaluate** appropriately.
(7) Exercise rehabilitation program under proper supervision or at home for motivated patients.

(E) **Prognosis of acute MI:**
(1) **Mortality is ≤ 5% among patients ≤ 75 years of age** because of defibrillation, thrombolytic drugs, angioplasty, bypass surgery, and sophisticated CCU management.
(2) Patients with **non-Q-wave** infarctions **can develop syndrome of incomplete or nonsustained thrombotic coronary artery occlusion.**
(3) Early prognosis is better in **non-Q-wave** infarction than Q-wave infarction.
(4) **Mortality rate** after infarction is **higher in non-Q-wave** infarction than Q-wave infarction because of reocclusion, reinfarction, and sudden cardiac death.

80. **Surgical treatment of coronary artery disease**:
(A) **Indications of coronary artery bypass grafting (CABG)**:
(1) **Patients unresponsive to intensive medical therapy for chronic angina, acute MI, or occlusion of left main coronary artery (> 70% diameter).**
(2) **Chronic ischemia:**
(a) **'Silent'** ischemia: Asymptomatic patients **with exercise ECG reveals ischemia with coronary artery occlusion.**
(b) **Chronic stable angina: This is the largest group of patients (men in sixth decade of life) for CABG.** Patients are receiving beta-blockers, calcium channel blockers, vasodilators, aspirin, and

coronary arteriography reveals 2 to 3 vessels are blocked, **most commonly 3 vessels.**

(3) **Acute myocardial ischemia:**

(a) Unstable angina: Patients complain of pain at rest, at night, or continuous pain with ECG ischemic changes (**not** infarction) even with medications.

(b) **Evolving** myocardial infarction: Patients with **3 vessels** coronary disease are the candidate for CABG (**single** vessel disease is treated with thrombolytic therapy and/or PTCA). **CABG can be done within 6 hours of the onset of chest pain.**

(c) **Subendocardial infarction**: Clinical presentation and angiographic findings are same as unstable angina.

(d) **Postinfarction angina**: Patients had transmural myocardial infarction and CABG can be performed **within hours to days** of the completed MI.

(e) **Myocardial infarction with cardiogenic shock**: Patients usually have **at least 40% of LV infarction** and they should be **stabilized** with **medications and mechanical devices, careful evaluation of LV function and anatomy of distal coronary vessels before emergency CABG.**

(f) **CABG with other cardiac surgeries: Elderly** patients with aortic valve disease, ventricular septal infarction, ruptured, or dysfunctional papillary muscles, LV aneurysm or rupture, pseudoaneurysm.

(B) **Basic of surgical treatment of coronary heart disease**:

(1) Coronary artery bypass operation, a conduit **is sutured distal to the obstructing lesion in the artery** and **connected proximally to either the aorta** or naturally by in situ connection such as internal thoracic artery to the subclavian artery. **The best available conduit is the internal thoracic (mammary) artery**. The **reversed autogenous saphenous vein graft** is a reliable and flexible conduit. **Recently**, right internal throacic artery, right gastroepiploic artery, and even the radial artery have been used.

(2) Post operative complications of CABG patients:

(a) Most common complication is acute atrial fibrillation (30% of cases).

(b) Perioperative myocardial infarction (new ECG Q waves or elevated CK enzyme in 2 to 5% of cases).

(c) **Postoperative stroke (< 2% of cases)** is an important cause of morbidity. It can be prevented by **using single aortic cross-clamp during anastomosis** to prevent showering of platelet emboli to the brain and **postoperative use of aspirin** to prevent platelet stickiness in the grafts.

(3) **Reoperation of coronary bypass**:

(a) Currently used **'no touch'** technique with early **onset of femorofemoral cardiopulmonary bypass. and improved retrograde cardioplegia myocardial protection**, the risk of reoperation has decreased significantly.

(b) Use of **internal thoracic artery bypass graft to at least the left anterior descending artery significantly delays** reoperation.

(c) Indications for reoperation: It is the same as primary operation but ischemia should be well documented because risk of reoperation is higher (5 to 8%) and benefit is somewhat reduced than primary operation.

(4) **Late results of CABG:**

(a) Operative mortality is **2 to 5%.**

(b) **Long term graft patency is better with internal thoracic artery** (95% at 5 years) than saphenous vein (75 to 80% at 5 years).

81. **Most common cause of myocardial and cerebral infarction, and principal cause of death in USA** and western Europe: **Atherosclerosis**. It is a lipid rich lesion of the **medium, large muscular, and elastic arteries**. (**Arteriosclerosis** is a generic term for thickened and stiffened arteries of **all sizes**; **Monckeberg's arteriosclerosis** is a focal calcific arteriosclerosis; arteriolosclerosis is a disease of small vessels).

82. **Atherosclerosis**:

(A) **Most common artery** which develops atherosclerosis is the **aorta**, other arteries are coronary, internal and external carotid, cerebral, femoral, popliteal, and tibial. **Abdominal aorta is the most common site**, in thoracic aorta lesions most commonly occur around orifices of branches and bifurcations.

(B) **Two forms of atherosclerosis**:

(1) **Early lesion or fatty streak:** It is **the most common form**, occurs in all **ages**, lesions are confined to **intima**. Fatty streak contains two cell types (**foam cells** contain macrophages filled with lipids in the form of cholesteryl esters; other cells are **T lymphocytes** mainly CD8 + with some CD4 + cells).

(2) **Advanced lesion or fibrous plaque**: It is located in the intima, causes eccentric thickening of the artery, and occlusion of the lumen.

(C) Risk factors for atherosclerosis:

(1) **Hyperlipidemia (plasma cholesterol > 220 mg/dL**, **in USA 200 mg/dL** is the upper limit of normal). Elevated **cholesterol** is associated with increase of **LDL**. There is an **age-related increase in plasma triglyceride levels** which is associated with **increase of VLDL**. Hyperlipidemia could be due to genetic reason. **Most common form of hyperlipoproteinemia is secondary to diabetes, renal disease, alcoholism, hypothyroidism, and dysglobulinemias.**

(2) **Homozygous familial hypercholesterolemia (FH):** It is **rarer** than secondary and genetic hyperlipidemia. **In genetic hyperlipidemia, plasma cholesterol levels** (500 to 1000 mg/dL or higher) **and LDL levels** are very high **due to faulty or missing LDL receptors.** Normally LDL attached to normal receptors and inhibit the enzymes for cholesterol synthesis. **In FH disease** there is **no** inhibition, so liver and peripheral tissues **continue to produce large amount of cholesterol**.

(3) **High density lipoprotein (HDL): Elevated HDL cholesterol is protective** against ischemic heart disease and **abnormally low levels of HDL can increase the ischemic heart disease. HDL is elevated** by **regular strenuous exercise, decreased by cigarette smoking, and diet rich in some fish oils (eicosapentaenoic acid).** HDL transfers cholesterol out of the cells.

(4) **Cigarette smoking enhances** the atherosclerosis and sudden death.

(5) **Hypertension** (BP > 160 systolic, > 95 diastolic) **enhances atherosclerosis.**

(6) **Diabetes mellitus and glucose intolerance: Both insulin-dependent and non-insulin-dependent diabetics have higher incidence of myocardial infarction.** Lower extremity gangrene is the result of atherosclerosis in diabetics. Diabetics form modified proteins termed **advanced glycosylation end products (AGE's).** LDL can be modified and AGE-LDL may play a role in atherosclerosis **like** oxidized LDL (ox LDL).

(7) **Obesity**: When the body weight **is > 20% above normal, particularly persons < 50 years of age** are associated with hypertriglyceridemia, hypercholesterolemia, hypertension, and diabetes.

(8) **Genetic factors:** Atherosclerosis is higher in individuals **with homozygous familial hypercholesterolemia and familial combined hyperlipidemia**, other factors are diabetes and hypertension.

(9) **Physical activity: Sedentary individuals are more susceptible to atherosclerosis and sudden death** than active individuals.

83. **Treatment of hypercholesterolemia** (cholesterol levels > 200 mg/dL or triglyceride levels > 250 mg/dL, or both indicates hyperlipidemia):

(1) **Weight** should be brought to normal.
(2) **Diet should be low in saturated fat, cholesterol, and calories is the best approach.**
(3) **Eliminate or limit alcohol intake.**
(4) **Patients with severe cholesterolemia > 350 mg/dL or triglyceridemia > 400 mg/dL or both usually** indicates genetic disorder, so **patients families and first-degree relatives should be examined. Remember, both oxidized LDL and glycated LDL (in diabetes) form free radicals.**
(5) If dietary approach is **not** successful, then use bile acid-binding resins, nicotine acid,or HMG-CoA-reductase inhibitors (statins). These are **contraindicated** before puberty and during pregnancy.
(6) Future therapy is antioxidant.

84. **Sinus rhythm**:
(A) **Clinical features**:
(1) Sinus bradycardia: Resting heart rate < 50 to 60/minute.
(2) Sinus tachycardia: Resting heart rate > 100/minute.
(B) **ECG findings**: Normal atrial rate and P wave vector (upright P wave in leads III and aVf, normal PR interval), heart rate is < 50 or > 100/minute.
(C) **Management**:
(1) Sinus bradycardia without symptom: No treatment.
(2) Acute sinus bradycardia with symptoms: IV atropine.
(3) Chronic sinus bradycardia with symptoms: Use electronic pacemaker.
(4) Sinus tachycardia: Treat according to the underlying cause, usually extracardiac.

85. **Atrial premature complexes (APC's):**
(A) **Clinical features**: APC's occur in normal or diseased heart (atrial flutter, atrial fibrillation, or paroxysmal supraventricular tachycardia).
(B) **ECG findings**: Premature P waves, abnormal P wave morphology, and prolonged PR interval.
(C) **Management**:
(1) Patients with normal heart plus APC's: General hygienic measures, rest, reduce or avoid the use of alcohol, tobacco, or caffeine.
(2) APC's plus intermittent or sustained atrial arrythmias: Digoxin or class I, II, or IV antiarrythmic drugs to prevent arrythmias. (**Class I** drugs are lidocaine, mexiletine, tocainide, disopyramide, moricizine, procainamide, quinidine, encainide, flecainide, indecainide, propafenone; **class II drugs** are beta-blockers such as acebutalol, propanolol; **class III drugs cause prolong repolarization** such as

amiodarone, bretylium, sotalol; **class IV drugs are calcium channel blockers such as diltiazem, verapamil**).

86. **Paroxysmal supraventricular tachycardia (PSVT)**:
   (A) **Clinical features**: PSVT can occur in normal or diseased heart. PSVT can begin abruptly, cause palpitation, and can terminate abruptly. **Cough, Valsalva maneuver, or facial immersion can stop the PSVT**. When PSVT is rapid (180 to 220 beats/minute**), the systemic BP falls, diastolic pressure of both ventricles rise** even without heart disease. **Salt and water retention** is a complication of rapid and prolonged SVT.
   (B) **ECG findings**: Regular, rapid rate of 150 to 230 beats (minute, QRS duration < 100 msec, abnormal P wave in a fixed relationship to each QRS complex, P wave often superimposed on T wave or the QRS complex, and the R-R interval **is regular except** in the first or last few cycles.
   (C) **Management**:
      (1) **Vagal stimulation (e.g., Valsalva maneuver or carotid sinus massage), adenosine or verapamil is effective** in 90% of cases.
      (2) **PSVT with hypotension or cardiac failure**: Use DC cardioversion.
      (3) **To prevent recurrence of PSVT due to AV nodal reentry: First drug of choice is digoxin**, if fails then use class I antiarrythmic drugs.
      (4) WPW syndrome with recurrent symptomatic tachyarrythmias: Catheter ablation is preferred to drugs.

87. **Atrial flutter**:
   (A) **Clinical features**: It is either due to **intrinsic heart disease** (rheumatic, coronary, myocardial, ASD, MS or MR, TS or TR, chronic ventricular failure) or **extrinsic factors** (thyrotoxicosis, alcoholism, pericardial inflammation from pneumonia or pericardial infiltration from bronchogenic carcinoma). In all these conditions plus systemic emboli are more common in atrial fibrillation than atrial flutter.
   (B) **ECG findings**: Rapid atrial rate (250 to 350 beats/minute), narrow QRS, ventricular rate (125 to 175/minute) i.e., **2:1 AV conduction ratio**. Characteristic **saw-toothed** appearance best seen in leads II, III, and aVf.
   (C) **Management:**
      (1) The treatment of choice is **atrial pacing or DC cardioversion**.
      (2) IV verapamil or beta-blockers can be **used temporarily** to control heart rate while arrangement are made for DC cardioversion.
      (3) **To prevent recurrence** use class I antiarrythmic drug with or without digoxin.

88. **Atrial fibrillation**:

(A) **Clinical features**: It is due to myocardial, pericardial, or adverse extrinsic influence like atrial flutter. It may be paroxysmal, chronic, stable rhythm or occurs abruptly with serious heart disease results in palpitations, angina pectoris, or pulmonary edema. Chronic atrial inflammation causes left atrial thrombi and systemic emboli. '**Lone atrial fibrillation' means isolated atrial fibrillation without heart disease or other systemic illness**.

(B) **ECG findings: Presence of fibrillatory waves best seen in leads II, III, aV_F or V_1; absence** of P waves; **irregular atrial activity at a rate of 350 to 600/minute; rapid, irregularly irregular ventricular rhythm (150 to 200/minute).**

(C) **Management**:
  (1) Atrial fibrillation with symptomatic hypotension: Immediate cardioversion is indicated.
  (2) To control the heart rate: Use of IV **digoxin** is adequate. Verapamil or beta-blockers can be used with digoxin to control the heart rate but can aggravate cardiac failure and cause hypotension.
  (3) **Avoid** digoxin and verapamil in WPW syndrome because they can increase ventricular rate and produce ventricular fibrillation.
  (4) The goal of chronic treatment of atrial fibrillation is to control ventricular rate, maintain sinus rhythm, and prevent thromboemboli.

89. **Multifocal atrial tachycardia**:

(A) **Clinical features**: It is mostly due to overtreatment with theophylline or catecholamines in chronic obstructive pulmonary disease.

(B) **ECG findings**: Frequent APC's, different P wave morphology and marked variability in P-P interval.

(C) **Management**:
  (1) To improve ventilation and antibiotics to treat lung infection.
  (2) Reduce the dose of bronchodilators.
  (3) Verapamil may control arrythmia.
  (4) Remember, digoxin does **not** work.

90. **Sinoatrial block:**

(A) **Etiology**: It is due to intrinsic sinus node disease, adverse drug effect, or electrolyte disturbance. **Most offending drug is digoxin**. Class I antiarrythmic can cause SA block in patients with pre-existing sinus node disease.

(B) **ECG finding:**
  (1) First-degree SA block: It is a delay in conduction from SA node to atrium. ECG is **normal** but diagnosed by electrophysiologic studies.

(2) Second-degree SA block: It is diagnosed by ECG finding**. Type I** is identified by Wenckebach periodicity of **P-P intervals**, P-R interval is constant**; Type II** is identified by P-P interval suddenly lengthens to **almost twice the usual P-P interval**.

(3) **Third-degree SA block**: It causes atrial arrest.

(C) **Clinical features of sick sinus syndrome**: The symptoms are intermittent, varied, and may not correlate with ECG finding. **Syncope, dizziness, and palpitations are common. Bradycardia-tachycardia syndrome** can cause cerebral thromboembolism. CHF and cardiac angina can be aggravated.

(D) **Management**:

(1) Persistent symptomatic sinus bradycardia: Use pacemaker.

(2) Atrial tachyarrythmias: Use digoxin.

(3) After pacemaker to control tachyarrythmias: Use Class I antiarrythmic drugs.

(4) Bradycardia-tachycardia syndrome: Pacemaker can improve symptoms but it can cause cerebral thromboembolism.

(5) Atrial fibrillation plus sick sinus syndrome: Treatment of atrial fibrillation can cause severe bradycardia. Temporary ventricular pacemaker should be used during conversion of atrial fibrillation with slow ventricular rate to sinus rhythm.

91. **Nonparoxysmal AV junctional tachycardia (Important):**

(A) **Clinical features**: It is associated with **acute inferior myocardial infarction, digoxin toxicity, acute carditis such as acute rhematic fever, viral myocarditis, or surgical trauma.**

(B) **ECG findings**: QRS complex is normal or slightly abnormal, junctional focus fires 70 to 130/minute. If the AV junctional focus captures the atria, the retrograde P may be positioned 0.10 second or less in front of QRS, simultaneous with the QRS, or 0.20 second or less after the QRS.

(C) **Management**:

(1) To treat the underlying conditions.

(2) In digoxin toxicity, immediate therapy of digoxin toxicity should be undertaken.

(3) In post open heart surgery or acute inferior MI: No therapy is needed because of transient episodes.

92. **AV block**:

(A) **Clinical features**:

(1) **First-degree AV block** is asymptomatic but soft first heart sound may be present.

(2) **Second-degree AV block** is usually **asymptomatic unless the ventricular rate becomes very slow**. It may cause **characteristic pulse intervals**, change of intensity of first heart sound and intermittent prominent A waves.

(3) **Incomplete heart block** with sinus rhythm, the pulse is regular, slow, and full; markedly varied intensity of first heart sound and intermittent cannon A waves in the jugular venous pulse.

(B) **ECG findings**:

(1) **First-degree AV block**: Prolonged PR interval.

(2) **Second-degree AV block**: (Two types).

(a) Type I (AV nodal): Characteristic **Wenckebach periodicity (PR) interval prolongs with each cycle until a P wave fails to conduct to the ventricles. The longest R-R interval is less than twice the shortest R-R interval.**

(b) **Type II block**: Sudden failure of P wave to conduct to the ventricles without lengthening of PR interval. It is found in bundle branch disease and site of block is distal to the AV node.

(C) **Management**:

(1) **First-degree AV block**: No treatment is needed.

(2) **Type I second-degree block**: Usually resolves **without** the use of temporary pacemaker. When **type I block is due to chronic AV junctional disease**, block can progress slowly to complete AV block. Symptomatic patients need pacemaker.

(3) Type II second-degree block: It is due to chronic bundle branch disease and often progress to complete heart block. Symptomatic patients need pacemaker.

(4) **Symptomatic** second and third-degree heart blocks: Pacemaker should be implanted.

93. **Ventricular premature complexes (VPC's):**

(A) **Clinical manifestations**: VPC's can occur in young persons, increase in frequency with increase in age. VPC's without heart disease have good prognosis. VPC's with heart disease can cause cardiac death. The frequency of **VPC in acute MI increases with the size of the infarct. When VPC's are caused by drug toxicity (e.g., digoxin, quinidine, or TCA)** the lethal rhythm disturbances should be controlled with discontinuation of the drugs.

(B) **ECG findings: The QRS is wide, premature; ST segment and T wave are opposite in direction to the QRS complex; no** premature P wave before QRS complex; the RV interval plus the VR interval is equal to two R-R interval in sinus rhythm.

(1) **Bigeminy**: When every other QRS is a VPC.

(2) **Trigeminy**: When every third QRS is a VPC.
(3) **Pair or couplet**: Two successive VPC's.

(C) **Management:**
(1) Asymptomatic patients with VPC's: Do **not** need treatment.
(2) Symptomatic VPC's: **Beta-blockers** (class II antiarrythmic drug) **are the drug of choice.**
(3) Symptomatic VPC's after acute MI or after cardiac surgery: Use IV lidocaine or procainamide.

94. **Ventricular tachycardia (VT)**:

(A) **Clinical features**: **VT is most common with coronary artery disease, two weeks after acute MI (myocardial infarction) about 10% of patients have VT detected by a 24 hour continuous ECG monitoring** (Important). Patients with **class III or IV** heart failure **develop VT in 40 to 50% of cases in a 24 hour ECG.**
Most episodes of VT is usually brief (3 to 5 consecutive VPC's) **and asymptomatic,** but may increase the mortality. Sustained VT is rare, can progress to ventricular fibrillation, and has poor outcome**. The symptoms depend upon the heart rate and LV function. Remember,** blood pressure and mental status are not useful to distinguish between VT and PSVT.

(B) **ECG findings:** The characteristic of VT is **three or more VPC's in succession at a rate of 100/minute or greater**. Unsustained VT last <15 to 30 seconds. Two findings strongly suggest VT in a tachycardia with wide QRS complex: **Ventricular captures and fusion complexes**. Sinus impulses may capture the ventricle during VT, producing either a **normal QRS** (ventricular capture), or a QRS intermediate in contour between normal and VT (fusion complex).

(C) **Management of VT**:
(1) **Symptomatic unsustained VT: Beta-blockers are the drug of choice** same as VPC's.
(2) **Sustained VT in chronic heart disease**: Acute episode is treated with **IV lidocaine or procainamide** when patients are hemodynamically stable, **use DC cardioversion** in unstable patients.
(3) **Baseline studies** should include 48 hours of continuous ECG monitoring, exercise testing, endocardial electrical stimulation, and cardiac catheterization with coronary angiography.
(4) The first drug of choice is **dl-sotalol**.
(5) **Implantable defibrillator is the treatment of choice** when drug is **not** effective.
(6) In some cases, surgery is the best treatment of choice.

(7) The evaluation of long-term treatment is done by noninvasive methods (24 hours ECG continuous monitoring, exercise testing) and invasive method is endocardial electrical stimulation.

95. **Accelerated idioventricular rhythm (AIVR):**
(A) **Clinical manifestations**: AIVR is usually **asymptomatic**, it is found in 30% cases of acute MI (inferior or anterior infarcts), or after coronary reperfusion.
(B) **ECG findings**: Three or more consecutive QRS complexes of ventricular origin with a rate between 50 and 100/minute. Fusion QRS complexes may be present in the beginning or end of AIVR.
(C) Treatment: No treatment is needed because patients are asymptomatic.

96. **Ventricular flutter and fibrillation**:
(A) **Clinical diagnosis**: Both are catastrophic, patients are **unconscious**, required CPR immediately, without CPR patients cannot survive. **Both are associated with acute myocardial infarction or ischemia, severe hypokalemia, severe hypothermia, electrocution, and drug toxicity (Important). Remember, most victims of ventricular fibrillation who are resuscitated have advanced coronary atherosclerosis and poor ventricular function** (not the above mentioned conditions). Ventricular flutter either converted to sinus rhythm or ventricular fibrillation.
(B) **ECG findings**:
(1) Ventricular flutter is diagnosed when ventricular tachyarrythmia has **large sinusoidal or zigzag QRS's and the rate is between 240 and 280/minute.**
(2) Multiform VT or torsades de pointes is diagnosed by the periodic twisting of the points of the QRS complexes.
(3) Ventricular fibrillation is diagnosed **by absence of QRS complexes and T waves**, but presence of low-amplitude baseline undulation with variability in amplitude and periodicity.
(C) **Management:**
(1) **Ventricular fibrillation**: Defibrillation should be done STAT. Most patients do not have recurrence.
(2) **Recurrent ventricular fibrillation after defibrillation**: Use lidocaine, bretylium, or propranolol to stabilize the rhythm.
(3) Ventricular fibrillation **without** transient or reversible causes (MI, drug toxicity, hypokalemia, hypothermia): The long term evaluation for treatment is the same as ventricular tachycardia (**noninvasive method** of 24 hours continuous ECG monitoring and exercise testing**, invasive**

method is endocardial electrical stimulation; **noninvasive method is better than invasive method**).

(4) VT can be induced by programmed ventricular stimulation. **Uninduced patients have high recurrence rate.**

(5) Multiform VT (torsades de pointes) due to drug toxicity,hypokalemia, or hypomagnesemia: Ventricular pacing, correct hypokalemia, IV magnesium or catecholamine infusion, avoid the drug causing toxicity and class I antiarrythmic action.

97. **Most common cause of sudden cardiac death: Coronary artery disease (75% of cases);** other causes are ventricular hypertrophy or dilatation, diseases of the heart valves, and primary electrophysiologic abnormalities. **Remember, cocaine is an important cause of sudden cardiac death.** **The long QT syndrome** is an important electrophysiologic abnormality which causes sudden cardiac death.

98. Most common **autopsy finding of coronary artery in sudden cardiac death: More than 90% narrowing of at least one coronary artery is found (in 75% of cases).** More than **75% narrowing of three vessels or old myocardial infarction is found (in 66% of cases). Proximal left anterior descending coronary occlusion is an important cause of sudden cardiac death**.

99. **Few important points in sudden cardiac death**:

(1) Death occurs **within 1 hour** of the onset of acute symptoms**, most common age group between 45 and 75**.

(2) Sudden cardiac death, stroke, and myocardial infarction **occur more frequently between 6 A.M. to 12 noon** when a **hypercoagulable state** with **increased platelet aggregability or coronary vasoconstriction exists**.

(3) It is more common during physical exertion.

(4) **Coronary artery disease is the most common cause**.

(5) **Proximal left anterior descending coronary artery** is most commonly involved.

(6) **More than 90% of sudden cardiac deaths are most commonly due to ventricular tachycardia/fibrillation (80% of cases),** and bradyarrythmia or ventricular asystole (20% of cases).

(7) **Treatment of sudden cardiac arrest: Chest compression, clear the airway, mouth-to-mouth ventilation, electrical cardioversion/defibrillation** to treat ventricular tachycardia/fibrillation, **pacing** for bradyarrythmia/asystole, **and drug therapy**.

After successful resuscitation, patients are admitted to CCU for further management to provide **hemodynamic support, prevent a second cardiac arrest, and evaluate cause of the first attack**.

100. **Few important points in arterial hypertension (BP is 140/90 and above):**

(1) It is the most common CVS disease in USA.

(2) **Please remember that a single elevated BP reading** does **not** make the diagnosis of hypertension but patient should be followed.

(3) The diagnosis of hypertension in adults is made when **the average of the two or more diastolic BP measurements** on at least two subsequent **visits is ≥ 90 mm Hg or when average** of multiple systolic BP reading on two or more subsequent **visits is consistently > 140 mm Hg**.

(4) **Isolated systolic hypertension** means systolic BP ≥ 140 mm Hg.

(5) **Most common type of hypertension is essential, primary, or idiopathic hypertension** (95% of all cases).

(6) **Secondary** hypertension is a hypertension of known underlying cause (5% of all cases).

(7) **Malignant** hypertension means diastolic BP usually > 140 mm Hg plus papilledema.

(8) **Accelerated** hypertension means markedly elevated BP plus hemorrhages and exudates in the retina (grade 3 Kimmelstiel-Wilson retinopathy). **Untreated patients may progress to malignant hypertension.**

(9) **Both acclerated and malignant hypertension cause widespread degenerative vascular changes results in following syndrome which** includes sudden onset, fulminant course, extreme BP elevations, grade 3 or 4 K-W retinopathy, encephalopathy, hematuria, and renal dysfunction.

(10) **Complicated hypertension** means complications are due to high BP such as stroke, CHF, myocardial infarction, arterial aneurysm, and renal failure.

(11) **White coat hypertension means** elevation of BP when measured by physician or any health care professional but BP **is normal** when measured outside the health care setting. It is **diagnosed by 24 hour ambulatory or home BP monitoring.**

(12) Hypertension is more common between age **65 and 74**, **blacks** are more affected than whites, **men** are more affected than women.

101. **Classification of hypertension**:

(1) **Mild hypertension (stage I)**: Systolic (140-159 mm Hg), diastotic (90-99 mm Hg).

(2) **Moderate hypertension (stage II)**: Systolic (160-179), diastolic (100-109).

(3) **Severe hypertension (stage III)**: Systolic (180-209), diastolic (110-119).

(4) **Very severe hypertension (stage IV)**: **Systolic (≥ 210),** diastolic (≥ 120).

102. Diagnosis of hypertension:

(A) **Initial evaluation**:

(1) Determine baseline BP.
(2) Assess the degree of target organ disease.
(3) Identify the other CVS risk factors.
(4) To determine any secondary cause of hypertension.
(5) Characterize the patient (gender, race, age, lifestyle, and concomitant illness).
(6) Determine the appropriate therapy.

(B) **Blood pressure measurement**:

(1) Most important is the accurate measurement of BP, patients should be seated comfortably for at least 5 minutes with his or her arm bare.
(2) **In each visit, BP should be measured 2 or 3 times**, one BP reading should be in standing, **and at least 2 minutes should be allowed between readings.**
(3) **Patients with white coat hypertension without** evidence of target organ damage, usually do not need any pharmacologic therapy and **patients with evidence of progressive target organ disease** pharmacologic therapy may be beneficial but should be given very carefully to avoid overtreatment.
(4) **Pseudohypertension: In elderly patients, loss of arterial wall compliance can result in falsely elevated BP**. Osler maneuver can identify the problem. (**Osler maneuver**, BP cuff is inflated above the level of systolic BP, if the pulseless radial or brachial artery is palpable that means the arterial wall is thickened causing pseudohypertension).

(C) Selection of patients for evaluation of secondary hypertension (< 5% of all cases of high BP): Some cases of secondary hypertension are curable. The diagnostic evaluation should be done in the following patients:

(1) Routine history, physical examination, and laboratory investigation suggests secondary cause.
(2) Sudden worsening of BP.
(3) Patients unresponsive to drug therapy.
(4) Patients are younger than 30 years.
(5) Older patients develop new onset of hypertension.

(D) The following things should be done to all patients of high BP before the therapy:

(1) **Complete medical history**: Past and the present should be obtained including lifestyle.

(2) **Complete physical examination should** include BP reading, fundus examination, CVS, abdomen, neurological, AV fistulas under the scar, and other pertinent systems.
(3) **Laboratory investigation should include** routine CBS; urinalysis for proteinuria and hematuria; serum BUN, creatinine, k, glucose, cholesterol, triglyceride, and uric acid levels; chest X-ray for heart size, rule out coarctation, pulmonary edema; serial ECG and echocardiograms.

103. **Treatment of hypertension**:
(1) Antihypertensive treatment is indicated when **diastolic BP ≥ 95 mm Hg** and in those with **lesser** elevation 90 to 94 mm Hg plus high risk of developing CVS complications.
(2) **The initial goal is to lower diastolic BP to levels <90 mm Hg and systollic to levels 140 to 160 mm Hg**.
(3) Excessive reduction of **diastolic BP < 85 mm Hg increases the risk** of ischemic heart disease due to coronary hypoperfusion, particularly in patients with pre-existing coronary artery disease. It is **called J curve hypothesis. Remember, it has no effects on cerebral and renal perfusions**.
(4) Try to correct the underlying CVS risk factors in all patients.
(5) Patients with **stages 2 to 4 hypertension**, even partial BP reduction reduces CVS morbidity.
(6) **Patients with diastolic BP 90 to 94 mm Hg and low risk**: Careful monitoring of BP with nonpharmacologic therapy should be done initially; **if the diastolic BP remains > 90 mm Hg despite nonpharmacologic therapy for 3 to 6 months period then antihypertensive therapy should be started**.
(7) **Nonpharmacologic therapy should be instituted to all patients with hypertension, it may reduce the doses of medication** required to control the BP.
(8) Patients with ISH (systolic > 160 mm Hg)**: Antihypertensive therapy** should be instituted because it reduces BP and CVS morbidity and mortality, particularly myocardial infarction and stroke.
(9) Patients with **high normal BP** (systolic 130-139 mm Hg, diastolic 85-89 mm Hg) **without risk factors**: Careful monitoring and nonpharmacologic therapy should be done.

104. **Lifestyle modification in hypertension**:
(A) **Weight reduction**: It is **the most effective among all nonpharmacologic therapy**. It reduces BP and CVS risk, improve self-image and sense of

well-being. **Remember, patients should avoid appetite suppressants** (e.g., phenylpropanolamine can elevate BP).

(B) **Alcohol restriction**: Acute and chronic alcohol consumption raise the BP. (Moderate alcohol consumption reduces the CVS risk in general population but effects on hypertensive population needs further investigation).

(C) **Exercise: Regular isotonic exercise** (jogging, swimming, or bicycling) causes modest reduction in BP in persons with mild to moderate hypertension. **Current recommendation** for reducing BP and overall CVS risk include **aerobic** exercise maintaining 70 to 80% of **maximal heart rate (220–age)** for 20 to 30 minutes three times a week. Patients should work gradually toward this goal.

(D) **Restriction of dietary sodium**:

(1) **Restriction of dietary sodium can reduce BP in patients with low renin activity**, such as elderly and black patients. **It is called salt-sensitive hypertension.**

(2) Sodium restriction can **minimize** diuretic-induced hypokalemia and helps to **control the BP in patients on diuretic**.

(3) **In some patients** sodium restriction have **no** beneficial effects or **may increase the BP. It is called salt-resistant hypertension.**

(4) Moderate sodium restriction (4 to 6 grams of salt per day) would be beneficial in some hypertensive patients. Do **not** add salt during food preparation or at the table and avoid processed food containing salt preservatives.

(5) **Salt substitutes** (sodium is replaced by potassium) are useful in hypertensive patients **with normal renal function**.

(6) Do **not** decrease calcium and k intake.

(E) **Dietary calcium supplementation**:

(1) Increase dietary calcium (≥1 gram/day) reduces the BP, particularly in patients **with salt-sensitive hypertension** (no response in salt-resistant hypertension).

(2) Calcium supplementation also prevent osteoporosis and GI malignancy.

(F) **Dietary k supplementation**:

(1) BP is reduced with dietary k supplementation.

(2) Higher the sodium intake, more effective k supplementation to reduce BP.

(3) Adequate potassium (K) intake (100 mEq/day) by eating enough fresh fruits, vegetables, or using K supplements prn.

(4) K supplementation **should be avoided** in patients with renal insufficiency, diabetes, or receiving **potassium-sparing diuretics (spironolactone).**

(5) **Hypokalemia** (diuretic use or poor dietary intake) **should be treated**, particularly in patients on digoxin or have coronary artery disease, as it causes arrythmia.

(6) Potassium-sparing diuretic may be used in patients **who develop hypokalemia** either before diuretic therapy or **after non-potassium-sparing diuretic.**

(G) **Dietary magnesium supplementation**: It is **not** recommended to increase dietary magnesium to reduce BP.

(H) **Special diets: Vegetarian diet, increase total fiber** intake, **decrease** total fat intake, **increase polyunsaturated fats** relative to saturated fats, and **increase fish oils which may lower the BP** (preliminary study) and reduce CVS risk.

(I) Cessation of smoking and restriction of caffeine:

(1) **All patients should quit smoking** because of high incidence of malignancy and CVS disease.

(2) Quitting smoking or caffeine does not decrease the BP.

(3) Do **not** take tea, coffee, or smoke immediately before the BP is checked.

(4) **Caffeine and nicotine raise BP acutely**, but **neither cigarette** smokers **nor** coffee drinkers have increased incidence of sustained high BP.

(J) **Relaxation and reducing stress**: They can reduce BP only a bit, so no clinical benefit in treating hypertension.

(K) Overall recommendation in essential hypertension:

(1) Weight loss for overweight patient.

(2) Reduce dietary sodium and increase dietary calcium and k.

(3) Regular exercise.

(4) Stop smoking.

(5) Moderation of alcohol consumption.

(L) **Treatment of Mild Hypertension Study (TOMHS)** demonstrate well motivated patients **with stage 1 and 2 hypertension, modifying life style effectively is the initial therapy of choice than antihypertensive drug therapy (Important).**

The same modifying lifestyle therapy is also effective in the primary prevention of essential hypertension.

105. **Pharmacologic therapy for essential hypertension in addition to continued lifestyle modifications:**

(A) **Initial selection of medication:**

(1) **Diuretics and/or beta-blockers reduce the cardiovascular morbidity and mortality** but have **adverse** metabolic effects. These are the first drugs of choice.

(2) ACE inhibitors, calcium channel blockers, and alpha1-receptor blockers have **favorable metabolic profiles and/or cardiovascular and renal protective** effects but have **not** been tested or shown to reduce CVS morbidity and mortality.

(B) If the BP is **not** adequately controlled, then do the following:

(1) **Increase drug dose**, or.

(2) Substitude **another** drug, or.

(3) Add a second drug from a **different class**.

(C) If the BP is still **not** adequately controlled, then add a **second or third drug** and/or diuretic if not already taken.

106. **Few important points in managing essential hypertension:**

(1) **ACE inhibitors** reduce LV hypertrophy, decrease mortality from CHF, reduce CVS morbidity and mortality in patients with asymptomatic LV dysfunction.

(2) **ACE inhibitors**, like calcium channel blockers, do not alter circulating lipid/lipoprotein levels and also **reduce** insulin resistance.

(3) **ACE inhibitor such as captopril preserves renal function, reduces the need for dialysis and transplantation**, and **reduces mortality rate in patients with insulin-dependent diabetic nephropathy**.

(4) **Alpha-adrenergic blockers have bebeficial effect on the serum lipid profile, decreasing total and/or LDL cholesterol and increasing HDL (protective) cholesterol.** They are also used in **benign prostatic hypertrophy, decrease insulin resistance, and may reduce LVH and platelet aggregability and stimulate synthesis of tPA (tissue plasminogen acivator).**

(5) **Diltiazem** (sustained release preparation of calcium channel blocker) is more effective in reducing BP in **male veterans group** than other antihypertensive drugs.

(6) ALLHAT (The Antihypertensive and Lipid-Lowering Treatment for Prevention of Heart Attack Trial) **is currently under study** to address the issue of vasoprotective effect independent of BP lowering effect.

(7) **Step-down therapy or slowly withdrawal of antihypertensive medication** in patients with stage 1 or 2 hypertension whose **BP has been controlled for 1 year or more. This therapy is most effective in patients with modified lifestyle therapy.**

(8) **Thiazide diuretics** reduce BP in all patient groups, particularly in blacks and elderly. They should be used **cautiously** in diabetes, gout, hypercalcemia, or hyperlipidemia.
Side effects of thiazide diuretics: Impotence, decreased libido, fatigue, muscle cramps, and hypomagnesemia.

(9) **Loop diuretics (furosemide, bumetanide) are useful in hypertensive with CHF, other edematous states, or renal insufficiency (Important).**

(10) **Potassium-sparing diuretics** are used in patients **with low k** prior to diuretic therapy or develop after non-potassium-sparing diuretic therapy. **They are also magnesium-sparing diuretics and prevent hypomagnesemia which is common after thiazide diuretic therapy. Potassium-sparing diuretics may be used very carefully in patients with** diabetes, renal insufficiency, receiving ACE inhibitors, or oral potassium salts because of potential hyperkalemia.

(11) **Beta-blockers** (propranolol, atenolol, carteolol, naldolol, metaprolol, betaxolol) are **more effective in younger than elderly, whites than blacks, and they are initial drug of choice in hypertension plus coronary artery disease, particularly high BP with rapid heart rate and wide pulse pressure (due to sympathetic hyperactivity).**
Side effects of beta-blockers: Decrease HDL cholesterol, increased triglycerides, bradycardia, AV blocks, CHF in susceptible patients, CNS effects (**impotence, decreased mental** acuity, fatigue); **beta-2 bockers exacerbate bronchospasms, peripheral vascular constriction, and Raynaud's phenomenon; they can be used carefully in COPD for bronchospasms and insulin-dependent diabetes for masking symptoms and delaying recovering from hypoglycemia.**

(12) **Labetolol (alpha particularly alpha-1 and beta** adrenergic antagonist): It is **effective in labile hypertension** with marked neurogenic component. **It is used safely in COPD and peripheral vascular disease patients**, and **no** effects on serum lipid levels.

(13) **Calcium channel blockers (nifedipine, diltiazem, verapamil, nicardia, amlodipine, isradipine): Please remember these drugs can increase serum digoxin levels, particularly with verapamil**. They are more effective in **blacks and elderly**, and should be **used cautiously with beta-blockers because of common synnergistic negative inotropic and chronotropic properties (Important). Adverse effects are less common with sustained release.**
Side effects of calcium channel blockers: Sexual dysfunction and CNS effects. Dose adjustment should be done in patients with hepatic disease (metabolized in the liver) **but can be used safely in renal disease**.

(14) **ACE (angiotensin-converting enzyme) inhibitors (captopril, enalapril,lisinopril,quinapril, benzapril, fosinopril, ramipril, perindopril): Most common side effect is nonproductive cough, particularly at night (25% of cases) (Important);** other side effects are high k levels, angioedema, and ARF (acute renal failure).

ACE inhibitors do **not** have the following adverse effects: CNS, sexual dysfunction, and metabolism (do not increase lipid and uric acid levels and glucose intolerance).

ACE inhibitors reduce after load and are the drug of choice in patients with hypertension and CHF, particularly effective **in hypertensive with diabetes** (decrease proteinuria and stabilize renal function in diabetic nephropathy). They are also **effective in hypertensive due to renovascular disease** but **any patients with renal artery stenosis they precipitate acute renal failure. Try to avoid use of ACE inhibitors in renal artery stenosis in solitary kidney, bilateral renal artery stenosis, or post transplantation renal artery stenosis (Important).**

(15) **Centrally acting drugs (clonidine, reserpine, methyldopa, gaunabenz, guanfacine): Mechanism of action**: They stimulate adrenoceptors in the brainstem and hypothalamus, therefore inhibit sympathetic outflow from CNS results in decrease in BP, heart rate, and peripheral vascular resistance. **Side effects**: Most common side effects are **dry mouth, drowsiness, and fatigue. Less** frequent side effects are orthostatic hypotension, sexual dysfunction, hepatitis, **positive Coombs' test, decreased mental activity, and local rash by transdermal clonidine**. **Withdrawal syndrome is due to abrupt withdrawal of centrally acting agents particularly clonidine:** It is characterized by headache, vomiting, anxiety, and rebound hypertension that may need emergency therapy.

(16) **Alpha-adrenergic receptor blockers (prazosin, terazosin, doxazosin):** Due to the development of **longer-acting alpha-antagonists** with **minimal side effects and positive effects on serum lipid levels**, they can be **used as initial drug in patients** with **COPD, diabetes, hyperlipidemia, and peripheral vascular disease.**

Side effects: Dizziness, mild fluid retention, headache, and weakness. **Orthostatic hypotension** can be avoided by giving small dose at bedtime. (They **do not have CNS** side effects such as fatigue, dry mouth, and sexual dysfunction).

(17) **Vasodilators (hydralazine, minoxidil): The combination of vasodilator plus diuretic and beta-blocker is effective in treating patients with severe, refractory, essential, or renal hypertension.**

Side effects: Nasal congestion, tachycardia, fluid retention, palpitation, headache, and in **patients with coronary artery disease develop myocardial ischemia.**

(a) **Hydralazine**: It causes **lupus reaction** which resolves after discontinuation of therapy or sometimes require several years for complete resolution **(Important).**

(b) **Minoxidil: Hirsutism, unexplained percardial effusion, skin rash, and fatigue (Important).**

107. **Hypertensive crisis and its management**:

(A) **Hypertensive urgencies**: BP is >200/120 mm Hg but **absence** of target organ damage such as fundus, renal, CVS, or neurologic system. **Treatment**: Do **not** require immediate BP reduction; **oral initiation of maintenance therapy without acute oral loading for effective and sustained BP reduction, then early follow-up is needed for efficacy and compliance.**

(B) **Hypertensive emergencies**: BP is >200/120 mm Hg and presence of target organ damage such as fundus, renal, CVS, or neurologic system. **Treatment**: Immediate admission to an intensive care plus parenteral antihypertensive medication.

(C) **Clinical manifestation of hypertensive crisis**: Headache, dizziness, blurred vision, palpitations, chest pain, and shortness of breath. **Physical examination reveals fundoscopic changes** (hemorrhage, exudates, papilledema, arteriolar narrowing, arteriovenous nicking); **signs of LV dysfunction** (tachycardia, gallops, cardiomegaly, jugular venous distension, pulmonary edema); **signs of increased incranial pressure** (confusion, somnolence, stupor,seizures, neurologic deficits); **renal insufficiency and microangiopathic hemolytic anemia. Patients may be present with stroke, aortic dissection, LV failure, myocardial ischemia,subarachnoid or intracranial hemorrhage.**

(D) **Laboratory investigations** should include CXR, ECG, complete blood count with smear (hemolysis), serum electrolytes, and urinalysis.

(E) **Treatment of hypertensive crisis**:

(1) The goal is **prompt and gradual reduction in BP, ideally BP should be reduced to 150 to 160/100 to 110 mm Hg and maintained at that level for few days.** Rapid or excessive reduction cause hypoperfusion to the organs, particularly heart (myocardial ischemia). BP should be returned to normal slowly.

(2) **Ischemic stroke: Use nitroprusside, labetalol** (**avoid** beta-antagonists, methyldopa, clonidine, diazoxide).

(3) **Hypertensive encephalopathy: Use nitroprusside, labetalol, diazoxide** (**avoid** beta-antagonists, methyldopa,clonidine).

(4) **Intracerebral hemorrhage: No treatment, or nitroprusside, labetalol** (**avoid** beta-antagonists, methyldopa, clonidine, diazoxide).

(5) **Subarachnoid hemorrhage: Use nimodipine, nitroprusside, labetalol** (**avoid** beta-antagonists, methyldopa, clonidine, diazoxide).

(6) **Myocardial ischemia or infarction: Use IV nitroglycerin, labetalol, calcium antagonists, nitroprusside (avoid** hydralazine, diazoxide).

(7) **LV failure: Use nitroprusside, IV nitroglycerin (avoid** beta-antagonists, labetalol).

(8) **Postoperative crisis: Use labetalol, nitroglycerin, nicardipine, nitroprusside (avoid** trimethaphan).

(9) **Acute renal insufficiency: Use nitroprusside, nicardipine, labetalol (avoid** beta-antagonists, trimethaphan).

(10) **Hyperadrenergic states (cocaine overdose, clonidine withdrawal, diet pills, amphetamines, pheochromocytoma):** Use phentolamine, labetolol, nitroprusside; for clonidine withdrawal use clonidine.

(11) **Eclampsia: Use magnesium sulfate, hydralazine, labetalol, calcium channel blockers (avoid** diuretics, ACE inhibitors,and trimethaphan).

108. **Pulmonary artery (PA) hypertension (elevation of pulmonary artery pressure above the normal range)**:

(1) Normal PA pressure is at sea level: **12 to 15 mm** Hg (systolic 20, diastolic 12, mean 15). **It is approximately 1/12 of the value of systemic BP**.

(2) PA pressure is **elevated in high altitude due to hypoxic arteriolar vasoconstriction.**

(3) **Calculation of pulmonary artery pressure (Ppa)**:
Ppa = CO X PVR +Ppv.
(CO = cardiac output, PVR = pulmonary vascular resistance, Ppv = pulmonary venous pressure). **Normal PVR = 120 dynes.sec.cm^{-5}, normal left atrial pressure = 5 mm Hg ; normal PA pressure = 15 mm Hg; difference between PA pressure and LA pressure = 10 mm Hg.**

109. **Causes of increased pulmonary artery (PA) pressure**:

(A) **Physiologic causes are the following**:

(1) Normal individuals **during severe exercise** cause **slight** increase in PA pressure **because pulmonary vascular resistance (PVR) falls with increase cardiac output**.

(2) High altitude causes increases PA pressure due to hypoxic pulmonary arteriolar vasoconstriction (**means increase PVR**).

(B) **Nonphysiological causes are the following**:

(1) **Increased viscosity** of blood due to increased RBC's.

(2) **Increased intrathoracic pressure** which is directly transmitted to pulmonary vessels. Patients on mechanical ventilator with positive end-expiratory pressure (PEEP) cause increased intrathoracic pressure.

(3) **Increased resistance to pulmonary** blood flow (e.g., pulmonary emboli).

(4) **Loss of pulmonary arterial cross-sectional areas** (e.g., pulmonary fibrosis, vasculitis, tumorous infiltration, pulmonary resection).
(5) **Hypoxia and acidosis** cause increased PA pressure.
(6) Vasoactive chemical compounds (e.g., pyrrolizidine alkaloids) increase PA pressure.
(7) **Increased pulmonary venous (PV) pressure (results in increased PA pressure) is due to PV thrombosis** (e.g., mitral stenosis, LV failure, sickle cell anemia, PV occlusive disease).

110. **Diagnosis of pulmonary hypertension**:
(1) **Most accurate noninvasive diagnostic study is doppler echocardiography but physician must take history and perform physical examination to decide which patients need doppler echocardiography**.
(2) **History and physical examination**:
(a) Patients with **mild to moderate** pulmonary hypertension are **asymptomatic**, **severe** hypertension causes **exertional dyspnea, easy fatigability, syncope, cough, hemoptysis, and rarely**, hoarseness due to compression of left recurrent laryngeal nerve by a dilated pulmonary artery.
(b) Physical examination reveals **increased loudness of the pulmonic component of the second heart** sound, **diastolic murmur of pulmonary regurgitation, left** parasternal heave or lift means RV dilatation; evidence of RV failure (ascites, hepatomegaly, peripheral edema, jugular venous distension, increased loudness of S_3 on inspiration).
Please remember, these physical findings may be **absent** in **patients with severe emphysema and increased thoracic AP diameter due to chest expansion.**
(3) **ECG: RVH is the first suggestion of pulmonary hypertension but RVH is often the late finding. Chronic RV pressure** causes right axis deviation and an R/S ratio >1.0 in lead V_1.
(4) **Echocardiography and doppler study**: Pulmonary arterial systolic BP > 30 mm Hg by doppler study (or cardiac catheterization). **Echocardiogram shows RV dilation/hypertrophy, RA dilatation, and paradoxical septal wall motion associated with RV volume overload. It is the best noninvasive diagnostic study.**
(5) CXR, CT/MRI, or radionuclear ventriculogram: **Enlarged RV and/or pulmonary arteries.**

(6) **Cardiac catheterization and angiography: Pulmonary angiography is the most accurate method of diagnosing pulmonary embolism.** Quantitative estimation of RV failure can be done.

111. **Treatment of pulmonary hypertension:**

(A) **General measures**:

(1) To reduce pulmonary vascular resistance directly.

(2) **Supplementing inspired oxygen, inspired air should be** cool, dry, and free of inhaled irritants.

(3) To correct acid-base abnormalities.

(B) **Specific measures for treating pulmonary hypertension:**

(1) **Diltiazem** (calcium channel blocker) can lower pulmonary vascular resistance by dilating pulmonary vessels if vasoconstriction persists. **Remember, only few patients** have vasoconstriction when first seek for medical advice.

(2) **Life long anticoagulation** for patients high risk for pulmonary embolisms.

(3) **Patients with acute pulmonary embolisms**: IV heparin is followed by oral warfarin for 3 to 6 months.**Thrombolytic therapy or surgical embolectomy** for patients with massive, life-threatening embolism.

(4) **COPD plus pulmonary hypertension**: Inspired oxygen, bronchodilators, and antibiotic for infections.

(5) **High altitude pulmonary hypertension**: Supplemental inspired oxygen or return to sea level.

(6) **Kyphoscoliotic pulmonary hypertension**: Corrective orthopedic surgery.

(7) **Sarcoidosis induced pulmonary hypertension**: Use corticosteroids.

(8) **Mitral stenosis and reactive pulmonary hypertension**: Relieve mitral valve obstruction improves pulmonary pressure.

(9) **Pulmonary veno-occlusive disease**: Cardiopulmonary or pulmonary transplantation should be done.

112. **Laplace formula in cardiac failure**:

$$T = \frac{Pr}{2}$$

(T= tension develop in the wall of the heart during systole; P= mean pressure the cardiac wall is supporting; R= mean radius to ventricular chambers.). Higher the tension is higher the cardiac failure, tension is directly proportional to radius; **larger radius in dilated heart produce higher tension and cardiac failure; smaller radius in normal heart has normal tension**.

113. **Cardiac transplantation**:

(A) **Indications for cardiac transplantation**:

(1) **Most common underlying disease** leading to cardiac transplantation in USA is **ischemic heart disease (IHD) with congestive heart failure (CHF).**

(2) **CHF is the primary indication** of cardiac transplantation. **CHF is the most common cause of hospital admission in medicare population in the USA.**

(3) Idiopathic dilated cardiomyopathy is the second most common disease leading to cardiac transplantation. (CHF secondary to IHD have a higher mortality than CHF secondary to nonischemic causes).

(4) Sarcoidosis (especially limited to restrictive cardiomyopathy) and valvular heart disease when risk of cardiac surgery is extremely high.

(5) Cardiac transplantation **should be limited to those patients who will benefit the most, with improvement in both quality of life and duration of life.** This is based on the following facts:

(a) Cardiac transplantation is **not** a surgical cure for advanced heart disease.

(b) It has high morbidity and mortality in operative and postoperative medical management.

(c) Shortage of cardiac donors.

(B) Evaluation for cardiac transplantation:

(1) Assessment of immunologic state of potential recipient: A **high PRA** (a higher percentage of the panel that is positive) predicts a higher chances of **posttransplant rejection and death. A very high PRA may preclude transplantation**.

(2) **Associated comorbid conditions (such as** irreversible hepatic, renal, or pulmonary failure; irreversible pulmonary artery hypertension; systemic illness with poor prognosis etc.) are contraindications of cardiac transplantation. Near-absolute contraindications are HIV, active severe infection, and neoplasms (except excisable skin cancer).

(3) Patient and family education regarding **prognosis, complications, medical expenses, and follow up after cardiac transplantation**.

114. **Few important points in cardiac transplantation**:

(1) Donors are usually **less than 40 to 50 years of age**, older donors may have higher incidence of IHD.

(2) Heart must be **obtained for use while still functioning** from donors declared brain dead.

(3) Donor heart ischemic time (the time that the donor heart is not beating) should **be as minimum as possible**, preferably < 4 hours **because longer time has higher death after transplantation.**

(4) Immunosuppressive therapy should begin with preoperative administration of azathioprine and often cyclosporine. Intraoperative corticosteroids often should be given and should be continued post operatively. **Cyclosporine and azathioprine are started soon after surgery initially IV then by mouth**. Use of OKT3 (anti-T cell monoclonal antibodies) or ATGAM, RATG (polyclonal antibodies are controversial).

(5) Chronic immunosuppressive therapy includes three drugs (prednisone, azathioprine, and cyclosporine).

(6) **Immunosuppressed** patients should **not** receive Sabin oral polio and MMR (measles, mumps, rubella) vaccination.

(7) **Close contacts** of immunosuppressed patients should not receive Sabin oral polio because of viral shedding **but** contacts may receive MMR.

(8) Immunosuppressed patients **can receive the following vaccinations**: Diptheria, pertussis, tetanus, intramuscular Salk polio, pneumococcus, and Haemophilus influenzae. **Use of influenza vaccine is controversial, may offer some protection.**

(9) The following prophylactic drugs are used:
   (a) Clotrimazole or nystatin for oral candida infections.
   (b) Acyclovir for herpes zoster.
   (c) Gancyclovir for CMV.
   (d) Trimethoprim-sulfamethoxazole or pentamidine for Pneumocystis carinii.
   (e) Pyrimethamine and sulfadiazine (or clindamycin in sulfa-allergic patients) for Toxoplasma gondii.

(10) **The symptoms of rejection** are nonspecific such as lethargy, malaise**, low-grade fever, fatigue, and mood changes. Depressed cardiac function with or without hemodynamic changes indicates acute rejection. Patients may have dyspnea, low BP** (especially if previously hypertensive), **and new S_4 and S_3 heart sounds in rejection.**

(11) The following drugs may be used in rejeciton: Prednisone, IV methylprednisolone, OKT3 ATGAM, plasmapheresis, methotrexate, or chronic cyclophosphamide.

(12) **Most common cause of death in the first year after cardiac transplantation is infection lung and blood-borne infections** are most common. **Bacterial infection (46% of cases) is most common, usually highest around 1 week after transplantation.**
Viral infection (40% of cases, mostly due to CMV) is highest around 1 to 1½ months. **Fungal infection** (7% of cases) occurs within the first month

after transplantation. **Protozoal infection** (6% of cases) occurs from 2 to 5 months after transplantation.

(13) Solid organ transplant recipients have **higher incidence of malignancy** than general population (e.g., squamous cell skin cancer, Kaposi's sarcoma, other sarcomas, lymphoma, cancer of the vulva, perineum, kidney, and hepatobiliary tumors).

(14) **Complications of cyclosporin**: Hypertension, renal toxicity (decreased GFR and increased creatinine), renal tubular acidosis (treated with oral bicarbonate), hepatic dysfunction, hyperuricemia, gout, and **rarely** hemolytic-uremic syndrome (HUS).

(15) **Complications of corticosteroids**: Glucose intolerance, hyperlipidemia, and osteoporosis.

(16) **Complications of azathioprine: Leukopenia is most common**, other **less** common bone marrow suppressive effects are thrombocytopenia, red cell aplasia, reticulocytopenia, and megaloblastic anemia appears 7 to 14 days after the onset of therapy.

(17) Postcardiac transplantation 5 year survival is 75 to 80% in USA.

115. **Heart-lung transplantation:**

(A) **Indications in adults**:

(1) Severe primary lung disease plus secondary severe RV failure.

(2) Primary end-stage cardiac disease plus secondary irreversible pulmonary arterial hypertension.

(B) This procedure is **technically easier than** heart transplantation because it involves only right atrial, aortic, and tracheal anastomosis.

HEMATOLOGY AND ONCOLOGY

1. **Most common cause of anemia in clinical practice**: **Normocytic anemia due to marrow failure (low or normal absolute reticulocyte counts).** Other cause of anemia are acute blood loss and hemolysis (both **have high absolute reticulocyte counts**).

2. **Most common causes of normocytic marrow failure or anemia due to decreased cell production**: Iron deficiency, anemia of chronic disease, and anemias secondary to renal, hepatic, endocrine disorders (hypopituitarism is characteristic,primary adrenal insufficiency, **few patients** of thyrotoxicosis and hyperparathyroidism), **and primary marrow disorders**.

3. **Iron deficiency anemia**: It is usually **hypochromic, microcytic (MCV < 80 fl., normal MCV = 80-100 fl). Remember hematocrit falls before MCV becomes subnormal,** so in iron deficiency anemia initial MCV may be normal, blood smear may be normal **except mild anisocytosis and few microcytic cells.**

4. **Most common causes of iron deficiency anemia**: **Loss of blood** (commonly from gastrointestinal or uterine source) **is the most common cause in developed countries. Imbalance between** demand and supply frequently cause iron deficiency anemia in **normal pregnancy**.

5. **Diagnosis of iron deficiency anemia and anemia of chronic disease**: **The most useful screening test is the serum ferritin level**.
   (1) **Iron deficiency anemia: Low serum** ferritin level, **elevated** TIBC (total iron binding capacity); **low** serum iron level.
   (2) **Anemia of chronic disease: Normal or elevated** serum ferritin level, **decreased** TIBC; low serum iron level (same as iron deficiency anemia).
   (3) **Many patients may have iron deficiency complicated by chronic disease**: TIBC may be **normal or low**. **In both conditions**, the percent saturation of serum transferrin (i.e., the serum iron divided by the TIBC X 100) **is low**. The test is useful when the **value is > 25% that indicates absence of iron deficiency anemia.**
   (4) **Iron deficient patients suffering from** inflammation, malignancy, liver disease, or renal failure: **Serum ferritin level is low**. Presence **of elevated or high normal serum ferritin level** in the above mentioned diseases indicates **absence of iron deficiency anemia** (**Important for Board examination**). (**Serum ferritin** is an acute phase reactant, **it is elevated out**

of proportion to the amount of iron stores in acute and chronic inflammatory disorders, malignancy, liver, and kidney diseases).

6. **Different diseases and blood smears**:
   (1) **Renal failure: Burr cell (echinocytes)**.
   (2) **Liver disease, abetalipoproteinemia: Spur cells (acanthocytes).**
   (3) **Myelofibrosis: Treadrop cells**, nucleated RBC's.
   (4) **Autoimmune hemolysis**, hereditary spherocytosis: **Microspherocytes**.
   (5) **Hemoglobin SS, SC, S-thalassemia: Sickle cells**.
   (6) **Microangiopathic or traumatic hemolysis: Red cell fragments (schistocytes).**
   (7) **Hemoglobin C, SC, thalassemia, liver disease: Target cells**.
   (8) **Cobalamin and folate deficiencies: Hypersegmented neutrophils and macro-ovalocytes are characteristic features.**
   (9) Hereditary elliptocytosis: Elliptocytes.
   (10) **Iron deficiency anemia, thalassemias: Hypochromia, microcytosis**.

7. **Definitive results** for iron stores in the body (Important):
   (1) **Deficient iron stores are confirmed** by **low** ferritin, **high** TIBC.
   (2) **No deficiency in iron stores are confirmed** by high ferritin or high normal values of ferritin.
   (3) These **are all equivocal results**: Low normal ferritin, low serum iron, low or normal TIBC, low percentage.

8. **Common cause of microcytic marrow failure anemias**: Iron deficiency, anemia of chronic disease, thalassemias (**rarely**, aluminium toxicity, thyrotoxicosis).

9. **Causes of macrocytic marrow failure anemias**: **Alcoholism, hypothyroidism**, cobalamin and folate deficiencies, liver disease, artifactual MCV elevations, primary marrow disorders (also cause **normocytic** marrow failure) **and drugs** such as zidovudine (antiviral); hydroxyurea, alkylating agents, and cytosine arabinoside (anticancer); azathioprine (immunosuppressive); methotrexate, pyrimethamine, trimethoprim, pentamidine, triamterene (dehydrofolate reductase inhibitors).

10. **Drugs causing bone marrow suppression or aplasia: Antimetabolites, alkylating agents, phenytoin, sulfonamides**, chloramphenicol, phenylbutazone, and **insecticides**.

11. **Few important points in megaloblastic anemia**:

(1) Serum cobalamine level is usually **low in megaloblastic anemia** but it may be **normal in some patients with or without clinical maifestations**.
(2) **Serum cobalamine level should be done** in all **patients with clinical features** of atrophic glossitis, neurologic **disorder related to cobalamin deficiency** and patients **without** clinical features but positive blood smears (hypersegmented).
(3) **MCV is elevated** before the lowered hematocrit in cobalamin or folate deficiency.
(4) Patients **with less obvious clinical features**, serum cobalamin **values are low-normal or low**: Next helpful investigations are measurement of **methylmalonic acid** and **total homocysteine in serum, both are elevated in cobalamin deficiency.**
(5) Folate deficiency **has elevated homocysteine** (like cobalamin) **but normal methylmalonic acid value**.
(6) **The red blood cell folate** concentration is a **better indicator of tissue folate stores**. It is usually **low** in folate deficiency but in **some patients it may be normal**, or it may **be low in primary cobalamin deficiency** (50% of cases). **The determination of methylmalonic acid can distinguish between folate (normal value) and cobalamin (elevated value) deficiency (please remember this point).**

12. **Most common cause of cobalamin deficiency: Pernicious anemia.** Its specific diagnostic test is the **determination of antibodies to intrinsic factor in serum**.

13. **Macrocytosis** in chronic alcoholic intoxication is due to: It is due to **direct effect of chronic alcohol**. It is **not** due to associated liver disease, reticulocytosis, vitamin B_{12}, or folic acid deficiency.
Treatment: Abstinence from alcohol (**not** the vitamin B_{12} or folic acid).

14. Most common cause of **elevated MCV in nonalcoholic patients: Drug-induced macrocytosis.**
(1) **Mechanism of action**: Drugs **interfere with the DNA synthesis** by erythroid precursors.
(2) Drugs which cause **macrocytosis without anemia** and **normal** reticulocyte count. **Low** hematocrit develops after prolonged high-dose. Sulfasalazine and azathioprine may cause mild elevation of reticulocyte count.

15. **The following tests result indicate hemolysis**:
(1) **Blood (plasma/serum):** Decreased haptoglobin, increased unconjugated bilirubin and LDH (lactate dehydrogenase).

(2) **Urine: Presence of hemosiderin and hemoglobin.**

16. Common causes of hemolytic anemia in adults:
    (1) **Antibody-induced**: Autoimmune hemolysis (warm antibodies), hemolytic transfusion reaction, cold agglutinin disease.
    (2) **Membrane protein anchoring abnormality**: Paroxysmal nocturnal hemoglobinurea.
    (3) **Mechanical fragmentation**: Intravascular coagulation, malignant hypertension, malfunctioning valve prosthesis, thrombotic thrombocytopenic purpura, and cancer chemotherapy.

17. **Investigations in hemolytic anemia**: Physician must decide **which laboratory test is appropriate after the history, physical examination, and blood smear evaluation**. The following few examples are important:
    (1) A previously healthy middle-aged woman appears with sudden onset of severe anemia, smear reveals many microspherocytes: Initial investigation should be **Coombs' test**.
    (2) A man with H/O malignant hypertension appears with signs of hemolysis, smear reveals many RBC fragments: **No further investigation is needed to diagnose microangiopathic hemolytic anemia** secondary to damage to small blood vessels.
    (3) A young black woman with H/O episodic bone pain, blood smear reveals sickle cell**: First investigation of choice is hemoglobin electrophoresis** to diagnose sickle cell disease.

18. **Most common cause of aplastic crisis**: **Virus**. It causes aplastic crisis in many hemolytic anemia, including sickle cell disease. **Parvovirus B19 infection of red cell marrow precursor (CFU-E) causes an aplastic crisis without compensatory reticulocytosis.**

19. **Bone marrow examination in anemia patients**:
    (1) Bone marrow examination (aspiration or biopsy) is **not needed in > 90% of patients.**
    (2) Bone marrow examination is indicated in the following conditions:
        (a) Primary bone marrow disease.
        (b) Pancytopenia of unknown cause.
        (c) Suspected tumor infiltration, myelofibrosis, or granulomatous infections: Biopsy is better than aspiration.
        (d) Severe unexplained anemia.
        (e) Monoclonal gammopathies.
        (f) Suspected combined anemias (iron plus B_{12} deficiencies).

20. **Blood transfusion in chronic anemic patients:**
    (i) There is **no** absolute number to give blood transfusion. Try to avoid blood transfusion.
    (ii) Never give blood transfusion **to avoid** diagnostic evaluation for more definitive diagnosis and treatment.
    (iii) Blood transfusion depends upon **patients symptom and functional status**.
    (iv) Blood transfusion **may be required** in elderly anemic patients before colonoscopy or barium enema.

21. **Decreased MCV with normal hematocrit:**
    (i) Heterozygous alpha-or beta-thalassemia (Important).
    (ii) Some patients of polycythemia (Vera or hypoxia).
    (iii) Previously high hematocrit which falls to normal.
    (iv) Rarely in self-limited or treated iron deficiency anemia.

22. **Increased MCV with normal hematocrit**:
    (i) Chronic alcoholism.
    (ii) Cobalamine or folate deficiency.
    (iii) Drugs (zidovudine, azathioprine, hydroxyurea, cytosine arabinoside, alkylating agents methotrexate, trimethoprim, pyrimethamine, trimethoprim, pentamidine, triamterence).
    (iv) Myelodysplasia (e.g., sideroblastic anemia or refractory anemia following antimetabolite treatment).
    (v) Young adult develops congenital Fanconi's anemia (marrow aplasia)
    (vi) Reticulocytosis in compensated hemolytic disease.

23. **Aplastic anemia**: It is most commonly occurs in young adults approximately **25 year of age** except the patients on cancer chemotherapy.
    (A) **Severe** aplastic anemia: It means patients have two of the following three values:
        (i) **Absolute neutrophil count** (percentage of polymorphs, plus band forms multiplied by the total WBC count) **< 500 per cubic millimeter**.
        (ii) Platelet count <20,000 per cubic millimeter.
        (iii) Reticulocyte count < 1%.
    (B) **Important etiologic agents**:
        (i) Most common is idiopathic.
        (ii) Radiation injury.
        (iii) Drugs: Cytotoxic drugs (alkylating agents, antimetabolites, antimiotics) used for cancer chemotherapy; antibiotics (chloramphenicol).
        (iv) **Infections**: Hepatitis (most commonly non-A, non-B, and non-C) is the most common infection preceding aplastic anemia.

(v) **Immunologic disease:** Eosinophilic fascitis; **pure red blood cell aplasia associated with thymoma**.

(C) **Clinical manifestations**:

(i) **History**: Most common early symptom is the bleeding (**easy bruising, nose bleeds, oozing from the gums, or heavy menstrual bleeding**, and sometimes petechiae).

(ii) **Physical examination: Petechiae, pallor, ecchymoses are frequently present;** (**absence** of lymphadenopathy and splenomegaly); **Cafe-au-lait spots and short stature are found in Fanconi's anemia**; peculiar nails in dyskeratosis congenita.

(D) **Diagnosis of aplastic anemia**: Combination of **pancytopenia with fatty, empty bone marrow**.

(E) **Treatment:**

(i) **Bone marrow transplantation** from sibling donor is the best treatment of choice in patients < 20 years old. It is **not** recommended for patients **older than 45 years** because of opportunistic infections and interstitial pneumonitis. Management of patients between **20 to 45 years** depend upon the general clinical condition, transfusion history, and medical insurance coverage. **Most patients do not find suitable donor**.

(ii) **Immunosuppressive therapy: Antithymocyte globulin (ATG) therapy is effective in 50% cases** of autologous bone marrow function. Unresponsive patients should be treated with **3 to 6 month course of cyclosporine. The combination of ATG plus cyclosporine** is superior to ATG alone **as initial therapy of severe aplastic anemia**.
Complications after long term immunosuppressive therapy: Relapse, myelodysplasia, paroxysmal nocturnal hemoglobinuria (**positive Ham test**: abnormal sensitivity of RBC to complement), or acute leukemia. **ATG can cause serum sickness** about 10 days after onset of therapy. Patients should be treated **with methylprednisolone** to control the immune reaction of heterologous protein infusion.
Complications of cyclosporine therapy: Nephrotoxicity, high BP, seizures, and Pneumocystis carinii pneumonia.

(iii) **Other therapy:**

(a) Patients with moderate disease, severe pancytopenia, and failure of immunosuppressive therapy: Use **nandrolone decanoate** (weekly IM injection for 3 months) or **oxymetholone** (by mouth).

(b) Antibiotic for infection: Broad-spectrum antibiotic, combination of **aminoglycoside, cephalosporin,** and **semisynthetic** penicillin; or alternative monotherapy with **ceftazidime. Add vancomycin when indwelling catheter is contaminated**. Remember, **therapy is empiric** and should **not** wait for cultures.

(c) **Handwashing technique** for prevention of infection.
(d) Nonabsorbed antibiotic for gut decontamination may be useful but **rarely tolerated** for GI side effects.
(e) **Total reverse isolation** is **not** helpful because it is difficult, expensive, and does **not** reduce mortality from infection.
(f) **Blood and platelet transfusion** to maintain the adequate levels. **Never** give blood products from family members; **single-donor platelets (after removal of leukocytes) are the best product**.
(g) **Avoid aspirin and NSAID's** that inhibit platelet function.

24. **Myelodysplasia (cytopenias plus dysmorphic or abnormal bone marrow findings)**:
(1) **Etiology:** Radiation, benzene, radiomimetic alkylating drugs; **chromosomal association (5q-syndrome)**.
(2) Clinical features: (**Idiopathic** variety is most commonly found in **elderly, 68 years; drug related** variety is **not** age related). Asymptomatic (50% cases) or symptomatic (50% cases) patients appear with **anemia, pallor, dyspnea, weakness, and fatigue**. (**Remember, fever and weight loss indicates myeloproliferative** than myelodysplastic process)
Sweet's syndrome (febrile neutrophilic dermatosis) may be present.
(3) **Diagnosis**:
(a) Blood: **Anemia** with or without bicytopenia or pancytopenia, macrocytosis, **platelets are large and lack** granules, **neutrophils** may lack granules, show Pelger-Huet, ring or segmented nuclei and contain Dohle's bodies; total WBC count is **normal or low** (**except** monocytosis is found in chronic myelomonocytic leukemia)
(b) **Bone marrow:** Usually normocellular or hypercellular; may be hypocellular. The **specific diagnosis depends upon the presence of ringed sideroblasts,** the **percentage of blasts,** and **increased immature** myelomonocytes. Chromosomal analysis should be done from bone marrow.
(4) **Treatment: (Not satisfactory)**:
(a) Sometimes sideroblastic patients respond to pyridoxine.
(b) Androgens and corticosteroids may improve blood counts but do **not** increase the survival.
(c) To improve blood counts, use **granulocyte or granulocyte-macrophage colony-stimulating growth factors** results in increased WBC counts, reduced blast cells, but decreased response to platelet and reticulocyte counts.
(d) Supportive therapy: Same as aplastic anemia (discussed in item number 23).

25. **Most common cause of death in myelodysplasia**: **Due to complications of pancytopenia** (**not** due to leukemic transformation).

26. **Normocytic normochromic anemia (MCV 80 to 95 fl)**: It is found in early stages of most anemias, early stage of blood loss, anemia of chronic renal insufficiency (due to **inadequate erythropoietin** production from **renal interstitial cells**), anemia of liver disease in less advanced stages (advanced stages cause **macrotic** anemia), and anemia of endocrine abnormalities (hypothyroidism, hypopituitarism; **remember Cushing's disease causes erythrocytosis due to androgen stimulation of the bone marrow; Addison's disease** has **RBC mass reduction** but it is **not** evident due to concomitant **reduction of plasma volume due to deficiency of mineralocorticoids**).

27. **Clinical features, diagnosis, and treatment of iron deficiency anemia**:
   (A) **Clinical features: Fatigue** is disproportionately higher than degree of anemia. (Fatigue is due to **decreased** iron-containing enzymes and decreased energy production in muscles; **iron therapy cures the fatigue**). The other **less common** clinical manifestations are glossitis, angular stomatitis, atrophy of gastric mucosa with achlorhydria, atrophic rhinitis with foul nasal discharge, **koilonychia** (brittle fingernails), chlorosis (greenish discoloration of the skin). **Elderly women** may develop **dysphagia** due to esophageal web (**Plummer-Vinson or Patterson-Kelly syndrome** may change to malignancy later on). Iron therapy may **not cure the web** which may need **esophageal dilatation for relief of the symptoms**.
   (B) **Diagnosis of iron deficiency anemia:**
      (1) **Hypochromic, microcytic anemia; Low** MCV, MCH, and MCHC; reticulocyte baseline count.
      (2) **Serum: Low ferritin, low iron, increased TIBC; increased levels free erythrocyte protoporphyrin** (iron is incorporated into the protoporphyrin ring in final step of heme synthesis).
   (C) **Treatment of iron deficiency anemia:**
      (1) Recognition of anemia, identification of the causes (**benign cause of aspirin induced GI bleed** or serious cause of **occult malignancy**), and treatment of the underlying conditions **are the most important**.
      (2) **Ferrous sulfate is the treatment of choice**. It is best absorbed in empty stomach but best tolerated with meals. If patients cannot tolerate then use ferrous gluconate.
      (3) **Very rare condition** when patients **cannot** tolerate or absorb iron from GI tract, then use **parenteral form (IM or IV) of iron-dextran**

complex (side effects are anaphylaxis, arthralgias, myalgias, and adenopathy). **A small test dose** should be given to rule out the hypersensitivity reaction.
Formula: Dose (ml) = 0.0476 x wt (kg) x (normal hemoglobin-observed hemoglobin) + (1 ml/5 kg) to maximum of 14 ml to replete iron stores.
Total dose should be diluted with normal saline (1:20 dilution) and **infused slowly over several hours and watch for side effects**.

28. **Step by step responses of iron therapy in iron deficiency anemia (Important)**:
    (1) **First**, improvement in symptoms (fatigue and lassitude).
    (2) **Second**, maximum **reticulocytosis after 7 to 10 days**.
    (3) **Third, rise** of hemoglobin levels after 2 to 2½ weeks, normal hemoglobin level about 2 months.
    (4) **Finally, normal** ferritin levels suggest discontinuation of iron therapy.

29. **Anemia of chronic disease (ACD)**: It is a hypochromic anemia without iron deficiency due to **deficient delivery of iron to developing RBC's even with increased iron stores**.
    (1) **ACD is the most common anemia in hospitalized patients. (Iron deficiency anemia is the most common anemia in general population)**.
    (2) **Clinical manifestations:** ACD itself does **not** produce symptoms. The anemia is mild and patient is **asymptomatic unless** it is superimposed upon underlying disease condition. ACD may help in diagnosing **underlying occult disease**.
    (3) **Diagnosis of ACD**:
        (a) **Normochromic normocytic anemia** (60 to 70% cases); microcytic anemia (30 to 40% cases) may confuse with iron deficiency anemia.
        (b) **Elevated serum ferritin** (low in iron deficiency anemia) and **elevated** ESR (normal in iron deficiency anemia).
        (c) Increased bone marrow iron stores (decreased in iron deficiency anemia)
    (4) **Treatment of ACD:**
        (a) To treat the underlying condition.
        (b) Most patients do **not** need any other therapy (Erythropoietin **and P-RBC may be helpful** but are **not** needed because symptoms of ACD is **not** severe; do **not** give iron which causes iron overload).

30. **Sideroblastic anemias:** It is an **uncommon cause of hypochromic anemia**.
    (1) **Characteristic features: Paradoxical finding of hyperferremia and a nearly total transferrin saturation plus hypochromic anemia**.

(2) **Different types** of sideroblastic anemia:
   (a) Hereditary: X-linked recessive, clinical manifestations of **hypochromic, normocytic anemia** in **early adulthood**.
   Treatment: Larger dose of pyridoxine.
   (b) **Idiopathic refractory type (acquired)**: **Unknown** cause, clinical manifestations of **hypochromic, mildly macrocytic** anemia in **elderly patients** as **predominently erythroid manifestation** of myelodysplastic syndrome.
   Pseudo-Pelger-Huet anomaly: Idiopathic sideroblastic **anemia plus leukopenia due to WBC developmental defects**.
   Treatment: Blood transfusion is the only effective therapy plus chelation (deferoxamine) prn. **Very limited** success with pyridoxine, androgen; erythropoietin.
   Associated diseases: Cancer, rheumatoid disease, and endocrine disorders. Remember, treatment of underlying condition **does not correct** the sideroblastic anemia.
   (c) Sideroblastic anemia due to drugs or toxins: Intake of large amounts of alcohol over several weeks can cause this anemia.
   Mechanism of actions: Alcohol interferes with pyridoxine metabolism and produces toxic effect on mitochondria.
   Treatment: Abstinence from alcohol. Bone marrow changes usually persists for 7 to 10 days after withdrawal of alcohol.

31. **Most common cause of cobalamine deficiency in USA**: **Pernicious anemia**. It is due to gastric mucosal defects results in **inadequate intrinsic factor,** and **subsequently inadequate absorption of cobalamine**.

32. **Megaloblastic anemias**:
   (A) **Etiology:** Cobalamine deficiency (most common), folate deficiency, drugs, and **rarely** enzyme deficiencies. Drugs are **5-FU** (flurouracil) and **leucovorin** (5-formyltetrahydrofolate), both inhibits **thymidylate synthase enzyme**.
   (B) Cobalamine deficiency and diets: It is present **only** in animal products (**not** present in plants). Persons who do **not** eat meat, fish, eggs, milk, cheese or any other animal products, **are likely to develop cobalamine deficiency unless supplemented with multivitamin tablets; cobalamine is absorbed by the intrinsic factor in the stomach which also contains cobalamine-binding protein** secreted from saliva.
   (C) **Folate deficiency and diets:** It is found in **both plants and in animal products**. **Most common cause of folate deficiency is the decreased intake; other causes are** chronic **alcohol consumption, triamterene** (impair the utilization of folate), **pregnancy, hyperthyroidism, chronic**

hemolytic disease, exfoliative skin diseases and hemodialysis. Clinical manifestations appear after (approximately) 4 months of decreased intake.

(D) **Clinical manifestation of megaloblastic anemia (all causes produces similar clinical and laboratory finding):**

(1) **Hematologic manifestations**: **Anemia develops slowly over many months and patients remain asymptomatic until the hematocrit is <20%**, high MCV (>100 up to 140 fl); **low** reticulocytes, neutrophils, and thrombocytes; peripheral smear **reveals hypersegmented neutrophils,** macro-ovalocytes, and variation size and shape of RBC's.

(2) **Bone marrow:** Hypercellularity, megaloblastic morphologic changes, giant bands, and metamyelocytes.

(3) **Neurologic manifestations:** It may occur **early or late due to loss of myelin with axonal degeneration**. Patients appear with **paresthesia,** ataxia; **impaired** pain, touch, position, or vibration sense; memory loss, disorientation; **decreased** reflexes and muscle strength; Babinski's sign and spasticity; urinary and fecal incontinence and impotence; decreased vision or optic altrophy.

(4) **Psychiatric manifestations:** Depression, listlessness, acute confusional state, paranoia, insomnia, hallucinations, delusions, psychosis, suicide, and personality changes.

(E) **Diagnosis of megaloblastic anemias:**

(1) **Cobalamine deficiency: Decreased or low normal serum cobalamine** (normal 200-900 pg/ml), **elevated serum levels** of **methylmalonic acid** (**normal** 70-270 nm) and **homocysteine** (normal 5-16 micro M); **normal** serum folate (normal 2.5-20 ng/ml).

(2) **Folate deficiency: Decreased or low** normal serum folate, **elevated** serum homocysteine levels; **normal** serum methylmalonic acid and cobalamine values.

(F) **Treatment of megaloblastic anemia**:

(1) Cobalamine deficiency: IM or SC (subcutaneous) injection of **either cyanocobalamin (1000 micrograms) or hydroxocobalamine**. Patients who **cannot** take injection, oral cobalamine should be given to those patients only. Injections should be given **weekly for 8 weeks and then monthly for life**.

(2) Patients with neuropsychiatric abnormality may **have normal** MCV, **normal hematocirts** or both **up to 50% cases with cobalamine deficiency. The higher the severity of neuropsychiatric abnormality, the lower the degree of anemia (inverse corelation)**.

(3) **Folate deficiency:** Oral folic acid tablet (1 to 2 mg daily dose).

(4) Cobalamine or folate deficiency: **Rarely** RBC transfusion are required (try to **avoid** the transfusion) and should be given very slowly to avoid CHF. **Only additional therapy** is to give antibiotics in bacterial overgrowth or dietary changes in celiac disease.
(5) **Drugs or other causes**: Avoid or reduce the doses of drugs. Some patients may respond to **pharmacologic doses of pyridoxine or thiamine**.

33. **Few important points in hereditary spherocytosis (HS)**:
   (1) **Autosomal dominant** (75% cases), rest are combination of autosomal recessive and new mutations
   (2) Molecular defects in vertical connections among **spectrin, ankyrin, protein 4.2, and protein 3**.
   (3) **Anemia, jaundice, and splenomegaly** are the characteristic clinical features.
   (4) The following complications can occur:
      (a) Hemolytic crisis is most frequent, mild, and clinically **not** significant.
      (b) Aplastic crisis occurs **less** frequently but **more severe results in heart failure and require transfusion. Remember** aplastic crisis is usually **caused by parvovirus B19**.
      (c) **Megaloblastic crisis** occurs when dietary intake of folic acid is **not** adequate due to **increased demand by erythroid** bone marrow in HS or other hemolytic anemias.
      (d) **Gallstones in HS is due to increased bilirubin production, most common after fifth decades (55 to 75% cases)** and 40 to 50% cases between second and fifth decades.
      (e) Other rare complications: Gout, chronic erythematous dermatitis, or indolent ankle ulcers. **All of them disappear after splenectomy**.
      (f) **Extramedullary tumors** (usually in the thorax) **which can bleed severely if biopsy is done, so diagnosis is made by MRI. Tumors do not disappear after splenectomy (Important)**.
      (g) Spinocerebellar degeneration and familial myocardiopathy are **rare association**.
   (5) **Diagnosis of HS:**
      (a) **Most reliable diagnostic test is incubated osmotic fragility (OF) which is almost always abnormal in HS**.
      (b) Presence of **spherocytes** in the smear is the second most reliable finding. **Remember,** spherocytes could **be artifact** in normal blood smear and it is also found in **other disease condition such as immunohemolytic anemias (warm antibody type)**.

(c) **Most dependable sign of hemolysis is high reticulocyte count** (than presence of jaundice). **Elevated reticulocyte count is always present with or without anemia in HS**. (Important to remember for examination).

(d) **Increased MCHC** (mean corpuscular hemoglobin concentration) **level 36 or more** is present in 50% cases of HS.

(6) **Treatment of HS:**

(a) **Splenectomy cures almost all cases of spherocytosis. Recent study shows** that **partial splenectomy** is effective because it can relieve hemolysis and also maintain residual **splenic phagocytic** function.

(b) **All splenectomized patients must receive polyvalent pneumococcal vaccine (given several weeks before surgery**); Immunization with **meningococcal vaccines and Haemophilus influenzae B vaccine** (if **not** given previously) should also be given. Prophylactic antibiotic (**penicillin-VK or equivalent, 250 mg orally twice daily in adults**) should be given possibly for life.

(c) **Folic acid:** It is given **before splenectomy** to prevent folate deficiency.

(d) **Postsplenectomy changes in blood: Howell-Jolly bodies are the most characteristic finding;** target cells, acanthocytes, and siderocytes are present. **Please remember, spherocytosis persists because basic RBC defect is not changed but conditioned microspherocytes disappear**.

(e) Ischemic heart disease may increase after splenectomy.

34. **Indications of splenectomy in HS:**

(1) All patients with severe disease (hemoglobin ≤8 grams/dl, reticulocytes ≥ 10%) and moderate disease (hemoglobin 8 to 11 grams/dl, reticulocytes ≥8%), if they **have reduced vitality due to anemia** or **compromised perfusion of vital organs** or **developed extramedullary hematopoietic tumor**.

(2) **Splenectomy is controversial** in **asymptomatic** patients with **moderate HS**.

(3) Do **not** perform splenectomy: Mildly symptomatic patients with compensated hemolysis (hemoglobin 11 to 15 grams/dl, reticulocytes < 6 to 8%).

35. **Most common enzyme defect associated with hemolytic anemia**: **G6PD (glucose-6- phosphate dehydrogenase) deficiency**.

36. **G6PD deficiency**:

(A) **Clinical manifestations:** Patients appear with **jaundice, hemoglobinuria** (red-brown to black urine), **hemoglobinemia** (pink to brown plasma), abdominal or back pain, **symptoms of anemia** (palpitation, dizziness,

headache, dyspnea), and in **secere** case **renal tubular necrosis and renal failure**.
Patients may **be asymptomatic without** hemoglobinuria but **hemoglobin may be only 3 to 4 grams/dl (Important)**.
Patients (both Gd^{A-} and Gd^{MED}) are **completely asymptomatic without hemolysis** and **normal** blood smear **between hemolytic episodes (Important)**.

(B) **Causes of hemolysis in G6PD deficiency**: Most important cause is **infection** (every kind of infection), other causes are **fava beans** (Italian broad beans), **drugs** such as anitmalarials, sulfonamides and sulfones, nitrofurans, antihelminthics, analgesics (aspirin, **acetaminophen, the later is safe alternative**), probenecid, vitamin K, BAL, naphthalene, methylene and toluidine blue.

(C) **Two types (Gd^{A-} and Gd^{MED}): Gd^{A-}** is common in African populations, cause **moderate** hemolysis, rarely need transfusion, **infection stimulates the hemolysis but not the drugs**.
Gd^{Med} is common in Mediteranean populations, cause **severe** hemolysis, may need transfusion, **both drugs and infections** stimulate hemolysis.

(D) **Genetics in G6PD deficiency:** X-linked disease (males have one type and females have two types). **Patients are protected** from **Plasmodium falciparum malaria**.

(E) **Diagnose of G6PD deficiency:**

(1) Definitive diagnosis is made by the **assay of the enzyme** depends on **direct spectrophotometric measurement of NADPH production**. It is more sensitive **than screening test**. The sensitivity can be increased by comparing the level of G6PD to other age-dependent enzymes.

(2) Screening test are **less** sensitive, it is **based on NADPH-mediated dye decolorization or on the reduction of methemoglobin in the presence of methylene** blue.

37. **Few important points in paroxysmal nocturnal hemoglobinuria (PNH)**:

(1) **Chronic intravascular hemolysis** is a more common clinical presentation.

(2) PNH is a **primary bone marrow disorder** that affects all the cells (RBC, WBC, platelet, pluripotent hematopoietic stem cells).
Rarely, PNH can evolve into acute leukemia.

(3) Patients appear with **abdominal, musculoskeletal, and bone pain** associated with **hemolysis, hemoglobinuria,** or **thrombosis of hepatic veins (Budd-Chiari syndrome)** or **other veins** (cerebral, portal, splenic, mesenteric). **Thrombosis are common cause of death**. Acute intestinal infarction may occur.

(4) **Diagnosis of PNH**:

(a) Ham's test: **Hemolysis of cells in PNH** (cells are incubated in acidified serum) but **no hemolysis of normal cells**.
(b) Sugar-water test: **Hemolysis of cells in PNH** (patients serum is mixed with 5% dextrose in water and incubated with patient's cells) but **no** hemolysis in normal cells.

(5) **Treatment of PNH:**
(a) **Prednisone** can decrease the rate of hemolysis in **some** patients.
(b) Anemic patients respond to **androgens, including the anabolic steroid danazol**. Androgens may increase the platelet counts.
(c) Bone marrow transplantation is **not** effective in PNH.
(d) Oral iron replacement therapy should be attempted (acute iron replacement can cause **hemolysis**), parenteral iron is given in severe loss of iron.
(e) Anticoagulation therapy is used for thrombosis.
(f) Acute intestinal infarction may require surgical resection.

38. **Autoimmune hemolytic anemia is most commonly due to**: **IgG**; other type is IgM-induced autoimmune hemolytic anemia (or cold hemagglutinin disease). IgG-induced autoimmune hemolytic anemia is either idiopathic or due to underlying disease conditions such as immunoprolilferative disorders (SLE, chronic lymphocytic leukemia, and non-Hodgkin lymphoma). IgG-induced automimmune hemolytic anemia is either idiopathic (or primary) or due to underlying disease conditions (or secondary) such as **mycoplasma pneumoniae,** SLE, chronic lymphocytic leukemia, and non-Hodgkin lymphoma.

39. **Few important points in autoimmune hemolytic anemia (both IgG and IgM)**:
(1) Patients appear with **symptoms of weakness, malaise, and light-headedness due to anemia**; other common symptoms are **pallor, fever, jaundice, dark urine, and abdominal pain**.
(2) Physical examination findings depend upon the underlying disease conditions (**mild** splenomegaly in severe autoimmune hemolytic anemia, **massive** splenomegaly in lymphoma, and **hepatosplenomegaly plus lymphadenopathy** in non-Hodgkin lymphoma).
(3) **Diagnosis**:
(a) **The definitve diagnostic test is positive result or direct Coombs' test** (**Important for Board examination**).
(b) **Blood test:** Anemia, reticulocytosis, smear shows spherocytes, polychromasia, erythrophagocytosis, and nucleated RBC's.
(4) **Treatment:**
(a) Many patients do **not** need any treatment because hemolysis is mild.

(b) Treatment of underlying disease also control the hemolytic anemia.

(c) Patients with significant anemia need the following therapeutic intervention: **glucocorticoids (prednisone) should be the first drug of choice in IgG-induced hmeolytic anemia** but it is **not** effective in IgM-induced hemolytic anemia because of large **anit RBC** antibody. Patients with **cold-hemagglutinin** (**or IgM**) **disease respond best to avoid cold and control the underlying disease; Splenctomy** is indicated in patients **unresponsive to glucocorticoid or require > 10 to 20 mg prednisone daily or higher doses in every other day therapy**.
Immunosuppressive drugs are used in treating autoimmune hemolytic anemia. **Most commonly used drugs are thiopurines** (6-mecaptopurine, azathioprine, and thioguanine) and alkylating agents (cyclophosphamide and chlorambucil).**These drugs reduce the production of antibody and take at least 2 weeks to achieve therapeutic response**. These drugs may be used 3 to 4 months for reasonable clinical treatment.
Indications for immunosuppressive therapy: Persistent uncontrolled hemolytic anemia despite prednisone and splenectomy or patients who are resistant or intolerant of prednisone and poor surgical candidate for splenectomy.
Blood transfusion is **rarely** required because anemia is developed gradually. **In cold agglutinin disease, blood should be prewarmed (to 37°C) like and other fluids for infusion (Important)**.
Intravenous gamma globulin may be effective in IgG variety but **not** effective in IgM-induced cases.

40. **Evan's syndrome:** Autoimmune hemolytic anemia plus thrombocytopenia. Many patients have **chronic lymphadenopathy or dysgammaglobulinemia**. **Treatment: Prednisone** is effective in acute episode but is **not** needed between relapses. **Splenectomy** is indicated in patients unresponsive or inadequate response to steroids.

41. **Most common drug-induced immune hemolytic anemia: Methyldopa type (or levodopa)**; other types are **hapten type** (high dose of penicillin) and **quinidine type** (quinidine, quinine, sulfonamides, chlorpromazine, and stibophen).

42. **Signs and symptoms of drug-induced immune hemolytic anemia and diagnosis**:

(A) **Signs and symptoms**: Same as autoimmune hemolytic anemia. Quinidine can cause severe intravascular hemolysis.

(B) **Diagnosis:** By history and in vitro assay. **Positive Coombs' test** in hapten type, quinidine type, and 25% cases of methyldopa type. **Methyldopa type have positive antierythrocyte antibodies in almost all patients** and 15% have positive antinuclear antibody.

43. **Few important points in unstable hemoglobins (or reduced solubility hemogloibins or more oxidative damage hemoglobins)**:
    (1) **Rare**, caused by **both** alpha and beta globin, the beta globins **is more symptomatic** than alpha.
    (2) Hemolysis is precipitated by **oxidative stress,** such as **infection** or exposure to oxidizing drugs (e.g., quinine).
    (3) Patients appear with chronic hemolytic **anemia,** unexplained **jaundice**, **premature biliary tract disease due** to gallstones produced by hemolyzed RBC's, **unexplained reticulocytosis**, dark urine, leg ulcers, or transient jaundice.
    (4) Diagnosis is made by the **presence of Heinz body** (intracellular precipitated hemoglobins). Sometimes Heinz body may be **absent** in **less** acute hemolysis and it is removed by the spleen. Two provocative tests are: the heat instability test (**unstable hemoglobins precipitate to 50°C**) or isopropanol instability test (unstable hemoglobins precipitate due to insolubility in 17% isopropanol).
    (5) **Please remember**, hemoglobin electrophoresis should be done but it is **not** the sole criteria to rule out or rule in a hemoglobinopathy.
    (6) **Treatment:** Avoid the drugs causing hemolysis, **few patients** may need blood transfusion, **severely morbid patients** need splenectomy especially if hypersplenism has developed, **treat infection** which precipitates hemolysis.

44. A male smoker who is working either as tunnel toll booth collectors or casisson workers came for routine physical examination, CBC study **reveals erythrocytosis**. He has positive family history of unexplained **erythrocytosis**. **Definitive diagnostic test**: P_{50} curves shows **lower than normal P_{50} values** (i.e., **shift to the left** means hemoglobin reaches 50% saturation at **lower** partial pressure of oxygen and poor tissue oxygen delivery). Hemoglobin electrophoresis should be done but may **not** be helpful.
    Most likely dagnosis: **High-affinity hemoglobins (Hb Zurich)**. **Most common cause of a low P_{50} value is carbon manoxide poisoning. Most common cause of hemoglobin-carbon monoxide is cigarette smoking.** Chronic carbon monoxide exposure occurs in tunnel toll booth workers or caisson workers.
    Treatment:
    (1) Stop smoking, change the job enviroment.

(2) No treatment is needed for mild erythrocytosis.
(3) **Rarely,** phlebotomy is required for patients with **high** hematocrit and viscosity.

45. A **male** patient appears with **unexplained cyanosis or anemia but completely asymptomatic**. Routine CBC reveals **low hematocrit (pseudoanemia)**.
Definitive diagnostic test: P_{50} curves shows **higher** than normal P_{50} values (i.e., shift to the right means **tissue oxygen delivery is efficient** even with low hematocrit).
Most likely diagnosis: Decreased-affinity hemoglobins (Hb Kansas).
Treatment:
(1) No treatment is needed because patients are asymptomatic.
(2) Cyanosis is a **cosmetic** problem: Do **not** give blood transfusion.

46. **Few important points in methemoglobinemia:**
(1) Inherited forms: M hemoglobins (here **histidine is replaced by a tyrosine** which stabilizes iron in ferric state) and **rare** cause is hereditary methemoglobinemia (due to methemoglobin reductase deficiency).
(2) **Acquired** form or **toxic methemoglobinemia** are **due to nitrates (most common),** aniline dyes, phenacetin, vitamin K_3, acetaminophen, nitroprusside, sulfa drugs, benzocaine, procaine.
(3) Patients appear with **unexplained cyanosis, altered metal status**, but **normal** arterial Po_2. **History of ingestion of nitrites as a suicide attempt** by persons **having knowledge in chemistry, pharmacology or medicine**.
(4) **Diagnostic study**:
  (a) Laboratory detection of methemoglobins **is the confirmation test**.
  (b) **Inherited M hemoglobins** is diagnosed by hemoglobin electrophoresis.
  (c) Gross blood has **brownish color**.
  (d) Hereditary methemoglobinemia is diagnosed by enzyme assay.
(5) **Treatment:**
  (a) **Methylene blue is used as an emergency management of toxic methemoglobinemia.**
  (b) No treatment is needed for mild intoxication.
  (c) Patients with M hemoglobins are asymptomatic: No treatment is needed.
  (d) Patients with reductase deficiency: Usually no treatment is needed but **cyanosis is improved** by the treatment with **oral methylene blue (causes blue color urine) or riboflavin (preferred drug)**.
  (e) **Follow up therapy for toxic methemoglobinemia:** The most important is to find the causative agent and remove it from the environment.

47. **Few important points in thalassemias:**

(1) Hemoglobin consist of **heme plus globin**.
(2) Globin moiety has **alpha and beta chains**.
(3) Deficiency of alpha chain causes **alpha-thalassemia** and beta chain causes **beta-thalassemia**.
(4) Patients who are **silent carrier** (alpha or beta): Hematologically normal.
(5) Patients with thalassemia trait (alpha or beta): Patients are **asymptomatic**, and CBC reveals **mild anemia with microcytosis and hypochromia**.
(6) **Patients with severe beta-thalassemia (cooley's anemia)**: Patients appear with severe anemia, growth retardation, hepatosplenomegaly, bone deformities. **It is subdivided into tow groups**:
   (a) Thalassesmia major: Patients must need repeated **blood transfusions plus** chelation **therapy with deferoxiamine**, some patients **may require splenectomy**. Absence or low Hb A, large amount of Hb F, and Hb A_2 (4 to 10% of total hemoglobin, normal <2.5%) are found in electrophoresis study.
   (b) **Thalassemia intermedia**: Patients **usually** do **not** need blood transfusion and are able to maintain hemoglobin 6 to 7 grams/dl without transfusion. They have **normal** growth and development and many patients survive into adulthood. **They have large amount of Hb F, significant amount of Hb A_2,** and **variable amount of Hb A** (Important). Patients may have severe osteoporosis, disabling arthritis, secondary hemochromatosis (due to increased iron absorption in GI tract), and spinal cord compression with paraplegia (due to large masses of erythroid tissues compression).
   Treatment:
      (1) **Splenectomy** may be required in patients with hypersplenism.
      (2) Local radiation therapy reverses the spinal cord compression.
      (3) Any or all of these complication may necessiate **blood transfusion** therapy which may also prevent facial dusfiguration.
   (c) **Hemoglobin H disease (alpha thalassemia):** Patients appear with moderately severe **hemolytic anemia**, **jaundice**, and **splenomegaly** but can maintain regular job and family. Electrophoresis may reveal **beta-4 globin up to 10 to 30% of the total hemoglobin**.
   Treatment:
      (1) Folic acid, treat infections, judicious use of blood transfusion; avoid iron salts and oxidant drugs.
      (2) **Splenectomy may be needed** when there is definitve evidence of **hypersplenism** (leukopenia, worsening anemia, thrombocytopenia) but may develop postsplenectomy complications such **as thrombocytosis and pulmonary embolisms**.

Remember, **acquired form of HbH disease** may occur in various forms of myeloproliferative and myelodysplastic disorders
Treatment: To treat the underlying disease.

(d) Hydrops fetalis is the **most severe form of alpha-thalassemia**, patients only have Hb Bart's (gamma 4) and Hb H (beta 4) (**Not** important for examination).

(e) Future therapy for thalassemias:
   (1) Allogenic bone marrow transplantation may be effective in **homozygous beta-thalassemia**.
   (2) Gene therapy: Introduction of **normal** beta or gamma globin genes into the **pluripotent stem cells of thalassemic patients**.
   (3) Manipulation of the hemoglobin F to hemoglobin A switch may be promising.
   (4) Hydroxyurea is under investigation, butyrate also stimulates Hb F production.

48. **Hemoglobin electrophoresis findings in different thalassemias**: (**Electrophoresis findings in normal individual is Hb A > 95%, Hb A_2 1.5 to 3.5%, Hb F < 2%**).
   (1) Silent carrier (normal MCV) = Normal,Hb A_2↓
   (2) Alpha-thalassemia trait (low MCV) = Normal, Hb A_2↓
   (3) Hemoglobin H disease (Heinz bodies, target cells) = Hb H↑ (beta 4, 10-30%).
   (4) Hydrops fetalis (increased nucleated RBC's) = Very high Barts (gamma 4) hemoglobin.
   (5) Heterozygous beta-thalassemia (low MCV, stippling) = ↑Hb A_2 with or without Hb F↑.
   (6) Homozygous beta-thalassemia (nucleated RBC's, target cells) = Very high Hb F (in both thalassemia major or intermedia).

49. **Different diseases, Hb electrophoresis, and CBC findings**:

Diseases	Hb (gm/dl)	MCV (fl)	Hb A (%)	Hb A_2(%)	Hb F (%)	Reticulocytes (%)
(i) Normal	13-17	80-100	>95	1.5-3.5	<2	0.5-1.5
(ii) Hb SS	↓↓↓ (7-8)	→ (86)	Absent (0)	→ (3)	↑↑ (5)	↑↑↑ (10)

(iii) Hb-S, beta-(0)-thal	↓↓ (8-9)	↓↓↓ (69)	Absent (0)	↑↑↑ (5)	↑↑ (6)	↑↑ (7)
(iv) Hb-S, beta-(+)-thal, type I	↓↓ (8-9)	↓↓↓ (64)	3-5	↑↑↑ (5)	↑↑ (7)	↑↑ (9)
(v) Hb-S, beta-(+)-thal, type II	↓ (10-11)	↓↓ (70)	8-15	↑↑↑ (5)	↑↑ (5)	↑↑ (7)
(vi) Hb-S, beta-(+)-thal, type III	↓ (11-12)	↓↓ (70)	18-24	↑↑↑ (5)	↑↑ (5)	→ (1)
(vii) Hb-S-HPFH	→ (14-15)	Low normal (82)	Absent (0)	→ (2)	↑↑↑↑ (26)	↑ (2)

50. **Clinical manifestations of sickle cell disease**:
    (1) Typical presentation is asymptomatic anemia **except during painful crisis**.
    (2) Approximately 33% cases admitted to the hospital > 6 times per year due to pain related conditions, another 33% cases admitted for the same reason but 2 to 6 times per year, another 33% cases rarely have pain. Frequency of pain is **highest in third and fourth decades**.
    (3) **Most common sites of pain** are in the **back, chest, extremities,** and abdomen but can affect may part of the body.
    (4) Pain is mostly **due to vaso-occlusion** and can cause depression, apathy, and despair.
    (5) Precipitating factors causing pain: dehydration, cold, infection, stress, **alcohol,** or menstrual period.
    (6) **Physical examination may reveal fever, tenderness, swelling, vomiting, tachypnea, and hypertension**.

51. **Growth and development in sickle cell disease:**
    (1) Usually the weight is **low** but height is normal.
    (2) Skeletal maturation may be delayed.
    (3) **Incidence of retarded sexual maturation** is **more in Hb SS and sickle cell-beta-o-thalassemia** than in Hb SC or sick cell-beta-+-thalassemia. It is associated with **elevated gonadotropin levels** for the stages of sexual development. **It also causes delayed menarche**.
    (4) Retarded sexual maturation **in males** could be due to primary hypogonadism, hypopituitarism, or hypothalamic hypofunction.
    (5) Impaired development may be due to the effect of hemolysis on increasing BMR.

52. **Infections in sickle cell disease**:
   (1) Most common organism causing osteomyelitis **is Salmonella species**, next common organism is **S. aureus**.
   (2) Joint infection is **less** common and is often due to **S. pneumoniae**.
   (3) **Most common organisms causing pneumonias are Mycoplasma pneumoniae, Chlamydia, and Legionella. Acute chest syndrome is due to bacterial pneumonias**.
   (4) Most common organism for septicemia and meningitis (most commonly in children) is **S. pneumoniae**.

53. **Different complications in sickle cell disease**:
   (1) **Hepatobiliary system:** Pigmented gallstones (70% cases), hepatomegaly, hepatic parenchymal atrophy, hemosiderosis, periportal fibrosis, and cirrhosis. Viral infection can cause acute hepatitis.
   (2) **Renal system**: It causes medullary, proximal tubular, distal tubular, and glomerular abnormalities. **Hb SS disease with hematuria should be evaluated by ultrasonography to rule out any serious abnormalities** (Important). Patients may appear with high BP, hyperuricemia, proteinuria, high k, and low hematocrit.
   (3) **Cardiac system:** Acute myocardial infarction may occur.
   (4) **Eye:** Sickle retinopathy which is treated with laser photocoagulation. Ocular disease is **more common in Hb SC disease and sickle cell-beta-(+)-thalassemia** than Hb SS disease and sickle cell beta-(0)-thalassemia.
   (5) **Pripism:** It is a painful unwanted erection due to engorgement **of corpus cavernosa** (**not** involving corpus spongiosum and glans **expcept** in few patients, **this tricorporal priapism is diagnosed by nuclear scan** and it may results **in impotence**).
   Treatment: Monitor intercavernous pressure, **IV hydration and analgesia,** if **no** response in 12 hours then do **partial exchange transfusion**. If no response within next 12 hours, then do **Winter procedure (fistula between glans penis and corpora cavernosa** by inserting a large bore needle through the glans). **Diethylstilbestrol may prevent the recurrence**.
   Complication: Up to 45% patients develop some degree of impotence.
   (6) **Pulmonary system:** Acute chest syndrome is due to pneumonia.
   (7) **Skin: Leg ulcers develop near the medial or lateral malleolus with or without tranuma** (Important Board **question, may be given as a picture**). Ulcers may cause osteomyelitis, systemic infection, or tetanus. It is more common in **male, resistant to healing,** and more likely to recur.
   Treatment: Remove nonviable tissues, apply **wet-to-dry dressing or Duoderm hydrocolloid dressing**, put zinc oxide-impregnated Unna boots

after debridement. Bed rest, elastic wraps, and leg elevation to promote healing and reduce the edema.

The myofascial syndromes includes soft tissue swelling, subcutaneous edema results in 'peau d'orange' appearance. It is due to dermal or subdermal vaso-occlusion and is treated symptomatically.

(8) **Bones: Osteonecrosis** causing vertebral compression, shortening of cuboidal bones, of the hands and feet; **acute aseptic or avascular necrosis ; bone infarction causes 'hand-foot syndrome'.** Bone marrow infarction (**low** reticulocytes count, **low** hematocrit, leukoerythroblastic picture, or pancytopenia) is **diagnosed by bone scan. Bone infarction** is diagnosed by **bone scan or MRI. The best study to diagnose osteonecrosis is MRI**. Patients may have arthritic pain, effusion, and swelling are either due to periarticular infarction or gouty arthritis. It is treated **with NSAID's**.

(9) **Nervous system:** Transient ischemic stroke (TIA), cerebral infarction, cerebral hemorrhage, seizures, and unexplained coma. **Cebral thrombosis is the most common cause of CVA (cerebrovascular accident)** and **is due to large vessel occlusion** rather than microvascular occlusion commonly found in Hb SS disease.

Patients who are high risk for CVA: Severe anemia, **high** reticulocyte counts, higher WBC counts, **lower Hb F levels, and sickle cell anemia rather than** Hb SC disease or sickle cell-beta thalassemia.

Diagnosis: CT scan or MRI of the brain; **Please remember, subclinical cerebral infarction can be diagnosed by MRI and transcranial doppler flow study**. In hemorrhage, angiography is done after partial exchange transfusion to aviod complications from injected contrast material.

Treatment:

(a) **Hemorrhage:** Partial exchange transfusion should be done.

(b) **Thrombosis: Partial exchange transfusion should be done promptly; chronic direct transfusion to maintain Hb S level < 30% to prevent recurrent thrombosis and improves arterial stenosis. Chronic transfusion therapy** should be continued for **indefinite period of time** for patients whose cerebral flow **abnormalities recur soon after discontinuation of therapy** or **persistent flow abnormality even after 5 years of transfusion**.

(c) **To prevent recurrence of thrombosis:** The **best treatment is chronic transfusion therapy**.

(10) **Obstetric and gynecologic problems:** Most important complication is pregnancy which can lead to premature birth and fetal death. Prophylactic transfusions do **not** improve fetal outcome. **Maternal complications** inculde infection, painful crisis, severe anemia, and death.

Recommended method of birth control: Low-dose estrogen containing oral contraceptives is the safest; injection of medroxyprogesterone every 3 months or barrier method may be used.

54. **Sickle cell trait**: Hb A and Hb S is usually 60:40. **Hematuria** is a common complication among African American, **splenic infarction** can occur at high altitude, and higher incidence of **sudden death in military recruits during basic training** is due to exercise-induced vaso-occlusion and rhabdomyolysis. Patients are usually **asymptomatic,** if any patients is symptomatic **then diagnosis must be verified** because **rare hemoglobinopathy** (Hb S Antilles or Hb Quebec-CHORI) may appear as symptomatic 'sickle cell trait'.

55. **Hemoglobin SC disease:** Patients are **less** symptomatic than Hb SS disease **except proliferative sickle retinopathy (Important)**. Hb SC disease patients have **less** painful crisis, **less** anemia, **mild** reticulocytosis, and more survival.

56. **Sickle cell-beta-thalassemia:** Hypochromic, microcytic anemia. **The clinical feature of sickle cell- beta (+)- thalassemia is more benign** than that of sickle cell-beta-(0)-thalassemia **except proliferative retinopathy which is more frequent in beta (+) disease**, that means sickle cell syndrome with higher **hematocrits have more frequent ocular complications**. Patients appear with leg ulcers, acute chest syndrome, aplastic crisis, priapism, and splenomegaly, **with less frequency in beta (+) disease than beta (0) disease**.

57. **Sickle cell anemia plus alpha-thalassemia:** Patients have **decreased** incidence of leg ulcers and CVA but **increased** incidence of **osteonecrosis and acute painful crisis**.

58. Sickle cell- HPFH (hereditary persistence of fetal hemoglobin): Patients with sickle cell- deletional HPFH are **not** anemia and do **not** develop vaso-occlusive crisis.

59. **Diagnosis and treatment of sickle cell anemias**:
    (A) **Diagnosis:**
        (1) **Hemoglobin electrophoresis is the best diagnostic study. Please remember, 'sickle cell prep' has no value**.
        (2) **Other laboratory tests:** Sickle cells are **normochromic except** with coexistent iron deficiency anemia or thalassemia. **WBC and platelet counts, and are elevated** in sickle cell anemia but **not** in Hb SC disease or sickle cell-beta-(+)-disease. **The hemolytic anemia of** Hb SS disease results in **elevated** LDH, unconjugated bilirubin, and reticulocytes

count; **decreased** haptoglobin, hemoglobin, PCV, and RBC levels. Howell-Jolly bodies indicate hyposplenia.

60. **Therapy of sickle cell anemias**:
   (1) **Health care maintenance: Folic acid** (1 mg PO daily), **counseling** (genetic, psychosocial, and disease related), routine **retinal** examination, and for sexually active women low-dose estrogen oral contraceptive and routine pelvic examination.
   (2) **Infections:**
      (a) Acute chest syndrome: Use cefuroxime plus erythromycin.
      (b) Ostemoyelitis (Salmonella, S. aureus): Antibiotics for 2 to 6 weeks; surgical drainage or sequestrectomy may be needed.
      (c) Meningitis: Antibiotics for 2 weeks.
   (3) **Hydration:** Adequate hydration by PO or IV also relieves the pain.
   (4) **Pain therapy:** Analgesics, use narcotics (**IV morphine** is recommended for prompt relief of pain and patient-controlled analgesia), psychosocial support, local anesthetics, NSAID's, antidepressive drugs (prn), **and adequate hydration**. (Do **not** use oxygen and transfusion of blood for pain) (**Important point**).
   (5) **Hypoxia:** Give oxygen therapy.
   (6) **Transfusion therapy:**
      (a) **Indications:** To improve oxygen-carrying capacity and blood-volume replacement such as (**splenic sequestration, aplastic crisis**); to protect from imminent danger such as (**septicemia, metabolic acidosis, acute chest syndrome**); to improve rheologic properties of blood such as (**priapism, probably preoperative**, and **most important is prevention of recurrence of CVA**).
      (b) **Contraindication:** Routine acute painful crisis.
      (c) **Types of transfusion: Simple transfusion** is to improve blood volume and oxygen-carrying capacity; **chronic transfusion** is to improve blood viscosity and reduce iron burden; (**one unit of** red cells transfusion increases **Hb levels 1 grams/dL and hematocrit levels 3%**); **partial exchange transfusions** (500 ml of blood out, 300 ml of normal saline in, then 500 ml of blood out, followed by 4 to 5 units of P-RBC in) are used for acute emergencies.
   (7) **Chelation therapy: Deferoxamine is** used with elevated total body iron and serum ferritin levels > 2000 microgram/ml.
   (8) New therapeutic potential:
      (a) **Membrane active agents that improve sickle cell hydration**: Cetiedil citrate, imidazole compounds (clotrimazole).

(b) **To improve rheologic properties of sickle cells**: Pluronic F-68 or poloxamer 188. It also inhibits the adherence to endothelial cells.
(c) **Hydroxyurea can reduce the pain in adult patients** (recent study reports). It stimulates Hb F synthesis, improves rheologic properties of sickle cells, and inhibitor of ribonuleotide reductase.
(d) **Recombinant human erythropoietin** can potentiate the effects of hydroxyurea.
(e) **Valproic acid** can stimulate Hb F production and may be used in selected patients.
(f) Do **not** use butyric acid for inadequate efficacy and neurotoxicity. No improvement in Hb F or hemolysis.
(g) Bone marrow transplantation (BMT) is reserved **only for severe disease**.
(h) **Gene therapy** may provide promise to the future.

61. **Irradiated RBC's transfusion**: It is used to prevent GVHD (graft-versus-host disease). It is used in patients who are severely immunocompromised by chemotherapy (malignancy both hematologic and solid tumors), Hodgkin disease, non-Hodgkin lymphoma, and bone marrow transplantation recipient.

62. **Leukocyte-reduced RBC's transfusion**: It is used in patients with **H/O two or more febrile, nonhemolytic transfusion reaction** to prevent the recurrence. WBC counts should be $< 5 \times 10^8$ /unit to avoid febrile reaction, and $< 5 \times 10^6$ /unit to reduce the incidence of alloimmunization. It can **also reduce the transmission of CMV infection** but the amount of WBC reduction is **not** certain.

63. **Washed RBC's transfusion**: Washed RBC's are used to prevent severe allergic or anaphylactic reaction.

64. Types of blood transfusion and amount:
(A) **Types**: **Rh-negative** patients should received **Rh-negative whole blood, Rh-positive patients** may receive either **Rh-positive or Rh-negative blood**. If ABO type is known, give the **same type** of red cells (blood) and if it is **unknown** then give **O type** red cells (blood). So, **O, Rh-negative blood is perfect for an emergency when** blood type is **not** known.
(B) To improve **Hb from 4 gm/dL to 10 gm/dL how much red cells are needed**: Answer is **6 units** (because **one unit of red cells transfusion increases Hb level 1 gram/dl** and **hemacrit levels 3%**) of red cells transfusion should be done.

65. **Complications of blood transfusion**:

(A) **Acute reactions**:

(1) **Acute hemolytic reactioon**: **Fever is the first sign**, other clinical manifestations are vomiting, chest pain, back pain, dyspnea, wheezing, hemoglobinuria, hemolysis, intravascular coagulation, hypotension, and renal failure. Most common cause is clerical error or blood given to the wrong patients.

Treatment: First is to stop the transfusion, send the blood back to the blood bank for **analysis**. The goal is to correct hypotension, control bleeding, and prevent renal damage. **IV fluids, mannitol, or other diuretics** increase renal blood flow and maintain urine output.

(2) **Nonhemolytic febrile reaction**: Patients appear with **chills** and **fever** (at least 1°C elevation) **about 1 hour after the** onset of transfusion. Patients may have **high diastolic BP or frank rigors**.

Treatment: To stop the blood transfusion, send blood for analysis, antipyretics, and suyportive measures. After the second reaction (occurs < 15% cases), subsequent **transfusion should be 'leukocyte-reduced' by third-generation filters (Important)**.

(3) **Acute lung injury form blood transfusion**: Patients would develop symptoms (dyspnea, cough, blood-tinged sputum, hypoxemia, and cyanosis) **within 6 hours after infusion of plasma-containing materials**.

Treatment: Oxygen, respiratory support, mechanical ventilation, and **if the pulmonary capillary wedge pressure and systemic BP are low, fluid therapy may be given**. Patients usually improves within 48 hours.

(4) **Allergic reactions:** Urticaria and pruritus are due to interaction between donor plasma proteins and **recipient IgE antibodies**.

Treatment: Antihistamines; blood transfusion may be continued after hives subside.

(5) **Anaphylactic reactions**: It is due to **reaction of anti-IgA antibodies against IgA in donor plasma**. It may be foound in some IgA-deficient patients. Patients appear with **generalized urticaria,** facial flushing, **laryngeal or facial edema, bronchospasm**, vomiting, diarrhea, or **hypotension**.

Treatment: IV epinephrine; if subsequent transfusion are needed, then blood components **should be washed to remove IgA** (Important).

(6) Bacterial sepsis (gram-negative organisms produce more severe symptoms than gram-positive organisms): **Most common gram-negative organism is Yersinia enterocolitica**. Patients appear with chills, vomiting, or rigors initially, followed by low BP, fever, shock, and DIC.

Treatment: Stop the transfusion, send the blood for Gram-stain and culture (**remember**, sepsis can occur with negative Gram-stain), and **broad spectrum antibiotics**.

(7) **Volume overload:** Patients can develop CHF due to impaired myocardial function.

(B) Delayed reaction (from **days to years** after transfusion):

(1) Graft-versus-host disease (**4 to 30 days after transfusion**): Pancytopenia, infection, and hemorrhage occur (mortality 90% cases). **Prevention: Gamma radiation** to the blood and blood components.

(2) **Post-transfusion purpura: Severe thrombocytopenia 5 to 9 days after transfusion due to unknown cause**. Patients should be treated with **IV gamma globulin infusion or plasma exchange**.

(3) **Chronic transfusions** (60 to 200 units of blood) cause endocrine, liver, and cardiac dysfunctions.
Treatment: Deferoxamine, some cases need exchange transfusion.

(4) **Delayed** hemolytic transfusion reaction (3 to 21 days after transfusion): Positive direct antiglobin test and < 20% appear with signs of hemolysis.

66. **Disease transmitted by blood transfusion**:

(1) **Hepatitis C infetion** produces symptoms **7 to 8 weeks after** transfusion. It can cause chronic hepatitis, subsequently may develop cirrhosis, hepatocellular cancer, or liver failure (usually after 10 years).

(2) **Retroviral infections:** Risk of HIV-1 (< 1 per 420,000 transfusion), no new cases of HIV-2 since 1992 in USA. HTLV-I induces adult T-cell leukemia/lymphoma and tropical spastic paraparesis. HTLV-II is **not** linked to specific illness. HTLV-I and II are transmitted **through blood cells**.

(3) **Other diseases** are CMV, malaria, (very rarely) syphilis, chagas disease, Toxoplasma, E-B virus, parvovirus, Bartonella, and Babesia.

67. **Leukocyte adhesion deficiency (LAD):** Patients appear with recurrent and gangrenous soft tissue **infections of subcutaneous tissues or mucous membrane** caused by **S. aureus, Pseudomonas,** other gram-negative entericv rods, or candida infections.
Diagnosis: Measurement of surface CD 11/CD 18 in stimulated and unstimulated neutrophils using monoclonal antibodies against CD 11/CD 18.
Treatment: Supportive; Bone marrow transplantation is the treatment of choice in severe LAD patients. **Trimethoprim-sulfamethoxazole** is used as proplylaxis in recurrent infections.

68. **Chediak-Higashi syndrome (autosomal recessive)**: Clinical features include **neutropenia** causing infections, **mild bleeding disorder** due to platelet defect, **peripheral neuropathies**, and natural killer cells abnormalities. Most serious clinical problems are due to **abnormalities** in neutrophil chemotaxis, degranulations, and **bactericidal activities**. These patients can **develop acclerated phase of this disorder at any time due to proliferation of polyuclonal T-cells** in the liver, spleen, and bone marrow results in **hepatosplenomegaly, high fever (without bacterial infections),** lor pancytopenia with increased susceptibility to infections.
Diagnosis: Demonstration of giant granules in neutrophils and eosinophils.
Treatment: Antibiotic for infection, **prophylactic antibiotics** (trimethoprim-sulfamethoxazole), **ascorbic acid. Bone-marrow transplantation is the treatment of choice for acclerated phase of the disease**.

69. **Chronic granulomatous disease (CGD):** X-linked and autosomal recessive; inability of phagocytes to generate superoxide anion (O_2^-) due to absence of the component of the NADPH oxidase system; lack of cytosolic factors (47-KD protein or 67-KD protein).
Clinical manifestations: **Any patients with recurrent lymphadenitis, CGD should be ruled out**; other features are **pneumonias, skin infections, bacterial hepatic abscesses and osteomyelitis in multiple** site or in small bones of the hands or feet.
Diagnosis: NBT test (nitroblue tetrazolium) reveals **failure to reduce NBT** because phagocytic cells of CGD **cannot** produce superoxide anion (O_2^-).
Treatment: Long term **antibiotic prophylaxis** (trimethoprim-sulfamethoxazole), long-term **interferon-gamma, aggressive antibiotic** therapy, **surgery if needed**. Somatic gene therapy may be promising in future.

70. **Most common inherited disorder of neutrophil function**: Myeloperoxidasse deficiency (MPO). MPO causes **delay** in the **microbicidal** activity **of neutrophils initially, eventually effective killing of bacteria occurs**.
Clinical manifestations: **Asymptomatic or increased Candida infection in some patients with diabetes mellitus**.
Diagnosis: Peroxidase stain of the blood reveals **missing peroxidase activity** in neutrophils and monocytes (**but** normal activity in eosinophils).
Treatment: No treatment is needed.

71. **Neutropenia** (peripheral neutrophil coount is $< 2.0 \times 10^9$ per liter):
(A) **Clinical manifestations**: It depends upon the variety of systemic diseases. Patients are usually asymptomatic when neutrophil count is **$> 1.0 \times 10^9$ per liter** or those whose neutropenia is **acute and self-limited**. The risk of

bacterial infection increases slightly when neutrophil count is < 1.0 x 10^9 per liter but is **severely increased at levels < 0.5 x 10^9 per liter**. Most common sources of infection are lung, GU, GI, throat, and skin.

(B) **Diagnosis: WBC count and its differential count** plus blood smear examination; try to find out the underlying cause; **bone marrow examination** should be done in **neutropenia due to sepsis or toxin**. In pancytopenia or bicytopenia, bone marrow examination should include **biopsy along with aspirataion**. Bone marrow examination is **not** needed for vitamin B_{12} or folate deficiency.

(C) **Treatment:**

(1) To treat the underlying cause (antibiotic for infection, stop the drug or toxin causing neutropenia.

(2) Immunosuppressive therapy: **Glucocorticoids or cyclosporin**. (Do **not** use lithium carbonate which increases neutrophil count in normal individual but **no** response in neutropenia and produce toxicity).

(3) Recombinant human granulopoietic factors: Both **GM-CSF and G-CSF produce neutrophilic leukocytosis, GM-CSF also increases eosinophils and monocytes. It is particularly effective in patients develop neutropenia after cancer chemotherapy**.

(4) **Bone marrow transplantation** is needed in severe aplastic anemia, myelodysplastic syndromes.

(5) **Infected neutropenic patients:**

(a) **Afebrile** and **no** sign of sepsis: Diagnostic work up in the outpatient clinic to avoid hospital nosocomial infections.

(b) **Fever plus severe nutropenia**: Patients should be hospitalized; cultures of blood, urine, and other appropriate sites should be obtained; **IV broad-spectrum antibiotics should be given full course** followed by **7 to 14 days of oral antibiotic therapy** if the patients have severe **infections plus necrosis, slow response** to initial antibiotic therapy, **recurrent infection,** and **no** organism is identified plus **no** improvement in clinical p;ictures after 3 days of empiric treatment. **If the patient is critically ill, then amphotericin B should be added** particularly in acute leukemia, diabetes, prolonged antibiotic therapy, dysphagia, esophagitis, endopthalmitis, or receiving immunosuppressive therapy.

72. Lymphocytopenia (peripheral blood lymphocyte count < 1.5 x 10^9 per liter):

(A) Clinical manifestations: It depends upon the underlying disease condition.

(B) **Treatment**:

(1) No specific therapy; treat the underlying cause.

(2) Hypogammaglobulinemia with lymphocytopenia: Give IV immunoglobulin.
(3) Adenosine deaminases deficiency (a cause of severe combined immune deficiency): **Give adenosine deaminasse conjugated to polyethylene glycol**.

73. **A patient with sepsis does not have eosinopenia, most likely diagnosis: Adrenocortical insufficiency** or **primary myeloproliferative syndrome**.

74. **Causes of eosinopenia and basophilopenia:** Stress, acute infections, severe injury (e.g., burns), and widespread neoplasms.

75. **Causes of eosinopenia**: Glucocorticoids, epinephrine, and prostaglandins.

76. **Neutrophilia (neutrophil counts > 7.5 x 10^9 /liter)**:
(A) **Few common causes are the following: Inflammatory response to acute or subacute infection is the most common cause. Other causes are** chemical effects; glucocorticoids, epinephrine, lithium chloride; chronic myeloproliferative disorder, chronic meylogenous leukemia, polycythemia rubra vera, essential thrombocytosis.
(B) **Diagnosis:** Try to find the underlying cause.
(1) **Leukoerythroblastosis:** Bone marrow aspiration and biopsy are important.
(2) **Neutrophilic leukocytosis only:** Observation of the course of neutrophilia and try to find the linkage with underlying condition.

77. **Few important values of blood cells**:
(1) Leukocytopenia: Total leukocyte count < 4.5 x 10^9 per liter.
(2) Leukocytosis: Total leukocyte count > 11.0 x 10^9 per liter.
(3) Leukemoid reaction: Total leukocyte count >25 to 30 x10^9 per liter.
(4) Lymphocytosis: Total lymphocyte count > 5.0 x 10^9 per liter.
(5) Lymphocytopenia: Total lympocyte count < 1.5 x 10^9 per liter.
(6) Neutrophilia: Total neutrophil count > 7.5 x 10^9 per liter.
(7) Neutropenia: Total neutrophil count < 2.0 x 10^9 per liter.
(8) Monoytosis: Total monocyte count > 0.50 x 10^9 per liter.
(9) Eosinophilia: Total eosinophil count > 0.4 x 10^9 per liter.

78. **Polycythemia vera** (myeloproliferative disease characterized by persistence elevation of Hb and hematocrit):
(A) **Clinical manifestations:** Thrombohemorrhagic complications are the most common presentation. The disease may transform into postpolycythemia

myeloid metaplasia (20% cases) or acute myeloid leukemia (5 to 15% cases).

(B) **Diagnosis:** Patients should **have all three major criteria** or the **first two major** criteria plus **any two of the minor** criteria.

(1) **Major criteria**:

(a) Increased red cell mass (males ≥36 ml/kg, females ≥32 ml/kg).

(b) Normal arterial oxygen saturation (≥ 92%).

(c) Splenomegaly.

(2) **Minor criteria**:

(a) Leukocytes > 12,000/microl.

(b) Platelets > 400,000/microl.

(c) Leukocyte alkaline phosphatase > 100, or vitamin B_{12} > 900 pg/ml, or unbound B_{12} binding capacity > 2200 pg/ml.

(C) **Treatment of polycythemia vera**:

(1) **Phlebotomy is the treatment of choice** to decrease the red cell mass (remove 500 ml of blood weekly to maintain hematocrit of 42% or less). Phlebotomy alone can cause thrombosis.

(2) Concurrent treatment with **myelosuppressive drug (hydroxyurea) can prevent the thrombosis** particularly in patients **older than 70 years**, H/O thrombosis, frequently require phlebotomy, or thrombocytosis > 600,000 per microliter. **The goal** is to maintain the hematocrit < 42%, platelet count < 500,000 per microliter, and WBC couont > 3000 per microliter. **Hydroxyurea should be continued until** the phebotomy is **not** needed **or thrombocytosis resolved**.

(3) In advanced stage of the disease (spent phase), the hematocrit and platelet counts may decrease to normal: Specific therapy may **not** be needed.

(4) **Interferon-alpha is an effective therapy**.

79. Essential thrombocythemia (platelet count is $\geq 6 \times 10^5$ per microliter): It is a chronic myeloproliferative disorder.

(A) **Clinical manifestations:** Most common presentation is **asymptomatic** with incidental finding of high platelet count in peripheral blood, or symptomatic (25% casses) with either **thrombotic or hemorrhagic manifestations such as acute strokes, transient cerebral ischemic attacks**, GI tract hemorrhages, angina, MI, sagittal vein thromboses, ecchymoses, epistaxis, digital microvascular ischemia, deep vein thrombosis, and Bud-Chiari syndrome (splanchnic vein thrombosis). Patients may appear with vasomotor disturbances, paresthesias, acrocyanosis, and **erythromelalgia** (pain in palms and soles, erythema, warmth due to microvascular obstruction of platelets).

(B) **Diagnosis:**

(1) Platelet count > 6 x 10^5 per microliter.

(2) Normal iron stores and normal red cell mass.

(3) No philadelphia chromosome.

(4) Absence of conditions associated with reactive thrombocytosis.

(5) Bone marrow collagen fibrosis must be absent, or in the absence of splenomegaly and leukoerythroblastic picture, must be restricted to < 1/3 of the biopsy ares.

(C) Differential diagnosis from reactive **thrombocytosis**: Reactive thrombocytosis have **known cause** and **elevation** of acute-phase reactants (including Creactive protein and fibrinogen) **unlike** essential thrombocythemia; reactive thrombocytosis **does not have the following**: Chronic increase in platelets, splenomegaly, thrombosis, hemorrhage, bone marrow reticulin fibrosis and megakaryocyte clusters, and spontaneous colony formation (erythroid or megakaryocyte colony) but essential thrombocythemia **does have** the above mentioned features.

(D) **Treatment**:

(1) **Current recommendation is to treat all patients who are older than 50 years, especially those who have cardiovascular** risk factors or a history of thrombosis:

(a) **Hydroxyurea is the initial drug of choice**. (It inhibits radionucleotide reductase and its **side effects** include reversible neutropenia, mild GI symptoms, nail atrophy, maculopapular rash, hyperpigmentation).

(b) **Anagrelide** (**not** approved by FDA) is also effective, it **inhibits** megakaryocyte maturation and its side effects include palpitation, tachycardia, dizziness, diarrhea, and fluid retention. **The goal is to** keep the platelet count between 100,000 and 400,000 per microliter, and WBC count > 3000 per microliter.

(c) **Interferon-alpha** is used when there is **no** response with **hydroxyurea or anagrelide (experimental)**.

(d) **Occasionally** radioactive phosphorus (leukemogenic potential) may be used in elderly patients, or noncompliant patients.

(2) Management of young patients (12 to 40 year):

(a) Symptomatic patients: The goal is to keep the platelet < 5 x 10^5 per microliter to prevent recurrence of serious events. **Use hydroxyurea, if fails interferon-alpha**.

(b) Asymptomatic patients: No recommendation is made for or against of **specific** therapy.

(3) **Management of pregnant patients:** No therapy is needed because complications are **rare** and deliveries are **uncomplicated**.

80. **Agnogenic myeloid dysplasia:** It is a **chronic myeloproliferative disorder** characterise by significant bone marrow **fibrosis plus the clonal myeloproliferative process**.
   (A) **Clinical manifestations:** Symptomatic patients (80% cases) appear with **anemia (most common)**, mechanical effects of the **enlarged spleen**, and **abnormal bleeding**. Anemia causes weakness, palpitation, or fatigue. **Painful enlarging spleen** is often associated with **cachexia**. **Hypermetabolism** is present and causes low-grade fever, night sweats, and weight loss. Purpura, ecchymoses, or **bleeding is due to low plataelet, platelet dysfunction, acquired Factor V deficiency, or DIC.** Patients may have Factor VIII deficiency and increased fibrin split products.
   (B) **Diagnosis:** Presence of **splenomegaly, teardrop poikilocytes** in peripheral blood smear (produced by spleen and a sign of extramedullary erythropoiesis), **leukoerythroblastic** response in blood, and **bone marrow fibrosis** are diagnostic features.
   (C) **Chromosomal defect:** Clonal cytogenetic abnormalities include 20q -, 13q-, and trisomy 21 may be present (33% cases).
   (D) **Treatment:**
      (1) Only symptomatic therapy is available, **no** medication can cause cure.
      (2) Patients with normocytic normochornic anemia: **Oxymetholone (androgens) is the drug of choice**.
      (3) Patients with hemolysis: Add **prednisone along with oxymetholone,** if fails then perform **splenectomy**.
      (4) Patients with Factor V deficiency: Use FFP (fresh frozen plasma).
      (5) **Indications of splenectomy**: Mechanically painful splenomegaly, refractory hemolytic anemia, refractory thrombocytopenia, and portal hypertension.

81. **Chronic myelogenous leukemia (CML) and chromosome**: **Philadelphia (Ph^1) chromosome** is present in bone marrow cells (> 95% cases) (**Important**).

82. **Few important points in chronic myelogenous leukemia(CML)**:
   (1) **No** definite etiologic agent is found, but **exposure to ionizing radiation increases the risk of CML**.
   (2) **Radiation therapy of ankylosing spondylitis and cervical cancer** increase the risk of CML.
   (3) CML is **not a frequent secondary** leukemia following treatment of other cancers with radiation and/or alkylating agents.
   (4) **No** increase incidence of CML among workers in the nuclear industry.

(5) **Remember,** benzene exposure does **not** cause CML but does cause AML (acute myelogenous leukemia).
(6) CML have **increased frequency** of Cw3 and Cw4 human leukocyte antigens.
(7) CML occur most frequetly **between 45 to 50 years**; **poor prognosis** above 60 years; **less** common in **adolescent**.
(8) **Molecular finding in CML: The Philadelphia chromosome** results from balanced translocation **between the long arms (q) of chromosomes 9 and 22 (chromosome 22 is short** because more chromosomal material is lost than gained from chromosome 9). **The P 210 protein** (tyrosine kinase) may stimulate uncontrolled proliferation of CML. The fusion of **BCR/ABL gene and the P 210 protein** is found in many patients of CML.

83. **Clinical manifestations, diagnosis, and treatment of chronic myelogenous leukemia (CML)**:

(A) **Clinical manifestations:** Most patients are **asymptomatic and diagnosed by routine blood test**, or mildly symptomatic. **Fatigue, malaise, weight loss, loss of appetite, and sense of fullness in left upper quadrant due to splenomegaly are the most common presentation in symptomatic patients**. GI ulcerationo and bleeding could be from **elevated** blood histamine level due to basophil cell mass.
Physical examination: Most common sign is splenomegaly (large size), other rare signs are lymphadenopathy, infiltration of skin and other tissues.
All symptoms subside as WBC count falls and the splenomegaly decreases after appropriate therapy.
More than 90% patients have benign course but some patients can develop **acclerated phase or blast crisis**.
Acclerated phase or blast crisis: **Increase in blast cells** (> 15%) or **basophils** (> 20%) in the blood or bone marrow, **severe anemia** (Hb < 7 grams/dL), **thrombocytopenia** (< 100,000 per microliter); presence of extramedullary leukemia, or new chromosomal changes plus philadelphia chromosome.

(B) **Laboratory findings of CML**:
(1) **Elevated WBC count** (10,000 to > 1,000,000 per microliter), **mostly neutrophils** with a left shift to blast cells; **elevated eosinophils and basophils are common; few** cases have mild monocytosis (**monocytosis is common in myelomonocytic leukemia**).
(2) **Bone marrow** is **hypercellular** with marked myeloid hyperplasia. The myeloid-crythroid ratio is 15:1 to 20:1.
(3) **Elevated both helper and suppressor** T cells (**not** B cells).
(4) **Thrombocytosis** (>450,000 per microliter) **is present** (in 50% cases).

(5) **Usually normochromic, normocytic anemia**; nucleated RBC may be present (25% of cases).
(6) **Markedly decreased** LAP (leukocyte alkaline phosphatase) scores in neutrophils.
(7) Elevated levels of LDH, uric acid, lysozyme, **vitamin B_{12} (> 10 times normal), transcobalamines I and III**.
(8) **Elevated** colony forming cells in the blood but **normal** in the bone marrow.

(C) **Diagnosis of CML**:
(1) **The presence of myeloid leukocytosis, splenomegaly, decreased LAP levels in neutrophils, bone marrow hyperplasia and hypercellularity** strongly suggests the diagnosis.
(2) **The best diagnostic study is cytogenetic analysis which reveals presence of Philadelphia chromosome (>95% cases) plus this clilnical findings** confirms the diagnosis of CML.
(3) If philadelphia chromosome **is absent,** then look for **BCR/BAL gene** which is present in 40-50 % patients with **negative** Philadelphia chromosome.
(4) Some patients (10 to 15% cases) may have **loss of Y chromosome, and trisomy 8**.

(D) **Differential diagnosis**:
(1) **Leukemoid reaction**: WBC counts < 50,000 per microliter, toxic granulation vacuolation, Dohle bodies in the granules, absence of basophilia, normal or nicreased LAP level, plus history and physical examinations of leukemoid reaction.
(2) Myelodysplastic or myeloproliferative syndrome: **Agnogenic myeloid dysplasia** with or without myelofibrosis have **splenomegaly, neutrophilia, thrombocytosis**.

(E) **Treatment of CML:**
(1) **Palliative therapy: Oral busalfan plus hydroxyurea** because overdose of busulfan can cause prolonged myelosuppression. They control the WBC and platelet count and spleen size but **rarely** eliminate the philadelphia chromosome from bone marrow cells **which occurs with cytogenetically directed therapy**.
(2) **Cytogenetically directed therapy**:
(a) Interferon therapy: Both human leukocyte interferon and recombinant alpha-interferon produce hematologic and cytogenic remissions.
(b) **Chemotherapy**: Same drugs used in AML have been used to suppress Philadelphia chromosome which was successful in > 50% cases. Chemotherapy is presently under research protocol.

(c) **Allogenic bone morrow transplantation**: It is more effective in patients < 30 years, absence of graft-versus-host disease (GVHD), and transplantation **within 1 year of diagnosis**.

(3) Treatment of accelerated CML and blast crisis of CML:

(a) Splenectomy sometimes correct thrombocytopenia.

(b) Same drugs used in AML should be used.

(c) Patients with lymphoid blast crisis phenotype should be treated with vincristine, corticosteroids, asparaginase, and/or anthracyclines.

(d) Allogenic marrow transplantation.

84. **Hairy cell leukemia (HCL) (rare, mostly in male, median age 50 years)**:

(A) **Clinical manifestations**: Fever, anemia, weight loss, abdominal discomfort due to enlarged spleen.

Physical examination: Most common finding is **splenomegaly** (75 to 80% cases); other finding is lymphadenopathy. Retroperitoneal lymphadenopathy is diagnosed by CT scan.

(B) **Blood tests**: Anemia (<10 grams/dL), **leukopenia (<4000 per microliter),** neutropenia (<1500 per microliter), thrombocytopenia (<100,000 per microliter), and monocytopenia (<100 per microliter).

(C) **Diagnosis of HCL:** Clinical features and blood tests are suggestive of HCL. Peripheral smear **reveals hairy cells** (cells with cytoplasmic projections). **Hairy cells exhibit a strong acid phosphatase (isoenzyme 5) cytochemical reactiono in 95% cases** Hairy cells express CD 19, CD 20, CD 22, and FMC 7 (**not** CD 21 or CD 5). **Bone marrow biopsy** (aspiration is **not** helpful) demonstrates **hairy cells plus hypercellularity**.

(D) **Treatment of HCL**:

(1) **Splenectomy** is **now** recommended for patients with splenic infarcts or massive splenomegaly.

(2) Interferon: Human leukocyte interferon (HuIFn) or r-IFn apha is the treatment of choice.

(3) **Investigational drugs**: **Pentostatin** (2-deoxycoformycin) is and adenosine deaminase inhibitor, and **2- chlorodeoxyadenosine** (2-CDA) is an adenosine analogue have shown significant improvement; **Granulocyte colony-stimulating factor** (G-CSF) can correct granulocytopenia in HCL.

85. **Most common leukemia in the western coountries: Chronic lymphocytic leukemia (CLL)** (1/3 of all cases of leukemias).

86. **Few important points in chonic lymphocytic leukemia (CLL)**:

(1) Etiology is **unknown**; **no** association with ionizing radiation and viruses; **farmers** have higher incidence of CLL than in any other occupation.
(2) **Family clustering in CLL** is more common than in any other leukemias; **please remember, first-degree relatives of patients have 2 to 4 folds higher risk of** CLL than general population.

87. **Clinical features, diagnosis, and treatment of chronic lymphocytic leukemia (CLL):**
(A) **Clinical features: Most patients are asymptomatic** and **routine blood test shows absolute lymphocytosis in the peripheral blood smear**. Patients may have **nonspecific symptoms** such as fatigue, lethargy, loss of appetite, reduced exercise tolerance or weight loss. **Patients may have noticed enlarged cervical lymph nodes. Sinopulmonary infections are most common during early** infection, as **the disease progresses** patients develop fever, night sweat, infection (bacterial, fungal, or viral), neutropenia, T-cell deficiency, and hypogammaglobulinemia.
Physical examination: Cervical lymphadenopathy (rubbery, discrete, mobile, later on become matted) **is the most common finding (66% cases). Pulmonary symptoms and signs are present. Less** likely involves liver, spleen or CNS. **CNS is involved by opportunistic infections (cryptococcosis or listeriosis). Later in the disease,** massive adenopathy causes **obstructive jundice, intestinal obstruction, obstructive uropathy, leg edema due** to obstruction of lymphatic or venous system.
(B) **Diagnosis of CLL:**
(1) **Absolute lymphocytosis (usually 40,000 to 150,000 per microliter**; may reach as high as 1 x 10^6 per microliter in late stages; may be as low as 5000 per microliter) in **the peripheral blood smear**; **some patients** have anemia (< 11 gram/dL) and thrombocytopenia (<100,000 permicroliter).
(2) If the lymphocyte count is between 5,000 to 15,000 per microliter, **supportive documetation of clonality** (kappa or lamda light-chain excess or immunoglobulin gene rearrangement) **should be done for the diagnosis**.
(3) Bone marrow lymphocytosis (<30% lymphocytes) is present and bone marrow biopsy is performed.
(4) Hypochromic, microcytic anemia with normal reticulocytes count is the **most common**; up to 10% cases can have **autoimmune hemolytic anemia which is diagnosed by positive direct Coombs' test, reticulocytosis, elevated unconjugated bilirubin,** and **low serum haptoglobin level**.

(5) Four patterns of lymphocytic infiltration on bone marrow biopsy occur: Nodular (15%), infiltrative (30%), mixed nodular and infiltrative (30%), and diffuse (35%). Diffusse infiltration means advanced disease.

(6) Decreased levels of IgG, IgA, or IgM. It is more common in advanced (up to 70% cases) than early stage (25% of cases).

(7) Cytogenetic abnormalities in **CLL include trisomy 12 (40%)**, 14q + abnormalities (25%), and abnormalities in the long arm(q) of chromosome 6 and 11.

(C) **Treatment of CLL:**

(1) **Chlorambucil** (less commonly, cyclophosphamide) is the **first drug used in CLL**.

(2) **Corticosteroids** (prednisone) is often used simultaneously with chlorambucil.

(3) COP regimen: Cyclophosphamide, oncovin (vincristine), and prednisone are also used. This regimen is **not** more effective than chlorambucil.

(4) CAP regimen: Cyclophosphamide, adriamycin (doxorubicin), and prednisone or with vincristine is also effective.

(5) Prednisone is also indicated in **Coombs' positive autoimmune hemolytic anemia** and is some cases of immunemediated thrombocytopenia in CLL.

(6) **Radiation therapy**: It is restricted to external localized nodal masses or an enlarged spleen.

(7) **Experimental treatment:** Two adenosine analogues (fludarabine monophosphate and 2-CDA), and pentostatin (deoxycoformycin) which is an adenosine deaminase inhibitor have future potential to treat CLL.

88. **Most common causes of death in CLL**:

(1) CLL is more common in **elderly patients**, death is due to **intercurrent illnesses** of this age group.

(2) CLL patients < 60 years of age, death is either **due to result of CLL or one of its complications,** particularly **infections (most commonly due to gram-negative becterial** infection or fungal infection).

89. **Few important points in acute leukemias**:

(1) ALL (acute lymphocytic leukemia) is most common **in children (not** important for Board examination).

(2) **AML (acute myelogenous leukemia) gradually increases with age**, 50% patients are under 50 years of age (Important).

(3) Incidence of **all leukemias**: **AML (46%)**, ALL (11%), CLL (chronic lymphocytic leukemia, 29%), CML (chronic myelogenous leukemia, 14%).

(4) Etiology of acute leukemia **is unknown in most cases**.

(5) Ionizing radiation can cause **AML, CML,** and ALL.
(6) **HTLV-I** (human T cell lymphotropic virus type I) can cause **adult T cell leukemia (ATL)**. HTLV-II virus has been linked to a syndrome resembling hairy cell leukemia but its link to cancer is uncertain.
(7) **Benzene** causes marrow hypoplasia and acute leukemia.
(8) **Alkylating agents** (chlorambucil, melphalan, nitrogen mustard) can cause **AML,** which is also caused by prolonged exposure of epipodophyllotoxins.
(9) Myelodysplastic syndrome can occur before development of secondary AML.
(10) Most frequent chromosomal abnormality in **AML** (80% of cases) is **gain of chromosome 8** or **loss of part or all of chromosome 7 or 5**.
(11) **Acute promyelocytic leuykemia** almost always has a translocation involving chromosome 15 and 17.
(12) **Acute myelomonocytic (M4)** leukemia with abnormal eosinophilia is associated with inversion of **chromosome 16**.
(13) **Adults with ALL** have Philadelphia chromosome [t(9;22)] up to 20% cases.

90. **Clinical manifestations, diagnosis, and treatment of acute leukemias**:
(A) **Clinical manifestations**: Most patients have **anemia** causing pallor, fatigue, headache, and in predisposed cases cause angina or cardiac failure. **Thrombocytopenia** (33% cases) causing petechiae, ecchymoses, epistaxis, gum bleeding, or hemorrhage. **Granulocytopenia** causes infections (mostly bacterial).
ALL usually infiltrates **normal** organs more than AML, results in **enlarged** lymph nodes, liver, spleen; bone pain, leukemic leptomeningitis (seizures and palsies). ALL frequently relapses into the CNS. Patients with acute **promyelocytic leukemia** (M3) causes subclinical or clinical DIC. Acute **monocytic or myelomonocytic** leukemics are the forms of AML, most commonly cause **extramedullary infiltration. Mediastinal masses** usually produce by **T cell ALL**.
(B) **Diagnosis of acute leukemias**:
(1) WBC count is usually **5,000 to 50,000** (50% cases), **<5000** (in 25% cases), and **>50,000** (in 25% cases).
(2) Anemia plus thrombocytopenia (<20,000 per microliter).
(3) Presence of **blast cells** in peripheral smear.
(4) **The diagnosis is confirmed by bone marrow aspiration and biopsy reveal hypercellular marrow and 30 to 100% blast cells**, other findings are **fibrosis** (especially with M7 AML) or **bone marrow necrosis**.
(5) Elevated uric acid (especially in ALL) and increased LDH in serum.

(C) **Treatment of acute leukemias:**

(1) Acute leukemias could be cured with chemotherapy and bone marrow transplantation.

(2) Antileukemic therapy should begin as soon as possible, **usually within 48 hours**.

(3) **Before therapy**, infection should be controlled with anitbiotic and hemorrhage should be controlled.

(4) **To prevent uric acid nephropathy,** patients should be **hydrated** and receive **allopurinol**.

(5) **To alleviate psychological shock, at least one** conference with the patient and family members should be arranged **before treatment**.

(6) **Emergency treatment:**

(a) **Platelet transfusion** to maintain the platelet > 20,000 per microliter.

(b) **Bleeding due to DIC:** Use low-dose IV heparin.

(c) **Fever and granulocytopenia:** IV broad spectrum antibiotic after appropriate cultures.

(d) CNS vascular injury and hemorrhages: Leukapheresis, hydroxyurea, and immediate whole-brain irradiation.

(e) Uremia and anuria due to elevated serum uric acid levels: To prevent these complications institute **hydration**, urinary alkalinization with **acetazolamide** and **allopurinol** to prevent uric acid production; institute **dialysis** for renal failure.

(7) **Treatment of ALL:**

(a) **Remission induction**: Vincristine, prednisone, and most experts add L-asparaginase and/or daunorubicin **can produce complete remission**. Failure to achieve complete remission is either due to resistance of the leukemic cells to the drugs or to progressive infections.

(b) **Post remission chemotherapy**: High-dose methotrexate, cyclophosphamide, and cytarabine are used. **Most commonly used maintenance** therapy are daily **6-mercaptopurine** and **weekly or bi weekly methotrexate**.

(c) **CNS prophylaxis:** Intrathecal methotrexate alone, or it is combined with 2400 cGy to the cranium, or 2400 cGy to the craniospinal axis.

(d) **Treatment of relapsed ALL** (most relapses occurs in marrow and within 2 years, other places are CNS, or testes): Same therapy as initial induction should be given; for CNS or testes involvement **additional specific therapy** to those sites should be instituted.

(e) **Marrow transplantation**: It is used after high-dose of chemotherapy, marrow should be from HLA-identical sibling or HLA-matched unrelated donor, or autologous marrow.

(8) **Treatment of AML**:

(a) Remission induction: Combination of **anthracycline** (daunomycin or idarubicin) **and cytarabine** produce complete remission in 60 to 80% cases of AML.

(b) **Post remission therapy:** Repeated couses of daunomycin and cytarabine at convetional doses, high-dose cytarabine or other agents are useful. **Unlike ALL**, low-dose therapy has **no** benefit, CNS prophylaxis does **not** improve the survival.

(c) **Treatment of recurrent AML**: Daunomycin-cytarabine combination or high-dose of cytarabine.

(d) Treatment of acute promyelocytic leukemia (APL): All-trans-retinoic acid (ATRA) should be used alongwith other therapy because of recurrence when used alone.
ATRA complication: Characteristic hyperleukocytosis plus respiratory distress and pulmonary infiltrates.

(e) **Bone marrow transplantation:** It is the **treatment of choice in patients with initial relapse** and **should be used in most patients while in first remission**.

(9) Supportive care:

(a) **Infections** (**most common organisms are S. epidermidis, Pseudomonas aeruginosa, E. coli, and Klebsiella aerobacter**): **Cephalosporin plus a semisynthetic penicillin** or **a semisynthetic penicillin plus an aminoglycoside**. Antibiotics should be continued until the patients become afebrile and granulocyte counts become normal. **If fever persists** despite appropriate antibiotics, **catheter should be removed** and **granulocyte** transfusion for leukopenia. To reduce the infection **selective GI decontamination** (ciproploxacin or combination of trimethoprim-sulfamethoxazole plus colistin) is useful.
Fungal infection should be considered in patients with recurrence of fever or persistence of fever and granulocytopenia while **receiving broad-spectrum antibiotics**, patients should be treated empirically with **amphotericin. To prevent Pneumocystis carinii** infection, use prophylactic **trimethoprim-sulfamethoxazole**. **To prevent CMV infection** in CMV- seronegative patients, use CMV-seronegative blood products. **Herpes simplex and herpes zoster** should be treated with acyclovir. To **prevent transfusion induced graft-versus-host dieases** (rash, fever, falling blood counts, elevated LFT's), all blood products **should be irradiated before transfusion**.

91. **Non-Hodgkin lymphomas:**

(1) Male > female, increase in frequency throughout adulthood, and **unknown** etiology.
(2) Associated with **Burkitt's lymphoma** (Africa), adult T cell leukemia/lymphoma (Japan), and intestinal lymphoma (Middle East).
(3) Burkitt's lymphoma have specific **chromosomal breakage and translocation** (c-myc oncogene on chromosome **8** and the immunoglobulin havey-or light-chain gene on chromosome 14, 2, or 22).
(4) Clinical manifestations of **low grade lymphomas**: History of waxing and waning or **slowly progressing lymphadenopathy**; affected nodes are **mobile, rubbery, not** painful, **no** overlying skin infiltration; **commonly involved bone marrow;** may have hepatosplenomegaly with **normal** LFT's with mild elevation of alkaline phosphatase; **normal** blood cell counts; **extranodal involvements** include **pleura, lung,** skin, GI tract, and breasts; enlarged lymph nodes may cause lymphedema, epidural spinal cord compression, or ureteral obstruction.
(5) Clinical manifestations of **intermediate and high grade** lymphomas: **Sudden rapid enlargement of lymph node masses**; lymph nodes may be rubbery and mobile or hard and fixed with overlying skin infiltration and **may have inflammatory changes**; large **lymph node masses may be present** in mediastinum, retroperitoneum, and mesentry; **hepatosplenomegaly** may be present with abnormal LFT's or obstruction; **not** commonly involved bone marrow (unlike low-grade); extranodal involvement include **stomach, SI,** lung, bone, CNS (meninges), and skin; Waldeyer's ring may be associated with extranodal involvement of the stomach or SI, or both.
(6) **Miscellaneous clinical manifestations: Mycosis fungoides** (rare helper T cell skin lymphoma), true histiocytic lymphoma, and composite lymphoma. Most important subgroup is Ki-1 lymphoma (diffuse large cell lymphoma) which can mimic Hodgkin disease. **HTLV-I associated adult T cell leukemia/lymphoma** appears with generalized lymphadenopathy, hepatosplenomegaly, lytic bone disease, dermatologic infiltration, bone marrow involvement, and hypercalcemia.
(7) **Diagnosis of non-Hodgkin lymphoma**: It is done by **interpretation of tumor tissue preferably lymph nodes**, B cell and T cell typing, clinical presentation, and HTLV-I or HIV antibody determination. **Staging** should be done to determine the **extent of the disease**. Pathologic confirmation should be done such as GI biopsy, skin biopsy, pleural cytology or **some cases** laparatomy or thoracotony which is usually **not** done for Hodgkin disease.
(8) Treatment for **low-grade** lymphomas:
    (a) Patients with **stage I or II (localized disease):** Local radiation therapy.

(b) Patients with **stage III or IV (advanced stage):** It is **controversial.** Single agent or multiagent chemotherapy with or without radiation may be effective. Cyclophosphamide or cholorambucil or combination of cyclophosphamide, vincristine, prednisone with or without procarbazine or doxorubicin (Adriamycin) is useful.
Another approach is to defer initial treatment until disease progresses because disease may be indolent, slow progressing, or therapy would **not** cure the disease.

(9) Treatment for **intermediate-grade and high-grade lymphomas:**

(a) **Combination chemotherapy is the best treatment of choice**. Most commonly used combination drugs are MACOP-B (methotrexate, Adriamycin, cyclophosphamide, oncovin, prednisone, bleomycin) plus co-trimaxazole. The **recently used CHOP therapy is the gold standard** (cyclophosphamide, hydroxydaunomycin/Adriamycin, oncovin, prednisone).

(10) Special treatment for involvement of different parts of the body:

(a) **Primary brain lymphoma**: Whole-brain irradiation with or without chemotherapy.

(b) **SVC syndrome**: Chemotherapy and/or irradiation therapy.

(c) **GI involvement:** To avoid perforation or bleeding, **surfical resection of the involve segment should be done** before chemotherapy. **Gastric lymphomas** do **not** need surgical resection, it is **treated with combination chemotherapy and/or irradiation therapy**.

(d) Tumor mass > 10 cm: Supplementary irradiation therapy is sometimes used **along with or after** chemotherapy; **surgical resection is only effective in intra-abdominal Burkitt's lymphoma**.

(e) **Tumor lysis syndrome:** Rapid urate production is treated with allopurinol. Patients also have high k and phosphate, low calcium.

92. **Few important points in Hodgkin disease:**

(1) Peak incidence in **third decade** of life, same-sex **sibling have 10 times more risk** of developing the disease.

(2) It is associated with infectious mononucleosis and Epstein-Barr virus (EBV).

(3) Among the four subtypes, **NSHD** (nodular sclerosing Hodgkin disease) **is the most common** and it affects young **females** with early-stage supradiaphragmatic presentation; **second most common** is MCHD (medium-cellularity Hodgkin disease) and it affects mostly **males** with generalized lymphadenopathy or extranodal involvement and systemic symptoms; rare two types are LPHD (lymphocytic-predominant Hodgkin disease) and LDHD (lymphocyte-depletion Hodgkin disease).

(4) **The Reed-sternberg (R-S) cell is the diagnostic tumor cell.**

93. **Clinical manifestations of Hodgkin disease**:

(1) Most common presentation is **supradiaphragmatic lymphadenopathy (>80% cases)**, mostly present in anterior mediastinum; **rest are** below the diaphragm.

(2) **Mediastinal presentation**: **It remains silent** (unlike non-Hodgkin lymphoma) **until the tumor becomes very large;** symptoms include **cough, chest discomfort, tightness, or wheezing**; the **symptoms increase when lying supine (due to tracheal compression) but decreases in upright position**. **Remember,** it usually does **not** cause SVC (superior vena cava) syndrome, phrenic nerve paralysis or laryngeal nerve involved hoarseness (**unlike** non-Hodgkin lymphoma).

(3) Reginoal lymph node presentation (cervical, supraclacvicular, axillary lymph nodes are commonly involved): **Remember,** it does **not** usually involve posterior mediastinal, Waldeyer's tonsillar ring, preauricular, occipital, popllitaeal, and mesenteric lymph nodes (**unlike non-Hodgkin lymphoma**). **(Important) A 35 year old man appears with cervical lymphagenopathy which is partially improved with antibiotic:** Always rule out Hodgkin lymphoma because superimposed reactive lymphadenopathy may respond to antibiotic.

(4) **Extranodal involvement:** Isolated extranodal involvement **indicates non-Hodgkin disease except when associated with HIV disease**. Hodgkin disease does **not** have only isolated extranodal involvement such as skin nodue or gastric involvement. It is always associated with lymphadenopaathy.

(5) **Generalized lymphadenopathy is uncommon; so always rule out** non-Hodgkin lymphomas, viral, fungal, mycobacterial, bacterial, and autoimmune disorders.

(6) **Systemic mainfestations of Hodgkin disease**: Chronic pruritus; lymph node pain with alcohol consumption; hematologic abnormalities (**elevated** WBC, polymorphs, eosinophils, and thrombocytes); **systemic B symptoms** (fever, night sweat, or weight loss).

94. **Diagnosis of Hodgkin disease**:

(1) **History** of B symptoms (fever, night sweats, and weight loss) and **pruritis** are important. Presence of pruritus has adverse outcome.

(2) **Physical examinations** include location of lymphadenopathy, hepatosplenomegaly, cardiac or respiratory symptoms, or inspection of Waldeyer's ring.

(3) **Imaging studies: CXR, CT scan with IV contrast,** gallium radionuclide scan and bipedal lymphogram are useful. They are **not** able to detect splenic involvement.

(4) **Laboratory studies**:
Blood: CBC and its differential count, platelet counts, ESR; liver and renal function test. Patients usually have anemia (mild to moderate), moderate to marked leukemoid reaction, thrombocytosis; eosinophilia associated with pruritus; **HIV-related Hodgkin lymphoma can have absolute lymphopenia** (< 1000 cells per cubic millimeter) which indicates poor prognosis.

(5) Bone marrow biopsy: It is important in staging process but bone marrow involvement is **rare**.

(6) **Staging laparatomy**: It is **not** done routinely. It is the **most definitive method for detectiong occult infradiaphragmatic** Hodgkin **because splenic involvement is not usually diagnosed by imaging studies**.

95. **Treatment of Hodgkin disease**:

(A) **Early-stage disease**:

(1) **Radiation therapy alone** to clinically staged patients with favorable prognostic factor. **Side effect of radiation therapy**:

(a) **Acute side effects:** Dry mouth, alteration in taste, pharyngitis, fatigue, dry cough, nausea, and dermatitis.

(b) **Lhermitte's sign:** Electric shock sensation radiating down the backs of both legs when the head is flexed. It occurs **after 3 weeks to 3 months** completion of therapy, resolves spontaneously, and this **sign is due to transient demyelinization of the cervical spinal cord**.

(c) **Late effects:** Subclinical hypothyroidism should be treated with L-thyroxine; **most frequent solid tumors after radiation or chemotherapy are lung cancer, breast cancer, stomach cancer, and melanoma; mediastinal irradiation** can increase the **risk of coronary artery disease**.

(2) **Chemotherapy**:

(a) **MOPP therapy** (nitrogen mustard, oncovin, procarbazine, prednisone) is most commonly used.

(b) **The best therapy is ABVD therapy** (Adriamycin, bleomycin, vinblastin, DTIC) and may be **more effective and less toxic than MOPP therapy.**

(c) MOPP-ABVD therapy.

(d) MOPP-ABV hybrid therapy.

(B) **Advanced-stage disease:** The principal mode of therapy in the stage is **combination chemotherapy. Toxicities of combination chemotherapy**:

(1) **ABVD:** Fatigue, hair loss, neutropenia; transient azoospermia (**not** permanent fertility) in men, temporary dysmenorrhoea in women. **Bleomycin causes pulmonary toxicity. Vinblastin** causes phlebitis and peripheral or autonomic neuropathy.

(2) **MOPP: Thrombocytopenia (myelosuppression) permanent infertility** in most males and many older females; **vincristine** causes autonomic and peripheral neuropathy; **after 10 years (5% cases), secondary myelodysplasia or acute myeloid leukemia**.

(C) **Relapsed Hodgkin disease**:

(1) Hodgkin disease may be **cured** even **if the initial treatment is not successful**.

(2) **Patients relapse after radiation therapy**: **ABVD is the treatment of choice.**

(3) **Patients relapse** early after completion of combination chemotherapy: High dose (HD) chemotherapy plus autologous stem cell transplantation (HD-ASCT) is the preferred treatment of choice. Chemotherapentic drugs are CBV (cyclophosphamide, BCNU, and VP-16).

(D) **Treatment in special circustances**:

(1) Hodgkin disease in pregnancy: Usually **no** treatment is needed because this disease **remains clinically silent or symptomatic** for many months. If treatment is needed, then use **field irradiation** with shielding uterus, **vinblastin alone**, or even combination chemotherapy.

(E) **Treatment recommendations**:

(1) Stage I and II A, good-risk patients with low chances of abdominal involvement: **Primary irradiation (no laparatomy)** is the treatment of choice.

(2) **Stage I and II A moderate-risk** with > 10% chances of abdominal involvement: Primary irradiation and may require staging laparotomy to confirm the diagnosis.

(3) **Stage III A with minimal splenic** involvement: Radiation therapy alone or alternative therapy with ABVD or MOPP-ABV hybrid plus extended-field irradiation.

(4) **Stage Ix or IIx disease**: ABVD or MOPP-ABV hybrid, after remission followed by extended-field consolidation.

(5) Stage III A: ABVD or MOPP-ABV hybrid plus extended-field radiation.

(6) Stage III B and IV (advanced stages) ; ABVD or MOPP-ABV hybrid or combined with involved or extended-field irradiation.

96. **Monoclonal gammopathy of undetermined significance (MGUS) (median age 64 years):**

(1) **Presence of M-protein in** persons **without** evidence of multiple myeloma, amyloidosis, macroglobulinemia, or other related disease.
(2) **Absence** of lytic bone lesions, anemia, hypercalcemia, and renal insufficiency.
(3) **MGUS is charcterized** by **serum M-protein** concentration < 3 grams/dl ; < 5% plasma cells in the bone marrow; absence or only small amount of M-protein in the urine.
(4) Most of the patients (75% cases) medical problems are **not** related to the monoclonal gammopathy.
(5) Anemia, low or high WBC count, high calcium, low platelet, and renal insufficiency may be present but **are not** due to monoclonal protein.
(6) The M-protein mostly consists of **IgG**.
(7) Most common cause of death (47% cases) is **not** related to underlying condition.
(8) Approximately 24% patients can develop **complications** such as **multiple myeloma (16%)**, and other conditions, anytime between 2 to 29 years after the diagnosis of M-protien.

97. **Disease associated with monoclonal gammopathies**:
(1) **Dermatologic disease:** Lichen myxedematosus, pyoderma gangrenosum, and necrobiotic xanthogranuloma.
(2) Leukemias: **CLL**, chronic myelomonocytic, hairy cell, or adult T cell leukemia.
(3) Lymphoproliferative disease.
(4) Neurologic disease: Peripheral neuropathy (more sensory involvement than motor involvement), but normal cranial nerves and autonomic functions.

98. **Few important points in multiple myeloma (or Kahler's disease)**:
(1) Etiology is **unknown**; exposure to benzence, radiation, insecticides, herbicides may have a role; men > women, median age 61 years (**rarely** occur < 40 year).
(2) Most cases plasma cells are CIg^+, CD 38^+, and PCA-1^+; IL-6 is an important growth factor for myeloma cells; c-myc, H-ras, and p53 genes may involved in the pathogenesis of this disease.
(3) Chromosomal structural changes is found in chromosomes 1, 11, 14, monosomies, and trisomies.
(4) Clinical manifestations: **Most common is bone pain in the back or chest (66% cases),** pain is **enhanced by movement**, so does **not** occur in night **except in change of poition**; other findings are **reduced height** due to vertebral collapse, **fatigue, weakness, and anemia**. Presence of **fever means infection** (Respiratory or UTI, gram-positive or gram-negative

organisms). Patients may have **renal insufficiency** (due **to myeloma kidney** from light chains or **hypercalcemia**), **bleeding disorder** due to low platelet counts or coating of platelets with M protein, or amyloidosis (10% cases).

(5) **Radiologic findigns: Puched-out lytic lesion, osteoporosis,** or **fractures** are most commonly found in **vertebrae, skull**, thoracic cage, pelvis, proximal humeri and femora; CT scan or MRI is diagnostic when X-ray findings are negative and patients have pain.

(6) **Diagnostic criteria: Bone marrow** should have > 10% **plasma cells** or **plasma cytoma plus at least one of the following findings**: Serum M-protein > 3 grams/dl, M-protein in the urine, and lyting bone lesions.

(7) **Complications**:

(a) **Neurologic: Radiculopathy** in the thoracic or lumbosacral area is the most common neurologic finding due to nerve compression from vertebral collapse.

(b) **Renal: Bence Jones proteinuria** (75% cases) and **elevated serum creatinine** (50% cases). **Characteristic finding is presence of large waxy laminated casts** in distal and collecting tubules due to precipitation of monoclonal light chains.

(c) **Infections:** Most common organisms are **Diplococcus pneumoniae** and **S. aureus.**

(d) Bleeding and rarely thrombosis

(8) **Treatment:**

(a) The combination chemotherapy (**melphalan and prednisone** or a combination of **alkylating agents**) is the best treatment of choice for symptomatic patients.

(b) Pain is controlled by **analgesic** plus chemotherapy; radiation therapy is used only in **disabling pain** unresponsive **to above mentioned therapy Complications of prolonged chemotherapy**: Myelodysplastic syndrome or acute leukemia.

(c) **Alpha-2-interferon** can prolong the plateau state but **not** the survival.

(d) Bone marrow transplantation may be useful in some patients.

(e) **Treatment of refractory cases**: VAD (Vincristine, Adriamycin, dexamethasone) is the treatment of choice.

(f) Treatment for hypercalcemia: Hydration with isotonic saline plus prednisone.

(g) Treatment for renal insufficiency: **Furosemide**; **hemodialysis** in symptomatic azotemia; plasmaphresis may reverse renal function but **not responsive in severe cases**.

(h) Treatment for infections: **Appropriate antibiotics** for infections; **prophylactic penicillin** for recurrent infections; IV gamma globulin is also helpful; **immunization with pneumococcal and influenza vaccines should be given to all patients**.

(i) **Treatment for bony lesions**: Remain active, avoid trauma; fixation of fractures or impending fractures of long bones with an **intramedullary rod** and methyl methacrylate are useful.

(j) Treatment for hyperviscosity: Plasmapheresis.

(k) Treatment for extradural plasmocytoma: Radiation and dexamethasone.

99. **POEMS syndrome (osteosclerotic myeloma)**:

(1) It is characterized by **polyneuropathy, organomegaly (hepatomegaly), endocrinopathy, M-protein, and skin changes**.

(2) Hyperpigmentation, hypertrichosis; gynecomastia, atrophic testes, clubbing of the fingers and toes.

(3) Most common presentations are chornic inflammatory demylenating papilledema but normal cranial nerves.

(4) Laboratory values ; Thrombocytosis, normal or elevated hemoglobin; < 5% plasma cells in bone marrow; most patients have λ protient.

(5) Diagnosis is confirmed by demonstration of monoclonal plasma cells from biopsy of an osteosclerotic lesion.

(6) Treatment:

(a) Localized lesions: Radiotherapy.

(b) Widespread osteosclerotic lesions: Melphalan and prednisone are used.

100. **A 60 year old man** appear with H/O **bleeding (oozing) from oronasal area, weakness, fatigue**; patient may also complain of blurred vision, loss of weight, recurrent infection, dyspnea, and cardiac symptoms (CHF).

Physical examination reveals pallor, hepatosplenolmegaly, lymphadenopathy, retinal changes (hemorrhages, exudates, venous congestion with vascular segmentation or sausage formation), diffuse **pulmonary infiltrates**, and sensorineural peripheral neuropathy.

Laboratory findings: Normocytic, normochromic anemia; low serum cholesterol; **characteristic serum electrophoresis** (tall, narrow peak or dense band and gamma mobility), **large IgM M protien (<3 grams/dl)**, and lymphoid-plasma cell infiltration of the bone marrow **are diagnostic features**.

Most likely diagnosis: Waldenstorm's macroglobulinemia (primary macroglobulilnemia).

Treatment:

(1) **Chlorambul is used initially in symptomatic patients**.

(2) **Patients with relapse:** Use combination of alkylating agents such as M2 protocol (vincirstine, BCNU, melphalan, cyclophosphamide, and prednisone).

(3) Previously untreated patients mostly respond to fludarabine or 2-chlorodeoxy-adenosine.
(4) Transfusion is given for anemia, plasmapheresis is used for viscosity.

101. **Hyperviscosity syndrome:**
(1) **Signs and sumptoms:** Chronic nasal bleeding, oozing form the gums, postsurgical or GI bleeding, retinal hemorrhages and papilledema causing blurring or loss of vision. Patients may develop **CHF** (congestive heart failure), dizziness, **ataxia, nystagmus, dilplopia, decreased hearing, somnolence, and coma**.
(2) **Diagnosis:** Viscosity > 4 centipoises (cP) but the relation between viscosity and symptoms is **not** accurate.
(3) Treatment: **Plasmapheresis** should be done daily until the patient is asymptomatic (3 to 4 liters of plasma should be **replaced by albumin**).

102. **Primary amyloidosis (AL):** Most commonly involves **males**, median age **is 64 years**.
(A) **Clinical manifestations: Most common** presentations are **loss of weight**, **weakness or fatigue**. Patients may **develop CHF** (dyspnea, pedal edema) or **peripheral neuropathy. Hoarseness and jaw claudication** may be present.
Physical examination reveals hepatomegaly (25% of cases), **nephrotic syndrome** (33% of cases), **carpal tunnel syndrome**, CHF, postural hypotension, or peripheral neuropathy.
(B) **Diagnosis of AL**: **Physical findings** plus **presence of M-protein in the serum or urine electrophroesis** strongly suggests AL. **Diagnosis is confirmed by appropriate biopsy. Bone marrow plasma cells are modestly increased.** Other fingings are **proteinuria (80% cases), renal insufficiency (50% cases)**; low albumin and elevated cholesterol and triglyceride in nephrotic syndrome; prologed prothrombin time (PT), thrombin time (TT) and decreased Factor X level may be present.
(C) **Treatment:**
(1) **Melphalan and prednisone or clochicine are effective**.
(2) **Nephrotic syndrome:** Diuretic, salt-restriction; dialysis prn.
(3) **Orthostatic hypotension:** Elastic stockings or leotards is helpful; fludrocortisone may be helpful but it causes fluid retention.
(4) **CHF:** Diuretic, salt-restriction; digoxin may be used with caution because of increased drug sensitivity, heart block, and arrythmias.

103. **Most common causes of moderate and transient splenomegaly**: **Systemic infections. Infectious mononucleosis due to Epstein-Barr virus always have splenomegaly, Rocky Mountain spotted fever, HIV disease-related**

complex (ARC). Other few important causes are SLE, acute and chronic leukemias, myelodysplastic disorders, non-Hodgkin lumphoma, and Banti's syndrome (chronic congestive splenomegaly, pancytopenia, GI bleeding due to portal hypertension, splenic vein hypertension due to cirrhosis or portal or splenic vein thrombosis).

104. **Idiopathic thrombocytopenic purpura (ITP)**:

(1) Most common in **women, < 40 years of age, gradual onset** of the disease **without a preceding illness** and with a chronic course.

(2) Patients may appear with petechiae, ecchymoses, epistaxis, or menorrhagia in women. Splenomegaly is usually **absent**.

(3) **Diagnosis** is made by thrombocytopenia plus clinical presentations; determination of antiplatelet antibodies (IgG) is **not** needed to confirm the diagnosis in most cases; bone marrow examination is done **only** when blood tests and clinical presentations **cannot** confirm the diagnosis of ITP, (bone marrow is **normal** with increased megakaryocytes).

(4) **Treatment of ITP**:

(a) **Asymptomatic patients with platelet counts > 40,000 per microliter**: Observation with periodic evaluation of the patients condition.

(b) Patients with < 20,000 platelets are usually symptomatic: **Prednisone or a similar corticosteroid is the treatment of choice.**

(c) **Patients with > 30,000 platelets plus bleeding** (may have acquired platelet dysfunction): Prednisone or similar corticosteroid is used.

(d) **Steroid unresponsiveness** (< 50,000 platelet count after 4 weeks of treatment), and **steroid failure** (subnormal platelet counts after 6 weeks of treatment).

(e) **Intravenous gamma globulin** is used in patients with active bleeding or waiting for major surgery. It increases the platelet count within **3 to 5 days in most** patients and is the most rapidly active agent.

(f) Splenectomy improves the platelet counts (>70% cases of ITP) within a few days or maximum within 2 weeks. Spleen is the major site of platelet destruction and antiplatelet antibody formations.

(g) Chronic ITP patients with ineffective splenectomy: **Danazol** induces remission in 40% cases; IV **vincristine and vinblastine** can raise the platelet count within 1 to 2 weeks; **immunosuppressive therapy (cyclophosphamide and azathioprine**) can increase platelet counts in **refractory ITP (60% responsivenesss); pulsed high-dose dexamethasone** is also effective in refractory ITP.

105. **Thrombotic thrombocytopenic purpura (TTP)**:

(1) TTP is a **rare** disease, unknown etiology.

(2) **TTP is characterized by fever (98% of cases)** severe thrombocytopenia, microangiopathic hemolytic anemia (>96% of cases), neurologic abnormalities (>92% of cases), renal involvement (proteinuria, hematuria, casts, and azotemia; 88% of cases). **Remember, symptoms frequently wax (platelet aggregation)** and **wane** (platelet **disaggregation**) such as **aphasia, stupor one moment and become alert in the next moment**.
(3) TTP can occur due to pregnancy and oral contraceptives.
(4) **Diagnosis of TTP is straight forward in most cases**; when diagnosis is **not** certain then **biopsy** of the gum, skin, or bone marrow is helpful.
(5) **Treatment of choice is large-volume plasmapheresis** (about two plasma volumes) with replacement infusion of normal plasma.

106. **Drugs inhibit platelet function:**
(1) NSAID's block platelet synthesis of prostaglandins (PGE).
(2) Aspirin irreversibly acetylates PGE synthetase results in impairment of platelet function.
(3) High doses of beta-lactam antibiotics (penicillin and related compounds) can cause reversible abnormality of platelet function. Platelet function becomes **normal after 2 to 3 days of discontinuation** of the drug.

107. **Treatment of thrombocytopenia in different diseases**:
(A) **Liver failure: DDAVP** improves bleeding time in moderately severe liver disease with platelet count > 90,000 per microliter.
(B) **Renal failure:**
(1) **Low hematocrit (< 24%) prolong the bleeding time in uremia: Transfusion of packed red blood cells** to raise the hematocirt above 26% improves the bleeding time. Coagulation profiles are normal.
(2) The causes of bleeding in uremic patients are due to **hemostatic abnormality** or structurial lesion (**rarely** due to thrombocytopenia): Patients with hemostatic abnormality should be **dialyzed** (peritoneal or hemodialysis) which can reverse the hemostatic defect; if the **bleeding time is prolonged and patient is bleedinhg, use low-dose estrogens, DDAVP** (1-deamino-8-D-arginine vaspressin), **or cryoprecipitate**. Platelet transfusion is **useless**.
(C) **Paraproteinemias (multiple myeloma or Wadlenstorm's macroglobulinemia;** prolonged bleeding time and bleeding can be severe): Plasmapheresis and/or chemotherapy can stop bleeding be lowering paraprotein levels.

108. **Hemophilia A (Factor VIII deficiency)**: It is a X-linked recessive disease. Males are affected. Females are carries.

(A) **Clinical manifestations**: **Most common presentation is hemarthrosis of** knees, elbows, or other joints with **progressive destruction of the joint**; other manifestations are **airway obstruction** from bleeding into the neck or pharynx, **partial intestinal obstruction** from hemorrhage into the intestinal wall, **intestinal ischemia and necrosis** from mesenteric bleeding, **painless hematuria or ureteral colic** from clot formation, bleeding into muscles and retroperitoneum are usually underestimated; subdural or other intracranial hemorrhages **are rare but** represent major cause of morbidity and mortality. Minor (dental extraction) or major surgery causes significant bleeding.

(B) **Severity of the disease: Mild** (5 to 25% normal Factor VIII activity), **moderate** (1 to 5% normal activity), and **severe** (< 1% normal activity).

(C) **Diagnosis: Normal PT, prolonged APTT, normal** (or slightly prolonged) **bleeding time** (severely prolonged bleeding time in von Willebrand disease), **deficiency of Factor VIII c**, (deficiency of Factor VIII Ag or von Willebrand factor in von-Willebrand disease).

(D) **Treatment:**

(1) The patient should be educated and motivated in a major way in his **medical care at home with** the backup of a **primary care physician, a nurse coordinator,** plus multidisciplinary team of hematologist orthopedic surgeon, infectious disease specialist, dentist, social worker, financial coounselor.

(2) **The patients should go to work or to go school full time**, minimum ER visits, and hospital admission for medical illness, major trauma, or elective surgery.

(3) Patients should **carry identification about their disease to alert caregivers in an emergency**.

(4) **Primary care physician should** follow up these patients, receiving long term replacement therapy, day to day basis; but regular evaluation about 6 to 12 months interval.

(5) **The clinic visit should include complete** physical examination particularly to the joints, and inhibitor screen, LFT's, tests for antibodies to hepatitis viruses and HIV.

(6) **Replacement therapy**: Concentrated Factor VIII in the form of cryoprecipitate or lyophilized purified protein or F VIII is made by recombinant DNA techniques. (**Infusion of 15, 30, and 60 units/kg should raise the plasma levels to 25%, 50% and 100% respectively**)

(7) **Desmopressin** can raise F VIII level transiently and **EACA** to minimize mucosal bleeding.

(8) **Mild early diagnosed hemarthrosis**: Self-managed with a single infusion to attain F VIII level of **25 to 50% of normal**.

(9) **Severe hemorrhage:** F VIII infusion for 2 days after cessation of symptoms and signs of bleeding.

(10) **Major trauma or surgery**: F VIII level should be maintained **> 70% of normal until bleeding stops** then maintained in the range of **25 to 50% normal for 10 to 14 days**.

(11) **Muscle hematomass:** F VIII level should be maintained **40 to 60% normal for 4 to 6 days**.

(12) Patients have low F VIII levels despite replacement therapy: Patients have either **not** received enough F VIII or developed inhibitor that neutralizes infused F VIII.

(13) **Treatment of hemarthrosis: Immobilization** of the affected joint, application **of ice packs;** first **infusion of F VIII, aspiration** is performed only when there is pressure necrosis or worry about infection; **rehabilitation therapy** begins after the relief of pain and swelling; patients **with joint disease** should be treated but orthopedic surgeon (artificial joint or synovectomy is useful in severe chronic joint injury).

(14) **Dental care:**

(a) Frequent dental examination to maintain dental hygiene.

(b) Local anesthetic **by needle puncture or dental extraction should be done after F VIII infusion** prophylactically.

(c) Desmopressin, EACA or tranexamic **is also helpful** in prevention of rebleeding after tooth extraction.

(15) **Analgesics**: **Acetaminophen and codeine are the drug of choice; never give aspirin;** in selected cases **ibuprofen** can be used for chronic joint pain, **then mointor bleeding time** after several days of ibuprofen, if prolonged then stop the medication.

(16) F VIII inhibitor: It develops in childhood but create problems throughout life. Inhibitor are removed by plasmapheresis or neutralized by F VIII infusion (large amount).

109. **Von Willebrand disease (V-W disease)**: **It is an autosomal dominant disease** except type 3 which is autosomal recessive. It occurs in both males and females.

(A) **Clinical manifestations**: Patients may appear with **severe hemorrhages** or **asymptomatic,** diagnosed by laboratory testing due to positive family history. **Bleeding problems are mostly superficial such as epistaxis, easy bruising; less** commonly heaturia, GI bleeding, and hemarthrosis. **Postoperative bleeding is a serious problem.** Patients with **mild** disease, bleeding **only occurs after trauma, surgery, or dental extractions**. Excessive menstruation or postpartum bleeding is common in women.

(B) **Diagnosis**: Low F VIII Ag or von-Willebrand factor, prolonged bleeding time.

(1) **Type 1 disease**: Prolonged APTT, prolonged bleeding time, and low level of F VIII and von-Willebrand factor that parallels the level of F VIII, **diminished** or **absent** platelet aggregation when ristocetin is added to the patient's platelet-rich plasma. Patients with **severe** disease may **have < 1%** of normal von Willebrand factor **in plasma and platelets** and F VIII level < 5% of normal. Severe disease more commonly **recessive** disorder. **Recessive** disease is sometime called **type 3**.

(2) Type 2 disease: **Prolonged** bleeding time, **abnormal** ristocetin-induced platelet aggregation, but **normal or slightly** decreased levels of von-Willebrand factor and F VIII. These patients have **qualitative abnormalities of von Willebrand factor**. Type 2M disease have **decreased activity of ristocetin cofactor** even though **multimer pattern is normal. Type 2B disease have platelets to aggregation by ristocetin in the patient's platelet-rich plasma**. It may be due to **defects** in the patient's von Willebrand factor or in the patient's platelets (**pseudo von Willebrand disease**) or defect in **glycoprotein Ib** which is function **as receptor of** von Willebrand factor on the platelet cell surface. Type 2N (rare type, **autosomal hemophilia**) have von Willebrand factor which functions **normally** in platelet adhesion **but cannot bind and stabilize** F VIII, and **normal** platelet dependent function. **Von Willebrand factor** is **secreted** by endothelial cells and megakaryocytes. **Endothelial cells injury can increase von Willebrand factors** which is **increased** with the **aging and vigorous Valsalva maneuver,** and this factor is **decreased** in **hypothyroidism** and people with **type O blood** (than type A and B). **To avoid the wrong diagnosis, serial studies** of von Willebrand factor levels **over several months** and **to other family members are helpful**.

(C) Genetics:

(1) **Type 1 disease** may be due **to defect in von Willebrand factor gene**, but a defect in another gene **cannot** be excluded.

(2) Type 2 disease is due to mutation of von-Willebrand factor.

(D) **Treatment**:

(1) **Cryoprecipitate** (F VIII and von Willebrand factor) **corrects both the deficieny of** F VIII and prolonged bleed time of **type 1 von Willerbrand disease**. (Most F VIII concentrates does **not** have enough von Willebrand factor **except** F VIII concentrates of intermediate purity which contain multimeric von Willebrand factor). Management protocol is similar as described in hemophilia.

(2) **Desmopressin** is also useful and it releases von Willebrand factor and plasminogen activator from endothelial cells. It is given by infusion with saline over 15 minutes or by nasal spray. It is **contraindicated in type 2B disease because thrombocytopenia is the complication** after desmopressin therapy. Overuse causes fluid retention and hyponatremia. Desmopressin stimulates fibrinolysis (**fibrinolytic agent**).

(3) EACA or tranexamic acid suppresses baseline fibrinolysis (**antifibrinolytic agent**). It is used for **oral surgical procedures** and therapy should begin in the evening before the procedure and end when all wounds are healed. Its use **in major surgery is** controversial because of antifibrinolytic property.

(4) **Treamtment during menstruation: Hormone therapy** can suppress excessive menstrual blood loss.

(5) **Treamtment during pregnancy**: The levels of F VIII, von Willebrand factor, and ristocetin cofactor activity may become **normal** during pregnancy. These tests should be repeated in **third trimester** for replacement therapy during delivery. **Cryoprecipitate is indicated** if the F VIII level is **low.** If the F VIII level **is > 50%** but the bleeding time is **prolonged,** cryoprecipitate is given **if there** is **postpartum blood loss**.

110. **Complications of replacement therapy in von Willebrand disease**:

(1) In **severe** von Willebrand disease, the complications are same as in hemophilia.
(2) Chronic arthropathy is **less** common than hemophilia.
(3) **Rarely** develops **antibody** against von Willebrand protein.
(4) Patients should be vaccinated for hepatitis B.
(5) Monitor for acquired HIV or hepatitis viruses.

111. **Few important findings in different types of von Willebrand disease**: **All types have porolnged bleeding time**.

(1) Type 1 (classic): Reduced [F VIII-c, **von Willebrand antigen (vW-Ag), ristocetin cofactor (R-Cof),** and **ristocetin-induced platelet aggregation(RIPA)**]; **normal** multimer structure; autosomal dominant.
(2) Type 3: Same as above **except variable** multimer structure; **autosomal recessive**.
(3) **Type 2 A: Normal or reduced** [F VIII-C, vW- Ag]; **reduced** [R-cof, RIPA]; **abnormal** multimer structure; **autosomal dominant**.
(4) **Type 2 B: Same as** type 2A **except increased RIPA; normal or reduced R-Cof**; autosomal dominant.

112. **Hemophilia B (Factor IX deficiency)**: X-linked recessive disorder, affects only males. It is **less** severe than F VIII deficiency.

(A) **Clinical manifestations**: Patients can develop muscle hematomas, hemarthrosis of large joints with crippling joint deformities, and GI bleeding or may remian **asymptomatic** until surgery or trauma.

(B) **Diagnosis:** Prolonged APTT that can be corrected by normal serum. **Patients plasma cannot correct prolonged APTT of a patient with known F IX deficiency will confirm the diagnosis**.

(C) **Treatment:**

(1) **Mild to moderate bleeding: Fresh-frozen plasma** can stop the bleeding. **EACA is** used as an adjunct to plasma transfusion for **dental work or mucosal bleeding**.

(2) Moderate to severe bleeding (muscle hematomas or large hemarthrosis): **Infusion of commercially prepared F IX concentrate. Two types** of concentrates are available-highly purified F IX concentrates and prothrombin complex concentrates.

(D) **Complications of therapy**:

(1) Prothrombin complex concentrate (contains **six vitamin K dependent factors** II, VII, IX, X, **protein C and S**): **Thromboembolism** particularly when used in **high doses** with liver disease or after surgery. Low dose heparin may be used in postsurgical patients.

(2) EACA greatly **increases the risk** of **thromboembolism** and should **not** be used along with F IX replacement therapy.

(E) **Detection of carrier:**

(1) It is best done by F IX genetic markers and polymorphism.

(2) F IX activity assay, F IX levels may be low.

113. Most common cause of **unexplained thrombosis**: **Abnormal Factor V which is resistance to APC (20 to 50%)**; other causes are **protein C deficiency** (2 to 5%), protien S deficiency (2 to 5%), or antithrombin III deficiency (1 to 2%).

114. **Abnormal Factor V resistance to APC**: Patients develop **thrombosis** due to Leiden mautation of Factor V results in resistance to APC.

Diagnosis of Leiden mutation: PCR (polymerase chain reaction) amplification of Factor V genes followed by restriction fragment analysis.

Treatment:

(1) Long term **anticoagulation for** patients with thrombotic episode or other risk factors.

(2) **Asymptomatic family members** should be counseled for their **higher risk of thrombosis**.

115. **Deficiency of antithrombin III (AT III):** AT III levels are 50% of normal.
Signs and symptoms: **Most comon manifestation is lower-extremity thrombophlebitis with or without pulmonary embolism**, other findings are **chronic leg ulcers and venous insufficiency**.
Diagnosis: It is made by **an activity assay** which should be done **after patients are recovered from thrombotic events** (because ongoing thrombosis and heparin therapy lower the AT III levels).
Treatment:
(1) **Acute thrombosis**: **Heparin is used**.
(2) **Patients are resistant to heparin when AT III level is very low:** Use FFP (fresh frozen plasma) or AT III concentrate. **Warfarin should be started immediately**.
(3) **Prophylactic use of anticoagulants** should be used to avoid fatal outcome.

116. **Protein C deficiency**:
(1) Heterozygous deficiency (protein C level is 50% of normal): **Patients develop venous thrombosis or remain asymptomatic**.
(2) Homozygous deficiency (protein C level is < 1% of normal): Massive venous thrombosis, ischemic necrosis of skin and digits in **neonates**.
Diagnosis: It is made by decreased level of protein C antigen in the plasma.
Treatment:
(1) **Long term anticoagulation (warfarin) should be** reserved for patients with thrombotic episode or have other risk factors.
(2) **Asymptomatic family members** should be counseled **to avoid** smoking, prolonged immobilization, and obesity because of **higher risk of thrombosis**.
(3) It is preferred to start warfarin while the patients are receiving heparin but **heparin can cause thrombocytopenia or thrombocytosis in some patients**.

117. **Protein S deficiency:** Autosomal dominant; affected patients protein S level is 50% of normal.
Signs and symptoms: Venous thrombosis.
Diagnosis: Decreased protein S antigen level.
Treatment: Same as protein C deficiency.

118. **Anticoagulation therapy during pregnancy**: **Heparin** is used **between 6 and 12 weeks**, and **after 38 week because** coumarin anticoagulants cause **facial and skeletal malformations** when used **between 6 to 12 weeks**. Use of

coumarin drugs in 2nd and 3rd trimester may **cause CNS malformations** probably **due to sporadic intracranial hemorrhages**.

119. **Few important points in coumarin anticoagulations**:
   (1) Warfarin and other anticoagulants competitively inhibit the effects of vitamin k.
   (2) Do **not** use aspirin in **any form**.
   (3) Patients should wear bracelet or neck tag that they are receiving oral anticoagulant.
   (4) **Over-treatment** with oral anticoagulation can cause **severe GI, GU,** and **intracranial** bleeding, or **hematoma formations after trauma**, or **patients may appear** with purpura, slight gum bleeding, or mild hematuria.
   (5) Treatment of over-anticoagulation includes **FFP or vitamin K** (**IV infusion** corrects PT in **4 to 6 hours**, **oral or IM** injection corrects PT within **8 to 24 hours**).
   (6) **More than 5 mg vitamin K** administration develops **warfarin resistance**, a round of reanticoagulation should be done.
   (7) **The best therapy** for patients on anticoagulation is to give **plasma** or **small doses (1 to 2 mg)** of vitamin K while close monitoring the **INR (patient's PT/normal PT) ISI** and clinical condition.
   (8) The coumarin compounds in **rat poisons are stronger than warfarin and can cause extreme resistance to vitamin K for weeks and months**.

120. **DIC (disseminated intravascular coagulation)**: DIC is divided into **four** clinical syndromes and these are the following:
   (A) **Compensated DIC: Patient develop thrombosis but no** bleeding. Patients with serious underlying disease (such as infection, malignancy, trauma) usually **have increased production and consumption of platelets, fibrinogen, and other coagulation proteins**.
   Laboratory finding: **Normal** PT, **normal or mildly reduced platelet counts**, elevated plasma fibrinogens.
   Treatment:
      (1) **Heparin or other anticoagulant** is used as prophylaxis or treatment of **thrombosis of large vessels**.
      (2) Trousseau syndrome of migratory venous thrombosis in cancer patients: **Long-term regimen of heparin is the drug of choice** (because warfarin is **not** effective).
   (B) **Defibrination syndrome:** Patients develop **thrombosis and bleeding** due to massive utilization and depletion of fibrinogen and **platelets in sepsis, shock, burn, cancer, and obstretic complications**.

Laboratory findings: Prolonged PT, severe depletion of platelets and fibrinogens, **elevated fibrin degradation products; decreased** (F V, VIII, II other vitamin K dependent factors, AT III, plasminogen);

Treatment:

(1) Underlying disease condition should be treated aggressively.

(2) Patients should receive **platelet concentrates, cryoprecipitates** (contain fibrinogen), **FFP** (contains AT and other plasma proteins). **The goal is to achieve platelet count** >50,000 per microliter, **fibrinogen** concentration > 100 mg/dL, **INR** (1.5 or less), **AT III concentration** (>40% normal).

(3) Use of heparin is controversial. **Low dose heparin should not** increased PT, APTT, or enhance bleeding diathesis. **Low dose heparin can be used in uncontrollable bleeding or unresponsive patients**.

(4) Patients with purpura fulminans with severe deficiency of protein C: Give protein C concentrates.

(5) Severely ill patients have higher risk of vitamin K deficiency: Give parenteral vitamin K.

(C) **Primary fibrinolysis**: Patients develop **bleeding** due to the release of plasminogen activators. It is associated with **primary fibrinolysis or cancer prostate, hemangiomas, acute promyelocytic leukemia, or injection of venoms**. Patients can have ecchymoses, mucosal bleeding, and severe bleeding from injection sites.

Laboratory findings: Prolonged PT and thrombin time, platelet counts are **appropriate** for the state of bone marrow, **normal** antithrombin levels.

Treatment:

(1) **Cryoprecipitate** to keep plasma fibrinogen > 100 mg/dL.

(2) **EACA** may be effective in reducing bleeding if the activity of **alpha-2-antiplasmin** is < 35 to 40% of normal.

(3) Low dose heparin may be used with EACA which can develop thrombosis.

(D) Microangiopathic thrombocytopenia: Patients develop **widespread microthrombi, severe depletion of platelets, microangiopathic changes in RBC's and ischemic necrosis of the tissues. It is found in patients with** sepsis, cancer, vasculitis, immune complex disease, malignant hypertension, vascular malformations, eclampsia, and intravascular aspergillosis. Patients **develop TTP** (thrombotic thrombocytopenic purpura). Most common organisms are **Shigella dysentariae or E. coli** (0157: H7, it has shigella like toxin).

Treatment:

(1) FFP and glucocorticoids.

(2) Plasmapheresis is needed.

(3) If plasmapheresis fails, then use drugs inhibiting platelet aggregation, splenectomy, and vincristine.

(E) **Snake bites**: Vipers and rattlesnakes can cause DIC. Laboratory findings are more severe than clinical manifestations.
Treatment: Anitvenoms; platelets or FFP transfusion; general supportive measures.(Low platelets and fibrinogens may persist for weeks).

121. **Few important points in cancer**:
(1) Most common site of **cancer in male** is **prostate**.
(2) Most common cancerous cause of death in male is **lung** cancer.
(3) Most common site of **cancer in female is breast**.
(4) Most common cancerous cause of **death in female** is lung cancer.
(5) **Cancer can be prevented by the following**: Stop smoking, moderation alcohol intake, diet (decreased fat, increased fiber), and increase physical activity.

122. **Drugs causing cancer**:
(1) Alkylating agents, MOPP therapy, melphalan, treosulfan: Leukemia.
(2) Androgen anabolic steroids: Liver cancer.
(3) Azathioprine and cyclosporine: Non-Hodgkin lymphoma.
(4) Chlornaphazine: Bladder cancer.
(5) Phenacetin-containing analgesics: Renal pelvic tumors.
(6) Diethylstilbestrol: Vaginal and cervical cancer.
(7) Steroid contraceptives: Liver and cervical cancers.
(8) Postmenopausal estrogens: Endometrial cancer.
(9) Debriosquine (antihypertensive): Lung cancer.

123. **Infectious agent causing cancers**:
(1) Hepatitis B and C (p53 gene mutation): Primary hepatocellular cancer.
(2) Epstein-Barr virus: Burkitt's lymphoma and nasopharyngeal cancer.
(3) HIV-I: Kaposi' sarcoma and non-Hodgkin lymphoma.
(4) HTLV-I: T-cell leukemia.
(5) Human papillomaviruses: Cervical cancer.
(6) Helicobacter pylori: Gastric cancer.
(7) Clonorchis sinensis: Cholangiocarcinoma of liver.
(8) Schistosoma haematobium: Bladder cancer.

124. **Few important points in cancer prevention intervention:**
(1) Oral contraceptives (estrogen progesterone combinations): Reduces the endometrial cancer and epithelial ovarian cancers (independent of parity).

Combination therapy is preferred for postmenopausal hormonal replacement therapy.

(2) Diethylstilbestrol and LHRH agonists: Used in treatment of metastatic prostate cancer.

(3) Inhibitors of 5-alpha-reductase: It is useful in high-risk patients or in primary prevention.

(4) Retinoblastoma and polyposis coli have **specific mutations,** so important in genetic screening.

(5) Breast cancer gene(s) and cell-cycle/tumor –suppressor gene (MTS- 1) p16 also help ingenctic screening.

125. **Occupatinal exposures and cancers**:

(1) **Nasal sinuses: Wood dusts**, isopropyl alcohol manufacture, boot and shoe manufacture.

(2) **Bladder: Benzidine**, 4-aminobiphenyl, auramine manufacture, beta-naphthylamine, and magenta manufacture.

(3) **Lung: Aluminium, arsenic, asbestos,** bischloromethylether, coal, coke production, chromium compounds, radon, mustard gas, nickel compounds, tar, oils, and soots.

(4) **Liver: Vinyl chloride**.

(5) **Skin:** Mineral oils, arsenic, tar, oils, and soots.

(6) **Leukemia: Benzene** (Important).

(7) **Pleura:** Erionite, asbestos.

(8) **Peritoneum:** Asbestos.

126. **Myasthenia gravis (MG)**:Remember **thymoma** is the **most common cancer seen in MG**. MG can be present **at any time** during malignancy. Patients with MG (50% cases) **have gross or microscopic thymomas**.

(A) **Pathophysiology**: MG is an **autoimmune disorder** producing **antibodies against acetycholine receptor** on the motor endplates.

(B) **Diagnosis:** Clinical manifestations (episodic **muscle weakness,** especially ocular and bulbr muscles; **normal** deep tendon reflexe and sensation; improvement of muscle strength with anticholinesterase such as edrophonium or neostigmine is called **Tensilon test**); presence of **autoantibodies** against the acetylcholine receptors; **EMG** reveals progressive decrease in amplitude upon repeated electrical stimulation; **documentation of thymomas** by radiologic studies.

(C) **Treatment:**

(1) **Pyridostigmine or neostigmine** improve the clinical symptoms.

(2) **Thymectomy** is helpful in most patients.

(3) Other treatments are **steroids,** plasmapheresis, or cytotoxic drugs.

(D) **Prognosis**: **Remember** it depends upon the **stage of the thymoma but does not** depend upon the **duration** of MG before surgery and presence of associated syndrome of MG.

(E) **Remember,** comprehensive physical **examination is important** particulary breast, pelvis, and rectum **to rule out cancer**.

127. **Eaton-Lambert syndrome (ELS)**:

(A) **Clinical manifestations: Proximal muscle weakness in the legs, arm, and pelvic girdle (spare ocular and bulbar muscles) plus reduced or absent** deep tendon reflexes; **autonomic dysfunctions** (dry mouth, peripheral paresthesias, impotence);

(B) **Associated cancer: Small cell cancer of the lung is the most common** (Important). ELS can predict the **future** (up to 4 years) occurrence of cancer.

(C) **Diagnosis:** Clinical manifestations, EMG reveals increase muscle response to each stimulation, poor response to Tensilon test, and absence of acetylcholine receptor antibodies.

(D) **Treatment:**

(1) Treat the underlying cancer.
(2) **Guanidine hydrochloride** improves the symptoms by increaseing acetylcholine release.
(3) **Plasmapheresis or plasma exchange**.
(4) Immune therapy with **azathioprine and glucocorticoids**.
(5) Do **not** use 4-aminopyridine which causes confusion and seizure.

128. **Paraneoplastic cerebellar degeneration (PCD)**: **It is the most common** among CNS paraneoplastic syndrome.

(A) **Clinical manifestations**: Progressive ataxia, nystagmus, and dysarthria; PCD **can predict future cancers** such as gynecologic tumors, breast cancer, bronchogenic cancer, and lymphoma.

(B) **Diagnosis:** Clinical manifestations plus **presence of autoantibodies** (**anti-Yo** against the Purkinje cells, **anti-Hu** against the cerebral cortex) **in serum or CSF**.

(C) **Treatment:**

(1) Treat the underlying cancer.
(2) Plasmapheresis.
(3) **Immunosuppression** with steroids, gamma globulin, and pulse cyclophosphamide.

129. **Paraneoplastic eye syndróme (PES)**:

(A) **Clinical manifestations: Opsoclonus-myoclonus** (diplopia,oscillopsia, blurred vision; myoclonus of the head, trunck, limbs; hyperreflexia, ataxia, equivocal Babinski reflexes) and **cancer associated retinopathy** (bilateral vision loss, optic atrophy).

(B) **Associated findings:**

(1) Opsoclonus-myoclonus is associated with **breast and gynecologic cancers**.

(2) Cancer associated retinopathy is associated with **recoverin** (autoantibody to retinal antigen).

130. **Sweet's syndrome (SS) or acute febrile neutrophilic dermatosis**:

(A) **Clinical manifestations: Fever, neutrophilia, and rash** (tender red or bluish firm papules or nodules, or coalesce to from irregular border) **present over the upper extremities asymmetrically**.

(B) **Associated cancer:** SS is most commonly associated with **hematologic cancer (acute leukemia).**

(C) **Diagnosis:** Clinical manifestations and skin biopsy reveals **diffuse infiltration of mature neutrophils** in the superficial dermis.

(D) **Treatment:**

(1) SS is a **self-limited** condition.

(2) **Steroids are the drug of choice**.

(3) Potassium iodide or colchicine is useful.

(4) Treat the underlying disease.

131. **Dermatomysitis (DM) and polymyositis (PM)**:

(A) **Clinical manifestations**: Both of them appear with symmetrical **proximal uscle weakness**; sometimes dysphagia due to involvement of **esophageal striated muscles. DM has characteristic skin rash** but PM does **not** have skin rash. Both can exist **without cancer** but **altered immune system can cause cancer**.

(B) **Diagnosis: Myositis on muscle biopsy,** abnormal EMG, and **elevated serum muscle enzymes**.

(C) **Pathophysiology:** Recent study shows DM is **due to humorally mediated capillary necrosis.** PM is due to **T cell-mediated inflammation** and destruction of muscle fibers.

(D) **Treatment:**

(1) **Immunosuppressive therapy is useful**.

(2) Treatment of underlying disease may or may **not** improve the DM/PM.

(E) **Recurrence of cancer:** Patients with pre existing cancer, **appearance of DM/PM indicates recurrence of cancer (Important)**.

132. **Most common cancer which is associated with acanthosis nigricans (AN): Adenocarcinomas of the GI tract.**
Clinical manifestations of AN: Characteristic hyperpigmented skin lesion in the intertriginous areas; oral lesions are found in cancer associated AN.
Diagnosis: Clinical manifestations plus skin biopsy reveals hyperkeratosis, increased melanin, and papillary hypertrophy.
Treatment:
(1) Topical steroids, retinoids, and podophyllin may be useful.
(2) AN may or may not improve with the treatment of underlying cancer.

133. **Most common cancer which is associated with erythema gyratum repens (EGR)**: Lung and breast cancers.
(A) **Clinical manifestations of EGR: Characteristic rapidly enlarging serpiginous, whirled concentric erythematous bands** on **the trunk and extremities;** pruritus (50% of cases).
(B) **Diagnosis**: Clinical manifestation of EGR plus eosinophilia (biopsy finding is nonspecific)
(C) **Treatment of EGR:**
(1) Treatment of underlying cancer (chemotherapy or irradiation) results in resolution of the lesions.
(2) Radiation therapy to the skin lesions.
(3) Topical/systemic steroids are useful.

134. **Most common cancer which is associated with Bazex's syndrome (BS) or acrokeratosis paraneoplastica**: **Squamous cell cancer of the upper aerodigestive tranct**.
(A) **Clinical manifestations of BS: Symmetrical distal erythematosquamous eruptions in the ears, nails, nose, fingers, palms, soles, toes, knees, elbows,** cheeks, trunk, scalp (descending order of involvement), and dystrophy of nails.
(B) **Etiology of BS:**
(1) **Growth factor puduction** by the tumor.
(2) **Immunoglobulin depositon** in the basal layer and basement membrane.

135. **Most common cancer** which is associated with acquired icthyosis (AI): **Hodgkin disease**.

136. **Most common cancers which are associated with tripe palms (TP) or acathosis nigricans of the plams**: **Bronchogenic cancer and gastric cancer**.

137. **Most common cancer which is associated with Leser-Trelat (LT) syndrome: Adenocarcinoma of the GI tract. Clinical manifestations of LT syndrome:** Multiple seborrheic keratoses is most commonly present in elderly patients.
Etiology: It is due to production of **cytokines** such as tumor-specific epidermal growth factor, insulin-like growth factor, and transforming growth factor-alpha.

138. **Most common cancer which is associated with pulmonary osteoarthropathy (POA) ; Non-small cell lung cancer**.
   (A) **Clinical manifestations of POA: Clubbing, synovitis, and periostitis**; painful, red, swollen joints of lower extremities but pain is noted in the distal tibia/fibula, and radius/ulna.
   (B) **Diagnosis of POA:** Bone scan confirms the diagnosis; X-ray reveals periosteal elevation.
   (C) **Treatment of POA:**
      (1) Aspirin or NSAID's is used for arthritis.
      (2) Atropine may be used.
      (3) Vagotomy can produce analgesia.
      (4) Treat the underlying cancer with chemotherapy or radiation therapy is also useful.

139. **Most common cancer which is associated with paraneoplastic nephrotic syndrome (PNS): Hodgkin disease**.
PNS is charecterized by **lipoid nephrosis** which may be due to **deficient T lymphocyte function**.

140. **Paraneoplastic endocrine syndromes**: Hypercalcemia and SIADH (syndrome of inappropriate antidiuretic hormone secretion).
   (A) **SIADH:**
      (1) **Etiology: Most common** cause in cancer patients is **small cell cancer of the lung**. Drugs causing SIADH are the following: Vincristine, vinblastin, cyclophosphamide; TCA and narcotics.
      (2) **Clinical presentations:** Asymptomatic hyponatremia or abnormal neurologic findings due to hyponatremia. Patients are usually **euvolemic**.
      (3) **Diagnosis:** Low serum sodium and osmolality, high urine osmolality (greater than serum osmolality), and increased excretion of urinary sodium.
      (4) **Treatment:**
         (a) Treat the underlying disease.

(b) Fluid restriction.
(c) Hypertonic saline (3%) is used in life threatening condition.
(d) Demeclocycline is used, it causes nephrogenic diabets insipidus.

(B) **Hypercalcemia**:

(1) **Etiology: PTHrP** (parathyroid hormone-related peptide) **is the most common cause in cancer patients.**
(2) **Clinical manifestations**: Cardiac dysfunction **due to prolonged QT interval,** constipation, vomiting, cachexia, **polyuria,** dehydration, fatigue, muscle weakness, and coma.
(3) **Diagnosis: Normal or low** PTH level, **normal or low** 1,25-dihydroxyvitamin D level, **mild metabolic alkalosis**; elevated urinary cyclic AMP levels; **low** serum phosphorus and **high** serum calcium; **high** urinary calcium and phosphorus.
(4) **Treatment:**
(a) **Hydration** inproves dehydration, increase GFR and calcium excretion.
(b) **Furosemide** is given after adequate hydration, it promotes calcium excretion.
(c) **The best therapy** is to treat the underlying desease.
(d) **To inhibit bone resorption**: Use bisphosphonates (etidronate, pamidronate), mithramycin, glucocorticoids, calcitonin, and gallium nitrite.
(e) **Please remember, there is no need to reduce nutritional calcium because GI absorption does not** have an **important** effect.

141. **Complications of anticoagulation therapy in patients with cancer (Important)**:

(1) Hemorrhage because tumor invades blood vessels.
(2) CNS metastasis.

142. **Treatment of coagulation abnormalities in cancer patients**:

(1) **The best** therapy is to treat underlying cancer.
(2) Initial therapy with **heparin** followed by **warfarin**.

143. **Paraneoplastic hematologic abnormalities**:

(A) **Coagulation abnormalities**: both thrombosis and hemorrhage can occur.
(B) **Paraneoplastic leukemoid reaction (PLR): Peripheral WBC count** > 20,000 per microliter without evidence of infection or leukemia. It is a diagnosis of exclusion.
(C) **Cancer-associated erythrocytosis (CAE) and anemia (CAA)**:

(1) **CAE: Most common cause is the kidney** (benign or malignant) **disease** such as renal cell cancer, cystic kidney, hydronephrosis, and Wilms' tumor. CAE is also found in hepatoma, sarcomas, cerebellar hemangioblastoma.
Etiology: Increased endogenous erythropoietin levels in most cases; some patients may have increased androgens and PGE (prostaglandins).

(2) **CAA**: It is the **most common finding in cancer patients**.
Etiology: Chemotherapy, radiation therapy, nutritional deficiency, chrnoic disease, blood loss, bone marrow invasion; red cell aplasia (**in thymoma**), autoimmune hemolytic anemia (**in B cell lymphomas** and **rarely** with solid tumors).

Treatment of chemotherapy induced anemia: Recombinant erythropoietin (effective in 30 to 40% cases).

(3) **CAT (cancer-associated thrombocytosis)**: It is due to overproduction oflthrombopoietin (s) and is found in Hodgkin disease, non-Hodgkin lymphoma, leukemias, and other solid cancers.

144. **Stauffer syndrome:** Hepatic dysfunction, fever, weight loss, It is **most commonly** found in **nonmetastatic renal cell cancer**.
Etiology: Autoimmune phenomenon to hepatic cells or substances released by the tumor causing hepatic dysfunction.
Diagnosis: Hepatomegaly, **elevated LFT's, PT, and Platelet counts**. Liver biopsy reveals **Kupffer cell hyperplasia** plus nonspecific inflammatory findings.
Treatment:
(1) Nonmetastatic lesion: To treat the primary cancer (in the kidney).
(2) Metastatic lesion should be ruled out for management.

145. **Tumor related cachexia:**
(1) **Etiology: Tumor-secreted factors like TNF-alpha is called cachexin. It inhibits lipogenic enzymes and causes wasting syndrome. Other causes are** alteration of taste and smell, decreased caloric intake, increased metabolic acitivity, treatment-related vomiting and loss of appetite, malabsorption, or GI obstruction.
(2) **Treatment:**
(a) Treat underlying cancer.
(b) Supplemental nutrition.
(c) High doses of progestational hormone (megestrol acetate) also improves the appetite.

146. **Few important points regarding tumor markers**:

(1) **Colorectal cancer**: Serum CEA (carcinoembryonic antigen). **Elevated CEA, level means that tumor has increased capacity for invasion and metastasis. Declining CEA levels** in patients undergoing treatment means **good response** but **serial levels are more important than a single value. Please remember after early therapy CEA level may rise initially, no** intervention is needed but **continuous monitoring should be done**. **CEA elevation occurs before (several months)** the clinical and radiological findings but it does **not** separate curable from incurable patients of colon cancer. **CEA is also elevated in adenocarcinomas of lung, stomach, pancreas, and breast. CEA is also elevated in medullary cancer of thyroid and squamous cell cancer of head and neck**. **CEA is nonspecific and should not be used as screening test**.

(2) **Prostate cancer: PSA** is used as a screening test probably in combination with DRE (digital rectal examination) and TRAS (transrectal ultransonography).

(3) **Ovarian cancer: CA 125** (monoclonal antibody that recognizes antigens secreted by ovarian an other cancers) **is used** as a screening test in high-risk groups in combination with **pelvic examination and ultrasonography**.

(4) **Hepatoma: AFP** (alpha feto protein) is used as a screening test in high-risk patients in combination with **ultrasonography**.

(5) **Breast cancer:** CA 15-3, CEA **cannot** be used as screening tests because they are **neither specific nor increase in early breast cancer. Rising levels** indicate **recurrent disease** or first sign of progressive disease.

(6) **Testicular cancer:** HCG (human chorionic gonadotropin) and AFP **cannot** be used as **screening test**. Normal HCG and AFP should **not** be present in males or nonpregnant females, **presence of HCG and AFP indicates cancer**. (HCG is secreted by the placenta and AFP is secreted by fetus). **Very high level of AFP is found in nonseminomatous tumor (treated with chemotherapy)** and about 15% of **seminomatous tumors (treated with radiation therapy)** elevated levels of HCG.

(7) **Carcinoid:** 5-HIAA is a tumor marker, helpful in diagnosis and response.

(8) **Multiple myeloma:** Beta-2-microglobulin is the **most important prognostic factor in this disease**. It is an useful marker but **cannot** used as a screening test.

(9) **Neuroblastoma** ; VMA is a tumor marker, helpful in diagnosis and responses.

(10) **Non-Hodgkin lymphoma** LDH is an important marker and prognostic factor **but cannot** be used as screening test.

147. **Most common cancer causing tumor-associated Cushing's syndrome: Small cell lung cancer** (SCLC) secretes ACTH, CRF (corticotropin-releasing

factor), ADH, calcitonin, GRF (growth hormone releasing factor), and GRP (gastrin-releasing peptide).

148. **Hormones secreted by different tumors**:
   (1) **Somatostatin: Medullary thyroid cancer** (also secretes ACTH, GRF, GRP).
   (2) **Calcitonin: Small cell lung cancer**.
   (3) **VIP:** Ganglioneuroma (also secretes ACTH, GRF).
   (4) **HCG: Non-small cell lung cancer,** sarcomas, testicular (embryonal) cancer.
   (5) **PTH RP (parathyroid hormone-related peptide)**: Squamous cell cancer (lung, head, neck), bladder and renal cancer, lymphomas, adenocarcinomas. **All causes hypercalcemia**.
   (6) **ADH: Small cell lung cancer**.
   (7) **ACTH: Small cell lung cancer,** melanoma, prostate cancer, medullary thyroid cancer, ganglioneuroma, pheochromocytoma, islet cell tumors of pancreas, carcinod tumors (lung, GI tract, pancreas, thymus, ovary).

149. **Oncogenic osteomalacia syndrome: Bone pain muscle weakness and X-ray picture of osteomalacia** are present in benign osteoblastomas, giant cell osteosarcomas, hemangiomas, or **rarely** SCLC and prostatic epithelial tumor.
   Treatment:
   (1) To treat the underlying condition.
   (2) Replacement therapy with phosphorus and vitamin D.

150. **Paraneoplastic syndromes affecting the CNS (remote effects of cancer):**
   (A) **Brain and cranial nerves:**
      (1) Dementia-limbic encephalitis.
      (2) Optic neuritis.
      (3) Retinal degeneration.
      (4) Subacute cerebellar degeneration.
      (5) Brain stem encephalitis.
      (6) Opsoclonus-myoclonus.
   (B) **Spinal cord:**
      (1) Subacute motor meuropathy.
      (2) Myelitis.
      (3) Necrotizing myelopathy.

151. **Therapaeutic radiation causing injury to the nervous system**:
   (A) **Primary injury:**

(1) **Immediate injury** (minutes to hours): Acute encephalopathy due to increased ICP and cerebral edema from radiation-induced alteration in **blood-brain barrier**.

Treatment: Corticosteroid. This effect is **absent** in spinal cord irradiation.

(2) **Early delayed (6 to 16 weeks):**

(a) **Brain**: It occurs transiently after **prophylactic irradiation** of the brain in patients **with small cell lung cancer**. Patients appear with **somnolence, nausea, vomiting, sometimes fever. Whole brain irradiation** for brain tumor causes **lethargy** and **focal neurologic sign**. CT or MRI shows worsening condition.

Treatment: Corticosteroids, or resolve spontaneously without therapy.

(b) **Spinal cord**: Early delayed myopathy or Lhermitte's sign (electric shock-like sensation radiating to the different parts of the body when the neck is flexed):

Treatment: It resolves spontaneously, no treatment is needed.

(3) **Late delayed (months to years)**:

(a) **Brain:** Dementia, focal signs; diagnosis by CT scan or MRI.

Treatment: Corticosteroids may help; focal lesions need surgery.

(b) **Spinal cord**: Transverse myelopathy, **Brown-Sequard syndrome (weakness and loss of propioception** in the extremities of **one side** and **loss of pain and temperature** sensation on **the other side)**.

Pathology: Necrosis of the spinal cord.

Treatment: Corticosteroids may be helpful.

(c) **Cranial or peripheral nerves: Blindness** from optic neuropathy and **paralysis of upper extremity** from brachial plexopathy secondary to radiation therapy **for lung or breast cancer**.

Pathology: Fibrosis and ischemia of the plexus.

Treatment: No therapy is available.

(B) **Secondary injury (years after therapy):**

(1) **Radiation-induced tumors: Meningiomas, sarcomas**, or rarely gliomas. Malignant or atypical nerve sheath tumors of the brachial, cervical, or lumbar plexus.

(2) **Atherosclerosis** and cerebral artery occlusion and infarction:

(3) **Endocrinopathy:** Hypothyroidism is commonly present; hyperthyroidism or hyperparathyroidism from radiation can cause encephalopathy.

152. **Sezary syndrome (or leukemic variant of mycosis fungoides):**

(1) **Skin lesions:** Exfoliative dermatitis, edema, redness, and thickening **of the skin with ectropion and leonine facies**; mostly spares body folds.

(2) **Other features:** Hepatosplenomegaly, lymphadenopathy, Sezary cells in blood with high WBC counts. (**Sezary cells are atypical T lymphocytes**).
(3) **Complications: Staphylococcal or Pseudomonas infection is the most common cause of death (50% of cases)**.

153. **Pautrier's absesses: Atypical lymphocytes** accumulate in the epidermis to from these absesses. It is founf in cutaneous T-cell lymphomas (mycosis fungoides, Sezary syndrome, and adult T-cell lymphoma).

154. **Skin lesion in adult T-cell lymphoma** which is associated with retrovirus, HTLV (human T-cell lymphoma virus): **Flesh-colored papules, nodules, tumors are common (70% cases)** and generalized erythroderma may be present. These skin lesions are diffusely spread over the trunk.
Non skin lesions: Lymphadenopathy, hepatosplenomegaly; hypercalcemia and 'punched-out' **osteolytic lesions** in the axial bones and long bones.

155. **Kaposi's sarcoma**: It is a multifocal, vascular malignant tumor. AIDS patients with Kaposi's sarcoma have **characteristic widely distributed, red-brown macules, papules, and nodules** over the upper part of the body; lesions in the **oropharyngeal macosa and along the skin cleavage lines**.

156. **Acquired hypertrichosis lanuginosa** (malignant down): It is **characterized** by sudden onset of **excessive growth fetal hair** (lanugo is fine, long, underpigmented hair) **over the face, limbs, and trunk**. It is associated with **cancer** of the breast, pulmonary, pancreatic, GI tract, uterine, and lymphomas.

157. **Leser-Trelet sign:** It is characterized by the sudden **appearance and growth of multiple seborrheic keratoses** in elderly patients with underlying **cancer** of the lung, mycosis, fungoides, adenocarcinoma of the bowel, and Sezary's syndrome.

158. **Bezex syndrome (or acrokeratosis paraneoplastica):** It is an **unique cutaneous marker** of the upper respiratory tract cancer particulary **squamous cell cancer** of oral,pharyngeal, esophageal, laryngeal,and bronchial areas, mostly found in males. The charcteristic of rash:
(1) **Asymptomatic tumor:** Scaling, red to violaceous, **psoriasis like patches** are found **over the bridge of the nose, fingers, and toes**.
(2) **Initial symptomatic tumor:** Lesions extends into the palms and soles results in **honeycomb appearnace**.

(3) **Last stage of untreated tumor**: Psoriasis extends over the face, trunk, arm, knees, and scalp, and **severe dystrophy of the nails**.

159. **Gardner's syndrome:** It is charcterized by **sebaceouos cysts** of the face and scalp, **multiple epidermoid, osteomas** of bones of the face and head, **polys** of colon and rectum, and **fibrous tissue tumors** of the skin (fibromas, fibrosarcomas, desmoid tumors).
Associated cancerous lesion: Adenocarcinoma of the bowel is the most common.

160. **Torre's Syndrome**: Autosomal dominant; it is characterized by **multiple sebaceous gland tumors, adenomas, and hyperlasias;** and **basal cell cancers**. This syndrome is associated with **cancer** of the colon, GU tract, duodenum, ampulla of Vater, and uterus.

161. **Cowden's disease** ; It is characterized by the **numerous hamartomas** of **the skin, mucous membrane, and internal organs**. It is assciated with the **cancer of the breast and thyroid**. Skin lesions are keratotic, **warty papules and nodules on the hands, arms, and central area of the face**. Cobblestone lesions may be present on the palate, gums, tongue, and larynx.

162. **Chediak-Higashi syndrome**: Autosomal recessive; light coloration of skin and hair; can **develop leukemias and lymphomas**.

163. **Bloom's syndrome**: Autosomal recessive; telangiectatic redness of the skin exposed under the sun and stunted growth; can develop leukemias and lymphomas.

163. **Wiskott-Aldrich syndrome**: Atopic dermatitis, petechiae due to thrombocytopenia, immunologic defects in both the humoral and cell-mediated systems; can develop **malignant lymphomas (79%)** or leukemias.

164. **Peutz-Jeghers syndrome:** Numerous brown macules on the lips, perioral reigion, hands and feet; associated with hamartomatous polyps of the small intestine and stomach; polyps **rarely** change to malignancy.

165. Nevoid basal cell cancer syndrome may be associated with: Medulloblastoma or fibrosarcoma of the jaw.

166. **Ataxia-telangiectasia**: Autosomal recessive; progressive cerebellar **ataxia**, **telangiectasica** over the ears, nose, eyelids, butterfly areas of the face, and

conjunctiva; severe immunologic deficiency, **sinopulmonary** infections; can develop Hodgkin and non-Hodgkin lymphoma or leukemia (10% cases).

167. **Oncogene and neoplasms:**

(1) HER-2/neu: Breast and ovarian cancers.
(2) c-myc: Burkitt's lymphoma.
(3) n-myc: Neuroblastoma.
(4) c-abl: Chronic myelogenous leukemia.
(5) bcl-2: Follicular lymphoma.

168. **Toxic effects of radiation therapy to normal tissues**:

(1) Bone marrow: Aplasia.
(2) Brain, spinal cord: Infarction, necrosis.
(3) Heart: Pericarditis, myocarditis.
(4) Lung: Pneumonitis, fibrosis.
(5) Intestine: Ulceration, fibrosis.
(6) Liver: Hepatitis.
(7) Kidney: Nephrosclerosis.
(8) Skin: Dermatitis, sclerosis.

169. **Anticancer drugs and their uses**:

(1) Melphalan: Multiple myeloma.
(2) Nitrogen mustard, procarbazine: Hodgkin disease.
(3) Chlorambucil: Chronic lymphocytic leukemia.
(4) Busulfan: Chronic myelocytic leukemia.
(5) Cyclophosphamide: Lymphoma, bladder and breast cancers.
(6) Dacarbazine: Melanoma, Hodgkin disease.
(7) Nitrosoureas (carmustine, lomustine): Brain tumors, lymphoma.
(8) Ifosfamide: Soft tissue sarcomas.
(9) **Hydroxyurea**: Chronic myelocytic leukemia.
(10) **Methorexate** (folic acid antagonists): ALL, breast, bladder, head, and neck cancer; choriocarcinoma.
(11) 5-Flurouracil: GI and breast cancer.
(12) 5-Flurodeoxyuridine: Intra-arterial or intraperitoneal therapy for colon cancer metastasis.
(13) Cytosine arabinoside, 6-mercaptopurine, 6-thioguanine: Acute leukemia.
(14) Fludarabine: Chronic lymphocytic leukemia.
(15) Deoxycoformycin: Hairy cell leukemia, T-cell lymphoma.
(16) 2-Chlorodeoxyadenosine: Hairy cell leukemia.
(17) Vincristine: Lymphoid cancer.
(18) Vinblastine: Hodgkin disease and testicular cancer.

(19) Doxorubicin: Lymphoma, sarcomas, breast cancer.
(20) Daunorubicin, idarubicin: Acute leukemia.
(21) Actinomycin D: Choriocarcinoma, rhabdomyosarcoma, Ewing's sarcoma, Wilms' tumor.
(22) Bleomycin: Lymphoma, head and neck cancer.
(23) **Mitomycin: GI cancer**.
(24) Asparaginase, VM-26: ALL (acute lymphocytic leukemia).
(25) Taxol: Ovarian and breast cancers.

170. **Side effects of few cancer drugs**:
(1) Flutamide: Gynecomastia.
(2) **Megestrol acetate**: Fluid retention.
(3) **Diethylstilbestrol:** Fluid retention, hypercalcemia, acclerated coronary artery disease, uterine bleeding, feminization.
(4) **Dexamethasone:** Osteoporosis, Cushingoid appearance, cataracts, GI ulcers, and immunosuppression.
(5) **Prednisone:** Hyperglycemia, fluid retention, low serum k, depression, euphoria.
(6) **Tamoxifen:** Hot flashes, fluid retentioon, retinal degeneration.
(7) **Hydroxyprogesterone:** Thromboembolism, weight gain.
(8) Fluoxymesterone: Cholestatic jaundice with oral therapy.
(9) Testosterone: Virilization.
(10) Aminoglutethimide: Dizziness.

171. **Interferon-alpha used in different cancers**: Hairy cell leukemia, chronic myeloid leukemia, follicular B-cell lymphoma, cutaneous T-cell lymphoma, carcinoid syndrome, Kaposi's sacrcoma, multiple myeloma, renal cell cancer, metastatic melanoma.

172. A 58 year old male cancer patient appears with fever (38°C) and neutropenia (absolute neutrophil count< 1000 per cubic millimeter).
Most likely diagnosis: Infection and septic syndrome.
Immediate management:
(1) **Appropriate cultures** should be obtained immediately. Blood culture should be obtained from peripheral site and central catheter (if placed).
(2) Removal of the indwelling central catheter is **not** always needed but should be considered.
(3) **Catheter tip** should be send from Gram stain and culture.
(4) Sputum culture and Gram stain is done if patient is producing sputum.
(5) Removal of the urinary catheter is indicated and urine culture should be send, urinalysis should be performed.

(6) Other appropriate studies like CXR, culture of the localized lesion should be done.
(7) Remember, spinal tap should **not** done unless clinically indicated.

Immediate treatment:

(1) Broad-spectrum antibiotics should be started immediately after cultures are obtained. Anitbiotics should cover **Pseudomonas** and **other gram-negative organisms**; **S. aureus and S. epidermidis for indwelling catheter infection**.
(2) **Antibiotics: Ceftazidime is the drug of choice**, or semisynthetic penicillin (pipercillin or mezlocillin) plus aminoglycoside (gentamicin or tobramycin); **vancomycin is the drug of choice for S. aureus and S. epidermidis infections; clinamycin should be added to cover anaerobic infection in patients with mucositis, perianal or periodontal infection.**
(3) **Antifungal: Amphotericin B is the drug of choice** for suspected fungal infection (oral thrush or esophagitis), or **oral fluconazole** also can be used. Fungal cultures should be obtained before treatment.
(4) Patient receiving prolonged antibiotic therapy: **Clostridium difficile** infection and **vitamin K deficiency** should be considered and treated appropriately.
(5) **Recombinant hematopoietic cytokines such** as granulocyte colony stimulating factor (G-CSF) and granulocyte macrophage colony stimulating factor (GM-CSF) can be used in neutropenia.

173. **Few important points in treatment of cancer patients in different conditions**:

(1) Massive hemoptysis with respiratory compromise: Patients should be admitted to ICU, correction of coagulopathy and thrombocytopenia, blood transfusion, **bronchoscopy is the best diagnostic procedure, radiation therapy or surgical resection is** useful; **less useful** therapeutic measures are: Nd: YAG laser is used in nonmassive hemoptysis; endobronchial tamponade should **not** be used in RUL hemorrhage; **embolization can** cause **spinal cord damage**.
(2) Cardiac tamponade: It occurs due to **noncancerous cause** in cancer patients or effects of disease progression. **Rapid accumulation** of fluid (150 to 250 ml) (normal <50 ml) cause **tamponade**.
Treatment: Pericardiocentesis is the life saving procedure; fluid is send for cultures and cytology; radiation, chemotherapy, or surgery is used for cancer patients.
(3) **Hemorrhage cystitis** (cyclophosphamide and ifosfamide produce this symptom due to metabolites such as chlorethylazeridine, chloracetic acid, and acrolein): To maintain **high urinary output** to dilute the metabolites, **correct coagulation** defects, systemic use of **sodium 2-mercaptoethane-**

sulfonate (mesna) prevents mucosal irritation by detoxifying the metabolites within the bladder; if conservative therapy fails, then bladder is irrigated with **N-acetylcysteine**, if fails then irrigation with **formalin solution**, or **alum** or **prostaglandin E2 and F2**.

174. Most common cancers are associated with pregnancy: **Cervical cancer**, next is breast cancer. Breast cancer in pregnancy is difficult to diagnose because of **painless lump, physiologic changes,** and high **false negative mammogram(75% cases)**. Most breast cancers are ER-negative (hormone independent) although estrogen is elevated during pregnancy but **abortion** is **not** indicated unless patients have decided not to continue pregnancy.
Treatment of breast cancer:
(1) Do **not** use methotrexate (folate antagonist) which is highly teratogenic.
(2) First trimester chemotherapy: CAF therapy (cyclophosphamide, doxorubicin or Adriamycin, and 5-FU).
(3) Second and third trimester: CMF therapy (cyclophosphamide, methotrexate, and 5-FU) or chemotherapy may be delayed until the delivery if possible.
(4) Early stage cancer: Primary surgery alone may be effective.

1. Acute myelogenous leukemia:

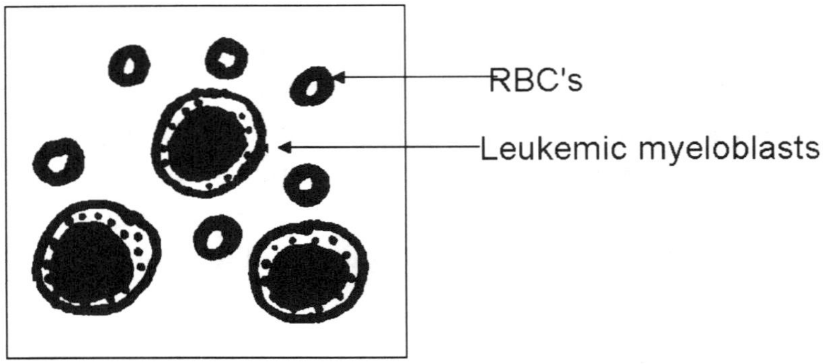

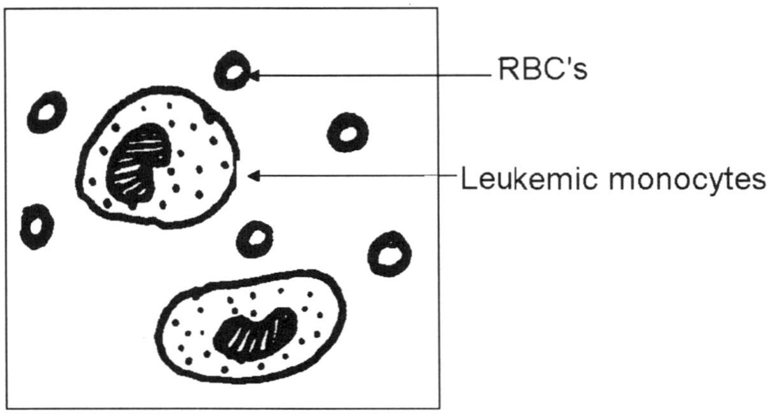

2. Chronic myelogenous leukemia:

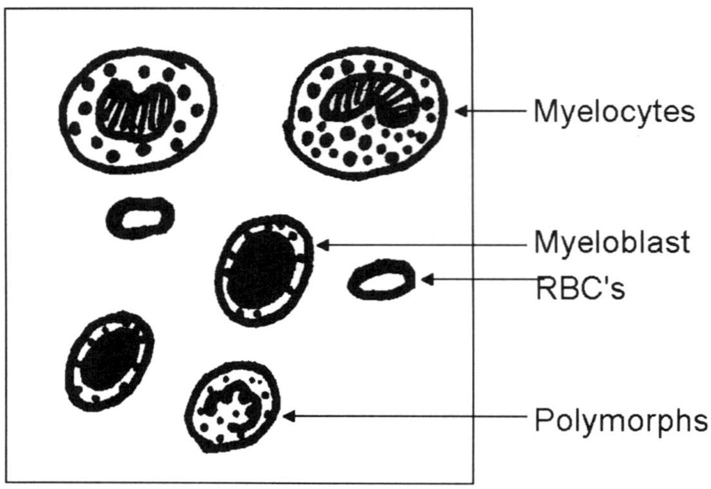

3. Acute lymphocytic leukemia:

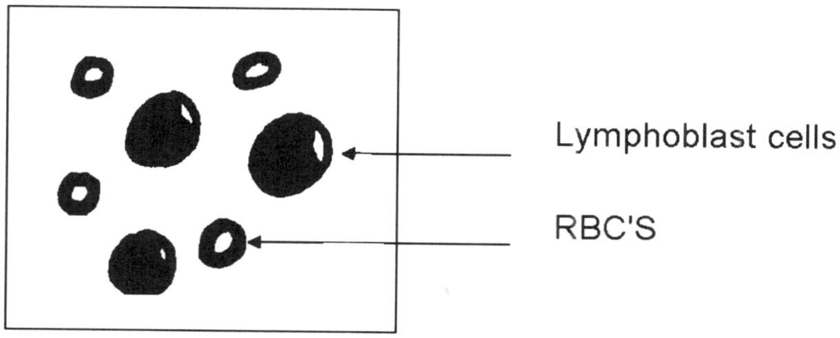

4. Chronic lymphocytic leukemia:

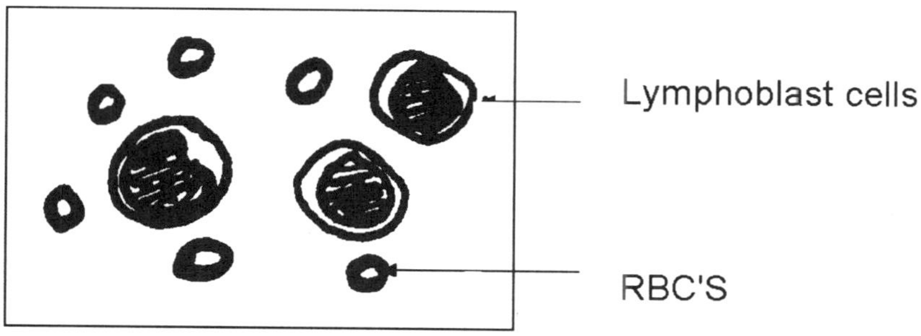

5. Infectious mononucleosis:

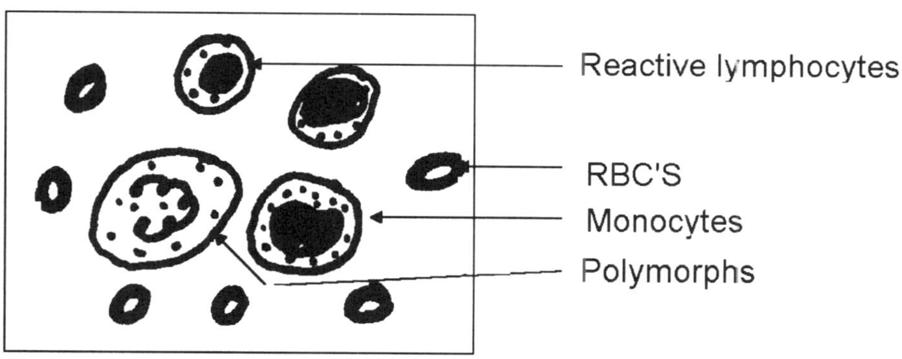

6. Myeloproliferative disease

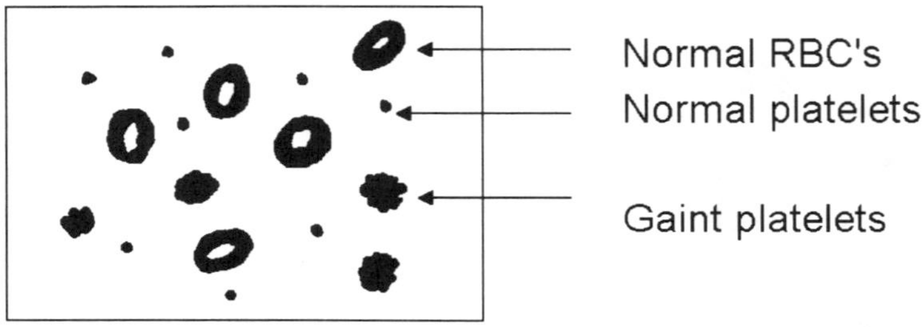

7: Hereditary spherocytosis:

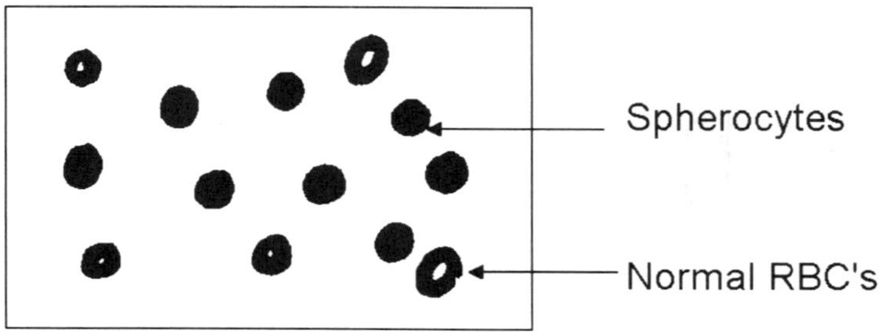

8: Autoimmune hemolytic anemia:

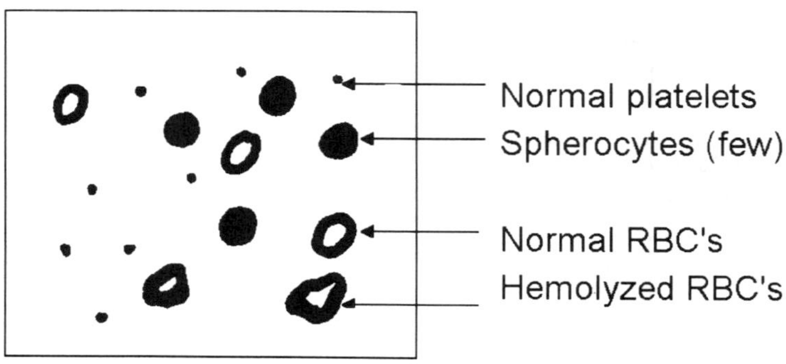

9. Homozygous sickle cell disease:

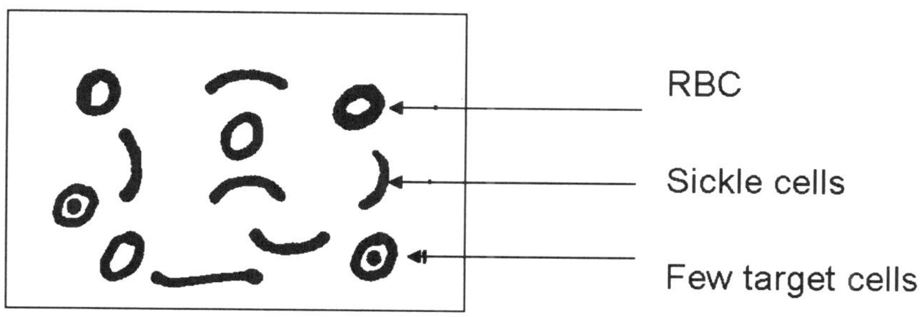

10: Homozygous SC disease:

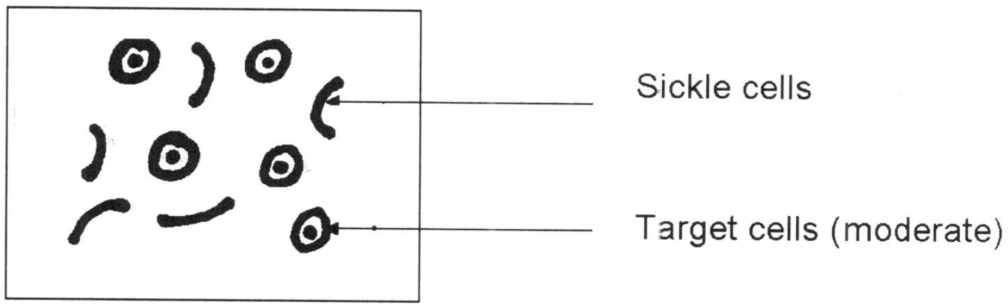

11: Hemoglobin C disease:

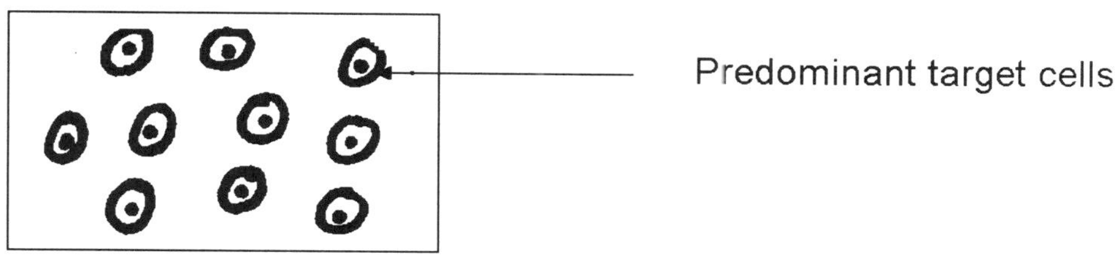

12: Iron deficiency anemia:

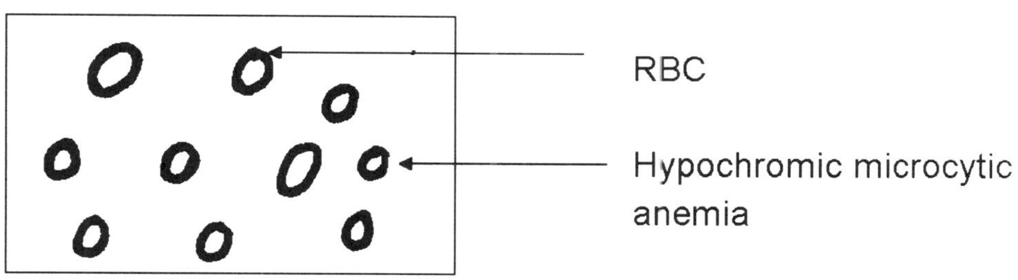

13: Acanthocytosis:

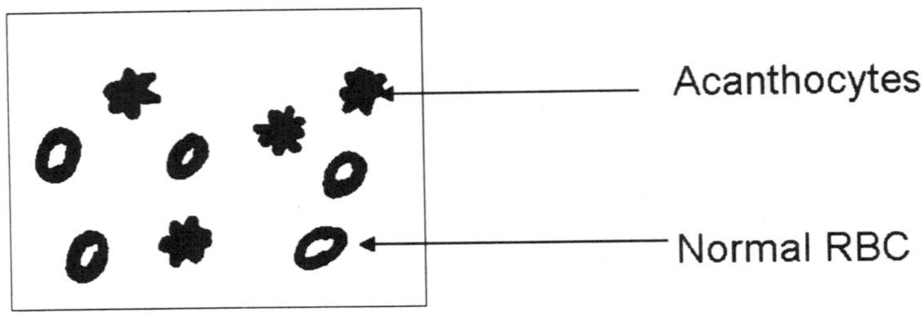

14: Elliptocytosis:

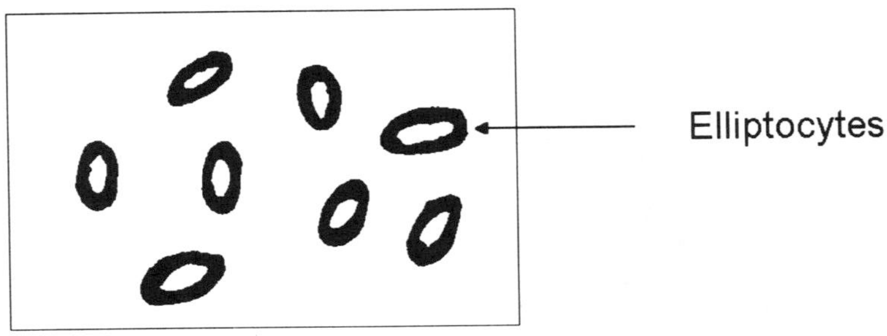

15: Metastatic neuroblastoma (bone narrow)

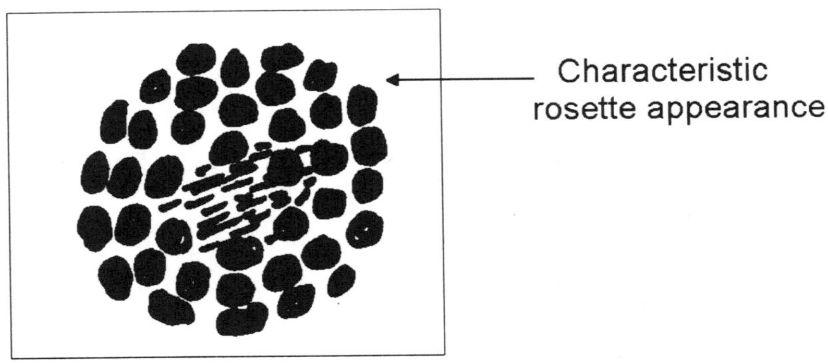

16: Howell-Jolly bodies:

It indicates poor function of the spleen

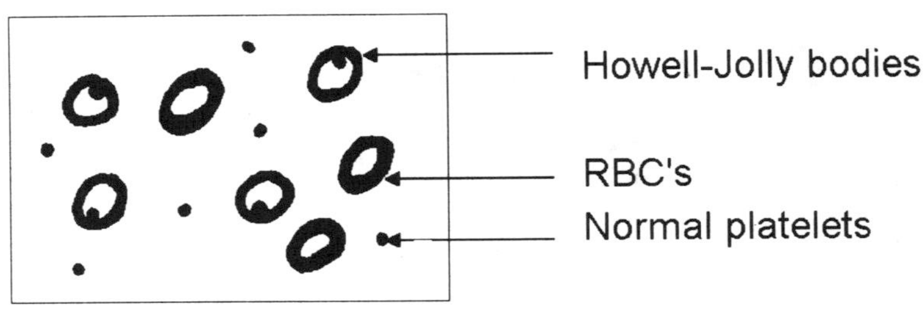

Nutritional Diseases

1. Few important **toxicities** of vitamins:
   (1) **Vitamin A toxicity (Important)**:
      (a) **Acute toxicity: Increased intracranial pressure,** hepatocellular necrosis, and skin exfoliation.
      (b) **Chronic toxicity: Pseudotumor cerebri**; hyperlipidemia, hepatocellular necrosis, ataxia, alopecia, cheilitis, and dermatitis.
      (c) **Excessive ingestion of carotenoids**: Benign, yellowish discoloration of the skin (**normal** conjunctival color); retinopathy (large doses of canthaxanthin).
   (2) **Vitamin K toxicity**:
      (a) **Rapid IV infusion of K_1**: Dyspnea, flushing, and CVS collapse **due to dispersing agentis in the solution**.
      (b) **Pregnancy:** Infants may develop hemolytic anemia, jaundice, and kernicterus.
   (3) **Vitamin D toxicity:** Metastatic calcifications, altered mental status, and renal damge.
   (4) **Vitamin E toxicity:** Hemorrhage stroke, impaired leukocyte function.
   (5) **Vitamin B_1 (thiamine) toxicity:** Lethargy, ataxia, and reduced GI tract motility.
   (6) Vitamin B_2 (riboflavin) toxicity: None.
   (7) Vitamin B_3 (niacin) toxicity: Flushing, hyperglycemia, hyperuricemia, and parenchymal hepatic injury.
   (8) Vitamin B_6 (pyridoxin) toxicity: Photosensitivity and peripheral neuropathy.
   (9) Vitamin B_{12} toxicity: None.
   (10) Vitamin C toxicity: Nephrolithiasis, urinary acidification.
   (11) Biotin toxicity: None.
   (12) Folate toxicity: Neuropathy, enhance seizure activity in patients prone to seizure.
   (13) Pantothenic acid toxicity: Diarrhea (in doses > 10 grams/day).

2. **Toxicity of trace elements**:
   (1) Copper: Vomiting, diarrhea, epigastric gain in acute mild toxicity; severe cases cause hepatic necrosis and coma.
   (2) **Fluorine**:
      (a) Acute ingestion >30 mg/kg: Death occurs.
      (b) Chronic toxicity: Dental fluorosis, exostoses, tendinous calcification, and brittle bones.
   (3) **Iodine toxicity**:

(a) **Large doses**: Hypothyroidism by blocking thyroid hormone synthesis.
(b) Patients receiving (>100 microgram/day): Hyperthyroidism may occur.

(4) **Iron toxicity**: Hemosiderosis is mild (iron accumulates in reticuloendothelilal system) and **hemochromatosis** is severe(iron accumulates in liver, pancreas, heart, and synovium).

(5) **Selenium toxicity:** Loss of hair and nails, peripheral neuropathy, diarrhea, and altered mental status.

(6) **Zinc toxicity:**
(a) **Acute ingestion**: Epigastric pain, vomiting, and diarrhea.
(b) **Inhalation of zinc fumes**: Hyperpnea, weakness, and diaphoresis.
(c) **Chronic ingestion**: Low HDL cholesterol levels, gastric erosions, and impaired cellular immunity. It also cause **copper deficiency** because zinc and copper compete for intestinal absorption.

3. **Keshan's disease**: It is characterized by **cardiomyopathy** which can be prevented **by selenium supplementation (but cannot** be treated with selenium**)**.

4. **Few important functions of vitamins**:
(1) Vitamin C, beta-carotene (Provitamin A): Antioxidant.
(2) Vitamin A: Epithelial differentiation (induction and maintenance), maintenance of cell-mediate immunity.
(3) Vitamin D: Modulates epithelial proliferation and enhances differentiation.
(4) Vitamin B_6: Modulation of steroid activity.
(5) Niacin: Reduces LDL and increases HDL cholesterol.
(6) Folate: Reduces homocysteinemia and neural tube defects.

5. **Drugs causing deficiency of micronutrients:**
(1) INH: Pyridoxine deficiency (impairs B_6 utilization).
(2) NSAID's: Iron deficiency (GI blood loss).
(3) Penicillamine: Zinc deficiency (increases renal excretion).
(4) Sulfasalazine, methotrexate: Folate deficiency (impair absorption and inhibit folate dependent enzymes).
(5) Cholestyramine: **Vitamin D and folate** deficiency (decreases absorption and increases adsorption of nutrients).
(6) Omeprazole: Vitamin B_{12} deficiency (stimulates bacterial growth, decreases absorption and gastric acid).
(7) Levodopa, dextroamphetamine, fenflluramine: Deficiency of all micronutrients (due to anorexia).

6. Most common cause of protein-energy malnutrition (PEM) in developed countries: **Secondary** PEM; it is due to **decreased intake of calories and protein**, **increased nutrient losses, or increased nutrient requirements**.

7. Clinical manifestations of secondary PEM (protein-energy malnutrition), diagnosis and management:

(A) **Clinical manifestations**: It occurs mostly in cancer and COPD (chronic obstructive pulmonary disease). Weight loss could be mild, moderate, or severe. **In severe cases all body fat disappears and muscle mass wastes away**.
Laboratory finding: Serum albumin levels are normal or mildly decreased (**rarely** decrease <2.8 grams/dl).
Patients with **trauma, burns, and sepsis can** appear as **kwashiorkor-like secondary PEM** such as dependent edema, ascites, and anasarca.
Laboratory finding: Serum albumin level are <2.8 grams/dl.
Patients with indolent chronic disease can **have combinations** of marasmus-like secondary PEM and Kwashiorkor-like secondary PEM.

(B) **Diagnosis of PEM**:

(1) Most important is weight loss (>10% weight loss in acute illness is clinically significant).

(2) **Laboratory tests**: Most important is **serum albumin levels**; other are prealbumin, transferrin, retinol-binding protein; BUN, total lymphocyte counts, anergy to skin test antigens, urinary excretion of creatinine; skinfold thickness and mid-arm muscle circumference.

(3) History and physical examination.

(C) **Treatment:**

(1) **Severe PEM: First phase to correct fluid and electrolyte abnormalities** (**low** serum K, calcium, phosphorus, and magnesium; and **hyperchloremic metabolic acidosis**) and **treat acute medical problems such as infection with antibiotics**.
Second phase is to provide adequate nutritional substrate to **begin repletion. Nutrition** is given **gradually** to avoid overfeeding. Initially patients should receive **maximum 0.8 gram of protein per kilogram actual body weight per day and 30 kcal/kg acute** body weight/day. Subsequently protein is increased **1.0 to 1.5 grams/kg/day** and calories is increased to **35 to 40 kcal/kg/day**.

Micronutrients should be given adequately.

(2) Patients with extremely **severe PEM (cancer) should be fed very cautiously**.

(3) Nutrition is given either enterally or parenterally.

(4) Physical therapy and other measures to improve functional status is important.

(5) To treat the underlying disease and to solve the social problems.

(D) **Prevention:** Early identification of PEM and appropriate nutritional therapy can prevent PEM.

8. **Few important points in anorexia nervosa (AN)**

(1) AN occurs mostly in young, affluent, **white females**.

(2) AN depends upon biologic factors (increased risk in twin and sibling), sociocultural factors, and psychological factors

(3) Patients have **intense fear of gaining weight**.

(4) Patients weight is about **15% below** the normal expected weight, **look emaciated**.

(5) **Primary or secondary amenorrhea** (**absence** of at least **three consecutive** menstrual cycle).

(6) Patients can have **congnitive deficit** (defect in abstract reasoning and conceptual thought), **sense of ineffectiveness** (unable to function separately from other family members).

(7) **Physical examination**: Patients pulse, BP, and temperature are **decreased**; severe **loss of subcutaneous fat, visible bony prominences**, acrocyanosis, **jaundice** (hypercarotenemia is either due to excessive intake or inadequate metabolism). Remember, **AN patients do not have higher incidence of infection**.

(8) **Endocrine abnormalities**:

(a) **Gonadal:** Decreased FSH and LH in females; libido and infertility in males.

(b) **Thyroid: Clinically insignificant** mild hypothyroidism develop (low T_3 levels, high reverse T_3 levels) and does **not** require any treatment.

(c) **Growth hormone**: Human growth hormone (hGH) levels are **normal or mildly elevated**, and decerase in somatomedin levels.

(d) **Adrenal:** Plasma cortisol levels are **normal or mildly elevated, decreased** urinary excretion of 17-hydroxycorticosteroids, **normal** ACTH and 24-hour cortisol production.

(9) **Hematologic abnormalities**: **Low** WBC, platelet, and hematocrit; **decreased** WBC function; **no increased incidence of infection**.

(10) **GI abnormalities: Decreased gastric** emptying, **increased GI tract transit time**; may have pancreatic fibrosis or jejunal dilatation.

(11) **CVS:** Decreased cardiac wall thickness and chamber size, decreased BP and cardiac oxygen consumption; **ECG reveals** decreased QRS amplitude, prolonged QT interval, nonspecific ST segment changes, and U wave; cardiac arrythmias (ectopic atrial, ventricular, or junctional beat;

tachycardia, sinus arrest); **sudden death** may occur in severely emaciated patients.

(12) **Diagnosis of AN:** History and physical findings confirm the diagnosis.

(13) **Treatment of AN:**

(a) **General medical care:** Physician should encourage the patient to take **personal responsibility of the treatment plan; involving the family** in the treatment plan; remaining objective, consistent, and honest to maintain patient's trust; serving as liaison and patient advocate with **different consultants**.

(b) **Nutritional care**:

- **Mild degree weight loss** (weight 80% of ideal or better): Nutritional and psychological counseling is usually adequate. The physician's role to monitor clinical deterioration perodically, education about physical development and it is relation to diet, personal support.
- **Moderate degree weight loss** (weight 65 to 80% of ideal): No hospitalization is needed; nutritional support (e.g., Ensure plus) may help; some cases may need **cisapride, metoclopramide, or bethanicol** to improve gastric emptying and to tolerate larger meals.
- **Severe degree weight loss (weight is < 65% of ideal)**: Hospitalization is needed; oral replacement or tube feeding into the duodenum for noncompliant patients; **extra 400 to 600 calories above daily caloric need** with the goal to gain **no more** than 1 to 2 kg weight per week.
- **Severe degree weight loss, not toleration oral or tube feeding**: Parenteral nutrition (peripheral or central vein).
- **The goal** of enteral or parenteral therapy: To increase **the body weight slowly**, stop nutritional intervention when body weight becomes 80% of ideal because nutritional supplements **interfere with the natural appetite** and **it is psychologically disturbing to the patients**.

(c) **Pharmacologic therapy**: **No treatment is ideal**, but **short-term use** of chlorpromazine, amitryptiline, cyproheptadine, and lithium carbonate may be effective.

(d) **Psychologic therapy: Behavioral modification** is an effective method of short-term weight gain; **family therapy** is the best method of long-term benefit.

9. **Most common cause of death in AN patients**: Inanition and **severe electrolyte disturbances** (suicide is **only 1%**). Short-term progtnosis is good, it is a life-long behavioral disorder with periodic exacerbations.

10. **Few important points in bulimia nervosa (BN)**:
   (1) Bulimia means patients who **binge and purge**.
   (2) BN is most common in **young (<30 year) women (>95% cases)**.
   (3) **Unlike anorexia nervosa**, BN patients have **normal** body weight, **less distortion** of body image, **more acceptance** in treatment.
   (4) Most BN patients do **not** seek medical advice (<33% cases discuss with the physician).
   (5) Clinical manifestations:
      (a) **Psychological and behavioral features**: Binge-purge cycle, feeling of frustration, loneliness, Patients look healthy and more outgoing than AN. Some patients of BN have used drugs, sexual promiscuity, and kleptomania. Patients seek medical attention because of feeling of **guilt, anxiety, or depression. First-degree relatives of BN patients can have major affective disorders**.
      (b) **Medical features**: Parotid or salivary gland swelling due to vomiting; conjunctival hemorrhage from retching, Russell's sign (bruising of the knuckles due to rubbing against upper incisor during the induction of vomiting).
      Complications of vomiting: Esophagitis, aspiration pneumonia, or Mallory-Weiss tears (tearing of lower gastroesophageal junction); cathartic colon with degeneration of Auerbach's plexus due to stimulant laxative overuse.

Laboratory findings of BN: Most common is **hypokalemic** (due to loss of potassium, hydrogen, and chloride ions) results in cardiac arrythmias, tetany, seizures, or renal injury.

   (6) **Diagnosis:** History and physical examination, and exclusion of other diseases.
   (7) **Differential diagnosis**:
      (a) **Kleine-Levin syndrome: Sleep disorder** with oversleeping and overeating.
      (b) **Kluver-Bucy syndrome**: Bilateral temporal lobe damage associated with indiscrimate sexual behavior, excessive eating, and pica.
   (8) **Treatment:**
      (a) **The best therapy** is the **combination of cognitive-behavior and antidepressant therapy**.
      (b) Psychotherapeutic approach includes cognitive-behavioral therapy in which patients can **identify abnormal behaviors** and **try to correct** it.
      (c) Antidepressant therapy **decreases** binge eating and **increases** the sense of well-being.

11. **Few important points in obesity**:

(1) **BMI** (body mass index) **above 25** cause health risk (**mean BMI is 22.4 kg per square meter for men and 22.5 for women**).
Formula: BMI = kg/(height in meters)^2. **BMI is the most useful index for obestiy**.
(2) **Measurement of skin fold thickness** in four (biceps, triceps, subscapular, and suprailiac) places are very useful.
(3) **Etiology:** Mostly unknown, **but most important is energy intake exceeds energy expenditure**; genetic factor.
(4) **Clinical manifestations**: **Obese patients have higher incidence** of diabetes mellitus (NIDDM), insulin resistance; hypertension; hypertriglyceridemia, high LDL and low HDL cholesterols; LVH, LV dilatation, CHF, and sudden death; chronic hypoxia, cyanosis, hypercapnia; obstructive or central apnea; venous stasis and pulmonary thromboembolism; cancer (endometrial, breast, gallbladder, and bililary system in women; colon, rectum, and prostate in men); cholesterol gallstones, cholecystitis, and fatty liver; arthritis; skin deseases (intertrigo, fungal, and yeast infections).
(5) **Mortality is higher with upper body obesity** than lower body obesity.
(6) **Endocrine disease** (<1% of all cases of obesity) are **Cushing's disease** (pituitary), Cushing's syndrome (adrenal), hypothyroidism, hypothalamic disease, polycystic ovarian syndrome (hirsutism, obesity, and irregular menses or amenorrhea).
(7) Severely obese men can develop mild hypogonadotropic hypogonadism.
(8) **Obese young women develop pseudotumor cerebri** (benign intracranial hypertension). Patients have headache, blurred vision, and papilledema **but normal** intracranial findings.
(9) **Treatment:**
   (a) Diet: About **1100 calories** with adequate vitamins and minerals, high quality protein (at least 0.8 to 1.2 grams/kg body weight), fat should be < 30% total calories, encourage high fiber diet, and avoid refined sugar.
   (b) Very low calorie diets (VLCD): Intake of 300 to 700 calories, adequate vitamins and minerals, high quality protein (either PSMF diet: protein supplemented modified fast) or both protein and carbohydrates. Most patients regain weight rapidly.
   Side effects: **Orthostatic hypotension** (due to loss of sodium and impaired norepinephrine secretion), cholecystitis, gallstones, dry skin, hair loss, and fatigue.
   (c) **Exercise** is helpful but food intake should **not** be increased along with exercise. **Energy expenditure must be more than intake**.
   (d) **Behavior modification**: Change of eating habit is most important **but** psychotherapy and psychoanalysis are **not** very helpful.

(e) **Drug therapy:** Short-term use of drugs along with diet and exercise may be useful. Drugs used are **amphetamine** (**decrease appetite by** stimulating central hypothalamic neurochemical pathways, elevates mood, and increases arousal by increasing norepinephrine and dopamine at the synapses), **fenfluramine** (decrease brain serotonin), and **mazindol** (acts through dopaminergic mechanism). **Try to avoid drug therapy**. **Side effects: Amphetamine** can cause agitation, sleep disorder, and psychosis; **fenfluramine** can cause sedation, depression,and diarrhea.

(f) **Goal of treatment: To lose 10 to 15% of present weight** (do **not** try to achieve ideal weight), maintain that weight for months before further reduction can be attempted.

(g) **Surgery:** It is still experimental and unsatisfactory but it can done in some patients with **severe obesity** (>100% over desirable weight), failed weight control programs, and developed complications (cardiac failure, phlebitis, arthritis, sleep apnea).

Surgical methods: Make small fundic pouch or reservoir; vertical banded gastroplasty.
Complications of surgery: Dilatation of gastric pouch and stoma; obstruction of stoma and gastric dehiscence.

12. **Most difficult problem in the treatment of obesity**: **To maintain the reduced body weight**. Prevention of obesity is very important because **overweight in early adult life is more dangerous than** in older ages.

13. **Most important stimulus for intestinal growth and function**: **Presence of nutrients within the GI tract**.

14. **Indications for enteral nutrition in adult medical patients**:
    (1) Severe dysphagia.
    (2) Protein-energy malnutrition with anticipated significantly reduced oral intake for at least 7 days.
    (3) Anticipated significantly reduced oral intake for 10 days.
    (4) Massive small intestinal resection.
    (5) Low output (<500 ml/day) enterocutaneous fistula.

15. **Complications of enteral mutrition**:
    (1) **Gastrointestinal: The most common complication of enteral nutrition is diarrhea** (stool volume > 200 ml/day) which is due to hyperosmolality, lactase deficiency, or high fat contents.
    Treatment: To treat the underlying cause; **reduce the feeding flow rate temporarily** improves the diarrhea.

(2) **Infections: Aspiration pneumonia is the most common infectious complication**, it can occur **without** episodes of vomiting, patients appear with new onset of tachypnea, tachycardia, hypoxemia, fever, or positive CXR.
Prevention of aspiration: Elevation of head side of the bed to 30 degrees, periodic measurement of gastric residuals, inflation of ET tube cuffs. **Silent aspiration** can be detected by checking **tracheal aspirate for glucose** with the use of oxidant reagent strips.
(3) **Mechanical: Obstruction**(pylorus or SI), **leakage** around the tube, **esophageal reflux, TE fistulas, rupture of varices,** sinusitis, otitis media, and nasopharyngeal irritation.
(4) **Metabolic: Hyperglycemia** (10-30% cases), **overhydration** (20-25% cases), trace elements and vitamin K deficiency.
Treatment:
(a) **Hyperglycemia:** Reduce the infusion rate, insulin, or both.
(b) **Overhydration:** Reduce the infusion rate, use 1.5 to 2 kcal/ml formula, rarely diuretic.

16. **The caloric requirement** of majority of the hospitalized patients: **Normal energy expenditure**, between **100 to 120%** of **predicted caloric expenditure**.

17. **The complications of over feeding or excess calories in hospitalized patients**: It **increases** oxygen consumption, CO_2 production, minute ventilation, and work of breathing; **hyperglycemia** inhibits the WBC and complement function; **abnormal LFT's**.

18. **Guidelines for estimating daily caloric, protein, and lipid requirements in hospitalized patients**: Physician must decide the **appropriate volume first, then caloric requirements, then estimate, protein and fat requirements,** remaining calories should be given as **carbohydrates (Important)**.
(A) **Moderate to severely stressed** patients **in ICU**:
(1) **Calories = Basal Harris-Benedict equation**:
(a) Females = 655+(9.6 x Wt, kg)+(1.7 x Ht, cm)-(4.7 x age, yr.).
(b) Males =66 +(13.7 x Wt, kg)+(5.0 x Ht, cm)-(6.8 x age, yr.)
Caloric need is calculated from **current weight**, even in over weight patients.
(2) **Protein** = 1.5 g/kg of (ideal) body weight. (Ideal) body weight is measured by:
Females = 45.4 kg for 1.5 meters and 2.3 kg per additional 2.5 cm.
Males = 48.1 kg for 1.5 meters and 2.7 kg per additional 2.5 cm
(3) Lipid = 30% of total calories during 24 hours.

(B) **Mildly to moderately** stressed patients in hospital ward:
   (1) **Calories** = Basal Harris –Benedict to Harris-Benedict plus 20%.
   (2) **Protein** = 1.0 to 1.5 g/kg of (ideal) body weight.
   (3) **Fat** = 30% of total calories during 24 hours.

19. **Caloric availability:**
   (1) Protein = 1gram provides 4.0 kilocalories.
   (2) Carbohydrate = 1 gram (dextrose monohydrate) provides 3.4 kilocalories.
   (3) Fat = 10% solution (1.1 kcal/ml) or 20% solution (2.0 kcal/ml) of intravenous fat emulsion.
   Minimum daily glucose requirement is the amount necessary to meet the need of brain glucose (100 to 150 grams/day).
   Stop or reduce lipid infusion when serum triglyceride levels > 400 mg/dL.
   Essential fatty acid deficiency **can be prevented** if approximately **5% of total calories is** provided as fat (ideal is 30% of total calories).

20. **Few other important points in parenteral nutrition:**
   (1) Malnutrition is an indication for parenteral nutrition.
   (2) **Electrolytes** (Na, k, cl, ca, p, Mg and sulfur), **trace elements** (zinc, copper, manganese, and chromium), and **multivitamins** (three fat solube vitamins A,D,E **except** K; and nine water solube vitamins) should be added in parenteral nutrition.
   (3) **Prothrombin time** (PT) should be measured peridically to see whether vitamin K supplementation is needed (elevated PT in vitamin K deficiency).
   (4) Soruce of carbohydrate **is dextrose** (10 to 70% solutions), **crystalline amino acids** is the source of nitrogen for protein synthesis, and IV fat emulsion containing **long-chain fatty acids** derived from safflower and/or soybean oil, egg yolk phospholipid, and glycerin to make it isotonic.
   (5) **PPN** (peripheral parenteral nutrition) is usually given in medically stable patients requiring short-term (7 to 10 days) parenteral nutrition.
   (6) **CPN** (central parenteral nutrition) is needed for patients who are **moderately to severly stressed** or **require longer** parenteral nutrition.
   (7) Osmolarity of PPN solution should **not** exceed 1000 mOsm/liter because it causes infiltration and phlebitis of the peripheral veins.
   (8) **CXR** should be obtained to confirm the catheter tip location in the distal SVC (superior vena cava) before the initiation of CPN.
   (9) **Monitoring parenteral nutrition:**
      (a) Vital signs; to determine the volume measure hemodynamic data, fluid balance, creatinine, urea, and sodium.
      (b) Weight increase **> 0.25 kg over 24 hour** indicates fluid gain.

(c) Biochemical monitoring includes CBC; electrolytes, BUN, creatinine, glucose; AST, ALT, bilirubin, alkalline phosphatase, phosphorus, calcium, and albumin.

(d) Monitor serum triglyceride level before lipid infusion (stop or reduce when triglyceride level is >400 mg/dL).

(e) If glucose levels **exceed 180 to 200 mg/dL, regular insulin** may be added into the solution or given separately.

(f) **Sudden discontinuation** of PN can cause **hypoglycemia** due to exaggerated insulin response. A **50% reduction of PN infusion for 1 hour prior** to discontinuation of PN does **not** cause hypoglycemia.

(10) **Patients with excess total body water and salt, use volume restricted TPN:** Use concetrated commercial solution (10% amino acids, and **70% dextrose in 1 liter can** will provide **70 grams of protein and 200 grams of dextrose, and 960 total calories**). Medications such as **histamine receptor antagonists and insulin** are added to PN.

21. **Complications of parenteral nutrition (PN)**:

(A) **Mechanical: Pneumothorax is the most common** due to faulty central vein cannulation technique.

(B) **Infections: Most common organisms are S. epidermidis, S. aureus, and yeast. Catheter is the most common source of infection, followed by bacteremia and fungemia**; organisms arise from patient's own skin flora, **invade the intracutaneous tract** during the catheter insertion and there after.

(C) **Subclinical venous thrombosis**: It usually occurs after long-term infusion, patients appear with **swelling in the arm and neck** of same side of the catheter.

Prevention: Very low doses of heparin (5000 to 6000 U in PN/day) or **warfarin** (1 mg/day) should be used for long term PN.

(D) **Metabolic:** Fluid and electrolyte abnormalities. **Hyperinsulinemia** promotes. Renal tubular **reabsorption of sodium** (results in increase of ECF volume), and **decreases** plasma values of K, phosphorus and magnesium. **Insulin promotes passage of K from extracellular space to intracellular space, results in hypoxalemia (Important)**. Insulin and glucose promote cellular uptake and use of phosphorus; insulin stimulates the tissue uptake of magnesium results in hypomagnesemia.

(E) **GI complications:** Most common is hepatic abnormalities which are **benign and temporary**. Elevation of **AST and ALT** occurs **1 to 2 weeks** after the onset of therapy, resolve spontaneously without any change in PN. Elevation of **bilirubin and alkaline phosphatase** occur **2 to 3 weeks after** the onset of therapy.

Most common biliary complication is gallbladder sludge (when GI tract is not used), others are acalculous cholecystitis and cholelithiasis.

(1) **Etiology of PN-related hepatobiliary complications**: **Unclear;** but factor causing the complication are **PN solutions (total high calories,** or **excessive dextrose,** or **fat-free PN)**, **cholestasis**, and **nutritional deficiencies** (such as carnitine, taurine, and essential fatty acids).

(2) **Management of PN related hepatobiliary complications**:

(a) **Abnormal LFT's** does **not** always represent true liver function, so **stop or alteration of PN solution** is **not** always necessary.

(b) **Exclude the other causes** such as extrahepatic **obstruciton** (ultrasonography or hepatobiliary scan), **medication**, or **infection (treated with antibiotics** after cultures are taken).

(c) **Avoid** excessive calories.

(d) Use dextrose, protein, and fat simultaneously.

MUSCULOSKELETAL AND CONNECTIVE TISSUE DISEASES

1. **American college of rheumatology (ACR) revised classification criteria for rheumatoid arthitis (RA)**:
   (1) Morning stifness (≥ 1 hour).
   (2) Swelling (soft tissue) of three or more joints.
   (3) Swelling (soft tissue) of hand joints (**PIP** = proximal interphalangeal, **MCP** = metacarpophalangeal, or **wrist**).
   (4) Symmetric swelling (soft tissue).
   (5) Subcutaneous nodules.
   (6) Serum rheumatiod factor.
   (7) Erosion and/or periarticular osteopenia, in hand or wrist joints (x-ray findings).
   Criteria (1) to (4) must have continuously present for 6 weeks or longer and must be observed by a physician. **Four of the seven criteria must be present to diagnose rhumatoid arthritis**.

2. **Clinical manifestation of rheumatiod arthritis (RA)**:
   (1) **Most patients develop joint pain and/or stiffness gradually over several weeks to months, one or more small joints of the hands, wrist,** knee, or shoulders and/or metatarsophalangeal joints are **usually the first manifestation. The joint involvement is characteristically symmetric, polyarticular, involving** proximal interphalageal (PIP) and metacarpophalangeal (MCP) **excluding distal interphalangeal joint (DIP) (Important)**.
   (2) Approximately 20% of patients can develop acute onset such as patients had **no** symptoms in the night before, awaken with **acute rheumatoid arthritis symptoms**.
   (3) **Criteria for clinical remission in RA:**
      (a) Duration of morning stiffness < 15 minutes.
      (b) Absence of fatigue.
      (c) Absence of joints pain.
      (d) Absence of joint pain or tenderness on motion.
      (e) Absence of soft tissue swelling in joints or tendon sheaths.
      (f) ESR is < 30 mm/hour for females or < 20 mm/hour for males.
   (4) **Classification of functional capacity of the joints**:
      (a) Class I: **Normal** joint activities.
      (b) Class II: **Moderate** restriction but can perform most daily activities.
      (c) Class III: Marked restriction and **cannot** perform most daily activities.
      (d) Class IV: Confined to bed or wheelchair.

(5) **Joint mainfestations and differential diagnosis of RA**:

(a) **Hands**: Distal interphalangeal joints (DIP) are **not** involved, remember osteoarthritis and psoritatic arthritis commonly involves DIP; **ulnar deviation of MCP joint; swan-neck deformity** is due to hyperextension of PIP joint plus flexion of DIP joint; **Boutonniere deformity** is due to flexion contractures of the PIP joint and hyperextension of DIP joint.

(b) **Wrists: Carpal tunnel syndrome** (is due to compression of median nerve by proliferating synovium) **causing paresthesias or pain** in the thumb, index, middle finger, and radial side of the ring finger; wasting of thenar muscles may be present;
Positive Tinel's sign: Tapping over the median nerve (wrist area) causes paresthesias.
Positive Phalen's maneuver: Forced flexion of both hands (90° angle to the forearm) cause pain and/or paresthesias in the distribution of median nerve.

(c) **Knees:** Effusion produces 'bulge sign' along the medial **side of patella; quadriceps** atrophy and popliteal cysts (Baker's) may be present.

(d) **Feet:** Metatarsophalangeal joints (MTP) are most commonly involved.

(e) **Neck (Important): Atlantoaxial joint (c_1 on c_2) subluxation is present (up to 30% cases); vertigo or syncope** may be due to compression of vertebral artery or vertebrobasilar insufficiency.

(f) **Remember,** RA does **not** involve sacral, lumbar, and thoracic spine; but sacroiliitis is common in spondyloarthropathies.

(g) **Cricoarytenoid joints:** Synovitis causes hoarseness, dysphagia, anterior neck pain; or sudden onset of stridor or dyspnea is an emergency.
Treatment: Corticosteroids (intraarticular or parenteral) and/or tracheostomy in serious cases.

(6) **Extra-articular manifestations**:

(a) **Felty's syndrome:** It is a **traid** consist of **chronic rheumatoid arthritis, splenomegaly,** and **neutropenia**. It may be associated with hepatomegaly, lymphadenopathy, thrombocytopenia, anemia, fever, and weight loss. **Most serious clinical problems are recurrent infections with gram-positive organisms** but do **not** correlate with the severity of neutropenia.

(b) **The large granular lymphocyte syndrome:** It mimics Felty's syndrome. **It is a premalignant disorder of T lymphocytes**. Do **not** perform splenectomy which hasten the onset of malignancy.

(c) **Eye: Sjogren's syndrome is the most common** ocular complication, it causes **corneal dryness** and corneal damage. Dry mouth and parotid gland enlargement may be present along with corneal dryness. **Scleritis** is painful and any cause visual impairment. Episcleritis is less painful, self-limited mild eye redness.

(d) **Skin: Subcutaneous nodules** (20 to 25% cases) occur mostly in **periarticular structures** and areas subject **to pressure** (elbows, Achilles tendons, extensor and flexor tendons of the hands and feet); palmer erythema and skin fragility (easy bruising) are common. **Rheumatiod vasculitis** is manifested **either** by **small, splinter-shaped brown** infarcts in the nail folds and digital pulp, or **severe necrotizing vasculitis of small** and medium size arteries.

(e) **Lungs: Most common presentation is asymptomatic pulmonary nodules** or nodules could be infected or rupture into the pleural space (pneumothorax).
Caplan's syndrome: Rheumatoid lung plus pneumoconiosis produces distinct but similar intrapulmonary nodules like RA.

(f) **Heart:** Most common finding is **pericardial disease (constrictive pericarditis** results in dyspnea, peripheral edema, and right-sided cardiac failure).

(g) **Neurologic findings:** Peripheral nuropathies (**carpal tunnel syndrome** from median nerve compression, **tarsal tunnel syndrome** from anterior tibial nerve compression); patchy sensory loss with wrist or foot drop; cervical myelopathy from atlantoaxial subluxation.

3. **Different body fluids composition in rheumatoid arthritis**:
   (1) **Pericardial fluid: Low** glucose, low complement activity; elevated LDH and immunoglobulin level.
   (2) **Pleural fluid (exudate):** WBC counts < 500 per microliter; **low** glucose, low C3 and C4; elevated LDH; presence of RF (rheumatoid factor) and immune complexes.
   (3) **Synovial fluid:** Poor mucin clot test; WBC counts are between 5000 to 20000 per cubic millimeter, 50 to 70% neutrophils; **low levels of complement; glucose levels are normal usually but very low values occur sometimes without any superimposed infections (arthritis)**.

4. **Diagnosis and treatment of rheumatoid arthritis (RA)**:
   (A) **Diagnosis of RA**:
   (1) **Hypochromic, microcytic anemia with hematocrit values 30 to 35%**.
   (2) **Low** serum iron and TIBC level. (Anemia does **not** respond to iron therapy but **does respond to erythropoietin in severe cases**).
   (3) **Normal** CBC and differential; **elevated platelet counts** due to chronic inflammation; eosinophilia is found in severe cases; elevated ESR.

(4) **Presence of RF (rheumatoid factor) is found in >80% cases, it is a diagnostic finding (Important)**.

(5) **Low ANA titer (antinuclear antibody)** is found in 30 to 40% cases (Important).

(6) **Remember**, HLA-DRB1 alleles (DR4, DR1) from DNA typing has **no** diagnostic value because **these genes are present in normal population**.

(7) Analysis of synovial, pleural, and pericardial fluids in RA was discussed in item number 3.

(B) **Treatment of RA**:

(1) NSAID's (nonsteroidal anti-inflammatory drugs): **Salicylates** (aspirin) **are the drug of choice**; most patients require 3 to 6 grams of aspirin per day to maintain the **aspirin level of 20 to 30 mg/dL**; coated aspirin is well tolerated.

Side effects of salicylates: Deafness, ringing in the ears, or GI intolerance. **Other NSAID's drugs** are also effective such as **ibuprofen**, ketoprofen, flurbiprofen, oraprozin; naproxen, nabumetone; indomethacin, sulindac;; meclofenamate sodium, piroxicam, diclofenac, diflunisal, and etodolac. These drugs are **not more effective than salicylates** but they can used when patients **cannot tolerate salicylates** or change of one drug to another is often beneficial in some patients and minimize the side effects.

Side effects of other NSAID's: Silent GI bleeding (minimal and tolerable).

(2) **Disease-modifying therapy**: Antimalarials, penicillamine, gold, sulfasalazine, and methotrexate, **all these drugs are slowly acting**. **Recently methotrexate** is considered effective therapy in RA and is being used widely.

Side effects of all these drugs:

(a) **Antimalarials:** Loss of vision and retinal lesioons; opthalmologic follow up twice a year is recommended.

(b) **Penicillamine:** It can induce autoimmune diseases such as myasthenia gravis, SLE, or Goodpasture's syndrome; renal (proteinuria) and bone marrow toxicities (low WBC and platelets count).

(c) Gold salts: Pruritic skin rashes, painful mouth ulcers; bone marrow suppression (low WBC and platelets count) and renal damage (proteinuria) in severe cases.

(d) **Methotrexate:** Hepatotoxicity, possible cirrhosis; oral ulcers; lifethreatening pneumonitis; bone-marrow suppression; leukocytoclastic vasculitis and enhance formation of reumatoid nodules plus systemic nodulosis. **Folic acid (1 mg/day) should be added with methotrexate** to reduce its toxicity.

(e) **Sulfasalazine:** Try to avoid it for its hematologic toxicity.

(3) **Long-term corticosteroid therapy:** It is used **only** in patients with aggressive joint disease and unresponsive to above mentioned therapy. **Local steroid injections are the treatment of choice for Baker's (popliteal) cyst of the knee.**

(4) **Surgery: Reconstructive orthopedic surgery of the knee and hip joints have an excellent outcome.**

5. **How to remember synovial fluid findings in different disease**:
   (A) **WBC counts**:
      (1) < 3000 = Osteoarthritis, traumatic arthritis. Both of them have <25% polymorphs.
      (2) 3,000 to 50,000 = Rheumatoid arthritis, gout or pseudogout, Reiter's/psoriatic arthritis. All of them have >70% polymorphs.
      (3) 50,000 to 300,000 = Septic arthritis. More than 90% are polymorphs.
   (B) **Glucoses levels in synovial fluids**:
      (1) 5 to 10% less than serum = Osteoarthritis, traumatic arthritis.
      (2) **10 to 25% less** than serum = Rheumatoid arthritis, gout or pseudogout, Reiter's/psoriatic arthritis.
      (3) **70 to 90% less** than serum = Septic arthritis.
   (C) **Total protein levels** in synovial fluids:
      (1) 1.8 to 3.0 grams/dL = Osteoiarthritis, traumatic arthritis.
      (2) > 3.0 gram/dl = All **other** disease mentioned above.
   (D) **Complement levels in synovial fluids**:
      (1) Normal = Osteoarthritis, trumatic arthritis, gout, or pseudogout.
      (2) Low = Rheumatoid arthritis.
      (3) High = Septic arthritis, Reiter's/psoriatic arthritis.
   (E) **Culture:** Only positive in septic arthritis.
   (F) **Microscopic features:**
      (1) Microbes (Gram stain) = Septic arthritis.
      (2) MSU and CPPD crystals = Gout or pseudogout.
      (3) **The following are nonspecific and nondiagnostic findings**: RA cells in rheumatoid arthritis; Reiter's cells in Reiter's arthritis; cartilage fibrils in osteoarthritis and traumatic arthritis.

6. **Adult-onset Still's disease (or arthritis of systemic onset)**:
   (A) **Clinical manifestations:** It is characterized by high **fever with salmon-colored rash,** lymphadenopathy, hepatosplenomegaly, polyserositis; leukocytosis, thrombocytosis, anemia, and very high serum ferritin levels.

(B) **Laboratory features:** RF (rheumatoid factor) and ANA (antinuclear antibody) **are absent**.

(C) **Treatment**:

(1) Salicylates or other NSAID's.

(2) Short course of prednisone may be needed.

(D) Prognosis: Good in majority of the patients.

7. **Spondyloarthropathies:**

(1) **These disorders include** ankylosing spondylitis, Reiter's syndrome, reactive arthritis, enteropathic arthritis, and psoriatic arthritis. **All of them are** hetergenous but have **common** clinical, radiological, and genetic features.

(2) **Criteria for diagnosing spondyloarthropathies:** Diagnosis require score of 6 or more.

(a) **Score 1 for each of the following within bracket** = (Lumbar pain at night or morning stiffness); (buttock pain); (psoriasis, balanitis, or inflammatory bowel disease); (nongonococcal urethritis/cervicitis within 1 month of onset of the disease).

(b) **Score 2 for each of the following within bracket** = (Asymmetric oligoarthritis); (heel pa;in or enthesitis); (sausage-like toe or digits); (iritis); (sacroilliitis, bilateral grade 2 or unilateral grade 3); (HLA-B 27 positive or positive family history of a spondyloarthropathy); (response to NSAID's in < 48 hours).

8. **Few important points in ankylosing spondylitis**:

(1) Men > women; it is the **most common inflammatory disorder of the axial skeleton**.

(2) **First symptom** is the gradual onset of low back pain and/or stiffness. It is mostly **symmetrical bilateral sacroiliits**, only 30% have asymmetric oligoarthropathy.

(3) **Acute uveitis** (unilateral orbital pain, loss of vision) is more common **in HLA-B 27 positive individual**.

(4) Diminished (< 4 cm) chest expansion (circumference) between expiration and inspiration (normal >5 cm).

(5) **Laboratory findings:** Elevated ESR or C-reactive protein, anemia of chronic disease, mildly elevated alkaline phosphatase, or sometimes elevated IgA; HLA-B27 is postive 95% cases but it is **rarely** needed to confirm the diagnosis because x-ray findings are conclusive, **so it is needed when x-ray finding** is **not** conclusive.

(6) **X-ray findings**: Sacroiliitis, generalized osteoporosis, bamboo spine; CT scan or MRI is **rarely** needed to make the diagnosis.

(7) **Diagnostic criteria**: Young age of onset, strong family history of low back pain, low back pain lasting > 3 months, prolonged morning stiffness, and symptomatic improvement with activity or exercise.

9. **Few important points in Reiter's syndrome**:
(1) **Traid** includes arthritis, urethritis, and conjunctivits are found in only 33% cases.
(2) Peak during **third decade** of life; postvenereal Reiter's syndrome is more common **in male** and postdysenteric Reiter's syndrome is equal in both sexes.
(3) It is the **most common cause of acute inflammatory arthritis in young men**.
(4) Many patients will **not** have enteric or urethral inflammation, such patients are named as 'incomplete Reiter's' or SARA (sexually acquired reactive arthritis).
(5) This syndrome is usually appear within 1 to 4 weeks after microbial exposure.
(6) Arthritis **most commonly involves the lower extremities** (first metatarsophalangeal joints, toes, ankle, and knees).
(7) Low back pain and other axial involvement are found in 50% of cases.
(8) Other features are: **fever,** anorexia, weight loss, and fatigue.
(9) X-ray findings are **positive only** in chronic and severe disease (only 20% of severe cases have positive sacroiliitis).
(10) **Extra- articular manifestations (Important)**: **Enthesitis** (heel pa;in); **GU symptoms** (transient mucopurulent urethral discharge, urethritis, balanitis, crevicitis, vaginitis); Skin (**most common is keratoderma. blennorrhagicum** which appears as **painless papulosquamous eruption on the soles or palms**); eye (conjunctivitis, uveitis).
(11) X-ray findings (feet, ankles, knees): Joint space narrowing, juxta-articular osteopenia, and soft tissue swelling.
(12) Recurrent attacks and prolonged disease free interval is common.
(13) Death is **rare** but it is due to **cardiac** (prolonged PR interval, complete heart block, arotitis, and aortic regurgitation) **or amyloidosis**.

10. **Few important points in reactive arthropathies**:
(1) It is an **acute, nonsuppurative, sterile inflammatory arthropathy developing after an infectious process** (e.g., Reiter's syndrome is one of the most common example).
(2) **Most common** microbial pathogens are Shigella, Salmonella, Yersenia, Chlamydia, and Campylobacter.

(3) Reactive arthritis initially appears as **an asymmetric oligoarthritis after 1 to 4 weeks of documented infection**.
(4) **Inflammatory extra-articular process** is an important finding.
(5) It responds to anti-inflammatory and immunosuppressive drugs.
(6) It is mostly **self-limited but can** cause **serious and chronic joint damage**.
(7) **Shigella flexneri** is the most common among Shigella **species** (**not by Shigella sonnei**) to produce Reiter's syndrome; **diarrhea usually resolves** before the occurrence of joint symptom.
(8) **Salmonella typhimurium is the most common** among Salmonella species to produce reactive arthritis within 3 weeks of infection. About **60% patients have positive HLA-B27, HLA-B7, or HLA-B60**.
(9) Arthritis is similar in **both** Salmonella and Shigella infections.
(10) Yersinia enterocolitica is **rare** is USA; it causes acute self-limiting GI illness plus arthritis (50% cases); **HLA-B27 positive individuals have more chronic, severe sacroiliitis and ocular inflammation; arthritis is predominantly oligoarticular** affecting the **lower extremities and hands;** chronic low back pain and sacroiliitis are found in 33% cases, HLA-B27 negative individuals have erythema nodosum and glomerulonephritis; elevated IgA antibody titers; treatment includes **antibiotic** therapy (for positive stool culture) plus similar treatment of other arthropathies.
(11) **Chlamydia** (10% of all cases of reactive arthritis): **The diagnosis** is suggested by the presence of **genitourinary infection, arthritis** of at least one joint, detection **IgG or IgA anti-Chlamydia antibodies** or positive Chlamydia culture. **Positive anti-chlamydia antibodies** (**rarely** positive culture) are found in > 50% cases of Reiter's syndrome, SARA, or nongonococcal urtheritis. HLA-B27 positive < 50% cases.
Treatment: Doxycycline, minocycline, or lymecycline (for 12 weeks) is given.

11. **AIDS patients and reactive arthritis:**
(1) AIDS patients can develop **severe form** of Reiter's syndrome but the incidence or prevalence is same as non-HIV positive.
(2) Most AIDS patients are HLA-B27 positive and appear with incomplete signs and symptoms of Reiter's syndrome.
(3) AIDS patients can have asymmetrical polyarthritis or intermittent oligoarthritis of lower extremities.
(4) **Rarely** causes uveitis or axial disease.
(5) Enthesitis (heel pain), fascitis, urethritis, and conjunctivitis are **early** and prominent presentation.
(6) **Treatment:** Poor reponse to NSAID's; some patients respond to isotretinoin.

12. **Few important points in psoriatic arthritis**:
    (1) Most patients have **established** skin disease; 5% of all cutaneous psoriasis develop arthritis.
    (2) Age of onset **30-55 years**, equal in both sexes but males have more psoriatic spondylitis.
    (3) **Cutaneous psoriasis** is associated with HLA-B13, HLA-Bw17, and HLA-Cw6; **axial involvement and sacroiliits** is associated with HLA-B39, HLA-B27; and **peripheral arthropathy** is associated with HLA-Cw6, HLA-Bw38, HLA-DR4, and HLA-DR7.
    (4) **Etiology:** Unknown; but stress, trauma, infection (streptococcus or staphylococcus), or expression of heat shock protein may be the factor.
    (5) Psoriatic arthritis has **gradual** onset and **progressive** disease.
    (6) **Five forms of psoriatric arthritis are** present and **one form can change to another; most common form** (30 to 50% of cases) involves both large or small joints (**sausage digits or dactylitis** of the fingers or toes); **second variant (10 to 15% cases) is associated with nail changes** (pitting, onycholysis, transeverse ridge, subungual hyperkeratosis and/or white discoloration); third variant is symmetrical polyarthritis **without** rheumatoid factor or rheumatoid nodule; fourth variant (20% cases) is psoriatic spondylitis and 50% of them are HLA-B27 positive; fifth variant (5% cases) is **erosive destructive polyarticular** arthritis of the hands, feet, and spine.
    (7) Extra-articular presentation and laboratory findings are **same as Reiter's syndrome** but **less** conjunctivitis, mitral valve prolapse, and myopathy.
    (8) X-ray findings are the same as Reiter's syndrome.
    (9) **Diagnosis is made by skin psoriasis, nail changes, and joint involvements**.

13. **Few important points in enteropathic arthropathy**:
    (1) It is associated **ulcerative colitis or Crohn's disease** ; peripheral arthritis **follows** the intestinal lesions and often parallels intestinal inflammation.
    (2) Arthritis involves both **peripheral** (20% cases, associated with erythema nodosum) and **axial** bones.
    (3) **Axial** arthritis **mimic** ankylosing spondylitis and it can occur **before** or **at the same time** with the colitis).
    (4) HLA-B27 **negative is most common** in enteropathic arthropathy (Important).

14. **Treatment of spondyloarthropathies**:

(1) **NSAID's are the drug of choice** (**not** salicylates), all the drugs are useful but **sustained release indomethacin is the drug of choice** particularly in ankylosing spondylitis and/or Reiter's syndrome. **Phenylbutazone** is very effective but used in **only severe cases** because of its complication of aplastic anemia. NSAID's can exacerbate the colitis in some patients.
(2) **Conrticosteroids:** It is mostly used for **local** intra-articular injection, **topical application** for conjunctivitis or uveitis, sometimes local intralesional injection for enthesitis (heel pain); **systemic use of steroids is only for severe disease**.
(3) Slow-acting antirheumatic drugs (SAARD's) (e.g., **sulfasalzine, methotrexate**): These drugs are used in patients unresponsive to NSAID's and have delayed onset of action (2 to 6 months).
Sulfasalazine is **most effective** in Reiter's syndrome, reactive and enteropathic arthritis; **methotrexate** is most effective in both cutaneous and articular disease; **azathioprine** is used in patients **unresponsive to** other SAARD's.
(4) Patients with psoriatic arthritis: Both methotrexate and sulfasalazine are effective; some patients may benefit from the use of gold salts, antimalarials, etritinate, or cyclosporine.
(5) **Surgery**: Total hip or knee replacement is very successful; arthroplasty is helpful in postoperative heterotopic bone formation.

15. **Most common organism causing nongonoccal bacterial arthritis**: **S. aureus**; next non-group A beta-hemolytic streptococci, Streptococcus pneumoniae; and gram-negative and anerobic infection (common in immunosuppressed, prior joint disease, osteoarthritis, or prosthetic joint).

16. **Clinical manifestations, diagnosis, and treatment of nongonococcal bacterial artheritis**:
(A) **Clinical manifestations:** Most commonly involves **single joint** (80-90% cases) particularly **knee**. Patients appear with **fever, chills; warm, swollen, painful joints** ; inflammatory signs may be absent in patients receiving corticosteroids or immunosuppressive drug or in severely ill patients.
(B) **Diagnosis: Arthrocentesis is best diagnostic procedure;** Gram stain and culture of the fluid; joint fluid examination reveals **WBC counts > 100,000 per cubic millimeter,** polymorphs > 90 to 95%, **low** glucose, and **high** protein; plain x-ray is **not** very helpful in early disease; bone scan, CT scan, or MRI may be helpful in **suspected** cases.
(C) **Treatment:**
(1) Appropriate antibiotics (**methicillin is the drug of choice for S.aureus,** vancomycin is used for methicillin-resistant S. aureus; first-or third-

generations cephalosporin or an aminoglycoside for gram-negative organisms) for 2 to 4 weeks or more.

(2) Drainage of the joint is very important. **Closed-needle aspirationo** is the procedure of choice **except** hip or shoulder involvement or unresponsive patients or suspected osteomyelitis, in those cases **arthroscopic surgery is preferred** than open surgical drainage.

17. **Clinical manifestationos, diagnosis, and treatment of gonococcal arthritis**: DGI (disseminated gonococcal infection) is the frequent type of septic arthritis in lower socioeconomic class.

(A) **Clinical manifestationos: Most common presentation is** monoarthralgia, oligoarthralgia, or polyarthralgia (migratory or additive joint involvement) usually in **knees, wrists, hands, and ankles** joints. Tenosynovitis with or without arthritis is found in 66% cases. Gonococcal skin **rash** (66% cases of DGI) is **nonpainful macules, papules, or pustules** may progress to **central necrosis** (may develop up to 48 hours after antibiotic therapy) usually present in extremities.

Most common presentation is DGI patients is asymptomatic gonococcal genitourinary infection.

(B) **Diagnosis**:

(1) **Definitive diagnosis** of DGI is made by **positive culture** of N. gonorrhoeae in synovial fluid, blood, or skin lesions but it is **rarely** positive.

(2) Most commonly diagnosis is made by positive culture of genitourinary tract (urethra, cervix), less commonly from rectum or pharynx.

(3) **Nonspecific findings:** High ESR and WBC counts, inflammatory synovial fluid.

(C) **Treatment:**

(1) **Ceftriaxone** (1 gram IM or IV every 24 hours) **is the drug of choice** or another beta-lactamase resistant cephalosporin is used because of **penicillin-resistant organism**.

(2) Penicillin or ampicillin (IV) is used if the organism is sensitive.

(3) Parenteral therapy should be continued for 2 to 4 days or until patients improve, **then switch to oral therapy**.

(4) Joint effusion should be tapped everyday, if indicated.

18. **Lyme disease causing arthritis:** H/O tick bite; **Borrelia burgdorferi** is the causative organsim; **asymmetrical arthritis** (mostly monoarticular or oligoarticular involves large joints particularly **knee**) occurs in **late** persistent or stage 3 infection; associated with HLA-DR4.

Diagnosis: Positive antibodies (IgM) against B. burgdorferi in the serum is diagnostic.
Treatment: Doxycycline ; unresponsive patients may need vaccination.

19. **Few important points in viral arthritis**:
   (1) Human parvovirus B 19 (DNA virus) can cause **rheumatoid like syndrome** (symmetrical polyarthralgia and polyarthritis) and **adult erythema infectiosum;** but rarely presence of RF (rheumatoid factor), joint effusion, and subcutaneous nodules are helpful to exclude other disease.
   Diagnosis: Specific IgM antibodies in the serum is diagnostic.
   (2) **HIV infection** most commonly causes oligoarticular arthralgia (intermittent with moderate intensity) particularly knees, shoulders, and elbows.
   Treatment: Anti-inflammatory drug plus AZT (zidovudine) reduce the joint symptoms; **unresponsive** patients may be treated with **methotrexate** and other immunosuppressive **drug along with AZT plus prophylactic antibiotic** (Rheumatic manifestations also occur in HTLV-I and HTLV-II infections).
   (3) Hepatitis infections (HBV is most common; less frequently HAV and HCV infections): HBV (hepatitis B virus) develop acute arthritis in smaller joints symmetrically (in prodromal phase) along with fever and urticarial rash; **arthritis disappers when jaundice** appears about 3 weeks later.
   HBV and HCV infections can cause **a syndrome** includes **polyarteritis nodosa and mixed essential cryoglobulinemia**.
   Treatment: Analgesic and/or anti-inflammatory drug is used most commonly; patients with **serious rheumatic syndrome** need prednisone, cytotoxic drug, and interferon-alpha with or without plasma exchange.
   (4) Rubella infection causing arthritis is most common in **adult women and adolescent. Migratory polyarthralgia develops within few days** of the appearance of skin rash in natural rubella or **2 to 4 weeks after rubella vaccination**; acute episode subsides within 3 to 21 days.
   Diagnosis: Rubella virus can be isolated from blood and synovial fluid; synovial fluid **shows inflammatory** changes **with monocytosis**.

20. **Fungal arthritis**: It is **rare** but can occur in imunosuppressed patients. The organisms most commonly involved are:
   (1) **Immunocompromised patients:** Candida, Aspergillus, Cryptococcus, and histoplasma.
   (2) **Other patients:** Coccidioides immitis, Histoplasma capsulatum, Sporothrix schenckii, and Blastomyces dermatitides.
   Diagnosis : Identification of fungus in synovial fluid or tissues.

Treatment: Amphotericin B plus newer triazole antifungal drugs (e.g., fluconazole and itraconazole) **with or without** surgical debridement are effective therapy.

21. **Criteria for classification of systemic lupus erythematosus (SLE)**: SLE is diagnosed if any 4 or more of the 11 criteria are present, serially or at the same time, during any interval of observation:
    (1) **Malar rash: Fixed erythema** (flat or raised) over the malar eminences, sparing nasolabial folds.
    (2) **Discoid rash:** Erythematous raised patches, keratotic scaling, follicular plugging.
    (3) **Phostosensitivity:** Skin rash due to sunlight.
    (4) **Oral ulcers:** Painless oral or nasopharyngeal ulcers.
    (5) **Arthritis:** Nonerosive arthritis (redness, swelling, effusion) in two or more peripheral joints.
    (6) **Serositis:** Pleuritis (pleuritic rub), pericardial rub and ECG finding in pericarditis.
    (7) **Kidney:** Persistent proteinuria (>0.5 gram/day or >3+), cellular casts (RBC, Hb, granular, tubular, or mixed).
    (8) **CNS:** Psychosis or seizure (**without** uremia, ketoacidosis, electrolyte imbalance, or drug).
    (9) **Hematologic:** Hemolytic anemia, WBC (<4000), lymphocyte counts (<1500), thrombocyte counts (<100,000 **without** offending drug).
    (10) **Immunologic disorder:** Positive LE cell preparation or anti-DNA or anti-Sm or **false-positive** VDRL or RPR for at least 6 months.
    (11) **Antinuclear antibodies (ANA's): Positive** especially to DNA, Sm, RNP, Ro, La, and others are characteristic to SLE (**except** drug-induced lupus syndrome).

22. **Few important points in SLE**:
    (1) Unknown etiology, women > men (8 to 13: 1).
    (2) Genetic risk factors: High incidence in first-degree relative (5-12%) and monozygotic twin (14-55%); **increased frequency with HLA-B8, DR2, DR3, C2, C4** (C4A), CR1 deficiency, DQA1, DQB1, TCR gene.
    (3) Characteristic clinical course of remission and relapse (acute or chronic).
    (4) **Most sensitive** test is **ANA** (99%) and **most specific test** is anti-**Sm** (99%) (antibodies to Sm nuclear antigen).
    (5) SLE with renal disease has anti-DNA and anti-Sm; anti-RNP with Raynaud's; anti-Ro with photosensitivity.
    (6) **Anti-La (SS-B)** is present in SLE and Sjogren's syndrome; **anti-Ro (SS-A)** is present in SLE, Sjogren's syndrome, primary photosensitivity and

primary biliary cirrhosis; **anti-RNP** is present in SLE, rheumatoid arthritis, Sjogrens's syndrome, scleroderma and MCTD.

23. **Clinical manifestations of SLE**: It has highly variable onset and course.
    (1) **General symptoms: Fatigue (90%) is the most common** and **fever (80%)** is due to infection.
    (2) **Musculoskeletal:** Arthralgia and arthritis **are most common** (95% cases), characterized by **migratory, asymmetric involvement of the fingers, hands, wrists, and knees joints; morning stiffness** only lasts for few minutes (>15 minutes for rheumatoid arthritis); **avascular necrosis of femoral head** (often bilateral) is common, appears with groin pain, MRI is diagnostic (x-ray may be negative), and risk factor is steroid (prolonged use and high doses).
    (3) **Mucocutaneous lesions: The classic butterfly rash** over the nose and checks (>50% of cases), **photosensitive rash** (>50% of cases); rash may last for hours or days and then reappears; discoid lesion (25% of cases), subacute cutaneous lupus erythematosus (SCLE, 10% of cases); **premature hair loss (telogen effluvium)** in scalp (71% of cases) is most common.
    (4) **Vascular lesions: Raynaud's phenomenon** (15 to 30% of cases) characterized by blanching of nail beds, fingers, and toes (due to vasospasm of small and medium size arteries); **livedo reticularis** (due to spasm of dermal ascending arterioles) is seen in forearms and legs; **urticara or purpura** (20% of cases) due to vasculitis of postcapillary venules.
    (5) **CVS: Most patients have pericardial effusion; pericarditis** (48% of cases); **myocaraditis and CHF** (8 to 78% of cases); **younger patients with coronary artery disease** (may be due to immune complex or IC deposition along blood vessels, hypertension, steroid-induced lipid abnormalities); valvular disease (25% of cases; **most common is mitral valve prolapse**); Libman-Sacks verrucous endocarditis (verrucae are typically present near the edge of the valve); thrombophlebitis (>10% of cases, most commonly occurs in lower extremities).
    (6) **Pulmonary: Most patients have pulmonary involvements such as pleurisy, coughing, dyspnea, postivie CXR findings** (pleural thickening and effusion), and **abnormal pulmonary function tests. Coughing is due to infection (Important). Pulmonary edema** is due to cardiac or renal failure, or fluid overload in steroid recipients. Acute lupus pneumonia (5 to 12% of cases) appears with fever, cough, dyspnea, and hemoptysis. **Characteristic of pleural fluid in SLE: Low** complement and protein levels; glucose levels **same** as plasma levels (low in rhumatoid arthritis); **few** WBC counts (mostly monocytes); and **presence of LE cells**.

(7) **Renal: Chronic lupus nephritis** (50% of cases, characterized by either urinary or clearance abnormality); diffuse proliferative glomerulonephritis (43% of cases); minimal or mesangial nephritis (type II; 24% of cases); focal proliferative nephritis or membranous nephritis (15% of cases). Renal biopsy confirms the type of nephritis. **UTI is very common**. NSAID's can cause azotemia.

(8) **GI tract involvement (50% of cases): Dysphagia** (25% of cases) may be due to stress (normal radiologic finding) or scleroderama-overlap syndrome (positive esophageal study) or hiatal hernia or gastro-esophageal reflux; **mesenteric vasculitis should be ruled out in patients with intermittent or acute abdominal** pain, diagnosed by angiography; other findings are abnormal LFT's (no hepatomegaly but abnormal LDH, SGPT); pancreatitis.

(9) **Hematologic findings: Anemia** (50% of cases) **is most commonly due to chronic disease** (normocytic, normochromic anemia, low reticulocyte count, normal iron stores) or chronic GI bleeding (due to NSAID's, steroids) or hemolytic anemia (low Hb, high reticulocyte counts, **positive Coombs' test**). A positive Coombs' test with **both immunoglobulin and complement** on RBC's **indicates hemolysis** but positive Coomb's test with **only** complement does **not** indicate hemolysis.

Most common is WBC counts between 4000 and 4500 (<50% of cases), predominantly granulocytopenia (due to antineutrophil antibodies, immune complexes). Active disease may have low lymphocyte counts (due to complement fixing IgM or cold reactive antiboidies).

Most common is platelet counts between 50000 and 150000 (<50% of cases) and it is due to idiopathic thrombocytopenic purpura (ITP), DIC, myeloproliferative disease, abnormal platelet production and distribution, or anti-platelet antiboides. The symptomatic bleeding (petechiae, purpura, gum or nose bleeds) **occurs with < 20,000 platelets count**.

Most patients have SLE when they appear with both hemolytic anemia and ITP (Evan's syndrome). In SLE patients with ITP IgG sensitized platelets are destroyed by splenic macrophages (Fc receptors). Other features are elevated ESR (most patients); lymphadenopathy (50% of cases); false-positive VDRL or RPR (25% cases; FTA-ABG, TP1 confirmatory tests are negative); splenomegaly (10 to 20% of cases); antibodies to clotting factors (F VIII, IX, XI, XII, XIII) and antiphospholipid antibodies (25% of cases).

(10) **Neuropsychiatric problems**: Most patients have this problem such as **fatigue, anxiety, depression, insomnia, anorexia**. Other features are psychosis (24% of cases), seizures (15 to 20% of cases), stroke (15% of cases).

(11) **Eye findings:** Rash over the eyelids, conjuncitivitis, and keratoconjunctivitis are common; retinal cotton wool exudates near the disc is **rare**.

(12) **Women**:

(a) Menses: Some patients have excessive menstrual bleeding which may be due to lupus anticoagulants, hormonal abnormalities, NSAID's or steroid uses.

(b) **Pregnancy**: Fetal loss (50% of cases), premature delivery, preeclampsia, or increased mortality of fetus due to renal disease.

24. **Diagnosis and treatment of SLE**:

(A) **Diagnosis**:

(1) **Most physicians use SLE criteria to** make the diagnosis but this criteria is developed for classificationo of SLE (**not** for individual diagnosis):

(a) **SLE is most likely: 4 out of 11** criteria are present.

(b) **SLE is probable: 3 out of 11** criteria are present.

(c) **SLE is possible: 2 out of 11** criteria are present.

(2) **Best screening test:** ANA (99% sensitivity and 80% specificity). Patients with **negative ANA** have 0.14% probability of SLE and **positive ANA** have 15-35% predictive value.

(3) **Determination to antibodies helps to confirm the diagnosis:** Anti-Sm (99% specificity), anti-ds DNA (95% specificity), PCNA (95% specificity), anti-RNP (87-94% specificity).

(4) **Maximum predictive value of SLE:** Anti-Sm (97%), anti-ds DNA and PCNA (95%).

(5) **Complement levels:** Reduced CH 50 (total hemolytic complement), C4 and C3. They are helpful in diagnosis as well as to asses the disease activity.

(6) Elevated immune complexes (IC's) in SLE.

(7) Active SLE: **Low complement levels, high anti-DNA and IC's level**.

(B) **Treatment of SLE:**

(1) Remember, **not** all patients need steroids which may cause more harm than good.

(2) Assurance should be given to patients that **most SLE is mild**; support of the family, friends, and organizations are important.

(3) **Prevention**:

(a) **Avoid drugs** (sulfonamides, penicillin, high doses birth control pills) which exacerbate lupus.

(b) **Exercises** is recommended because it reduces the fatigue.

(c) Photosensitive patients should use sunscreen and avoid photosensitive drugs (tetracyclines and psoralens).
(d) Post menopausal women: Estrogen is recommended to reduce osteoporosis and coronary artery disease.
(e) Immunizatioon: Flu and pneumococcal vaccines should be given.

(4) **Treatment of lupus nephritis**:
(a) **Mesangial or focal glomerulonephritis:** Bed rest, short course of prednisone (30 mg/day).
(b) **Diffuse proliferative glomerulonephritis: Prednisone** (1 mg/kg); in azotemia (creatinine > 1.2 mg/dL) use **immunosuppressive therapy either azathioprine or cyclophosphamide; pulse steroids may be used acutely** until the immunosuppressive drugs start working which is usually 7 to 10 days.
(c) **Acute membranous glomerulonephritis:** High does of prednisone of pulse steroid is used; if unresponsive then use immunosuppressive drug.
(d) Hypertension: **ACE** (angiotensin-converting enzyme) **inhibitors** to control BP and helps in proteinuria; then calcium channel blockers, then beta-blockers, then vasodilators.
(e) Diuretic: It reduces edema and high BP.

(5) Treatment of acute organic brain disease: **High does of prednisone** (1 to 2 mg/kg) **plus antipsychotic** drug; prednisone **should be decreased rapidly** to avoid infection once the psychosis has improved (remember **steroid may also induce psychosis**, so close clinical observation and /or EEG, MRI, SPECT scans, CSF protein, and antibrain antibodies may be detected); **seizures** are treated with phenytoin, phenobarbital, or carbamazepine. Function CNS disease should be treated with antianxiety or antidepression drug.

(6) Treatment of the APL syndrome: Low levels of antibodies do **not** cause symptoms; high levels of antibodies should be treated with **low-dose aspirin; coumadin** is used in symptomatic patients.

(7) **Treatment of acute severe lupus:** Split doses are recommended, then switch to **daily morning dose,** after that every other day with reducing doses is recommended.

(8) **Antibiotic** for infection (presence of fever indicates infection).

(9) **Fever:** NSAID's, then antimalarials, then sterodis.

(10) **Rashes:** Sunscreen, then topical steroids, then antimalarials, then injection.

(11) **Oral ulcers:** Antimalarials.

(12) **Arthralgia or myalgia:** NSAID's, then acetaminophen, then amitriptyline.

(13) **Arthritis:** NSAID's, then antimalarials, then alternate day steroids or methotrexate.
(14) **Serositis:** Indomethacin, then steroids.
(15) **Pulmonary involvements:** Steroids.
(16) **Raynaud's phenomenon:** Stop smoking, caffeine, and decongestants; then warm clothing; then biofeedback, then long acting nifedipine, then prazocin.
(17) **Thromobocytopenia and hemolytic** anemia: Steroids, then IV gamma globulin, then immunosuppressive drug, then finally splenectomy.

25. **Most common cause of death in SLE: Infection**.

26. **Recommonedation of SLE patients on NSAID's and antimalarials**:
   (1) NSAID's: Watch for GI bleeding and renal toxicity.
   (2) Antimalarials: Perform opthalmologic examination every 6 months.

27. **Drugs inducing lupus**: Hydralazine and procainamide are most common.

28. **Important features in drug induced lupus**:
   (1) Most common age is around 50; equal in both sexes; does **not** occur in black population.
   (2) Abrupt onset of clinical manifestations: **Most common is arthralgia/arthritis (95% of cases); other features are fever, myalgia, malaise, and pleuropericarditis (50% cases);** skin rash (10 to 20% of cases); renal problem (5%); does **not** cause CNS and hematologic problems.
   (3) **Diagnosis: Normal** complement and immune complexes (**unlike** nondrug induced lupus); **presence of ANA** (95% of cases), **anti-LE cells** (90% of cases) **anti-histone** (90% of cases), and anti-ss DNA; are common; **rare** presence of anti-ds DNA, anti-Sm, and anti-RNF.

29. **Diseases associated with positive ANA's: SLE, Sjogren's syndrome, rheumatoid arthritis, juvenile arthritis, scleroderma,** infectious mononucleosis, liver disease, vasculitis, aging, and drugs.

30. **Most important cause of sclerosing peritonitis: CAPD (continous ambulatory peritoneal dialysis).** Patients appear with signs and symptoms of **intestinal obstruciton;** diagnosis is made by ultrasonography which reveals **hemoperitoneum and peritoneal calcification**. Few cases of this fibrotic syndrome have been reported with **propranolol and other beta-blockers (practolol** is **not** used anymore).

31. **SAPHO syndrome**: Synovitis, acne, pustulosis, hyperostosis, and osteomyelitis. This **syndrome is associated** with **mediastinal fibrosis**.

32. **Mediastinal fibrosis (superior and anterior mediastinum):**
    (1) **Etiology:** Histoplasmosis, TB, SAPHO syndrome, and drug use (**methysergide** cause mediastinal hemorrhage and fibrosis).
    (2) **Signs and symptoms:** Obstruction of superior vena cava (puffy face, nonpitting edema of the face, neck, and upper extremities; distended veins in the neck and upper extremities; obstruction of pulmonary veins cause hemoptysis; constrictive pericarditis due to pericardial fibrosis.
    (3) **Diagnosis:** MRI, CT scan, or angiography.
    (4) **Treatment:** Corticonsteroid is usually effective; SVC bypass surgery for SVC obstruction; some patients of SAPHO syndrome spontaneously improves slowly due to collateral circulation.

33. **Retroperitoneal fibrosis:**
    (1) **Etiology:** Trauma, after surgery, SLE, vasculitis, scleroderma, cancers (renal, uterine, and other), carcinoid, drugs (beta-blockers, ergotamine, hydralazine, methyldopa).
    (2) **Signs and symptoms (peak in fifth and sixth decades)**: Most common symptom is **abdominal pain, anemia, high ESR,** low-grade fever, weight loss, and signs of obstruction of intestine (most common) or inferior vena cava or **late finding is urinary tract obstruction** until azotemia or renal insufficiency, although **ureter is most commonly involved** in fibrosis.
    (3) **Diagnosis: Intravenous pyelography** reveals displacement of ureters towards midline and obstruction; ultrasonography, CT or MRI; biopsy at the time of surgery.
    (4) **Treatment:**
        (a) Surgery to relief the obstruction is the treat of choice.
        (b) Progesterone and tamoxifen can cause regression in fibrosis.
        (c) Steroids and azathioprine may be useful in some cases.
    (5) **Death:** Most commonly due to renal failure.

34. **Causes of erythromelalgia** (a syndrome of episodic **burning pain and redness of the feet and hands** provoked by increased environmental temperature or fever): Thrombocythemia (high platelet count > 500×10^9 per liter) is the most common cause; other causes are diabetes mellitus, drugs (nifedipine, bromocriptine).

35. **Most common articular tumors**: **Synovial chondromatosis and osteochondromatosis** Patients appear with **episodic pain or swelling** of a knee, hip, elbow, or shoulder; **joint may lock** due to detached plaques forming loose bodies. Radiography may reveal multiple opacites. **Arthroscopy** confirms the diagnosis and helps in treatment.

36. A middle aged man appears with pain and swelling of the **left knee joint**. MRI reveals soft tissue swelling, pressure erosions, and subchondral cyst. Synovial fluid is serosanguinous.
Most likely diagnosis: **Pigmented villonodular synovitis (PVNS) (unknown cause**).
Treatment: Synovectomy

37. **Tietze's syndrome:** Patients complain of unilateral chest pain. Physical examination reveals **swelling and tenderness of** one or more **costosternal junctions** Biopsy reveals **chronic inflammatory fibrosis**.
Differential diagnosis: Costochondritis has **no** signs of inflammation.
Etiology: Idiopathic, prolonged coughing, or hyperventilation.
Treatment: Triamcilone injections into the painful areas are sometimes curative.

38. **Tennis elbow**: **Patients usually never play** tennis but complain of burning or aching pain at the **outer** elbow, along the **back** of the forearm, or momentary grip paralysis during grasping and lifting (forceful extension of wrist).]
Diagnosis: MRI reveals tear or area of degeneration at the origin of common externsor tendon from lateral epicondyle of humerous.
Treatment: Triamcilone injecitons into the painful scar, manipulation, or partial tenotomy.

39. **Golfer's elbow:** Patients usually never play golf but complain of pain at the **inner side** of the elbow during resisted flexion of the wrist.
Treatment: Triamicinolone injections at the site of pain or massage.

40. **Carpal tunnel sundrome:** Patients complain of **parestesias and pain** in the palmer side of thumb, index, middle, and half of ring finger due to pressure on the median nerve.
Diagnosis: Confirmed by electrophysiologic nerve tests, and MRI detects the etiology and helps in treatment.
Treatment: Splinting of the wrist, injections of corticosteroids, and surgical release of transverse carpal ligament; oral pyridoxine may be useful.

41. **de Quervain's disease**: It is due to stenosing tenosynovitis of the abductor policis longus and extensor policis brevis at **medial stytoid process.** Patients complain of pain at the medial side of elbow or radiate into the hand or shoulder. It is more common during pregnancy like carpal tunnel syndrome.

42. **Bursitis: Subdeltoid bursal** (largest bursa) inflammation causes pain, tenderness, and restricted movements of shoulder joint. **Trochanteric bursitis** (chronic strain on weak quadricep muscles) causes pain along the lateral side of thigh and low back pain.
    Treatment and diagnosis: Intrabursal injeciton of **lidocaine** is diagnostic and curative.

43. **Fibromyalgia (fibrositis):** It is **a chronic,** widespread musculoskeletal pain and tenderness **involving multiple sites without** any connective tissue or musculoskeletal disease. **It is also associated with disturbed sleep, headeaches, and irritable bowel syndrome.** It is most common in **women in developed coountries**.
    Treatment: Low dose amitryptiline can decrease pain and improve sleep in some patients. This is a **benign** condition, so physician should **not** use too much medications.

44. A patient with known diabetes mellitus appears with the painless swelling of feet.
    Physical examination reveals nontender swelling of the tarsometatarsals and metatarsophalangeal joints.
    Radiological finding reveals sclerosis, loss of joint space, multiple irregular bodies due to chip fractures, and new bone formation (similar findings may be seen in osteomyelitis, cancer, and calcium pyrophosphate deposition disease).
    Most likely diagnosis: Charcot's joint (or neuropathic joint disease). Diabetes mellitus is the most common cause of this disease, next is syphilis.
    Treatment: To control the underlying disease; stabilization of the joint with orthotic devices are **not** very helpful, and **surgical fusion is also difficult**.

45. **Multicentric reticulohistiocytosis** : **Symmetric polyarticular arthrits** (also includes distal interphalangeal joints **unlike** rheumatoid arthritis), may progress to **destructive arthritis plus skin nodules** (red to purple) in any part of **the skin, fever, and weight loss.** It may be associated with cancer.
    Treatment: Alklylating agents are more effective than prednisone; methotrexate is also helpful.

46. **Hypertrophic osteorthropathy (HO)**: Most common cause is **intrathoracic cancer particularly squamous cell cancer** (next is pulmonary infection). HO is characterized by **periostitis** of the distal tubular bones (tibiae, ulnae, femora, radii) **plus digital clubbing,** other less common features are joint swelling (30% of cases), gynecomastia, and **thickening and furrowing of the facial skin**.
Treatment: To treat the underlying cause.

47. An elderly patient appears with **sudden onset of polyarthritis** like rheumatoid arthritis (RA) but denies any family history of RA.
Most likely underlying disease: Cancer.

48. An elderly women appears with pelvic pain, weight loss, and **palmar fascitis**.
Most likely diagnosis: Ovarian cancer.

49. **Sjogren's syndrome (SS)** : It is characterized by the clinical features of **keratoconjunctivitis sicca and xerostomia** due to chronic immune mediated inflammatory disorder results in lymphocytic infiltration of the lacrimal and salivary glands.
   (1) **Clinical manifestations: Dry eye symptoms** (including burning, itching, or foreign body sensation) usually **worsen at the end of the day**, other features are blurred vision, conjuctival redness, mucinous discharge, and photophobia;; **dry mouth**, difficulty in chewing and swallowing, **positive cracker test** (**cannot** swallow saltine crackers without fluid); other features include polymyositis, arthralgia, nondeforming arthritis; **lung** (chronic bronchitis, lymphocytic intersital pneumonitis); **renal** (nephritis, type I RTA); liver (hepatomegaly, primary biliary cirrhosis); **vascular** (**Raynaud's phenomenon, vasculitis**); endocrine (hypothyroidism due to Hashimoto's thyroiditis); **nervous system** (peripheral neuropathy, multiple sclerosis, stroke, dementia, transverse myelitis); and reticuloendothelial system (splenomegaly, lymphadenopathy).
   (2) **Diagnosis of SS:**
      (a) Eye exam: Documentation of keratoconjuctivits sicca.
      (b) **Biopsy of the labial salivary gland** confirms the diagnosis by demonstrationg **focal lymphocytic infiltrations**.
      (c) Leukopenia, normochromic and normocytic anemia, and high ESR.
      (d) **ANA (antinuclear antibodies) positive (75% of cases)**; antibodies to Ro (SS-A) (50-66% of cases); antibodies to La(SS-B)(25-33% of cases);**positive RF** (rheumatoid factor, 50-75% cases); polyclonal hyperglobulinemia.
   (3) **Treatment of SS**:

(a) **Dry eyes:** Artificial tears, lubricant ointments (at bedtime), **sometimes** need surgical punctal occlusion to block tear drainage.
(b) **Dry mouth:** Saliva substitutes; pilocarpine hydrochloride to stimulate salivary flow; nystatin or clotrimazole vaginal troches for oral candidiasis; prevention and treatment for dental caries.
(c) Patients with extraglandular manifestations: Systemic corticosteroids, hydroxychloroquine.
(d) Patients with secondary SS: Treatment should be given for associated connective tissue disease.
(e) Patients with lymphoma: Lymphoma should be treated appropriately.

(4) **Prognosis**:
(a) **Patients with primary SS**: They can develop non-Hodgkin lymphoma (B cell derived, mostly are IgMk; translocation of bcl-2 t (14;18) protooncogene).
(b) **Young women with primary SS particularly with antibodies to Ro (SS-A)**: Higher risk of delivering a **child** with neonatal SLE and congenital heart block.
(c) Eye and oral lesions: Nonprogressive.

50. **Clinical manifestations, diagnosis, and treatment of systemic sclerosis (SS or scleroderma)**:

(A) **Clinical manifestations**:
(1) **Diffuse cutaneous SSc:** Patients (fourth decade) appear with **sudden onset of swollen hands, feet, and face, associated with Raynaud's phenomenon** (epsiodic onset of pallor of the digits, nose, or ears following stress or exposure to cold associated with cyanosis followed by pain, tingling, and erythema). The fingers and toes have nonpitting edema and are cold to touch, dusky or cynotic. Patients may have **interstitial lung disease, myocardial diseases, diffuse GI abnormalities, oliguric renal failure, absence of anticentromere antiboides (ACA).**
(2) **Limited cutaneous SSc:** Women or men who are working with vibrating machine, plastics or in mining) between **third and fifth decade,** appear with 10 to 15 year history of **numbness,** and **dead or wooden sensation associated with pallor of the second and third fingers**; subsequent development of **Raynaud's phenomenon in fingers 2 to 5** particularly in the winter or hard crusting lesions on the fingertips followed by **taut skin to the digits (sclerodactyle)** after years of Raynaud's phenomenon. Patients may have **skin calcifications telangiectasia, trigeminal neuralgia, pulmonary hypertension**, and

dilated nailfold capillary loops without capillary dropout. **Presence of anticentromere antibodies (ACA).**

(3) **Systemic sclerosis:**

(a) **Skin:** Skin tautness over the wrists, elbows, mouth, shoulders, and thorax are very important findings.

(b) **GI: Most common is esophageal hypomotility** (diagnosed by radionuclide esophageal delayed transit time or light barium swallow study), or heart burn; insignificant gastric hypomotility.

(c) **Pulmonary:** Pleural effusion, pulmonary hypertension, interstitial lung disease with fibrosis, or COPD.

(d) **Cardiac:** Silent pericardial effusion, shortness of breath, and ankel edema develop **slowly ; asymptomatic patients may have intramyocardial reperfusion defect by thallium scan (95% of cases) while most patients have normal coronary angiography (remember thallium scan should be recommended for asymptomatic diffuse SSc patients)**, and ECG and electrophysiologic abnormalities (80% cases).

(e) **Renal: To detect early hypertension** by frequent measuring BP and its treatment with ACE inhibitors (captopril, enalapril); **24-hour urine collection for protein excretion and creatinine clearance at least yearly** and its management appropriately.

(f) **Raynaud's phenomenon:** Pallor is the most important among triphasic responses (pallor, cyanosis, rubor).

(g) **Articular and musculoskeletal:** Stiffness and swelling of the fingers, wrists, knees, and ankles; or indolent myopathy, or symmetric small joint polyarticular synovitis.

(h) Male patients with SSc patients can develop **impotence**.

(i) Dry eyes and dry mouth are very important.

(4) Systemic sclerosis **without** skin manifestations.

(B) **Diagnosis of systemic sclerosis:**

(1) **Diffuse SSc:** It is characterized by Raynaud's phenomenon, nonpitting edema, and taut skin (other causes of Raynaud's phenomemnon produce pitting edema), presence of systemic manifestations, and **absence** of ACA (anticentromere antibodies).

(2) **Limited cutaneous SSc (lc SSc):** Clinical manifestations plus presence of ACA antibodies.

(3) Systemic sclerosis sine scleroderma (ss SSc): Systemic manifestations **without** skin involvement.

(C) **Treatment:**

(1) **No** therapy can stop the progression of cutaneous or visceral disease.

(2) ACE inhibitors to control the high BP.

(3) Appropriate management for renal involvement.
(4) D-Penicillamine can cause skin softening after 2 years of therapy but it produces toxicities. **Colchicine** is less toxic and produces skin softening.
(5) Warm clothing is useful; avoid cold, stress, or exhaustion in Raynaud's phenomenon.
(6) Nitroglycerin ointment to apply locally over the digital arteries to produce vasodilatations in Raynaud's phenomenon.
(7) **Nifidepine** is used most frequently in Raynaud's phenomenon, other drugs are verapamil, nicardipine, and diltiazem.
(8) Patients with gangrene: Immediate hospital admission for epidural sympatheic block and further management.
(9) To stabilize lung function in alveolitis-positive SSc patients: Use prednisone and cyclophosphmide.

51. **Hypersensitivity vasculitis**: It is a hypersensitivity reaction to an antigenic stimulus (drug or infectious agent).
(A) **Clinical manifestations:** The characteristic lesions are **palpable purpuras** (due to extravasation of RBC's into the tissues); other skin findings may be found are macules, papules, vesicles, bullae, ulcers, subcutaneous nodules, or urticaria; **arthralgias** of multiple joints; **colicky abdominal pain** with occasional passage of blood and mucous; microscopic hematuria without significant renal function impairment. **Some patients** produce serum sickness (by serum protiens) and serum sickness-like reaction (due to penicillin) characterized by **fever, urticaria, lymphadenopathy, and arthralgias**. Low levels of C3 and C4, and high levels, of C3a.
(B) Diagnosis:
(1) Demonstration of vasculitis by biopsy confirms the diagnosis.
(2) Wegener's granulomatosis is diagnosed by presence of antibodies against the cytoplasm of neutrophils (c- ANCA).
(C) **Treatment:**
(1) Most patients do **not** need treatment because it is self-limited.
(2) If disease persists or causes organ dysfunction: Prednisone is the drug of choice.
Patients unresponsive to prednisone: Use cyclophosphamide.

52. **Polyarteritis nodosa:** It is more common in **men,** in fifth and sixth decades. It causes segmental nodules of medium-sized muscular arteries. Classic variety does **not** involve the lungs, but lungs are involved in allergic angiitis and granulomatosis of Churg-Strauss.
(A) **Clinical manifestations:** Early findings are fever, weight loss, pain in the viscera and/or musculoskeletal system.

(1) **Kidney:** Polyarteritis (most common) and/or glomerulitis results in intermittent proteinuria, microscopic hematuria and **hypertension. It is the most common cause of death in classic variety (66% of cases)**, and 33% cause of death in allergic angiitis and granulomatosis.

(2) **GI systems: Abdominal pain (most common),** mucosal ulcerations, perforations, or infarction with melena or bloody diarrhea. Liver involvement may cause hepatomegaly **with or without jaundice** and extensive hepatic nevcrosis **but normal spleen**.

(3) **CNS and peripheral nervous system:** Seizures, retinal hemorrhages exudates with or without localizing sign; multiple mononeuropathy; asymmetric sensorimotor perpheral neuropathy.

(4) **Cardiac:** Involvement of coronary arteries and their branches cause **myocardial infarction** plus renal causes of high BP cause LV failure.

(5) **GU:** Asymptomatic, or gross hematuria with dysuria due to mucosal bladder ulceration.

(6) **Musculoskeletal:** Migratory arthralgias **without** swelling and myalgias are common.

(7) **Skin: Most characteristic but less** common findings are **cutaneous and subcutaneoous nodules** (appear in crops and groups); other findings are purpura, urticaria, and severe subcutaneous hemorrhages.

(8) **Lung:** It is involved **only** in allergic angiitis and granulomatosis. Patients appear with **asthma** plus eosinophilia, hemoptysis, and/or pleuritic pain. **It is the most common cause of death (50% of cases)**.

(9) **Untreated patients:** Progressive destruction of vital organs (kidney, lung, heart, and CNS).

(B) **Diagnosis:**

(1) Leukocytosis (mostly polymorphs) is found in polyarteritis nodosa, with eosinophilia is common in allergic angiitis and granulomatosis; elevated ESR; (low serum compliment levels only in hepatitis B antigenemia); **diagnosis is confirmed by tissue biopsy** (subcutaneous tissue, muscle, testis, epididymis, liver, or kidney, if clinically involved).

(C) **Treatment:**

(1) Corticosteroids are the drug of choice (NSAID's are **not** effective).

(2) Cyclophosphamide is also effective.

(3) Patients with polyarteritis nodosa associated with hepatitis B virus infection: Use this regimen of **cytokine, interferon alpha-2b,** and **plasma exchange plus short-term steroids** and **antiviral treatment with Vira-a** can cause long-term remission and seroconversion of hepatitis, or **alternative therapy** with cytotoxic drugs and steroids are effecive.

53. **Wegener's granulomatosis** (WG): It is a **necrotizing granulomatous vasculitis** involving **small arteries and veins** of the **upper and lower respiratory tracts and kidneys**.

(A) **Clinical manifestations: Classic presentation** includes **sinusitis, rhinitis with nasal ulcerations, serous otitis media, hemoptysis, and constitiutional symptoms; fulminant cases** appear with progressive renal and respiratory failure; **mild cases** appear with arthralgias,polymyalgia rheumatica-type symptoms or inflammation of eyes. **Constitutional symptoms** of fever, anorexia, weight loss, fatigue, myalgias, and arthralgia are **nonspecific but are commonly present**.

Renal: Asymptomatic microscopic heaturia, proteinuria with or without renal insufficiency, hypertension, and nephrotic syndrome.

Musculoskeletal: Polymyalgias, myalgias, arthritis (mono, oligo, or poly), myositis.

Eye: Conjunctivitis, scleritis, episcleritis, uveitis, retinal vasculitis, corneoscleral ulcerations.

Skin: Palpable purpura (most common in lower extremities), subcutaneous nodules, petechiae, vesicles, and Raynaud's phenomenon.

Neurologic: Mononeuritic multiplex, peripheral neuropathy, cranial neuropathy, and CNS vasculitis.

CVS: Pericarditis, pancarditis, arrythmias, cardiomyopathies, and coronary arteritis.

(B) **Diagnosis: Clinical manifestations** of multisystem illness particularly involving upper and/or lower respiratory tract, glomerulonephritis, and vasculitis in an organ.

The diagnosis is confirmed by open lung biopsy demonstrating **necrotizing granulomatous vasculitis**.

Normocytic normochromic anemia with high ESR and positive rheumatoid factor (30-40% cases).

cANCA and **more sepcific antibodies against PR-3 are helpful in diagnosis. X-ray and CT scan** of the chest and sinuses **are also helpful in diagnosis.** The spectrum of angiocentric immunoproliferative lesions (AIL) may be a prelude to lymphoma.

(C) **Treatment: Cyclophosphamide and corticosteroids are the drugs of choice. Alternate therapy** for patients with cyclophosphamide toxicities (hemorrhagic cystitis, infections, bone marrow toxicity, infertility, bladder cancer, lymphoma, leukemia). Altermate drugs are **methotrexate (most commonly used)**; azathioprine, pulse monthly cyclophosphamide, cyclosporine, IV immunoglobulin and immune modulators are also used in some patients.

Antibiotic should be used to cover infections (staphylococcal and other organisms) due to nerotic tissues.

54. **A 55 year old women** appears with history of **pain and morning stiffness** (>60 minutes) of the **neck, shoulder girdle, and pelvic girdle for > 1 month duration**. Initially pain may **subside** and return later after a period of inactivity. The patient also have low-grade fever and mild weight loss. **The patient rapidly improves after prednisone therapy.**
Laboratory tests: ESR is markedly elevated, with normochromic anemia.
Most likely diagnosis: Polymyalgia rheumatica.
Treatment: Corticosteroid (perdnisone) is the drug of choice; NSAID's may be given during withdrawal of steroid therapy if patient has mild symptoms.

55. **Giant cell (temporal) arteritis**: It is found in elderly persons; affects large and medium size arteries.
    (A) **Clinical manifestations: Headache (most common), scalp tenderness** over the arteries of the head or other sites, **may have diplopia** (or amaurosis fugax), **visual loss** (transient or permanent due to narrowing or occlusion of opthalmic or posterior cilliary arteries), jaw claudication, mononeuropathy or polyneuropathy, or polymyalgia rheumatica (up to 40% cases).
    Physical examinations: The **temporal,** occipital, or cervical arteries may be **tender, enlarged, or erythematous. Bruits or pulse deficits** may be found over the carotid, brachial, or subclavian arteries. Patients with eye symptoms may have **papilledema, hemorrhages, and exudates**.
    (B) **Diagnosis: Temporal arterial biopsy is confirmatory,** it should be done from most clinically abnormal arterial segment. Elevated ESR and platelet counts.
    (C) **Treatment: Prednisone is the drug of choice**; cyclophosphamide, azathioprine, methotrexate,and dapsone may be used.
    (D) **Complication:** Aortic aneurysm is a late complication.

56. **Idiopathic inflammatory myopathies:** It is a **rare** disease, **unknown** cause, produces symmetrical proximal muscle weakness and nonsuppurative inflammation of skeletal muscles. It is found more in women between age 15 and 44.
    (A) **Clinical manifestations:** Gradual onset of symmetrical **weakness** (sometimes pain and tenderness) of **shoulder and pelvic girdles, proximal muscles** (leg, arm, neck flexors, or pharyngeal muscles), fatigue, morning stiffness, with or without dysphagia.

Lung: Hypoventilation due to muscle weakness results in aspiration and infection.
Heart: CHF from hypoxia, cardiomyopathies.
Gottron's patches: Raised, red to violet, scaly patches over the knuckles, elbows, and knees. It is found in **dermatomyositis which is characterized by heliotrope rash on the upper eyelids**.
Associated with: Polymyositis or dermatomyositis may be associated with **breast or lung cancer** (most common); or ovarian or stomach cancer.

(B) **Diagnosis: Elevated CPK (creatine phosphokinase) levels (most sensitive) is characteristic;** elevated LDH, aldolase, AST, and ALT; EMG: demonstrate inflammatory myopathy.
Muscle biopsy: Fiber necrosis, phagocytosis, and inflammatory exudate.
Circulatory autoantibodies: MSA, anti-Jo-1 is common in polymyositis (less in dermatomyositis); anti-SM and anti-double-stranded DNA for SLE; anti-SSA and anti-SSB for Sjogren's syndrome; anticentromere for CREST syndrome; and anti-PM-1, anti-Ku, anti-SCL 70 for scleroderma.

(C) **Treatment: Bed rest** in active disease condition; **physical therapy** is important to maintain function and avoid contractures; **stop smoking; elevelation of head side** of the bed to avoid aspiration; **antacids or H_2 antagonists** to raise gastric pH.
Prednisone is the drug of choice; unresponsive or inadequately responsive patients should be treated be azathioprine, methotrexate; only refractory patients should be treated with cyclophosphamide, chlorambucil, cyclosporin, and IV immunoglobulin.

57. **Most common systemic amyloidosis in USA**: **Primary amyloidosis**, which is associated with plasma cell myeloma (20%) or plasma cell dyscrasias (80%) plus involvement of skin, subcutaneous tissue, liver, spleen, **nerve**, heart, lung, and kidney.

58. **Clinical manifestations of amyloidosis**:

(A) **Primary (AL) amyloidosis: Fatigue and weight loss** are most common (50% of cases); **less frequent other features are** dyspnea, peripheral edema, paresthesias, hoarseness, hepatomegaly, **orthostatic hypotension**, macroglossia, **carpal tunnel syndrome**, peripheral neuropathy, CHF, pinch purpura, albuminuria, and nephrotic syndrome. It depends upon the organ involvements.

(B) **Secondary (AA) amyloidosis**: It usually involves the liver, spleen, and kidney; some patients may develop osteomyelitis, TB, bronchiectasis, JRA, rheumatoid arthritis, ankylosing spondylitis, Crohn's disease, and familial Mediterranean fever.

(C) **Familial (ATTR) amyloidosis**: It is associated with the presence of abnormal plasma prealbumin protein (**transthyretin**), and involves heart, bowel, and kidney.

(D) **Dialysis related** (beta-2-microglobulin) amyloidosis (AB_2M): It develops after prolonged (>8 years) use of hemodialysis or peritoneal dialysis due to deposition of **beta-2-microglobulin** amylolid in the bone, periarticular tissue, and **carpal tunnel tissue**. Beta-2-microglobulins are **not** removed by dialysis membranses, moreover this membrane **stimulates the production IL-1 and activation of compliments** which stimulates beta-2-microglobulins production.

(E) Beta protein amyloidosis (Alzheimer's disease or AD): **AD is the most common cause of dementia over age 65**. The cerebrovascular deposition of **beta-protein** is an important cause of **nontraumatic/nonhypertensive brain hemorrhage in the elderly**.

(F) **Differential diagnosis**:

(1) POEMS syndrome (polyneuropathy, organomegaly, endocrinopathy, monoclonal gammopathy, and skin findings): It is due to plasma cell dyscrasia, mimic amyloid disease **but no amyloid** deposits.

(2) Immunotactoid glomerulopathy (fibrillary renal deposits): Proteinuria, hypertension, and microscopic hematuria; glomerular depostis of IgG, IgM, C3, C4, inverted Y, and K light chains.

(G)**Diagnosis:** It is confirmed by detection of **amyloid deposits** in tisue preparation stained with Congo red; **avoid** liver biopsy due to bleeding complications; bone marrow aspiration and biopsy are done to **count the number of plasma cells** and can be stained for amyloid.

(H) **Treatment:**

(i) Melphalan and prednisone together; use diuretic for fluid retention.

(ii) Prevention and treatment of amyloidosis **of familial Mediterranean fever**: Use low-dose **colchicine**.

(iii) **Highly permeable dialysis membrane (experimental)** is available to prevent dialysis-related A beta-2 M which is very common in localized amyloidosis.

(iv) No preventive therapy is available yet.

59. **Bechet's disease (BD)**: It is **rare** in USA; patients appear with mouth ulcers (most common), genital ulcers, skin lesions, uveitis, self-limited arthritis (knees, ankles), phlebitis, arteritis, and aseptic meningitis (in all cases of neurologic BD).

Treatment: Anticoagulants for thrombosis; **prednisone** for serious cases like CNS involvements; **cyclosporin** is better than colchicine to reduce eye problems: **azathioprine** can preserve the visual acuity and reduce the arthritis and oral-genital ulcers; **methotrexate may be used**; **oral retinal protein S** is useful in retinitis; chlorambucil can reduce the disease progression but long-term use may cause cancer.

60. **Gout: Types: Primary and secondary**. Most common cause of **primary gout is idiopathic (>99%)** with normal urinary excretion (80-90% of primary gout) and increased urinary excretion (10-20% of primary gout), idiopathic has **polygenic** inheritance; **other primary type** is (<1%) x-linked and is due to inherited metabolic defect.
The secondary type is due to G-6-PD deficiency (autosomal recessive), renal problems, and chronic hemolysis. Men are mostly affected around 45 years of age and women are mostly after menopause. Men have asymptomatic hyperuremia for 20 to 30 years before the clinical manifestation.
(A) **Clinical manifestations**:
(i) **Acute gouty arthritis**: **Most commonly involved joint is metatarsophalangeal joint of the great toe**; followed by **ankle**, heel, knee, wrist, finger and elbow. The joint suddenly (within minutes to hours) become hot, tender, painful, dusky red; severe cases may have fever, high ESR, and high WBC counts suggest infection. Desquamation of inflammed skin occurs when acute attack subsides.
(ii) **Chronic trophaceous gout**: Initially appear with **superficial yellowish-white infiltrates** on the **palms, soles and fingertips** followed by fusiform or nodular enlargement of the **Achilles tendon** or **distension of olecranon bursa**; presence of tophi on the **helix or anthelix** of external ear is characteristic but **less** frequent; tophi are usually painless but it **causes punched out bony lesions** and **disabling joint disease**; skin over tophi causes ulceration and exudation of chalky or pasty **`milk of urate'**.
(iii) **Gouty nephropathy**: It causes renal failure with inherited metabolic disorders which cause **excessive urate production.** Progressive deterioration in renal function is **not** due to hyperuricemia but **due to hypertension, renal calculi, pyelonephritis and aging.** Acute renal failure may be due to bilateral ureteral obstruction by uric acid deposits, this can be **prevented** by **high urine volume, with alkalinization**, and with **allopurinol**.
(B) **Diagnosis of gout**:
(i) Clinical manifestations are characteristic.
(ii) **The diagnosis is confirmed by demonstrating** brilliant, negatively bire-fringent, **needle-shaped MSU crystals**.
(iii) Synovial fluid analysis: Gram stain and culture should be done to rule out infection; WBC counts 5000 to > 50000 per cubic millimeter.

(iv) Determination of 24 - hours urinary excretion of uric acid: Values > 600 mg per 1.72 square meters/day is considered over production, values > 800 need further investigations. It causes renal stone.
Treatment of excessive uric acid excretion: **Allopurinol is used** (do **not** use uricosuric drug)

(c) **Treatment of gout**:

(i) Acute gout: The goal is to terminate acute inflammatory attack.

(a) NSAID's (indomethacin, ibuprofen) are the drug of choice.

(b) Colchicine orally (preferred) or IV if cannot take by mouth.

(c) When NSAID's and colchicine are contraindicated such as postoperatively: Use IV prednisone or local injection into the join; triamcinolone or dexamethasone can be used.

(d) Do **not** use hypouricemic drugs that have **no** benefits and can initiate recurrent attacks. This drug should not be used until the acute attack resolves.

(ii) **Interval gout**: The goal is to prevent recurrent attacks.

(a) Colchicine orally is used as prophylaxis.

(b) Use hypouricemic drug.

(c) **High fluid intake** (promote uric acid excretion); **moderate protein and low fat diet**; **avoid** excessive alcohol; treat high BP if present.

(iii) **Long term therapy of gout**: The goal is to prevent attacks, resolve tophi, and keep serum urate levels $\leq$ 6 mg/dL.

(a) Colchicine orally 1-2 weeks before the onset of hypouricemic therapy and for many months afterwards to prevent recurrent attacks during early phase of hypouricemic therapy.

(b) **Allopurinol** may be needed in some patients; or **uricosuric agents** (probenecid or sulfinpyrazone).
Side effects: Headache, rash, GI upset; reduced effectivity if creatinine clearance < 80 ml and ineffective if < 30 ml.

(c) High fluid intake (especially at night); **acetazolamide** at bedtime to keep urine pH >6 ; moderate protein and low fat diet; avoid excessive alcohol; treat high BP if present.

(iv) **Asymptomatic hyperuricemia**: **Allopurinol therapy should be given** before articular or renal problems in **patients with strong family history of trophaceous disease or gout and renal problems**. No therapy **is needed** for asymptomatic hyperuricemia in family members of patients with gout and general population **because <20% of them will develop gout and patients should be treated during acute attacks (Important)**

61. Calcium pyrophosphate dihydrate (CPPD) crystal **deposition disease (or pseudogout syndrome)**: It is **most common** in **elderly patients** of **80 years and above**; most commonly involved joints are **knees, wrists, second and third metacarpophalangeal joints.**
X-ray: Chondrocalcinosis is present. **Synovial fluid findings**: **WBC counts** up to **100000** per cubic millimeter with **80 to 90% polymorphs**.
Treatment: **Aspiration of crystals and NSAID's are very helpful**; **intra-articular injection of steroids are needed** in some refractory cases; **intravenous colchicine** can reduce the frequency of acute attacks; **last resort is joint replacement**.

62. **Apatite crystal deposition disease**: It involves the joints or bursae especially **shoulders, knees, hips**, and **digits including** the first metatarsophalangeal joints. **Milwaukee shoulder is an extremely severe arthritis**. **X-ray** shows soft tissue calcifications with or without bone erosions. **The definitive diagnosis of crystal type by electron microscopy**. **It can be associated** with scleroderma, other connective tissue disease, high-dose vitamin D therapy, CNS injury, or repeated corticosteroid injections.
Treatment: **NSAID's or colchicine** is used for acute arthritis or periarthritis. **Aspiration** of crystals and **local injection with corticosteroids** are also effective.

63. A patient of renal failure on dialysis (peritoneal or hemodialysis) for long time, **demonstrates** signs of spinal cord compression, and X-ray reveals **soft tissue calcifications** or **chondrocalcinosis.**
Most likely diagnosis: **Vertebral oxalate crystals** cause spinal cord compression.
Diagnosis is confirmed by demonstration of **typical bipyramidal crystals in joint fluid or biopsy specimens**. Avoid vitamin C which can enhances this crystal formation.

64. Diseases can cause CPPD (**calcium pyrophosphate dihydrate**) deposition: Hyperparathyroidism, myxedematous hypothyroidism, hemochromatosis, hypophosphatasia, hypomagnesemia and onchronosis.

65. Most common cardiac defect in relapsing polychondritis: **Aortic insufficiency** due to involvement of aortic root; **sometimes aortic aneurysms.** Other features of **relapsing polychondritis** (inflammation and destruction of **cartilages of pinnae of ears, nose and tracheal rings**) are inflammation of **ear cartilage (most common);** inner or middle ear involvement's can cause

hearing loss or vertigo; saddle nose; hoarseness or upper respiratory obstruction; conjunctivitis, episcleritis, iridocyclitis, and proptosis.

Diagnosis of relapsing polychondritis:

No definitive test but high ESR, anemia, high WBC counts; antineutrophil cytoplasmic antibodies (ANCA's) are present.

Treatment of relapsing polychondritis:

(i) Mild cases: NSAID's are useful

(ii) **Moderate to severe cases**: **Prednisone** is the drug of choice. Cyclosporine and immunosuppressive drug are helpful. **Dapsone** may be helpful. **Tracheostomy** or stents for tracheal collapse.

Most common causes of death: **Infection and systemic vasculitis** cause more death than airway obstruction.

66. Most common joint disorder or chronic disease in the elderly: **Osteoarthritis (degenerative bone disease)**. It is most common above 65 years of age. **Women are most commonly affected above 55** and **men are most commonly affected younger than 45**, Etiology is **unknown but runs in the family.**

67. **Osteoarthritis (OA):**

(a) **Clinical manifestations:** Initially patients are **asymptomatic** with **positive** radiological and pathological finding. Even in later stages there is poor **correlation between** clinical findings and cartilage and bone destructions.

First symptom is the pain in a single joint which is **relieved by rest** initially; **later on multiple joints stiffness** which follows **a period of inactivity** (in the morning and after sitting for a while); in **severe disease pain is persistent** and patients are unable to sleep and perform normal activities even with therapy;

Physical examination: Most commonly involved joints are the **metatarsophalangeal** (MTP) joint of the big toe, proximal **interphalangeal (PIP)** and **distal interphalangeal (DIP) joints**, and **carpometacarpal (CMC)** joint of the thumb, lumbar and cervical spine, hip and knees (**sparing ankle**). **Joint has tenderness, crepitus, restricted movements, swelling and may be subluxation.** This disease is not always progressive.

(i) **Hands:** **Heberden's nodes** (bony enlargement of **DIP joints** due to marginal osteophytic spurs) are most common in women; **washerwoman's hands** (pain while wringing out clothes) due to involvement of CMC joint of the thumb.

(ii) **Knees:** Idiopathic OA in knees are the common cause of painful ambulation, most common in women with overweight.

(iii) **Hips: Most patients with hip pain have lumbar spine OA (Important);** hip OA is diagnosed by **loss of internal rotation and then limited range of motion.**

(iv) **Feet: Most commonly involved joint is first MTP joint with swelling and deformity (bunion);** More common in **women** than men.

(v) **Spine**: Localized pain, referred pain along the nerve roots (radiculopathy), nerve root compression may cause muscle **weakness, hyporeflexia, paresthesia, or hypesthesia.**

(b) **Diagnosis of OA (osteoarthritis):**

(i) **Normal** ESR, hemoglobin, and WBC counts.

(ii) Synovial fluid has **no** evidence of inflammation (WBC counts <3000 per cubic millimeter)

(iii) **Absence** of RF (rheumatoid factor) in most patients.

(iv) **X-ray reveals** presence of **osteophytes** at the margins of involved joints, narrowed joints, **narrowed** joint space due to loss of cartilage, and evidence of bony reactions (subchondral sclerosis and bone systs). X-ray is **not** sensitive because patients may have **normal** X-ray with destroyed cartilage.

(v) **MRI is the best method to diagnose cartilage injury.**

(vi) **Scintigraphy and ultrasonography** may be used.

(c) **Treatment of OA (osteoarthritis):**

(i) **For pain: Acetaminophen is the drug of choice** or other simple analgesics.

NSAID's is not used initially GI side effects, decreased renal functions in elderly patients **but low-dose NSAID's can be used in patients but low-dose NSAID's can be used in patients unresponsive to simple analgesics.**

(ii) Intra-articular injections (**not** more than 3 or 4 times/year) can reduce joint symptoms. Repeated use may cause cartilage breakdown.

(iii) Do **not** use systemic steroids.

(iv) **Experimental therapy: Topical** application of capsaicin (substance-P inhibitor) can reduce pain; **Intra-articular injection of hyaluronan**.

(v) **Physical therapy and exercise program are** very important in OA patients. **Isometric exercise is better than** isotonic because it produces **less stress on the involved joints.**

(vi) **Heat and cold are used** along the physical therapy.

(vii) **TENS** (transcutaneous nerve stimulation) to reduce back pain is useful in some patients.

(viii) **Periods of rest** throughout the day; **using cane** to reduce the joint load; **cushioned shoes; back pain** is reduced by muscle strengthening **exercises plus well-fitted brace.**

(ix) **Joint replacement** surgery is the **most advance** and ultimate therapy of choice.
(x) Some patients may benefit from osteotomy.
(xi) **Arthroscopic surgery** is used to remove loose bodies and repair intrinsic defect of the knee; arthroscopic lavage to remove cartilage debris with saline is also used.

68. **Rotator cuff lesions**: **Rotator cuff tendinitis is the most common cause of shoulder pain and is usually due to over use of the arm in overhead activities**. Pain occurs most commonly on active abduction, particularly the initial 90 degrees of motion, pain is in the lateral aspect of the shoulder frequently at night.

Physical examination: Positive **'drop sign'** i.e., patients arm are passively placed at full abduction, then slowly **adducted from 120 to 60 degrees which causes severe pain and arm will reflexly drop.**

Diagnosis:

(i) **X-ray reveals sclerotic and cystic changes** of the humeral greater tuberosity; narrowing or obliteration of the acromiohumeral space due to attrition or complete tear of the cuff.
(ii) **Arthrography is the best** study to document complete ruptures and often incomplete tears.
(iii) MRI and ultrasonography are useful.
(iv) Intralesional injection of local anesthetic agent is also diagnostic: **Patients should have significant relief of pain and capable of active, painless abduction except in complete repture of rotator cuff** in which pain will be relieved but patients will **not** be able to do active abduction.

Treatment:

(i) Complete tear: Surgical management
(ii) **Initial management:** Heat, physical therapy, and NSAID's
(iii) **Patients unresponsive to initial management:** Use intralesional injection of corticosteroid.
(iv) **Recalcitrant cases of impingement**: Acromioplasty
(v) Job modification if needed.

69. **Bicipital tendinitis**: Pain in the **anterior aspect of the shoulder especially** while actively using biceps. Positive **Yergason's sign** (means tenderness in the anterior shoulder) is diagnostic.

Treatment: Initial treatment **with rest and NSAID's. Physical therapy and intralesional** corticosteroids are used for refractory cases. **Surgery** is used for complete rupture and some intractable cases of tendinitis.

70. **Subacromial or subdeltoid bursitis**: Pain in the **lateral aspect** of the shoulder (like rotator cuff tendinitis) but it causes **tenderness during passive abduction and direct palpation beneath the acromion process** (unlike rotator cuff tendinitis).
X-ray reveals calcification in chronic subacromial bursitis.
Treatment: Rest, physical therapy, and NSAID's. Unresponsive patients should be treated with intralesional injection of corticosteroids.

71. **Frozen shoulder or adhesive capsulitis:** It may be associated with diabetes mellitus, TB, upper extremity injury, cervical spine disease, chronic pulmonary disease and coronary artery disease. Patients initially complain of **pain in the shoulder**, followed by **painless progressive loss of** passive range of motion in all directions, **finally** shoulder **'thaws' with the return of range of motion after several years.** It is usually **unilateral**.
Diagnosis: **The diagnosis is confirmed by arthrography** which reveals **reduced** articular volume and **loss of the axillary pouch.**
Treatment: NSAID's, physical therapy, and judicious use of intraarticular corticosteroids are used for pain.

72. **Reflex sympathetic dystrophy syndrome**: It is similar to adhesive capsulitis but more **diffuse pain** and vasomotor instability of the hand, arm, and wrist. It is associated with diseases **similar to** adhesive capsulitis or **trauma of the upper extremity**. It is usually bilateral and **responds more to early therapy.**
Treatment: **Non-narcotic analgesic, aggressive physical therapy; short, rapid tapering (over 3 weeks) course of corticosteroids**. Intra-articular injection of corticosteroids and Stellate ganglion blocks may be helpful.

73. **Glenohumeral joint arthritis**: Presence of tenderness on passive rotation of the fully **adducted shoulder**. It may be a part of polyarthritis.
Milwaukee shoulder: It is an isolated severe destructive degenerative **glenohumeral** arthritis found in elderly patients.

BONE AND BONE MINERAL METABOLISM

1. **Most common type of metabolic bone disease**: **Osteoporosis**. It is characterized by a **parallel decrease in bone mineral and bone matrix**, results in **decreased in amount but normal composition** of the bone.

2. **Osteoporosis:**
   (A) **Genetic factors and bone density**:
   Genetic factors are responsible **up to 80%** of the variance in peak bone mass. Genetic difference in bone density is due to a **gene closely linked to the vitamin D receptor gene, probably the receptor gene itself**.
   Other factors can affect the peak bone density are **gender** (men>women), **race** (black>Caucasians); delayed puberty and delayed menarche cause **decreased bone density;** physical activity enhances bone density; moderate calcium supplementation can increase prepubertal bone accretion.
   (B) **Clinical manifestations of osteoporosis**:It is **asymptomatic** unless associated with fractures. Vertebral compression **fractures (middle and lower thoracic, and upper lumbar regions are most common sites)** can occur with sneezing, lifting a object, or bending. Patients complain of acute **back pain** which may radiates to the flank or anteriorly. Pain subsides gradually over several weeks by **recurrence of pain is due to new fractures.**
   Dowager's hump: It is a characteristic finding which includes **cervical lordosis and dorsal kyphosis.**
   Complications of osteoporosis: Hip fractures (femoral neck and intertrochanteric types) are **the most serious complication**. It is most commonly due to fall on the side or can occur before a fall.
   Complications of hip fractures: Pulmonary thromboembolism or nosocomial infections.
   (c) **Diagnosis**:
   (i) **Dual energy X-ray absorptiometry (DXA) of the lumbar** spine is the **best diagnostic method of choice. Lateral spine DXA is more sensitive** than anterior - posterior spine DXA for **diagnosis of osteoporosis**.
   (ii) Quantitative computed tomography (QCT) of the spine is more sensitive than DXA but QCT has **high radiation** and **very** expensive. QCT is **not** recommended routinely.
   (D) **Treatment**:
   (i) Secondary osteoporosis: To correct the underlying cause
   (ii) No treatment can reverse the established osteoporosis.

(iii) **Early** intervention can prevent osteoporosis and **later** intervention can stop its progression once osteoporosis has developed.

(iv) Acute vertebral compression: Analgesics, muscle relaxants, rest, heat and massage. Orthopedic back brace or corset my be helpful.

(v) Physical therapy is useful.

(vi) Both weight-bearing and non-weight-bearing exercises enhance the bone mass.

(vii) Precaution to prevent falls

(viii) Pharmacologic treatment goal is to prevent further bone loss and reduce the fracture.

(ix) Postmenopausal women should consume **1000 to 1200** mg calcium / day, **calcium can retard the bone loss**, but **cannot arrest or prevent the bone loss completely**.

(x) Estrogen replacement therapy (orally or topically) prevent bone loss (cortical and trabecular) in estrogen-deficient women. It should used with calcium

Side effects of estrogen therapy: **Endometrial cancer**, breast cancer (higher dose and >15 years of therapy); (women with intact uterus to prevent endometrial cancer **estrogen should be combined with progestin**)

Advantage of estrogen therapy: Decreases the risk of coronary artery disease by lowering LDL cholesterol and raising HDL cholesterol.

(xi) **Calcitonin** (only available parenterally in USA, given subcutaneously preferably at bedtime): It inhibits bone resorption and approved for use in postmenopausal women. It has analgesic effects, so useful in pain with fractures or skeletal deformity. **Side effects**: Nausea, local inflammatory reaction, and flushing.

(xii) Etidronate (biphosphonates): It can prevent spinal bone loss in recently menopausal women. (**Not** FDA approved for osteoporosis).

(xiii) Vitamin D and its metabolites: Small dose of vitamin D plus calcium can **reduce** the risk of hip and other nonspine fracture, but **its use for osteoporosis is controversial**. It should be **reserved** for patients unable to receive other therapy.

(xiv) **Future therapy**: **Tamoxifen** (antiestrogen) can prevent spinal bone loss in postmenopausal women; **PTH** can **prevent or reverse** estrogen deficiency.

3. **Most common causes of osteoporosis in men**:
Androgen deficiency (most common), ethanol abuse, gastric resection, and prior glucocorticoid use. In **adult men**, castration or treatment with long-acting GnRH analogues causes osteoporosis due to androgen deficiency. **Peak bone**

mass is reduced in Klinefelter's syndrome, idiopathic hypogonadotropic hypogonadism, or constitutionally delayed puberty.

Treatment of androgen-deficiency osteoporosis Androgen replacement therapy.

Contraindication of androgen therapy: Prostatic cancer.

4. **Glucocorticoid-induced bone loss**: Excess glucocorticoid could be **exogenous** therapeutic use or **endogenous** Cushing's syndrome. Glucocorticoid inhibits osteoblast activity and **inhibits** vitamin D independent **intestinal calcium absorption**. Bone formation is inhibited partially by **inhibition of secretion of IGF-1 in bone**. Bone loss is mostly irreversible.

   Treatment:

   (i) Try to reduce the exogenous glucocorticoid doses as low as possible.

   (ii) Physiologic **vitamin D** (400 IU/day) should be given to all patients receiving glucocorticoids.

   (iii) **Calcium supplementation** (1000 mg/day) should be given **except** in excessive urinary calcium excretion.

   (iv) **Calcitrol can be useful** but it causes hypercalcuria and/or hypercalcemia. It is good for patients with **low** urinary calcium excretion.

5. **Paget's disease of bone (osteitis deformans)**:

   (A) **Etiology**: Unknown; positive family history (10% of cases); weak association with HLA Dqw1 (in USA) and A9 and B15 (UK); **paramyxoviridae infection** in osteoclasts.

   (B) **Pathophysiology: Increased osteoclast numbers and sizes, increased** (5 to 10 folds) metabolic activity of bone surfaces.

   (C) **Clinical manifestations**: Asymptomatic (95% of cases) or symptomatic patients appear with **bone pain, skeletal deformity**, and **fracture**. Onset of symptoms are gradual **except** in fracture. **Most common sites involved are pelvis, lumbar spine and femur. Multiple sites are involved more commonly** than single site in **asymmetric distribution. Most common site of fracture** is **femur** followed by tibia and radius-ulna. Neurologic complications include **deafness, vertigo and tinitus. Spinal syndromes** due to **spinal cord in compression** from enlarged vertebrae **mostly in thoracic level. High-output cardiac failure** is noted in extensive disease. **Remember**, **new-onset of pain** in patients with long-standing **Paget's disease without fracture indicates tumor** (benign or malignant gaint cell tumor or **rarely** sarcoma)

   (D) **Diagnosis of Paget's disease**:

   (i) **Radiologic findings:**

Early phase: Osteoporosis circumscripta of **skull** or V-shaped advancing front in long bones.
Second mixed phase: **Patchy osteolysis and sclerosis** are the most common X-ray findings.
Third phase: Bone sclerosis is predominant.
Long bones: Cortical thickening and enlargement of long bones.
Pelvis: Positive X-ray in 66% of cases.
Hip: Narrowing of the joint space.

(ii) **CT scan:** It can **detect** the cause of pain at the spine and **osteosarcoma**.

(iii) **Biochemical findings**:

(a) Extracellular calcium homeostasis is almost **normal** despite severe increase of bone turnover.

(b) Hypercalcuria and **rarely** hypercalcemia may be present due to prolonged immobilization or fracture.

(c) Increased **urinary excretion of pyridinoline is more sensitive and specific** than hydroxyproline excretion.

(d) Elevated alkaline phosphatase indicates degree of skeletal involvements but values are **normal** in 10% of symptomatic patients like **normal** hydroxyproline levels (>10% of cases)

(e) **Treatment of Paget's disease:**

(i) **Salcatonin** (synthetic salmon calcitonin) subcutaneous injection **is most commonly used** (nasal spray available in Europe)
Life-long therapy is indicated because disease recurs once treatment is stopped.
Remember this point, calcitonin treatment cannot reverse deafness but it can reverse osteolytic lesions; improves cardiac output, neurologic symptoms and bone pain.
Side effects of calcitonin: Nausea or flushing.

(ii) **Biphosphonates: Etidronate** can suppress the disease process and relieves the pain but does **not** produce radiologic improvement.

(iii) **Surgical therapy**: Most commonly done for **fractures, hip joint involvements**; osteotomy is useful in fissure fracture with pain or deformity; elective surgery is done along with medical management; hip pain **uncontrolled** by medical therapy should be treated with **replacement arthroplasty** (treatment of choice)

6. **Most common causes of osteonecrosis in adults**: Long-term glucocorticoid therapy and ethanol abuse (dose-dependent effects).

7. **Osteonecrosis** (or bone infarction):

It is an **ischemic** aseptic, or avascular necrosis of bone.

Signs and symptoms: **Asymptomatic** or **acute pain** due to skeletal collapse or chronic arthralgias.

Diagnosis:

(i) **MRI** can detect **marrow edema** which is found in **early osteonecrosis**.

(ii) **Late** radiologic findings are **patchy areas** of **osteopenia and osteosclerosis**.

(iii) **Crescent sign**: It is **linear subchondral radiolucency** and **indicates bony collapse.**

(iv) **Bone scintigraphy** detects skeletal reconstitution with or without fracture.

Treatment:

(i) Do **not** bear weight in an affected limb

(ii) **Trephine** insertion for decompression, **arthotomy** to remove debris; other procedures are transpositional osteotomy, arthroplasty, or joint replacement may be needed.

8. **Camurati Engelmann disease (progressive diaphyseal dysplasia)**: Autosomal dominant; **new bone formation** in periosteal and endosteal areas of the long bone **diaphyses**.

   Clinical manifestations: Large head with prominent forehead, proptosis, tender thickened bones, thin limbs with little subcutaneous fat or muscle., Cranial nerve palsies and raised intracranial pressure may occur.

   Diagnosis: X-ray of femora and tibiae (most commonly affected bones) reveal symmetric, irregular **cortical hyperostosis of diaphyses**. Routine biochemical tests are **normal.** Serum alkaline phosphatase, urinary hydroxyproline leves and ESR can be **elevated**. Histopathology reveals newly formed woven bones. Electronmicroscopic study of muscles reveals myopathy and vascular abnormalities.

   Treatment: Low-dose glucocorticoid therapy can relieve bone pain and **normalize** histologic findings.

9. **Osteopetrosis (marble bone disease)**:

   (A) **Two types**: **Autosomal recessive or malignant** type **that kills children** if untreated; autosomal dominant or benign condition that produces **few or no symptoms**. Defective gene is **not** known except CA II gene (carbonic anhydrase) defect in renal tubular acidosis with cerebral calcification.

   (B) **Clinical manifestations**:

   (i) **Benign type**: **Rarely** causes fracture, facial palsy, deafness, impaired hearing or vision, **mandibular osteomyelitis**, carpal tunnel syndrome, and osteoarthritis.

   (ii) Malignant type (**affects children**; **not important for examination**): Nasal stuffiness (malformed mastoid and paranasal sinuses), short stature, large head, frontal bossing, hepatosplenomegaly, CA II deficiency causes RTA, cerebral calcification and developmental delay.

(c) **Diagnosis**:

(i) X-ray reveals characteristic **generalized symmetric osteosclerosis**; severe cases appear with **alternating dense and lucent bands (Erlenmeyer flask deformity**); bone scintigraphy can detect fractures and osteomyelitis; MRI helps to asses the success of bone marrow transplantation.

(ii) **Benign osteopetrosis**: Normal biochemical indices of mineral homeostasis **except** PTH levels may be elevated.

(iii) **Malignant type**: Low calcium with secondary hyperparathyroidism and elevated serum calcitriol levels.

(iv) Elevated acid phosphatase and creatine kinase (brain isoenzyme) from osteoclasts.

(D) **Treatment;**

(i) Malignant type: HLA-identical bone marrow transplantation is useful.

(ii) **Large doses of calcitriol plus dietary restriction of calcium** (to prevent hypercalciuria and hypercalcemia), and **human interferon-gamma** (stimulates superoxide production and osteoclastic activity)

(iii) Prednisone with low calcium and high phosphate diet may be useful.

(iv) High-does glucocorticoid for pancytopenia and hepatomegaly.

(v) **Hyperbaric oxygenation** to treat osteomyelitis.

10. **Pyknodysostosis: Autosomal recessive; adult patients are usually** very short (up to 4 feet 11 inches), micrognathia causing chronic upper airway obstruction and **RV failure; x-ray reveals uniform osteosclerosis,** hypoplastic clavicles and wormian bones; **normal** serum calcium, alkaline phosphatase and inorganic phosphate level; **no** effective medical therapy is available, long bone fractures usually mend properly (internal fixation is not done for bony hardness).

11. Sudden enlargement of **hereditary multiple exostoses** (autosomal dominant; irregular bony protrusion from expanded long bone metaphyses); **Sarcoma (Important).**

12. **Maffucci's syndrome: Enchondromatosis** (dyschondroplasia, Ollier's disease) **plus multiple hemangiomas**. Both can turn into malignancy up to 15% of cases. (Enchondromatosis are **cartilaginous masses** from growth plates interfering normal bone growth)

13. **Fibrous dysplasia**: It is an expansile fibrous lesion(s) that can **fracture, deform or sometimes entrap nerves**. **Monostotic** disease is **common in early adulthood** or **adolescence** (polyostotic is common in children).
    (i) **Clinical presentations**: Skull and long bones are most commonly affected, Pregnancy can **enhance** the previously quiescent lesions.
    (ii) **Diagnosis**: Long bone x-ray reveals **thin cortices and ground-glass appearance** (characteristic findings).
    (iii) **Treatment:**
        (a) Pathologic fractures usually mend well.
        (b) Stress fracture is difficult to diagnose and treat.
        (c) No medical therapy is available.
        (d) Nerve compression from skull involvement may need surgery.

14. **Most common metastatic bony tumors**:
    (i) Men: Prostate cancer
    (ii) Women: Breast cancer
    (iii) Direct bony invasion: Lung cancer (ribs or vertebrae)

    Breast and prostate metastatic cancers are **mixed lytic and blastic**, but lung and renal cancers are **purely lytic.**

15. **Most common bone tumors:**
    (i) **Benign: Bone island** is the most common and least significant; patients are **asymptomatic**; slowly enlarge and spontaneously regress; found incidentally by x-ray (**not** detected by bone scan); observation is adequate.
    (ii) **Malignant**: **Multiple myeloma is the most common**; next is osteosarcoma. Osteosarcoma (peak second decade and fifth-sixth decades) is most common in **distal femur** and **proximal tibia**. It is highly malignant; x-ray reveals sunray appearance and bony erosions; treated with chemotherapy, amputation or limb-sparing surgery if possible; **most common site of metastasis is the lung**.
    (iii) Ewing's sarcoma: It is **highly malignant**, occurs in young adults. It is **characterized by clinical manifestations simulating** infection such as fever, chill and malaise.

        Treatment: Chemotherapy and surgery.
    (iv) **Chondrosarcoma**: It has **low or intermediate** malignancy, occurs between fourth to sixth decades.

        Treatment: Surgery can cause cure (85% of cases); radiation and chemotherapy are **not** effective.

DISEASE OF THE IMMUNE SYSTEMS

1. **Immune deficiency with thymoma**: Patients develop **hypogammaglobulinemia, benign thymoma, deficits in cell-mediated immunity** and poor antibody formations.
   Laboratory findings: High or low eosinophil counts, **low** platelet counts, anemia (hemolytic or aregenerative), pancytopenia, or progressive **low** lymphocyte counts **but normal percentages of immunoglobulin bearing B lymphocytes**.

2. **Insect sting allergy**: Remember, **it is IgE mediated.**
   (A) **Clinical manifestations:**
      (i) **Generalized or systemic**: **Fatal anaphylaxis** can occur **without** a history of sting allergy, other symptoms and signs are **urticaria-angioedema (most common, 78% of cases)**, dizziness-hypotension, dyspnea-wheezing, tightness-hoarseness of the throat or loss of consciousness.
      (ii) **Localized skin reaction**: It can occur **without** generalized manifestations. It increases in size progressively for **first 1-2 days** then spontaneously resolve over several days.
   (B) **Dignosis of insect allergy and anaphylaxis History** and **positive skin test** (intradermal injection produces wheal >5 mm diameter with at least 20 mm erythema develops within 20 minutes). RAST (radioallergosorbent test) is **less** sensitive than skin test but both **are equally** accurate when positive.
   (c) **Treatment:**
      (i) **Anaphylactic reaction: Subcutaneous epinephrine** can be repeated twice if needed; airway maintenance and IV volume expansion may be needed. If patients are **resistant to epinephrine**, then use **norepinephrine**.
      Venom immunotherapy is effective in all patients but <1 to 2% patients develop less severe systemic symptoms after challenge sting. Venom immunotherapy is **contraindicated** in patients **without positive skin test or RAST**.
      Side effects of venoms immunotherapy:
         (a) Early: Anaphylaxis
         (b) Late: Local skin reaction
      (ii) **Antihistamines and prednisone**: They are **not** helpful in acute life-threatening conditions **but reduce the duration and** severity of dermatologic manifestations.

3. **Anaphylaxis**: Remember, it is **IgE mediated.**

(A) **Clinical manifestations**: **Most common clinical manifestation is urticaria**, other initial symptoms are **skin erythema, pruritus, light-headedness**, vomiting, lump in the throat and **shortness of breath**. Fatal anaphylaxis usually involves the respiratory tract results in hoarseness, stridor, **angioedema of the larynx and epiglottis cause respiratory obstruction and death.**

CVS: Low BP, myocardial ischemia, ventricular arrythmia and CVS collapse.

GI: Nausea, vomiting, abdominal cramps and diarrhea

CNS: Delirium, seizures due to hypoxia and/or low BP

(B) **Diagnosis of anaphylaxis**: History of exposure to foreign antigen and clinical manifestations. **Diagnosis is confirmed** by **demonstration of IgE antibody by skin test or RAST**.

(C) **Prevention of anaphylaxis**: Avoid drugs which cause anaphylaxis (most common is **penicillin** which has cross reactivity with **cephalosporin** 15% cases). History of penicillin allergy is **not** reliable because about 80% patients with positive history of allergy have **negative skin test to major determinant (penicillin polylysine) or minor determinant (penicillin, penicilloic acid, penicillioylamine)**. **Please remember penicillin allergy is due to all the major and minor determinants (Important) and IgE antibodies to minor determinants. Patients with previous history of anaphylaxis should wear a Medic-alert bracelet.**

(D) **Treatment of anaphylaxis:**

(i) First to maintain adequate airway.

(ii) Epinephrine (subcutaneously) can be repeated every 20 minutes as needed.

(iii) **Tourniquet may be used** if the anaphylactic reaction is initiated by an injection into the arm or leg.

(iv) **Honeybee sting**: Remove the stinger without compressing the venom sac

(v) **Upper airway obstruction**: Emergency intubation or tracheostomy.

(vi) **Asthma or lower airway obstruction**: Epinephrine, inhaler (beta-2 sympathomimetic, or IV aminophylline).

(vii) IV line should be placed and arterial blood gas should be obtained. Oxygen is given for hypoxia.

(viii) For hypotension use IV fluid and use dopamine if unresponsive to IV fluid or H_2-receptor blocker.

(ix) IV antihistamine can reduce pruritus, urticaria, and angioedema.

(x) Corticosteroids have **no** value in **acute episode** but it is often given intravenously. It is very useful in **severe asthma** and **late reaction** (1 to 2 days often the initial attack)

4. **Drug allergy**: Most hy**persensitivity reaction to drugs are IgE mediated. The risk factors for developing drug allergy** depend upon the **ability of patients to respond immunologically to hapten-carrier complexes** and the balance of **drug-metabolizing enzymes (drugs first** undergo **oxidation** then **acetylation and** conjugation)
   (A) **Clinical manifestations**: **Most common manifestations** are **urticaria**, cutaneous exanthems, contact dermatitis, **drug fever** and high **eosinophil counts**. Patients **improve within 2 to 3 days after discontinuation of the drug.**
   (B) **Diagnosis of drug allergy**: Clinical manifestations plus specific diagnostic tests are: **Skin test which is more sensitive than drug-specific IgE levels in the serum** and **challenge test**. Challenge test should **not** be done in patients with possible anaphylaxis and this test is used when the **drug is very important for therapy** and **the history is vague or suggests mild symptom**.
   (C) **Treatment of drug allergy**:
      (i) **Discontinue the medication immediately**.
      (ii) **Diphenhydramine or hydroxyzine** can relieve pruritus and reduce the duration of symptoms.
      (iii) Corticosteroids are used **only** in prolonged or severe reaction.
      (iv) HIV infected patients are high risk for multiple drug sensitivities: Patients have delayed-onset **maculopapular rash and fever**. This reaction is due to **immune dysregulation** due to HIV infection. Successful rechallenge or densesitization with acyclovir, dapsone and trimethoprim-sulfamethoxazole has been done.
   (D) **Prevention: History of previous drug reaction** and **avoid those drugs**; skin tests can diagnose type I hypersensitivity reaction to some drugs (penicillin) and should be done routinely **before giving heterologous antisera;** desensitization is done only when the drug is considered very essential because it is a high-risk procedure. **It should be done by physician ready to treat severe side effects** and informed consent should be obtained before desensitization therapy.

5. **Few important point in different drug allergy:**
      (i) Patients with asthma and chronic sinusitis and polyposis should **avoid aspirin and NSAID's.**
      (ii) Angiotensin converting enzyme (ACE) inhibitors cause **angioedema of the face and oropharynx**. Angioedema is characterized by nonpruritic swelling **without** urticaria and angioedema is **not** related to ACE-

inhibitor induced cough. This drug reaction usually occurs **within 7 days of** therapy and **as long as 7 years after the onset of drug use**.

(iii) **Procaine and benzocaine are the most common local anesthetic causing true allergy**.

(iv) Most patients with insulin allergy have idiopathic urticaria or sensitivity to other drugs.

(v) Imipenem, aztreonam and ceftazidime (third-generation cephalosporin) have cross-reactivity with penicillin.

6. **Most common skin manifestation of mastocytosis (abnormal increased in mast cells in the bone marrow, spleen, liver, lymph nodes, skin and GI tract)**: Urticaria pigmentosa; other type is diffuse cutaneous mastocytosis.

7. **Mastocytosis**: Patients do **not** suffer from recurrent infections and have no involvement of respiratory and endocrine systems.

(A) **Clinical manifestations**: Flushing or frank anaphylaxis may occur in every variety.

(i) **Skin: Most common is urticaria pigmentosa (scattered small** reddish-brown macules or papules.
Positive Darier's sign: Urticaria or erythema forms around the macules after scratching or rubbing the lesions.

(ii) **GI**: Gastric **hypersecretion** results in gastritis and peptic ulcer disease; diarrhea and abdominal pain.

(iii) Liver and spleen: Portal hypertension and ascites are due to **fibrosis** of liver and spleen; **most common chemical finding is elevated alkaline phosphatase**.

(iv) **Bone: Bone pain is the most common symptom** and **proximal long bones are commonly affected**, then pelvis, ribs, and skull bones. Due to marrow invlovements patients develop anemia, low WBC and platelet count, high eosinophil counts. **Bone scan (scintigraphy) is the best diagnostic procedure** (better than X-ray)

(v) **Neuropsychiatry**: Memory loss, irritability, and depression.

(B) **Diagnosis of mastocytosis:**

(i) **The diagnosis is confirmed by biopsy (skin biopsy** because majority of patients have skin lesions) **and histologic findings.** Toluidene blue, Giemsa and enzyme stains are most useful to detect mast cells.

(ii) Patients without skin lesions, **should have bone marrow biopsy**.

(iii) To rule out carcinoid tumor, **suspected** patients of mastocytosis should have 24-hours urine for 5- HIAA (hydroxyindolacetic acid) which is **normal** in mastocytosis and elevated in carcinoid tumor.

(c) **Treatment:**

(i) **Hydroxyzine and doxepin** are used to reduce pruritus, flushing and tachycardia. These are H_1 - receptor antagnists; if failed then H_2-receptor antagonists such as **ranitidine or cimetidine**.
(ii) Disodium cromoglycate (or cromolyn sodium) inhibits mast cells degranulation and useful in mastocytosis.
(iii) **Epinephrine** is used for **anaphylaxis and H_1 - and H_2 - receptor antagonists** are used for **recurrent** anaphylaxis.
(iv) **H_2- receptor antagonists** are used for gastric hypersecretion and peptic ulcer disease.
(v) **Mild** malabsorption (diarrhea) is treated with **anticholinergics** and **severe** malabsorption may be treated with systemic steroids.
(vi) Portacaval shunt for portal hypertension.
(vii) Ascites may be treated with systemic steroids.
(viii) Mast cell leukemia: Chemotherapy is **not** very effective.
(ix) **Severe mastocytosis**: Splenectomy may be useful
(x) Indolent mastocytosis: **Never** use chemotherapy.

8. **Thymoma**: It is **rare but it** is the **most** common tumor of **anterior superior mediastinum**

Signs and symptoms: Dysphagia, chest pain, signs of SVC obstruction and tracheal impingement or **may be asymptomatic.**

Associated with: It is associated with myasthenic gravis (Important)

Diagnosis:

(i) **The definitive diagnosis** is done by **biopsy** and histology of thymic tissues.
(ii) CT scan or MRI can detect the **extent** of the tumor.
(iii) Direct tumor visualization by thoracotomy is useful in diagnosis and treatment.

Treament:

(i) Well-encapsulated thymomas: Surgical removal is the curative therapy.
(ii) Thymoma invaded the surrounding tissues: Surgical removal plus irradiation or chemotherapy.

9. **Few important points in urticaria:**

(i) **Aquagenic urticaria** is due to **chlorine** inside the water which causes urticaria when patients are exposed to water.
(ii) Solar urticaria **develops shorty after exposure to sun** and it **is IgE-mediated**. It is treated **with sunscreen lotion containing butyl methoxydibenzoyl methane**.
(iii) Chronic urticaria / angioedema therapy: **First** drug of choice is **H_1 antihistamines.** Hydroxyzine and cyproheptadine cause drowsiness **but well tolerated medications are** terfenadine, astemizol, cetirizine and

loratidine, **H_2- inhibitors may be added** to H_1 - inhibitors for inadequate clinical response. Other drugs may be effective are **doxepin** (TCA with anti - H_1 and anti H_2 activities), **ketotifen** (used in physical urticarias), and nifedipine (calcium channel blocker); if all three drugs are unresponsive then **use glucocorticoid (prednisone)**.

(iv) **Acute urticaria / angioedema** is treated with **epinephrine except** in patients with severe cardiovascular system disease. Long-acting epinephrine (Sus-Phrine) may be used.

10. **Complication of ACE - inhibitors (angiotensin converting enzyme) and interleukin -2 therapy: Both produces angioedema**.

(i) **ACE - inhibitors**: It can cause **life-threatening** angioedema within **hours to 1 week** after therapy due to breakdown of bradykinin and neuropeptide substance P.

(ii) **Interleukin - 2 (IV infusion):** It is used in cancer treatment. It produces angioedema **due to activation of T cells, those damage the endothelium directly**.

Treatment of both conditions: Discontinue the medications; **antihistamines and/or epinephrine**.

11. **Few important points in hereditary angioedema (HAE)**:

(i) HAE is more **severe at puberty** (than childhood), **unknown** etiology, autosomal dominant, abnormal gene for C1 inhibitor on **chromosome 11**.

(ii) HAE causes **brawny nonpitting edema usually in** the extremities and genitalia; it also involves mucosal surfaces particularly GI tract result in **abdominal pain** due to submucosal swelling ; earythema marginatum like rash (33% of cases). The clinical manifestations **progress over 36 hours and then regress in about 36 hours**.

(iii) **Diagnosis of HAE**: Low levels of C1 inhibitor antigen, or function and low levels of complement protein C4 and/or C2; **normal C1 and C3 level.**

(iv) **Treatment of HAE**: Patients **respond poorly** to epinephrine, antihistamines and glucocorticoids.

(a) Acute attacks: **Epinephrine** (nebulized and subcutaneous injections) may be repeated; **antihistamines for sedation; (future therapy** with purified C1 inhibitor infusion)

(b) **Long-term therapy**: Androgen therapy (**methyltestosterone** for men, and **danazol** for women; danazol causes masculinization); few **unresponsive** patients may be treated with aminocaproic acid (plasmin inhibitors)

12. **Acquired C1 inhibitor deficiency**: Clinical manifestations are the same as HAE (hereditary angioedema). The characteristic laboratory findings are **very low levels of C1, C4 and C2 (normal C1 in HAE); normal** plasma C1 inhibitor antigen level (**low** level in HAE), Patients **develop monoclonal** or **polyclonal autoantibodies to the C1 inhibitor**. **Associated diseases condition**: Multiple myeloma, anti-idiotypic antibody producing same symptoms. **Treatments**: **To treat the underlying** disease; some patients respond to **danazol** or **other anabolic steroids**; patients with anti - C1 INH autoantibody usually respond to **glucocorticoids**.

13. **Few important points in allergic rhinitis**:
   (i) **Autosomal dominant**; **high levels of allergen-specific IgE**; **gene located on chromosome 6**.
   (ii) **Clinical manifestations**:
      (a) **Acute allergic rhinitis**: **Swollen nasal mucosa** (pale and blue color; may be red and indurated in chronic allergen exposure), rhinorrhea, nasal obstruction, postnasal drip, cobblestone - appearance of posterior pharynx. Nasal secretions contain **eosinophils** demonstrated by Giemsa or Hansel's stains.
      (b) **Chronic allergic rhinitis**: Anosmia, sinusitis, sleep disturbances and secretory otitis media. It is associated with allergic asthma, atopic dermatitis (eczema), and allergic conjunctivitis.
   (iii) **Remember**, nasal eosinophilia is **not** diagnostic of allergic rhinitis because it is **also** present in **nonallegic rhinitis with nasal eosinophilia syndrome (NARES)**. NARES patients can have sinusitis (50% of cases), nasal polyps (33% of cases), and asthma (14% of cases).
   (iv) **Differential diagnosis**:
      (a) **Vasomotor rhinitis** (perennial nonallergic rhinitis): Chronic nasal congestion exaggerated by changes in temperature, humidity, alcohol or odor. Patients **do not have itching and sneezing**; but **do** have symptoms of **sinusitis, anosmia and headaches**. It is due to nasal autonomic nervous system dysfunctions.
      (b) **Atrophic rhinitis**: **Bad odor** in the nose, chronic nasal congestion, and atrophy of the nasal mucosa.
      (c) **Rhinitis medicamentosa**: **Beefy red nasal membranes**, chronic nasal obstruction, and it due to chronic use of vasoconstrictor nasal Spray.
      (d) **Unilateral rhinitis**: It is due to obstruction, tumor, polyp and foreign body.
   (v) **Diagnosis of allergic rhinitis**: History of exposure to allergens, clinical manifestations are suggestive; **diagnosis is confirmed by skin test (best method**), or RAST.

(vi) **Treatment of allergic rhinitis**:

(a) **Avoid the allergens** is the first step.

(b) Next step is to use **antihistamines. Oral antihistamines** that contains a **decongestant** (pseudoephedrine, phenylephrine, or phenyl propranolamine) have added benefits. It is **contraindicated in glaucoma**; **can cause** urinary retention, insomnia, palpitations; and should **not** be **used with monoamine oxidase therapy**.

(c) **H-$_1$ receptor antagonists** may be used but it causes sedation, dry mouth and urinary hesitancy.

(d) **H-$_2$** receptor antagonists (terfenadine, astemizole) can be used. **It can cause ventricular tachycardia and torsades de pointes when used** with **ketoconazole, itraconazole** or **macrolide antibiotic** (Important).

(e) Do **not** use **H-$_1$** and **H-$_2$** receptor antagonist **together**.

(f) **Nedocromil** is more effective than cromolyn, both inhibit mast cell degranulation in allergic rhinitis.

(g) **Topical intranasal steroids are recommended** (do **not** use oral or IV because of its complications). **It is more effective than cromolyn**. Treatment failure is due to mucous or debris **inside the nose** which **should be cleaned with saline nasal spray or washes before steroid therapy**.

(h) **Nonallergic rhinitis with rhinorrhea**: Intranasal application of ipratropium bromide (a congener of atropine) is usually effective.

HIV AND THE ACQUIRED IMMUNO DEFICIENCY

1. **Most common mode of transmission of HIV sexual contact**; other are parental exposure to blood or blood products and perinatally from infected mothers to their newborns.

2. **Few important points in sexual transmission of HIV infection:**
   - (i) Most important factor is that the partner should be HIV- infected.
   - (ii) It is transmitted through vaginal, anal and less commonly, oral intercourse.
   - (iii) No sexual activity involving the exchange of semen or blood, should be considered **without risk**.
   - (iv) **In homosexual men**, The risk acquisition of HIV infection is higher with multiple sexual partners, frequency of receptive anal intercourse, and rectal trauma.
   - (v) **In bisexual women and lesbians**, most cases of HIV infections are **due to injecting drug** use or **heterosexual contacts** (Important)
   - (vi) **Female to female** transmission is rare but mostly associated with **traumatic sexual activities**.
   - (vii) **Most common heterosexual transmission occurs through vaginal intercourse**; but women get infected from infected men through receptive anal intercourse.
   - (viii) HIV transmission from infected HIV patients with **low T-helper lymphocyte counts is higher** because of **increased quantity of HIV in blood and semen**.
   - (ix) **Increased risk** of HIV acquisition in women **with cervical infections** with Neisseria Gonorrhoeae or Chlamydia trachomatis or with cervical ectopy. Prevention and treatment of other sexually transmitted infections can reduce the **risk of HIV transmission (important)**.
   - (x) **Genital or anal ulcers caused by infections** such as Haemophilus ducreyi, Treponema pallidum, herpes simplex virus or other pathogenic organisms **increase the acquisition of HIV through sexual contact** mostly due to disruption of anal or genital skin and mucous membrane.
   - (xi) Consistent use of condom **reduces both heterosexual and homosexual HIV transmission** (>90%) in comparison to nonuse or inconsistent use of condom.
   - (xii) **Antiretroviral therapy** may reduce but **cannot** eliminate the risk of HIV transmission through sexual contact (preliminary study suggests).
   - (xiii) IV Zidovudine therapy to HIV positive pregnant women reduces the **risk of HIV transmission to newborns(8% of cases) and newborns are also treated for first 6 weeks of life**.

3. **Few important points in transmission of HIV through parenteral exposure of blood or blood products**:
   (i) **HIV is transmitted** through whole blood, plasma, blood cells and clotting factors.
   (ii) HIV is **not** transmitted through hepatitis B vaccine, hepatitis B immune globulin, immune serum globulin and Rho (O) immune globulin.
   (iii) Transfusion of whole blood packed cells or plasma from an HIV infected donor results in 100% transmission of HIV infection.
   (iv) Screening of all donated blood and plasma for HIV and heat treatment of clotting factors **minimized** the risk of HIV transmission
   (v) The problem is the **window period** (6 to 8 weeks between the recent onset of HIV infection and antibody formation) when the screening test of **donor blood will be falsely negative** (HIV transmission is about **1 in 36000 to 225000 units** transfused in USA).
   (vi) **Positive** HIV test in organ, tissue, or semen should **not** be used for transplantation or insemination.
   (vii) **Risk factors** for HIV infection depend upon the needle sharing, use of drug in shooting galleries, duration of injecting drugs and living in a community with high rate of HIV infection.

4. **Risk of seroconversion** following a needle stick or other parenteral exposure to the blood of HIV-infected persons: About 0.3%

5. **HIV and body fluids**:
   HIV is present in **virtually every body fluid and tissue. In most cases virus resides in lymphocytes present within the body fluids**.

6. **Most effective means of preventing HIV infection through vaginal or anal intercourse: Properly used latex condom plus nonoxynol-9 (spermicidal with some antiviral activity)**
7. **Prevention of HIV infection**:
   (A) **From sexual transmission**: (first five items **are safe sex** activities).
      (i) **Abstinence** is the best way of preventing HIV transmission.
      (ii) Monogamous sexual activity with confirmed seronegative partner.
      (iii) Intercourse with latex condom plus **nonxynol-9** (spermicidal with some **antiviral activity**).
      (iv) **Mutual** nontraumatic **masturbation (avoid ingestion of semen or vaginal secretion)**
      (v) Kissing (**except deep French kissing which is not safe**)
      (vi) Failure of condom effectiveness(5 to 15% of cases) due to improper placement, falling off during intercourse or rupture.

(vii) **Unknown partner should be serologically tested** and use safe sex technique or **avoid sexual activity** until the result of test is available.

(viii) Verbal claim of seronegativity could **be** misleading and **potentially dangerous**.

(ix) Avoid **unsafe** sexual activities which are the following

(a) Use of natural skin condom during intercourse

(b) Use of latex condom lubricated with petroleum-based lubricants

(c) **Unprotected** vaginal, anal or orogenital sexual activity

(B) **Prevention of HIV transmission through intravenous drug use:**

(i) **To prevent the use of intravenous drugs**

(ii) **Educational programs results in behavioral changes is most challenging**

(iii) Accessability of treatment in patients already using IV drugs.

(iv) Patients who do **refuse** treatment or unable to gain access to the treatment: Avoid sharing needles and works are the most effective ways; free needles and syringes for IVDU's ; clean needles and syringes with chlorine bleach.

(v) HIV antibody testing with pretest and posttest counseling

(C) Prevention of HIV transmission through blood products:

(i) **Heat inactivation process for cryoprecipitate and clotting factor concentrates e**liminated HIV from these products.

(ii) All blood and blood products should be tested for HIV antibody.

(iii) Self-deferral programs have limited success.

(D) Prevention of HIV transmission to health care workers **(universal precautions**):

(i) Handwashing should be done before and after patient contact and after removing gloves.

(ii) All blood, blood products, and body fluids should be **considered hazardous** and potentially infected.

(iii) Use gloves when hands are likely to come in contact with body fluids.

(iv) **Use gowns**, protective eyewear and mask when splashing, splattering or aerosolization of blood or body fluids is likely to occur.

(v) Sharps should be handled very carefully and disposed in impervious container.

(vi) Needles should not be recapped, bent, broken, or manipulated.

(vii) Blood spills should be handled with initial absorption of spill with disposable towel, cleaning the area with soap and water then disinfecting the area with household bleach.

(viii) Contaminated reusable instrument should be decontaminated appropriately.

(ix) Health care workers with **open lesions** should avoid direct patient contact and should not touch contaminated equipment.

(x) Pocket masks or mechanical ventilation devices should be available for areas where cardiopulmonary resuscitation procedures are done.

(xi) Remember, private rooms are **not** needed for routine care.

(xii) **AZT prophylaxis is recommended for massive or definitive exposure (doubtful cases should not take AZT**). It can reduces the risk by 30% ; informed consent should be obtained before AZT is given; AZT should be given as soon as possible and higher doses to achieve maximum effectivity; doses should begin within **2 to 4 hours after exposure, 200 mg AZT every 4 hours with or without a 4 A.M. dose, for 4 to 6 weeks** (this may vary in different institution)

(E) Prevention of HIV transmission from infected health care workers to their patients: Incidence of transmission is very low 1 in 42,000 to 420,000. **Routine use of universal precaution is sufficient at this point.**

(F) Future preventive therapy: Vaccination for HIV infection.

8. Few important preventive points in neurologic complications of HIV-1 infection:

(A) **Early HIV-1 infection:**

(i) **Less** common than late stage of HIV-1 infection ; nervous system is affected as early as **primary infection and seroconversion**.

(ii) **CNS**: Focal or diffuse encephalopathy, ataxia, myelopathy or meningitis can occur.

(iii) **Peripheral nervous system (PNS):** Mononeuropathy of cranial or segmental nerves, brachial plexopathy and polyneuropathy can occur.

(iv) CNS and PNS involvement can occur together

(v) **Clinically latent phase of infection**: **GBS** (Gullain- Barre syndrome) and CIDP (chronic idiopathic demylelinating polyneuropathy) can occur both have high CSF cell counts) and both of which **mimic** demyelinating polyneuropathies (normal CSF cell counts) **non-HIV-1-** infected patients. It responds to intravenous immunoglobulin, plasma exchange and corticosteroids.

(vi) **Early asymptomatic HIV-1 infection of the CNS**: IT occurs soon after the initial systemic infection and it reveals **mild elevation of CSF** cell count, protein, and immunoglobulin levels plus **anti-HIV-1 antibody synthesis** from **local intra-blood-brain** barrier.

(B) **Late HIV-1 infection:**

(i) Opportunistic infections: **Cerebral toxoplasmosis is most common in the brain (non-HIV-1** patients with organ transplantation usually develop cerebral Candida or Aspergillus infections) other infections are Cryptococcal meningitis, CMV encephalitis, polyradiculitis.

(ii) **Opportunistic neoplasms**: **Primary brain lymphomas is the most common**. It is multicentric; occurs when **blood CD4 + lymphocytes are low**; tumor cells always **positive for Epstein-Barr virus (EBV)**; responds to **radiation** therapy but poor **prognosis**. Systemic lymphomas usually **metastasize to the leptomeninges (not into the brain parenchyma).** Kaposi's sarcoma can metastasize to the brain very rarely.

(iii) HIV-1 can cause **aseptic meningitis**, AIDS-dementia complex, and predominant sensory polyneuropathy:

(a) **Meningitis and headache: Cryptococcal neoformans meningitis is the most common**. Patients may be symptomatic (headaches, vomiting, confusion) or **completely asymptomatic** with **normal** CSF cell counts, glucose, and protein level. So, **CSF examination should done routinely for Cryptococcal indentification** by India ink stain, antigen determination and culture. **Long-term treatment is needed** because it is difficult **to sterilize the CSF**.

The syndrome of **aseptic meningitis (acute or chronic**) could be due to **direct** HIV-1 infection of the leptomeninges, **most commonly occurs in the period of transition to AIDS**. Most commonly involved cranial nerve is **seventh** (**less** common are fifth and eighth nerves). **CSF examination reveals high monocyte counts**, **mildly elevated protein, normal glucose,** and **positive isolation of the virus**. The syndrome is **benign** but its progression to AIDS indicates **poor** prognosis.

(b) **Predominant nonfocal brain lesions**: Most common is **AIDS dementia complex** (characterized by **cognitive behavioral dysfunction but they are alert**). **MRI reveals** cerebral atrophy, increased signal in white mater or basal ganglia.

Treatment: Zidovudine (AZT) can prevent and **partly reverse** this clinical manifestations.

Differential diagnosis:

- Metabolic encephalopathies (hypoxia, sepsis), patients are lethargic (**not alert**) and confused.
- Toxoplasma usually causes focal encephalophathy (sometimes diffuse lesions)
- **CNS lymphomas** affect cognitive and motor functions **without** prominent focal symptoms or signs.
- Herpes simplex virus type 1 and 2 cause **subacute focal encephalitis**.

CMV brain infection causes diffuse lesions (autopsy) **with or without symptoms** (mild)

(c) **Predominant focal brain lesions**: Most common lesion is **cerebral toxoplasmosis,** next is **primary cerebral lymphoma** and **PML** (progressive multifocal leukoencephalopathy)

(i) **Cerebral toxoplasmosis**: Lesions, develop very repidly (**within few days**); presence of fever and reduced consciousness; focal or generalized multiple lesions; **MRI reveals 'ring-enhancing', spherical lesions in basal ganglia and cortex**; **rapid response with pyrimethamine and sulfa drug**; **brain biopsy** is **not** needed because of rapid response to treatment and **positive antibody to** toxoplasma (**only** atypical cases, unresponsive patients and negative toxoplasma antibodies will need brain biopsy)

(ii) **Primary CNS lymphoma**: Lesions develop within **days to weeks**; **absence** of fever and one or two lesions but diffuse in nature ; **MRI reveals 'weekly enhancing' lesions in the periventricular white areas** ; and reaponse to corticosteroids and chemotherapy.

(iii) PML (progressive multifocal leukoencephalopathy): Lesions develop within weeks; absence of fever and normal level of consciousness ; usually **multiple** lesions ; MRI reveals **'nonenhancing' lesions in the cortical white mater**.

(iv) **Rare** lesion are the following: Herpes simplex virus causes focal deficits; varicella-zoster virus can cause demyelinating focal disease like PML ; CMV rarely causes macroscopic lesion ; cryptococcoma almost always present with meningitis.

(d) **Myelopathies: Most common lesion** is diagnosed by MRI is **vacuolar myelopathy** which is included in **AIDS dementia complex**. Patients appear with **subacute or gradual** onset of **painless gait ataxia and spasticity** followed by bladder and bowel dysfunctions, **increased deep tendon reflexes and Babinski sign** but sensory or motor level is **not** very distinct (like transverse myelopathies)

(e) **Peripheral neuropathies**: Most common finding is **distal axonal neuropathy, characteristically sensory symptoms exceeds** both sensory and motor abnormalties. **Patients appear with 'burning feet' or severe painful paresthesias which is unresposive to AZT.**
Treatment: TCA (tricyclic antidepressants) **and analgesics.**
Toxic neuropathies are caused by the following **newer antiretroviral drugs**: Dideoxyinosine, dideoxycytidine, and d 4T.

CMV can cause **polyradiculopathy** (uncommon with pain, sacral sensory loss, followed by ascending flaccid paralysis ; CSF contains mostly polymorphonuclear leukocytes; **responsive to ganciclovir or foscarnet**.

(f) **Myopathy**: HIV-1 infection can cause both inflammatory or noninflammatory myopathies ; either **asymptomatic with elevated creatine kinase or severe proximal muscle weakness**. Steroid is useful in inflammatory polymyositis.

Remember, **ANZ can cause proximal weakness and loss of muscle mass** ; muscle biopsy reveals **excessive or abnormal mitochondria** ; patients respond with discontinuation of AZT.

9. **Few important points in pulmonary manifestations of HIV infection**
   - (i) **Acute bronchitis** is the most common pulmonary **disease (nonopportunistic)** in HIV patients.
   - (ii) PCP (Pneumocystis carinii) pneumonia is **the most common when CD4 + counts <200 cells per microliter** (but it is only 6% when CD4 + >200)
   - (iii) Patients with **higher** CD4 + counts appear with higher fever, oral thrush, lymphadenopathy, and weight loss.
   - (iv) **Lower** the CD4 + counts and **higher** the following infections: PCP, TB, bacterial pneumonias, fungal infections, Kaposi's sarcoma ; **but remember** CD4 + counts have **no** relation with the incidence of **acute bronchitis** (nonopportunistic disease)
   - (v) **Advanced HIV infection** causes fungal infections, lymphomas, Kaposi's sarcoma, and **nontuberculous mycobacterial infections**.
   - (vi) Remember, Mycobacterium avium complex and CMV, both either colonize or cause infection in lungs, so it is difficult to distingusish between real infection or colonization.

10. **Clinical manifestations of HIV-related pulmonary diseases**:
    (A) Diseases **usually not** associated with severe immune suppression:
    - (i) **Bronchitis**: In acute bronchitis patients appear with **cough and sputum for at least 2 days** ; CXR or CT scan reveals normal findings or **peribronchial thickening.**
    - (ii) **Bacterial pneumonia:** Most common organism is **Streptococcus pneumoniae** (67% cases), **next is** Hemophilus influenzae (15% cases), and third is **S.aures (particularly in pulmonary Kaposi's sarcoma)**. Patients have cough, purulent sputum, positive infiltrates and responses to antibiotics. Diagnosis is made by sputum Gram stain and culture, blood culture, or pleural fluid Gram stain and culture if present.
    - (iii) **Tuberculosis (TB):**

(a) **Early HIV disease**: Gradual onset of upper lobe pulmonary cavitary lesion with **fewer** systemic manifestations ; **positive tuberculin test, positive sputum smear and culture** ; respond to therapy well ; and infectious to others. Bronchoalveolar lavage (BAL) is done when sputum is not available. BAL culture is more sensitive than smear.

(b) **Late HIV disease:** Acute onset of predominantly **extrapulmonary or disseminated** lesions with diffuse or lower lobe pulmonary infiltrates plus adenopathy ; **negative** tuberculin test but **positive** sputum smear and culture if lungs are involved ; respond to therapy well and infectious to others. BAL culture (89%) is more sensitive than smear (20%) should be done when sputum is not available.

(iv) **Nonspecific interstitial pneumonitis (NIP**): It is common in adult, self-limited disease required **no** invasive diagnostic method, and no treatment is needed. LIP (lymphoid interstitial pneumonitis) is **rare** in adults. **Defininitive diagnosis** of NIP and LIP are made by **lung biopsy** (but transbronchial biopsy is not adequate to make the diagnosis)

(B) **Diseases associated with severe immune suppression:**

(i) **PCP pneumonia is the most common pulmonary disease** in advanced HIV infection. Patients appear with **cough, fever and/or shortness in breath. Please remember, evaluation for P.carinii is not indicated unless patients complain of cough and/or shortness of breath. CXR:** Most common finding is **diffuse interstitial infiltrate**; but **focal infiltrates (particularly upper lobe in patients recieving aerosol pentamidine**). cavitary lesions or nodules, **pneumatocele, or spontaneous pneumothorax may also be present.**

Treatment: Antipneumocystis therapy plus corticosteroid

(ii) **Nontuberculous mycobacterial disease**: Disseminated M.avium complex disease occurs in advanced HIV disease occurs in **advanced HIV disease when CD4 + lymphocyte count <50 cells per microliter.** Patients appear with fever, cough, weight loss, abdominal pain and diarrhea. It is difficult to distinguish between colonization and infection. CXR: **Nonspecific findings. Patients with diffuse infiltrates** by CXR, other **diagnosis should be excluded first because considering M.avium infecton.**

M.Kansasii more likely to cause diffuse infiltration than M.avium

(iii) Fungal infections: Most common organisms are **Histoplasmosis** and **coccidioidomycosis**. Both of them can cause disseminated infections with respiratory symptoms and acute repiratory failure. **Histoplasmosis is usually severe, febrile and wasting disease**.

CXR: Histoplasmosis appears with diffuse infltration (reticulonodular or alveolar) and **coccidioidomycosis** appears with localized or scattered nodular or diffuse infiltration.

Cryptococcosis infection may be asymptomatic or symptomatic with **fever**, fatigue and weight loss; **CXR may appear as** focal or diffuse infiltration, localized or scttered nodules, **with or without** pleural effusion and hilar adenopathy.

Aspergillosis can cause either **pulmonary** disease or **obstructive bronchial disease**. This infection occurs when patients have **neutropenia, smoking marijuana, use of broad-spectrum antibiotics and corticosteroids.** Patients appear with fever, cough and bronchial casts in productive cough. **CXR reveals focal infiltration, cavitary lesions and pleura-based thickening**.

(iv) **CMV infections:** It **rarely** causes pulmonary infection. The diagnosis is established by isolation of CMV in culture and specific histopathologic findings

(v) **Neoplastic disease**: **Kaposi's sarcoma (KS) is the most common in advanced HIV infection**. KS is more common with both pulmonary and mucocutaneous lesions together.

Definitive diagnosis of KS: The characteristic bronchoscopic finding are **endobronchial lesions** appear as **flat, red or pruple submucosal lesions mimic** submucosal bleeding. It is difficult to do biopsy because of submucosal location. **Bronchoscopic typical finding is diagnostic. (Only few** cases requirebiopsy to confirm the KS when characteristic lesions are **absent**). These lesions are visible anywhere from vocal cord to distal airway.

CSR findings of KS: Lesions are mostly central and consist of **bronchial wall thickening and nodules. Kerly B lines are present (71% of cases),** pleural effusion (52% of cases), and hilar and mediastinal adenopathy (15% of cases) are present.

The **second most** common cancer in HIV patients is **non-Hodgkin lymphoma**., the most common CXR findings are patchy **parenchymal infiltrates, nodules, and solitary masses**. The diagnosis is done by **biopsy** (transbronchial, needle aspiration, thoracoscopic, or open)

11. Diagnostic approach for **pulmonary infections** in **suspected or positive HIV patients**.

Patients have **cough, shortness of breath, with or without fever** and **CD 4 + count ≤300**. Sputum could be either **nonpurulent or purulent**. **PCP infections** usually do **not** cause purulent sputum. **IDU's plus HIV** have higher

incidence of bacterial pneumonias and **tuberculosis** than **non** IDU's plus HIV patients.

(A) **First investigation of choice is chest x-ray**

(i) **Normal CXR** with **purulent** sputum: Symptomatic therapy with or without antibiotics.

(ii) **Normal CXR** with **nonpurulent** sputum: **Pulmonary function test with measurement of diffusing capacity for carbon monoxide (DLco) should be done:**

(a) DLco >75%= Symptomatic therapy with or without antibiotics.

(b) DLco <75%= Induced sputum for AFB, P.carinii, and mycobacterial culture should be done

- Positive P.carinii or AFB = Appropriate therapy should be given.
- Negative P.carinii or AFB = Perform bronchoscopy with BAL (bronchoalveolar lavage)
- BAL positive P.carinii, AFB, or fungus = Appropriate therapy should be given.
- BAL positive Kaposi's sarcoma = Appropriate management for KS.
- BAL nagative = Repeat BAL, transbronchial lung biopsy (Tb Bx) should be done.

(iii) **Diffuse infiltrates in CXR** = Induced sputum for AFB, P.carinii and mycobacterial culture **should be done** and subsequent.

(iv) **Focal infiltrates in CXR without purulent Sputum** = Induced sputum for AFB, P.carinii and mycobacterial culture should be done and subsequent managements are same as above.

(v) **Focal infiltrations plus purulent sputum**: Sputum Gram stain and culture, blood culture should be done. **Most likely diagnosis is bacterial pneumonia or tuberculosis.** Patients should get antimicrobial therapy.

12. Prevention of lung disease in HIV patients:

(i) **Prevention of PCP**: Trimethoprim-sulfamethoxazole, dapsone and pentamidine aerosol for patients with HIV with CD4 + lymphocyte counts <200 cells per microliter.

(ii) **Prevention of tuberculosis**: Tuberculin test should be done, if positive ($\geq$ 5 mm induration) **give INH prophylaxis irrespective of the CD4 + lymphocyte counts ; INH should also be given if HIV patients are exposed to a person with infectious tuberculosis irrespective of tuberculin** test results; do **not** give INH to **nonexposed HIV patients who are anergic to tuberculin test**.

(iii) **Prevention of pneumococcal infection**: Pneumococcal vaccine has **no** proven benefit yet but **this vaccine can be given. Moreover, trimethoprim- sulfamethoxazole can reduce pneumococcal infections along with PCP**.

(iv) **Prevention of M.avium complex disease**: Prophylactic **rifabutin** can reduce the infection by 50%. **It is recommended in HIV patients with CD4 + count is <100 cells per microliter.** Rifabutin can cause **resistance** of **M.tuberculosis when rifabutin and rifampin is given to patients with undiagnosed tuberculosis.**

13. **Gastrointestinal manifestations of AIDS:** Most of these complications occur when T4 lymphocyte count is <200 per cubic millimeter.

(A) Oral lesions:

(i) **Most common lesion is oral candidiasis** (80 to 90% of cases in advanced stages).
Diagnosis: Clinical ; KOH preparation (yeast and pseudohyphae) if necessary.
Treatment: Nystatin, clotriamazole troches, ketocontazole or fluconazole.

(ii) Oral hairy leukoplakia (OHL): It is found **exclusively** in HIV patients; **involves Epstein-Barr virus** ; usually **asymptomatic on the tongue** and sometimes pain or voice changes.
Treatment: **Acyclovir**

(iii) Herpes simplex virus (HSV): Painful vesicles on an erythematous base.
Treatment: Acyclovir

(iv) Kaposi's sarcoma oral lesions: **Typical erythematous purplish raised lesions predominantly on the palate** or anywhere inside the mouth, **mostly asymptomatic** and sometimes symptomatic.
Treatment: Radiation therapy for symptomatic patients only.

(v) Gingivitis or periodontitis is common.
Treatment: Topical chlorhexidine or systemic metronidazole.

(vi) Apthous ulcers: Respond to topical or systemic corticosteroids.

(B) **Esophageal lesions:**

(i) Most common is **candidiasis ;** most patients have thrush, **odynophagia indicates esophageal lesions** ; caused by HSV, CMV, or apthous ulcers.
Diagnosis: Endoscopy (grayish white plaques), smear, and biopsy confirms the diagnosis.
Treatment: C.albicans is treated with systemic corticosteroiod.

(C) **Gastric lesions:** Gastric achlorhydria is commonly present, rarely Kaposi's sarcoma and opportunistic lesions.

(D) **Small and large intestinal lesions.**

(i) **Diarrhea-wasting syndrome (diarrhea plus severe weight loss)** is included in AIDS- defining diagnosis. Acute and/or chronic diarrhea is most common; small intestine is most commonly involved ; most common organisms causing chronic diarrhea (intermittent or continuous loose or watery stools for more than 1 month) are **Cryptosporidium**, Microsporidia, mycobacterium avium and CMV.

(a) **Cryptosporidium causing diarrhea.** It usually causes **intermittent** diarrhea for months ; SI **biopsy** reveals villous atrophy, crypt hyperplasia and intraepithelial lymphocytes ; **malabsorption** of D-xylose and absence of fecal WBC's by presence of **oocysts in the stool.**

Complications: papillary stenosis and obstruction of common bile duct.

Treatment: No therapy is effective.

(b) **Microsporidium causing diarrhea**: Most common organism is **Enterocytozoon bieneusi** ; diagnosis is made by **SI biopsy** with electronmicroscopic study, histologic findings are the same as cryptosporidium infection **but has unique morphology,** and organism **is located within the cytoplasm of the enterocytes**.

(c) **M.avium causing diarrhea:** Most patients have M.avium bacteremia ; SI biopsy reveals **acid-fast M.avium, bacilli and mimic Whipple's disease**.

Treatment: Clarithromycin plus ethambutol ; clarithromycin with clofazimine ; or clarithromycin plus ethambutol plus clofazimine.

(d) **CMV causing diarrhea**: Most commonly causes **diffuse colitis with superficial ulcerations** but can involve any part of GI tract (mouth to rectum) ; symptoms include **bloody diarrhea** and **abdominal pain** ; diagnosis is made by **intestinal biopsy** which reveals typical **viral inclusions**.

Treatment: Ganciclovir and foscarnet may be useful.

(e) **Isospora belli** (1 to 3% of cases) causes **chronic diarrhea**, diagnosed by large acid-fast **oocysts** in stool, and treated with **trimethoprim-sulfamethoxazole.**

(f) **Incidence of Entamoeba histolytica** and **Giardia lamblia** infection are the **same as** immunocompetent host.

(g) **Bacteria causing diarrhea**:

Salmonella typhimurium is the most common organism and is treated with ampicillin or amoxicillin, trimethoprim-sulfamethoxazole, third-generation cephalosporins and quinolones. **Clostridium difficile infection is also common (Important). Other organisms are Shigella and Campylobater jejuni.**

(ii) **Tumors of GI tract**: Most common lesion is **Kaposi's sarcoma** (skin lesions are associated with GI lesions in 40 to 50% cases) **diagnosis is made by endoscopic finding of raised red nodules** but histologic confirmation is **difficult** due to depth of pathologic finding (Important), most patients are **asymptomatic** or rarely symptoms include diarrhea, protein-losing enteropahty, subacute intestinal obstruction, and rectal ulcer.

(iii) AIDS enteropathy: Morphologic changes (villous blunting, reduced villous-crypt ratio and low number of mitotic activity) without superimposed opportunistic infections.

Malabsorption with abnormal D-xylose and 14 C - glycerol - tripalmitin absorption tests.

Diagnosis of diarrhea in AIDS patients:

(i) Initial evaluation includes bacterial stool cultures (Salmonella, Shigella and Campylobacter jejuni) ; direct stool examination for ova and parasties; Clostridium difficile toxin assay.

(ii) Patients with unexplained, persistent, disabling diarrhea may require radiographic contrast study, CT scan and/or endoscopy. Extensive use of endoscopy may not be necessary in case of AIDS enteropathy, Cryptosporidium, and Microspordium infections for which treatment is not available.

Treatment of diarrhea in AIDS patients:

(i) Salmonella: Ampicillin or amoxicillin, quinolone, trimethoprim-sulfamethoxazole or third-generation cephalosporin.
(ii) Clostridium difficile: Metronidazole or vancomycin.
(iii) Campylobacter species: Erythromycin or quinolone
(iv) Isospora: Trimethoprim-sulfamethoxazole
(v) Cryptosporidium: Paromomycin (experimental)
(vi) Microsporidia: Albendazole (experimental)
(vii) Giardia lamblia: Quinacrine or metronidazole
(viii) E.histolytica: Metronidazole plus diloxanide
(ix) Nonspecific antidiarrheal drugs may be used: Imodium (or loperamide), bismuth salts, indomethacin, or somatostatin.
(x) Natritional therapy: Patients with chronic diarrhea should get small, frequent meals (low in fiber, lactose, fat, and residue) plus caffeine. Supplemental enteric (polymeric formulas) feeding, or use elemental formuls for severe GI disorders.

14. **Gray bowel syndrome:** It includes enteric and **perirectal infections**. It is more common in (immunocompetent) **homosexual men** than in HIV infected patients.
    (i) **Most common organisms** in **homosexual men** in the small intestine (Giardia) ; colon (**Chlamydia tracthomatis** is the most common, Campylobacter, Shigella, E.histolytica) ; **anus plus rectum (Neisseria gonorrhoeae is the most common,** Treponema pallidum, Condylomata accuminatum, Herpes simplex), and **oral cavity (N.gonorrhoeae is the most common**, herpes simplex)
    (ii) Most common organisms in HIV infected persons in the **SI (Cryptosporium is the most common,** Isospora, Microsporidia, M.avium, CMV, and **Salmonella is the most common among bacterial infections); colon CMV)** ; oral cavity (Candida albicans is the most common, oral hairy leukoplakia, herpes simplex, apthous ulcers, necrotizing gingivitis, and Kaposi's sarcoma) ; and esophagus (**C.albicans is the most common,** CMV, herpes simplex, apthous ulcers)
    (iii) **Herpes simplex virus (HSV) infections are** found in both (homosexual and HIV infected) categories **but HSV infections in HIV infected persons are** more severe, prolonged, and may be **resistant to acyclovir.**

15. **Most common organisms causing biliary obstruction in AIDS patients**: **Cryptosporidia, CMV.**

16. **Most common organisms causing cholestatic changes in AIDS patients:** M.avium,TB, histoplasmosis, and lymphoma.

17. **Most common organisms causing liver disease in AIDS patients**: Hepatitis B and C viruses.

18. **Few important points in HIV patients with abdominal surgery**:
    (i) HIV patients tolerate the procedure well.
    (ii) Most common condition required surgery is CMV peritonitis with perforation.
    (iii) Lymphoma of the intestine usually **involves terminal ileum** results in obstruction and bleeding.
    (iv) Patients with cholangiopathy (CMV or Cryptosporidium) may respond to **endoscopic retrograde cholangiopancratography.**

19. **Most common skin cancer in AIDS patients: Kaposi's sarcoma.** In AIDS patients it frequently involves the **mucosa**. **Lesions** are single or disseminated,

macules or nodules, **light tan to deep purple color** and arranged in follicular, linear, or Zosteriform pattern.

Other common skin lesions in AIDS patients are transient macular roseola-like rash, candidiasis, seborrheic, dermatitis, dermatophytosis, scabies, **herpes simplex and zoster ;** molluscum contagiosum and human papillomavirus in cosmetically sensitive region ; Reiter's syndrome ; **vesicular lesions of bacillary angiomatosis due to Rochalimaea henselae/quintana;** psoriasis and atopic dermatitis.

20. **Few important points in eye complications of AIDS patients**:

(i) **Most common eye complication** is the **retinal microvascular disease (up to 40% cases)**. Patients have **asymptomatic cotton-wool spots or small retinal hemorrhages** which usually **resolve spontaneously or remain nonprogressive** and **do not** need any therapy. It is difficult to distinguish from **early** CMV retinitis which is usually progressive. **It is more common than CMV retinitis.**

(ii) **Most common is the CMV retinitis, usually occur when CD4 + lymphocyte** (T helper) **counts <50 per microliter.** Patients appear with **white, cottage cheese-like retinal exudates** (with or without hemorrhages) **mostly located near the major blood vessels, one eye is more affected than the other.**

Diagnosis of CMV retinitis: Typical retinal findings **(not by viral cultures which is neither specific nor sensitive)**

Treatment: Ganciclovir or foscarnet. Foscarnet causes **more survival** than ganciclovir. Both inhibits CMV replications. Ganciclovir is **phosphorylated** to active ganciclovir **triphosphate within the CMV infected cells** but **foscarnet** is a pyrophosphate **analogue,** so does not need any change to become active against CMV. **If organism develops resistant to this drug, use higher doses or both the drugs together.**

(iii) **Toxoplasma chorioretinitis in AIDS patients.** It is **rare** and is due to spread of **toxoplasmosis from nonocular sites to eyes (not** by **reactivation of congenitally acquired cysts which are found in imunocompetent persons).** It causes white or yellow multifocal exudates in both retinas and **is always associated with toxoplasma encephalitis, so CT scan of head should be done.**

Diagnosis: Toxoplasma gondii IgG titer.

Treatment: Pyrimethamine plus sulfadiazine, or pyrimethamine plus clindamycin (same doses to treat encephalitis)

(iv) Herpes simplex virus (HSV) or varicella-zoster virus (VZA) retinal necrosis: It is a **painful** lesion **(unlike** CMV and toxoplasmosis which are painless) and associated **with keratitis or iritis**, and **loss of vision. Retina**

appears confluent, gray or pale mostly in the periphery and **retinal detachment** is **extremely common.**
Diagnosis: Viral culture of skin lesions
Treatment: IV acyclovir can prevent further retinal necrosis.

(v) **Progressive outer retinal necrosis syndrome:** It is a **clinical variant of VZV retinitis** and common in patients with CD4 + lymphocyte counts **<100 cells per microliter.**
Retina appears with **multifocal, deep lesions that progress to confluence.**
Treatment: Poor response to IV acyclovir therapy.

(vi) **Syphilitic retinitis: Nonspecific** retinal changes (focal or posterior retina), associated with **rash, hearing loss, visual field defect.**
Diagnosis: FTA-ABS is confirmatory, VDRL is nonspecific.

21. Retinal hemorrhages in HIV - patients - Varicella - zoster virus, herpes simplex virus, CMV, toxoplasmosis and rarely in syphilis.

22. **Side-effects of antiviral drugs:**
    (i) **Ganciclovir**: Granulocytopenia, thrombocytopenia, and azoospermia
    (ii) **Foscarnet**: Nephrotoxicity, nephrogenic diabetes insipidus, genital ulcers, ionized hypocalcemia (seizure or arrythmia with overdose), low serum (K,calcium, phosphate and magnesium)

23. **Most common cause of optic neuropathy: CMV infection**. **CMV causes swellin**g of optic nerve head **(papillitis)** and optic disc results in loss of vision. It causes optic neuritis (intraorbital or retroorbital). **Other causes of optic neuropathy** are herpes simplex, VZV, syphilis and streptococcal meningitis (arachnoiditis)
Diagnosis: It is made from associated clinical manifestations and laboratory findings.
Treatment: Specific therapy fails to improve significant vision loss in optic neuropathy.

24. **Most serious eye complication of cryptococcal meningitis (arachnoiditis)**: Retrobulbar optic neuritis and sometimes blindness.
Please remember, exclusive retrobulbar lesion cannot be diagnosed by opthalmoscopic examination because retina is normal.

25. **Eye lesions in Kaposi's sarcoma:**
    (i) **Eyelid: Periorbital edema** (due to lymphangitic Kaposi's sarcoma) without other eye lesions.

(ii) **Conjunctiva:** Bright **red subepithelial nodules (small lesions mimic subcojunctival hemorrhages).**

(iii) **Orbital lesions.**

Treatment of all lesions in Kaposi's sarcoma: Local irradiation therapy.

26. **Most common hematologic disorders in AIDS patients**: **Anemia (60%) is most common,** next neutropenia (50% of cases), and thrombocytopenia (40% of cases). Anemia is mostly normochronic and normocytic due to chronic disease (iron studies are normal). **Please remember**, **only thrombocytopenia** occurs in **early or asymptomatic phase** ; anemia and neutropenia are **found** in late stage or symptomatic phase **(Important). HIV infection should be ruled out in asymptomtic patients with thrombocytopenia. Thrombocytopenia** is **not** a **criteria for advanced HIV infection (CDC guidelines).**

27. **Effect of parvovirus in bone marrow of HIV infected patients**: **Anemia is most common among cytopenia plus presence of characteristic gaint pronormoblasts**.

28. **Treatment of thrombocytopenia in HIV infected patients**: **AZT (zidovudine) is the drug of choice. It increases the platelet counts threefolds within 12 weeks of therapy**. Failure of AZT indicates the following therapy:
Interferon-alpha, corticosteroids, danazol, IV gamma globulin, anti-RhD therapy, vincristine, or splenectomy. **Corticosteroids** can be used for **short-term** only because it can exacerbate **fungal infection**, HIV infection and kaposi's sarcoma.

29. **Most common cause of neutropenia in AIDS patients**: **Myelosuppressive therapy (in AIDS patients). Impaired hematopoiesis** is the major cause, other causes are **increased destruction of WBC's due to antibody against neutrolphils. Myelosuppressive drugs are trimethoprim-sulfamethoxazole, pyrimethamine-sulfadiazine, ganciclovir, or acyclovir,** and very **rarely AZT** treatment has to be stopped for neutropenia. (**Remember, ddI or ddC** does **not** cause this problem).

30. **Anemia in AIDS patients is due to** :
    (1) **Chronic disease process (normocytic, normochronic anemia with normal iron stores).**
    (2) **Positive Coombs' test** in most patients with AIDS and 33% of cases in **asymptomatic** HIV infected persons (anti-i antibodies or other specific antibodies but **true hemolysis is rare in HIV-infected** persons).

(3) **Sometimes** decreased vitamin B_{12} levels cause macrocytic anemia (but true B_{12} deficiency is **rare**).
(4) **Impaired erythropoiesis** is the **most common** cause in HIV-infected persons but the serum erythropoietin levels are **low without** renal abnormalities.
(5) **Parvovirus induced RBC's aplasia** in HIV-infected persons usually respond to gamma globulin therapy (**Important**).
(6) **AZT induced anemia is** due to **dose-related and idiosyncratic reaction (Important)**.
(7) Antiretroviral drugs, dideoxyinosine (**ddI**) and dideoxycytidine (ddC) do **not** cause anemia.
(8) Recombinant **erythropoietin therapy** is most effective when pretreatment serum erythropoietin levels **<500 mU per milliliter**.

31. **Treatment of leukopenia in HIV-infected persons**:
(1) **Myeloid growth factors** are **G-CSF** (granulocyte colony stimulating factor) and **GM-CSF** (granulocyte macrophage colony stimulating factor) are useful.
(2) Treatment with AZT, interferon-alpha, or ganciclovir may be successful along with G-CSF and **GM-CSF** (use low doses myelotoxicity).
(3) GM-CSF augments the **antiretroviral effects** of **AZT in monocytes**, and increased the **uptake and phosphorylation of AZT results** in increased concentration of AZT within the cells.

32. **Few important points in Kaposi's sarcoma (KS) in HIV-infected persons**:
(1) **KS is the most common cancer in AIDS** patients and is **most common in homsexual and bisexual men than in any other group**.
(2) **Increased incidence of KS in patients receiving immunosuppressive therapy,** particularly after hepatic and renal transplantation, and resolution of KS **after discontinuation** of immunosuppressive therapy.
(3) SLE and pemphigus vulgaris are associated with KS.
(4) **Recently** herpes virus genome has been associated with KS and cytokine (interleukin-6) may be elaborated by KS.
(5) KS involves skin, lymph nodes, and viscera (trachea, lungs, and GI tract).
(6) **KS** can cause **lymphedema** involving the lower extremities, head and neck; and can involve lung and pleura results in severe respiratory problems.
(7) AIDS patients do **not** die of KS **except** pulmonary KS cases die of infections.
(8) KS patients with symptomatic visceral disease, edema, or rapidly evolving **extensive skin lesion**: Patients should receive **chemotherapy such as** doxorubicin, etoposide, vinblastin, bleomycin, and vincristine.

Combination of doxorubicin, bleomycin, and vincristine are most useful. **Patients with borderline marrow function should receive bleomycin and vincristine** (these drugs are **less** myelotoxic) along with AZT.

(9) Anthracycline drugs are also effective in KS.

(10) KS patients **without** rapidly progressive disease: Patients can be managed by **observation**, single agent **interferon-alpha**, local irradiation, local cryotherapy, intralesional chemotherapy, or combination of therapies; single agent interferon-alpha may be toxic because of higher doses, so **low dose of interferon-alpha plus** AZT are equally effective.
Side effects of interferon-alpha: Flulike symptoms; anemia and leukopenia can be treated with erythroid growth factor (erythropoietin) and myeloid growth factors (G-CSF, GM-CSF).

33. Few important points in **non-Hodgkin lymphoma** of HIV-infected patients:

(1) **B-cell lymphoma** occurs in **immunosuppressed persons,** immunosuppressive therapy in **organ transplantation,** and **Wiskott-Aldrich syndrome**.

(2) **The chromosomal defect** in B-cell lymphoma include translocation of loci encoding the immunoglobulin gene with c-myc oncogene. **Genetic evidence of Epstein-Barr virus** is present in 50% cases of B-cell lymphomas **in AIDS** patients and almost 100% in all primary CNS lymhomas in AIDS patients.

(3) Most common histologic type is **small immunoblastic** type (75% of cases); and diffuse large cell type (25% of cases).

(4) **Most patients of** B-cell lymphoma have extranodular diseases **involving GI tract, liver, CNS, soft tissues, or bone marrow. Primary CNS lymphoma** is immunoblastic and is a **solitary lesion**. CNS involvement with systemic lymphoma is **meningeal**.

(5) Most patients have stage III (involving both sides of diaphragm **without** visceral involvement) or stage IV (visceral involvement) disease in AIDS patients with B-cell lymphoma.

(6) The prognosis is **poor** and patients do **not** tolerate aggressive chemotherapy.

(7) Radiation therapy results in tumor response in most patients and prophylactic CNS radiation is also effective.

34. **Most common HIV associated nephropathy (HIVAN): Focal and segmental glomerulosclerosis (FSGS)** (80 to 90% of cases).

35. Clinical manifestations, diagnosis, and treatment of HIVAN (HIV associated nephropathy):

(A) **Clinical manifestations:** Proteinuria, rapidly progressive irreversible azotemia, and nephrotic syndrome. ESRD (end-stage renal disease) develops within **4 to 16 weeks** from the time of onset of proteinuria (heroin associated nephropathy or HAN develops ESRD in 20 to 40 months and **accelerated hypertension is characteristic of HAN**) and **absence of hypertension, peripheral edema, and anasarca** in HIVAN **despite** large proteinuria and hypoalbuminemia. **Nephropathy can occur months or years before the onset of clinical symptoms of early symptomatic HIV patients**.

(B) **Diagnosis of HIVAN**:

(1) Estimation of **quantitative** protien excretion and **creatinine clearance in 24-hour urine**.

(2) The decision of renal biopsy should be made on a case-by-case basis.

(C) **Treatment of HIVAN:** The therapeutic response is poor.

(1) **Zidovudine** can slow the progression of azotemia.

(2) **Corticosteroids** can partially reverse the progression of azotemia and can prevent the need for dialysis in some patients.

(3) Nutritional support: High-protein and high-calorie diets.

(4) Dose adjustment of nephrotoxic drugs are very important.

(5) Hemodialysis can only prolong the survival.

(6) CAPD (continuous ambulatory peritoneal dialysis) is better than hemodialysis because it does **not** cause leukopenia, and causes **less anemia in hemodialysis patients due to hemodialysis membranes**. CAPD causes **peritonits**.

(7) Do **not** perform renal transplantation.

36. Most common fluid and electrolyte disorder in HIV infected patients: **Hyponatremia is most common. Hypovolemia is the most commoon cause of hyponatremia. Hypovolemia** is most commonly due to **GI fluid loss. Euvolemic hyponatremia is due to SIADH** (syndrome of inappropriate ADH) release which is found in **PCP infections, cancer, or CNS disease**. Hypofunction of adrenal gland (<5% of cases) results in hyponatremia, hyperkalemia, renal salt wasting, hypovolemia, **non-anion gap metabolic acidosis**.

37. **Drugs causing fluid and electrolyte disorder in HIV infected patients**:

(1) **Amphotericin B: Hypokalemia,** hypomagnesemia, renal insufficiency, and RTA (renal tubular acidosis).

(2) **Foscarnet:** Decreased levels of ionized calcium and rarely renal insufficiency.

(3) **IV pentamidine: Hyperkalemia** and **non-anion gap metabolic acidosis**.

(4) Chemotherapeutic drugs used in malignancy: Direct nephrotoxicity, vomiting, or diarrhea causes fluid and electrolyte abnormalities.

38. **Few important points in cardiac disease of HIV infected patients**:
(1) **Most patients are asymptomatic; no** specific cardiac lesion is found but **myocardial disease (>90% of cases) is most common**, and pericardial disease (20% of cases).
(2) Most common clinical manifestation in symptomatic patients are hepatomegaly, jugular venous distension, rales, heart murmur, S3 gallop due to right sided cardiac failure. Cardiac tamponade is common in advanced pericardial disease.
(3) Echocardiography usually reveals ventricular enlargement, pericardial effusion, and ventricular hypokinesis. Right ventricular enlargement from pulmonary hypertension is due to **severe or recurrent opportunistic infections**.
(4) Supportive therapy includes diuretic, reduce afterload as needed, correct cardiac arrythmias; pericardial disease needs appropriate volume management, **avoid** severe diuresis or preload reduction; and specific therapy according to underlying disorder should be instituted.

39. **Most common endocrine abnormality in HIV infected patients:**
Hypogonadism results in **decreased libido** (50% of all male patients) and **impotence** (30% of cases) are due to **low serum testosterone levels**.
Diagnosis: Serum FSH and LH level are **low normal** or inappropriately normal; after stimulation with gonadotropin-releasing hormone FSH and LH level become normal, **indicating hypothalamic hypogonadism in most cases**; other study shows elevated FSH and LH indicating primary testicular dysfunction.
Drugs causing low testosterone levels or decreased spermatogenesis: Ganciclovir, acyclovir, and ketoconazole.

40. **Most common endocrine gland involved in HIV infected patients**: Adrenal gland is most commonly involved **but mostly asymptomatic (>92% of cases)**, only 8% of cases show adrenal hypofunction. Most common findings are adrenal lipid depletion and adrenal necrosis. CMV invasion occurs up to 50% of cases.
Diagnosis of adrenal insufficiency: Basal 8 A.M. **plasma cortisol levels are higher in advanced HIV patients than in asymptomatic HIV patients or normal individuals but** other ACTH-dependent steroids (deoxycorticosterone, 18-hydroxy-deoxycorticosterone, and compound B) are **not** elevated and **reveals blunted response with ACTH stimulation indicating adrenal**

insufficiency. Plasma cortisol levels 20 or less microgram per deciliter 60 minutes after ACTH stimulation indicates adrenal insufficiency or high risk for adrenal insufficiency. Plasma ACTH levels may be **normal or subnormal** even with **low plasma cortisol** levels indicates primary pituitary or CNS disorder.
Treatment: Same as in any other patients with adrenal insufficiency.

41. **Most common thyroid disorder in HIV infected patients**: **Most patients remain asymptomatic despite invasive disease** but hypothyroidism is a **reversible cause** of fatigue, failure to thrive, altered mental status, **it should be always ruled out despite its incidence. Remember, ketoconazole rarely causes hypothyoridism.**

42. **Few important points in metabolic abnormalities of HIV infected patients**:
    (1) IV pentamidine is the most common cause of hypoglycemia and renal insufficiency is a predisposing factor. Aerosolized pentamidine also causes hypoglycemia. Drugs can directly act on beta cells to cause hypoglycemia.
    (2) **Hyponatremia** due to hypovolemia is the most common electrolyte abnormality.
    (3) **Hypercalcemia** is found in HIV-related leukemia and lymphoma.
    (4) **Hypocalcemia** is due to **amphotericin B and foscarnet** which also cause **hypomagnesemia.**
    (5) **Isolated elevation of triglycerides** is found in 50% of cases in both symptomatic and asymptomic AIDS patients.

43. **Few important points in rheumatologic disease (musculoskeletal) in HIV infected patients**:
    (A) Arthralgias: Generalized arthralgias are found in 33% of cases. **Initial zidovudine** therapy can cause **arthralgia and myalgia; self-limited condition, usually resolves within 4 to 6 weeks of treatment. The 'painful articular syndrome'** characterized by severe articular pain of 2 to 24 hours, unknown etiology, and unresponsive to NSAID's or narcotic analgesics.
    Treatment of HIV associated arthralgia except painful articular syndrome: NSAID's are the drug of choice.
    (B) **Myopathies** : Polymyositis-like illness (proximal muscle weakness, wasting, and myalgias) and **elevated CPK levels** (**>5 times normal**); biopsy reveals necrosis, fibrosis, **inflammation** but less extent than non-HIV patients.

Zidovudine long-term therapy can cause myositis includes muscle weakness, myalgias, myopathy but **less** inflammatory cells in biopsy, and elevated CPK levels.
Treatment:
(1) Discontinuation of zidovudine can reverse the process.
(2) Corticosteroids may be helpful in some patients but **no** specific therapy is available.

(C) **Reiter's syndrome:** It can precede or occur at the same time of HIV infection but most cases follow the onset of immunodeficiency, mostly HLA-B27 positive.
Treatment: NSAID's are **not** very effective; **no treatment** is available; methotrexate and azathioprine can cause Kaposi's sarcoma and opportunistic infections.

(D) **Sjogren's syndrome**: Dry eyes and dry mouth are characteristic in this syndrome, mostly in males, **absence** of anti-Ro/SS-A and anti-La/SS-B antibodies, **presence of HLA-DR 52 and DR 5** (instead of characteristic A1, B8, DR3, DR2, DQ1/DQ2 antigens) and **predominance of CD8+ lymphocytes** (instead of CD4+ cells) **infiltrating salivary glands which is characteristic of AIDS-related Sjogren's syndrome**.
Treatment: Symptomatic therapy only.

(E) **Septic arthritis:** Most common organisms are **C.neoformans, H.capsulatum**, S.schenkii, mycobacteria and pyogenic organisms.
Diagnosis and treatment: Same as in any other non-HIV patients.

(F) HIV-associated arthropathy (HIVAA): Mono-or polyarticular arthritis (severe) involves knees and ankles last from 1 week to 24 weeks **but no** extraarticular involvement; **non inflammatory** synovial fluid; **absence** of rheumatiod factor, ANA, anti-DNA, and antibodies against RNP, Sm, Ro/SS-A, La/SS-B; **no** predominant HLA pattern
Treatment: **NSAID's may be useful or intraarticular injection of steroids.**

(G) **Vasculitis:** Most common is necrotizing vasculitis of the polyarteritis nodosa. It involves the medium size vessels of the nerves, muscles, and skin.
Drugs causing hypersensitivity vasculitis are penicillin, griseofulvin, amitryptyline, and trimethoprim-sulfamethoxazole. **Rifampin can cause uveitis** when used along with fluconazole and clarithromycin.

44. **Antiretroviral therapy of HIV-infected adults**:
(A) **No previous antiretroviral therapy**:
(1) Asymptomatic (CD4 cell count > 500) = No treatment.
(2) Asymptomatic (CD4, 200-500) = Zidovudine or no treatment.

(3) Symptomatic (CD4, 200-500) = Zidovudine.
(4) Asymptomatic (CD4, < 200) = Zidovudine.
(5) Symptomatic (CD4, < 200) = Zidovudine, (some experts prefer to **add** didanosine or zalcitabine).

(B) **Previous antiretroviral therapy**:
(1) Stable (CD4, ≥ 300) = Continue zidovudine.
(2) Stable (CD4, < 300) = Continue zidovudine or switch to didanosine.
(3) Progressing (CD4, 50-500) = Switch to didanosine or zalcitabine.
(4) Progressing (CD4, < 50) = Switch to didanosine or zalcitabine.

(C) **Intolerant to zidovudine**:
(1) Stable or progressing (CD4, > 500) = Stop the treatment.
(2) Stable or progressing (CD4, 50-500) = Switch to didanosine or zalcitabine.
(3) Stable or progressing (CD4, < 50) = Switch to didanosine or zalcitabine.

45. **Prophylaxis of opportunistic infections**:
(A) Pneumocystis carinii pneumonia: Sulfamethoxazole-trimethoprim.
(B) Mycobacterium avium complex (MAC): Rifampin.
(C) Toxoplasma encephalitis: May be sulfamethoxazole-trimethoprim.
(D) Cryptococcal meningitis: Fluconazole.

46. **Few important points regarding physicians responsibility in counseling HIV-infected patients**:
(1) **The most important component of counseling is education about HIV disease**, its **transmission, and its treatment.** This process should continue **along with physician-patient relationship**.
(2) Patients with substance abuse, physician must advice patients to seek for drug treatment programs.
(3) **Physicians must treat recidivous patients firmly** and without judgement.
(4) Physicians must **reinforce positively to recovering addicts**.
(5) **Physicians should aware of AIDS service organization in their community** that provide support services such as patient education, transportation, shelter, food, medications, case management, or support groups to their clients.
(6) Some patients may need **formal psychiatric referral**.

METABOLIC DISEASES

1. **Treatment of hyperlipidemia**: (Total blood cholesterol is **high** >240 mg/dL, borderline is 200-239 mg/dL, and **desirable is < 200 mg/dL; LDL is high > 160 mg/dL,** borderline is 130-15g mg/dL, **desirable is < 130 mg/dL; HDL level should be > 35 mg/dL**).

   (A) **Treatment of hypercholesterolemia**:

   (1) All patients should be managed in the same way irrespective of the causes.

   (2) **First** is the **dietary restriction of cholesterol and saturated fat** result in suppression of hepatic LDL receptor activity and reduction of both cholesterol and LDL levels.

   (3) Solube **dietary fibers (oat bran)** also lower plasma cholesterol by binding bile acids in the intestine like **bile acid-binding resins** and subsequent **loss** in the stool. **Sometimes** bile sequestrant therapy causes **increased production of VLDL** (plasma triglycerides) along with decreased LDL levels, but **VLDL subsequetly increases the LDL levels,** finally suboptimal lowering of LDL levels.

   (4) **The second agent** is added along with bile acid-binding resin for synnergistic activity such as **nicotinic acid** (inhibits the release of lipoproteins from the liver) and HMG-CoA reductase inhibitor (**directly inhibits** cholesterol biosynthesis results in **decreased** new lipoprotiens production and reduction of hepatic sterol pools). **HMG-CoA reductase inhibitor plus bile acid-binding resin** can lower LDL levels **>50%** and **addition of nicotinic acid can lower LDL levels 70% or more** when used along with the first two drugs.

   (B) **Treatment of mild hypertriglyceridemia**:

   (1) Mild hypertriglyceridemia patients should be treated **initially** with **nonpharmacologic therapy such** as weight reduction in obese patients, low-fat diets, increased physical activity, restriction of alcohol, **use of gemfibrozil** (lowers VLDL but increases LDL), use of **niacin** (lowers VLDL and increases HDL), and some experts are using **statin** as initial therapy for patients with **familial combined hyperlipidemia**.
   Side effect of combined use of statin and gemfibrozil: Myositis may occur.

   (C) **Treatment of marked hypertriglycerdemia (>350 mg/dL)**, (the chylomicronemia syndrome **consists of plasma triglyceride levels >1000 mg/dL plus clinical manifestations** such as abdominal pain with or without pancreatitis, eruptive xanthomas, lipemia retinalis, recent memory loss, paresthesia of the dorsum of the hands and feet, erythematous flush of the face and chest or sometimes symmetric arathralgia without physical joint findings ; **low serum sodium levels due to high serum chylomicron levels** is called **pseudo hyponatremia**): The treatment is the **total elimination of dietary fat until** the triglyceride levels are safe; pancreatitis patients should be kept NPO (nothing per orally) which reduces serum triglyceride level significantly.

2. **NCEP (National Cholesterol Education Program) recommendations are the following**:
   (1) Total cholesterol levels should be measured in all adults over **age 20** (**nonfasting state**) at least **once every 5 years**. HDL cholesterol (>35 mg/dL) should be measured at the same time.
   (2) **Desirable** total cholesterol levels are < 200 mg/dL, LDL levels are < 130 mg/dL, and HDL levels are > 35 mg/dL.
   (3) **Ideal or optimal cholesterol levels (160 to 180 mg/dL) are much lower than normal** values **(desirable < 200 mg/dL)** which are 90-95**th** percentile of the bell-shaped curve of normal population.

3. **Alcaptonuria:** Rare hereditary disease; **absence** of homogentisic acid oxidase enzyme activity results in **accumulation of homogentisic acid which cause black pigmentation** of the cartilage (costal, laryngeal, tracheal) and other connective tissues; urine is initially **clear** but becomes **dark** when alkaline or prolonged exposure to the air; patients appear initially with slight **pigmentation of the sclerae or the ears around 20 to 30 year of age and arthritis if hips, knees, or shoulders**; high incidence of **generalized atherosclerosis**, chronic mitral and aortic valvulitis with calcification, and **myocardial infarction is a common cause of death**; radiologic finding reveals **degenerative arthritis** of hip, shoulder, knee, and lumbar vertebral bodies; diagnosis is **confirmed by identification of homogentisic acid in the urine** (**normally** phenylalanine and tyrosine are converted to homogentisic acid); treatment includes **ascorbic acid** (protects lysyl hydroxylase from inhibition by homogentisic acid) and NTBC (2-2 nitro-4-trifluoromethylbenzoly-1,3-cyclohexanedione) prevents excess formation of homogentisic acid and **please remember** dietary restriction of phenylalanine and tyrosine **are detrimental**).

4. **Homocystinuria**: Most common cause is **cystathione beta-synthase enzyme deficiency**; clinical manifestations include **ocular lens dislocation (anteroinferior** type; Marfan syndrome has **posterosuperior** dislocation), **thromboembolism** (arterial and venous occlusion of small and large vessels), **skeletal abnormalities** (defective fibrillin gene causes skeletal and eye abnormalities) and mild to moderate mental retardation in untreated patients;

diagnosis is made by **quantitative** elevation of homocysteine in urine and plasma, confirmed by (liver) tissue biopsy or assay of culture fibroblast cells or lymphocytes to determine the enzyme deficiency.

Treatment:

(1) Cystathione beta-synthase deficiency: **Folic acid is given before pyridoxine therapy;** dietary restriction of **low methionine is indicated in patients with inadequate response** to pyridoxine; **betaine** (N, N, N-trimethylglycine) cause remethylation of homocysteine by an alternate pathway and may be useful in patients unresponsive to pyridoxine; **dipyridamole and low-dose aspirin** may be used as adjuvants; **preoperative hydration plus pyridoxine** can prevent thromboembolic complication > 95% of cases.

(2) Methylenetetrahydrofolate reductase deficiency: Betaine, folinic acid, methionine, addition pyridoxine (B_6) and cyanocobalamine (B_{12}); milder adult variety can be treated with decreasing homocysteine.

(3) Cobalamine metabolic disorders: Hydroxycobalamine may be more effective than (large dose of) cyanocobalamine.

5. **Marfan syndrome**: Autosomal dominant; mutation in the gene (FIBN1) located on **chromosome 15q 21**; tall stature, mitral valve prolapse, posterosuperior subluxation/dislocation of the lens, arachnodactyly; aortic dissection and rupture is the most life threatening complication and most common cause of death if untreated; lens subluxation is usually nonprogressive after adolescence, may need artificial lens if vision is impaired.
   Treatment: Beta-blockers may slow the progression of aortic enlargement, try to maintain the normal BP, replacement of aorta with aortic valve (human cadaver homograft or composite graft with prosthetic valve) is performed when aortic root diameter reaches approximately 55 to 60 mm (normal 20 to 37 mm).

6. **Ehlers-Danlos syndrome:** Ten different types, most common is type III (autosomal dominant) which is **familial hypermobility** characterized by soft skin, **no** scarring, severe large and small joint hypermobility, **joint discomfort and early onset** of degenerative joint disease; **few uncommon types are type IV (arterial) characterized by arterial, bowel, and uterine ruptures,** severe bruising but **normal skin and joint extensibility**, autosomal dominant; VI (ocular) characterized by ocular fragility and keratoconus, hyperextensible skin and joints, autosomal recessive; type VIII (periodontal) characterized by generalized periodontitis, soft, hyperextensible skin, easy bruising and hypermobile joints, autosomal dominant.
   Treatment: Only type VI responds to ascorbic acid; type IV may need surgery because of arterial and visceral rupture; **no** specific therapy for other types.

7. **Pseudoxanthoma elasticum:** It is a connective tissue disorder; **mostly autosomal recessive**; characterized by skin lesions (**initially** yellow is papule like plucked chicken skin apearance, **followed** by thickened, lethary skin, and **finally** becomes redundant, lax, and inelastic skin); **bilateral eye lesions** (appear **after** skin lesions, around third or fourth decade, **angioid streaks** are grayish or brownish-red streaks radiating across the fundus; **hemorrhages** and **exudates** in Bruch's membrane and loss of vision); **vascular lesions** (**most frequent complication is recurrent GI tract bleeding; most devastating complication is coronary occlusion or cerebral hemorrhages**; high BP, weak pulses, and claudication).
   Treatment: No specific therapy is available; vitamin E and C, or a low calcium diet has **no** proven benefit; **plastic surgery is helpful for cosmetic reason**; genetic counseling is important.

8. **The porphyrias**: It is due to deficiency of specific enzymes in **heme** biosynthetic pathway results in accumulation of heme pathway intermediates. Three important types are the following:
   (A) **Acute intermittent porphyria (AIP)**: Autosomal dominant; patients appear with diffuse, crampy **abdominal pain** (most common), high BP, tachycardia, fine tremors, peripheral neuropathy (mostly motor), weakness of proximal muscles, tendon reflexes initially hyperactive followed by hypoactivity in advanced stages, CNS (anxiety, insomnia, hallucination, depression, hyponatremic seizures due to increased ADH secretion); **chronic cases have higher incidence of hepatocellular cancer** (**not** due to hepatitis B or C).
   Precipitating factors: Progesterone, P-450 inducing drugs, dietary restriction.
   Diagnosis: Urinary porphobilinogen.
   Treatment: Heme, glucose.
   (B) **Porphyria cutanea tarda**: Patients appear with chronic blistering skin lesions; precipitating factors are alcohol, iron, hepatitis C virus, estrogens, and halogenated hydrocarbons; diagnosis is made by elevated plasma or urine porphyrins; treated with phlebotomy and low-dose chloroquine.
   (C) **Erythropoietic protoporphyria:** Patients appear with acute onset of painful skin and swelling; diagnosed by elevated plasma or RBC's porphyrins; treated with beta-carotene.

9. **Hyperammonemia: Most common cause is liver failure in adults**, less commonly is due to toxic ingestion; it is due to urea cycle defects, **high ammonia levels (> 1000 microgram N/dL**; normal is 15-45**) plus**

accumulation of glutamine are toxic to the CNS, uptake of fluid into astrocytes causing cerebral edema; death is due to cerebral downward herniation through foramen magnum; two enzymes defect are found **in adults** (carbamoyl phosphate synthetase or CPS and ornithine transcarbamoylase or OTC); **diagnosis** of CPS deficiency (autosomal recessive) is made high levels of ammonia, low levels of citrulline, normal or elevated bicarbonate levels and confirmed by **liver biopsy**; diagnosis of OTC deficiency (x-linked recessive) is made by high ammonia levels, very **high level of orotic acid in the urine,** and confirmed by liver biopsy; carrier female can be detected by an allopurinol challenge test.
Treatment: Lever transplantation is the definitive treatment of choice; future treatment is artificial liver and gene therapy.

10. **Wilson disease: Autosomal recessive;** gene is located on **chromosome 13q 14.3**; it is a hereditary disorder of **hepatocellular degeneration** characterized by **accumulation of copper in the body** particularly **liver, brain, kidneys, and corneas;** patients appear with hepatic symptoms (**jaundice**, malaise, and anorexia **like** viral heptitis), **transient hemolytic anemia** (due to massive release of copper from the liver), neurologic symptoms (chorea, dystonia, **wing-beating tremor of upper extremities, Kayser-Fleischer ring (golden brown or greenish is a characteristic feature in the Descemet's membrane of the cornea**); psychological symptoms (intellectual deterioration, unstable behavior, organic dementia, or schizophrenia like symptoms).
Diagnosis: Low levels of serum ceruloplasmin (< 20 mg/dL), high levels of liver copper (>250 microgram per gram of dry weight), high levels of urinary copper (>100 mircrogram per 24 hours).
Detection of asymptomatic siblings: Low levels of serum ceruloplasmin in 95% of homozygotes and 20% of heterozygotes, if the level is low then measure liver copper content (>250 microgram per gram of dry weight indicates Wilson disease). **Asymptomatic homozygotes should be treated but** heterozygotes will never become symptomatic, so **no** treatment is needed.
Treatment: D-Penicillamine is the drug of choice; pyridoxine is also given.
Side effect of D-penicillamine: Fever, rash, low WBC counts, low platelet counts, and adenopathy. The drug should be stopped. When symptoms have cleared then use **prednisone plus penicillamine**. If patients **cannot** tolerate penicillamine, then use **trientine** or **zinc acetate; liver transplantation is curative** for fulminant hepatic failure.

11. **Hemochromatosis: Autosomal recessive; primary or hereditary** hemochromatosis is due to mutation in a gene on short arm of **chromsome 6;** associated with **HLA-A3 antigens; secondary hemochromatosis** is found in

homozygous beta-thalassemia (most common) and multiple blood transfusion; patients may be asymptomatic or appear with **fatigue (most common),** arthralgias, abdominal pain, impotence, amenorrhea, weight loss, hyperpigmentation, alopecia, cardiac arrythmias and cardiomegaly, swollen-tender joints, ascites, hepatosplenomegaly, spider telangiectasia, testicular atrophy, or hypothroidism. (**Normal adult men** absorb **1 mg of iron** per day, **normal adult women** absorb **2mg of iron** per day; in **symptomatic hemochromatosis** iron accumulation is **15 to 40 grams**). Yersinia enterocolitica or Vibrio vulnificus may cause severe peritonitis or septicemia. **Diagnosis: Elevated serum iron concentration, elevated serum transferrin saturation >60 up to 100% (normal 20 to 50%), elevated** serum ferritin (>500 microgram per liter); **definitive diagnosis by liver biopsy (iron stain by Perls' Prussian** blue method and hepatic iron concentration **>200 micromol per gram of** tissue in **homozygous** hemochromatiosis, **<100 in heterozygous** hemochromatosis or alcoholic cirrhosis, **normal <40 for men and <33 for women)**.
Treatment: Repeated phlebotomy is the treatment of choice;; chelation therapy is effective **except** in hereditary hemochromatosis in which dietary manipulation is **not** effective.

12. **Hypophosphatemia (<2.6 mg/dL; normal** 2.7 to 4.5 mg/dL): Two types are **transient** low phosphorus with normal body stores (**phosphorus goes into the cells due to ingestion of carbohydrate and respiratory alkalosis**) and **sustained low phosphorus** with reduced body stores (**moderate** variety is due to **decreased** renal tubular absorption and intestinal absorption, and extracorporeal losses from dialysis; **severe** variety is **due to prolonged use of phosphate binding antacids (most common),** parenteral alimentation, severe respiratory alkalosis, nutritional recovery syndrome, recovery phase of severe burns, alcoholism and alcohol withdrawal, and poorly controlled diabetes mellitus).
    (1) **Moderate hypophosphatemia** (serum phosphorus 1 to 2.5 mg/dL): Decreased renal absorption of phosphorus in **hyperparathyroidism, glucocorticoid or alkali** administration, increased ECF volume, magnesium loss, and Fanconi's syndrome.
    (2) **Severe** hypophosphatemia (serum phosphorus <1 mg/dL): Most common cause is prolonged use of phosphate-binding antacids **(Important)**.
    (3) Clinical manifestations of hypophosphatemia: **CNS** (irritability, ataxia, seizures, coma), **neuromuscular** (rhabdomyolsis, muscle weakness or paralysis), congestive cardiomyopathy, **hypoglycemia, transient jaundice,** impaired renal tubular function, **impaired** RBC's, WBC's, function and platelet aggregation; bone (osteomalacia, resorption).

(4) **Treatment**:
   (a) **Normal** body stores in transient hypophosphatemia: **No** phosphate replacement, only to treat the underlying cause.
   (b) **Moderate** hypophosphatemia: Reduce urinary losses and sodium diuresis; **discontinue** phosphate binders; increase GI absorption; high-phosphate foods (skimmed cow's milk 1 mg p/ml), oral supplements of sodium salts (Phospho-Soda), and K salts (Neutra-Phos).
   (c) **Severe hypophosphatemia:** IV phosphorus (2.5-5 mg/kg) Q6H, until the serum phosphorus is 2 to 2.5 mg/dL; hypocalcemia with renal failure needs IV phosphorus but lower doses than mentioned above.

13. **Hypermagnesemia** (>2.1 mEq/L; **normal** serum magnesium is **1.3 to 2.1** mEq/L): Most common cause is **large oral intake of magnesium in the form of laxatives or antacids** in patients with advanced renal failure; other causes are advanced renal failure; hypothyroidism, and hypofunction of adrenal glands. **Clinical manifestations:** Asymptomatic until the magnesium is >4 mEq/L, first sign is decreased deep tendon reflexes; when serum magnesium levels are **10 to 15 mEq/L,** deep tendon reflexes are **absent**, flaccid **quadriplegia, respiratory depression, dilated** pupils, **low BP and heart rate, rarely** cardiac arrest and complete heart block.
    Treatment:
    (1) **Severe cases: IV calcium** (5 to 10 mEq) which is a direct antagonist to magnesiun.
    (2) **Hemodialysis** (magnesium-free dialysate) is the best treatment of choice.
    (3) Patients with reasonable renal function: Use **furosemide plus 0.5 N saline** to maintain urine volume and produce diuresis which enhances magnesium excretion.

14. Hypomagnesemia (<1.3 mEq/L; symptoms begin when <1.0 mEq/L plus **associated low K and low calcium**) : It is due to **GI causes** (steatorrheic conditions, severe diarrhea, familial magnesium malabsorption), **renal causes** (**intrinsic** causes are Bartter's syndrome, familial or sporadic magnesium loss, nephrotoxic agents; extrinsic causes are DKA, diuretics, increased volume, urinary loss of calcium), and other causes are **alcoholism, burns,** parathyroidectomy, thryotoxicosis, and lactation.
    (1) **Clinical manifestations:** Muscle fasciculations, tremors, tetany, weakness, positive Chvostek's and Trousseau's signs.
    (2) **Treatment:**
       (a) Mild (1 to 1.2 mEq/L) asymptomatic: No treatment is needed **if patients take normal diet**.
       (b) Severe (<1 mEq/L) symptomatic: IM or IV $MgSO_4$.

(c) Tetany or seizures: IV $MgSO_4$ push over 10 minutes.
(d) Chronic oral therapy (steatorrheic states and renal magnesium loss): Oral magnesium oxide (stop when develops diarrhea).

DERMATOLOGY

1. **Contact dermatitis:** Most common causes are poison ivy (or poison oak) and **hand dermatitis** (soap, chemicals, hand lotions). It can also occur in face, neck, forearms, feet, trunk. It appears with redness, edema, vesicles, bullae or oozing.
   (A) **Management of poison ivy**: Non-contagious; debridement of blilsters, Burow's solutions wet pack; hydrocortisone (1%) lotion or fluorinated corticosteroid, chlorpheniramine (for itching); severe cases steroid injections may be given; severe cases of poison ivy needs oral prednisone therapy.
   (B) **Management of contact dermatitis**: Non-contagious; avoid the irritants; use gloves; use mild soaps (Dove, Neutrogena); Burow's solution soaks; fluorinated corticosteroids locally; severe cases may need short course of **oral** prednisone.

2. **Atopic dermatitis (or eczema)**: Most common sites **cubital** and popliteal fossae; dry, thickened (lichenification), excoriated skin.
   Management: Avoid excess soap and water during bathing; use coal tar solution (LCD), fluorinated corticosteroids locally, chlor-trimeton (drowsiness), antibiotic (erythromycin) for superimposed infection; systemic steroids in severe and resistant cases.

3. **Nummular eczema**: **Coin shaped (nummular)**, papulovesicular lesions or the arms and legs, followed by lichenification (thickening) and bacterial infection.
   Management: Avoid excess soap and water during bathing; **avoid foods** containing excessive iodides and bromides (chocolate, seafood, tomatoes, melons, salted nuts, cheese **except** cottage cheese; increase protein-rich foods; **corticosteroid ointment** and **benadryl**; resistant cases need oral prednisone, coal tar solution and PO erythromycin.

4. **Drug eruptions**: History of drug intake is important.
   (i) **Urticaria**: Penicillin, sulfur drugs, ACE inhibitors, barbiturates, oral contraceptives.
   (ii) **Vesicular or bullous**: Sulfonamides, penicillin, phenylbutazone.
   (iii) **Pigmentary lesions**: Oral contraceptives, atabrine, chlorpromazine.
   (iv) **Seborrheic dermatitis-like rash**: Gold, ACTH
   (v) **Pityriasis rosea-like rash:** Bismuth, gold, barbiturates, antihistamines
   (vi) **Scarlet fever-like rash:** Arsenic, barbiturates, morphine, codeine, Salicylates, Sulfur drugs.

(vii) **Psoriasis exacerbation:** Beta-blockers, lithium, ACE inhibitors, antimalarial drugs.

(viii) **Purpuric rash:** Salicylates, barbiturates, organic arsenic, dicumarol, Chlorthiazide diuretics, Sulfur drugs and prolonged use of corticosteroids.
Management: Elimination of the drug is the treatment of choice; itching can be relieved with starch baths and nonalcoholic calamine lotion or white shake lotion; exfoliative dermatitis or severe erythema multiforme needs corticosteroids and other supportive therapy.

5. **Erythema multiforme bullosum (common in adults):** Unknown etiology; **chronic large vesicles and bullae usually overlying** red, **irislike macules** (characteristic bull's eye lesion) appear on the arms, legs and face for several days to months.
Management: **Corticosteroids** (orally and injection) **are the drug of choice**; refer to dermatologist; severe cases need hospitalization; local care with potassium permanganate crystalls with **lukewarm** water in bathtub, talcom powder in bed sheet, polysporin or bactroban antibiotic ointment in infected areas.

6. Erythema multiforme (common in young adolescents): Characteristic **bull's eye lesions** on the lips, extremities and face for 2 to 4 weeks; associated with **mild fever, arthralgias**.
   (i) Steven-Johnson syndrome: Severe erythema multiforme, high fever; extensive bullae, purpura and ulcers of the mucous membrane (mouth, eye) followed by ulcers of skin after 2 to 3 days.
   (ii) **Erythema Chronicum migrans**: Characteristic of **lyme** disease (Ixodes dammini is deer tick and vector for the spirochete), treated with doxycycline or ampicillin.
   (iii) **Bechet's syndrome**: Triad of genital, oral and eye ulcerations; mostly found in males; last for years with recurrence.
   (iv) **Reiter's syndrome**: Triad of conjunctivitis, urethritis and arthritis; mostly found in males; last about 6 months.
   (v) Erythema **multiforme-like rash due to drugs:** Phenacetin, pencillin, quinine, mercury, arsenic, barbifurates, phenytoin, sulfur drug.
   Management: Corticosteroids (prednisone) orally are the drug of choice; bed rest, adequate fluid intake; acetaminophen for fever; severe cases such as Steven Johnson syndrome may need hospitalization, IV fluid therapy.

7. **Erythema nodosum**: Most common in **young women**; **erythematous nodules appear in successive crops in anterior tibial regions and preceeded**

by fever, malaise and arthralgias; due to streptococcal infections, fungal infections, sarcoidosis, pregnancy, syphilis, drugs (contraceptive pills, iodided, bromides, sulfur drugs), and rarely tuberculosis.
Management: Treat the underlying cause; **rest**, **local heat application and aspirin** are very helpful; eruption may be self-limited along with the treatment of underlying disease; some cases may need naproxen or NSAID's; chronic disabling cases may need short course of corticosteriods.

8. **Stasis dermatitis (or venous dermatitis) and ulcers**: Most common in older persons with varicose veins; **primary lesions** appear with **red**, **scaly**, **pruritic patch followed by vesicular and crusted lesions with edema due to** scratching and secondary bacterial infection; **secondary lesions** cause hyperpigmentation, in fections eczematoid and stasis ulcers.
Management: Rest, elevation of the leg (4 inches) by lying in bed (not by sitting in a chair, which is not helpful); Burow's solution wet pack; antibiotic plus corticosteroid ointment mixture; **severe cases** may need hospitalization, strict bed rest, leg elevation, elastic bandage, prolong use of wet pack, **prednisone** and short course of **antibiotic**; ulclers should be treated with **occlusive dressing** (bactroban ointment, Telfa dressing, ace elastic bandage), **multivitamins plus mineral** supplement including zinc and magnesium, prednisone, erythromycin, lying down prone with maximum elevation of legs.

9. **Pigmented purpuric eruption**; Less common lesion; occur in middle-aged adults; grouped petechial lesions that begin on the legs and extend up to the thighs.
Management: **Combination** of hesperidin complex plus vitamin C is effective in some cases; or occlusive dressing with corticosteroid cream; for resistant cases use prednisone orally.

10. **Urticaria (or hives)**: It may be **acute or chronic**; **immunologic** variety is due to type **I hypersensitivity reaction** with polyvalent antigen with IgE molecules most acute than chronic, **nonimmunologic** variety is due **to release of histamines** (such as lobster, crayfish, chemicals, morphine, codeine, physical agents and **pencillin and its derivatives (most common) either ingested, inhaled, injected or rarely with local application**)
Treatment: **First is** to continue the medicine; **mild cases** are treated with colloid bath (starch or oatmeal), Sarna lotion OTC, hydroxyzine, diphenhydramine, betamethasone sodium phosphate; **severe cases** are treated with benadryl injection, epinephrine subcutaneously, prednisone orally, chronic hives (>6 months duration) are treated with hydroxyzine, terfenadine,

cimetidine, mild sedatives (meprobamate, chlordiazepoxide); avoid foods causing urticaria.

11. **Dermatitis herpetiformis** (not due to **herpes**): **Rare autoimmune** disease; **chronic (months to years)** pruritic, papular, vesicular, bullous lesions **typically distributed over** the scalp, sacral area, forearm, elbows, thighs and scapular areas; may be associated with **nontropical sprue**; skin biopsy reveals IgA and Complement (C3) in the dermis.
    Management: Refer to dermatologist; sulfapyridine or dapsone; control itching with benadryl and other drugs; **use corticosteroids** for acute lesions; **diets which are gluten free, low in iodine and bromine** may be useful.

12. **Pemphigus vulgaris**: Rare disease; unknown etiology; paraneoplastic pemphigus is associated with underlying cancer; primary lesions are charcterized by vesicles, bullae over the underlying denuded red skin and mucous membrane, positive **Nikolsky sign (skin easily separate with gentle pressure)**; **secondary lesions are** due to bacterial infections results in mousy odor and crusty lesions.
    Management. Refer to dermatologist; mild cases are treated with **oral prednisone**; **local lesions** are treated with potassium permanganate crystals with lukewarm water in bathtub, talc powder in bedsheet, antiboitic (polysporin or bactroban) ointment; supportive therapy with vitamins, iron, and oral antibotics are also helpful; dapsone, methotrexate may be used in some cases; **severe cases** need hospitalization:

13. **Epidermolysis bullosa**: The simple form is autosomal dominant; commonly **misdiagnosed as athlete's foot**; **tense, slightly itching bullae at the sites of pressure,** heals without scarring; commonly occurs in **summer**.
    The dystrophic form is autosomal recessive; severe disease with hemorrhagic bullae, leaves scar results in amputation; death is due to infection or metastatic squamous cell cancer; treated with supportive therapy and future gene therapy.

14. **Acne**: It is common in **young adults** characterized by comedones (blackheads), pustules, cysts and scarring occurs more commonly on the face and neck.
    Management: Dial or neutrogena soap; sulfur ppt (6%), resorcinol (4%) local application; Benzamycin lotion (benzoyl peroxide plus erythromycin); tretinion gel(Retin A); local antibiotics (clindamycin 1% or erythromycin 2%); remove comedones; ultlraviolet therapy in subsequent visit; for **scarring acne** use tetracycline orally, vitamin A, intralesional corticosteroid, short course of oral

prednisone, oral isotretinion (Accutane is teratogenic to pregnant women); residual scarring severe acne may need surgical dermabrasion.

15. **Rosacea**: Uncommon lesion, occurs in fourth to sixth decade, characterized by pustular butterfly rash over the face, long-standing cases develop rhinophyma (bulbous, hypertrophic nose)
Treatment: Dial soap, oral tetracycline, metronidazole gel, sulfur ppt and resorcinol locally.

16. **Seborrheic dermatitis** (or dandruff): It is common around puberty; etiology is **unknown** but pityrosporum ovale fungus is a common cause; red, scaly (dry or greasy) lesions are most commonly found in the scalp.
Treatment: **Selenium sulfide** (2-1/2%) shampoo, triamcinolone spray at night, low-strength corticosteroid cream or ketoconazole (2%) cream (corticosteroid-sparing drug)

17. **Psoriasis: Unkown cause**; positive family history (30% cases); **acute form of psoriasis occurs** in young adults after streptococcal throat infection is called guttate psoriasis; characterised by **chronic, recurring, non-contagious, whitish, scaly patches most commonly seen in elbows, knees and the scalp.** The disease can disappear sometimes but no cure has been found.
Treatment:
(i) **Scalp lesions:** Tar shampoo, **triamcinolone** containing FS shampoo, triamcinolone spray at night.
(ii) **Body lesions**: Fluorinated corticosteroids locally; coal tar solution (LCD) plus sulfur, ppt plus white petrolatum locally; calcipotriene ointment; occlusive dressing after fluorinated corticosteroid cream is helpful for extremities.
(iii) Severe cases: Ultraviolet therapy plus oral psoralen are very effective; coal tar solution is also used.

18. **Tinea versicolor**: Rarely contagious; characterized by **tannish colored, irregularly shaped scaly patches** (asymptomatic), located mostly on the **upper chest, back, neck and extremities**; caused by Pityrosporum or Malassezia furfur.
Treatment: Selenium sulfide suspension to apply locally.

19. **Lichen planus:** Unkonwn etology; noncontagious chronic pruritic discese with **violaceous flat-topped** papules usually seen or **the flexor aspect of wrists and the legs**; mucous membrane lesions on the cheeks or lips are whitish.

Treatment: Corticosteroid cream, chlorpheniramine antihistamine, avoid excessive bathing with soap; occlusive dressing with corticosteroid is helpful for extremities.

20. **Pityriasis rosea**: Unknown cause; most common in young adults; characterized by **larger 'herald patch' like patch of ringworm precede the generalized papulosquamous oval erythematous lesion** by 2 to 10 days; noncontagious disease.
    Treatment: Colloid bath (oatmeal preparation), calamine lotion, cyproheptadine for itching, ultraviolet therapy; unresponsive patients need hydrocortisone locally and severe cases need oral prednisone.

21. **Job's syndrome**: Chronic cutaneous abscesses, eczema and severe elevation of IgE.

22. **Wiskott-Aldrich syndrome**: X-linked recessive; eczema, purpura, pyodermas; increased IgA and decreased IgM.

23. **Chediak-Higashi syndrome**: Defect of lysosomes; subgroup of oculocutaneous albinism.

24. **Ataxia-Telangiectasia**: Autosomal recessive; type IV immunodeficiency; telangiectasias plus ataxia; absence of IgA.

25. Nonbullous autoimmune cutaneous diseases:
    (i) Vitiligo: Loss of pigmentation either localized or widespread; autoantibodies to melanocytes and melanocyte antigen may be present; may be associated with thyroid desease, diabetes mellitus, Addison's disease, alopecia areata, and pernicious anemia.
    (ii) Autosensitization dermatitis (id reaction): Etiology is unknown (may be immune reaction); symmetric eczematous or vesicular eruption occurs distant from localized inflammation of the skin.
    (iii) **Alopecia areata:** Type IV delayed hypersensitivity reaction; nonscarring well defined areas of scalp hair loss; or total hair loss (alopecia totalis), or total body hair loss (alopecia universalis); may be associated with atopy, pernicious anemia, vililigo, Addison's disease or thyroid disease.

26. **Dermatomyositis**: Periorbital heliotrope, erythema over the joints; usually absence of autoantibodies.

27. **Scleroderma**: Selerosis of skin; ANA positive in systemic form (increased interleukin 8 may be present), ANA negative in localized form or morphea.

28. **SLE**: Butterfly rash over the face; ANA positive (99% of cases), anti-DNA positive (70% of cases), low complement.

29. **Rheumatoid arthritis:** Subcutaneous nodules, vasculitis; positive IgM RF (rheumatoid factor).

30. **Sjogren's syndrome**: Pruritis, dry skin, decreased sweating, dry mouth, dry eyes; presence of anti- SS-A and anti-SS-B.

31. **Bullous pemphigoid**: Large tense bullae, urticarial or circinate lesions; may be associated with underlying malignancy; positive IgG and C3 in the basement membrance.

32. **Senile pruritus**: Purritus with or without dry skin and excoriation; occurs on the scalp, legs, sacral areas, and shoulders.
Treatment: Corticosteroid ointment, chlorpheniramine or diphenhydramine (itching) or injection of triamcinolone.

33. **Lichen simplex chronicus (or localized neurodermatitis or lichenified dermatitis):** Usually single areas of chronic, itching **(worse at night),** thickened, scaly, dry skin over the feet, neck, scrotum; chronic patients have nervous habit.
Treatment: Burow's solution pack, corticosteroid ointment; occlusive dressing with steroids is useful; severe cases need intralesional injection of corticosteroid.

34. **External otitis or otitis externa**: Dermatitis of external ear; may due to seborrheic (most common) or contact or atopic dermatitis or pseudomonas or fungus infection.
Treatment: Corticosteroid ointments, Burow's solution packs..

35. **Pruritus ani:** Itching, redness, excoriation, followed by lichenification (thickening) of the anal area; may be due to prolonged use of antibiotics (with or without fungus), nervousness itching of lichen simplex chronicus, psoriasis and rarely localized cancer.
Treatment: Corticosteroid cream or oinement, benadryl and Burow's solution wet packs.

36. **Folliculitis of the beard (or barber's itch)**: Bacterial infection (staphylococcal) spread rapidly with shaving.
Treatment: Oral erythromycin, local antibiotic plus hydrocortisone cream mixture, change the blade daily, do not shave closely, use dial or other antibacterial soap.

37. **Furuncle (or boil):** S.aureus infection of hair follicle; common in oily skin, dark skin, poor hygiene, diabetes, diet rich in sugar and fat.
Treatment: Incision and drainage, dicloxacillin orally, Burow's solution wet pack.

38. **Carbuncle**: Multiple opening furuncle due to S.aureus infection of adjoining hair follicles.
Treatment: Same as furncle.

39. **Sweat gland infections: Two types:**
    (i) Apocrinitis: Single apocrine gland infection in axilla usually associated with change of deodorant.
    Treatment: Same as furuncle.
    (ii) Hidradenitis suppurativa: Chronic, recurring, pyogenic infection of apocrine gland, mostly in the axilla; hereditary component of follicular occulusion; associated with acne conglobata and dissecting cellulitis of the scalp.
    Treatment: Oral antibiotic (dicloxacillin) for several weeks, hot packs locally; severe cases need plastic surgery or marsupilization operation to drain the sinuses or canals.

40. **Erysipelas: Subcutaneous tissue infection with beta-hemolytic streptococci results in characteristic type of cellulitis** (red, warm, tender, raised, brawny**, well defined areas),** most commonly occurs in the face and around the ears after ear piercing; associated with **fever and malaise**. It comonly recurs.
Differential diagnosis: Cellulitis does not have well defined border and **rarely** recurs.
Treatment: Bed rest, dicloxacillin or erythromycin orally, antipyretics, local cool wet dresing and semi-isolation for hospitalized patients.

41. **Chancroid**: Small, superficial or deep erosion with surrounding redness and edema over the genitalia, caused by **hemophilus ducreyi**, incubation peroid **1 to 5 days;** heal spontaneously within 1 to 2 weeks even without treatment, **rarely** form buboes (enlarged lymph nodes)

Treatment: Sulfonamide, erythromycin or third-generation cephalosporin; fluctuant bubo should be aspirated by large needle but should **never be incised.**

41. **Syphilis**: It is caused by Treponema pallidum.
   (i) Primary syphilis: Primary chancre most commonly occurs on the genitalia, average incubation period is 3 weeks (2 to 6 weeks), lesion heals even without treatment within 1 to 4 weeks; initially serologic test may be negative, subsequently becomes positive; Treponema pallidum is visible with dark field examination and present in CSF only 25% cases.
   (ii) Early latent syphilis: Only positive serology but no other signs of syphilis, it is between primary and secondary stages.
   (iii) **Secondary syphilis:** Macular, papular, pustular or squamous lesions over the body, palms and soles; positive serologic tests (except in AIDS), abnormal CSF fluid in 30% cases and visible spirochete under the darkfield examination.
   Treatment: Penicillin

42. **Lyme disease**: Borrelia burgdorferi spirochete is transmitted by Ixodes tick bites; erythematous circular rash appear 2 to 30 days after tick bites with peripheral enlarging and central clearing plus fever, chills, myalgia and headaches.
   Treatment: Doxycycline or amoxicillin; ceftriaxone is used for late stage cardiac or neurologic manifestations.

43. **Geonorrhea**: Purulent discharge from the urethra or local sites, caused by Neisseria gonorrhoeae, metastatic bacteremia causes arthralgia, fever and skin lesions (hemorrhagic vesicopustules most commonly present on the fingers).
   Treatment: Ceftriaxone, Spectinomycin or penicillin.

44. **Actinomycosis**: Chronic, granulomatous, suppurative infection with draining sinuses near the jaw, thorax or abdomen; caused by Actinomyces israelii (normal inhabitat of the mouth with poor dental hygiene); presence of sulfur granules (colonies of the organism) inside the pus.
   Treatment: Pencilillin (resistant cases use broad-spectrum antibiotics with or without penicillin); incision and drainage; good oral hygiene.

45. **Herpes Simplex**: Group of vesicles most commonly seen on lips, mouth ; genital region or eye (keratitis or corneal ulcers)
   Treatment: **Acyclovir (Zovirax) PO or locally; Burow's solution** ; sunscreen preparation for sun-induced herpes simplex; for pain and superficial inflammation use antibiotic plus corticosteroid mixture.

46. **Herpes Zoster**: Multiple groups of **painful vesicles** followed by crusted lesions along distribution of peripheral nerves ususlly in the thorax, face, neck; low-grade fever and malaise may be present; caused by same virus causing the chicken box.
Treatment: **Acyclovir orally**;local use of hydrocortisone lotion; for eye involvement refer to an opthalmologist; analgesic for pain; severe cases need oral acyclovir plus famciclovir; post-herpetic pain is treated with capsaicin cream locally, prednisone orally, sedative capsule at bed time; disseminated cases (AIDS patients) need hospitalization, IV acyclovir.

47. **Warts (Verrucae)**: It is causes by human papilloma virus (DNA), commonly found in fingers, hands, palms, soles and genital regions.
Treatment: Electrosurgery to destory the warts; liquid nitrogen (painful therapy); salicylic acid locally.

48. **Erythema infectiosum (or Fifth disease)**: It is caused by **parvovirus B19**; in adults joint invlovement and itching are more common (in children slap cheeks appearance).

49. **Tinea infection of the feet** (or athlete's foot): Acute form has **blisters** on the feet or feet; **chronic** form has dry, scaly, itchy lesions; superimposed bactrial infection is common; diagnosed by KOH preparation and culture. Tinea infections of nails (onychomycosis), groin (tinea cruris) and body (tinea corporis) are also found.
Treatment: Miconazole, econazole or clotriamazole cream locally; Burow's solutions soak; antifungal powder; systemic fungal therapy (griseofulvin) for **beard, nails, hands and groin (not** for feet).

50. **Candidias** (or moniliasis): It is caused C.albicans; can invlove nails, between fingers, neck, genital areas, mouth (oral thrush); diagnosis by KOH preparation and cultures.
Treatment: For nails (antifungal solution of Lotrimin or Mycelex; avoid soap and water); for skin (Mycostatin plus hydrocortisone cream); for vulvovaginitis (Mycostatin vaginal tablets or Monistat-Derm lotion)

51. **Scabies:** It is caused by Sarcoptes scabiei ; excoriated, itchy; lesions are common on the **lower abdomen**, back, pubic and axillary areas, legs and arms (**uncommon** site is webs of fingers); may be sexually transmitted disease.

Treatment: **Permethrin cream or Lindane lotion apply from the neck down and keep it 24 hour.** May repeat after 1 week; clean and washing all clothes (sterilization not needed); bathing after 24 hours.

52. **Vitiligo**: Depigmented lesions most commonly found on the face, dorsum of hands and feet; unknown cause, may be associated with thyroiditis.
Treatment: Psoralen (topical or oral) plus ultraviolet light therapy is effective; avoid sun light; early stages may respond to local steroid (betamethasone) cream.

53. **Chloasma (melasma):** Irregular, hyperpigmentation of the skin, commonly seen on the face, forehead and sides of the neck; unknown cause.
Treatment: **Retin-A cream or gel, NeoStrata gel** (both have sunscreen preparation).

54. **Hirsutism**: Excessive growth of terminal hair in a male sexual growth pattern; may be idiopathic or drug-induced (danazol, androgens, progesterone)
Treatment: Spironolactone is useful in idiopathic variety; oral flutamide and oral contraceptive may be useful.

55. **Hypertrichosis**: Excessive growth of hair (not in a male sexual growth pattern); may be found in dermatomyositis, poprphyrias, Cushing's disease, hypothyroidism, insulin-resistant diabetes, and POEMS syndrome.
Treatment: Shaving, bleaching, plucking, depilatories, and electrolysis.

56. **Androgenic hair loss** (male and female pattern hair loss): Nonscarring diffuse hair loss due to excess androgens.
Treatment: Topical minoxidil (Rogaine), hair transplantation and scalp reduction. Finasteride (Propecia) can be used for male baldness (effective 83% of cases). It inhibits the formation of dehydrotestosterone which causes male baldness.

57. **Telogen effluvivum**: Excessive hair loss during resting phase or telogen phase (normally maximum hair loss occurs in anagen or growth phase); postpartum alopecia is a telogen effluvivum with delayed androgen release.
Treatment: Treat the underlying cause, no specific treatment, hair regrows in 6 months.

58. **Alopecia areata**: Nonscarring usually patchy, sometimes diffuse hair loss of unknown cause.

Treatment: Topical corticosteroids and topical anthralin are useful; intralesional corticosteroids and psoralens with ultraviolet light have also used.

59. **Trichotillomania**: Nonscarring, patchy, hairloss mostly in the periphery of the scalp; due to hair permanents, hair dyes, hair straighteners, tight ponytails and tight braiding.
Treatment: Clomipramine is effective in some patients.

60. **Geographic tongue**: Irregular shaped, pale red patches over the trunk; unknown etiology; some patients complain of burning and tenderness while eating sour or salty foods.
Treatment: No effective therapy; for burning and tenderness use Kenalog in Orabase.

61. **Apthous stomatitis**: Painful, superficial ulcers inside the mouth; unknown cause.
Treatment: Tetracycline oral suspension (250 mg in 5 ml of water) keep inside the mouth for 2 minutes, then swallowed four times a day; or toothpaste swisth therapy after each meal and at bedtime.

62. **Photodermatitis or Sunburn**: Acute painful, erythematous, vesicular skin rash usually on the face, body;develops **within 2 to 12** hours after exposure to the sun and maximum lesions up to 24 hours. **Late reaction** to sunlight may cause actinic **or senile keratoses** usually after 50 years of age. Excessive sun exposure may cause malignant melanomas, basal and squamous cell cancers.
Treatment: Acute cases are treated with Burow's solution wet dressing, calamine or pramsone lotion, systemic analgesic and systemic corticosteroid may be used; Silvadene cream for extensive burn; blisters can be drained but should not be debrided; corneal sunlight injury should be referred to an opthalmologist.

63. **Basal cell cancer of the skin:** It is the most common skin cancer, almost never metastasize; most commonly occurs on the head, neck and then trunk; very slow growing tumor with bleeding, but sometimes grow rapidly; occurs on skin exposed to the sun.
Treatment: Surgical excision of the tumor is curative (100% cases of early lesions)

64. **Squamous cell cancer of the skin**: Rapidly growing nodule with central ulcer and raised border; highly malignant cancer; most commonly occurs on the lower lip, ears, tongue and dorsum of the hands.

Treatment: Surgical and/or radiation therapy.

65. **Keloid**: Abnormal overgrowth of fibrous tissue following injury, surgery, burn; more common in African American; most common in back and upper chest.
Treatment: Unsatisfactory result; excision and intralesional corticosteroid are helpful or silicon sheeting therapy.

66. **Maligant melanoma of the skin**: It is the most common cause of skin cancer death in USA; black or purple nodule (flat, pedunculated) or may be brown, pink, red or **no color**; bleeding **and ulcer are common ; any sudden change of recent onset or long standing lesions whould raise** the suspicious of malignant melanoma.
Treatment: Surgical excision, lymph nodes removal, chemotherapy and immunotherapy.

67. **Seborrheic keratoses**: It is most common in **elderly persons**; lesions are flesh-colored, tan, brown or coal black; oval shaped (average size 1 cm in diameter), most found on the face, scalp, neck, back, and upper chest ; hereditary and age are important factors.
Treatment: Liquid nitrogen freezing therapy is the treatment of choice; curettement followed by application of trichloroacetic acid or electrosurgery.

SPORTS MEDICINE

1. **Best fluid therapy recommended for sports: Cool plain water is the best;** cool dilute flavored beverages are more likely to be consumed by the athlete; fluid should be ingested **during and after sports** because there is significant delay between the onset of thurst and dehydration. Do **not** use glucose and electrolyte solutions which are hyperosmolar, results in decreased gastric emptying. Cool water increases gastric emptying.

2. **Recommendations of pregame meal**:
   (i) **Avoid high-fat foods** which delays gastric emptying.
   (ii) **Avoid simple carbohydrate** which stimulates insulin secretion results in impairment of hepatic glycogenolysis and free-fatty-acid mobilization.
   (iii) **Plenty of fluids should be taken** (2 to 3 cups with the meal and 1-1/2 cups 1 hour later)
   (iv) **Avoid caffeine** which is a diuretic and also causes jitteriness.
   (v) **Avoid alcohol** which is a diuretic and also causes CNS depression.
   (vi) Liquid meal which is balanced and easily digested.
   (vii) Meal should be taken **3 to 4 hour before sports** for adequate digestion.

3. An athlete approached to an internist to gain weight, a realistic weight gain should be **2 lbs per week**; slow weight-gain is recommended because that causes increased lean body weight; rapid weight gain is due to fat stores; no more than **extra 1500 calories per day is recommended**.
   Similarly is an athlete will benefit from weight loss program that should **be done gradually.**

4. **Few important points in nutrition of athletes:**
   (i) Good, balanced diet (meat, dairy, bread, cereal, fruits and vegetables) is adequate for athletes.
   (ii) Protein intake is about **15% total calories**, recommended protein intake is **0.8 mg/kg day except** during strenuous exercise (1.8 to 2.0 mg/kg/day)
   (iii) Extra vitamins, minerals and iron will **not** increase athletic performance but deficiency of iron and magnesium cause decreased athletic performance.

5. Drug that are **not** banned by IOC, NCAA, or other professional organization: **NSAID's, oral proteolytic enzymes** which enhances healing and recovery from traumatic injury, injection of glyco-aminoglycans also enhances healing, dimethyl sulfoxide (DMSO) has anti-inflammatory property.
   USOC has banned the use of narcotics, IM or IV corticosteroid and injection of anesthetic. Under certain condition intra-articular or superficial skin

injection may be allowed **(no** cocaine or epinephrine; plus medical justification and notification are necessary) but **only** the NCAA did **not ban the use of codeine and heroin and other narocotics.**

6. Most commonly used agent to increase energy by athlete: **Caffeine which is a CNS stimulant.** Urine levels >12 microgram/ml is prohibited by the IOC and >15 microgram/ml is prohibited by the NCAA.

7. IOC banned the following agents or drugs that should **not** be used by athletes Cocaine, marijuana, alcohol, amphetamines, anabolic steroids, diuretics, beta-blocker, growth hormone other stimulants, human chorionic gonadotrophin, local anesthetics, beta-2 agonists and related compounds/substances such as bicarbonate/phosphate loading. (Bicarbonate raises muscle pH, clearing lactate ions quickly and thereby delaying hydrogen ion-induced muscle fatigue; phosphate improves tissue oxygen unloading by increasing 2,3 - DPG results shift of oxygen dissociation curve to the right.

8. Definitive therapy of high-altitude sickness (>6400 feet or >2000 meters; truncal ataxia, diplopia, slurred speech, and psychologic changes): **Immediate descent** (atleast 1000 feet) can have significant beneficial effect.

9. **Most common complication of scuba diving**: **Barotrauma** causes external and middle air squeeze and compression of tympanic membrane results in rupture, pain, vertigo, vomiting and panic; due to **too rapid ascent**; breath holding can cause pneumothorax and pulmonary interstitial emphysema. Other type of sickness is called decompression sickness due to release of nitrogen bubbles into various tissues: type I sickness includes throbbing, tearing pain of large joints, skin itching or burning; type II sickness involves the spiral cord and CNS (diplopia, hemiplegia, seizures). Type II sickness occurs usually within 10 minutes to 1 hour, and type I sickness begins within 1 hour up to 12 hours.

10. **Asthma and sports**: It is **not** a contraindication for sports. Aerosolized beta-2 agonist given 15 to 20 **minutes before exercise/sports is recommended**; (oral route is less effective; inhaled corticosteroid is not helpful). To prevent bronchospasm, regular supplementation with inhaled chromoglycate or corticosteroid is helpful. **Unstable asthmatic patients should be stabilized before participating in sports.**

11. **Diabetes mellitus and sports**: It is **not a** contraindication for sports but **uncontrolled** diabetes should **not** participate in sports. Exercise has proinsulin

effect. Frequent doses of **short-acting insulin** are preferable than long-acting insulin **and doses should be reduced upto 10 to 20%** for strenuous exercise for 40 to 60 minutes and **even up to 50% reduction of short and intermediate acting** insulin for prolong strenuous exercise such as marathons, or piking.

12. **Epilepsy and sports:** The following sports **are contraindicated such as** climbing, boxing, aviation, and hang gliding. **The following sports are allowed** such as swimming, sailing, water skiing, canoeing, gymnastics **under close supervision**. The bathtub is more dangerous than a swimming pool. Coaches and team members should know about the diagnosis. **Avoid** precipitating factors such as head trauma, fatigue, hyperventilation, alcohol or drugs. **Most** common cause of convulsion in an adolescent seizure patient is **failure to take medicine in a timely fashion (same as in diabetes)**

13. **Arthritis and sports**: Exercise should begin at very low intensity and then increase slowly; allowed to perform isometric and dynamic exercises; limited exercise only during pain and tenderness.

14. **HIV infection patients and sports**: Asympatic patients can participate in sports and symptomatic patients are too sick to participate in sports. The **following** sports are **contraindicated** such as **wresting, boxing and martial arts to avoid direct contact with blood**. They should have normal life-styles with sports and regular exercise programs.

15. **Cardiovascular disease and sports**: The patients should have **prescribed** exercise program individualized. **Regular exercise decreases** hypertension, obesity and hyperlipidemia.

16. **Chronic obstructive pulmonary disease (COPD) and sports**: **Prescribed** exercise for COPD patients increase the ability to do **more exercise** and diminish oxygen consumption. Initial exercise should be brief and then slowly increased.

17. **Cystic fibrosis and sports**: Exercise, appropriate sports and antibiotic therapy are extremely beneficial. Athletes should consume adequate **salts** and **fluid** to compensate for electrolyte abnormalities.

18. **Most common sites of sports injury in elderly**: **Knee (31% cases)**, next is foot (18%); most common causes is **tendinitis (23%)**, next is patellofemoral pain syndrome (10%).

19. **Average Caloric needs**:
    (i) Young adults women: 1700 Kcal/day
    (ii) Older women >75 years: 1400 Kcal/day
    (iii) Young adults men: 2700 Kcal/day
    (iv) Older men>75 years: 1800 Kcal/day

20. **Distribution of calories should be**:
    Carbohydrates (50 to 60%), fats (<30%), and proteins (10 to 20%).

INDEX